LEGAL
MEDICINE

LEGAL MEDICINE

American College of Legal Medicine Textbook Committee

S. Sandy Sanbar, M.D., Ph.D., J.D., F.C.L.M.
Chairman (1984 to 2001),
Project Director (1994 to 2001),
Past President, ACLM (1989 to 1990)

Allan Gibofsky, M.D., J.D., F.A.C.P., F.C.L.M.
Past President, ACLM (1994 to 1995)

Marvin H. Firestone, M.D., J.D., F.C.L.M.
Past President, ACLM (1993 to 1994)

Theodore R. LeBlang, J.D., F.C.L.M.
Publications Committee Chairman, ACLM (1994 to 2001)

Bryan A. Liang, M.D., Ph.D., J.D., F.C.L.M.
Board of Governor's, ACLM (1999 to 2001)

Jack W. Snyder, M.D., J.D., M.F.S., M.P.H., Ph.D.
President, ACLM (2000 to 2001)

Fifth Edition

American
College
of
Legal
Medicine

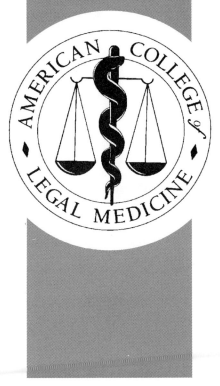

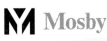 Mosby

A Harcourt Health Sciences Company

St. Louis   London   Philadelphia   Sydney   Toronto

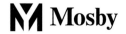

Mosby

A Harcourt Health Sciences Company

Acquisitions Editor: Liz Fathman
Developmental Editor: Ellen Baker Geisel
Project Manager: Carol Sullivan Weis
Project Specialist: Christine Carroll Schwepker
Designer: Mark A. Oberkrom

Mosby, Inc.
A Harcourt Health Sciences Company
11830 Westline Industrial Drive
St. Louis, Missouri 63146

Printed in the United States of America

Library of Congress Cataloging in Publication Data

Legal medicine / American College of Legal Medicine Textbook Committee, S. Sandy Sanbar . . . [et al.].--5th ed.
    p. cm.
    "American College of Legal Medicine"
    Includes bibliographical references and index.
    ISBN 0-323-01060-1
    1. Medical laws and legislation--United States. I. Sanbar, Shafeek S. II. American College of Legal Medicine. III. Title.

KF3821 .L44 2001
344.73'041--dc21   2001018005

01 02 03 04 05 TG/MVY 9 8 7 6 5 4 3 2 1

Contributors

GEORGE J. ANNAS, J.D., M.P.H.
Edward R. Utley Professor and Chair,
Health Law Department,
Boston University,
Schools of Public Health and Medicine,
Boston, Massachusetts
Chapter 1: Legal Medicine and Health Law Education
Appendix 1-3: Introduction to Health Law
Appendix 1-4: Human Rights and Health

RICHARD R. BALSAMO, M.D., J.D.
Vice President and Medical Director,
CIGNA HealthCare of Illinois,
Chicago, Illinois
Chapter 19: Risk Management

W. EUGENE BASANTA, J.D., LL.M.
Professor and Associate Dean,
School of Law,
Southern Illinois University,
Carbondale, Illinois
Appendix 1-2: M.D./J.D. Dual Degree Program

STEVEN B. BISBING, Psy.D., J.D.
Private Practice,
Clinical and Forensic Psychology,
Mental Health Consultation and Analysis, Inc.,
Takoma Park, Maryland
Chapter 4: Competency and Capacity: A Primer

BARRY H. BLOCH, J.D.
Raleigh, North Carolina
Chapter 45: Coproviders and Institutional Practice

MAX DOUGLAS BROWN, J.D.
Vice President and General Counsel,
Office of Legal Affairs,
Rush-Presbyterian-St. Luke's Medical Center;
Associate Professor,
College of Health Sciences;
Associate Professor (Conjoint Appointment),
Rush University College of Medicine;
Adjunct Professor,
Loyola School of Law,
Chicago, Illinois;
Adjunct Assistant Professor,
Business School of Dominican University,
River Forest, Illinois
Chapter 19: Risk Management

JASON C. BUCKEL, J.D.
Formerly McGuireWoods, LLP,
Richmond, Virginia
Chapter 30: Children as Patients

FILLMORE BUCKNER, M.D., J.D., F.C.L.M.
Clinical Professor,
Department of Obstetrics and Gynecology,
University of Washington School of Medicine,
Seattle, Washington
Chapter 22: Medical Records and Disclosure about Patients
Chapter 49: Telemedicine and Electronic Mail

JOHN R. CARLISLE, M.D., LL.B., F.C.L.M.
Lecturer, Osgoode Hall Law School,
York University;
Deputy Registrar,
College of Physicians and Surgeons of Ontario,
Toronto, Ontario, Canada
Chapter 24: Ethics and Bioethics

GENIFER Y. CHAVEZ, M.D., J.D., M.P.H., M.A., F.C.L.M.
Department of Medicine,
Tucson Medical Center,
Tucson, Arizona
Chapter 39: Public Health Law

DAVID P. CLUCHEY, M.A., J.D.
Professor of Law,
University of Maine School of Law,
Portland, Maine
Chapter 15: Antitrust

EDWARD DAVID, M.D., J.D., F.C.L.M.
Neurology Associates of Eastern Maine,
Bangor, Maine
Chapter 15: Antitrust

JOHN R. FEEGEL, M.D., J.D., M.P.H.
Professor (Courtesy),
Department of Criminology,
University of South Florida,
Tampa, Florida
Chapter 11: Liability of Health Care Entities for Negligent Care

MARVIN H. FIRESTONE, M.D., J.D., F.C.L.M.
Neuropsychiatric Consultant,
Brain Injury Rehabilitation Unit,
Division of Mental Health and Rehabilitation,
Palo Alto V.A. Medical Center,
Stanford University School of Medicine;
Former Professor,
Schools of Medicine, Law, and Health Services Administration,
George Washington University,
Washington, D.C.
*Chapter 8: Medical Staff Peer Review
    in the Credentialing and Privileging of Physicians*
Chapter 43: Psychiatric Patients and Forensic Psychiatry

SAL FISCINA, M.D., J.D.
Rockville, Maryland
Glossary: Selected Health Care and Legal Terminology

JUDITH A. GIC, R.N., J.D.
Private Practice,
New Orleans, Louisiana
Chapter 13: Nursing and the Law

LEONARD H. GLANTZ, J.D.
Professor of Health Law,
School of Public Health,
Boston University,
Boston, Massachusetts
Appendix 1-3: Introduction to Health Law

RICHARD S. GOODMAN, M.D., F.A.A.O.S., F.A.L.M.
Consultant, Department of Orthopaedics,
North Shore University,
Long Island Jewish Medical Center,
New Hyde Park, New York
Chapter 40: Sports Medicine

MICHAEL A. GRODIN, M.D., F.A.A.P.
Professor and Director,
Law Medicine and Ethics Program,
Health Law Department,
Boston University,
Schools of Public Health and Medicine;
Medical Ethicist,
Boston Medical Center,
Boston, Massachusetts
Chapter 1: Legal Medicine and Health Law Education
Appendix 1-3: Introduction to Health Law
Appendix 1-4: Human Rights and Health

CHARLES G. HESS, M.S., M.D.
Clinical Instructor of Pediatrics,
Baylor College of Medicine;
Former Chairman of Pediatric Sections,
Heights Hospital,
Memorial Hospital Northwest,
Houston, Texas
Chapter 47: Physician as an Employer

FREDDIE ANN HOFFMAN, M.D.
Mountain Lakes, New Jersey
Formerly, Deputy Director, Medicine Staff,
Office of Health Affairs,
U.S. Food and Drug Administration,
Rockville, Maryland
*Chapter 48: Health Professionals and Regulated
    Industry: The Laws and Regulations Enforced
    by the U.S. Food and Drug Administration*

EDWARD E. HOLLOWELL, J.D., F.C.L.M.
Adjunct Professor of Medical Jurisprudence,
School of Medicine,
East Carolina University,
Greenville, North Carolina;
Hollowell, Peacock & Meyer,
Raleigh, North Carolina
Chapter 45: Coproviders and Institutional Practice

MATTHEW L. HOWARD, M.D., J.D.
Department of Head and Neck Surgery,
Kaiser Permanente Medical Center,
Santa Rosa, California;
Assistant Clinical Professor,
Department of Otolaryngology,
University of California School of Medicine,
San Francisco, California
Chapter 20: Physician-Patient Relationship

JAMES R. HUBLER, M.D., J.D.
Clinical Instructor,
Department of Surgery,
University of Illinois;
Attending Physician,
Department of Emergency Medicine,
Assistant Director,
Central Illinois Center for Emergency Medicine,
Peoria, Illinois
*Chapter 18: Health Insurance and Professional Liability
    Insurance*

MARSHALL B. KAPP, J.D., M.P.H.
Frederick A. White Distinguished Service Professor,
Department of Community Health,
Wright State University School of Medicine,
Dayton, Ohio
Chapter 33: Geriatric Patients

CAROLYN S. LANGER, M.D., J.D., M.P.H.
Instructor in Occupational Medicine,
Department of Occupational and Environmental Health,
Harvard School of Public Health,
Boston, Massachusetts
Chapter 38: Occupational Health Law

THEODORE R. LeBLANG, J.D., F.C.L.M.
Professor and Chairman,
Department of Medical Humanities,
Southern Illinois University School of Medicine,
Carbondale, Illinois
Appendix 1-1: Program of Law and Medicine
Appendix 1-2: M.D./J.D. Dual Degree Program

BRADFORD H. LEE, M.D., J.D., M.B.A., F.A.C.E.P.,
F.C.L.M.
Seymour Johnson Air Force Base,
Goldsboro, North Carolina
Chapter 17: Countersuits by Health Care Providers

ELLEN L. LUEPKE, J.D., L.L.M.
Barnes & Thornburg,
Chicago, Illinois
Chapter 44: Practice Organizations and Joint Ventures

BRYAN A. LIANG, M.D., J.D., F.C.L.M.
Arthur W. Grayson Distinguished Visiting Professor of Law
and Medicine,
Southern Illinois University,
Carbondale, Illinois
Chapter 5: Alternative Dispute Resolution
and Application to Medical Disputes

WENDY K. MARINER, J.D.
Professor of Law,
School of Public Health,
Boston University,
Boston, Massachusetts
Appendix 1-3: Introduction to Health Law

JOSEPH P. McMENAMIN, M.D., J.D.
Attorney, Litigation,
McGuireWoods, LLP,
Richmond, Virginia
Chapter 30: Children as Patients

BRUCE C. NELSON, J.D.
Partner, Litigation,
Piper, Marbury, Rudnick & Wolfe,
Chicago, Illinois
Chapter 46: Liability Exposure Facing Managed Care
Organizations

TIMOTHY E. PATERICK, M.D., J.D., M.B.A.
Department of Cardiology,
Mayo Clinic;
St. Luke's Hospital,
Department of Cardiology,
Jacksonville, Florida
Chapter 31: Coronary Artery Disease
and Practice Guidelines

JOSEPH D. PIORKOWSKI Jr., D.O., J.D., M.P.H.,
F.C.P.M., F.C.L.M.
Clinical Assistant Professor,
Department of Surgery,
Georgetown University Medical Center;
Adjunct Professor of Law,
Georgetown University Law Center,
Washington, D.C.
Chapter 10: Medical Testimony and the Expert Witness

PETER H. RHEINSTEIN, M.D., J.D., M.S.
Senior Vice President for Medical and Clinical Affairs,
Cell Works, Inc.,
Rockville, Maryland
Chapter 48: Health Professionals and Regulated
Industry: The Laws and Regulations Enforced
by the U.S. Food and Drug Administration

MIKE A. ROYAL, M.D., J.D., F.C.L.M.
Clinical Adjunct Professor,
Department of Medicine and Anesthesiology/Pain
Management,
Oklahoma University College of Medicine,
Pain Evaluation and Treatment Center,
Tulsa, Oklahoma
Chapter 36: Patients with Human Immunodeficiency
Virus Infection and Acquired Immunodeficiency
Syndrome

MARK E. RUST, J.D.
Barnes & Thornburg,
Chicago, Illinois
Chapter 44: Practice Organizations and Joint Ventures

S. SANDY SANBAR, M.D., Ph.D., J.D., F.C.L.M.
Clinical Assistant Professor,
Department of Medicine,
Oklahoma University School of Medicine;
President,
Royal Oaks Cardiovascular Clinic;
Law of Medicine,
Sanbar Law Firm,
Oklahoma City, Oklahoma
Chapter 1: Legal Medicine and Health Law Education
Chapter 6: Selected Health Care Statutory Provisions
Chapter 7: Education and Licensure
Chapter 28: Physician-Assisted Suicide

ROBERT E. SCHUR, J.D.
Contracts Manager,
Vice President,
Administration Services,
Colorado State University,
Fort Collins, Colorado
Chapter 2: Contracts
Chapter 3: Agency and Partnership
Chapter 8: Medical Staff Peer Review in the Credentialing
and Privileging of Physicians

†**JANET B. SEIFERT**, J.D.
Glossary: Selected Health Care and Legal Terminology

BRUCE H. SEIDBERG, D.D.S., M.Sc.D., J.D., D.A.B.E., F.P.F.A., F.C.L.M.
Private Dental (Endodontics) Practice,
Liverpool, New York;
Dental-Legal Consultant,
Lecturer, Risk Management Skills and Legal
Aspects of Dentistry,
Child of Dentistry, Crouse Hospital;
Senior Attending Dentist,
Former Director, Center GPR,
St. Joseph's Hospital Health Center;
Former Associate Professor,
SUNY School of Dentistry,
Syracuse, New York
Chapter 14: Dental Litigation: Triad of Concerns

MELVIN A. SHIFFMAN, M.D., J.D., F.C.L.M.
Private Medical Practice,
Medicolegal Consultant,
Tustin, California
Chapter 34: Oncology Patients

MICHAEL A. SHIFLET, J.D.
Frasier, Frasier, and Hickman, LLP,
Tulsa, Oklahoma
*Chapter 36: Patients with Human Immunodeficiency
Virus Infection and Acquired Immunodeficiency
Syndrome*

JACK W. SNYDER, M.D., J.D., M.F.S., M.P.H., Ph.D.
Senior Vice-President and Chief Medical Officer,
DIANON Systems, Inc.,
Stratford, Connecticut
Chapter 32: Domestic Violence Patients

STAN TWARDY, J.D., LL.M.
Private Legal Practice,
Oklahoma City, Oklahoma
Chapter 16: Crimes by Health Care Providers

CLARK WATTS, M.D., J.D.
Clinical Professor,
Division of Neurosurgery,
University of Texas Health Sciences Center;
Attending Physician,
Department of Neurosurgery,
Southwest Methodist Hospital,
San Antonio, Texas;
Adjunct Professor of Law,
University of Texas School of Law,
Austin, Texas
Chapter 35: Brain-Injured Patients

CYRIL H. WECHT, M.D., J.D., F.C.L.M.
Clinical Professor of Pathology,
University of Pittsburgh School of Medicine;
Adjunct Professor of Law,
Duquesne University School of Law;
Director of Forensic Pathology,
Department of Pathology,
St. Francis Central Hospital,
Pittsburgh, Pennsylvania
Chapter 1: Legal Medicine and Health Law Education
Chapter 41: Forensic Use of Medical Information
Chapter 42: Forensic Pathology
Chapter 50: Human Experimentation and Research

MILES J. ZAREMSKI, J.D., F.C.L.M.
Lecturer in Health Law,
University of Chicago School of Law;
Assistant Clinical Professor Department of Family Medicine,
Chicago Medical School,
North Chicago, Illinois;
Chair, Health Care Law Department,
Chicago, Illinois;
Kovitz, Shifrin & Waitzman,
Buffalo Grove, Illinois
*Chapter 46: Liability Exposure Facing Managed Care
Organizations*

JAMES G. ZIMMERLY, M.D., J.D., M.P.H., LL.D. (Hon.)
Associate Professor,
Department of Epidemiology and Preventive Medicine,
University of Maryland Medical School,
Baltimore, Maryland;
Adjunct Professor of Law,
Georgetown University Law Center,
Washington, D.C.
*Chapter 18: Health Insurance and Professional Liability
Insurance*

†Deceased.

Preface

Since its founding in 1955, the American College of Legal Medicine (ACLM) has devoted itself to addressing problems that exist at the interface of law and medicine. As the foremost established organization in the United States concerned with medical jurisprudence and forensic medicine, the ACLM serves as a natural focal point for those professionals interested in the study and advancement of legal medicine.

Central to the mission of the ACLM is education in legal medicine, and this text has been prepared with the hope and expectation that the more knowledge that can be available concerning the relevant legal concepts, principles, and rules, the more effective an individual can become as a medical or legal practitioner.

The fifth edition of this text is updated and expanded. It includes new chapters dealing with nursing and the law, dentistry and the law, coronary artery disease, and public health law, as well as exhaustive updates on physician-assisted suicide, peer review, and managed care organizations.

This text attempts to highlight those areas of professional endeavor in a health care institution that constitute potential pitfalls and problems of a legal nature. The field of legal medicine is extremely broad and far-reaching, with new developments of a significant nature occurring constantly. The text is structured to explore and illustrate the legal implications of medical practice and the special legal issues attendant to organized health and medical care.

On behalf of the ACLM, we extend our deep appreciation to all the authors and contributors of the textbook chapters. Their contributions represent true labors of love to the ACLM and a monumental work in the field of legal medicine. The editors are saddened by the passing of our colleague, Janet Seifert, who worked tirelessly for many editions of this text. Her previous chapters and current glossary of terms have been and will continue to be a valuable resource for many editions.

Finally, we wish to express our thanks to the staff of Harcourt Health Sciences, especially Liz Fathman, Medical Editor; Ellen Baker Geisel, Developmental Editor; and Carol Weis, Project Manager, as well as Christine Schwepker, Project Specialist, and Mark Oberkrom, Designer.

American College of Legal Medicine
Textbook Committee

S. Sandy Sanbar, M.D., Ph.D., J.D., F.C.L.M.
Allan Gibofsky, M.D., J.D., F.A.C.P., F.C.L.M.
Marvin H. Firestone, Ph.D., M.D., J.D., F.C.L.M.
Theodore R. LeBlang, J.D., F.C.L.M.
Bryan A. Liang, M.D., Ph.D., J.D., F.C.L.M.
Jack W. Snyder, M.D., J.D., M.F.S., M.P.H., Ph.D.

Contents

Introduction

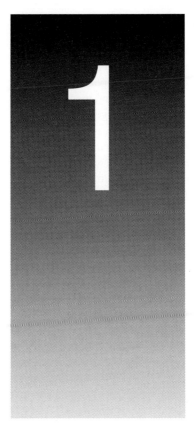

Legal medicine and health law education

S. SANDY SANBAR, M.D., Ph.D., J.D., F.C.L.M.
GEORGE J. ANNAS, J.D., M.P.H.
MICHAEL A. GRODIN, M.D., F.A.A.P.
CYRIL H. WECHT, M.D., J.D., F.C.L.M.

Law and medicine are separate professions, and attorneys and physicians often see their professions in conflict. There are, however, more similarities than differences between the two professions. And there are areas of mutual concern and overlap that demand the application of both legal and medical knowledge for the good of society. These areas have historically been united under the broader term of *health law.* This chapter introduces readers to a field that has been known by at least three different names by reviewing some historical highlights in its development and explaining how it is approached in legal, medical, and continuing professional education. What emerges is a field in evolution that has moved from almost exclusive concern with forensic pathology and psychiatry in country-specific settings to now encompass the bioethics, organization, and management of health care delivery and the growing global movement toward human rights in health.

LEGAL MEDICINE

The roots of legal medicine can be traced back to the sixteenth century in Italy and the late eighteenth century in Britain. Published treatises generated from Italy and Britain guided the development of legal medicine in Germany, France, and the United States. *Medicine legale,* or legal medicine, is a French term that first appeared during the late eighteenth and early nineteenth centuries.[1] The French legal medicine subject was broad and included medical evidentiary matters and medical areas of legal significance, for example, the criminally insane and the rehabilitation of criminals.

Harvard University established a separate professorship in legal medicine in 1877. In 1942 Dr. Alan R. Moritz, then the occupant of that professorship, defined legal medicine as

the application of medical knowledge to the needs of justice. Although by definition this would appear to be a broad and scientifically heterogeneous field, the practice of legal medicine is concerned chiefly with what might be most adequately described as forensic pathology.[2]

In 1975 another prominent Harvard professor of legal medicine, Dr. William J. Curran, who founded the Law-Medicine Institute at Boston University Law School in 1955 (now the Health Law Department of Boston University School of Public Health), defined the term *legal medicine* as

the specialty areas of medicine concerned with relations with substantive law and with legal institutions. Clinical medical areas, such as the treatment of offenders and trauma medicine related to law, would be included herein.[3]

The introduction of the term *medical jurisprudence* in America was the result of developments in Britain. In 1788 Dr. Samuel Farr of Britain published the *Elements of Medical Jurisprudence.* Until that time, the British did not systematically study or teach legal or forensic medicine, and no comprehensive British work on the subject was available.[4]

In 1789 Dr. Andrew Duncan was appointed professor of the Institutes of Medicine at the University of Edinburgh, and he began to give lectures in medical jurisprudence and public hygiene.[5] Duncan was the first in Britain to provide systemic instruction in legal medicine. He used the term *medical jurisprudence* to encompass both "medical police and juridical medicine." Dr. James S. Stringham of New York, who was at Edinburgh earning his medical degree in 1799, brought the term with him to America.

In 1804 Stringham defined medical jurisprudence as "that science which applies the principles and practice of the different branches of medicine to the elucidation of doubtful questions in courts of justice."[6] In 1975 Curran argued that the unfortunate title of "medical jurisprudence should at long last be relegated to the lexicographer's scrap heap. It was incorrectly applied to the medical side of the field in the first place. It is now either inappropriate or too pretentious a term for the legal aspects of the subject."[7] More recently the term *health law* has gained wide acceptance and is used in textbook and course titles in most law schools and law firms to denote the field, as well as in some medical schools and almost all schools of public health.

LEGAL MEDICINE IN AMERICA

Numerous excellent articles on the history of legal medicine have been published in the medical and legal professional journals, some of which are referred to in this chapter. Five extensive and authoritative references of articles on the general history of legal medicine are those by Gilbert H. Stewart (1910),[8] Sir Sydney Smith (1954),[9] Chester R. Burns (1977),[10] William J. Curran (1980),[11] and James C. Mohr (1993).[12] Some of these publications also include discussions of the history of medical ethics. This chapter focuses on the history of legal medicine and the early legal medicine scholars in America.

In the United States, legal medicine started to develop at the beginning of the nineteenth century. Stringham studied medicine first in his native city of New York and subsequently at Edinburgh, Great Britain, where he graduated with the doctor of medicine degree in 1799. In 1804 Stringham instituted a course of lectures in legal medicine at Columbia College of Physicians and Surgeons in New York. He was the first systematic teacher of legal medicine in America. In 1813 he was appointed professor of medical jurisprudence at the College of Physicians and Surgeons, a post he held until his death in 1817.

Dr. Benjamin Rush is credited with emphasizing the significance of the relationship between law and medicine in the early 1800s. As the nation's first surgeon general and a signatory of the Declaration of Independence, Rush established American legal medicine with his published lecture "On the Study of Medical Jurisprudence," which he delivered to medical students at the University of Pennsylvania, Philadelphia, in 1811.[13] The lecture dealt with homicide, mental disease, and capital punishment.

The work of Stringham and Rush inspired the teaching of medical jurisprudence in other American medical schools. Among the early teachers were Dr. Charles Caldwell in Philadelphia and Dr. Walter Channing at Harvard. In 1819 Dr. Thomas Cooper, a legal officer of distinction and president of the College of South Carolina, published *Tracts on Medical Jurisprudence.* This volume contained almost all available literature written in English on legal medicine.

In 1815 Dr. T. Romeyn Beck was appointed lecturer on medical jurisprudence at Western Medical College, New York State. In 1823 Beck published the *Elements of Medical Jurisprudence,* which defined the field of legal medicine for about half a century of American medical practice. Beck's two volumes included impressive topics, such as rape, impotence and sterility, pregnancy and delivery, infanticide and abortion, legitimacy, presumption of survivorship, identity, mental alienation, wounds, poisons, persons found dead, and feigned and disqualifying diseases.

In 1838 Isaac Ray published *A Treatise on Medical Jurisprudence of Insanity.* In 1855, the year that Beck died, Francis Wharton, an attorney, and Dr. Moreton Stille, a physician, collaborated to publish *A Treatise on Medical Jurisprudence.* In 1860 Dr. John J. Elwell, a physician and an attorney, published a book entitled *A Medico-Legal Treatise on Malpractice, Medical Evidence, and Insanity Comprising the Elements of Medical Jurisprudence,* which highlighted the issue of malpractice in the medical jurisprudence literature. Elwell's book presented excerpts from contemporary cases for the purpose of teaching physicians what to expect from malpractice litigation. Dr. John Odronaux, also a physician and an attorney, published *Jurisprudence of Medicine* in 1867 and *Judicial Aspects of Insanity* in 1878. In 1894 Randolph A. Witthaus and Tracy C. Becker published *Medical Jurisprudence, Forensic Medicine and Toxicology.*

For medical students and physicians, medical jurisprudence assumed the position of central importance in U.S. schools of medicine throughout most of the 1800s. During the course of the nineteenth century, the institutions, laws, and judicial decisions in America reflected the increasing influence of sound medicolegal principles, especially those pertaining to mental disease and criminal lunacy.

After the Civil War, however, things changed drastically; legal medicine became temporarily dormant. American Professor and Dean Stanford Emerson Chaille expressed his view of the deplorable condition of medical jurisprudence in the United States. Chaille demonstrated how the teaching of medical jurisprudence had deteriorated by noting that in some medical colleges the course had been dropped altogether, in others it had been attached to some other subject, and in many colleges the teaching of medical students was entrusted to an attorney with no formal training in the medical field.[14]

Even in the early twentieth century the teaching of medical jurisprudence was relegated to a position as an occasional subject taught outside the mainstream. However, by the middle of the twentieth century, legal medicine underwent a renaissance, as evidenced by the establishment of the American College of Legal Medicine (ACLM), the founding of the Law-Medicine Institute at Boston University, and the rekindling of contemporary interest in a vast array of legal medicine issues, medical ethics, physician and patient rights, and business and professional aspects of medical practice.

In 1867 the Medico-Legal Society was organized in New York. It was the first society in the world to be organized for the purpose of promoting the principles that an attorney could not be fully equipped for the prosecution or the defense of an individual indicted for homicide without some knowledge of anatomy and pathology and that no physician or surgeon could be a satisfactory expert witness without some knowledge of the law.[15]

THE AMERICAN COLLEGE OF LEGAL MEDICINE

In 1955, recognizing the growing impact of legislation, regulations, and court decisions on patient care and the general effect of litigation and legal medicine on modern society, a group of physicians and surgeons, some of whom were educated in the law, organized what would later become the ACLM. The college was incorporated on September 23, 1960, by nine doctors of medicine, three of whom were attorneys. Of the 36 physicians who were designated "founding fellows," 10 had earned law degrees.

The ACLM is the oldest and most prestigious U.S. organization devoted to problems at the interface of medicine and law. Its membership is made up of professionals in medicine, osteopathy, and allied sciences, including dentistry, nursing, pharmacy, podiatry, psychology, and law. The ACLM has published a scholarly journal, the *Journal of Legal Medicine,* since 1973. In 1988 the ACLM also published the first edition of this textbook, *Legal Medicine;* subsequent editions were published in 1991, 1995, and 1998.

THE AMERICAN SOCIETY OF LAW, MEDICINE, AND ETHICS

In 1972 a physician and two attorneys founded the American Society of Law and Medicine (Ethics was added in 1992; ASLME) as a successor organization to the Massachusetts

Society of Examining Physicians. Its founding president was cardiologist Dr. Elliot Sagall, who also cotaught the law and medicine course at Boston College Law School with George J. Annas, an attorney. The organization quickly became the largest medicolegal organization in the world dedicated to continuing education, as well as the publisher of the two leading medicolegal journals, the *Journal of Law, Medicine, and Ethics* and the *American Journal of Law and Medicine;* the latter is published as a law review at Boston University Law School. The ASLME also has sponsored international meetings in locations around the world in an effort to bring physicians, attorneys, ethicists, and others interested in health law together.

HEALTH LAW IN LAW SCHOOLS

From World War II until the late 1960s, the field of legal medicine was defined by law school courses that were almost exclusively concerned with issues of forensic psychiatry and pathology and were properly considered advanced courses in criminal law. In the late 1960s some law and medicine courses began concentrating on broader medicolegal issues faced in the courtroom, including disability evaluation and medical malpractice. These courses were properly considered either advanced tort or trial practice courses.

In the 1970s the concerns of at least some law and medicine courses expanded to include public policy, including issues of access to health care and the quality of that care. At the same time, advances in medical technology created new legal issues to explore—from brain death and organ donation to abortion and in vitro fertilization. These issues were increasingly incorporated into law and medicine courses, which were themselves becoming known by the broader term of *health law.*

Teachers of health law in law schools and medical schools, together with health law teachers in schools of public health and schools of management, began meeting on a regular basis in 1976 when the first national health law teachers meeting took place at Boston University under the auspices of the law school's Center for Law and Health Sciences (the successor organization to the Law-Medicine Institute).[16] The purpose was to help define the expanding field and develop necessary teaching materials. In 1987 the American Association of Law Schools sponsored its first teaching workshop on health law.[17] Although this narrower group only recently convened, its program and proceedings offer useful insight into the current state of health law in law schools. As the organizers of the workshop saw it, law and medicine (fields primarily concerned with medical malpractice, forensic medicine, and psychiatric commitment) had become subdivisions of the new field of health law.[18] Health law itself has three additional subdivisions: economics of health care delivery, public policy and health care regulation, and bioethics. These three subdivisions are actually three different approaches to the same subject matter—the health care industry.[19] Health law is applied law, much the way medical ethics is applied ethics.

Health law should be studied by all law students for at least the following five reasons:

1. No other applied legal field can match the "magnitude, complexity, and universality of health care."[20]
2. Health law introduces attorneys to the problems confronted by members of another great profession in the United States, medicine.
3. Changes in medicine directly affect what humans can do and how humans think about humanity itself (and therefore what rights and obligations humans should have).
4. As issues of public health and safety capture center stage in American culture, the prudent use of law to protect health and safety assumes a role of central importance.
5. Issues of social justice and resource allocation are presented more compellingly in the medical care context than in any other.[21]

Other reasons could be added to this list, of course. Health care accounts for almost 15% of the gross national product, and cost increases continue out of control. Most importantly, constitutional law questions now focus on medical issues, such as abortion, the right to die, and free speech in the physician-patient relationship. Legal jobs in health care exist in a wide variety of settings, including local, state, and federal regulatory agencies; private health care facilities; health maintenance or managed care organizations and insurance companies; and law firms, to name just the major employers. And, a factor that is perhaps more important to most who teach health law, there is no more intrinsically fascinating area of law than law applied to the health care field. Entire courses in law schools have been based on a single medical development, such as organ transplantation, and a single specialized medical activity, such as human experimentation.

Health law provides a uniquely critical and intrinsically fascinating field to which to apply law, as well as a field that can be fruitfully approached from a wide variety of perspectives. Rand Rosenblatt, for example, has suggested that health law can be approached from the traditional law and medicine avenue and from three more modern perspectives: a law and economics approach, a social justice approach, and a bioethics approach. A fourth approach is a public health approach, and a fifth approach of course tries to integrate (or at least expose) all of these approaches.[22] Each approach deserves comment.

Law and economics have provided many law school teachers with an overarching approach to all legal problems. To oversimplify, the basic viewpoint from which health law is approached is that private property regimes presumptively serve to maximize social welfare; in a many-seller market, goods are available at marginal costs; private contracts should be enforced; relationships among noncontracting parties must

be governed by explicit legal rule; and income distribution is and should be primarily a function of productive capabilities. Even some of its harshest critics concede that the law and economics movement "provides the most coherent and intelligible realization of the liberal social theoretical agenda."[23]

A different approach to health law is taken by the critical legal studies (CLS) approach. Like the law and economics rubric, the CLS rubric is used here as oversimplified shorthand for a course that is approached from an ideological perspective that dominates the discussion. Unlike the law and economics school with its market model, CLS has no single, coherent set of principles to apply to any given industry. Nonetheless, those who describe CLS as a "social justice" approach imply that it is concerned with questioning the assumptions of capitalism (or at least looking "critically" at those assumptions).[24] Such an approach to the health law industry does not ignore how society got where it is and does not assume that traditional race, class, and gender power relationships are proper or deserve to be privileged and given presumptive validity.

Adherents of the law and economics and the CLS schools are at home with theoretical and macroeconomics levels but not with medical ethics. When it comes to dealing with the real problems of real physicians and patients, they each have much less to say. Perhaps that is why members of both of these politically hostile camps agree (mistakenly, the authors think) that issues of medical decision-making, such as autonomy and the physician-patient relationship (the natural focus of a medical school course), should be relegated to a separate course called *bioethics*.

The fourth approach, the public health approach, has yet to receive much attention in law schools and is currently used primarily in schools of public health.[25] Nonetheless, as issues of public health, such as teen pregnancy, drug abuse, drunk driving, smoking, acquired immunodeficiency syndrome (AIDS), nuclear energy, the quality of the environment, and worker health and safety, continue to dominate the news and public policy development such courses will naturally find a home in the law school. When this happens, the pioneering work that has been done in the school of public health context will find a ready home in the development of courses that take a public health approach, including the issues of social justice and resource allocation.[26]

HEALTH LAW CONTENT

Regardless of the teaching approach taken, the available teaching material is especially rich. As the health care delivery system rapidly changes, it provides a real-world laboratory for examining the influences of law—from the courtroom (e.g., medical malpractice and termination of treatment) and constitutional litigation (e.g., the right of privacy) to legislation (e.g., various proposals for Medicare reform and national health insurance) and regulations (e.g., the Food and Drug Administration, the revised drug safety rules, and state rules regarding licensing of physicians and facilities). New medical technologies present new legal challenges that are so intrinsically fascinating that they routinely appear on the front pages of newspapers and news magazines and have no trouble holding the attention of law students.

The cases of Karen Ann Quinlan, Nancy Cruzan, and Mary Beth Whitehead are only a few examples of health law dramas played out in the courts. *Roe v. Wade,* the premier health law case, continues to be contested and contracted; and the right of privacy, so central to medicine and the physician-patient relationship, continues to play the key role in the politics of judicial appointments. Issues of organ transplants and implants, including the case of Barney Clark, also present particularly compelling case studies that naturally lead to broader policy discussions. Public health issues, including the use of drugs, alcohol, and tobacco; food consumption; the quality of the environment; the need for exercise; and the use of seat belts and motorcycle helmets, are of direct importance to the day-to-day lives of students. And, perhaps as important, health law permits direct study of (and possibly joint courses with) the other major profession in the United States, medicine. Relationships between the two professions have become increasingly adversarial, and increased knowledge may help restore more reasonable and socially constructive relationships. Finally, the advice attorneys give their clients in the health law field often has a direct impact on the lives and the manner of deaths of real people. Professional responsibility has an immediacy in this legal field that is lacking in most others.[27]

When no medical courses are offered in law school, unfortunately, self-education is the method used by attorneys involved in legal-medicine cases. Aside from the lack of time to prepare for medical case issues and acquire a medicolegal background, the foremost obstacle for an attorney is the move from the inductive reasoning of law to the deductive logic of the basic sciences. An additional problem is the diversity of medical knowledge required. A legal case may involve questions of anatomy, embryology, physiology, biochemistry, pharmacology, and pathology in a myriad of medical specialties and subspecialties. Attorneys, however desirous they may be of acquiring some medical training, lack the underlying basic science courses to support effective self-education.

Formal education is essential if the attorney is to be effective in evaluating medical evidence, both friendly and adversarial. An attorney who specializes in health law must possess a specific knowledge of pertinent medical services and specialties required in any particular case situation. Undertaking a medical issues case in spite of a lack of such knowledge could constitute legal malpractice.

M.D./J.D. DEGREES

In an effort to bridge the gap between law and medicine, some attorneys enroll in medical school or in dual-degree M.D./J.D. programs. The number of medical school courses

extraneous to a legal practice specializing in medicine also discourages attorneys from a formal medical education.

In 1993 Harry Jonas, Sylvia Etzel, and Barbara Barzansky, reporting on the educational programs in U.S. medical schools, noted that students can earn combined doctor of medicine and doctor of jurisprudence (M.D./J.D.) degrees in only 9 out of 125 degree-granting U.S. medical schools fully accredited by the Liaison Committee on Medical Education (LCME).[28] In contrast, students can earn combined doctor of medicine and doctor of philosophy (M.D./Ph.D.) degrees in 113 of the 125 U.S. medical schools. The majority of individuals who currently have M.D./J.D. degrees, however, earned their doctorate degrees separately, with most of them earning the M.D. first.

In 1985 Eugene Schneller and Terry Weiner published their findings regarding individuals who earned M.D./J.D. dual-degrees and noted that cross-professional education in law and medicine remains a relatively rare phenomenon in the United States.[29] They concluded that "without the development of institutionalized career lines and the acceptance of cross-disciplinary approaches to problem solving, M.D./J.D.s must negotiate their jobs and job descriptions within an occupational structure that rewards disciplinary efforts. The marginal status of the interprofessional specialist persists in the decade of the 1980s."[30] A combined M.D./J.D. program is probably not the most effective way to teach medical concepts to law students, and it is doubtful that many students are willing to pursue such a long period of training. Moreover there is more than enough to learn in either field.

These reasons probably explain the increasingly popular movement toward providing a health law concentration in many law schools and offering joint J.D./M.P.H. degree programs (such as those at Boston University and Georgetown University) for students interested in health law. Practicing attorneys need a working knowledge of the health care industry but do not need to know most of the material taught in medical schools. A well-developed health law program designed to fit into the law school curriculum can prepare an attorney to handle medical issues competently. Existing programs, such as health law concentrations at Boston University, Georgetown, Case-Western, St. Louis University, and Loyola of Chicago, are still few in number.

HEALTH LAW AND BIOETHICS IN MEDICAL SCHOOLS

Health law and medical ethics education is critical to the practice of both medicine and public health. Many health law dilemmas raise serious ethical concerns, and many ethical issues similarly raise serious legal questions. Medical ethics education and health law education are intimately intertwined, and the disciplines must be taught together in medical schools so that the student can learn about the cross-fertilization of the two.[31] Ethical principles, such as autonomy, beneficence, and justice, are intimately intertwined in legal analysis. Medical students should understand the similarities and differences in the ways medicine and law frame questions, address problems, and approach moral quandaries, as well as the various resources available to analyze these problems.

Medical students and physicians should learn that it is as problematic to never follow the law as it is to always mechanically follow what they consider to be the letter of the law. Physicians who do not understand how the law works often practice inappropriate defensive medicine, thinking that they are following the law or looking only to the law and the question of legal liability to decide what is "right." Most importantly a lack of a minimal understanding of the law can lead to inappropriate and misguided treatment of patients.

Medical ethics education dates back to the time of Hippocrates. The hippocratic schools and hippocratic ethics attempted to establish moral guidelines for the practicing physician. Throughout most of history, medical ethics was taught through apprenticeship in an attempt to inculcate values. The idea was to model the knowledge, skill, and behavior of seasoned physicians as part of a professionalization process. Before the 1970s such role modeling or mentorship was the primary method of teaching medical ethics. In the early 1970s, however, specific courses began to be taught in medical schools. These courses focused on the content, theory, and philosophy of medicine. In 1972 only 4% of medical schools had formal, separate, required courses for teaching medical ethics. By 1989 that number had risen to 34%, and close to three quarters of medical schools covered medical ethics within other required courses.[32] It wasn't until the late 1980s, however, that residency programs began providing separate education in medical ethics as well.

HEALTH LAW AND MEDICAL ETHICS

Several key elements have been proved necessary for a successful health law and medical ethics program. First, health law and medical ethics must be prominent within the curriculum, substantiating their importance. Ethics education should be relevant, rigorously taught, and horizontally and longitudinally integrated into the curriculum from the classroom through the clinical clerkships. It must be seen as part of and integral to the practice of medicine. It must be taught over time, space, departments, and courses. As such, interdisciplinary teaching is almost an imperative.

For ethics education to be successful there must be specific learning objectives. Those objectives must be content and method focused. Some objectives of health law and medical ethics education are to sensitize students to the value and nature of medical practice, to supply them with methods to identify and describe legal and ethical dilemmas, and to give them formal, procedural, and substantive methodologies for resolving such dilemmas. Ultimately the goal is to graduate medical students who are committed to being physicians with high moral character and an understanding of the law and to practicing moral medicine.

The goals of health law and medical ethics should be to increase legal knowledge and provide skills in ethical analysis, as well as to educate students about tolerance and diversity of ethical opinions. Case-based analysis should draw on the student's experience. Courses must teach the history of law and medical ethics and its use and abuse in areas such as human experimentation, consent to treatment, euthanasia, and rationing. Students should also be familiar with important legal cases that deal with informed consent, abortion, and refusal of treatment. Ethical behavior still must be learned through role modeling that continues through the clinical years, fostering collaboration between nurses, administrators, and attorneys and ultimately adding a broader humanistic approach to improve interactive skills.

Basic curriculum goals have been identified. Seven skills that medical students should master by the end of health law and ethics education are as follows:

1. The ability to identify the legal and moral aspects of medical practice
2. The ability to obtain a valid informed consent or a valid refusal of treatment
3. Knowledge of how to proceed if a patient is only partially competent or incompetent to consent to or refuse treatment
4. Knowledge of how to proceed if a patient refuses treatment
5. The ability to decide when it is legally and morally justified to withhold information from a patient
6. The ability to decide when it is morally justified to breach confidentiality
7. Knowledge of the legal and moral aspects of care of patients with a poor prognosis, including patients who are terminally ill.[33]

There is a consensus that teaching should focus on standard principles of biomedical ethics, such as autonomy, justice, and beneficence, as well as on broader, more complex notions, such as feminist, virtue-based, Marxist, casuistic, and narrative critiques.[34] There have been several suggested specific curricular content goals. Although law students need to learn many facts related to medicine, medical students primarily need to learn only how to think about legal and moral issues in their practice.

The health law and bioethics curriculum at the Boston University School of Medicine is one of the oldest and most extensive in the country. The curriculum begins in the first year, when an integrated 20-hour health law and medical ethics course is a requirement for all students. The course is taught by health attorneys and uses both lecture and seminar formats. The primary topics covered are a basic introduction to the legal system and bioethics, patients rights and informed consent, medical malpractice, confidentiality and privacy, reproduction and the law, death and organ transplantation, terminal illness and right to refuse treatment, human experimentation, medical student responsibilities, and the regulation of medical practice (Appendix 1-3).

The Boston University School of Medicine's health law and bioethics curriculum is integrated into other courses taken during the second year of medical school, such as drug law and research ethics in pharmacology and abortion in reproductive endocrinology. The clinical years also offer health law and bioethics faculty the opportunity to do general faculty inservice teaching, deliver formal grand rounds, participate in case conferences, consult to medical education (such as in the intensive care unit or a human immunodeficiency virus [HIV] clinic), and assist in creating policies. Specific health law and bioethics case studies have been developed for use in the third- and fourth-year clerkships and in the integrated problems seminar required of all students.

CONTINUING EDUCATION

Postgraduate medicolegal education should be an integral part of every specialty training program throughout each year of residency and fellowship. This can usually be accomplished with relative academic ease because the physicians (for the most part) are physically present in the hospital complex and can be convened at appropriate times. Moreover, because most residency training programs are located in large medical centers, there are often full- or part-time attorneys available at the center itself or within the close surrounding community who could be called on to give lectures and spearhead discussions on a variety of medicolegal subjects. In addition, staff physicians (hospital-employed and private practitioners), hospital administrative personnel, and other health care professionals can participate in these educational sessions.

Although much useful medicolegal information can be imparted to medical school students, many of these topics assume greater significance and critical importance to graduate physicians as they pursue their chosen careers in more focalized fashion. Broad philosophical concepts and generalized references then begin to have more immediate and identifiable applications to the actual daily practices of their designated specialties. This keener awareness of what is expected of them from the judicial system should be capitalized on to the fullest extent possible.

Regularly scheduled discussions of an informal nature should be augmented by more formal presentations given by experts on specific subjects. From time to time, visiting academicians and outstanding medical and legal practitioners are available in the community. They should be contacted in advance and invited to meet with staff and resident physicians to share their knowledge and experiences.

More formally structured programs should be implemented for appropriate specialties (forensic pathology instruction at the coroner's or medical examiner's office; forensic psychiatry at prisons, detention centers, and community mental health facilities; forensic aspects of orthopedic surgery and physical medicine at large trauma and rehabilitation centers, etc.).

Continuing medicolegal education for fully trained practicing physicians should be encouraged and facilitated by local medical and bar associations, specialty societies, and medical and law schools. Luncheons and dinner meetings with special speakers can be appropriate and pleasant forums in which to provide mandatory continuing medical education credits. Pharmaceutical companies, private foundations, insurance companies, large law firms, and some governmental agencies can be ethically solicited to sponsor such events. Many communities have annual interprofessional medicolegal meetings that can be used as vehicles to disseminate traditional information (e.g., preparing the treating physician for expert testimony) and newer concepts (e.g., physician-assisted suicide).

In 1982 the American Board of Legal Medicine was established to administer examinations to individuals with both legal and medical degrees. Since then, this Board has certified approximately 250 M.D./J.D.s in legal medicine. These examinations are given annually. Other specialty groups that may have some relevance to M.D./J.D.s are the American College of Physician Executives and the American College of Quality Assurance.

Although a law degree is not a prerequisite, formal legal training can be of great value to forensic pathologists seeking certification in that subspecialty by the American Board of Pathology and quite similarly to forensic psychiatrists seeking certification in their subspecialty by the American Board of Psychiatry.

HUMAN RIGHTS AND HEALTH

By the middle of the 1990s it was recognized that health law and medical ethics could constructively be combined in the growing area of international human rights, especially in the area of "human rights in health." The fiftieth anniversary of the Nuremberg physicians' trial, in which physicians and attorneys worked together to bring some of the Nazi physicians to justice, was observed in 1996.[35] The anniversary spurred the International Association of Bioethics to devote major portions of its biannual meeting to discussing health and human rights and an international commemoration meeting at the U.S. Holocaust Memorial Museum in late 1996. It also led to the foundation of Global Lawyers and Physicians (GLP), a new international organization devoted to bringing attorneys and physicians together to promote human rights in health around the world. GLP works with existing physician and attorney groups, such as Physicians for Human Rights and the Lawyers' Committee for Human Rights, toward realizing this goal.[36] There are a growing number of health and human rights courses, seminars, and student groups at schools of law, medicine, and public health (Appendix 1-4). A new course textbook focusing on the inextricable link between health and human rights also was recently published.[37]

CONCLUSION

As global interdependence grows and the metaphor of the global village approaches at least informational reality, the need for interdisciplinary study and real-world cooperation has taken on new meaning. Perhaps nowhere have both the need and opportunities for professional cooperation expanded as dramatically as in the field that was historically known as *legal medicine*. Physicians and attorneys must work together to both shape and respond to the new global realities in which country- and culture-based practices and laws are increasingly shaped by international events and the recognition of the impact of human rights on health. These exciting and challenging times demand both intensive health law and ethics education in medical and law schools, as well as constructive cooperation between the legal and medical professions in addressing the health-related problems of the world.

ENDNOTES

1. William J. Curran, *Titles in the Medicolegal Field: A Proposal for Reform,* 1 Am. J.L. Med. 1-11 (1975).
2. Alan R. Moritz, *The Need of Forensic Pathology for Academic Sponsorship,* 33 Arch. Pathology 382-386 (1942).
3. *Supra* note 1.
4. Sir Sidney Smith, *The History and Development of Legal Medicine,* in *Legal Medicine,* 1-19 (R.B.H. Gradwohi ed., C.V. Mosby Co., St Louis 1954).
5. *Id.*
6. Gilbert H. Stewart, *Legal Medicine,* 1-6 (Bobbs-Merrill Co., Indianapolis 1910).
7. *Supra* note 1.
8. *Supra* note 6.
9. *Supra* note 4.
10. Chester R. Burns, *Legacies in Law and Medicine* (Science History Publications, Canton 1977).
11. William J. Curran, *History and Development,* in *Modern Legal Medicine, Psychiatry, and Forensic Science,* 1-26 (William J. Curran et al. eds., F.A. Davis Co., Philadelphia 1980).
12. James C. Mohr, *Doctors and the Law: Medical Jurisprudence in the Nineteenth Century America* (Oxford University Press, New York 1993).
13. Benjamin Rush, *Introductory Lectures upon the Institutes and Practices of Medicine,* 363 (Bradford and Innskeep, Philadelphia 1811). *See* Curran, *supra* note 1.
14. *Id.*
15. *Id.*
16. George Annas chaired the first National Health Law Teachers conference, which was sponsored by Boston University's Center for Law and Health Sciences. Since 1976 the Health Law Teacher's Meeting has been held a dozen times, biannually until 1985 and annually since.
17. *Teaching Health Law: A Symposium,* 38 J. Legal Educ. 485-576 (1988).
18. 5. Law, *Teaching Health Law: A Symposium: Introduction,* 38 J. Legal Educ. 485, 486 (1988). The basic text for the standard law and medicine course is William J. Curran et al., *Law, Medicine and Forensic Science* (4th ed., Little, Brown and Company, Boston 1991).
19. R. Rosenblatt, *Conceptualizing Health Law for Teaching Purposes: The Social Justice Perspective,* 38 J. Legal Educ. 489 (1988).
20. C. Havighurst, *Health Care as a Laboratory for the Study of Law and Policy,* 38 J. Legal Educ. 499 (1988).
21. George J. Annas, *Health Law at the Turn of the Century: From White Dwarf to Red Giant,* 2 Comm. L. Rev. 551 (1989).
22. Standard texts include B. Furrow et al., *Health Law* (2d ed., West Publishing Co., St Paul, Minn. 1994) and *American Health Law* (Little, Brown and Company, Boston 1990).
23. M. Kelman, *A Guide to Critical Legal Studies,* 186 (Harvard University Press, Cambridge, Mass. 1987).
24. *Id.*
25. K. Wing, *The Law and the Public's Health* (3d ed., Health Administration Press, Ann Arbor, Mich. 1985).
26. Ten years ago one of us (George J. Annas) proposed devoting the entire last semester of law school to health law for all students. It is no secret to most law students and faculty that the final semester of the third year is often a lost semester. It is also no secret that law school curriculum is becoming increasingly detached from the real world, attorneys are becoming increasingly alienated from their work, and their fellow citizens are becoming increasingly alienated from them. *See, e.g.,* D. Bok, *A Flawed System of Law Practice and Teaching,* 33 J. Legal Educ. 570 (1983). *See also* H. Wellington, *Challenges to Legal Education: The "Two Cultures" Phenomenon,* 37 J. Legal Educ. 327 (1987) and J. White, *Doctrine in a Vacuum: Reflections on What a Law School Ought (and Ought Not) To Be,* 36 J. Legal Educ. 155 (1986). As already stressed, health law is applied law, and providing students with the opportunity to apply what they have learned in law school to a particular field of human endeavor gives them an opportunity to synthesize their knowledge and approach the world in an encompassing rather than a reductive mode. As Dean George Schatzki of the University of Connecticut Law School stressed in opening a 1989 health law symposium: "Law is concerned with making the world a better place to live in." (From *Welcoming Remarks, Conference on Law and Medicine: Unresolved Issues for the 1990s,* University of Connecticut School of Law, March 29, 1989.) When Dean Robert Clark of Harvard Law School was asked what he considered the "leading issues in the study of law today" he listed "health care regulations" first. (March 31 *New York Times* B6 [1989]). Dean Schatzki went on to list the four areas that are central to individuals' lives but are seldom dealt with in law school—family, work, recreation, and health. Health law is the only field that can cover all of these areas and thus play a key role in humanizing the law school curriculum and encouraging attorneys and law students to get involved in and help solve critical human problems.
27. There are a variety of curriculum options. One would be to have all students take a basic overview course on health law in the fall of the third year, with special emphasis on developing an understanding of the health care industry itself. The second semester would then consist of three or four courses, each approaching the industry from a different perspective (such as law and economics, social justice, bioethics, technology, public health, environmental law, occupational health and safety law, and law and medicine). Students would then participate in a writing seminar, a clinical project, or both, preferably with one or more medical students. Health law presents an opportunity to apply law and its rules and procedures to the most intrinsically fascinating and substantively influential industry in the United States. As the subject matter of health law—the fields of medicine, public health, and bioethics—continues to expand, so does the field of health law itself. Of course, once the health care system is under control, the final semester could concentrate on other real-world problems, such as the criminal justice system, education, energy, transportation, and the environment.
28. Harry S. Jonas et al., *Educational Programs in U.S. Medical Schools,* 270 J.A.M.A. 1061-1068 (1993).
29. Eugene S. Schneller & Terry S. Weiner, *The M.D./J.D. Revisited: A Sociological Analysis of Cross-Educated Professionals in the Decade of the 1980s,* 6 J. Legal Med. 337-359 (1985).
30. *Id.*
31. B. Blechner et al., *The Jay Healey Technique: Teaching Law and Ethics to Medical and Dental Students,* 20 American J. Law Med. 439 (1994).

32. S. Miles et al., *Medical Ethics Education: Coming of Age,* 64 Academic Medicine 705-714 (1989).
33. C.M. Culver et al., *Special Report: Basic Curricular Goals in Medical Ethics,* 312(4) New Engl. J. Med. 253-255 (1985).
34. M.A. Grodin ed., *Meta Medical Ethics: The Philosophical Foundations of Bioethics* (Kluwer Academic Press, Norwell, Mass. 1995).
35. M.A. Grodin & George J. Annas, *Legacies of Nuremberg: Medical Ethics and Human Rights,* 276 J.A.M.A. 1682 (1996).
36. George J. Annas & Michael A. Grodin eds., *The Nazi Doctors and the Nuremberg Code: Human Rights in Human Experimentation* (Oxford University Press, New York 1992).
37. Jonathan Mann, Sofia Gruskin, Michael A. Grodin, & George J. Annas eds., *Health and Human Rights* (Routledge, New York 1999).

APPENDIX 1-1   Program of law and medicine

SOUTHERN ILLINOIS UNIVERSITY, SCHOOLS OF MEDICINE AND LAW
THEODORE R. LeBLANG, J.D., F.C.L.M. (PROGRAM DIRECTOR)

BACKGROUND

The program of law and medicine, which began in the mid-1970s, is an academic program based in the department of medical humanities. Although teaching activity forming part of the various programs in the department is integrated throughout the 4-year curriculum, required instruction in legal medicine is concentrated during the clinical clerkship year. At this time students rotate through clerkships representing the major medical specialties. Students also participate in the multidisciplinary medical humanities clerkship.

The Department of Medical Humanities offers a curriculum designed to provide students with core knowledge in the humanities, emphasizing application of the content and methodologies of humanities disciplines to the practice of medicine. Substantive areas of teaching emphasis include ethics, health policy, law, medical history, philosophy, and psychosocial care. The 4-week medical humanities clerkship is divided into two segments—medical humanities A and B. Each segment lasts 2 weeks.

Medical humanities A is delivered during the junior year and focuses on the physician-patient relationship. Issues of confidentiality and privacy, informed consent, standards of care (malpractice), withholding and withdrawing life-sustaining treatment, assisted death, palliative care, organ donation, physician-patient communication, and psychosocial care are addressed in the context of lectures, panel discussions, case conferences, tutor group activities, and simulated patient interactions. Throughout the clerkship, teaching emphasis is placed on strengthening the physician-patient relationship.

Medical humanities B is delivered during the senior year and is composed of the following two content areas: (1) the physician's role in the administration of justice and (2) the physician's role in society, with emphasis on current changes in health care delivery. During the first part of the clerkship, students are exposed to an overview of the judicial process and the manner in which physicians serve as expert witnesses in civil and criminal trial proceedings. Systems of medicolegal investigation also are discussed, with emphasis on forensic pathology.

Students further explore issues involving regulation of medical expert testimony in the courts. Finally, a mock trial is staged, permitting students to observe the trial process in a courtroom setting. During the second part of the clerkship, students examine various important issues relating to health care in the United States. These issues include economic considerations bearing upon health care delivery; health care financing; access to and availability of health care; clinical, ethical, legal, and policy aspects of managed care; and the changing accountability of physicians in an evolving health care system.

Educational activities in the program of law and medicine are mastery based, with learning objectives that are designed to convey to each student relevant faculty expectations. Learning objectives are contained in modules, which are the basic leaning components of the curriculum. Modules are self-contained curriculum units, wherein faculty members designate specific learning objectives, required and recommended learning activities, and criteria for successful completion.

Presentation of legal medicine modules during the clerkship year familiarizes students with important legal principles at a time when these principles are particularly relevant to their clinical activities. Within the framework of the 4-week medical humanities clerkship, as previously described, approximately 40% of learning modules focus entirely or in pertinent part on issues arising at the interface of law and medicine. In addition to the modules that form part of the medical humanities clerkship, numerous additional modules focus on issues that are uniquely relevant to the medical specialties of internal medicine, obstetrics and gynecology, pediatrics, psychiatry, and surgery. These modules are integrated directly into the respective clinical clerkships.

In the internal medicine clerkship a multidisciplinary module on domestic violence focuses on clinical, legal, and psychosocial considerations relating primarily to partner abuse. In the obstetrics and gynecology clerkship one module focuses on the legal aspects of abortion. In the pediatrics clerkship an integrated module focuses on the legal aspects of child abuse and neglect. In the psychiatry clerkship a learning module focuses on issues involving the following topics:

civil commitment and patients' rights after involuntary hospitalization; concepts of insanity, competency, and testamentary capacity; confidentiality and privacy within the psychiatrist-patient relationship; and psychiatric malpractice, with emphasis on potential areas of liability, including the failure to warn third parties of a patient's dangerous propensities. In the surgery clerkship the applicability of advance directives is considered as part of clinical case problems. Thus throughout the clinical clerkship segment of the undergraduate curriculum, students participate in numerous required learning modules addressing important issues in legal medicine.

During the senior year, a diverse selection of electives is offered for students who wish to further their knowledge in areas of legal medicine. Included among these electives are the following: AIDS: Law and Ethics, Health Policy and Legal Issues in Aging, Legal and Ethical Issues in Organ and Tissue Donation and Transplantation, Negotiation and Dispute Resolution in Health Care, and Studies in Law and Medicine.

CURRICULUM DETAIL

Titles and descriptions of the various required and elective learning experiences that form part of the program of law and medicine are detailed in the following section.

Freshman year: confidentiality— legal and ethical issues

As soon as medical students begin their clinical experiences, they face ethical questions about protecting patient confidentiality and privacy. These questions will persist throughout their professional lives in one form or another. The purpose of this module is to give students a legal and ethical framework for thinking about whether to protect or breach confidentiality and privacy. The module focuses on dilemmas that participants face as students.

Sophomore year: introduction to family violence

With increasing frequency, physicians are confronted with problems of family violence in the context of patient care. Accordingly, students should be familiar with the basic clinical, legal, ethical, and psychosocial issues that may arise in treating victims of child abuse, partner abuse, or elder abuse. This learning experience provides students an opportunity to explore these issues in the context of lectures and small group, case-based discussions.

Junior year: medical humanities clerkship

LEGAL PERSPECTIVES ON THE PHYSICIAN-PATIENT RELATIONSHIP: OVERVIEW OF SOURCES OF LAW. Various societal expectations pertaining to the clinical practice of medicine have been codified in law. Predominantly this codification takes the form of state and federal legislation, as well as applicable regulations of state and federal agencies. Common law principles, which are articulated by state and

federal courts, also constitute an important source of law in this regard.

It is the purpose of this module to provide students with an overview of the sources and types of law that bear upon the physician-patient relationship. Certain illustrative Illinois statutes have been selected for discussion. In varying ways, each of these legislative enactments has an impact on the practice of medicine and the physician-patient relationship. Consideration of these statutes provides an excellent foundation for evaluating legal issues that arise in the context of clinical practice.

STANDARD OF CARE: LEGAL RIGHTS AND RESPONSIBILITIES IN THE PHYSICIAN-PATIENT RELATIONSHIP. The physician-patient relationship has at its core a set of rights and responsibilities attributable both to the physician and to the patient. These rights and duties establish the broad parameters of the relationship and are affected in various ways by established common law doctrines and pertinent statutory enactments. These bodies of law delineate the nature and scope of such concepts as medical malpractice, informed consent, physician-patient privilege, and privacy and confidentiality.

Because of the significance of these legal concepts in the context of the physician-patient relationship, it is essential to develop awareness of the specific meaning and applicability of these concepts and the legal bases on which they are founded. It is the purpose of this module to discuss the common law and statutory bases of medical malpractice against the background of specific case illustrations in which medical malpractice may have occurred in clinical situations. Emphasis is placed on consideration of the standard of care in the context of health care delivery and the physician-patient relationship.

INFORMED CONSENT: LEGAL RIGHTS AND RESPONSIBILITIES. Within the physician-patient relationship there is a set of legal rights and responsibilities applicable to both physician and patient. These rights and responsibilities provide a framework for consideration of the doctrine of informed consent. Under this legal doctrine, physicians are obligated to disclose to patients the nature of a proposed medical treatment or procedure, the anticipated benefits and material risks thereof, and any reasonably available alternatives. This disclosure obligation is evaluated based on application of principles of negligence and medical malpractice law, with emphasis on the standard of care.

It is the purpose of this module to discuss common law and statutory foundations for the legal doctrine of informed consent against the background of specific case illustrations that demonstrate applicability of this doctrine in clinical situations. Historical evolution of the informed consent doctrine also is traced with emphasis on medical ethics.

CONFIDENTIALITY AND PRIVACY: LEGAL RIGHTS AND RESPONSIBILITIES. Confidentiality within the physician-patient relationship facilitates full, frank, and candid disclosure of medical information from patient to treating physician. This exchange is intended to permit the physician to reach an appropriate diagnosis and achieve a satisfactory clinical outcome. Because of the personal nature of confidential patient information, in most situations physicians are ethically and legally obligated to protect such information from improper disclosure. Moreover, a statutory privilege exists to ensure that, as a general rule, physicians are not required to disclose confidential information in certain courtroom situations.

It is the purpose of this module to discuss the common law and statutory predicates of the legal doctrines of confidentiality and privacy against the background of specific case illustrations that demonstrate applicability of these principles in clinical situations. Related ethical and philosophical considerations also are addressed.

CLINICAL, ETHICAL, LEGAL, AND PSYCHOSOCIAL ASPECTS OF WITHHOLDING OR WITHDRAWING TREATMENT. Some physicians believe that they have an obligation to prolong life without regard to its quality or other considerations. Cardiopulmonary resuscitation and intensive care technologies have made it possible to prolong life in individuals who have little or no prospect of recovery. Death is kept at bay as if death is always undesirable and the physician's enemy. As a result, patients have sometimes been forced to endure a prolonged process of dying or to live what they or others judge to be a meaningless existence.

The ethical, legal, and psychosocial issues associated with these behaviors are complex. The purpose of this module is to familiarize students with a variety of issues, including the following: Do physicians really have an obligation to prolong life under all circumstances? Is withholding or withdrawing life support killing? If it is proper to withhold or withdraw care in some circumstances, who makes this decision? What criteria should be used to decide when medical care should be withheld or withdrawn? What mechanisms exist to ensure that the previously expressed desires of incompetent patients, with respect to withholding or withdrawing life-sustaining treatment, may be acted on by health care providers?

CASE STUDIES IN WITHHOLDING OR WITHDRAWING TREATMENT. This module focuses on the practical clinical problems associated with managing cases of terminal illness. In particular the module explores the professional attitudes and beliefs that contribute to difficulties surrounding terminal illness involving communicating and decision-making with patients, their surrogates, and other health professionals.

ASSISTED DEATH: LEGAL AND ETHICAL ISSUES. The growing controversy over whether physicians should assist patients in dying raises difficult ethical and legal questions. Those on each side of the debate claim that practices and policies defended by their opponents have a deleterious impact on physician-patient relationships. The purpose of this module is to examine those claims and place them in the context of the wider debate about physician-assisted death.

ORGAN DONATION. During the last 40 years the science of organ transplantation has advanced rapidly. Concomitant advances in medical procedures and medical technology have rapidly increased the number of patients who are medically eligible to receive donated organs as well. In an effort to respond positively to this demand, state and federal laws have changed repeatedly. Each change and proposal for change has raised questions about the rights and responsibilities of individuals, their families, physicians, and other health care professionals in supplying organs for potential recipients.

Physicians, because of their close relationships with patients, are sometimes looked to as a source of information about organ donation. They also manage care for the dying patients who will be organ donors. As such, they need to understand legal and ethical frameworks for organ donation.

OVERVIEW OF THE JUDICIAL PROCESS. Because of the significant potential for physician involvement in litigation either as a witness on behalf of a patient, an expert witness, or a party to a lawsuit, the physician must possess a general knowledge of the judicial process. The purpose of this module is to provide a broad overview of the judicial process with emphasis on pretrial, trial, and posttrial procedures. This module also addresses the appellate court process and its relationship to trial court activities. Federal and state court activities and litigation also are compared.

THE PHYSICIAN AS EXPERT WITNESS. Throughout the course of an active medical practice, a physician is likely to be called as an expert witness during the course of civil or criminal litigation. In the capacity of a medical expert the physician may be asked to give testimony regarding the nature and cause of injuries suffered as a consequence of an automobile accident or employment-related mishap. The physician expert also may be called on to testify regarding the standard of care in a medical malpractice case or regarding medical facts that bear directly on a criminal prosecution charging homicide or sexual assault.

In any of these situations the physician must be aware of the precise role played by the medical expert and the manner in which the medical expert's responsibilities may best be fulfilled. The purpose of this module is to examine the physician's role as a medical expert witness in civil and criminal proceedings, placing focus on pretrial and trial involvement.

THE PHYSICIAN AS EXPERT WITNESS: REGULATING THE MEDICAL EXPERT. Physicians make ideal expert witnesses; they are well-educated, well-respected members of society and have superior knowledge of complex scientific issues. A physician expert witness who can present to the jury an articulate, plausible opinion as to why a particular chain of events led to a particular result can help lead a jury to a particular decision.

Most physician experts perform their roles admirably. However, some, through inaccuracies or misrepresentations in their testimony, contribute to the ever-rising costs of health care services and malpractice insurance, diminish the public's confidence in the medical profession, and occasionally lead to the destruction of personal and professional reputations. This module explores what is being done to ensure that the physician who appears as an expert witness is a responsible participant in the administration of justice, as well as a practitioner who is promoting sound medicine.

FORENSIC MEDICINE: MEDICOLEGAL INVESTIGATION. Forensic medicine, broadly defined, has to do with an interaction between medicine and law and more specifically relates to medical problems that result in subsequent legal procedures. Forensic pathology is that branch of forensic medicine that involves the examination of deaths generally falling into the following categories: (1) physical injury, (2) chemical injury, and (3) unexpected "natural" death. The forensic pathologist is expected to aid in determining the cause, the mechanisms, and the manner of death.

Forensic pathology is conducted within the framework of a specific system created by state or local laws. The systems currently operating within the United States are the coroner's system and the medical examiner's system. Medicolegal investigation includes the circumstances of death, the postmortem examination, and a variety of laboratory procedures, including toxicology and trace analysis. Investigation of the circumstances of death is carried out by various law enforcement agencies, along with representatives of the coroner's or medical examiner's offices. The postmortem examination is generally carried out by a pathologist; however, in some instances practicing physicians perform postmortem examinations. Laboratory procedures may be performed in the pathologist's laboratory (usually a hospital laboratory), a state toxicology laboratory, and the so-called crime laboratory.

In Illinois there are three systems for handling medicolegal investigation. In Cook County, a medical examiner's system is responsible for all branches of the medicolegal investigation. A large number of remaining counties use the classic coroner's system. On the basis of the Illinois constitution, some more sparsely populated counties eliminate the coroner, and the county board appoints a "death investigator." The death investigator may be the local sheriff, a physician in the community, or some other community citizen.

MOCK TRIAL. The opportunity for the medical student to integrate substantive and procedural legal knowledge in the context of a clinical courtroom proceeding is an essential adjunct to a full and complete legal and medical learning experience. It is the purpose of this module to stage a mock trial that offers a realistic forum for consideration of substantive and procedural law.

To ensure maximum reality, the mock trial takes place in the Circuit Court of Illinois, Seventh Judicial Circuit. The landmark Illinois case of *Darling v. Charleston Memorial Hospital* is reenacted in an abridged fashion with an emphasis on demonstrating the major aspects of a complete civil trial.

MANAGED CARE: POLICY PERSPECTIVES. As a result of economic overhaul of the health care delivery system in the United States, managed care is now altering the nature and scope of private practice for nearly all physicians. These changes can be expected to have a significant impact on the physician-patient relationship and on individual physicians who must adjust to the changing environment and respond effectively to new challenges.

Various modules incorporate legal issues in evaluating health care delivery from the perspectives of cost, quality, and access. These courses include the following: Introduction to the U.S. Health Care System; Financing Health Care; Managed Care—Physician and Hospital Services; Clinical Decision Making and Quality of Care—Contemporary Challenges; Access to Health Care—EMTALA; Mental Health Care: Cost, Quality, and Access; and Health Care Access and Availability—Issues for Rural and Underserved Populations.

Internal medicine clerkship: domestic violence— interdisciplinary workshop. Medical humanities faculty members participate with internal medicine faculty members in the context of a domestic violence workshop, focusing primarily on spousal abuse. Clinical, legal, social, and psychosocial issues are explored in lectures, small group discussions, and simulated patient examinations that are observed and critiqued by faculty.

Obstetrics and gynecology clerkship: legal aspects of abortion. Illinois statutes, as well as U.S. constitutional laws, regarding abortion have undergone considerable change in response to related social, philosophical, cultural, religious, and political issues. The changes have become increasingly significant, and in the absence of a constitutional amendment the relevant decisions of the U.S. Supreme Court, on their face and through resulting state statutes, shall impact the parameters of the physician-patient relationship.

It is the purpose of this module to familiarize students with certain important Supreme Court decisions relating to abortion. This module also acquaints students with relevant Illinois laws that relate to abortion and traces the development of these laws.

Pediatrics clerkship: legal aspects of child abuse and neglect. Children have been victims of maltreatment throughout history, and child abuse remains a major concern for society today. As a result of the rapidly increasing numbers of abused and neglected children, practicing physicians are highly likely to be confronted with such children in a variety of contexts.

It is the purpose of this module to familiarize physicians with their statutory rights and responsibilities in the context of providing care and treatment to abused and neglected children. This module focuses on the Illinois Abused and Neglected Child Reporting Act. Emphasis also is placed on significant provisions of the Illinois Juvenile Court Act that pertain to cases of child abuse and neglect. In this regard the role of the physician as a participant in juvenile court proceedings and how the physician can effectively carry out this role are examined and discussed. Finally, this module addresses the issue of civil liability, which may result from a physician's failure to report instances of child abuse and neglect.

Psychiatry clerkship: psychiatry and law. The impact of law on clinical psychiatry has become increasingly apparent. Judicial decisions, state and federal legislation, and administrative regulatory schemes affect day-to-day clinical decision-making across a broad range of psychiatric settings and patient populations.

It is the purpose of this module to familiarize the student with significant statutory and common law developments at the state and federal levels that impact the nature and delivery of psychiatric patient care. Primary emphasis is placed on legal issues that involve hospitalization of mentally ill patients, patient's rights, confidentiality and privilege, psychiatric negligence, insanity, and fitness to stand trial.

Surgery clerkship: problem-based learning module. Medical humanities faculty members participate with Department of Surgery faculty in tutor group discussions with students that arise from problem-based learning modules that focus on specific patient cases. These cases examine issues relating to advance directives and surrogate decision-making in situations of terminal illness.

Senior year electives

AIDS: law and ethics. The purpose of the AIDS: Law and Ethics elective is to enable students to understand and think critically about the ethical and legal questions surrounding the AIDS epidemic. Those issues include but are not limited to testing, screening, reporting, partner notification, quarantine, and drug development. Students engage in research that results in an oral presentation and written research paper.

Health policy and legal issues in aging. In 2011 the first of the 76 million baby boomers will turn 65. The aging members of this huge generation will have enormous economic, social, and political consequences and put even greater strain on the country's already unstable health care delivery system. The Health Policy and Legal Issues in Aging elective is designed to enable students to develop an understanding of policy and legal issues concerning the care and treatment of America's aged population. Issues addressed may include the role of managed care in Medicare and Medicaid; the impact of changes in use of home health, assisted living, and nursing home services; proposed and recently adopted changes to the Medicare system; and special circumstances affecting older citizens living in rural areas. During the course of the elective, students engage in

research that results in an oral presentation and written research paper. Students also are responsible for completing assigned readings and participating in small group discussion.

Legal and ethical issues in organ and tissue donation and transplantation. The purpose of the Legal and Ethical Issues in Organ and Tissue Donation and Transplantation elective is to enable students to understand and think critically about the legal and ethical issues related to organ and tissue donation and transplantation. Topics include the following: gift versus market paradigms; use of anencephalic fetuses, prisoners, minors, and cadavers as sources of organs and tissue; rationing of scarce medical resources; and cost-effectiveness analysis of transplantation. The Uniform Anatomical Gift Act; the End-Stage Renal Disease Amendments to the Social Security Act; the National Organ Transplant Act; statutory and proposed definitions of brain death, routine inquiry, and required request; and other proposals are analyzed.

Negotiation and dispute resolution in health care. Negotiation occurs daily at all levels of the health care industry—from discussing treatment options with patients and insurance companies to resolving intraoffice conflicts to engineering multibillion dollar hospital mergers. Knowing how to effectively negotiate solutions to problems and disagreements is critical to a physician's ability to practice successfully in today's complex health care environment. This elective is designed to enable medical students to learn negotiation and dispute resolution techniques that can be used in medical and nonmedical settings. Students enrolled in this elective study the various forms of dispute resolution available outside the courtroom setting. Through assigned readings and role-playing exercises, students learn techniques that enable them to resolve conflicts by identifying and building on mutual interests.

Studies in law and medicine. The Studies in Law and Medicine elective enables students to develop the ability to analyze medical decisions from a legal viewpoint. It involves review of case law relating to health care delivery, the physician-patient relationship, and the physician's role in the administration of justice. The elective emphasizes a sophisticated analysis of national case law and a comparison of issues raised in previous medical humanities rotations.

Students attend lectures and seminars provided by various faculty, including attorneys from state agencies and professional organizations, representing the interests of health care providers. Students also examine medicolegal issues that are of specific interest to them.

APPENDIX 1-2 M.D./J.D. dual degree program

SOUTHERN ILLINOIS UNIVERSITY, SCHOOLS OF MEDICINE AND LAW
THEODORE R. LeBLANG, J.D., F.C.L.M. (PROGRAM DIRECTOR, SCHOOL OF MEDICINE)
W. EUGENE BASANTA, J.D., LL.M. (PROGRAM DIRECTOR, SCHOOL OF LAW)

PROGRAM OVERVIEW

Recognizing the heightened level of interaction between the professions of law and medicine in today's society, the Southern Illinois University (SIU) Schools of Medicine and Law offer an M.D./J.D. dual degree program to accommodate the increasing number of individuals seeking a carefully structured interdisciplinary education. The dual degree program is designed to lead to the concurrent award of degrees in law and medicine at the completion of a 6-year curriculum involving academic and clinical study.

CURRICULUM DESIGN AND PROGRAM CONTENT

The SIU program requires students to spend their first year at the School of Law in Carbondale, where they complete 31 credit hours of prescribed first-year course work. Students then enroll in the law school summer session and complete 6 credit hours of advanced course work, as well as a 1-hour legal research course offered during the summer intersession.

During the second academic year, students continue at Carbondale as full-time law students, completing an additional 32 credit hours of course work, with concentration in health law. Enrollment in a second summer session, during which students complete 6 credit hours of course work, is required. This session may include courses in legal research and clinical experience in state or federal agencies involved in the regulation of public health and the activities of the medical profession.

Students spend their third academic year enrolled as freshmen in the School of Medicine at Carbondale, where they complete all requirements of the first year of the medical school curriculum. Students then move to Springfield, where they continue as full-time medical students, completing the sophomore and junior years of the curriculum.

During the senior year of medical school, students are required to take a specially designed set of law, medicine, and health policy electives lasting 14 weeks full-time. In completing degree requirements for both the M.D. and J.D. degrees, this 14-week elective sequence fulfills 14 credit hours of course work required for attainment of the J.D. degree and 14 weeks of elective course work required for attainment of the M.D. degree.

M.D./J.D. ELECTIVE SEQUENCE

Eighteen weeks of electives are available to M.D./J.D. program students, from which they must select and participate in at least 14 weeks full-time. Descriptions of these electives are detailed here.

Forensic psychiatry subinternship

The forensic psychiatry subinternship provides a focused clinical experience in forensic psychiatry that builds on and enhances the basic clinical experience provided in the psychiatry clerkship. Emphasis is placed on clinical interaction with forensic patients and inpatients who have been involuntarily hospitalized under the provisions of the Illinois Mental Health and Developmental Disabilities Code.

Students act as subinterns at the Chester Mental Health Center (Chester). Supervision is provided by designated attending psychiatrists at Chester and consists of daily oral review of diagnosis, treatment, and management plans and individual supervisory sessions reviewing all aspects of patient care, with emphasis on forensic considerations and medicolegal interventions.

Activities and experiences include daily rounds, psychiatric evaluation and management of assigned patients, daily written progress notes and orders, and preparation of forensic reports based on psychiatric assessments of patients involved in criminal proceedings regarding their sanity and fitness to stand trial. Students also participate in treatment interventions with medicolegal ramifications, such as involuntary treatment, restraint, and seclusion.

Health policy formulation: the legislative and regulatory processes in Illinois

The Health Policy Formulation: The Legislative and Regulatory Processes in Illinois elective is designed to enable students to develop an understanding of health policy formulation in Illinois; emphasis is on the nature and scope of both the legislative and regulatory processes. Students are involved in reviewing proposed legislation and regulations having an impact on the development of health policy and the practice of medicine in Illinois. Students interact with the Illinois General Assembly with an objective of obtaining insight into the legislative process. When interest groups attempt to influence legislation affecting health policy, students interact with members of these groups to explore and evaluate their views.

Learning experiences also include interaction with regulatory personnel at state agencies that have jurisdiction over medical practice, health care delivery, public health, and health welfare programs. Students are afforded the opportunity to evaluate proposed regulations and to examine the assessment by the Joint Committee on Administrative Rules.

During the course of the elective, students undertake sophisticated analysis of proposed health laws and regulations. Students also attend seminars, lectures, and tutorials with state agency regulatory personnel, general assembly members and staff, and teaching faculty. In addition, students are responsible for completing assigned readings describing the legislative and regulatory processes in Illinois.

History of medical jurisprudence in American medical education

The History of Medical Jurisprudence in American Medical Education elective provides students with an overview of the development of medical jurisprudence as a special area for scholarly inquiry. Emphasis is on the early history of medical jurisprudence teaching in nineteenth century U.S. medical schools, but important European influences also are explored. Students trace the evolution of medical jurisprudence as a subject of study in medical schools from its era of central importance in the early 1800s to the resurgence of interest in law and medicine in contemporary curricula.

In exploring the history of medical jurisprudence, students pay particular attention to classic areas of medicolegal overlap, including medicine's role in assisting with legal definitions of paternity and insanity. The role of physicians as expert witnesses is discussed, and the history of toxicology as a forensic tool is explored. Attention also is paid to the development of a number of related legal issues as they have informed the curricula of American medical schools, particularly the emergence of malpractice as the central concern of medicolegal study.

Hospital and health care organizations: current legal issues

The Hospital and Health Care Organizations: Current Legal Issues elective is intended to provide students with an overview of legal issues that bear upon the structure, organization, and operation of health care organizations. By attending seminars, students gain insight into predominant aspects of the administration, management, and operation of health systems and associations. Additional learning activities focus on legal issues that form part of the policy agenda of the Illinois Hospital and Health Systems Association.

Issues in mental disability law

The Issues in Mental Disability Law elective provides the student with an opportunity to undertake in-depth scholarly study of some of the critical legal issues involving persons with mental disabilities. There is a general overview of mental disability law and a review of some of the major cases affecting mental health services.

The elective focuses on the following three issues: (1) the role of the psychiatrist in the implementation of the death penalty, such as participation in the insanity defense, competency to stand trial, and testimony concerning fitness to be executed; (2) the effect of the major "patient's rights" lawsuits on the quality of state mental health services, the impact of landmark court decisions on improving institutional

conditions, and Supreme Court case law that sets a standard for violation of constitutional rights in institutions; and (3) the development and implementation of the right to refuse psychotropic medication in Illinois and other states, with emphasis on major cases defining such a right and studies on the impact of such a right on the delivery of mental health services.

Each issue is examined with emphasis on the interaction between law and psychiatry. Death penalty cases involve a potential moral dilemma of a psychiatrist asked to perform an evaluation and thereby become part of a legal process he or she may find objectionable. The institutional quality cases reflect the effect of law on public policy, the state bureaucracy, and the daily treatment and living conditions of the patients. The right to refuse cases is the paradigm of a conflict between the "medical model" and the "rights model" in mental health service delivery.

Medicolegal investigation: advanced studies in forensic pathology

The Medicolegal Investigation: Advanced Studies in Forensic Pathology elective provides students with an in-depth understanding of the systems for medicolegal investigation. The role of forensic pathology in the context of medicolegal investigation is carefully explored. Student learning activities and experiences may include participation in and attendance at activities such as coroner's inquests, crime scene and laboratory investigations, postmortem examinations, criminal trial proceedings, and off-site visits to facilities that support medicolegal investigations (e.g., polygraph testing facilities and toxicology laboratories) or facilities where investigations may occur (e.g., investigations of death in prisons, jails, and mental health facilities). During the course of the elective, students are responsible for completing various assigned readings focusing on topics in forensic pathology, maintaining a daily record of activities, and preparing a one-hour formal oral presentation using photographs, graphics, and an annotated bibliography.

Regulation of the medical profession: current legal and policy issues

The Regulation of the Medical Profession: Current Legal and Policy Issues elective provides students with the opportunity to examine some of the key policy and legal issues confronted by state medical licensing boards in the context of regulating the medical profession. The role of the professional regulatory board with regard to the modern health care delivery system is examined in-depth. Discussion focuses on issues such as the role of licensing boards in managed care, prescribing practices and privileges, the impact of technology on physician oversight, and the changing supervisory role of physicians over allied health professionals. A seminar and tutorial teaching format is used, with emphasis on student research and class discussion.

Studies in medicolegal aspects of obstetrics and gynecology

The Studies in Medicolegal Aspects of Obstetrics and Gynecology elective is intended to provide students with an overview of medicolegal issues that have arisen in the context of clinical obstetrics and gynecology, with additional consideration of relevant research-related medicolegal issues. A seminar and tutorial teaching format is used, with emphasis on student research and group discussion.

Students are expected to read and evaluate assigned cases, focusing on important constitutional and common law issues involving such topics as abortion, maternal-fetal conflict, artificial human reproduction, the rights of newborns (including the anencephalic newborn), and other assigned topics. Relevant statutory law also is considered and discussed. Student activities include attendance at lectures, participation in interactive seminar discussions, and oral presentation of assigned research.

APPENDIX 1-3   Introduction to health law

BOSTON UNIVERSITY SCHOOL OF MEDICINE
GEORGE J. ANNAS, J.D., M.P.H.
LEONARD H. GLANTZ, J.D.
WENDY K. MARINER, J.D., M.P.H.
MICHAEL A. GRODIN, M.D., F.A.A.P.

Course	Learning objectives	Required readings	Lecture outline
Introduction to the American legal system	1. Explain the basic legal system and its purposes 2. Distinguish various types of laws and their applications to medicine 3. Read and analyze judicial opinions related to medicine	1. Wind, *The Law and the Legal System,* "Introduction" (pp. 4-15) 2. "Reading a Legal Case" (2 pages) 3. Massachusetts laws on physician licensure 4. The "Student Doctor" and "A Wary Patient" 5. *Legacies of Nuremberg*	I. Role and function of the law II. "Kinds" of law III. Application of various kinds of law IV. Judge-made law (including how a case is heard and appealed)
Medical malpractice litigation	1. Understand the basic concepts of negligence law and how these apply to physicians 2. Understand what is meant by "standard of care" and how it is established 3. Understand the liability of health care institutions 4. Understand the obligation of institutions to provide emergency care	1. *Darling v. Charleston Hospital* 2. *Helling v. Carey* 3. *Wilmington General Hospital v. Manlove* 4. Massachusetts Good Samaritan Statute 5. Massachusetts regulation on provision of medical services in emergencies 6. Annas, *Rights of Patients,* Chapters IV and XIV	I. The elements of negligence II. The concepts of the "reasonable person" and burden or proof III. The role of the "expert witness" IV. The difference between harm and negligence V. The legal liability of institutions: corporate and vicarious liability VI. The legal obligation to render emergency care
Informed consent	1. Understand the concepts underlying the theory of informed consent 2. Understand the difference between battery and negligence 3. Understand the difference between informed consent and informed consent forms	1. *Cobbs v. Grant* 2. "Neglected Aspects of Informed Consent," letter to the editor 3. *Truman v. Thomas* 4. *Informed Consent, Cancer and Truth in Prognosis* 5. Massachusetts statute on HTLV testing 6. Consent form for anti-HIV test 7. *Rights of Patients,* Chapters VI and VII	I. The legal concept of battery II. Consent and implied consent III. The creation of the legal theory of informed consent and its purpose IV. The application of informed consent in different contexts V. The purpose of consent forms VI. Defenses

Course	Learning objectives	Required readings	Lecture outline
Confidentiality and privacy	1. Distinguish privacy, confidentiality, and privilege 2. Explain elements of a lawsuit alleging breach of confidentiality 3. Determine when it is reasonable to breach confidentiality to protect others	1. *Rights of Patients,* Chapters X and XI 2. *Home v. Patton* 3. *Berthiaume v. Pratt* 4. *Tarasoff v. Regents of University of California* 5. Massachusetts general laws on medical records and confidentiality	I. The nature of the dilemma (the role of confidentiality and its rationale) II. *Home v. Patton* III. *Berthiaume v. Pratt* IV. *Tarasoff v. Regents of University of California* V. Conclusion
Reproduction and the law	1. Acquire a basic understanding of how the U.S. Constitution limits state power and protects individual rights 2. Understand the constitutional "right of privacy" 3. Understand how courts balance individual rights and state power 4. Understand the nature and limits of the constitutional right of privacy as it pertains to reproductive decisions	1. *Roe v. Wade* 2. *Planned Parenthood v. Danforth* 3. *Summary of U.S. Supreme Court Decisions on Abortion* 4. Mariner, *The Supreme Court, Abortion, and the Jurisprudence of Class* 5. *Rights of Patients,* Chapter VIII	I. Constitutional limitations on state actions II. Early right of privacy cases and contraception III. *Roe v. Wade* and the rights of physicians IV. The application of *Roe* in subsequent cases V. *Planned Parenthood v. Casey* and the future of abortion litigation
Death and organ transplantation	1. Define death 2. Determine which organ donation is appropriate 3. Distinguish the dead from the dying 4. Define competence (to consent to and to refuse treatment)	1. *Rights of Patients,* Chapters IX and XIII 2. "A Definition of Irreversible Coma," *JAMA* 3. *Notes on Brain Death and Organ Harvesting* 4. *Lane v. Candura* 5. *Matter of Quinlan* 6. "The Promised End: Constitutional Aspects of Physician-Assisted Suicide"	I. Definition of death (brain and respiration criteria) II. Relationship of brain death to organ transplantation III. Consent mechanisms for organ donation IV. Competence to consent to (and refuse) medical interventions *(Candura)* V. The persistent vegetative state as an example of dying *(Quinlan)* VI. Refusing treatment v. suicide prevention

Treatment of the dying	1. Distinguish various types of advance directives, especially living wills and health care proxies
	2. Recognize the barriers to patient autonomy near death
	3. Distinguish between refusing treatment and physician-assisted suicide
		1. *Rights of Patients,* Chapter XII
		2. Annas, "Nancy Cruzan and the Right to Die," *N Engl J Med*
		3. Massachusetts Health Care Proxy Form
		4. SUPPORT, "A Controlled Trial to Improve Care for Seriously Ill Hospitalized Patients," *JAMA*
		5. The Oregon Death with Dignity Act
			I. Patient rights at the end of life
			II. Documenting patient directives
			  A. The living will
			  B. The health care proxy (including the Massachusetts model)
			III. The SUPPORT study and its lessons
			IV. Physician-assisted suicide
			  A. What it is (and is not)
			  B. Why now
			V. Conclusion

HTLV, Human T cell leukemia/lymphoma virus; *HIV,* human immunodeficiency virus.

Appendix 1-4 **Human rights and health**

BOSTON UNIVERSITY SCHOOLS OF MEDICINE AND PUBLIC HEALTH
MICHAEL A. GRODIN, M.D., F.A.A.P.
GEORGE J. ANNAS, J.D., M.P.H.

COURSE DESCRIPTION

Human health is closely linked to the realization of human rights. Preventable illness, infant mortality, and premature death, for example, are closely tied to the violation of human rights. This course explores the relationship between human rights and health by examining relevant international declarations in historical context, exploring the meaning of "human rights" and "health," and analyzing specific case studies that illuminate the problems, prospects, and potential methods of promoting health by promoting human rights on the national and international levels.

Goals and objectives

By the end of this course the student will:
1. Understand the relationship between human rights and health
2. Be familiar with the Universal Declaration of Human Rights and the International Conventions on Human Rights
3. Understand the history, role, and function of nongovernmental organizations (NGOs) in addressing human rights problems
4. Be able to determine when human rights have been violated, know the organizations available for reporting and addressing human rights violations, and be able to suggest strategies to protect and promote human rights

Prerequisites

There are no prerequisites for this course.

Texts

The following texts are required:
E. Wiesel, *Night* (Bantam, New York 1982) ISBN 0553272535 (publication).
H.J. Steiner & P. Alston, *International Human Rights in Context: Law, Politics, Morals* (Clarendon Press, Oxford 1996) ISBN 098254261 (publication).
J. Mann, S. Gruskin, M. Grodin & G. Annas, *Health and Human Rights: A Reader* (Routledge, New York 1999) ISBN 0415921023 (publication).

Additional resources

Students are referred to the following Internet sites:
www.bumc.bu.edu/sph/internet.htm
www.glphr.org

Requirements

Students must complete a 20-page research paper (worth 80% of the final grade) addressing a specific problem in the area of human rights and health. The student must (1) define the nature, scope, and context of a human rights and health problem; (2) describe the impediments to addressing the problem; (3) identify allies; (4) prepare a proposed policy agenda for problem resolution. Students also are expected to give a 15-minute oral presentation of their proposals to the class (worth 10% of the final grade). Class participation, attendance, and preparation of readings also are considered (worth 10% of the final grade).

OUTLINE
Preassignment

Night (entire book)

Week 1
Discussion

Introduction to Health and Human Rights
The Link Between Health Status, Vulnerability, and Rights
Reading
Health and Human Rights Reader, pp. 1-71
International Human Rights in Context, pp. 1-116 (skim pp. 40-83)

Week 2
Discussion

Human Rights Instruments and Documents: The International Bill of Human Rights

Reading
Health and Human Rights Reader, pp. 480-481
International Human Rights in Context, pp. 117-160 (skim 132-144) and 1147-1290 (especially 1148-1171)

Week 3
Discussion

Mechanisms of Enforcement and Reporting

Reading
International Human Rights in Context, pp. 347-455 (skim 354-374 and 382-420) and 707-869 (skim 717-746, 766-778, 801-806, 818-836, 839-844, and 862-869)

1 Legal Medicine and Health Law Education **21**

Week 4
Discussion

Human Rights in Public Health Practice: Cultural and Ethical Relativism, Religion

Reading

Health and Human Rights Reader, pp. 336-372
International Human Rights in Context, pp. 166-240 (skim 177-181 and 226-240)

Week 5
Discussion

Nongovernmental Organizations: Amnesty International, Physicians for Human Rights

Reading

Health and Human Rights Reader, pp. 397-438
International Human Rights in Context, pp. 456-499

Week 6
Discussion

Human Rights in Extremis
Physician Involvement in Human Rights Violations
Armed Conflict and Torture

Reading

Health and Human Rights Reader, pp. 75-112.
International Human Rights in Context, pp. 1021-1109 (skim 801-806 and 1050-1070).

Week 7
Discussion

AIDS Policy and Research and Its Relation to Human Rights: Discrimination, Immigration, and Stigmatization

Reading

Health and Human Rights Reader, pp. 202-226 and 373-379

Week 8
Discussion

Women and Human Rights: Problems of Gender Discrimination, Empowerment of Women, and Population Control

Reading

Health and Human Rights Reader, pp. 253-280
International Human Rights in Context, pp. 885-968 (skim 240-255, 911-931, and 961-968)

Week 9
Discussion

Part I, Health and Human Rights in the Shadow of the Holocaust (Grodin)

Reading

Health and Human Rights Reader, pp. 281-335
Health and Human Rights Reader, pp. 380-384
International Human Rights in Context, pp. 1006-1020

Optional recommended reading

George J. Annas & Michael A. Grodin eds., *The Nazi Doctors and the Nuremberg Code: Human Rights in Human Experimentation* (Oxford University Press, New York 1992)
    Part II, Indigenous People and Human Genome Diversity Project (Annas)

Week 10
Discussion

Economics and Human Rights

Reading

Health and Human Rights Reader, pp. 130-144 and 181-201
International Human Rights in Context, pp. 870-883

Weeks 11 through 13

Student presentations

Week 14
Discussion

The Future of Health and Human Rights

Reading

Health and Human Rights Reader, pp. 439-450

PAPER TOPICS
General topics

Sexual rights and health in [country or region]
Refugees and internally displaced people in [country]
Mental health and human rights in [country]
Environmental, health, and human rights (focusing on specific environmental problem)
Universalism and cultural relativism (in specific context)
HIV/AIDS: new frontiers in prevention
Health professionals and the legacy of Nuremberg: where should we go from here?
Complex humanitarian emergencies: lessons from past failures (e.g., Somalia)
Homelessness: is it a human rights issue?
Women's health and human rights in [country]
Child labor: necessary evil for economic development?

Topics from past years

Truth-telling and patients' rights in Japan: the case of HIV
Child prostitution in Brazil
Rape as a war crime in Bosnia
Persecution of Coptic Christians in Egypt

Palestinian human rights in the West Bank

Economic sanctions in South Africa

Needle exchange program in Anchorage, Alaska

Group consent human genome diversity project

Child soldiers: the role of children in armed conflict

Trafficking: sale of women and children into forced prostitution in Thailand—effects on health

Corporal punishment in U.S. schools

Mandatory HIV testing of infants and women's rights

Dowry-related crimes in India

Canadian Red Cross tainted blood scandal

The Ogoni situation in Nigeria

HIV vaccine in developing countries

Routine episiotomy as violation of women's human rights

TB in developing countries in a context of human rights and health

Human rights: a new basis for public health?

Guatemalan human rights abuses: the 1996 Peace Accord

Environmental protection and disease prevention

Physicians' role in torture in Turkey

Human rights violation in orphanages in China

Capital punishment in U.S. death row inmates: human rights violations

Torture and the medical profession in Chile

Female genital mutilation in Egypt

Enforcing the Biological Weapons Convention

Environmental degradation as a human rights violation

HIV clinical trials in Africa

Involuntary sterilization

Women, reproductive rights, and pregnancy discrimination in Mexico

Disability rights in China

Effectiveness of the Truth Commission and human rights in El Salvador

Human rights of the elderly: a new convention on human rights

The media campaign to abolish the death penalty

Native American land claims

Embargoes including food and medicine as a political weapon

Human rights and China's orphan policy

Genocide and unaccompanied children in Rwanda

Chernobyl: environmental contamination from nuclear power plants

The Taliban's rule over women

Human rights: political asylum seekers and victims of torture

II

Legal Aspects
of Health Care

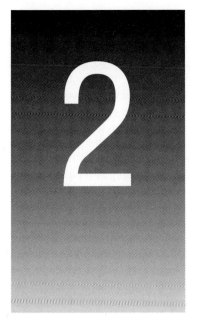

Contracts

ROBERT E. SCHUR, J.D.

BACKGROUND AND HISTORICAL DEVELOPMENT OF CONTRACT LAW

This chapter provides an overview of contract law as it relates to modern theory and practice of legal medicine.

What is a contract?

In modern law the term *contract* is a generic one, encompassing a variety of forms of agreement of varying enforceability under the law. In general, it is commonly understood to refer to any agreement, whether made orally or in writing, to exchange some thing or performance having value in return for another, coupled with an expectation that the other's promise must be kept under the law. In other words, it is an exchange of promises, the performance of which has value to the promisee and may lawfully be enforced if not given voluntarily. A commonly accepted legal definition found in the Restatement (Second) of Contracts section 1 reads as follows: "A contract is a promise or set of promises for the breach of which the law gives a remedy, or the performance of which the law in some way recognizes as a duty."[1]

The historical development of contract law

Contract law developed later than other areas of the law; it grew out of the development of commercial society rather than canonical or feudal systems. Modern contract law has roots in the thirteenth century, when European merchants created their own essentially private courts and used them in a procedure akin to modern commercial arbitration. This system was necessary because merchants could not rely on the law courts to enforce agreements. As mercantile interests expanded beyond simple dealings with a known, local group of individuals, the need for consistency and reliability increased. To members of a political unit, especially when dealing with those outside the unit, the advantages of a dependable method of enforcing contractual agreements were apparent.

Roman law influences

Part of the reason contract law developed relatively late was the profound influence that Roman codification of laws had on Western civilization. Roman law treated disputes regarding contractual obligations as problems of property. In other words, someone who had broken a promise to give some item was said to be in unlawful possession of the item. Thus a contract made up of promises to act at a later time (an executory contract) was not enforceable by law in Rome until late in that culture's history. As the Dark Ages descended on Europe and its once lively commercial society regressed to a more isolated and agrarian one, this late development of Roman law diminished in importance and was lost.

The beginning of modern contract law systems

The Roman foundations of contract law were rediscovered during the Renaissance that percolated out of northern Italy starting as early as the tenth century. Driven by the needs and practices of the merchant class, which became more important as the middle of the second millennium approached, contract law grew and contracts became enforceable everywhere. In the continental civil law countries of Europe, scholars, theorists, and academicians influenced the codification of contract law principles. The results were similar to the law that developed in England, where judges of the common law applied and distinguished decisions and rules enunciated in previous cases. This practice of following precedent, known as *stare decisis,* resulted in fairly consistent application of cohesive principles of contract interpretation and enforcement.

Where the common law and civil law approaches to contracts differ, it is usually in technique or procedure, with both designed to achieve the same end result. For example, civil law holds that an offer to enter into a contract is open for acceptance until there is a response (unless the terms of the offer state otherwise). Under the common law, an offer may be revoked at any time before it is accepted, but acceptance is effective when notice thereof is mailed by the offeree or when the offeree indicates acceptance by beginning performance.[2] Both rules respond to the need of the individual receiving the offer to be able to rely on the agreement once accepted; both rules balance this need with fairness to the individual making the offer. Differences in approach persist to this day but so do the similarities in policy aspirations, which are the goals of the contract law of both systems.

ELEMENTS OF AN ENFORCEABLE CONTRACT

The individual considering a contract faces concerns, some of which are common to all types of agreements. Will the other party fulfill his or her end of the bargain? What if disputes arise as to whether the agreement was fulfilled or as to what the agreement requires? If someone goes to court to sue on the basis of this contract, what will be the result? A preliminary consideration is whether the agreement contains the basic elements that a court will recognize as a contract and then as an enforceable contract.

Through the historical development of the common law, judicial decisions came to consistently require three principal elements—offer, acceptance, and consideration—in a contract before enforcement would be allowed. If the party requesting the aid of the law in enforcing the contract cannot prove that these elements were included, a remedy cannot be given as a matter of contract law (although other theories of law providing a basis for some recovery may apply). Other elements that usually are considered as a basis for enforceability include capacity of the parties to contract; legality of the subject matter; absence of duress, fraud, or unconscionability; and existence of a writing to prove the contract, where that requirement is imposed by statute (usually referred to as a *statute of frauds*).

Offer

The origin of a contractual commitment is the initial expression of willingness to enter a contract by one party, the offeror, to another, the offeree. An offer is a communication that creates the possibility of a contract; it must manifest intent of the offeror to be bound. It thus differs from a mere promise, which may be given in the absence of such intent. Disputes often arise over whether there was an offer. Does the physician who states at a medical meeting that he or she is looking for a partner state an offer? If so, does it follow that a physician who accepts the offer has thus bound both himself or herself and the offeror physician to a contract, despite the lack of any definite terms in the agreement? The first physician would likely argue with success that he or she was merely offering to discuss or negotiate partnership terms, or indicating a willingness to entertain offers, rather than intending to make an offer capable of being accepted.

The determination of whether an offer was made is, in the law, a practical one. The terms of the offer must be sufficiently firm to allow court enforcement. In the previous example, the terms and conditions of the partnership "offer" are so unclear that a court would be unlikely to be able to determine how to enforce the agreement. This legal principle also explains why in most instances advertisements are not held to be offers from which a contract is created when the target of the marketing effort expresses a willingness to purchase. Nevertheless, an advertisement that invites customers to purchase an item at a stated price may be considered an offer if there is sufficient indication that the advertiser intends that another may accept it by performing some act without further communication with the offeror.[3]

An offer is considered to be open for the time stated or for a reasonable time. The common law allows an offer to be withdrawn or revoked by the party making the offer at any time before acceptance in the absence of an express agreement to the contrary (e.g., stating that the offer will remain open for a period of 10 days, making it a "firm offer"). Usually the offeror can, for whatever reason or for no reason at all, withdraw or change an offer another party has not yet accepted. The law also presumes the offer closed on the death of the individual making the offer or on the destruction of something essential to the purposes of the offer. A prospective tenant cannot accept the offer of a lease after the building has burned to the ground and then expect the court to enforce that contract. An offer also is revoked by the rejection of that offer or by a counteroffer that varies the terms of the original offer. In such instances the counteroffer is treated exactly like a new offer, the parties' status is reversed, and the original offeror (now the offeree) may accept, reject, or counteroffer.

Acceptance

Before a court will enforce a contract, the court must find that an offer was accepted. There must be some act manifesting assent and willingness to be bound by the terms of the contract. The acceptance must be made in response to or at least with knowledge of the offer. Consider a physician who writes to a colleague, "I will buy your practice on the terms we discussed if you will fire your receptionist." The terms of the offer may indicate that acceptance may be made simply by rendering a performance (i.e., by firing the receptionist).

However, if the owner of the practice terminates the receptionist before this letter is received and thus has no knowledge that his or her conduct will manifest any intent to be bound, no contract is created; there must be some other manifestation of acceptance. An offer to contract that invites acceptance by another merely tendering performance, rather than first communicating the intent to accept, is referred to as a *unilateral contract.* The terms of the offer must clearly demonstrate the offeror's intent that performance be a satisfactory method of acceptance. Taking control of and using offered goods, for example, may constitute acceptance as intended by the offeror and thus create a contractual obligation upon the offeree to pay for the goods.

The common law rule was that the acceptance had to be in the terms set by the offer and had to be unequivocal. This strict rule has been modified over time such that the offer must be definite enough. For example, if an offer states, "Reply by wire," a letter may be sufficient to make a binding contract. Silence constitutes acceptance only when custom demands it and a continuing relationship exists that makes such an assumption fair.

Agreements to make a contract in the future (agreements to agree) are usually considered unenforceable by law. At times, professionals make a commitment to contract or to reduce an agreement to a written document at a later time, called a *gentleman's agreement,* which they intend to be binding despite the absence of a written document. In a suit based on such a contract, the court must determine whether there was merely an agreement to agree, which is not enforceable, or a binding (though perhaps unwritten) contract. For example, a physician who states to another that he or she will "be happy to sit down and discuss ideas for us to merge our practices" probably has created no obligation, whereas a physician who states, "I will buy your practice, and we will negotiate in good faith to determine the price," may have entered into a binding obligation if the other essential terms have been agreed on.

ORAL CONTRACTS: "AS GOOD AS THE PAPER THEY ARE WRITTEN ON?"

Contracts need not be in writing to be enforceable under the law. The difficulty of course lies in proving their existence and terms. The parties' intent to be bound and the details of the agreement must be clearly manifested by words or conduct that can be satisfactorily established to have occurred. In addition, the contract must be one that is capable of being orally created under the law, or in other words, one that is not subject to application of the state's statute of frauds, a law that defines certain contracts as unenforceable unless in writing. Typical examples are contracts for the sale of real property or goods in excess of a set amount, such as $500.

CONSIDERATION

Offer and acceptance alone do not make an enforceable contract. The law also requires the existence of consideration be-

fore finding a contract enforceable. Consideration is the quid pro quo that cements the deal. Something of value must have been exchanged or at least promised before the contract was formed. Consideration need not be a tangible thing; it may be nothing more than a promise to perform some act, deliver some thing in the future, or even refrain from doing something. As long as the item of consideration has value to the individual to whom it is promised and is not otherwise illegal or impossible it will generally support the formation of a binding contract. However, when the consideration has no value (i.e., is illusory) it will fail. For example, consideration will not be found if the promised performance is already owed as a legal duty. Think of a physician who stops to render medical assistance to an injured motorist. Under the state's law, he or she may be legally obligated not to abandon the patient once the effort to provide treatment has commenced; a promise by the injured individual, now a patient, to pay for the service will likely not be enforced because the treatment is not being rendered in exchange for that promise but in fulfillment of a preexisting legal duty. However, once the physician has met that legal duty (e.g., by stopping the patient's bleeding until the ambulance arrives and others have taken over care), further services offered in exchange for payment, such as follow-up care in the physician's office, certainly will be consideration enough to support a contract.

Some promises can be implied if necessary to validate consideration and to effectuate the parties' obvious intent. Thus, if the buyer and seller of a medical practice failed to include in their agreement language committing the buyer to pursue the practice and "work it" but did provide that the purchase price was to come from practice proceeds, the court may imply a promise to service and maintain the practice. However, where a stated promise is not of any real value, a court will not rewrite the promise. For example, if in response to an offer to sell custom-made splints the practitioner promises to buy "as many as I like," there is no consideration. The practitioner may purchase none. To imply consideration the court would have to change the agreement, and it will not do so.

Many contract documents contain recitations about consideration (e.g., "for and in consideration of $1 and other good and valuable consideration, receipt of which is hereby acknowledged"), but in fact nothing described changes hands. These statements are an attempt to dispense with the need for proof that consideration changed hands. In some jurisdictions, evidence to show that the consideration clause was a sham may be allowed by the court; in others the recitation stands alone.

PROMISSORY ESTOPPEL

A party acting on another party's promise may be protected in some instances even if the essential elements of a contract are not found. If B substantially changes his or her position in reliance on a promise made by A, such that B would suffer a significant detriment if A does not fulfill his or her promise, then B may argue that he or she is entitled to recover for A's failure to perform, so long as B's reliance on the promise was both foreseeable by A and reasonable. The theory of recovery in such cases is not really contract law at all; it is an exercise of the court's inherent power to do equity under the theory of promissory estoppel, meaning that the promisor should be "estopped" (i.e., not allowed to deny the existence and enforceability of the promise) once the promisee has detrimentally relied on it. Of course, detriment is just a form of consideration (the forbearance or loss of a legal right having value), and thus the distinction from contract law is one of formality rather than substance.

DEFENSES: REASONS OTHERWISE VALID CONTRACTS MAY BE UNENFORCEABLE

Some contracts are formed on all the essential requirements (offer, acceptance, and consideration were exchanged) but still will not be enforced by a court because of the existence of a legal defense. Defenses are not necessarily dependent on the specific language of the agreement; they may arise by operation of law. These defenses include illegality; violation of public policy; duress and undue influence; unconscionability; fraud and misrepresentation; lack of capacity; mistake; impossibility; and force majeure, or acts of God. In most cases, to prevail, the party seeking to avoid the contract must prove the existence of one of these defenses, which are discussed briefly here.

Illegality and violation of public policy

The rationale for court enforcement of contracts dissipates in the face of contracts and clauses that are damaging to society as a whole or injurious to the public. Courts will not enforce a contractual obligation to do something illegal. Obviously the court will not enforce a murder for hire contract or compel an individual to pay gambling debts where the gambling is illegal. Other examples may not be so obvious, however. For example, an employment contract may contain a "noncompete" clause that is void because it is against public policy (as is sometimes provided by a state statute or existing court decisions), even though the parties to the agreement were unaware that such law and policy existed. Or, the merger of two practice groups exercising control over the market for medical services may be invalidated because it unlawfully restrains trade.

Another example of an unenforceable contract clause frequently confronted by health professionals is the "liquidated damages" provision, which states that, if one party breaches the terms of the agreement, the other is liable to pay a specified sum as damages, regardless of whether actual injury can be proven. Such a clause may be enforced if it would be difficult to determine the amount of damages resulting from the breach and if the liquidated amount was a reasonable estimate at the time of contracting. However, if the amount is disproportionate to the actual injury suffered, it is characterized as a "penalty" and may not be enforced on the grounds that public policy disfavors the unjust enrichment of one party at the expense of another.[4]

Similarly, contract provisions designed to relieve a party of responsibility for its own negligent acts may be unenforceable because of public policy. This is one reason that contracts between patients and physicians or hospitals that prohibit the patient from suing for medical malpractice are generally not enforced, although agreements to submit any such complaints to arbitration frequently have been held to be binding.

Undue influence and duress

Contracts also may be unenforceable because great disparity exists in the positions of the two parties, particularly when one party has a fiduciary duty to the other. The physician-patient relationship may indeed imply such a duty, meaning that the patient is protected from being harmed by the physician even if he or she willingly entered into the agreement in the first place. Thus an agreement to pay for the physician's services may not be enforced if the physician takes unfair advantage by providing treatment that he or she knows is unnecessary.

The party defending against enforcement of a contract on the basis of duress must show that he or she acted under the threat of something wrongful or unlawful, thus negating the voluntariness of the agreement. Don Corleone's "offer you can't refuse" is an example of duress, but Snidely Whiplash's threat to foreclose on the mortgage is not.

The defense of undue influence addresses the mental capacity of the party asserting this defense at the time of the contract. It is more limited in scope and application than the defense of duress. The focus here is on whether the assent to the contract was real and knowing. If one party to the contract took unfair advantage of a mental infirmity of the other at the time the contract was entered, the defense of undue influence is applicable. It is akin to an inquiry into the mental state of an individual making a will. Fraud and duress focus on the behavior of the defendant in acquiring acceptance of an offer.

Unconscionability

Not all contracts in which there is a great disparity of terms are unenforceable. Many normal business agreements are "take it or leave it" and are obviously stacked in favor of the party authoring the contract. Contracts that on their face are strongly biased against the other party, particularly when contained in standard forms and presented to the buyer without opportunity for negotiation, are called *contracts of adhesion.* A court may not enforce such contracts if it is found that a substantial injustice will result, in other words, if the court finds that enforcement under the circumstances would be unconscionable.

Fraud and misrepresentation

To make a successful defense against enforcement of a contract based on fraud, the defendant must show that the plaintiff's assertions were made with knowledge of their falsity and with intent. If the inducement was truly fraudulent, such as the classic land sales of worthless properties, relief in the form of a suit in tort for fraudulent misrepresentation is available, as well as a defense to the contract.

Misrepresentation, however, can be an honest mistake, so the misrepresentation must be something that induced the defendant to agree to the contract. The court reviewing such a case considers whether the defendant acted reasonably in relying on the mistaken statements.

Lack of capacity and mistake

Lack of capacity is the legal principle that renders contracts with minors and incompetent individuals void and unenforceable. Capacity refers to a legal ability to commit meaningfully to a contract. Insane individuals, retarded individuals, and others may be incompetent to enter contracts. The defendant is required to show that, as a result of a certain mental state or infirmity, he or she was incompetent at the time the contract was made. Intoxication also may be a basis for a defense of incapacity, particularly if there is an additional showing that the other party to the contract knew (or should have known) that the defendant was incapacitated at the time.

Lack of capacity, like the other defenses, is much more likely to be successful if the plaintiff was at fault (i.e., he or she had knowledge of the defendant's incapacity and attempted to take advantage of the situation). In clear cases of incapacity, however, the contract may be found unenforceable even though this results in a hardship for the innocent party suing to enforce the agreement. The remedy or relief granted may be adjusted accordingly under these circumstances.

Mistake is another defense that is bolstered considerably by the misdeeds of the nonmistaken party. If the party seeking to enforce the contract knew that the other was mistaken about some critical underlying fact, the nonmistaken party may be seen as taking unfair advantage. Relief from a contract entered into mistakenly will not be granted, however, if the mistaken party acted unreasonably. In other words, there is a general understanding that parties to a contract must act responsibly, with reasonable caution to investigate where necessary and understand the agreement they are entering. An assertion of mistake is possible whenever one party is disappointed in a contract; therefore courts are not likely to grant relief simply on this basis. Failure to read a contract is not grounds for claiming that there was a mistake.

Impossibility and acts of God

Relief from enforcement of a contract based on impossibility or an act of God is granted rarely and only if economic hardships create the difficulties. Performance of the contract's terms must be impossible, not merely more difficult or expensive than a party would prefer. Impossibility almost always arises as the result of some change in conditions on which the parties relied. If the impossibility or act of God affects the consideration and makes it valueless, the contract can be found to have failed for lack of consideration. Where consideration was good and changed hands, the defense of impossibility is still available.

As an example, consider the case of a medical group that has an arrangement to provide emergency care at a hospital and contracts with an individual physician as a subcontractor or employee to provide emergency care. If the master contract with the hospital is terminated, the group may assert the defense of impossibility against the physician's suit to enforce his or her contract with the group. If the group's contract with the hospital was terminated because of some misdeed by the group's managers, the defense of impossibility may not be available. However, if the contract was terminated because the hospital burned down, clearly it is impossible for the group to perform and thus it may be relieved of its obligations.

REMEDIES: THE RELIEF GRANTED BY THE COURT

A court will grant a successful contract litigant the relief necessary and fair under the circumstances. Contract law is not criminal law and thus does not seek to punish the individual who commits a breach of contract but rather to place the parties in the positions they would have been in had the breach not occurred. The nonbreaching party to a contract cannot obtain more than that to which he or she would have been entitled under the agreement itself, regardless of the improper motive or behavior on the part of the other party. In some cases the court may enforce the "expectation interest" of the nonbreaching party (e.g., by awarding monetary damages in the amount, including profits, that would have been realized had the other party satisfactorily performed). In other cases the facts and circumstances allow the court to make an award sufficient only to ameliorate any loss or harm directly suffered by the plaintiff. In some circumstances the only remedy available is for the court to declare the contract canceled and to relieve a party from any further obligations thereunder. It is beyond the scope of this chapter to explain in detail all the reasons for a court's decision to provide a particular remedy, but in general, contract law seeks to enforce the bargain intended by the parties where possible and to avoid unjust enrichment or harm where it is not. The form of remedy and the measure of damages must be calculated to serve the interests of society, as well as to make the plaintiff "whole" by avoiding or ameliorating the harm suffered as a result of the breach. For these reasons, courts generally cannot award "punitive" damages or increased damages for bad faith of the breaching party (with certain exceptions, such as contracts of insurance breached by the insurer).

Consider the physician who has contracted with a stenography service to handle overflow typing of charts and correspondence for a certain period at $1 per page. If the service fails to perform, the physician must purchase the typing elsewhere and may have to pay more—say, $1.50 per page—for the duration of the contract period. The proper measure of damages is not the $1.50 per page that the physician now must pay but the $0.50 per page differential. The physician would have had to pay $1 per page under the terms of the contract, so only the difference is required to give the physician the benefit of the former bargain. If the physician failed to submit a required report on time because of the breach and thus lost the report fee, he or she may be able to recover the report fee as "consequential damages" if the loss was foreseeable to the typist at the time the contract was entered. However, such damages are unlikely to be awarded because the performance of typing is usually easy to obtain from another source. In such cases courts usually consider awarding consequential damages only if the contract clearly specifies that the parties anticipated the possibility of such harm occurring from a party's breach, and that party agreed to bear the risk of that type of consequential damage.

HOW TO READ A CONTRACT: SPECIFIC CLAUSES

The nonattorney can and should read his or her own contracts. Assistance of legal counsel is required in some situations, but those untrained in the law can understand most contract language. If an individual finds it impossible to understand what is meant by the language in a proposed contract, it may be a sign that the individual is not supposed to be able to understand it (i.e., the contract may be in the best interests of the party suggesting it). Although it is always advisable to retain the services of an attorney before entering into a contract involving significant sums or risks, the health care practitioner may benefit from a brief discussion of some typical contract clauses.

Most written contracts prepared by attorneys or businesspersons are organized in a common fashion. The reader should look for the caption or title of the agreement; recitals, which usually are nonbinding statements of background facts upon which the contract is based; commitments, or substantive terms; conditions, which define events that must be met as a prerequisite to certain of the parties' obligations; boilerplate, or legal terms found in most contracts of the same subject matter; and a place for signatures and attestations.

Restrictive covenants not to compete (noncompete clauses)

Noncompete clauses are common in health care contracts, particularly those between physicians and medical groups for employment or membership in the group. An important public policy disfavoring restrictions on trade or the practice of a profession may clash with the general freedom of parties to contract, making such clauses unenforceable in certain instances. Courts will not enforce restrictions on competition that are unreasonable, even if freely entered into. A noncompete clause may be considered unreasonable because it specifies a period that is excessive or a geographic area that is too broad, placing a hardship on the physician who leaves the employment or association with the group (and in theory damaging the public by stifling competition).[5] In some jurisdictions, noncompete clauses are never enforced if the relationship between the physician and the group was one of employee and employer as opposed to a true partnership or corporate shareholder arrangement.

Noncompete clauses often are accompanied by liquidated damages clauses, specifying that a breach will result in the loss of a specified monetary sum. As discussed earlier, such clauses are themselves subject to a requirement of reasonableness before they will be upheld.

Indemnification

To indemnify is to promise to answer for the debt or obligation of another or to hold the other harmless from any claim that may be brought by a third party not involved in the contract. A malpractice insurance contract is an indemnification agreement; the insurer and the physician are the parties to the contract, and the insurer pays for the costs of defense and the damages awarded in the event of a malpractice claim by a third party (the patient). Indemnification clauses are appearing in health care–related contracts with increasing frequency, often placing the burden on the weaker, individual party to indemnify the stronger, institutional party against certain losses or claims. Such clauses are dangerous in that they expose the indemnifying party to potentially unlimited damages and generally should be avoided.

Arbitration agreements

Arbitration is an alternative means of dispute resolution that is becoming increasingly popular in the health care arena. For example, one large nationally known health maintenance organization (HMO) has included mandatory arbitration clauses in both its employment contracts and its benefit terms for many years and has largely been successful in enforcing these clauses. Under these agreements the parties to the contract agree to submit any disputes to binding arbitration, thus waiving their rights to have disputes determined by a court of law. Although there are potential benefits to both parties in resolving their differences through private arbitration, sometimes the superior power of one party makes arbitration less than fair. Often the arbitration clause further restricts the plaintiff's rights to bring an action or complaint against the defendant by shortening the period within which a complaint may be filed (the "statute of limitations"), limiting access to information in possession of the other party before the hearing or trial (discovery), and limiting the type and amount of damages that may be awarded. Although physicians generally consider arbitration clauses beneficial when they restrict patients' rights to bring lawsuits for malpractice, the same clause in an employment agreement may not be so benign. Moreover, the idea that arbitration always saves money as compared with litigation in the courts may be misplaced; sometimes parties spend as much or more convincing paid arbitrators of their cause as they would have spent to convince a jury. Still, advantages, including potential cost savings, faster resolution of the dispute, more private proceedings, and the predictability that comes from having the initial decision be final (without a mechanism for appeal), certainly may be realized through the use of mandatory arbitration clauses. As with any contractual term, the important thing is to ensure that the individual fully understands the arbitration clause before accepting it.

CONTRACTING WITH HEALTH PLANS AND ORGANIZATIONS: SPECIAL CONSIDERATIONS

Health professionals confront increasing opportunities and necessities to contract with HMOs, preferred provider organizations (PPOs), and independent practice associations (IPAs), among other kinds of entities now found in the health care arena. These entanglements, though sometimes a matter of economic necessity, must be regarded with a cautious eye. Market conditions often lead to contracts that are highly disadvantageous to the physician, difficult to terminate once commenced, and potentially injurious to the individual's professional well being.

Consider the case of Dr. S. She has signed up with a PPO, and that organization's patients are being referred to her. Dr. S usually sends the biopsy specimens taken in her office to the laboratory of her choice, which is well known to her. The PPO has cut costs by making an arrangement with a discount laboratory service whose equipment, methodology, and employees are less than state of the art.

Dr. S now must submit her patients' specimens to the discount laboratory or payment by the patient's health plan will be denied, but Dr. S is risking the life and health of the patient, as well as her own professional liability and standing, by using the provider whom she knows or has reason to believe is unreliable. Dr. S complains, but the PPO refuses to accommodate by choosing another laboratory. Ultimately, Dr. S withdraws from the PPO and loses a substantial share of her business.

This sort of catch-22 is increasingly common but still extremely difficult to avoid. The physician considering contracting with any health care organization should ask numerous questions, such as the following:

"What happens if I want out?"

"What happens on termination of the relationship?"

"Will the PPO provide tail coverage or an extended endorsement for malpractice suits?"

"What is the organization's reputation among physicians and patients?"

"Which hospitals, laboratories, specialty groups, and other affiliated providers are associated with the organization?"

"Is there 'due process' in case of a forced revocation or restriction of panel membership or contract status under the participation plan?"

A contract allowing for the physician's easy exit from the organization on short notice probably offers the best protection.

Health care professionals also should beware of "evergreen" clauses in their contracts with such organizations. These provisions automatically renew the contract, year after year, if one party doesn't notify the other of the intent to terminate the arrangement by a specified date. Without the need to "re-up" every 1 or 2 years, it is harder to get out of an unfavorable plan or to avoid becoming involved in too many such arrangements at the same time.

Payment provisions are another frequent source of trouble for practitioners. The IPA or PPO may delay payment to the practitioner or force greatly reduced rates on its members. Payment provisions may be extremely confusing and are often overlooked by the physician who is more concerned with reading radiology reports than business contracts. Devices such as holdbacks, bonuses, and surcharges are easily misunderstood. How will these amounts be calculated? What expenses are charged against the withheld pool? Are the books open to individual physicians or the physician group's representatives? Are rights to earned compensation lost on withdrawal? Answering these questions and others may require careful, time-consuming investigation and legal review and negotiation of the contract terms.

In some parts of the United States where HMOs and PPOs are ubiquitous, brokers invite providers to sign agreements obtaining access to multiple plans. These agreements may be in the form of "power of attorney," giving extensive authority to the broker. Unlimited powers of attorney can enmesh the physician in multiple and varied commitments, without even the rudimentary notice provisions of responsible plans. Capitated physicians, usually the primary care providers, should ask what happens if there is an unexpectedly high use. Can the plan obtain catastrophic reinsurance?

Unjust dismissal and employment contracts

Suits over hiring and firing practices are burgeoning, affecting physicians as employees and employers. In most reported cases involving physicians as plaintiffs, physicians base employment or staff privilege claims on civil or statutory rights.[6] More often, physicians find themselves the target of these lawsuits brought by disgruntled or dismissed employees. This risk can be minimized or eliminated.

Problems most often arise over the dismissal of "at-will" employees. At-will employment can be terminated at any time by either party for any reason; the verbal or written contract provides for no fixed term and no procedures for termination. However, statutes and recent court cases in some jurisdictions limit at-will discharges. State and federal legislation creates a right to sue for termination of employment for one of several impermissible reasons.[7] Judges have allowed suits against employers in three types of cases—public policy, good faith and fair dealing, and violations of employee handbook provisions, which may be considered contractually binding on the employer.[8,9] Other courts have found that employee manual provisions do not give the employee the right to sue.[10]

CONCLUSION

Contracting is a process that begins with contract formation and ends either in successfully realizing the benefit of an individual's bargain or in suffering a personal or economic loss. The contracting minefield cannot be successfully navigated without a basic understanding of the elements of contract formation, the basic rights and defenses available to the parties, the remedies provided under the law, and typical traps for the unwary. The increasingly complex marketplace for health care services has created a myriad of opportunities and necessities for professionals to contract. Caution, preparedness, and counsel are needed to survive in today's health care world.

ENDNOTES

1. American Law Institute, 1979.
2. Restatement (Second) of Contracts § 50, 53 (1979).
3. *See* Restatement (Second) § 23, 29.
4. *See* Restatement (Second) § 356(1). Damages for breach by either party may be liquidated in the agreement but only at an amount that is reasonable in light of the anticipated or actual loss caused by the breach and difficulties of proof of loss. A term fixing unreasonably large liquidated damages as a penalty is unenforceable on grounds of public policy. *See especially* Illustration 2.
5. *Pathology Consultants v. Gratton,* 343 N.W. 2d 428, 434 (Iowa 1984). "Covenants not to compete are unreasonable restraints unless they are tightly limited as to both time and area."
6. *See, e.g., Zaklama v. Mt. Sinai Medical Center,* #87-5428, 6554, 11th Cir., April 12, 1988.
7. Examples include the Civil Rights Act, the Age Discrimination in Employment Act, and veterans' protections. State statutes may include service in the National Guard or jury duty; even local jurisdictions may have such laws.
8. For example, an employee may claim that he or she was terminated for refusing to obey an order to commit an illegal or otherwise impermissible act. Whistle blowers' suits fall under this category.
9. *Duldulao v. Saint Mary of Nazareth Hospital,* 505 N.E. 2d 314 (Ill. 1987).
10. *Garmon v. Health Group of Atlanta, Inc.,* 359 S.E. 2d 450 (Ga. App. 1987) (discharge procedures outlined in manual asserted to have been violated).

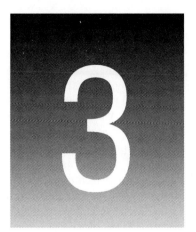

Agency and partnership

ROBERT E. SCHUR, J.D.

THE LAW OF AGENCY
PARTIES AND THE RELATIONSHIP
RIGHTS AND DUTIES BETWEEN PRINCIPAL AND AGENT
LIABILITIES OF PARTIES BASED IN TORT

THE LAW OF AGENCY

An agency is a consensual relationship between two persons whereby one person (the agent) is given a varying degree of authority to act for and on behalf of another (the principal). The *Restatement of the Law of Agency* defines the relationship as follows:

Agency is a fiduciary relationship that results from the manifestation of consent by one person to another that the other shall act on his behalf and subject to his control and consent by the other so to act.[1]

The liabilities, duties, benefits, and remedies attained through the agency relationship develop from both tort and contract law. Most agency relationships are formed by agreement, so that the usual defenses to the formation of a contract will, if successful, also negate the existence of an agency. However, other agencies arise as a result of the status of the parties or by operation of law and must be analyzed under other legal principles.

PARTIES AND THE RELATIONSHIP
The parties

To form an agency, the parties involved must have legal capacity. The power to act through another depends on the capacity of the principal to do the act himself or herself. For example, contracts entered into by a minor or an insane person are considered "voidable," that is, cancelable by or on behalf of the minor or insane party. Consequently the appointment of an agent by a minor or an insane person and any contracts resulting thereby are likewise voidable.

Capacity to be an agent is somewhat different from capacity required for contract formation or the execution of a will. An adult principal can appoint a minor agent. The fact that the agency agreement itself may be voidable does not in and of itself disqualify the agent from making a contract binding on the principal. An adult acting on behalf of a minor who could not make a binding contract directly may create such obligations, but they will be enforceable as against the adult agent rather than as against the minor principal.

Types of agencies, agents, and principals

Agencies may be classified in different ways. The relationship may be one of actual agency, in which valid authority, express or implied, has been given by the principal to the agent to act on the principal's behalf. An example of this is the retaining of a real estate broker to represent a seller in a particular transaction. Often, actual agencies are defined and created by the use of a written agency agreement (in this example, the listing contract).

An ostensible (or "apparent") agency arises when, in the absence of an actual agency, the conduct of the principal induces others to reasonably infer that an agency exists.[2] Most often an ostensible agency arises when the scope of an actual agency is exceeded by the agent, causing a third party to assume that the agent has authority where he or she does not. For example, P may appoint A to act on his or her behalf to sell a parcel of land to any buyer who qualifies and is willing to pay the asking price. A, in negotiating with buyer B, is unable to make a sale of the property in question but offers to sell another parcel, also owned by P, which is more to B's liking. By appointing A as his or her agent to sell one property, P may have created a reasonable assumption that A can act on his or her behalf to sell any property that P owns. If P fails to take reasonable precautions to limit the scope of A's actual authority, the resulting contract to sell the second property may be enforced in B's favor. This so-called agency by estoppel exists when a person by his or her conduct clothes another with indicia of authority by which a third party inferred that an agency relationship existed and relied on that inference when dealing with the agent.[3] The conduct of the principal leading to the creation of such an agency may be intentional or merely negligent, and the inference must be reasonable.[4] It is not a true agency because the consent element is lacking, but on equitable grounds the law prohibits the principal from denying the existence of the agency so as to cause harm to the party who acted in reliance.

An agent may deal on behalf of a principal whose existence and identity have not been revealed to a third party. The "undisclosed principal" is bound by contracts forged by the agent with a third party despite the secrecy of the agency relationship, but unlike an actual agent the agent of an undisclosed principal is also bound. An agent who deals for a principal whose existence (but not identity) has been revealed to the third party deals for a "partially disclosed" principal, rendering both the principal and the agent contractually liable to third parties. Some cases have held that, once the third party learns the identity of the principal, he or she must make an election as to whether the agent or the principal will be held responsible for the contractual obligations.

Agents are also commonly classified as *general* or *special*.[5] A general agent is authorized to transact all business or at least all business of a particular kind at a particular locale for his or her principal. A special agent is authorized to act for the principal only in a particular transaction.

A subagent is appointed by an agent, with the express or implied consent of the principal, to assist the agent in the conduct of his or her agency duties. This subagent is the agent of the agent, and because the agent has the authority to make such an appointment, the subagent also has authority to bind the principal. Moreover, the subagent is in a fiduciary relationship with both the agent and the principal.

One common characterization of agency is the "master-servant" relationship. A "servant" generally has limited authority, such as performing physical or ministerial tasks assigned by the "master." The master has the right to direct what is to be done, as well as how it is to be done. In most cases it is doubtful whether a servant could enter into a contract that would bind the principal without the presence of some expression of intent that the servant be clothed with such authority. So, in carrying out his or her duties, a delivery clerk is certainly the agent of the grocer, but no one would assume that he has authority to purchase a new truck on the grocer's behalf. On the other hand, the clerk's negligent handling of the old truck, causing accidental injury, will be imputed to his master based on the existence of the agency relationship under the doctrine of respondeat superior ("let the master answer").

The master-servant relationship is distinguished from that of the independent contractor. Like the servant, the independent contractor is hired to perform a specific task. However, the master or principal exercises less control over the performance of the act, allowing the agent to determine the means and methods of carrying out the purpose of the agency. Independent contractors commonly fall into some professional category. As such, this concept is important for the medical practitioner because he or she will encounter numerous situations in which the status of being independent impacts the determination of legal rights, duties, and liabilities. For example, a physician usually is considered an independent contractor of the hospital or other facility where he or she treats patients even if the hospital has the right to determine which patients the physician treats, where and when he or she treats them, and what equipment or facilities will be made available to accomplish these tasks. The hospital, it is claimed, neither controls the manner in which physicians apply their skills and knowledge to the patients' care nor assumes responsibility for errors in their judgment or technique.

An agency exists when individuals form partnerships, corporations, or any combination thereof. A general partner acts as agent for the partnership and for all the other general partners, with regard to partnership business. A corporate officer acts as agent for the corporation. A corporation or partnership may act as agent for an individual.

Formation of the relationship

An agency may be formed by a number of distinct methods. Such a relationship may be formed by an oral or written contract.[6] An agency also may result by implication from the circumstances (an "implied" agency). However, unlike an ordinary contract, in which consideration is required for formation, an agency may be gratuitous (lacking in any promise of compensation for the agent). Such a gratuitous agency does not affect the validity of contracts formed by the agent for the benefit of the principal.

Ratification is an affirmance by the principal of an unauthorized act of an agent, or purported agent, after the fact. Ratification relates back in time to the commission of the act, thus binding the principal just as if the agency had been authorized at the time.[7]

Termination of the relationship

An agency, once created, continues until terminated. Termination may occur in a number of ways. First is the termination of agency by lapse of time. Such terms may be specified in the agency agreement itself, where the relationship terminates as of a stated time. In the absence of a specified time, the agency is deemed terminable at will, and a reasonable time limitation may be implied from the facts and circumstances.

The agency agreement also may specify that the relationship is to terminate on the occurrence of a particular event. An agency also may be terminated by a material change in the circumstances underlying the agency agreement. This change in circumstances includes destruction of the subject matter of the authority, insolvency or bankruptcy of the agent or the principal, a drastic change in pertinent business conditions, and changes to the law that substantially affect the purposes of the agency. A breach of the agent's fiduciary duty may effectively terminate the agency. When either the agent or the principal unilaterally acts to terminate the agency, the principal is best advised to take reasonable steps to notify potential third parties that the agent no longer holds authority to bind the principal.

Finally, an agency may be terminated by operation of law, such as upon the death of either the agent or the principal or the loss of either party's legal or mental capacity. Where a partnership or corporation holds the position of agent or principal, dissolution of the partnership or corporation effects a termination.

RIGHTS AND DUTIES BETWEEN PRINCIPAL AND AGENT
Duties imposed on the agent

The law of agency attaches certain duties of performance to the agent. First, the agent is responsible to the principal as a fiduciary.[8] A fiduciary duty arises out of a relationship of trust and confidence. Fiduciary duties define many common agency relationships, including those of trustee and beneficiary, corporate directors and shareholders, attorney and client, and employee and employer. Breach of one's fiduciary duty often results in legal sanctions for the party at fault.

The agent owes the principal the utmost in loyalty and good faith. Therefore an agent must act only in the interests of the principal and not in the interests of himself, herself, or another. Thus an agent may not represent the principal in any transaction in which the agent has a personal or financial interest. To do so would be a conflict of interest.[9] This duty prevents an agent from competing with the principal concerning the subject matter of the agency. Moreover, an agent may not use information obtained during the course of the agency for his or her own benefit or retain a secret profit gained in the course of the agency; all profits belong to the principal. The principal's legal remedies include the right to demand an accounting and the right for disgorgement of profits.

The fiduciary duty also requires an agent to use reasonable efforts to notify the principal of developments or information reasonably calculated to be relevant to the affairs of the agency.[10] Knowledge of the agent is expected to include all information gained during the conduct of transactions for the principal, as well as information that (by the exercise of reasonable inquiry) the agent should have attained. Moreover, knowledge of facts material to the agency gained through transactions unrelated to the agency also may be imputed to the principal if this knowledge was present in the mind of the agent and used to the advantage of the principal during the agency. However, the agent is not required to notify his or her principal of facts gained while dealing for another principal (provided those facts were not used for the benefit of the first principal). With certain exceptions, knowledge gained by the agent after the termination of the relationship is not imputed to the principal unless it was gained from a third party who previously dealt with the agent during the pendency of the agency and who had no knowledge of the termination (there being an apparent authority). Moreover, the imputed knowledge of the principal is constructive knowledge and not ac-

tual; a principal cannot be held liable for a crime for which actual knowledge is an essential requirement, solely on the basis of imputed or constructive knowledge.

Violation of the fiduciary duty is both a breach of contract (agency) and a tort (fraud).[11] Thus the injured principal often has a choice of remedies. The agent may be held accountable for all damages proximately suffered by his or her principal. In tort situations in which malice or bad faith is proved, punitive damages also may be awarded. When the agent is found to have gained personally from the breach, the principal may void any transactions made with third parties that emanate from the violation of the fiduciary duty. For property held by the agent in violation of the duty, the law may impose a constructive trust on the property for its transfer to the principal.

The agency relationship imparts other duties on the agent as well. One is the duty to perform. This duty requires the agent to act in his or her conduct of the principal's affairs only as authorized and to obey all reasonable instructions and directions. The agent also is subject to the duty of care in his or her conduct of the agency and must act with reasonable care, diligence, and skill in the completion of his or her tasks.

Duties imposed on the principal

The principal also is subject to certain duties in the agency relationship. For example, the agent is owed reasonable compensation (unless of course it is a gratuitous agency) for services in the conduct of the agency. Furthermore, the agent is due indemnification from his or her principal for all reasonable expenses and losses incurred by the agent during discharge of authorized duties.[12]

A principal also owes the agent the duty of cooperation. To this end a principal must assist and provide to the agent any and all known information that is relevant to conduct of the agency. More important, this duty prohibits the principal from interfering in a way that would hinder or prevent performance by the agent. Consider the example of the physicians' group practice that contracts with a search firm to find a qualified ophthalmologist. The contract with the search firm is one of an exclusive agency. The search firm will be paid a finder's fee in the amount of a percentage of the hired specialist's first year compensation package. Later, certain members of the group, while at a medical seminar, locate and hire such an individual for the group. Under these circumstances, most courts would find for the search firm and award damages for the lost profits it would have made if it had located the new specialist. Such remedy is likely to be specified in the firm's contract as well.

If the principal breaches the contract of agency, the agent's remedies lie in an action in contract. Therefore most of the remedies available to a contracting party are likewise available to the agent. In addition, the agent may have the right to claim a retaining lien against the property of his or her principal that is in the lawful possession of the agent, as well as any other liens provided by law. Such liens usually extend also to a subagent as to property lawfully in the subagent's possession but only to the extent of the primary agent's rights in the property. Further remedies available to an agent include the rights to withhold performance, claim a setoff in any action brought by the principal, or demand an accounting by the principal. However, because the agency relationship is consensual in nature, there is generally no right by either the agent or the principal to the remedy of specific performance of the agency contract.

Powers vested in the agent

The power vested in an agent, if any, is to be strictly construed. As such, an agent is deemed to possess those powers that were expressly given or are reasonably required for the agent to perform his or her duties. Powers inherent in the agency, such as the power to sell land for a realty agency, are included.

In cases in which authority is present, an agent may provide warranties. Such warranties may be express or implied. A most important warranty of the implied type is the warrant of authority. An agent is deemed to impliedly warrant that he or she has the authority to act on behalf of the principal.

An agent is deemed to hold all powers that a reasonable third party would believe he or she holds. This principle is known as *inherent agency power* and holds true even if the principal expressly denied the agent such a power. The rationale behind this policy is the protection of innocent third parties. An example of such a power is the agent's power to make representations concerning the subject matter of the agency.

LIABILITIES OF PARTIES BASED IN TORT
Liability of the principal for the agent's acts

One who commits a tort is usually held liable to those harmed. This rule is true for an agent acting within the scope of his or her agency, and a principal may be held liable to third persons for the torts committed by the agent. This principle is called the *doctrine of respondeat superior.* Respondeat superior (Latin meaning, "let the master answer") is simply one form of vicarious liability. This doctrine developed in early common law when the servant was treated as property of the master. Because the master was deemed to have absolute control over the acts of the servant, the master might properly be held to answer for those acts, both rightful and wrongful. The basis for a finding of vicarious liability against the principal is the course and scope of employment of the agent. The tortious act must have been committed while the agent was engaged in work of the type that he or she was appointed to perform for the principal.

Today this doctrine has been retained in the law on the rationale of at least two theories. The first is based on the premise that, because the master or employer has the right of control and termination of the agency, the threat of holding him or her liable will cause him or her to act more prudently

in the selection, guidance, and supervision of agents. Moreover, it is the master who benefits from the acts of the agent, and the agent's acts may create increased risks to third persons. This rationale justifies placing the ultimate responsibility for the safety of others on the principal.

The second theory holds that public policy requires that an injured third person be afforded the most effective relief available. This doctrine assumes that the principal is generally wealthier than the agent and therefore more likely to be able to respond to damages. First year law students learn this as the "deep pocket" theory of recovery. In modern times probably nothing has encouraged our litigious society more than this doctrine. Plaintiffs seeking large recoveries have little chance of doing so against a mere employee. But the huge coffers of business, professional, and government treasuries or their insurance companies lie for the taking. As a result, a plaintiff can seek recovery against the principal, the agent, or both when injured.

Respondeat superior imposes on the principal a "strict liability" (i.e., liability without fault on the part of the principal), and it attaches notwithstanding the principal's due care in the selection of the agent or employee and in the subsequent supervision thereof. Such liability is both joint and several with that of the agent or employee. Of course, the plaintiff is not entitled to a double recovery. Recovery against either defendant bars recovery against the other.[13] When the principal is found to be vicariously liable, he or she is usually entitled to seek indemnification against the agent or employee for damages paid to the victorious third party.

Hospital as principal of the physician

Increasingly, plaintiffs injured by malpractice are bringing actions against both the negligent physician and the hospital where care was provided. Several legal theories support such a suit, including direct negligence in the operation of the hospital and insufficient supervision of residents who are employees of the institution. Most if not all jurisdictions hold that there is no hospital liability for the negligent acts of a physician absent a showing of a sufficient degree of control over the physician by the hospital. Thus the hospital may be liable for the acts or omissions of a physician in training but not for those of an attending physician because the latter is an independent contractor not subject to such control.[14]

In addition, if there is a showing that the professional in question is an employee rather than an independent contractor, the act in question must be shown to have occurred within the scope of employment. Among other requirements, to meet this showing, the act must be reasonably foreseeable by the employer.[15] When supervision and control are provided by a hospital or an attending physician over a resident, the suit will likely turn on the degree of control available. Presumably the more senior the resident, the less control may be exercised by the hospital and its employees. Nurses and other providers who are employed by the hospital or who answer to administrators are almost always considered agents for purposes of imputing liability. However, when the provider is beyond the control of the institution in performing his or her duties, employment alone may not sustain a charge of liability against the hospital.[16]

An important exception to the doctrine of respondeat superior is known as the *fellow servant rule*. This rule holds that a principal is not liable for injury done to one employee by another employee of the same principal in the same general enterprise. The rationale behind this doctrine is that a person who accepts appointment by a given principal assumes any risk that he or she might be injured by another appointed by the same principal and that he or she is in at least as good a position as the principal to discover such risks and protect himself or herself from them. These are poor justifications for such a rule, and the courts are not in favor of it, seeking generally to avoid its application. Today there are many exceptions to the applicability of the fellow servant rule (e.g., where the plaintiff seeks recovery based on the employer's negligence in hiring a fellow servant or where the servant is injured by a superior employee who is acting within his or her authority in supervision of an inferior servant).

ENDNOTES

1. Restatement (Second) of the Law, Agency, § 1, American Law Institute (1957).
2. *See* Restatement, Agency § 267.
3. *See* Restatement, Agency § 8B. The result is an agency created by operation of law. Such an agency also may be created by statute, such as where the law of state A directs that an out-of-state corporation doing business in state A automatically appoints the Secretary of State as its agent for service of process within state A.
4. There are some exceptions to this relation back doctrine, namely (1) where the principal, on the date of ratification or the date of the unauthorized act, lacked the capacity to do so; (2) where to do so would now be illegal; or (3) most important, where to do so would prejudice innocent third persons who have acquired rights in the transaction during the interim period.
5. *See* Restatement, Agency § 3.
6. Agency agreements made orally may be invalidated by the state's statute of frauds, whereby certain contracts are required to be in writing to be enforceable. Many states have enacted what generically may be called *equal dignity laws* providing that when the statute of frauds requires an agreement be made in writing the agent's authority also must be in writing. A written agency agreement is often in the form of a "power of attorney" appointing the agent as the principal's attorney-in-fact for a specific purpose (or in general to conduct the principal's business).
7. *Adamski v. Taco General Hospital*, 579 P. 2d 970, at 978 (Wash. App. 1978). Note that the term *reasonable* connotes an objective rather than a subjective standard. The proper test is what a reasonable person under the circumstances would believe.
8. *See* Restatement, Agency § 13.
9. Full disclosure of the conflict and written authority to act despite the conflict may relieve the agent from liability for breach of the agency agreement; however, this entails some risk for the agent, whose position as a fiduciary is not defeated by the disclosure.
10. *See* Restatement, Agency § 11, 381. The effect of this rule is that notice of all matters coming to the agent is imputed to the principal. Thus, as to third persons who dealt with the agent, the principal is deemed to know or have constructive knowledge of all that the agent should have told him or her. It would then seem useless for a principal to instruct his or her agent with the admonition, "I don't want to know of it!" *See also* Restatement, Agency § 272.
11. *See* Restatement, Agency § 399.
12. The scope of this right is usually defined by contract. Absent this, the courts will indemnify the agent where it is just to do so, considering the nature of the relationship, the transaction entered into, and the costs and losses involved. Note that there is no right of indemnification for unauthorized acts. Furthermore, there is likewise no right for costs and losses incurred for the commission of illegal acts.
13. Note that where the plaintiff entertains a suit against only the agent and is denied recovery by the court, this action will generally operate to release the principal as well because there can be no vicarious liability without primary liability. Still, the principal may be sued for his or her own negligence, such as in the hiring or supervision of the agent or employee.
14. *See, e.g., Kirk v. Michael Reese Hosp.*, 513 N.E. 2d 387 (Ill. 1987); *Gregg v. National Medical Health Care*, 699 P. 2d 925 (Ariz. App. 1985).
15. *Fock v. U.S.*, 597 F.Supp. 1325 (D.C. Kan. 1982).
16. *Foster v. Englewood Hospital Association*, 19 Ill. App. 3d 1055, 313 N.E. 2d 255 (1974).

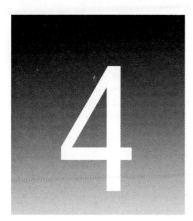

Competency and capacity: a primer

STEVEN B. BISBING, Psy.D., J.D.

COMPETENCY IN GENERAL
THE LAW IN GENERAL
COMMON COMPETENCY AREAS

COMPETENCY IN GENERAL

In American society there are few aspects of human endeavor that are not affected in some way by the law. Generally, for someone to "lawfully" engage in some endeavor and be held accountable for his or her actions he or she must be *competent.* Essentially, "legal" competency refers to "having sufficient ability . . . possessing the natural or legal qualifications [to engage in something as recognized by law]."[1] This definition is deliberately vague because the term *competency* refers to a broad concept that encompasses many different situations and legal issues. As a consequence the definition, requirements, and application of the term can vary greatly, depending on the act or issue in question. Regardless of the circumstance, however, the law seeks to underscore a basic assumption: only acts of a relatively rational person are to be afforded recognition by the public. In doing so the law attempts to reaffirm the autonomy of the individual and the general integrity and value of society.

Generally, competency refers to some minimal mental, cognitive, or behavioral trait, ability, or capability required to perform a particular legally recognized act or to assume some legally recognized role. Appendix 4-1 identifies a sample of different situations in which competency is typically an essential component. The term *capacity,* which is frequently interchanged with and mistaken for the word *competency,* refers to an individual's actual ability to understand, appreciate, and form a relatively rational intention with regard to some act.

Appendix 4-2 identifies several human acts for which capacity is legally defined for the purpose of determining whether a person's actions can be legally recognized as competent. As a distinction, the term *incompetent* is applied to an individual whose actions fail a legal test of capacity. When such a designation is made, the individual is considered by law to be mentally incapable of performing a particular legally recognized act (e.g., executing a will or making medical decisions) or assuming a particular legally recognized role (e.g., serving as a guardian or participating in a trial).

Several important distinctions about competency must be clarified. First, the adjudication of incompetence is subject or task specific. In other words, the fact that a person is adjudicated incompetent to execute a will, for example, does not automatically render him or her incompetent to do other things, such as consent to treatment or testify as a witness. Accordingly, determinations of competency should be made on a case-by-case basis with regard to a person's present mental capacity and the specific legal right or act that he or she wishes or is asked to exercise. Second, a finding of incompetency does not translate into and should not be interpreted as a finding of mental illness. The threshold question in any civil or criminal competency inquiry is the ability to understand and engage in whatever legal requirements are defined for a given act (e.g., make a contract, stand trial, or marry). A person may be actively delusional, mentally retarded, or deaf and mute yet still meet the legal specifications associated with certain competency tests. Third, legal incompetency is not synonymous with the need for psychiatric treatment. The fact that a patient is or is not competent has no bearing on his or her need for treatment nor does such a finding necessarily equate with finding an individual dangerous to self or others. Fourth, incompetency and insanity are two entirely distinct concepts, although they are commonly confused with one another. In addition to different legal requirements for their determination, they are viewed from opposite temporal contexts. Legal competency reflects an individual's present capacity to engage in an act at the time of an evaluation. Legal insanity and questions regarding criminal responsibility refer to a person's ability, mental state, or both at the time of the offense. Insanity is therefore a historical perspective.

THE LAW IN GENERAL

Generally the law recognizes only those decisions or choices that have been made by a competent individual. The reason for this is that the law seeks to protect the incompetent from the effects of his or her actions and from being taken advantage of because of his or her lack of capacity. Persons over the age of majority, which is now 18 years,[2] are presumed to be competent.[3] However, this presumption can be rebutted based on evidence of an individual's incapacity.[4]

The issue of competency, whether in a civil or criminal context, is commonly raised in cases involving two classes of parties—minors and persons appearing to be mentally impaired. In many situations minors are not considered legally competent and therefore require the consent of a parent or designated guardian. There are, of course, exceptions to this general rule, such as minors who are considered emancipated[5] or mature[6] and some cases of medical need[7] or emergency.[8]

The mentally impaired individual presents a slightly different problem in terms of competency. Lack of capacity or incompetency cannot be presumed based on either treatment for mental illness[9] or institutionalization.[10] Moreover, evidence of significant mental illness, such as acute psychosis or chronic schizophrenia, does not in and of itself render a person incompetent in any particular area or in all areas of functioning. Instead, such a condition should trigger an assessment to determine whether a person is incapable of making a particular kind of decision or performing a particular type of task as defined or required by law. When there is a question about a person's mental status with regard to the capacity to engage in some legal act, one commentator suggests that two questions be addressed[11]:

1. Is there evidence of mental illness or deficiency (e.g., alcohol induced, age related, organic, etc.)?
2. If so, does this condition prevent the person from satisfying the relevant legal test or criterion for competency?

Thus although it is not always obvious from the legal tests themselves (Appendix 4-2), there is typically a threshold condition of cognitive or mental illness or deficiency that serves as a qualifying consideration. However, such conditions, no matter how seemingly severe, should not trigger reflexive examinations intended to "confirm" a premeditated finding of incompetency. Respect for individual autonomy[12] demands that individuals be allowed to make decisions of which they are capable, even if they are seriously mentally ill. As a rule, therefore, a patient or person with a history of mental illness generally must be judicially declared incompetent before he or she loses the legal power to do what adults who are not mentally ill have the legal right or power to do.

COMMON COMPETENCY AREAS
Civil law

Consent to medical treatment. One of the most controversial and vexing areas of potential substitute decision-making concerns the medical treatment of individuals whose competency is in question. The doctrine of informed consent, as described in the following section, was developed to address this issue. Historically, concern about patient decision-making has centered around two essential

but sometimes conflicting purposes—individual autonomy and rational decision-making.[13] As one commentator aptly summarized, the interest in protecting autonomy in treatment-related decision-making is not merely a matter of the value that is placed on liberty or freedom for its own sake. Protection of autonomy also serves to humanize the physician-patient relationship and to restore the balance of authority between the physician and the patient on whose body or mind the proposed treatment would intrude.[14]

THE DOCTRINE OF INFORMED CONSENT. Under the doctrine of informed consent, health care providers have a legal duty to abide by the treatment decisions made by their patients unless a compelling state interest exists. The term *informed consent* is a legal principle in medical jurisprudence that generally holds that a physician must disclose to a patient sufficient information to enable the patient to make an "informed" decision about a proposed treatment or procedure.[15]

For a patient's consent to be considered informed, it must adequately address three essential elements—information, competency, and voluntariness. In general the patient must be given enough information to make a truly knowing decision, and that decision (consent) must be made voluntarily by a person who is legally competent. Each of these requirements must be met, or any consent given will not be considered informed or legally valid.

COMPETENT MEDICAL DECISION-MAKING. Only a competent person is legally recognized as being able to give informed consent. For health care providers working with patients who are sometimes of questionable competence because of mental illness, narcotic abuse, or alcoholism, this issue can be particularly important. The law presumes that an adult is competent unless he or she has been either judicially determined incompetent or incapacitated by a medical condition or emergency. The mere fact that a person is being treated for a mental illness[16] or is institutionalized[17] does not automatically render him or her incompetent. However, in addition to instances in which a patient's competency is manifestly suspect (i.e., he or she is acutely psychotic), there are several other circumstances in which competency considerations may be raised. First, and likely the most common, a patient of uncertain competency may refuse clearly necessary treatment; such a decision is especially questionable if the explanation for the refusal is illogical or indicates poor comprehension of the treatment information provided. Second, a physician may seek a consultation regarding the ability of a patient who is to undergo a significant medical procedure but is of questionable competency to give informed consent. This consideration may have more to do with protecting the physician against possible liability than with respect for patient liberty and autonomy. Third, a competency evaluation may be sought for a patient who has been legally found to be incompetent in one context (e.g., testamentary capacity) but "appears" to be competent in another context (e.g., giving informed consent to pursue a circumscribed course of treatment, such as drug therapy). Again, this practice may be motivated more by defensive medicine than deference to patient rights.

Notwithstanding the reasons that a person's competency to make medical decisions is questioned, the manner in which such a determination should be made is rarely described in the law and is not universally understood and practiced in the various health care professions. Instead, the treating provider (theoretically) is left to engage in a thoughtful analysis of the existing circumstances and arrive at a reasonable determination. From a legal perspective, the term *competency* is narrowly defined in terms of cognitive capacity.[18] Because there are no set criteria for determining a patient's competence, some commentators have likened "the search for a single test of competency to a search for a Holy Grail."[19] Regardless of the lack of a standard, health care providers should ensure that at a minimum the patient is capable of the following[20]:

1. Understanding the particular treatment being offered[21]
2. Making a discernible decision, one way or another, regarding the treatment being offered[22]
3. Communicating, verbally or nonverbally, that decision[23]

To assist with what can be a daunting determination for some health care providers to make on behalf of some patients and under some circumstances, asking the following straightforward questions can help in the assessment of a patient's capacity: What is the patient's primary health problem at this time? What intervention was recommended? If the recommended intervention is implemented, what is likely to occur? If the recommended intervention is not pursued, what is likely to happen? What is the basis of the patient's decision to accept or refuse the recommended intervention?[24]

Mentally ill patients who have been determined to lack the requisite competency to make a treatment decision, except usually in an emergency,[25] will have an authorized representative or guardian appointed to make medical decisions on their behalf.[26]

Capacity to contract. To execute any business transaction between two parties, the law recognizes that each party must have sufficient capacity to give free and relatively knowing consent to enter into an agreement or contract. Minors and the mentally incompetent historically have been recognized as being incapable of executing a legally recognized transaction because of their presumed lack of the requisite cognitive capacity.

This presumption can be traced back as far as Roman law, which held that "an insane person cannot contract any business whatever because he does not know what he is doing." Similarly the common law of contracts in England required that two persons who wished to enter into a business agreement had to reach a "meeting of the minds." If one of the parties lacked the necessary mental capability to reach such a meeting, the law would not recognize the contract.

In *Dexter v. Hall* the U.S. Supreme Court commented on the effect that mental illness could have on the legality of a contract.

[T]he fundamental idea of a contract is that it requires the assent of two minds. But a lunatic, or person non compos mentis ("not of sound mind"), has nothing which the law recognizes as a mind, and it would seem, therefore, upon principle, that he cannot make a contract which may have efficacy as such.[27]

As noted in the introduction, evidence of mental illness is not "per se" evidence of incompetency. Therefore for the "lunatic" in *Dexter* to legally be considered incapable of executing a contract, he or she would have to demonstrate a present inability to meet the applicable standards for doing so as defined by law.[28]

The lack of capacity to contract may be total or partial. In cases of total incapacity a person is unable to enter into any contractual obligation, and any attempt to do so would be considered void. For instance, a person whose property is under the supervision of a legal guardian as a result of a legal adjudication of incompetence is considered "totally lacking contractual capacity." Capacity to contract also may be partial, as is generally the case with minors, the mentally ill, and persons whose cognitive faculties have been impaired by drugs, alcohol, or medication.[29] The extent of the ability of such persons to legally contract depends on the nature of the transaction and the surrounding circumstances.

The interests of commerce underlie the basic values associated with requirements of competency in contracts. When the incapacity or mental unsoundness of one of the parties affects a contract, two contrary public policies come into play. From a business perspective there is a fundamental view that the security of the transaction should be upheld to promote the development of commerce and ensure that the reasonable expectations of the parties are met. However, there is a countervailing public policy grounded in notions of morality and fairness that states that persons who are unable to appreciate the consequences of their actions should not be held accountable for them.

At one time the law regarding contracts entered into by persons lacking capacity held that such contracts were void.[30] However, the overwhelming weight of modern authority is that such contracts are merely voidable at the incompetent person's election.[31] One exception to this rule is the party who is so mentally disabled that he or she has been adjudicated mentally incompetent and a guardian of the property had been appointed before a given transaction was entered into. In many states a contract made under such circumstances would be considered void.[32]

Generally, mental incapacity rising to the level of incompetency to contract is said to exist where a "party does not understand the nature and consequences of his acts at the time of the transaction."[33] This rather broad and flexible definition often leads to the implicit conclusion that, if the contract is fair and beneficial to the individual alleged to be incompetent, he or she was (would be considered) "sane"; otherwise the tendency is to find him or her incompetent.[34] The more contemporary view uses a cognitive test ("ability to understand") and may conclude that the contract is voidable if the party "by reason of mental illness or defect . . . is unable to act in a reasonable manner in relation to the transaction and the other party has reason to know of this condition."[35] This approach allows the incompetent person to disaffirm an agreement or contract that he or she might be capable of understanding but because of some infirmity was without power to resist entering into.[36]

Cases involving challenges to a party's competency typically involve one of two scenarios. In the first scenario there is evidence of a mental condition that impairs a person's cognitive ability (the ability to understand the nature and consequences of the proposed transaction). In the second scenario the evidence indicates that there are mental conditions that impair a party's motivation or ability to act rationally. When a party to a contract lacks cognitive capacity, the contract is voidable without regard to whether the other person knew or had reason to know of the mental impairment. However, when one party has impaired motivational control, the contract is usually held to be voidable only if the other party knew or had reason to know of the mental condition (e.g., alcohol or narcotics intoxication).[37]

Finally, there are two situations—restitution and necessity—in which the incompetency of a party may not necessarily void the provisions of an agreement. Sometimes a contract may be executed and its conditions performed before the issue of competency is raised. A person seeking to avoid a contract has the burden of proving why it should be voided.

Generally, if one party is incompetent and the contract is still to be executed[38] or if the contract is based on grossly inadequate provisions,[39] rescission or cancellation will be granted. If, however, the other party had no reason to know of the mental infirmity and the contract is not otherwise unfair, the right to void the agreement may be lost to the extent that the contract has already been executed.[40] In the latter situation, at the least the incompetent party would have the responsibility to place the other party in the status quo ante (or place he was in before the contract).

In such situations, mental incompetents, like minors, cannot void a contract in which "necessities of life" have been provided.[41] Whether a good or service is considered a necessity is a matter for the jury, but certainly food, shelter, and clothing qualify. Other provisions, such as medical assistance, legal services, and transportation, usually are evaluated based on the party's situation at the time of the contract.

Wills and testamentary capacity. A second area of business activity in which competency is a significant legal factor is the execution of a will. As with contracting, the competency to execute a will is not a matter of general competency but rather is related to specific legal requirements associated with formulating a will. For example, if the individual writing the will, or "testator," is judged to be without the requisite competency (referred to as *testamentary capacity*) at the time of writing the will, the will would not be admitted to "probate" and would not be judged legally valid. If this occurs, the will's terms or provisions have no legal effect. In these situations the distribution of the testator's estate is guided by any valid will that exists. If no other will is available, the rules of "intestate secession" (which favor the immediate family and relatives) are applied. If no immediate family is available, the estate can "escheat" (or revert) to the state.

The conveyance of property through some form of testamentary process has a long and colorful history. Before the sixteenth century there was no law recognizing the written conveyance of real property to third parties. Typically, property rights were passed from one person to another or from one family member (e.g., father) to another (e.g., eldest son) in the form of an oral agreement or understanding. Public declaration or formal written representation of this change of ownership was uncommon and generally had no legal effect even if executed. The basic integrity and good faith of the two parties involved provided the basis of any exchange of property. If a person died without settling his estate, personal or real, his personal possessions were considered to be "up for grabs" and the local authorities, acting in the name of the king or crown, typically seized his real property. In 1540 the first English Statute of Wills was passed.[42] This statute and its later amendments authorized wills of land, provided that they were in writing. No other formality was required.

Today the law recognizes that a person may dispose of his or her property in any way he or she sees fit as long as it does not violate state law. However, for a will to be considered valid, it, like a contract, must be executed knowingly and voluntarily. Challenges to the validity of a will frequently concern whether the testator had sufficient testamentary capacity when making the will or was free from any undue influences (i.e., the will was voluntarily made).

Any person wishing to execute a legally binding will must possess, among other things, testamentary capacity. Analogous to the fundamental criminal law concept of mental competency, testamentary capacity involves an individual having a certain level of understanding of what he or she is doing in deposing of his or her property. There are no hard and fast rules or requisite elements that define testamentary capacity. However, the majority of jurisdictions in the United States require some variations of the elements articulated in the early English case, *Banks v. Goodfellow*.[43] In *Banks* the court fashioned the following five-part test:

To make a valid will one must be of sound mind though he need not possess superior or even average mentality. One is of sound mind for testamentary purposes only when he can understand and carry in his mind in a general way:

1. The nature and extent of his property,
2. The persons who are the natural objects of his bounty, and
3. The disposition which he is making of his property.

He also must be capable of:

4. Appreciating these elements in relation to each other, and
5. Forming an orderly desire as to the disposition of his property.

If a will is challenged on the basis that the testator lacked the requisite capacity, a probate judge will generally inquire the following: Was the testator aware that he or she was making a will? Was he able to assess and appraise the amount and value of the property? Was he aware of his legal heirs? Finally, was there some organized or rational scheme to the distribution of the property?

In assessing each of these or similar criteria a probate judge will entertain any evidence by the challengers that indicates a contrary finding of fitness. As with all questions involving adults and issues of competency, a testator is presumed to possess the requisite capacity. Therefore the burden is on the challenger to prove that at the time the will was made the testator lacked the requisite capacity.

In determining whether testamentary capacity exists under the standards already articulated, the law does not require a high degree of capacity or extensive knowledge. As with many tests of competency, only a minimum level of functioning is required. For example, in *In re Estate of Fish,*[44] a New York appellate court held that a testator "did not need to know the precise size of estate" to be considered competent.

Similar to other areas of competency, the presence of an apparent disability, infirmity, or mental dysfunction, such as mental illness, alcoholism, or narcotics addiction,[45] does not automatically invalidate an individual's testamentary capacity. Although these conditions can cloud or impair a person's ability to think and reason, the extent of any adverse effect is variable and therefore must be assessed. Moreover, even a person who is or appears to be significantly impaired should not be presumed to lack testamentary capacity. For example, if the will is written during a "lucid interval," it can be deemed valid.[46] Similarly, evidence of personality quirks, abnormalities in perception, idiosyncrasies, or forgetfulness in and of themselves generally are not sufficient to support a claim of testamentary incapacity.

Guardianship. Guardianship can be defined as the delegation by the state of authority over an individual's person or estate to another party. Historically the state or sovereign possessed the power and authority to safeguard the estate of incompetent persons.[47] This traditional role still reflects the purpose of guardianship today. In some states there are separate provisions for the appointment of a "guardian of one's person" (for health care decision-making) and a "guardian of one's estate" (who has the authority to, for example, make contracts to sell one's property).[48] This latter type of guardian is frequently referred to as a *conservator,* although this des-

ignation is not uniformly used throughout the United States. Further distinctions found in some jurisdictions are general (plenary) and specific guardianships.[49] As the name implies, the latter type of guardian is restricted to exercising decisions about a particular subject. For instance, the specific guardian may be authorized to make decisions about major or emergency medical procedures while the disabled person retains the freedom to make decisions about all other medical matters. General guardians, in contrast, have total control over the disabled individual's person, estate, or both.[50]

DETERMINATION OF NEED. A guardian is necessary only when there is some question as to whether the individual is de facto (actually) incompetent. An interesting aspect of the guardianship proceeding is its relatively flexible and relaxed atmosphere. In most states any interested person can petition to have someone declared incompetent and subject to guardianship.[51] Often there is no requirement of a specific allegation in the petition, and notice to the respondent is limited to the fact that a hearing will be held.[52] At the hearing itself the respondent frequently has no right to counsel[53] or trial by jury.[54] In some jurisdictions the respondent is rarely present.[55] If counsel is appointed, he or she is often designated as a guardian ad litem and is free to act in what he or she believes is in the respondent's best interest.[56] Moreover, if the respondent is determined to be in need of a guardian, he or she usually bears the burden of challenging that issue at a later time if he or she is no longer in need of a guardian.[57] At a later hearing, such a person is placed in the awkward position of persuading the court that the situation has changed and he or she is now competent. This hearing is required even though the respondent has had no opportunity to manage his or her own affairs, which would be compelling evidence that competency has been restored and a guardian is no longer needed.

The informality and procedural permissiveness that define a guardianship proceeding are matched by the vagueness of the standards by which the need for a guardian is determined. For a general guardianship, most jurisdictions simply require evidence of deficient mental status (e.g., mental illness or senility) and incapacity to "care for oneself or one's estate."[58] Standards for specific guardianship are not much better than are those for general guardianship in providing concrete requirements or descriptions. Despite this lack of rigor in definition, some state courts require considerable evidence of incompetency and incapacity before they will order guardianship.[59] Other courts are less stringent in their scrutiny of the facts.[60]

SELECTION. Anyone can petition the court to become a guardian over the person or estate of another. A diversity of parties may be appointed, ranging from family members and relatives to government agencies and law enforcement authorities.[61] As a rule, the selection of one guardian over another is more likely than not a matter of policy or law.

ROLE. After appointment, the guardian is generally charged with the responsibility to safeguard an incompetent individual's interests pursuant to one of two decision-making models. In one model an objective test is employed. This test guides the guardian by framing his or her responsibilities in terms of the following question: What action will most effectively serve and protect the incompetent individual's best interests? The second, subjective, model uses a form of "substituted judgment." In this model the guardian asks to assume the role of the ward and should "act as he or she thinks the ward would have acted, if the ward had been competent."[62] In situations in which there is no relevant history or reliable information from which to hypothesize how a ward might have acted if competent, a guardian is usually left with no alternative but to employ a form of "best interests" test.[63] Under these circumstances it is likely that the guardian will objectively evaluate as much relevant information as is available and then determine a course of action that best serves the ward's interests.

Competency to testify. Competency to give testimony has generally been defined as follows: "[I]n the law of evidence, the presence of those characteristics, or the absence of those disabilities, which render a witness legally fit and qualified to give testimony in a court of justice."[64] The determination of whether a witness is competent to provide testimony[65] rests solely within the sound discretion of the trial court.[66] The test typically is composed of the following four separate inquiries[67]:

1. Whether, at the time of the event in question, the witness had the capacity "to observe intelligently"
2. Whether at the time of the trial the witness possessed the capacity to recollect that event
3. Whether the witness had the "capacity mentally to understand the nature of the questions put and to form and communicate intelligent answers"
4. Whether the witness had "a sense of moral responsibility, of the duty to make the narration correspond to the recollection and knowledge (i.e., to speak the truth as he sees it"

Often there are no statutorily defined requirements or standards for evaluating the competency of a witness to provide testimony. Instead, the courts (i.e., judges) apply traditional common law principles in making this determination.[68] Therefore there is no single, fixed standard of competency to be applied "across the board" to all witnesses.

Because perceptions and memories of events can vary widely and are prone to distortion and impairment by any witness, courts are especially vigilant to question any potential testimony that may be misleading. This concern is commonly raised with regard to the individual whose memory or perception of reality appears suspect because of developmental immaturity or mental or cognitive impairment. Thus in litigation, especially a criminal trial, the issue of competency to testify often arises if the prospective witness is a child, is mentally retarded, or is psychiatrically impaired (e.g., psychotic).

CHILDREN. Child witnesses present special challenges for the law. As observed by one court:

Not only does it pose problems in terms of the child's appreciation of the need to tell the truth with precision and accuracy, but the trauma attendant upon testimony in open court—subject to examination and cross-examination—before the unfamiliar faces of jurors, lawyers and judges may be particularly terrifying to a young child.[69]

In general there is a rebuttable presumption that children are not legally competent to testify. However, the age at which this presumption is rebuttable varies across jurisdictions. Notwithstanding this threshold there is no precise age that determines competence to testify.[70] The trial court has wide discretion in determining competence and selecting the method for arriving at that determination.[71] Competence of a minor will generally "depend on the capacity and intelligence of the child, his appreciation of the difference between truth and falsehood, as well as his duty to tell the truth."[72] To allow the testimony of a child, the court must determine that the child (1) possesses the intellect to differentiate truth and falsity and to appreciate the duty to tell the truth and (2) can recall the events in question.[73]

MENTALLY HANDICAPPED AND DISABLED INDIVIDUALS. Prospective witnesses who are intellectually handicapped, mentally ill, or mentally disabled as a result of drug or alcohol abuse may potentially testify, provided the court is satisfied that they are capable. For example, the determination of testimonial capacity of a witness who is intellectually limited or has learning difficulties generally proceeds in the same manner as the determination of testimonial capacity of a child witness. Expert testimony may be useful or required.[74]

When a witness is a known abuser of alcohol or illicit drugs, the court's determination is guided by whether the witness (1) was under the influence at the time of the events about which he or she will testify, (2) is under the influence while testifying, or (3) is mentally disabled as a result of long-term substance abuse. Because of the potentially technical nature of these questions, their assessment must be thorough,[75] and competency hearings rely on a variety of evidence, including the examination of medical records, lay and expert testimony, and the results of mental and physical examinations.[76]

A mentally ill person may be a competent witness.[77] As in the case of the substance-impaired witness, the court may conduct the usual examination of relevant evidence, such as the review of medical records, expert testimony, and the results of mental examinations, in making a determination.[78]

Criminal law

It is generally accepted in Western jurisprudence that incompetent individuals should not be permitted to proceed with a trial.[79] Conviction of an accused person while he or she is legally incompetent deprives him or her of liberty without due process of law.[80] Effective representation of a defendant with mental problems is a difficult task, demanding special skill and care in dealing with the defendant, as well as knowledge of a complicated body of statutory and case law. Consequently, every criminal attorney, judge, or other officer of the court must be alert to the possibility that a defendant's mental state—at the present time, at the time of the alleged offense, or both—may be relevant to the handling of his defense.

Standards and assessment of competency to stand trial. The legal standard for assessing pretrial competency is well established by the landmark case *Dusky v. United States.*[81] Throughout his or her involvement with the trial process, the defendant must have "sufficient present ability to consult with his attorney with a reasonable degree of rational understanding (and have) a rational as well as factual understanding of the proceedings against him."[82] These standards are general legal conclusions, and the precise meanings are deliberately ambiguous. The *Dusky* language suggests several fundamental elements. First, competency reflects a defendant's present ability to consult with counsel and to understand the proceedings. Second, the test of competency applies to the defendant's capacity rather than motivation or willingness* to relate to the attorney and understand the proceedings. Third, the criterion that the defendant must have a "reasonable" degree of understanding implies that the test for competency in a given case is flexible. As with other tests of capacity, "perfect" or complete understanding on the part of the defendant is not required.[83] Fourth, the court's focus on the defendant's "factual" and "rational" understanding suggests an emphasis on cognitive functioning. This final consideration reiterates the fact that evidence of a mental illness or the need for psychiatric treatment is not an automatic indicator of incompetency.[84] These factors are relevant only insofar as they affect or represent a sufficient impairment in the defendant's ability to meet the legal test of competency.

Numerous commentators have sought to identify specific reality-based factors that could be used in assessing the general standards established in *Dusky.*[85] These efforts typically focus on two areas—the defendant's comprehension of the criminal process, including the role of participants (e.g., attorneys, judge, and jury) in the process, and the defendant's ability to function in that process, primarily through consultation with defense counsel. For instance, one court noted that a defendant would be determined competent to stand trial if the following were found:

- The defendant possesses the "mental capacity to appreciate his presence in relation to time, place, and things."[86]
- The defendant has "sufficient elementary mental processes to apprehend (i.e., to seize and grasp with what mind he has) that he is in a court of justice, charged with a criminal offense."

- The defendant understands that there is a judge on the bench.
- The defendant "understands that a prosecutor is present who will try to convict him of a criminal charge."
- The defendant "understands that a lawyer will undertake to defend him against that charge."
- The defendant understands that "he is expected to tell his lawyer the circumstances, to the best of his mental ability (whether colored or not by mental aberration), the facts surrounding him at the time and place where the law violation is alleged to have been committed."
- The defendant understands that there will be a jury present to determine guilt or innocence.
- The defendant "has memory sufficient to relate those things in his own personal manner."[87]

The degree of a defendant's impairment in one specific area of functioning does not automatically equate with incompetency. The ultimate determination of incompetency is solely for the court to decide.[88] Moreover the impairment must be considered in the context of the particular case or proceeding.

[O]ne or another of the items will not be equal nor is it intended to be. Neither will the weight assigned to a given item by the court in reaching a finding on competency for a particular defendant necessarily apply to the next defendant. Considerations of the weight to be assigned a given item in the case of a particular defendant goes [sic] beyond the scope of what should be expected of the examining clinician. The task for the clinician is the providing of objective data, the import of which is the responsibility of the Court.[89]

Controversy exists regarding the general scope of the term *competency to stand trial* and its practical application in today's criminal justice system. Some commentators have suggested that the concept is overly broad, inadequate, and misleading in its current use.[90] For example, some defendants may be required to testify, decide whether to plead insanity, or make choices about plea options and plea bargains. Depending on the nature of the decision to be made, some commentators have argued that a given defendant may be competent to make certain decisions but not others. Although this analysis may be clinically valid and more realistic, it does not square with the present legal precedents on this issue. In a recent Supreme Court case, *Godinez v. Moran,* the majority held that the standard for the various types of competency (e.g., competency to plea, to waive counsel, and to stand trial) should be considered the same.[91]

While the decision to plead guilty is undeniably a profound one, it is no more complicated than the sum total of decisions that a defendant may be called upon to make during the course of a trial. . . . Nor do we think that a defendant who waives his right to the assistance to counsel must be more competent than the defendant who does not, since there is not reason to believe that the decision to waive counsel requires an appreciably higher level of mental functioning than the decision to waive other constitutional rights.[92]

---

*There is presently no single "test" that is given to a defendant and yields a valid finding of competency or incompetency.

Judicial evaluation. The judicial determination of competency must be an informed one.[93] Accordingly the court has broad discretion in both hearing a motion for a competency examination[94] and weighing evidence in making a final determination.[95] Because a careful evaluation of the accused's mental condition is required,[96] a hospital report that he or she is mentally competent to stand trial is not binding on the court,[97] especially if there is no supporting information or reasons regarding that conclusion.[98] The law often requires that a report or certificate be issued by a qualified mental health professional (e.g., psychiatrist), establishing that a person is competent to stand trial before the court.[99] This certificate does not preclude the expert testimony of a psychologist,[100] though less weight may be given to his or her testimony.[101] The determination of competency does not rest exclusively or primarily on the opinion of experts.[102] For instance, the U.S. Court of Appeals for the District of Columbia Circuit has stated that it would be useful for trial judges to question both the defendant and defense counsel about the ability of the accused to consult with his or her attorney because the attorney's own first-hand evaluation may be just as valuable as an expert's opinion.[103]

There are a number of checklists and psychometric tests designed to assist the clinician in assessing a person's competency to stand trial.[104] One of the more commonly used instruments is the Competency to Stand Trial Instrument (CSTI) designed by the Laboratory of Community Psychiatry.[105] The CSTI involves the consideration of 13 functions "related to what is required of a defendant in criminal proceedings in order that he may adequately cope with and protect himself in such proceedings."[106] The purpose of the CSTI is to standardize, objectify, and qualify relevant criteria for the determination of an individual's competency to stand trial. The presentation of these functions was written so it would be useful and acceptable to both the legal and medical professions. The 13 functions to be assessed include, among other factors:

- Appraisal of available legal defenses
- Unmanageable behavior
- Quality of relating to attorney and planning of legal strategy
- Understanding of court procedure
- Appreciation of charges and nature of possible penalties
- Capacity to disclose to attorney available pertinent facts surrounding the offense

All "competency-related" assessment instruments are essentially structured formats for interviewing the defendant. Generally a competency evaluation can be performed within the context of an outpatient interview. Actual psychological testing is not likely to be a cost-effective means of gathering relevant information, nor is it any more capable of directly answering the requisite competency questions.

Special considerations: the amnestic defendant. At face value, the defendant who has no memory of the criminal act of which he or she is accused appears to be incompetent on the grounds that the amnesia prevents reasonable consultation with counsel in preparing a defense.[1] However, as a general rule a claim of amnesia is not grounds for a finding of incompetency per se.[107] This rule is largely borne out of judicial mistrust of the authenticity of such claims. However, while generally rejecting outright such claims as an automatic determinant of incompetency, courts have labored to establish guidelines in determining the competency of the defendant claiming amnesia. Probably the most thoughtful analysis of this issue is found in *Wilson v. United States.*[108] In *Wilson* the defendant had no memory regarding the time of the alleged robbery because he suffered from permanent retrograde amnesia. This impairment was caused by injuries he suffered in an automobile accident that occurred as the police were pursuing him after the offense. The court concluded that the competency issue should be tested in accordance with the following criteria:

1. The extent to which the amnesia affected the defendant's ability to consult with and assist his attorney
2. The extent to which the amnesia affected the defendant's ability to testify on his own behalf
3. The extent to which the evidence could be extrinsically reconstructed in view of the defendant's amnesia (Such evidence would include evidence relating to the crime itself, as well as any reasonably possible alibi.)
4. The extent to which the government assisted the defendant and his counsel in that reconstruction
5. The strength of the prosecution's case (Most important here is whether the government's case is such as to negate all reasonable hypotheses of innocence. If there is any substantial possibility that the accused could, but for his amnesia, establish an alibi or other defense, it should be presumed that he would have been able to do so.)
6. Any other factors and circumstances that would indicate whether or not the defendant had a fair trial

For the clinician faced with a defendant claiming severe memory problems, the first objective is to determine whether the claim of amnesia is valid. If the claim is valid, the "customary" competency examination may proceed because all other functions associated with competency (e.g., communicating with counsel and understanding the legal proceedings) may be unaffected. Moreover, the amnestic defendant may be able to assist the defense by identifying and assessing other evidence depicting his or her conduct at the time of the crime.

Raising the competency issue. The competency of a defendant may be raised at any stage in the proceedings up until the time of sentencing.[109] However, prima facie evidence must be presented to support a request for a competency examination, particularly when the request comes on the eve of or the day of trial.[110]

Although questions regarding competency are usually raised by the defense attorney,[111] the court and the prosecutor have an obligation to ensure that a defendant whose competency is in question is not permitted to proceed with the trial until competency issues are resolved.[112]

ENDNOTES

1. *Blacks' Law Dictionary* 257 (7th ed., West Group, St. Paul, Minn. 1999).
2. *See e.g.,* Department of Health and Human Services, *The Legal Status of Adolescents 1980* 41 (DHHS, Washington, D.C. 1981).
3. *See e.g., Meek v. City of Loveland,* 276 P. 30 (Colo. 1929).
4. *See e.g., Scaria v. St. Paul Fire & Marine Insurance,* 227 N.W. 2d 647 (Wis. 1975).
5. J.T. Smith, *Medical Malpractice: Psychiatric Care* 178-179 (Shepard's/McGraw-Hill, Colorado Springs, Colo. 1986).
6. *See e.g., Gulf Southern Railroad Co. v. Sullivan,* 119 So. 501 (Miss. 1929).
7. *See e.g., Planned Parenthood v. Danforth,* 428 U.S. 52, 74 (1975) (abortion); Ill. Rev. Stat. ch. 91 1/2, para 3-501(a) (1983) (mental health counseling).
8. *See e.g., Jehovah's Witnesses v. King County Hospital,* 278 F.Supp. 488 (W.D. Wash. 1967).
9. *See e.g., Wilson v. Lehmann,* 379 S.W. 2d 478, 479 (Ky. Ct. App. 1964).
10. *See e.g., Rennie v. Klein,* 462 F.Supp. 1131 (D. N.J. 1978).
11. H. Weihofen, *The Definition of Mental Illness,* 21 Ohio St. L. J. 1 (1960).
12. *See e.g., Schloendorff v. New York Hospital,* 105 N.E. 92 (N.Y. 1914).
13. *See e.g.,* M.B. Stauss, *Familiar Medical Quotations* 157 (Little, Brown, Boston 1968) (quoting a 1649 Massachusetts Bay colony law that forbade physicians, midwives, and others from acting on mentally competent patients without their consent). Although the concept of informed consent has deep roots in the centuries-old individual liberty movement, its actual development as a legal doctrine did not occur until the 1960s. *See e.g., Salgo v. Leland Stanford Jr. Univ. Bd. of Trustees,* 317 P. 2d 170 (Cal. Dist. Ct. App. 1957); *Natanson v. Kline,* 350 P. 2d 1093, *rehg. den.* 354 P. 2d 670 (Kan. 1960).
14. J. Katz, *The Silent World of Doctor and Patient* 59-80 (Free Press, New York 1984).
15. *Supra* note 1, at 701.
16. *Supra* note 9.
17. *Supra* note 10.
18. *See e.g., Yahn v. Folse,* 639 So. 2d 261 (La. App. 1993). (An 82 year-old illiterate and hard of hearing woman was sufficiently alert [cognitively] and communicative to give valid consent to a medical procedure.)
19. Meisel, Roth & Lidz, *Tests of Competency to Consent to Treatment,* 134 Am. J. Psychiatry 279, 283 (1977).
20. *See also* Appelbaum & Grisso, *Assessing Patients' Capacities to Consent to Treatment,* 319 N. Engl. J. Med. 1635-1638 (1988) (proposing four different standards for assessing competency to consent to treatment).
21. Meisel, Roth & Lidz, *Toward a Model of the Legal Doctrine of Informed Consent,* 134 Am. J. Psychiatry 285 (1977).
22. M. Perlin, *Mental Disability Law: Civil and Criminal,* vol. 3, 80 (Michie Co., Charlottesville, Va. 1989).
23. *Supra* note 21, at 287 citing 139 Am. Law Rep. 1370 (1942); *but see, Lipscomb v. Memorial Hospital,* 733 F. 2d 332, 335-36 (4th Cir. 1984).
24. P.A. Singer & M. Siegler, *Elective Use of Life-Sustaining Treatments in Internal Medicine,* in *Advances in Internal Medicine* 66 (G.H. Stollerman, ed., Year Book Medical Publishers, Chicago 1991).
25. *See e.g., Frasier v. Department of Health and Human Resources,* 500 So. 2d 858, 864 (La. Ct. App. 1986).
26. *See e.g., Aponte v. United States,* 582 F.Supp. 555, 566-69 (D. P.R. 1984).
27. *Dexter v. Hall,* 82 U.S. 15 (1872).
28. *See generally,* J. Calamari & J. Perillo, The Law of Contracts 305-330 (4th ed. St. Paul, Minn., West Group, 1998) (capacity of parties).
29. *See e.g.,* Sharpe, *Medication as a Threat to Testamentary Capacity,* 35 N.C. L. Rev. 380 (1957).
30. *See e.g., Hovey v. Hobson,* 53 Me. 451 (1866).
31. *See* 2 Williston, *Contracts* §§249-252.
32. Restatement (Second) Contracts, §13.
33. *See e.g., Cundick v. Broadbent,* 383 F. 2d 157 (10th Cir. 1967), *cert. den.* 390 U.S. 948 (1968); *see also* Guttmacher & Weihofen, *Mental Incompetency,* 36 Minn. L. Rev. 179 (1952).
34. *See e.g.,* Green, *Proof of Mental Incompetency and the Unexpressed Major Premise,* 53 Yale L. J. 271 (1944); Green, *The Operative Effect of Mental Incompetency on Agreements and Wills,* 21 Tex. L. Rev. 554 (1943).
35. Restatement (Second) Contracts §15.
36. *See e.g.,* Danzig, *The Capability Problem in Contract Law,* 148-204 (Foundation Press, Mineola, N.Y. 1978); *but see* Hardisty, *Mental Illness: A Legal Fiction,* 48 Wash. L. Rev. 735 (1975).
37. *See generally* McCoid, *Intoxication and its Effect upon Civil Responsibility,* 42 Iowa L. Rev. (1956); 2 Williston, *Contracts* §§258-263.
38. *See e.g., Cundell v. Haswell,* 51 A. 426 (R.I. 1902).
39. *See e.g., Alexander v. Haskins,* 68 Iowa 73, 25 N.W. 935 (1885).
40. *See e.g.,* Restatement (Second) Contracts, §15(2).
41. *See e.g., Coffee v. Owens' Admiralty,* 216 Ky. 142 (1926).
42. E. Clark, L. Lusky & A. Murphy, *Gratuitous Transfers,* 372 (3d ed., West Publishing, St. Paul, Minn. 1985).
43. *Banks v. Goodfellow,* 5 Q.B. 549 (1870).
44. *In re Estate of Fish,* 522 N.Y.S. 2d 970 (App. Div. 1987).
45. 79 Am. Jur. 2d Wills §§77-101.
46. *See generally* 18 Am. Jur. P.O. F. 2d *Mentally Disordered Testator's Execution of Will During Lucid Interval* §1 (1979).
47. *See generally* Regan, *Protective Services for the Elderly: Commitment, Guardianship, and Alternatives,* 13 Wm. & Mary L. Rev. 569, 570-573 (1972).
48. R. Sales, D.M. Powell & R. Van Duizend, *Disabled Persons and the Law: State Legislative Issues* 461 (Plenum Press, New York 1982).
49. *Id.* at 462.
50. *Id.* at 461-462.
51. *Id.* at 463.
52. *Supra* note 47, at 605.
53. *Supra* note 48, at 463. (As of 1988, 10 states provide no statutory right to counsel.)
54. *Id.* (As of 1988, 22 states provide the respondent with the right to jury.)
55. *Id.* (As of 1988, only 38 states guarantee the right to be present and that right is often waivable with only a physician's certificate stating that the respondent is unable to attend.)
56. *Supra* note 48, at 463.
57. *Id.* at 464.
58. *Id.* at 469-474.
59. *See e.g., Plummer v. Early,* 190 Cal.Rptr. 578 (Ct. App. 1983). (Evidence that schizophrenic respondent was dirty, disheveled, and incontinent and spent the majority of his time in the backyard of his home was insufficient to warrant conservatorship or guardianship of person.)
60. *See e.g., In re Oltmer,* 336 N.W. 2d 560 (Neb. 1983).
61. *See generally* Hodgson, *Guardianship of Mentally Retarded Persons: Three Approaches to a Long Neglected Problem,* 37 Alb. L. Rev. 407 (1973).
62. *See e.g., In re Roe III,* 421 N.E. 2d 40 (Mass. 1981); *Rogers v. Commissioner of Mental Health,* 458 N.E. 2d 308 (Mass. 1983).
63. *See generally* Melton & Scott, *Evaluations of Mentally Retarded Persons for Sterilization: Contributions and Limits of Psychological Consultation,* 15 Prof. Psychol. Res. Prac. 34, 35-36 (1984).
64. *Supra* note 1, at 257.
65. Competency issues are frequently raised about a number of aspects of a witness' or defendant's conduct or litigation procedures (e.g., waive right to silence, counsel, or jury; stand trial; be sentenced; serve a sentence; and be executed).
66. *See generally Wheeler v. United States,* 159 U.S. 523, 524-525 (1895); *United States v. Benn,* 476 F. 2d 1201 (D.C. Cir. 1972); *In re B.D.T.,* 435 A. 2d 378, 379 (D.C. 1981).

67. J. Wigmore, *Evidence,* §478 (Chadbourn rev. 1979).
68. The four-part test enunciated by Wigmore would be a typical example of a common law rule or guiding principle.
69. *U.S. v. Comer,* 421 F. 2d 1149, 1152 n.3 (D.C. Cir. 1970).
70. *See e.g., Galindo v. U.S.,* 630 A. 2d 202 (D.C. 1993) (3-year-old found competent); *Wheeler v. U.S.,* 159 U.S. 523, 524 (D.C. Cir. 1895) (5-year-old found competent).
71. *U.S. v. Schoefield,* 465 F. 2d 560, 562 (D.C. Cir. 1972), *cert. den.* 409 U.S. 881 (1972).
72. *Id.*
73. *See e.g., Johnson v. U.S.,* 364 A. 2d 1198, 1202 (D.C. 1976); *In re A.H.B.,* 491 A. 2d 490, 492 (D.C. 1985).
74. *See e.g., U.S. v. Benn,* 476 F. 2d 1127, 1130-31 (D.C. Cir. 1972).
75. *U.S. v. Crosby,* 462 F. 2d 1201, 1203 (D.C. Cir. 1972).
76. *See e.g., U.S. v. Heinlein,* 490 F. 2d 725, 730 (D.C. Cir. 1973); *U.S. v. Butler,* 481 F. 2d 531, 533 (D.C. Cir. 1973).
77. *See e.g., In re Penn,* 443 F. 2d 663, 666 (D.C. Cir. 1970).
78. *See generally Vereen v. U.S.,* 587 A. 2d. 456 (D.C. App. 1991), *Collins v. U.S.,* 491 A. 2d. 480, 484 (D.C. App. 1985), cert. den. 475 U.S. 1124 (1986).
79. *See generally* W. Blackstone, *Commentaries on the Laws of England* (9th ed., Clarendon Press, Oxford 1773); *see also Frith's Case,* 22 How. St. Tr. 307 (1790).
80. *See e.g., Pate v. Robinson,* 383 U.S. 375, 378 (1966).
81. *Dusky v. United States,* 362 U.S. 402 (1960) (established the threshold test for determining a defendant's competency to stand trial).
82. *Id.* This standard also is applied to juvenile proceedings; *see e.g., In re W.A.F.,* 573 A. 2d 1264, 1267 (D.C. 1990).
83. The threshold for being found competent to stand trial is generally believed to be low; *see generally, Incompetency to Stand Trial,* 81 Harv. L. Rev. 454, 457-458 (1967).
84. Typically, evidence of a mental disease, condition, or defect is associated with the question of incompetence. However, a defendant may be adjudged incompetent to stand trial even if he or she lacks a mental disorder as defined by current mental health diagnostic standards, such as the American Psychiatric Association's *Diagnostic and Statistical Manual of Mental Disorders,* Fourth Edition (DSM-IV); *see generally, Wilson v. U.S.,* 391 F. 2d 460, 463 (D.C. Cir. 1968).
85. *See e.g.,* T. Grisso, *Competency to Stand Trial: Evaluations* 97-106 (Professional Resource Exchange, Sarasota, Fla. 1988). (See Appendix C: List of Defendant's Abilities and Trial Demands for Use in Pretrial Competency Evaluations and Appendix D: Information about Competency Evaluation Instruments.)
86. Competency is not met by a defendant's mere understanding or the fact that he or she has "orientation to time and place and [has] some recollection of events." *Supra* note 81.
87. *Weiter v. Settle,* 193 F.Supp. 318, 321-22 (W.D. Mo. 1961).
88. *United States v. David,* 511 F. 2d 355 (D.C. Cir. 1975).
89. *Id.* at 99 100.
90. *See e.g., Roesch & Golding, Defining and Assessing Competency to Stand Trial,* in *Handbook of Forensic Psychology* 378-394 (Weiner I.B. & Hess A.K., eds., J. Wiley, New York 1987).
91. *Godinez v. Moran,* 113 S.Ct. 2680 (1993).
92. *Id.* at 2686; *but see Id.* at 2691-2694 (J. Blackmon, dissenting). (The "majority's analysis is contrary to both common sense and long-standing case law;" competency cannot be considered in a vacuum, separate from its specific legal context; "competency for one purpose does not necessarily translate to competency for another purpose," noting that prior Supreme Court cases have "required competency evaluations to be specifically tailored to the context and purpose of the proceeding.")
93. *See Blunt v. U.S.,* 389 F. 2d 545 (D.C. Cir. 1967).
94. *Bennett v. United States,* 400 A. 2d 322 (D.C. App. 1979).
95. 18 U.S.C. §4241 (federal statute authorizing a psychiatric or psychological examination of a defendant on the issue of competency to stand trial and presentation of a report to the court).
96. *Supra* note 93.
97. *See e.g., Wider v. United States,* 348 F. 2d 358 (D.C. Cir. 1965).
98. *See e.g., Holloway v. United States,* 343 F. 2d 265 (D.C. Cir. 1964).
99. *See e.g., Bennett v. United States,* 400 A. 2d 322 (D.C. App. 1979). (If neither party objects, the court, without conducting a hearing, may enter an order adjudicating the defendant to be competent based on the certification of the examining psychiatrist.)
100. *See e.g., Jenkins v. United States,* 307 F. 2d 637, 643 (D.C. Cir. 1962).
101. *See e.g., Blunt v. United States,* 389 F. 2d 545 (D.C. Cir. 1957). (The lack of a general medical background may affect the weight given to a psychologist's testimony in a competency hearing.)
102. By analogy, testimony by lay witnesses as to their observations and opinions of the defendant's mental condition is admissible in support of the insanity defense. *Carter v. United States,* 252 F. 2d 608, 618 (D.C. Cir. 1957).
103. *United States v. David,* 511 F. 2d 355 (D.C. Cir. 1975).
104. *See generally,* T. Grisso, *Competency to Stand Trial Evaluations: A Manual for Practice* 101-105 (Professional Resource Exchange, Sarasota, FL 1988).
105. *Competency to Stand Trial and Mental Illness,* a monograph sponsored by the Center for Studies of Crime and Delinquency, National Institute of Mental Health, DHEW Pub. No. (HSM) 73-9105 (1973) (out of print).
106. *Id.*
107. *See generally* 46 A.L.R. 3d 544 (1972).
108. *Wilson v. United States,* 391 F. 2d 460, 463 (D.C. Cir. 1968).
109. *In Leach v. United States,* 334 F. 2d 945 (D.C. Cir. 1964). (A sentence was set aside and remanded with directions when a district court judge failed to consider evidence presented to him about the psychological unfitness of the individual he was sentencing. The appellate court specifically cited the lower court's failure to make any disposition of the prisoner's repeated request for a mental examination before sentencing. The appellate court noted that the trial court had psychiatric services at its disposal and this was precisely the situation in which to employ them.)
110. *See e.g., Thorne v. United States,* 471 A. 2d 247 (D.C. 1983).
111. An affidavit by defense counsel stating that he or she has serious doubts about the defendant's mental capacity to assist him or her intelligently is sufficient to require the granting of a motion for a mental examination. *Cannady v. United States,* 351 F. 2d 817 (D.C. Cir. 1965).
112. *See e.g., Winn v. United States,* 270 F. 2d 326 (D.C. Cir. 1959), *cert. den.* 365 U.S. 848 (1961).
113. *See e.g., In re Guardianship of Pamela,* 519 N.E. 2d 1335 (Mass. Sup. Jud. Ct. 1988).
114. *See e.g., McAlister v. Deatheridge,* 523 So. 2d 387 (Ala. 1988).
115. *See e.g., Daughton v. Parson,* 423 N.W. 2d 894 (Iowa Ct. App. 1988) (transfer of property set aside where the grantor did not have sufficient mental capacity to execute the deed).
116. *See e.g., Annas & Densburger, Competence to Refuse Medical Treatment: Autonomy vs. Paternalism,* 15 U. Toledo L. Rev. 561 (1984).
117. *See e.g., Weldon v. Long Island College Hospital,* 535 N.Y.S. 2d 949 (Sup. Ct. 1988).
118. *See e.g., Pace v. Pace,* 513 N.E. 2d 1357 (Ohio Ct. App. 1986).
119. *See e.g., Manhattan State Citizen's Group, Inc. v. Bass,* 524 F.Supp. 1270 (S.D. N.Y. 1981).
120. 42 U.S.C. §423(d)(1)(A) (1983 and Cumm. Supp. 1985 *et seq.*); *see also* 20 C.F.R. §404.1520-404.1574 (1983).
121. *In re Conservatorship Estate of Moehlenpah,* 763 S.W. 2d 249 (Mo. Ct. App. 1988).
122. *See e.g.,* D.C. Code §16-904 (d)(1)-(5) (grounds for annulment of marriage, including "insanity" at the time of marriage).
123. *See e.g., In re Marriage of Steffan,* 423 N.W. 2d 729 (Minn. Ct. App. 1988) (divorce decree binding where the wife's mental condition did not interfere with her comprehension).
124. *See e.g., In re Jason Y,* 744 P. 2d 181 (N.M. Ct. App. 1987).

125. *See e.g., In re J.O.L. II,* 409 A. 2d 1073 (D.C. 1979). (Defining factors used in the District of Columbia delineate whether an adoption by a petitioning party is in the "best interests of the child." Among these factors is the mental state of the petitioning party. Clearly, if the petitioner were incompetent, placement would not be in a child's best interests.)
126. *Dusky v. United Sates,* 362 U.S. 402 (1960).
127. *Drope v. Missouri,* 420 U.S. 162 (1975); *Pate v. Robinson,* 383 U.S. 375 (1966).
128. A defendant who has been found "competent" is not necessarily capable of making intelligent decisions on all issues, for example, the decision to waive an insanity defense. *Frendak v. United States,* 408 A. 2d 364, 379 (D.C. App. 1979).
129. *See e.g., Lyles v. U.S.,* 254 F. 2d 725 (D.C. Cir. 1975).
130. *See e.g., Nebraska v. Tully,* 413 N.W. 2d 910 (Neb. 1987) (defendant's confession and guilty plea held to be "knowingly, intelligently, and voluntarily made" despite IQ of 81 and diagnosis of mild mental retardation).
131. *See e.g., Faretta v. California,* 422 U.S. 806 (1975).
132. *See e.g.,* Note, *Mental Aberration and Postconviction Sanctions,* 15 Suffolk Univ. L. Rev. 1219 (1981); *State v. Hehman,* 520 P. 2d 507 (Ariz. 1974); *Commonwealth v. Robinson,* 431 A. 2d 901 (Pa. 1981).
133. *See e.g., In re Hews,* 741 P. 2d 983 (Wash. 1987).
134. *North Carolina v. Alford,* 400 U.S. 25 (1970).
135. *See e.g., Jurney v. Arkansas,* 766 S.W. 2d 1 (Ark. 1989).
136. *See e.g., Ford v. Wainwright,* 477 U.S. 399 (1986); Note, *The Eighth Amendment and the Execution of the Presently Incompetent,* 32 Stan. L. Rev. 765 (1980).
137. *See e.g., United States v. Thornton,* 498 F. 2d 749 (D.C. Cir. 1974); *Bethea v. United States,* 365 A. 2d 64 (D.C. App. 1976).
138. *See e.g., Fuller v. Texas,* 737 S.W. 2d 113 (Tex. Ct. App. 1987).

SUGGESTED READINGS

General

S. Brakal, J. Parry & B. Weiner, eds., *The Mentally Disabled and the Law* (3d ed., American Bar Foundation, Chicago 1985).

T. Grisso, *Evaluating Competencies: Forensic Assessments and Instruments* (Plenum Press, New York 1986).

G.B. Melton, J. Petrila, N.G. Poythress & C. Slobogin, *Psychological Evaluations for the Courts* (2d ed., Guilford Press, New York, 1997).

R. Reisner & C. Slobogin, *Law and the Mental Health System: Civil and Criminal Aspects* (2d ed., West Publishing, St. Paul, Minn. 1990).

Competency to stand trial

T. Grisso, *Competency to Stand Trial Evaluations: A Manual for Practice* (PAR Inc., Sarasota, Fla. 1988).

M. Perlin, *Mental Disability Law: Civil and Criminal* (3 volumes) (Michie Publishing, Charlottesville, Va. 1989).

Public Defender Service, *Criminal Practice Institute Trial Manual* (PDS, Washington, D.C. 1996).

Children and juveniles

S.J. Ceci & M. Bruck, *Jeopardy in the Courtroom: A Scientific Analysis of Children's Testimony* (American Psychological Association, Washington D.C. 1995).

T. Grisso, *Juveniles' Waiver of Rights: Legal and Psychological Competence* (Plenum Press, New York 1981).

Consent to research

Berg, *Legal and Ethical Complexities of Consent With Cognitively Impaired Research Subjects: Proposed Guidelines,* 24 J.L. Med. & Ethics 18 (1996).

Guardianship

J. Parry, *Incompetency, Guardianship, and Restoration,* in *The Mentally Disabled and the Law* (S. Brakal, J. Parry & B. Weiner eds., American Bar Foundation, Chicago 1985).

Parry & Hulme, *Guardianship Monitoring and Enforcement Nationwide,* 15 Ment. & Phys. Disability L. Rptr. 304 (May/June 1991).

Treatment decision-making

B. Winick, ed., *A Critical Examination of the MacArthur Treatment Competence Study: Methodological Issues, Legal Implications, and Future Directions,* 2 Psychol., Pub. Policy & L. 3-181 (1996).

American Bar Association, *The Right to Refuse Antipsychotic Medication* (American Bar Association, Washington, D.C. 1986).

B. Corsino, *Informed Consent: Policy and Practice* (Virginia National Center for Clinical Ethics, White River Junction, Va. 1996).

Redding, *Children's Competence to Provide Informed Consent for Mental Health Treatment,* 50 Wash. & Lcc L. Rev. 695 (1993).

APPENDIX 4-1   Some areas of law in which competency is an issue

CIVIL LAW

- Guardianship (care for one's self and property)[113]
- Contract[114]
- Make a will[115]
- Consent to treatment[116]
- Authorize disclosure of medical records
- Sue[117] or be sued[118]
- Testify in court
- Vote[119]
- Obtain a driver's license
- Act in public or professional capacity
- Receive benefits (e.g., Social Security)[120]
- Retain private counsel[121]

FAMILY LAW

- Marry[122]
- Divorce[123]
- Terminate parental relations with a child[124]
- Adopt[125]

CRIMINAL LAW

- Stand trial[126]
- Assume responsibility for a criminal act
- Raise the question of competency and order an examination[127]
- Waive the insanity defense[128]
- Make a distinction between insanity and competency[129]
- Make a confession[130]
- Waive the right to counsel[131]
- Be sentenced[132]
- Make a plea[133]
- Plead guilty[134]
- Provide testimony in court[135]
- Be executed[136]
- Entertain premeditation or "specific intent" of a crime[137]
- Consent to sexual intercourse[138]

APPENDIX 4-2   Some general tests of competency

Relevant act	General legal test regarding competency
Make a will	Understand the nature and object of the will, one's holdings, and natural objects of one's bounty
Make a contract	Understand the nature and effect of the proposed agreement or transaction
Marry	Understand the nature of the marital relationship and the rights, duties, and obligations it creates
Drive	Understand the pertinent laws of the state with regard to licensure; refrain from driving in a dangerous manner
Testify in court	Be capable of observing, remembering, and communicating about events in question; understand the nature of an oath
Be responsible for a criminal act	Possess sufficient capacity (cognitive) to understand and appreciate the criminality of one's acts and conform one's conduct to the requirements of the law
Stand trial	Possess sufficient capacity to rationally and factually understand the nature of the proceedings and be able to assist and consult with legal counsel
Make a confession	Possess sufficient capacity to make a knowing and intelligent waiver of certain constitutional rights and a knowing and voluntary confession
Be executed for a criminal act	Possess sufficient capacity to rationally and factually understand the nature of the trial proceedings and purpose of punishment
Consent to treatment	Possess sufficient mental capacity to understand the particular treatment choice being proposed and any relevant adverse effects associated with it

The specific and applicable language of these and other tests of capacity is generally defined by state or federal statute or administrative regulation. Their interpretation and practical usage are typically defined in case law, scholarly treatises, and commentaries.

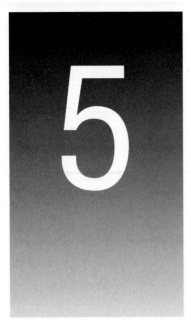

5

Alternative dispute resolution and application to medical disputes

BRYAN A. LIANG, M.D., Ph.D., J.D., F.C.L.M.

FORMAL ADJUDICATION
MEDIATION
ARBITRATION
HYBRID METHODS
OTHER FORMS OF ALTERNATIVE DISPUTE RESOLUTION
ALTERNATIVE DISPUTE RESOLUTION AND MEDICAL MALPRACTICE CLAIMS
ALTERNATIVE DISPUTE RESOLUTION AND OTHER MEDICAL DISPUTES
CONCLUSION

Disputes are as common in health care as in other industries and social circumstances that involve differing interests. However, resolving medical disputes using the formal adjudication process of court litigation is time consuming and expensive and may not suit the parties' needs. Thus, beyond formal adjudication, other alternatives may provide better opportunities to effectuate a resolution that is acceptable to the parties.

Over the past three decades, the alternative dispute resolution (ADR) movement has recognized the limitations of formal adjudication and has employed other mechanisms through which conflicts may be resolved. Each of these alternatives has important strengths and limitations. However, ADR methods, in combination with formal adjudication, offer a broad range of tools for the dispute resolution toolbox to address the concomitantly broad array of conflicts that may arise in health care.

Generally the binding or nonbinding nature of any ADR process is based on contract. The terms of the agreement dictate whether and which specific ADR process must be followed in an effort to resolve a dispute and whether the assessment is simply advisory or is legally binding on both parties.

This chapter reviews some of the main ADR methods and indicates the types of circumstances that appear to be most beneficial for each method's use. Each ADR method may vary when used in specific circumstances to resolve disputes, and the description of the methods herein represents only basic definitions. In addition, the controversial subject of ADR application to malpractice claims is discussed. Finally, application of ADR methods to non–malpractice, modern health care disputes is illustrated through the presentation and review of several case scenarios.

FORMAL ADJUDICATION

Formal adjudication is the use of the well-recognized court system to resolve disputes (i.e., litigation). Generally the important characteristics of the formal adjudicatory system include (1) the involuntary nature of the process (i.e., one party may be forced into adjudication by another party); (2) the imposition of a decision by a third-party, neutral decision-maker with no specialized knowledge of the subject matter of the dispute; (3) the use of a formal process as determined by rigid rules not designed by the parties; (4) the existence of an adversarial system in which each party presents proofs and arguments (in a majority of cases via attorneys) and each party attempts to discount or discredit the other party's proofs and arguments; and (5) the dispute process occurs and the conflict is resolved in a mandated public forum. Of critical importance, the decision is generally rendered for one party or the other (i.e., the resolution is mutually exclusive), meaning one party wins and one party loses.

Formal adjudication is most appropriate in circumstances in which resolution of novel legal issues, party vindication, declaration of activities that are illegal, and establishment of formal legal precedent are of paramount importance. For example, cases that involve the civil rights of parties; present difficult and untested issues in complex areas of law, such as antitrust assessments of new and unique business associations; or require a public policy stance, such as the legality of proposed regulations or orders, are generally appropriate for the court system to resolve.

MEDIATION

Mediation is a process by which a neutral third party assists disputing parties in negotiating a resolution. The mediator merely assists the parties; he or she has no formal power to impose any outcome on them. Usually the mediator does not evaluate the legal rights of either party and merely acts as a facilitator for communication between the parties. The parties generally select the mediator. The process usually is informal, with no set rules except those imposed by the parties or the mediator in an effort to further productive communications (e.g., no interruptions when one party is speaking).

Mediation is a voluntary process entered into by the parties in an effort to resolve their dispute. Generally, enforceability of these mediated resolutions is a function of private contract law; any agreement to mediate, as well as an agreement to abide by the mediated decision, is enforceable according to the terms of the contract.

The major advantages of mediation include the private nature of the process and the confidentiality of its results; the process focuses on improving communication between the parties so that interests, goals, and needs of each are identified and communicated to the other. This dynamic leads to the identification of common interests and hence to a mutually acceptable resolution of the conflict for the parties. Because the parties control the process without the constraint of rigid legal rules, creative and flexible solutions that can address each party's specific concerns regarding their dispute may be proposed and implemented. This process also gives the parties an opportunity to express emotion (in or outside the presence of the other party), shifts the focus of the conflict from past to future, allows the disclosure of interests important to the individual parties that each is reluctant to disclose to the other, and permits the parties to provide new information that may be helpful in resolving the dispute.

However, the dynamics of mediation may allow one party to take advantage of the other. Generally, mediation looks to identify joint interests and benefits between the parties. Thus the mediator's focus is to identify those benefits of the parties that overlap. This identification process often becomes the paramount goal of the mediator; once joint goals are identified, it is assumed that the parties will settle. Yet, even in circumstances in which joint benefits are identified, sometimes the dispute still cannot be resolved or is finally resolved using formal adjudication. These situations can be explained in part by the fact that one party may have some interests in common with the other but that unique interests of the party are valued more, such that no resolution to the dispute is preferable for that party. The party can thus game the system by appearing cooperative and by identifying joint benefits shared with the other party while surreptitiously blocking the resolution process. If the mediator does not recognize that unique party goals and interests may outweigh the joint benefits identified, the process may be frustrating and the time and resources of the party and mediator may be wasted.

ARBITRATION

Arbitration is a formalized system of dispute resolution in which parties provide proofs and arguments to a neutral third party who has the power to impose a binding decision on the parties. A common variation incorporates the use of multiple arbitrators (e.g., one is selected by each party and the chosen arbitrators chose a third). Arbitration is similar to formal adjudication except that the parties are allowed only limited pretrial discovery if any, the hearing is less formal, and the rules of evidence are not as rigidly applied in an arbitration proceeding.

Arbitration has been mandated by law for certain conflicts, such as labor disputes, and is used voluntarily by parties to resolve private disputes. When private parties agree to use arbitration, they must address a certain number of issues to ensure that the process will be useful. For example, the parties must decide on a method for selection of the arbitrator or arbitrators; stipulate who will pay for these services; set an objective standard by which the arbitrator or arbitrators will assess the conflict and claims of the parties (e.g., the law, trade or industry customs, or some combination); and specify the procedural rules that the arbitrator or arbitrators will follow. Unless otherwise indicated in the terms for arbitration, arbitration does not allow for pretrial discovery. Arbitration is most frequently used as a final, binding procedure.

There are several major advantages that may result from using arbitration. For example, arbitration allows the parties to draw upon arbitrators with specialized expertise relating directly to the conflict, the arbitrated decision is final, the dispute proceedings and the decision itself are private, the procedural rules are determined by the parties, and the cost for resolving the dispute is relatively low (in terms of time and money) as compared with formal adjudication. Of course, whether these advantages are realized depends on the specific conflict, the parties, and the arbitrator or arbitrators involved.

There is a strong public policy in favor of arbitration, and state and federal law makes agreements to arbitrate specifically enforceable.[1] Courts have agreed with the broad enforceability of arbitration[2] and have specifically held that the Federal Arbitration Act preempts state law to the extent that state law conflicts with the goals or policies of the federal statute.[3]

Unlike formal adjudication, once an arbitration decision has been made, there is no default mechanism through which the decision is enforced. However, the arbitration decision may be judicially confirmed by bringing the decision to a court; failure to abide by the arbitration decision at that point constitutes contempt of court. Both the Federal Arbitration Act and the Uniform Arbitration Act give courts jurisdiction to confirm (or refuse to confirm) an arbitration decision. The

Federal Arbitration Act indicates that generally the court must confirm an arbitration award except under the following circumstances[4]:

- Where the award was procured by corruption, fraud, or undue means
- Where there was evident partiality or corruption among the arbitrators
- Where the arbitrators were guilty of misconduct in refusing to postpone the hearing (on sufficient cause shown) or in refusing to hear evidence pertinent and material to the controversy or of any other misbehavior by which the rights of any party have been prejudiced
- Where the arbitrators exceeded their powers or so imperfectly executed them that a mutual, final, and definite award upon the subject matter was not made

Arbitration also may be part of an official state-sanctioned process. In these situations the government mandates that the parties go through arbitration before formal adjudication. Generally this "court-annexed arbitration" is provided for by state law and requires that a certain class of cases (e.g., automobile torts) or a certain monetary amount be at issue.[5] This requirement to use arbitration before accessing the formal adjudication system also applies to other ADR methods.[6] Some states exclude certain types of claims from arbitration, such as those involving personal injury, tort, and/or insurance contracts.[7]

HYBRID METHODS
Med-arb

"Med-arb" is a combination of mediation and arbitration. In this ADR process the parties agree to mediate their dispute first, using a neutral third party as a mediator. If mediation does not result in an agreement or settlement, then the mediator changes roles and becomes an arbitrator with the power to issue a final and binding decision with regard to the dispute. The primary advantage of using this hybrid method is its potential efficiency: The same neutral third party is used in both mediation and arbitration so that there is no need to educate him or her regarding the facts of the dispute and interests of the parties. However, a significant disadvantage of med-arb is that the parties may not substantively participate in the mediation stage because sensitive disclosures may be used against them if and when the neutral evaluator assumes the role of an arbitrator. Thus the third neutral party (as mediator) may have less information with which to work when attempting to help the parties craft a creative solution to their conflict. Indeed the dispute resolution dynamic may be so significantly altered by the specter of arbitration that the parties may spend their time trying to convince the mediator that they are "right" in anticipation of an arbitration decision.

An alternative to this standard med-arb is med-arb that results in only an advisory arbitration decision. This process attempts to mitigate the identified problems with med-arb involving binding arbitration. Because the mediator has no binding power to arbitrate a final decision, the parties have an increased incentive to substantively use mediation to resolve

their dispute. It also serves to allow the mediator as an advisory arbitrator to merely indicate what he or she believes the ultimate result would be at arbitration. However, the clear disadvantage of this process is its potential length; an extra step of binding arbitration may be required. Yet, approximately 85% of labor disputes in which this ADR method is used are settled.[8]

Mini-trial

The mini-trial is an evaluative process most often used for business and commercial disputes. Attorneys representing each party make summary presentations to a panel composed of a neutral advisor and high level executives from each party who have the power to accept a settlement. After the presentations, the executives try to settle the dispute through negotiation. If negotiation fails to result in a settlement, the neutral advisor provides an assessment as to what he or she considers to be the probable outcome of the dispute. Major beneficial characteristics of a mini-trial are that the process is voluntary and confidential; the parties agree to follow certain protocols or procedures; before the mini-trial, the parties agree to informally exchange important documents, provide summaries of witness testimony, and provide short statements regarding the dispute (and often provide that this information is confidential and inadmissible in any future proceeding); and a neutral third party who has expertise in the subject matter (e.g., a former judge) is chosen by consent of the parties (this neutral party may take a passive role in the process or be more active, such as taking on the role of a mediator). In some mini-trials, no third-party neutral advisor is included. At the presentation itself, the attorneys for each side attempt to provide a brief, cogent summary of their best case, usually within a specified time limit. Rigid rules of formal adjudication do not apply; questions, answers, and rebuttals may all be part of the process.

The basic dynamic involved in the mini-trial is that both parties' executive representatives are provided with the appropriate information to assess the merits of each party's position regarding the dispute. With this information, the parties may create a solution that makes business sense from their own perspectives while taking into account unique company needs and circumstances.

Summary jury trial

The summary jury trial is an evaluative process similar to a mini-trial, but it differs in several important ways. These differences stem from the goal of the process—determining what a jury might decide in the case. Hence, instead of a third-party neutral and corporate executives, a judge and an advisory jury drawn from the jury pool are used. Jurors are not told that their role is advisory until after they give their verdict. Attorneys for each side make summary presentations as in the mini-trial; however, the presentations usually are based on information that has been the subject of discovery and would be admissible at trial. Once the advisory jury has announced its decision, jury members answer questions regarding the verdict and their assessment and reaction to particular evidence and arguments. The attorneys and their respective executive representatives then attend a mandatory conference to discuss settlement. If no settlement occurs, the advisory jury verdict is not admissible in future final adjudication procedures.

A summary jury trial requires significant time and resources because it is similar to formal adjudication. This method is thus most useful when the dispute is unique or novel, when circumstances preclude an easy prediction of what a jury would decide, and when such unpredictability is what is preventing settlement.

However, there may be ethical concerns regarding summary jury trials. Summary jury trials use actual jurors taken from the jury pool to obtain only advisory jury verdicts. These jurors are not told that they are merely participating in a mock trial. Significant ethical issues arise because the process deceives individuals as to what they believe is their role—civic duty in a formal adjudication. Furthermore, this deception occurs while the disputing parties and the judge retain this knowledge for their own personal benefit (e.g., assessment of the potential for high jury award verdicts, reduction of court dockets).

OTHER FORMS OF ALTERNATIVE DISPUTE RESOLUTION
Early neutral evaluation

Early neutral evaluation is usually a court-annexed process that requires the parties to have their dispute assessed by an experienced third-party neutral evaluator on the basis of short presentations by both parties. It is thus a rights-based procedure like arbitration and formal adjudication. Usually the third-party neutral is a volunteer attorney chosen by the court. Once the presentations are made, the parties negotiate in an effort to settle the dispute. If the parties do not settle, the neutral evaluator assists them in simplifying and clarifying the case so that it will be more amenable to formal adjudication.

Private judging

With the advent and growth of ADR, a significant private market has emerged to render adjudicative services and decisions. Private judging (also known as *rent-a-judge*) is a reflection of this growth. Many of these participants are retired judges who provide informal adjudication or engage in other ADR processes. These private judges are paid by the parties involved and may be empowered by state statute to enter final judgments that have precedential value and are appealable to appellate courts, as are rulings made in formal adjudication.[9] California, Florida, and Texas have statutory provisions that require referral of certain court cases to private ADR providers paid for by the parties.[10]

"Rights-based" mediation

Generally, traditional mediation (also known as *interest-based mediation*) focuses on creating a mutually acceptable solution to resolve disputes and does not involve an evaluation of the legal strengths and weaknesses of each party's case. However, in rights-based mediation there is a focus on the legal rights of the parties, and thus the process is more akin to evaluative processes, such as early neutral evaluation. Often the line between rights-based mediation and interest-based mediation may be blurred because the third-party neutral mediator may, in an effort to assist the parties in creating a solution, assess the legal rights of the parties.

Screening panels

Screening panels usually are involved in state-mandated pretrial assessments of medical malpractice cases. Plaintiffs, before submitting their medical malpractice claims for trial, are required to have their case assessed by a special panel; this panel usually is composed of physicians or other medical professionals, attorneys, and laypersons. The panel hears the plaintiff's case and may issue a nonbinding opinion. Usually, either party can bring the case to court, regardless of the panel's assessment. Some states allow the panel's findings to be introduced as evidence in the court adjudication. Difficulties center around the administrative burdens these panels represent and the associated delays; furthermore, assessments may be made too early in the process, before discovery has been accomplished.

Settlement conference

In another form of ADR known as the *settlement conference* or *voluntary settlement conference,* a judge, a set of attorneys, or a "settlement master" (i.e., an independent party who assesses such conflicts) reads briefs and materials and hears presentations from both sides of a dispute, and then actively seeks to craft a settlement for the parties. As opposed to mediation, where the intermediary is merely a facilitator, in a settlement conference the intermediary is an active participant in the process. Often, after reading the submitted documents and hearing each side, the intermediary may caucus with each party independently and move between the parties in an effort to fashion a settlement. Courts use settlement conferences before formal adjudication to encourage parties to settle cases before they go to trial. Indeed, some courts will not set a case for trial unless a settlement conference has been held. The parties' major complaint regarding this form of ADR is that it is coercive. At times, parties feel pressured to settle and are later dissatisfied with the settlement.

ALTERNATIVE DISPUTE RESOLUTION AND MEDICAL MALPRACTICE CLAIMS

Although a wide variety of medical disputes are amenable to ADR methods, one type of conflict that has drawn significant attention to the use of ADR (specifically, arbitration) is the medical malpractice dispute. Those in favor of using ADR methods to resolve malpractice claims cite the associated reduction in cost, the involvement of a more informed decision-maker, the reduction in emotional trauma that results from formal adjudication, the ability for plaintiffs with "minor" injuries to have their claims heard, and the reduction in frivolous malpractice cases. State law often dictates how these contractual agreements must appear and the conditions under which they are valid,[11] subject to federal law.[12]

The difficulty with applying ADR to medical malpractice disputes is primarily twofold. First, any voluntary process requires participation by all parties and their attorneys. However, the parties may believe that a trial by jury will increase their chance at success. Defendants may be reluctant to participate because they will be reported to the National Practitioner Data Bank if any amount is paid to end the dispute. Second, malpractice cases involve complex issues of fact, and full and adequate assessment will most likely require extensive time and effort. Summary processes therefore do not easily lend themselves to malpractice disputes. Mandatory, binding arbitration could address the voluntary party and attorney participation problem, as well as provide for appropriate technical expertise; however, it too is limited by the summary nature of the assessment.

Although arbitration has its limitations, many institutional health care providers and managed care organizations (MCOs) now use mandatory arbitration in their contractual agreements with patients to resolve any patient care disputes. Broad-scale use of binding arbitration was pioneered by Kaiser-Permanente in California and has spread rapidly throughout the United States as managed care has become the predominant mode of medical care delivery. Patients' challenges to mandatory arbitration clauses generally have been rejected by the courts.[13] Significantly the Federal Arbitration Act,[14] as well as state laws in at least 40 states, provides a basis for enforcing these provisions.[15] However, because of the potential advantages for "repeat players," such as MCOs, these entities must meet specific legal requirements regarding their use of arbitrators and their participation in arbitration. California legislators have been particularly active in this area. California courts have held that arbitrators must exercise good faith in all adjudication procedures, including disclosure of previous relationships with a party in the dispute,[16] and that MCOs may not unduly delay arbitration proceedings.[17]

Because of the controversy surrounding the use of binding arbitration in malpractice disputes, the largest arbitration association in the United States, the American Arbitration Association (AAA), participates in the arbitration of medical malpractice disputes under mandatory binding arbitration clauses in managed care contracts only in limited circumstances. AAA participates in these arbitration proceedings only if the patient asks for arbitration or if the patient agrees to such a method for dispute resolution after the dispute arises.[18] With regard to the use of ADR in medical malpractice disputes, AAA, in conjunction with the American Medical Association and the American Bar Association, has drafted policy guidelines. These guidelines specify the following[19]:

- ADR can and should be used to resolve disputes over health care coverage and access arising out of the relationship between patients and private health plans and MCOs.
- ADR can and should be used to resolve disputes over health care coverage and access arising out of the relationship between health care providers and private health plans and MCOs.
- In disputes involving patients, binding forms of dispute resolution should be used only when the parties agreed to do so after the dispute arose.
- Due process protections should be afforded to all participants in the ADR process.
- Review of managed health care decisions through ADR complements the concept of internal review of determinations made by private MCOs.

It is not yet clear how or whether these policy guidelines will substantively affect the use of arbitration in malpractice disputes because of the significant number of non-AAA arbitrators available and the standard nature of these clauses in patient care contracts.

ALTERNATIVE DISPUTE RESOLUTION AND OTHER MEDICAL DISPUTES

Aside from the controversial use of ADR in medical malpractice conflicts, a large number of potential disputes in the health care arena are amenable to ADR processes. Because health care has become increasingly commercialized, ADR processes can address commercial disputes between facilities and those between facilities and medical providers in the same way that other commercial disputes are addressed. However, the provider's reputation, the health of a party, and the emotional concerns intimately related to illness, disease, and treatment make disputes in the health care arena unique. Factors such as the interface between the needs and capacities of the parties, whether their relationship is ongoing, third party involvement, and the parties' legal rights all play important roles in determining the particular ADR method or combination of methods that is appropriate for a particular health care dispute. Some circumstances, such as end-of-life situations, simply are not well suited to ADR or formal adjudication. However, by assessing each party's needs and goals in the context of the specific social and medical circumstances, as well as their underlying incentives, an appropriate dispute resolution strategy can usually be ascertained.

Examples of voluntary applications to several modern medical disputes outside the malpractice context follow.[19] These examples illustrate the process of choosing a particular ADR method but are not definitive statements on health law or policy.

Example 1: an interfacility dispute

Background. In the current health care climate, cost control has been a predominant consideration in the allocation of medical resources. As a result, federal, state, and local governments have used various strategies to minimize health care costs. One strategy has been to limit potential demand for expensive diagnostic technology by limiting the availability of such technology through requiring state-level approval before this type of asset can be purchased. However, if a health care facility can demonstrate to the state authority that there is sufficient patient need, there is no overlap between this form of capital investment and services derived therefrom, and there is available money to purchase and support the equipment, the facility may be granted a so-called certificate of need (CON), which is a permit that allows the facility to acquire such equipment. Such a grant is valuable because of the highly exclusive nature of the grant and the concomitant income arising therefrom.

Case scenario. In a local city, St. Francis Hospital has merged with Johnson City Hospital. Each hospital has been under pressure to expand services and improve reimbursements obtained from their patients' insurance. Both are located in the same urban area but in different neighborhoods. St. Francis is a nonprofit, private facility that caters primarily to middle class patients in its neighborhood. Johnson City Hospital is a nonprofit, private, inner-city facility established during the forgone days of prosperity in its community. Its current clientele consists of poor, disenfranchised patients who primarily are Medicaid program participants or are uninsured. Johnson City Hospital is a teaching hospital for the prestigious Physicians and Surgeons Medical School (P & S), which is located in the city. It is thus staffed with outstanding resident physicians (house staff) who supplement the hospital's retained attending physicians.

St. Francis and Johnson City merged just over 1 year ago. Subsequent to the merger, the hospital applied for and obtained a CON for a new magnetic resonance imaging (MRI) machine that would significantly enhance physicians' ability to diagnose disorders in emergency and other clinical situations. The hospital was granted the CON on the basis of Johnson City's locale (health care resources there are limited) and St. Francis' fiscal soundness, which would allow purchase and maintenance of the machinery.

The current dispute is over where to locate the MRI machine. Johnson City contends that the machine should be located at its facility because CON approval was based on its patients' medical needs. St. Francis' position is that the machine could not have been purchased without its funds, and thus the machine should be located at St. Francis. The state authority has expressed no opinion on the matter. There is vague talk of legal action by the parties. How can this dispute be settled?

From an ADR standpoint, before the methodology can be chosen, the goals of the parties must be ascertained. From Johnson City's point of view, the MRI machine should be located on its site primarily for financial reasons. Reimbursement for MRI procedures is relatively high compared with operational costs, and Johnson City has lost significant revenues by not having such services available. In addition, if Johnson City had the MRI machine, P & S would likely send more of its house staff to Johnson City. This action would reduce certain staff costs because P & S pays the salary of the house staff, and an increase in the number of house staff would reduce the need to employ other health care providers. Finally, Johnson City's patient population would be better served by having advanced diagnostic equipment, such as an MRI machine, available on site. When Johnson City physicians refer patients elsewhere for an MRI procedure, the patients often do not follow through with the referral to obtain the scan.

St. Francis has similar goals. It also wants to take advantage of the high reimbursement rate for MRI services. However, it also wishes to use the MRI machine as a marketing tool. The marketing department envisions hosting an event and running advertisements using the phrase "St. Francis and the Twenty-First Century: Bringing Advanced Health Care to the Community."

Alternative dispute resolution assessment. The continuing relationship between St. Francis and Johnson City mitigates against the desirability of formal adjudication. The nature of the dispute (not involving novel legal issues or the desire to establish precedent) also makes formal adjudication inappropriate.

Arbitration is a possibility. Advantages include involvement of an arbiter who has expertise in the area, thus ensuring that technical arguments can be made, and who can issue a final decision. Additional advantages include confidentiality, relatively low cost, and rapid resolution, as compared with formal adjudication. Most likely, both parties would find all of these characteristics agreeable. However, arbiters' decisions usually are based on objective standards because arbitration is a rights-based procedure. In this case there is no clear-cut, single objective standard: the CON application apparently does not decide the issue; the state authority has expressed no opinion; the law does not seem to apply; and a rights-based process may sully the future relationship between the parties. Furthermore, the possibility of either party withdrawing its support (Johnson City's patient base and St. Francis' money) would likely preclude acquisition of the MRI machine. Finally, arbitration does not fare well as compared with other ADR methods in terms of relative cost, speed, and ability to improve the parties' relationship by focusing on their joint interests. Thus there appear to be some significant disadvantages in using arbitration to settle this dispute.

Mediation provides potential for clarifying communication and allowing for a creative resolution of the dispute without the necessity of revisiting the divergent motivation for the CON application. The mediator also can take into account the possible internal pressures from the marketing department at

St. Francis. Because the mediation process can focus on the future of the relationship and the joint interests of the parties, it can provide a foundation for building consensus between the hospitals. As well, because these parties are relatively new partners, a creative solution could spur additional, innovative joint ventures while simultaneously providing for and integrating into the process a communications pattern that takes into account the important allocative decisions that affect an organizational entity with separate and distinct sites. Furthermore, an evaluative course of action, providing both parties with the opportunity for reflection and feedback, could be integrated into the process for each joint project so that important lessons are learned from each effort. These lessons of course could and should be applied to future projects. Thus mediation has many advantages in this situation.

Within this purview, it appears that evaluative hybrid methods would be inappropriate. For example, a summary jury trial, which is best for disputes involving a disparate view of the facts and the law by opposing parties, would be inappropriate because the parties do not disagree on the governing law. In addition, early neutral evaluation has similar limitations.

Thus in this interfacility dispute a mediation process might be proposed by appropriate representatives from the two hospitals. The mediation process fits best with the underlying sources of the dispute and addresses these issues from the perspective of an ongoing relationship with much promise for the future. It allows for the application of creative, mutually beneficial solutions. Because both parties have a strong incentive to come to the bargaining (or mediation) table (the valuable property interest that they jointly own, or the CON), the likelihood for a successfully mediated settlement is enhanced. Mediation also could provide for retrospective analysis of the conflict, which can teach important lessons to be applied in the future.

Although it meets some of the needs to clarify past miscommunications, arbitration does not look to the parties' future relationship. Moreover, it requires some relatively objective standard for dispute resolution that is not available. Finally, law-based processes (evaluative hybrids), as well as formal adjudication, seem inapplicable in this type of case because of the ambiguity of applicable legal rules.

Example 2: an intrafacility conflict—exclusive contracts and provider termination

Background. To procure necessary health care services, it is extremely common for health care facilities to contract for these services either with a single physician or with physician groups as independent contractors. This contractual arrangement thus allows the health care facility to offer 24-hour physician services in the particular specialty and avoids the necessity and the expense of providing health, retirement, and other benefits to these individuals.

In this regard, hospitals use an exclusive contract for hospital-based physician services. Hospitals typically contract with physicians for a specified time with the stipulation that, if given the amount of notice specified in the agreement, either the hospital or independent contractor physician may terminate the contract without cause.

Thus these contracts are double-edged swords. On the one hand, within the period for which the exclusive contract is applicable, the physician or physician group has the right and the power to charge for all physician services in the specialty, to the exclusion of other, nonexclusive contract physicians. On the other hand, the hospital has the power to terminate the relationship for any or no reason at all after giving the requisite notice as indicated in the contract.

Case scenario. Drake Hospital is a relatively large (450-bed) community hospital located in an affluent suburb. It serves primarily middle to upper class patients in the area and offers all of the major medical specialty services. Virtually none of the patients who come to Drake receive Medicaid benefits. Those who receive care from the hospital uniformly report satisfaction with its services. Patients generally find the new physical building, available parking, and courteous staff quite pleasing. The cafeteria is modern, and its food is delicious. Private physicians enjoy the facility's amiable atmosphere, delicious food, and private patient population.

Dr. Smith is a board-certified radiologist at Drake. After graduating from P & S and doing his residency training there, Dr. Smith entered private practice at Drake. Dr. Smith has worked at the hospital for the past 21 years under an exclusive contractual arrangement. Under the terms of the contract, Drake pays Dr. Smith a small salary; this salary is supplemented by charges to the hospital and referred patients' third-party insurers for rendered radiology services (as is normal practice). Dr. Smith also sees several of his own patients who come to Drake for specific radiologic procedures. For example, he performs and interprets chest x-ray films for a patient who was diagnosed several years ago with Hodgkin's disease and underwent curative radiation therapy but requires annual radiologic films to check for any recurrence. There have never been any allegations regarding the quality of care provided by Dr. Smith. Two years ago, Dr. Smith was awarded Drake Hospital's community service award for distinguished and long-term service to the hospital and its patients.

One month ago, Dr. Smith was in the radiology department reading room interpreting some MRI scans when a hospital administrator entered the room. The administrator asked to speak with Dr. Smith in private. When both were in Dr. Smith's office, the administrator told Dr. Smith: "As you know, in about 3 months your contract is up for renewal. We on the board have been happy with the work you've done, but we are not going to renew your contract. We just think it's time for some new blood."

After the administrator left, Dr. Smith sat alone and thought: "Why is this happening? This place is more than a workplace for me; this can't be happening. What can an older physician do for money? This shouldn't be happening; they don't have the right to sully my reputation. Should I contact an attorney? I'm going to challenge this somehow." Dr. Smith then finished up the MRI readings for the day and left for home.

Alternative dispute resolution assessment. The goals of the parties in this situation are not entirely clear. The hospital board wants to terminate Dr. Smith, and it appears that this action is well within its contractual and legal rights. A question is raised regarding why the board wants to terminate Dr. Smith, particularly in light of his service to the facility and the fact that they are happy with his work.

From Dr. Smith's perspective, termination results in the prospect of unemployment. Furthermore, concerns regarding reputation are evident. It is clear that Dr. Smith would like to stay at Drake if possible. He apparently has significant emotional ties to the hospital. However, it is also clear that Dr. Smith is contemplating legal action.

Because the goals of the hospital administration are unclear or unexpressed, there may be a lack of good communication between the parties. Perhaps the administrator was uncomfortable explaining to Dr. Smith that the board felt he was getting too old to maintain the rigors of a full-time practice. Or, although happy with Dr. Smith's services, the hospital board may have been offered a lower-cost contract by another radiologist or radiology group. Thus a method of dispute resolution that addresses this communication problem would be best.

From this assessment, mediation most likely would be an appropriate choice. The nature of the dispute seems to require the exchange of more information or the disclosure of new information. The parties must learn more about their respective interests. Given the apparent difficulty in communication, mediation may provide a sensitive and reasonable forum in which the dispute can be resolved.

Dr. Smith, however, appears to have conflicting goals that affect the choice of forum. On the one hand, Dr. Smith wishes to keep his radiology position at the hospital. Thus a continuing relationship is desired. However, it also appears that Dr. Smith has strong feelings that termination would be inappropriate. Furthermore, there is a concern that his reputation will suffer.

In contract disputes involving physicians, this potential effect on reputation is an important concern. There are few other professions to which this concept applies so broadly and to such a great degree. For Dr. Smith, reputation relates to patients, as well as to other physicians. If other physicians attempt to refer patients to Dr. Smith and he is required to inform them that he no longer has privileges at Drake, then there may be some implication of questionable competence or poor quality of care. Furthermore, if Dr. Smith attempts to find other work, the same reputational problems may arise. Although Dr. Smith sees some private patients at the hospital, the majority of his income is derived from hospital practice and referrals from other physicians. Accordingly, reputation becomes a significant concern to Dr. Smith as he considers actions involving (and possibly against) the hospital.

Thus, on one hand, a clearer understanding of the issues (the "why is this happening" factor), the desire to continue as the radiologist at the hospital, and the emotional ties might point toward a mediation approach. On the other hand, Dr. Smith's desire to maintain his reputation in the community (and with respect to other potential employers) would favor some other form of dispute resolution.

In this case a combination of mediation and arbitration might be optimal. Perhaps a mediation-advisory arbitration rather than a mediation-binding arbitration would be best because the latter form has some significant disadvantages as applied to this situation. First, there is a high probability that the hospital board members would not want to be completely candid when discussing their decision not to renew Dr. Smith's contract if they knew that there could be a binding decision later. Thus the mediator would have relatively little information with which to work when attempting to help the parties craft a jointly creative and beneficial solution. Furthermore, because subsequent arbitration may focus on whether one party is "right" (hence changing the dynamic so as to divert the dispute resolution process away from interest-based solutions to the conflict), the parties may be less likely to try to resolve the problem at the mediation stage. Indeed, the parties may make a significant effort to convince the mediator that one or the other is deserving of a favorable decision.

The hospital most likely would not wish to enter into a binding process and risk losing when it has a favorable legal position. Nevertheless, the hospital may wish to enter into an ADR procedure to avoid the legal costs of formal adjudication and eschew negative publicity. Moreover, certain "emotional" considerations may induce Drake administrators to treat Dr. Smith in a fair manner.

Mediation-advisory arbitration could address the disadvantages of mediation-binding arbitration. First, advisory arbitration is just that, only advisory. Advisory arbitration would preserve the creative solution emphasis and restore the mediation dynamic to the process rather than focus on a determination of who is "right." Perhaps the mediator could open the lines of communication between the parties, allowing the parties to participate actively in the dispute resolution process. If mediation fails, an advisory position (an evaluative process) could give Dr. Smith and Drake an objective assessment regarding the conflict and the outcome should the matter proceed to formal adjudication.

This process also could serve Dr. Smith's need to address his reputational concern; the settlement or possibly an acceptable advisory opinion could expressly state that the hospital's actions regarding Dr. Smith were not based on any quality of care concerns, or similar language to that effect. This statement would allow Dr. Smith to seek employment with other providers and show that a neutral third party had found (and the hospital had stated) that no quality of care issues triggered his change in status at the hospital.

However, a possible disadvantage of mediation-advisory arbitration is the potential length of the process. With both mediation and advisory arbitration, time may be spent on adjudicatory arbitration or formal court activity in addition to the extra step of advisory arbitration. However, empirical data suggest that there is a significant probability that the dispute could be resolved without resorting to formal adjudication.

Thus, in this physician termination scenario, mediation-advisory arbitration appears to be appropriate. Pure evaluative procedures, such as summary jury trial and early neutral evaluation, could be helpful if there were a different view of the legal rights of the parties. In this case the hospital has the authority to terminate Dr. Smith's contract. Arbitration, although possibly favorable to the hospital, would not serve Dr. Smith's interest-based concerns and, as a single method, would be inappropriate.

Example 3: provider and family end-of-life treatment conflicts

Background. The Patient Self-Determination Act of 1990 mandates that patients who are admitted to a hospital be given information regarding end-of-life directives and proxy decision-making in the event that the patient cannot personally make these decisions. In this capacity the patient can make preauthorized treatment choices regarding the types of medical care to be provided in the event that he or she has a terminal condition and becomes incompetent. For example, a patient can elect do not resuscitate (DNR) status for all incurable disorders. Furthermore, a patient can elect to transfer this decision-making capacity to another person (e.g., a family member or personal physician) in the event that the patient lacks the ability to make these decisions.

Case scenario. Mrs. Jones is an 89-year-old woman with many of the conditions associated with age. She has poorly controlled hypertension, non-insulin-dependent diabetes mellitus, renal disease, and a history of two heart attacks. She has been admitted to the hospital many times, most recently (4 months before the current admission) when she was diagnosed with pneumonia and spent 1 month in the intensive care unit. She recovered from the event but was weakened considerably by it.

After being discharged from the hospital, Mrs. Jones was cared for in her son's home. Her son and his family refused to send her to a nursing home. They believed that sending her to a nursing home "would be like saying we didn't want her." Mrs. Jones has enjoyed living with her son's family and has a good relationship with them, particularly her grandchildren. She believes that her current role in life is to "spoil my wonderful grandchildren as much as possible."

During past hospitalizations, Mrs. Jones has told her family and her personal family physician, Dr. Franklin, that she does not want "heroic efforts" to be made to save her life in the event that she loses her cogency. She signed an admission statement to that effect in accordance with the Patient Self-Determination Act when she was hospitalized 4 months ago. She also designated her son to serve as proxy if she could not make end-of-life decisions. Moreover, she refused to be placed on a ventilator in the intensive care unit, stating: "If I can't live without that thing, I don't want to live. Just give me antibiotics, and if that isn't enough, so be it." The hospital staff complied with her wishes, and Mrs. Jones subsequently recovered. She also stated, "If I don't know my family, I don't want to live. I mean, what would be the point?" The refusal of ventilator support was recorded on the medical chart; the latter statement was not.

Approximately 2 weeks ago, Mrs. Jones was hospitalized again. Her family brought her to the emergency room at the hospital where she had been admitted for pneumonia treatment 4 months earlier. Her current medical illness stems directly from her renal disease, and she was confused on admission, a normal medical finding in such clinical circumstances. She was admitted directly to the intensive care unit, where treatment that focused on addressing her renal condition was begun. Initially the treatment appeared to be working. Mrs. Jones became mentally clearer and recognized her family. She joked with her grandchildren and introduced the house staff to her family. However, within 1 week of admission, her condition worsened significantly, to the point where she no longer recognized her family and was somnolent and unreactive.

Dr. Franklin, who was seeing Mrs. Jones on a daily basis, noted that over the past 2 days she had suffered total renal failure, and despite 100% oxygen therapy, her blood oxygen levels dropped substantially so that her brain was provided with inadequate oxygenation. A scan obtained to determine her brain function indicated that Mrs. Jones no longer had any brain activity. Dr. Franklin checked Mrs. Jones' medical chart and found that she did not sign a new DNR or proxy agreement upon admission and the previous agreements had expired. Dr. Franklin thus went to Mrs. Jones' son to discuss the DNR status and withdrawal of life-support measures. Mrs. Jones' son, distraught over her condition, angrily stated that all efforts should be pursued, no DNR status was to be given, and he would "sue you for everything you've got and this hospital too if you let her die." Dr. Franklin believed Mrs. Jones' status should be DNR and that efforts to discontinue life-support measures should be undertaken in accordance with her wishes.

Alternative dispute resolution assessment. This conflict is difficult to address. Aside from the ethical dilemmas, the dispute is rife with emotional issues associated with the death of a family member. The goal of Mrs. Jones' son it appears is currently short term. He wants her to live, or more accurately he wants her to live with her previous quality of life. Because of the nature of the conflict—the tragedy of the end of a loved one's life—he is beginning to experience the traditional psychological stages (denial and anger) that those affected by loss go through. He is currently denying her condition and is angry about it; his emotionalism is blotting out his mother's own ideal as to what is appropriate treatment in this clinical situation. Thus his goals (and his lack of flexibility) are not likely to change until he reaches and passes through the other psychological stages of loss leading to acceptance.

Dr. Franklin's goals are more focused on Mrs. Jones' desires. Because Mrs. Jones made clear to her family and to Dr. Franklin that she would not want life-support treatment in the event of loss of cogency, Dr. Franklin raised this issue with the family. Moreover, Dr. Franklin believes that, in the unlikely event that Mrs. Jones survives her present illness, she will not leave the intensive care unit with any cogency or personality because of her lack of brain function and significant medical problems. Thus Dr. Franklin is attempting to follow the oral directions provided by Mrs. Jones regarding her choice of care in such a circumstance.

An ADR procedure that addresses these parties' needs is not immediately apparent. Although the emotional barriers that exist could perhaps be handled through mediation, efforts to gain the parties' trust, particularly that of Mrs. Jones' son, are likely to fail at this stage. Any attempt to consider cessation of treatment would alienate Mrs. Jones' son from the process. Aside from Mrs. Jones' son, the hospital also might be unwilling to participate because of a perceived liability risk if they allow termination of life support.

An arbitration process suffers from the same weaknesses. Certainly, voluntary arbitration would be unacceptable to Mrs. Jones' son in his current state. Furthermore, a mediation-arbitration procedure would be unacceptable because of the weaknesses of mediation already noted. An evaluative procedure, such as a mini-trial or summary jury trial, has potential advantages resulting from the use of and evaluation by a neutral third party. The process would include an analysis of the law in the area and a clarification and objective assessment of the relevant facts (including Mrs. Jones' previous communications to her son and Dr. Franklin). But again, this process also is likely to be futile because Mrs. Jones' son (in his emotional state) would not agree to the process. Moreover, if he did engage in the process, he would reject any decision or proposal that involved the cessation of medical treatment for his mother. In addition, the process would take some time because a number of evidentiary and other requirements, as well as the pragmatic concern of obtaining an appropriate adjudicator or jury, would have to be addressed.

Another possibility is to use an ombudsperson, perhaps with psychological training, to allow Mrs. Jones' son to vent his frustrations and to help him accept the reality of his mother's situation. However, once again, any consideration of a reduction in Mrs. Jones' care would result in her son rejecting this process. Anecdotal evidence also indicates that this method has a significant probability of failure.

Thus this highly charged, emotional situation involving a single party with a focused and inflexible (perhaps unrealistic) goal presents significant problems for any ADR process.

It appears that in this medical context the only reasonable solution would be for the hospital and Dr. Franklin to access the formal adjudication system. This solution, albeit weak, may be the only one available. To bring an emotionally torn individual to court because of the impending death of a loved one certainly will not help in that individual's progression through the grieving process. Furthermore, the position of the hospital and physician could appear to be draconian and lacking in compassion. It may be necessary to allow Mrs. Jones to stay in the intensive care unit until she dies. Such a solution is costly (in terms of dollars), inequitable (in terms of the patient's own directive), painful (in terms of the family grief), and potentially unfair (for other patients who would benefit more from the concentrated resources provided in an intensive care unit).

CONCLUSION

Disputes regarding medical care delivery are common. Many of these disputes can be addressed and resolved using ADR methods in combination with formal adjudication. An understanding of the various ADR methods, their strengths and weaknesses, their legal status, and the interests and goals of each party can usually but not always bring about an effective resolution to the dispute in the health care context.

ENDNOTES

1. *See, e.g.,* Federal Arbitration Act, 9 U.S.C.A. §§2 *et seq.; see also* Administrative Dispute Resolution Act, 5 U.S.C.A. §5581-5593; Ariz. Rev. Stat. Ann. §§12-1501 to 12-1518 (West 1994); Ark. Code Ann. §§16-108-201 to 16-108-224 (Mich. 1995); Del. Code Ann. tit.10 §§5701-5725 (1996); Fla. Stat. ch. 682.01-682.22 (1990); Idaho Code §§7-901 to 7-922 (1990); Iowa Code Ann. §§679A.1-679A.19 (1987); Kan. Stat. Ann. §§5-401 to 5-422 (1995); Ky. Rev. Stat. Ann. §§4417.145-417.240 (Michie 1996); Minn. Stat. §§572.08-572.30 (1996); Mont. Code Ann. §§27-5-111 to 27-5-324 (1996); Nev. Rev. Stat. §§38.015-38.360 (1995); N.J. Stat. Ann. §§2A:23A-1 To 2A:23A-19 (West 1996); Ohio Rev. Code Ann. §§2711.01 to 2711.16 (West 1992); Pa. Cons. Stat. §§7301-7320 (1982); R.I. Gen. Laws §§10-3-1 to 10-3-21 (1996); S.D. Codified Laws §§21-25A-1 to 21-5A-38 (Michie 1996); Tenn. Code Ann. §§29-5-301 to 29-5-320 (1996); Utah Code Ann. §§78-31a-1 to 78-31a-20 (1996); Vt. Stat. Ann. tit. 12, §§5651-5681 (1996); Wyo. Stat. Ann. §§1-36-101 to 1-36-119 (Michie 1986).

2. *See, e.g., United Steelworkers of Am. v. Warrior & Gulf Navigation Co.,* 363 U.S. 574 (1960); *Shearson/American Express v. McMahon,* 482 U.S. 220 (1987); *Mitsubishi Motors Corp. v. Soler Chrysler-Plymouth,* 473 U.S. 614 (1985); *Rodriguez De Quijas v. Shearson/American Express, Inc.,* 490 U.S. 477 (1989); *Gilmer v. Interstate/Johnson Lane Corp.,* 111 S.Ct. 1647 (1991); *Madden v. Kaiser Found. Hosps.,* 131 Cal.Rptr. 882 (Cal. 1976).

3. *See, e.g., Southland Corp. v. Keating,* 465 U.S. 1 (1984); *Volt Information Sciences, Inc. v. Stanford Univ.,* 489 U.S. 468 (1989).

4. Federal Arbitration Act, 9 U.S.C.A. §§2, 10.

5. *See, e.g.,* Cal. Health & Safety Code § 1373.19 (indicating that single arbitrator may assess claims for health services claim up to $200,000); Hawaii Arb. Rules, Rule 8 (Michie 1995) (monetary claims for amounts less than $150,000 must go to court-annexed arbitration except under certain circumstances).

6. *e.g.,* Cal. Civ. Code §4607 (contested custody cases must go to mediation); Tex. Code Ann., Civ. Prac. & Rem. Code §154.021 (court given discretion to send certain cases to ADR); Fla. Stat. Ann. ch. 44 (same).

7. *See, e.g.,* Ark. Code Ann. §16-108-201(b) (Michie 1997); Kan. Stat. Ann. §5-401(c) (1997); Mont. Code Ann. §27-5-114 (2) (1997); S.C. Code Ann. §15-48-10 (1998); Tex. Civ. Prac. Code Ann. §171.001 (1997).

8. S. B. Goldberg, *Grievance Mediation: A Successful Alternative to Labor Arbitration,* 5 Neg. J. 9-15 (1989).

9. *See Assami v. Assami,* 872 P.2d 1190 (Cal. 1994); Estate of Kent, 57 P.2d 901 (Cal. 1936); *Solorzano v. Sup. Ct.,* 22 Cal.Rptr. 2d 401 (Cal. 1993)

10. *See, e.g.,* Tex. Alcoholic Beverage Code §102.77 (parties must pay for arbitration costs); Fla. Stats. Ann. §44.103; Fla. Alt. Disp. Res. §718.1255 (mandating voluntary mediation and mandatory nonbinding arbitration).

11. *See, e.g.,* Cal. Civ. Pro. §1295 (describing wording, font, and color of enforceable medical malpractice arbitration agreement) subject to federal law.

12. *See, e.g., Perry v. Thomas,* 482 U.S. 483 (1987) (state laws that are unique to arbitration agreements are preempted by federal law governing arbitration).

13. *See, e.g., Coon v. Nicola,* 21 Cal.Rptr.2d 846 (Cal. Ct. App. 1993); *Buraczynski v. Eyring,* 919 S.W.2d 314 (Tenn. 1996); *Broemmer v. Otto,* 821 P.2d 204 (Ariz. 1991); *Wilson v. Kaiser Found. Hosps.,* 190 Cal.Rptr. 649 (Cal. Ct. App. 1983); *Dinong v. Kaiser Found. Hosp.,* 162 Cal.Rptr. 606 (Cal. Ct. App. 1980); *Madden v. Kaiser Found. Hosps.,* 131 Cal.Rptr. 882 (Cal. 1976) (all upholding use of ADR); *but see Colorado Permanente Med. Group v. Evans,* 926 P.2d 1218 (Colo. 1996); *Saika v. Gold,* 56 Cal.Rptr.2d 922 (Cal. Ct. App. 1996); *Beynon v. Garden Grove Med. Group,* 161 Cal.Rptr. 146 (Cal. Ct. App. 1980); *but see Rosenfield v. Sup. Ct.,* 143 Cal. App. 3d 198 (Cal. 1983); *Graham v. Scissor-Tail, Inc.,* 28 Cal. 3d 807 (Cal. 1990); *Cheng-Canindin v. Renaissance Hotel Assocs.,* 50 Cal. App. 4th 676 (Cal. Ct. App. 1996).

14. 9 U.S.C.A. §2

15. P. I. Carter, *Binding Arbitration in Malpractice Disputes: The Right Prescription for HMO Patients?* 18 Hamline Journal of Public Law and Policy 423-451 (1997).

16. *See, e.g., Neaman v. Kaiser Found. Hosp.,* 11 Cal.Rptr. 2d 879 (Cal. Ct. App. 1992) (overturning an arbitration decision on the basis of arbitrator nondisclosure of five cases of 300 where he acted as Kaiser Foundation Hospital's chosen arbitrator); *see also* Cal. Civ. Pro. §1281.9 (1998) (requiring arbitrator disclosure concerning previous experience with parties).

17. *See, e.g., Engalla v. Permanente Med. Group, Inc.,* 64 Cal.Rptr. 2d 843 (Cal. 1997) (remanding case after holding that MCOs may not unduly delay selection of arbitrators in medical malpractice cases).

18. G. H. Friedman, *AAA, ABA and AMA Issue Joint Resolution: Recommendations for Health Care Dispute Resolution* 15 Med. Mal. L. Strategy 1 (1998).

19. B. A. Liang, *Understanding and Applying Alternative Dispute Resolution Methods in Modern Medical Conflicts* 19 J. Legal Med. 397-430 (1998).

INTERNET REFERENCES

American Bar Association Section of Dispute Resolution
http://www.abanet.org/dispute

Alternate Dispute Resolution Resources
http://adrr.com

American Arbitration Association
http://www.adr.org

Chartered Institute of Arbitrators
http://www.arbitrators.org

Conflict Research Consortium
http://www.colorado.edu/conflict

CPR Institute for Dispute Resolution
http://www.cpradr.org

Georgetown University ADR resources page
http://www.ll.georgetown.edu/lr/rs/adr.html

Guide to Alternate Dispute Resolution
http://hg.org/adr.html

Institute for Conflict Analysis and Resolution
http://web.gmu.edu/departments/ICAR/

JAMS The Resolution Experts
http://www.jams-endispute.com

Law Forum: Alternative Dispute Resolution
http://www.lawforum.net/services/alternative.htm

Mediation Information and Resource Center
http://www.mediate.com

Program on Negotiation at Harvard Law School
http://www.pon.harvard.edu

Self-Administered ADR: Its Advantages and How it Works
http://www.cpradr.org/selfadm.htm

State Bar of Texas Alternative Dispute Resolution Section
http://www.texasadr.org/index.html

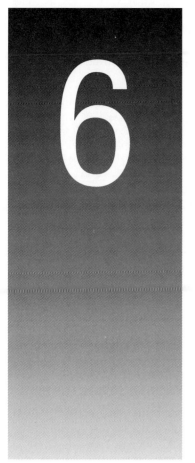

Selected health care statutory provisions

S. SANDY SANBAR, M.D., Ph.D., J.D., F.C.L.M.

ANTITRUST
THE FEDERAL FOOD, DRUG, AND COSMETIC ACT
MEDICAL DEVICES
LABORATORY REQUIREMENTS
HOSPITALS
HEALTH MAINTENANCE ORGANIZATIONS AND OTHER ORGANIZATIONAL STRUCTURES
THE SOCIAL SECURITY ACT
AREAS OF STATE JURISDICTION
QUESTIONS OF FRAUD
MILITARY PHYSICIANS
NATIONAL HEALTH SERVICE CORPS
THE PRISON SYSTEM
SPECIAL TYPES OF PATIENT EMPLOYMENT
ALTERNATIVE MEDICINE THERAPIES
RESEARCH AND MULTIDISCIPLINARY APPROACHES
PEER REVIEW
PHYSICIAN PAYMENT REVIEW COMMISSION
MISCELLANEOUS

At one time, the legal aspects of the practice of medicine were defined in terms of the common law. The chief areas of concern were negligence, breech of contractual agreements, and breeches in the confidentiality of the physician-patient relationship. However, times have changed.

Today there is a complicated regulatory web woven of laws at all levels of government. The statutory scheme touches on such diverse aspects as environmental concerns, antitrust law, product liability, and civil rights. Health care regulation is an ocean both broad in scope and deep in complexity. A WESTLAW search of "physicians" and "health care," for example, provides citations to more than 9900 separate federal statutes and regulations. Health care law is increasingly constitutional, statutory, and administrative law rather than common law doctrines.

This chapter provides a reference to certain types of federal and state statutes, giving health care practitioners a starting point for research into their specific concerns. Case law interpreting the statutes has been omitted, as has material touching on a number of overly broad or overly specialized topics.

The author gratefully acknowledges the assistance of Lisa Rower, J.D., in updating this chapter.

ANTITRUST

The major statutes in the area of antitrust law are the Sherman Act (15 U.S.C. section 21 et seq.) and section 7 of the Clayton Act (15 U.S.C. section 18). Guidance on allowable types of mergers for business entities in general, including health care institutions, can be found in the 1992 Merger Guidelines (4 Trade Reg. Rep. [CCH] paragraph 13,104 at 20,571). Section 4 of the Horizontal Merger Guidelines, dealing with efficiencies (72 ATRR 359), was revised by the U.S. Department of Justice and the Federal Trade Commission in April 1997. Guidelines for the health care field can be found in the Safe Harbor Regulations of the Medicare Anti-Kickback Provisions (42 CFR 1001 et seq., specifically at 1001.95 [1999] instead of 1001.952 [1991] [1001.952 gives exceptions]). Restrictions on physicians' ability to diversify the business aspects of their practices can be found in the Self-Referral Provisions (42 U.S.C. section 1395nn) and the Social Security Act (section 1877).

THE FEDERAL FOOD, DRUG, AND COSMETIC ACT

A major section of the regulatory structure related to health care is provided by the U.S. Food and Drug Administration. Of primary interest to the practicing physician is the Federal

Controlled Substances Act (21 U.S.C. section 801 et seq.), which details the allowable uses and the requirements for the possession, use, and recording of controlled substances, including narcotics. Information regarding the Substance Abuse and Mental Health Services Administration is codified at 42 U.S.C.A. section 290aa, et seq. Approval of new drugs is handled under 21 U.S.C.A. section 355. Cancer control programs under the National Cancer Institute are set forth at 42 U.S.C.A. section 284 et seq.

The Department of Health and Human Services is responsible for creating a board for the development of drugs and devices to treat rare diseases or conditions. This board is known as the *Orphan Products Board* (42 U.S.C.A. section 236).

Payment for covered outpatient drugs under the Social Security Act is covered at 42 U.S.C.A. section 1396r-8. Significant recent amendments to the act include the following:

Pub. L. 103-80, section 1, 107 statute 773 (August 13, 1993)	
Pub. L. 102-571, title I, section 101(a), 106 statute 4491 (October 29, 1992)	The Nutrition Labeling and Education Act Amendments of 1993 The Prescription Drug User Fee Act of 1992
Pub. L. 102-571, title II, section 201, 106 statute 4500 (October 29, 1992)	The Dietary Supplement Act of 1992
Pub. L. 102-353, section 1(a), 106 statute 941 (August 26, 1992)	The Prescription Drug Amendments of 1992
Pub. L. 102-584, 106 statute 4943 (November 4, 1992)	The Veterans Health Care Act
Pub. L. 103-18, section 662, 107 statute 53 (April 12, 1993)	Concerns the price of prescription drugs purchased by the Department of Veterans Affairs, other federal agencies, and Medicaid
Pub. L. 103-66, section 13602(a), 107 statute 613 (August 5, 1997)	Concerns changes in the drug rebate program

MEDICAL DEVICES

The general provisions regarding control of devices intended for human use are found at 21 U.S.C.A. section 360j. The practitioner also should note that significant questions regarding implantable medical devices arise in the area of patent law. The Social Security Act (42 U.S.C.A. section 1395m) sets forth special payment rules for durable medical equipment.

LABORATORY REQUIREMENTS

Laboratory requirements for all types of medical laboratories, including those in a physician's office, are specified under the Clinical Laboratories Improvement Amendments of 1988 at Pub. L. 100-578, 102 statute 2903, 42 U.S.C. section 263a. Under virtually all circumstances the Stark Law specifically prohibits physicians from sending laboratory work to a laboratory in which they retain an economic interest (42 U.S.C.A. section 1395nn). Hazardous substance release, liability, and compensation are covered at 42 U.S.C.A. section 9604. Patient radiation health and safety are discussed at 42 U.S.C.A. section 10003 et seq.

HOSPITALS

The regulation of hospitals has progressed to the point that it is proper to speak in terms of a hospital being a theoretically private but government-structured institution. Pertinent statutes are as follows:

The Hospital and Medical Facilities Act of 1964	42 U.S.C. sections 201nt, 247c, 291 et seq.
The Hospital and Medical Facilities Construction and Modernization Assistance Act of 1968	42 U.S.C. sections 201nt, 291a, 291b

Definitions on ambulatory and outpatient facilities are found at 42 U.S.C. section 291o. There are special rules, including grant funding to facilitate increased health care service, for rural areas (42 U.S.C.A. section 294d). The establishment of programs for improving trauma care in rural areas is covered by 42 U.S.C.A. section 300d-3.

Requirements for and assurances of quality of care in skilled nursing facilities are set forth at 42 U.S.C.A. sections 1395i-3 and 1396r. It is important to note that the Safe Harbor Regulations of the Medicare Anti-Kickback Provisions (42 CFR 1001 et seq.) also apply to hospitals.

HEALTH MAINTENANCE ORGANIZATIONS AND OTHER ORGANIZATIONAL STRUCTURES

The Health Maintenance Organization Act of 1973 (Pub. L. 93-222, Pub. L. 95-626) codified at 12 U.S.C. section 1721, 42 U.S.C. sections 201nt, 280c, 300e to 300e-14a, 2001, as amended, established the existence of health maintenance organizations (HMOs) and mandates their structure. Payments to HMOs and competitive medical plans under the Social Security Act are regulated at 42 U.S.C.A. section 1395mm. Federal mortgage insurance for group practice facilities and medical practice facilities is covered at 12 U.S.C.A. section 1749aaa-5.

THE SOCIAL SECURITY ACT

The Social Security Act can be found at 42 U.S.C.A. section 405 et seq. and 42 U.S.C. 1395c et seq. Rules for the exclusion of certain individuals and entities from participation in Medicare and state health care programs can be found at 42 U.S.C.A. section 1320a-7. Exclusion for filing invalid claims can result in civil monetary penalties and, in cases of persons knowingly and willfully making a false statement or representation of a material fact in any application for repayment, criminal prosecution.

The federal Anti-Kickback Law has been specifically held applicable to Medicare and Medicaid claims (42 U.S.C. section 1320a-7b). The provisions of this act also have been applied by the Internal Revenue Service (26 U.S.C. section 162) and the Securities and Exchange Commission to cases in their respective areas of responsibility (HLH, 26-7). The specific rules for determining disability and blindness under the act are found at 20 CFR section 404.1512 et seq.

AREAS OF STATE JURISDICTION

In a number of cases the federal statutes act to extend areas of traditional state law to actions taking place on federal land. For example, 42 U.S.C. section 13031 requires the reporting of child abuse taking place on federal land or in federal facilities. Another example is trauma care modifications to state plans for emergency medical services, found at 42 U.S.C.A. section 300d-13, which affects formula grants from the federal government to the states. State plans for medical assistance are included in the Social Security Act at 42 U.S.C.A. section 1396a et seq.

QUESTIONS OF FRAUD

Large sections of federal law, specifically including provisions under the Social Security Act, provide for the imposition of penalties for noncompliance with or attempts to defraud the federal government as part of a medical reimbursement effort. A number of such statutes are cited elsewhere in this chapter. Other applicable statutes include:

The False Claims and Civil Actions for False Claims Act	31 U.S.C. sections 3729-3733
The Program Fraud Civil Remedies Act of 1986	Pub. L. 99-509, 31 U.S.C. sections 3801-3812, amended to Pub. L. 103-272 section 4(f)(I)(Q), 1994, 108 statute 1362
The Major Fraud Act of 1988	Pub. L. 100-700

MILITARY PHYSICIANS

This chapter does not provide a detailed discussion of federal law relating to military duty by physicians. General rules are found at 10 U.S.C.A. section 1087. The standard for defense of medical malpractice suits is found at 10 U.S.C.A. section 1089. Basic relevant statutes on licensure, appointment, retention, and so forth can be found at 10 U.S.C. 1094, 50 Ap sections 454, 456.

Treatment of veterans and their medical benefits are covered at 38 U.S.C.A. section 7316 (defense of malpractice and negligence suits) and 38 U.S.C.A. section 7462 (major adverse actions involving professional conduct or competence).

NATIONAL HEALTH SERVICE CORPS

The provisions of the National Health Service Corps program can be found at 42 U.S.C.A. section 254h et seq.

THE PRISON SYSTEM

A number of federal statutes involve medical care provided to persons being detained or incarcerated. For example, 18 U.S.C.A. section 4244 covers hospitalization of a convicted person suffering from mental disease or defect. Claims under 42 U.S.C.A. sections 1981 and 1983 often result out of an incarceration context. Specifics on section 1983 claims by prisoners can be found in 42 U.S.C.A. section 1983, at heading XII, Medical Care of Prisoners, 841-890. The civil commitment of persons not charged with any criminal offense is covered at 42 U.S.C.A. section 3412.

SPECIAL TYPES OF PATIENT EMPLOYMENT

Statutes providing special treatment for certain types of employment are as follows:

5 U.S.C.A. section 7901	Services to government employees
5 U.S.C.A. section 8103	Compensation for work injuries
5 U.S.C.A. section 8904	Government employees' health insurance
22 U.S.C.A. section 4084	Health care program for foreign service
33 U.S.C.A. section 907	Medical services and supplies to longshoremen and harbor workers
26 U.S.C.A. section 9712	Coal industry health benefits
50 U.S.C.A. section 2051	Central Intelligence Agency retirement and disability system, retirement for disability or incapacity
46 U.S.C.A. section 11102 of the Merchant Seamen Protection and Relief Act	Provides for the maintenance of medicine chests aboard vessels

ALTERNATIVE MEDICINE THERAPIES

Information about grants for chiropractic demonstration projects is available at 42 U.S.C.A. section 295a. Provisions for the establishment of an Office of Alternative Medicine to evaluate alternative medical treatment modalities, including acupuncture, Asian medicine, homeopathic medicine, and physical manipulation therapies, formerly could be found at 42 U.S.C.A. section 283g (repealed). There do not seem to be any recent enactments dealing with this issue.

RESEARCH AND MULTIDISCIPLINARY APPROACHES

There are a number of advisory boards on specific disease types, including the National Heart, Lung, and Blood Institute; the National Diabetes Advisory Board; the National Digestive Diseases Advisory Board; the Office of Research on Women's Health; and the National Kidney and Urologic Diseases Advisory Board (42 U.S.C.A. section 285b-2 et seq.). Restrictions on fetal research are codified at 42 U.S.C.A. section 289g. Research grants for genetic diseases are provided at 42 U.S.C.A. section 300b-1. Research for acquired immunodeficiency syndrome is covered at 42 U.S.C.A. section 300cc-3 et seq.

PEER REVIEW

The peer review process is mandated at 42 U.S.C.A. section 299b-1, under the Forum for Quality and Effectiveness in Health Care. The administrator is authorized to enter into contracts with public and nonprofit private entities for the purpose of developing and periodically reviewing and updating guidelines for medical care. The general provisions for peer review are contained at 42 U.S.C.A. section 1320b-12. The obligations of health care practitioners and providers of health care services are set forth at 42 U.S.C.A. section

1320c-5. Promotion of professional review activities is covered at 42 U.S.C.A. section 11111 et seq.

PHYSICIAN PAYMENT REVIEW COMMISSION

42 U.S.C.A. section 1395w-1 (repealed) created the Physician Payment Review Commission, which made recommendations to Congress regarding adjustments to the reasonable levels at which physicians should charge for services. The provision for payment fee schedules is at 42 U.S.C.A. section 1395w-4. Determination of entitlement and provisions for appeal of a negative determination are at 42 U.S.C.A. section 1395ff et seq. Establishment of the Provider Reimbursement Review Board is at 42 U.S.C.A. section 1395oo.

MISCELLANEOUS

Subrogation of third-party claims by the United States is covered at 42 U.S.C.A. section 2651. The physician and his or her office manager must be aware of the requirements of the Equal Employment Opportunities Act (42 U.S.C.A. section 2000e et seq.). A prohibition against exclusion from participation in, denial of benefits of, and discrimination under federally assisted programs on the grounds of race, color, or national origin is imposed at 42 U.S.C.A. section 2000d.

Child abuse prevention and treatment and adoption reform are covered at 42 U.S.C.A. section 5106g et seq. and 42 U.S.C.A. section 13001b et seq. There is a specific reporting requirement for health care personnel, which is contained at section 13031.

APPENDIX 6-1   **Advanced health care directive statutes, by state**

State	Statute	State	Statute
Alabama	§ 22-8A-1 to § 22-8A-10	Nevada	§ 449.535 et seq.
Alaska	§ 18.12.010 to § 18.12.100	New Hampshire	§ 177.H.1 et seq.
Arizona	§ 36-3201 to 36-3262	New Jersey	—
Arkansas	§ 20-17-201 et seq., § 20-13-901 to 908	New Mexico	§ 24-7-1 et seq.
California	Health and S. § 7185 et seq.	New York	Pub. HE § 2980 et seq.
Colorado	§ 15-18-101 et seq.	N. Carolina	§ 32A.15 to § 32A.26, § 90.320 to § 90.323
Connecticut	§ 19A-570 et seq.	N. Dakota	§ 23-06-5-1, § 23-06-4 et seq.
Delaware	Title 16, § 2501 et seq.	Ohio	§ 2133.01, Durable Power § 1337.11 et seq.
Florida	§ 744.3115	Oklahoma	Title 63, § 3-101 et seq.
Georgia	§ 88.4101 et seq.	Oregon	§§ 97.050 - 97.090
Hawaii	§ 327F.2 et seq., § 327D.2 et seq.	Pennsylvania	§ 20 PS 5401 et seq.
Idaho	§ 39-4501 et seq.	Puerto Rico	—
Illinois	§ 755 ILCS 35/1 et seq., 210 ILCS 50/3.50	Rhode Island	Gen. Laws 23-4-11-1 et seq.
Indiana	§ 16-36-4-1 et seq.	S. Carolina	§ 44-66-10, § 44-77-10, § 44-66-110 et seq.
Iowa	§ 144A.1 et seq.	S. Dakota	§ 34-12D-1 et seq., § 34-12C-1 et seq., § 39-7-2 et seq.
Kansas	§ 65-28-101 et seq.		
Kentucky	§ 311.622 et seq.	Tennessee	§ 32-11-101 et seq., § 34-6-101 et seq.
Louisiana	§ 40:1299 et seq., §58.1	Texas	H+S 672.001 et seq.
Maine	Title 18A, §5801 et seq.	Utah	§ 75-2-1101 et seq.
Maryland	HG § 5-601 et seq.	Vermont	Title 18, § 5252 et seq.
Massachusetts	Chap. 201D-1 et seq.	Virginia	§ 54-1-2981 et seq.
Michigan	§ 700.496 et seq.	Washington	§ 70.122.010 et seq.
Minnesota	§ 145B.01 et seq.	W. Virginia	§ 16-30-1 et seq., §16-30B-1 et seq., § 16-30C-1 et seq.
Mississippi	§ 41-14-101, § 41-41-151 et seq.		
Missouri	§ 459.010 et seq.	Wisconsin	§ 154.01 et seq., § 155.01 et seq.
Montana	§ 50-9-102 et seq., § 50-10-101 et seq.	Wyoming	§ 35-22-101 et seq.
Nebraska	—		

APPENDIX 6-2 Controlled substances statutes, by state

State	Statute	State	Statute
Alabama	§ 20-2-1 to § 20-2-190	Nebraska	§ 28-401 et seq.
Alaska	§ 11.30 generally, § 11.71, § 11.73	Nevada	§ 453.021 et seq.
Arizona	§ 36-2501 et seq., § 32-1901 et seq.	New Hampshire	§ 172.1, § 318.B.1 et seq.
Arkansas	§ 5-64-101 et seq.	New Jersey	§ 24:21-1 et seq.
California	Health and S. § 11000 et seq.	New Mexico	§ 30-31-1 et seq.
Colorado	§ 18-18-101 et seq., § 18-18-605	New York	Pub. HE § 3302 et seq.
Connecticut	§ 21A-240 et seq.	N. Carolina	§ 90.86 to § 90.113.8
Delaware	Title 16, § 4701 et seq.	N. Dakota	§ 19-03-1-1 et seq.
Florida	§ 893.01 et seq.	Ohio	§ 3719.01 et seq.
Georgia	§ 79a.803 et seq.	Oklahoma	Title 63, § 2-101 et seq.
Hawaii	§ 329-1 et seq.	Oregon	§ 167.203, § 475.005, § 475.035 et seq.
Idaho	§ 37-2701 et seq.	Pennsylvania	35 PS 780.101 et seq.
Illinois	720 ILCS 570/1001 et seq., 720 ILCS 570/40	Puerto Rico	—
Indiana	§ 35-48-1 et seq.	Rhode Island	Gen. Laws 21-28-2-01 et seq.
Iowa	§ 124.101 et seq.	S. Carolina	§ 44-53-10 et seq.
Kansas	§ 65-655g et seq., § 65-4101 et seq.	S. Dakota	§ 34-20B-11 et seq.
Kentucky	§ 218A.010 et seq.	Tennessee	§ 39-17-401 et seq.
Louisiana	§ 40:961 et seq.	Texas	H+S 481.001 et seq.
Maine	Title 17A, § 1101 et seq.,Title 32, § 1081 et seq.	Utah	§ 58-37-2 et seq.
Maryland	HO § 27-277 et seq.	Vermont	Title 18, § 4201 et seq.
Massachusetts	Chap. 94c-1 et seq.	Virginia	§ 54-1-3401 et seq.
Michigan	§ 333.7101 et seq.	Washington	§ 69.50.101 et seq.
Minnesota	§ 151.01 et seq., § 152.01 et seq.	W. Virginia	§ 60A-1-101 to § 60A-7-707
Mississippi	§ 14-29-101 et seq.	Wisconsin	§ 161.001 et seq.
Missouri	§ 195.010, § 196.010 et seq.	Wyoming	§ 33-24-201 et seq.
Montana	§ 50, Chap. 32 et seq.		

APPENDIX 6-3 Medical licensure statutes, by state (statutes annotated)

State	Statute	State	Statute
Alabama	§ 34-24-50 to 84, -310-406	Missouri	§ 334.031 et seq.
Alaska	§ 08.64.107 360	Montana	Chap. 3, P. 3 (§ 301) et seq.
Arizona	§ 32-1421 et seq.	Nebraska	§ 71-1.102 et seq.
Arkansas	§ 17-93-400 to 500	Nevada	§ 630.160 et seq.
California	Bus. & P. § 2030 et seq.	New Hampshire	§ 329.10 et seq.
Colorado	§ 12-36-101 to 137	New Jersey	§ 45:9-12 et seq.
Connecticut	§ 20-8a, -10 et seq.	New Mexico	§ 61-6-11 et seq.
Delaware	Title 24, § 1701 et seq.	New York	Educ. Law § 6524 et seq.
District of Columbia	§ 2-3505 et seq.	N. Carolina	§ 90-6 et seq.
		N. Dakota	§ 43-17-17 et seq.
Florida	§ 455.01, Licensure and Sanctions 458.301 et seq.	Ohio	§ 4730.12
Georgia	§ 84.906 et seq.	Oklahoma	Title 59, § 481 et seq.
Hawaii	§ 453-4 et seq.	Oregon	§ 677-100 et seq.
Idaho	§ 54-1801 to 1841	Pennsylvania	Title 63, § 422.22, 422.25 et seq.
Illinois	225 ILCS 60/1 et seq.	Puerto Rico	Title 20, § 30 et seq.
Indiana	§ 25-22.5-1-1.1 et seq.	Rhode Island	Gen. Laws 5-37-2 et seq.
Iowa	§ 148.1 et seq.	S. Carolina	§ 40-47-140 et seq.
Kansas	§ 65-2802 et seq.	S. Dakota	§ 36-4-10 et seq.
Kentucky	§ 311.550 et seq.	Tennessee	§ 63-6-201 et seq.
Louisiana	§ 37:1271 et seq.	Texas	Civil Stat., Art. 4495b, 3.01 et seq.
Maine	Title 32, § 3269 et seq.	Utah	§ 58-11a-301 et seq.
Maryland	HO § 14-101 et seq.	Vermont	Title 26, § 1391 et seq.
Massachusetts	Chap. 112, § 2 et seq.	Virginia	§ 54.1-2930 et seq.
Michigan	§ 333.17011 et seq.	Washington	§ 18.71.021 et seq., § 18.120.010W
Minnesota	§ 147.02 et seq.	Virginia	§ 30-3-10 et seq.
Mississippi	§ 73-43-1 et seq., 73-25-1 et seq.	Wisconsin	§ 448.01 et seq.
		Wyoming	§ 33-26-303 et seq.

APPENDIX 6-4   Medical malpractice claims statutes, by state

State	Statute	State	Statute
Alabama	§ 6-5-480 et seq.	Montana	§ 27-6-103 et seq.
Alaska	§ 09.55.530-560	Nebraska	§ 44-2801 et seq.
Arizona	§ 32-1854, § 12-563 et seq.	Nevada	§ 41A.003 et seq.
Arkansas	§ 16-114-201 to 209	New Hampshire	§ 507C.1, § 507E.1 et seq.
California	Bus. & P. § 3527 et seq., 801, 802; CC 3333.1 to 2	New Jersey	§ 17:30D-1 et seq. (Liability Insurance Act)
		New Mexico	§ 41-5-1 et seq.
Colorado	§ 13-64-401 et seq.	New York	CPLR § 3017 et seq.
Connecticut	§ 52-184c	N. Carolina	§ 90.21.11 to .14
Delaware	Title 18, § 6801 et seq.	N. Dakota	§ 28-01-18, § 28-01-46, § 43-17.1 et seq.
Florida	§ 461.013 et seq., 766.101 et seq.	Ohio	§ 2305, § 2307, § 2317 et seq.
Georgia	§ 81a.109.1 et seq.	Oklahoma	Title 76, § 17 et seq.
Hawaii	§ 671-3 et seq.	Oregon	§ 18-470 et seq., § 30-080 et seq.
Idaho	§ 6-1001 et seq.	Pennsylvania	40 PS 1301.301 et seq.
Illinois	735 ILCS 5/2 et seq.	Puerto Rico	Title 20, § 52a, Title 31, § 2991 et seq.
Indiana	§ 27-12-1-1 to § 27-12-18-1	Rhode Island	Gen. Laws 9-19-32 et seq.
Iowa	§ 147.135 et seq.	S. Carolina	§ 40-47-60, § 40-47-190, § 40-47-260
Kansas	§ 60-3401, § 65-4901 et seq.	S. Dakota	Arbitration § 21-25-1 et seq.
Kentucky	§ 413.140 et seq.	Tennessee	§ 29-26-115 et seq.
Louisiana	§ 40:1299.39 et seq.	Texas	Civil Stat., Art. 4590i et seq.
Maine	Title 24, § 2501 et seq.	Utah	§ 78-14-1 et seq.
Maryland	HO § 14-101 et seq.	Vermont	Title 12, § 700 et seq., § 1908, § 1909
Massachusetts	CJ, § 3-2A-01 et seq.	Virginia	§ 55-7B-1 et seq.
Michigan	§ 600.1483 et seq., § 500.2477 et seq.	Washington	§ 655.001 et seq.
Minnesota	§ 145.682, § 573.02 et seq.	W. Virginia	§ 9-2-1501 et seq.
Mississippi	§ 11-1-59 et seq., 15-1-36	Wisconsin	§ 448.01 et seq.
Missouri	§ 383.010 et seq., 538.255 et seq.	Wyoming	§ 33-26-303 et seq.

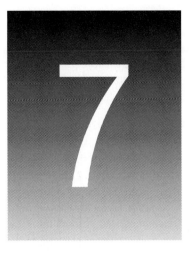

Education and licensure

S. SANDY SANBAR, M.D., Ph.D., J.D., F.C.L.M.

THE "RIGHT" TO BE A PHYSICIAN
MEDICAL SCHOOL ADMISSION CRITERIA
MEDICAL SCHOOL RETENTION AND GRADUATION
MEDICAL LICENSURE
CONCLUSION

Medical education—from admission to medical school to completion of postgraduate training—occurs in a definite legal framework. Both the student and the state enjoy certain legal rights and duties.

State licensure to practice medicine and surgery is also basic. The requirements for licensure and the ways in which that medical licensure may be lost or curtailed are many.

More than 400 years ago Shakespeare observed, "Oh, how full of briers is this working-day world."[1] This observation is still true for medicine today. This chapter points out the briers.

THE "RIGHT" TO BE A PHYSICIAN

There is no vested property or constitutional right to attend medical school. However, acceptance to a medical school class may not be based on any violation of the applicant's general civil rights nor may requirements be arbitrary or capricious. A medical school may not employ quotas but may employ some affirmative action in selecting students. The relationship of the medical student and the school is an enforceable contractual one. Some courts have held that a student admitted to medical school has a "liberty right or interest" mandating procedural due process necessary for administrative problems and substantive due process for disciplinary situations. The general rule is one of fair play in making rules regarding information, discipline, and punishment.

MEDICAL SCHOOL ADMISSION CRITERIA

Each medical school, public or private, can establish its own admission standards. The admission criteria must be uniformly applied to each candidate. The primary area of legal interest in medical school admissions is that of affirmative action admissions programs, which make race, gender, or

ethnic origin a factor of greater or lesser degree in the acceptance decision.

Early medical school admission cases focused on a variety of legal theories. The courts have allowed the return of entrance application fees under a theory of false pretenses when the standards used for admission were not in keeping with those advertised in the medical school's bulletin.[2] Professional schools have been ordered to award degrees to students who were denied admission or retention on an arbitrary or unreasonable basis.[3]

Judicial review

Judicial review of the medical school admissions process on constitutional equal protection grounds requires the existence of "state action" sufficient to trigger the provisions of the applicable constitutional provision or federal statute. In *Cannon v. University of Chicago* a female student's suit under the federal gender and age discrimination statutes was deemed as failing to state a cause of action because of a failure to prove the existence of state action.[4]

In a decision foreshadowing the *Bakke* decision, the Court of Appeals of New York held that a strict scrutiny standard of review applied to racial reverse discrimination in medical school admissions. The New York court did not discuss less restrictive alternatives available to the university because the cessation of the minority admissions program still would not have entitled the plaintiff to a place in the incoming class.[5]

The Bakke decision

The seminal legal decision involving medical school admission requirements is that of *University of California Regents v. Bakke.*[6] In that case Mr. Bakke was denied admission to the University of California, Davis Medical School because his credentials failed to meet the standards required for admission as a nonminority applicant. School policy established a quota-based affirmative action program, setting aside 16% of

The author gratefully acknowledges the past contribution from Daniel J. Gamino, J.D., and the assistance of Lisa Rowen, J.D., in updating this chapter.

the available places in the entering medical class for minority applicants, defined as "Blacks, Chicanos, and Asian Americans." Bakke's entrance scores were higher than those of certain persons accepted under the minority entry program. Thus, but for Bakke's race and ethnic origin, he most likely would have been accepted for entry into medical school.

Bakke sued, claiming a violation of the Equal Protection Clause of the U.S. Constitution and Title VI of the 1964 Civil Rights Act. No clear majority opinion developed from the U.S. Supreme Court's review of the case. Six separate opinions were written, with no more than four justices agreeing on any one chain of reasoning behind their decision. Evaluation of the *Bakke* decisions is thus somewhat difficult.

Four justices of the Court held that the university's plan was completely constitutional. Four held that the quota plan was in violation of Title VI but failed to reach the constitutional equal protection issue.

Justice Powell cast the swing vote. He considered Title VI primarily a codification of the constitutional equal protection standard, and thus the applicable standard of review was identical under either a constitutional or statutory evaluation. Powell, applying a strict scrutiny standard of review, considered race to be a valid factor in the evaluation of potential medical school candidates but stressed that the quota system was not necessary to achieve the university's desired goal and thus was not permissible. The four-justice group led by Justice Brennan agreed with Powell's approach (allowing the use of race as a factor in the admissions process) but considered the applicable standard of review to be an intermediate level of scrutiny, as is applied in gender discrimination cases, such as *Craig v. Boren*.[7]

The *Bakke* decision did not answer all questions. The decision established that affirmative action programs in a medical school admissions process could be structured to avoid constitutional legal protection violations and further that certain types of affirmative admissions programs, such as quota-based systems, were a violation of equal protection rights. The difficulty of *Bakke* was that the court failed to articulate a definitive standard of review for affirmative action admissions programs.

Reaction to Bakke

Reaction to the *Bakke* decision was mixed both during the case and after the decision was rendered. The National Conference of Black Lawyers and the National Lawyers Guild, for example, urged that the Supreme Court refuse to hear the case at all on the grounds of inadequate records regarding possible past racial discrimination by the university.[8]

The U.S. Supreme Court had previously refused to decide a similar case on the merits, declaring the matter moot because the student in question was about to complete his legal education.[9] On remand the Supreme Court of Washington upheld its earlier decision holding the minority admissions policy of the university to be valid.[10]

General rule

Generally, affirmative action minority placement programs for medical schools are permissible, as long as race is not used as the sole determining factor in the evaluation process. State action requirements must be established before a standard of review is applicable.

The Americans with Disabilities Act

The 1990 Americans with Disabilities Act (ADA) provides that "no qualified individual with a disability shall by reason of such disability be excluded from participating in or be denied the benefits of the services, programs, or activities of a public entity."[11] This mandate requires medical schools, both public and private, to make "reasonable accommodations" in evaluating applicants.[12] Case law on the ADA is nearly nonexistent. Requirements for accommodation may include granting candidates additional time to take entrance examinations, providing a reader for the sight-impaired or dyslexic candidate, and perhaps instituting a different standard of review for a disabled candidate's undergraduate transcript and grades.

MEDICAL SCHOOL RETENTION AND GRADUATION

The primary concern of most medical students is successful graduation. Numerous suits have occurred as a result of student dismissals on academic or disciplinary grounds. The nature of legal challenges raised in an attempt to prevent academic dismissals is quite varied.

Academic dismissal

Once accepted into the medical school program at a public institution, students are deemed to have a liberty or property interest in the continuation of their medical school education and in eventually receiving their medical degrees. Private medical schools, although not subject to Fourteenth Amendment due process itself, are subject to the standards set by accreditation requirements and any standard or procedures that have been internally adopted.

It is essential that the medical school administration pay attention to the due process requirement during an academic dismissal proceeding. Strict adherence to due process protects the student's rights and helps reduce the risk of future litigation by the student.

Academic dismissals (i.e., those based on poor academic performance or failure to complete the requirements for graduation) are evaluated differently than are disciplinary dismissals. The institution must give the student notice of the potential dismissal, but traditional legal procedures for fact-finding, such as for a hearing, are not legally required. Academic dismissals may arise from strict academic performance or clinical performance standards.

A key case on academic dismissals is *Board of Curators of the University of Missouri v. Horowitz*.[13] Therein the U.S.

Supreme Court ruled that in the case of academic dismissals notice of the impending dismissal was required to be given to the student, but a formal hearing was not mandatory. The Supreme Court based its decision on the long tradition of judicial deference to academic discretion and the belief that the academic evaluation of a student is more properly placed in the academic setting rather than the courtroom.

Post-*Horowitz* decisions have tended to uphold medical schools' decisions for academic dismissal over procedural due process challenges of medical school students. In most cases medical schools have provided procedural protections far beyond the scope required by *Horowitz,* including multiple forms of notice and multiple opportunities for academic hearings and inquiry before final dismissal on academic grounds. In *Sanders v. Ajir,* for example, the court held that a student going through the dismissal process on two separate occasions, with two levels of hearing on each occasion, had been afforded a level of procedural protection in excess of the requirements set by *Horowitz.*[14]

When academic hearings have been offered to a student before academic dismissal, court decisions have not required the same degree of formal procedural protection that has been required in other Fourteenth Amendment property or liberty settings. Most academic procedures do not provide for the presence of an attorney during hearings or for a formal transcript of the proceedings. Records consisting of the initial notice of dismissal and a summary of the final decision of the academic hearing committee are sufficient. The dismissal panel often questions witnesses, including faculty members, outside the presence of the student. Hearings are thus informal and nonadversarial. The hearings normally consist of the student making a statement to the appeals board and then answering questions.

Even in the post-*Horowitz* cases that have required a hearing, the court has required only that the student be given the opportunity to explain his or her poor scholarship and to provide any additional information that might lead to an expectation of future satisfactory performance.[15]

Disciplinary dismissal

In contrast to academic dismissal, disciplinary dismissal entitles the student to a greater standard of procedural protection. Disciplinary dismissal of students occurs on the basis of nonacademic considerations, usually specified in a formal academic code of conduct by the medical school. Reasons for disciplinary dismissal include plagiarism, cheating, and disruptive behavior. The legal requirements for due process in disciplinary dismissal cases include provision of notice to the student of the intended dismissal, an opportunity to be heard, and an opportunity to rebut the school's grounds for dismissal.

Disciplinary dismissal due process directly parallels protection afforded individuals before the deprivation of a liberty or a property interest. An example is *Goss v. Lopez.*[16] In *Goss*

the U.S. Supreme Court held that a high school student could not be suspended for improper behavior without being given notice of the charges against him or her, an explanation of the evidence, and an opportunity to present his or her side. The standard for procedural process is the *Matthews v. Eldridge* test, which weighs the strength of the private interest, the strength of the state interest, the risk of error under the current procedures used, and the probable value of additional or substitute procedural safeguards.[17]

Substantive due process claims

Substantive due process consists of the concept that the individual is entitled to a decision that is not arbitrary or capricious, when a liberty or property interest exists. Educational institutions cannot act in an arbitrary way or in a capricious manner. In a dismissal case the burden of proof is on the student to demonstrate that the decision was arbitrary or capricious, that is, that no real basis for dismissal existed or malice, bad faith, or ill-will existed on the part of the medical school or its acting employees. Exercise of discretion by the medical school in terms of retention based on academic failure has not been considered to be arbitrary or capricious action by the courts.

In contrast, the mandatory dismissal of a student for first-year academic failure, when three other students with an equal or greater number of failures were allowed to repeat the first year, was judged arbitrary by a New York court at the trial level, but the decision was reversed on an appeal.[18] In Michigan a court ruled against the medical school when a student was singled out on the basis of his initial score on the National Board of Nursing Examination (NBNE) and was deprived of his opportunity to retake the test along with 40 other students from the same school who had failed the same part of the examination.

Mere general allegations by a student that a particular grade or dismissal was improper usually fail to meet the requirements of proof to establish arbitrary, capricious action by the medical school. In contrast, if the student can demonstrate by objective evidence how he or she was singled out for disparate treatment from fellow students, the chances of proving arbitrary and capricious behavior on the part of the medical school are considerably enhanced.

Contractual relations between medical school and student

Related to the concept of substantive due process is the use of contractual claims by the student to establish procedural or substantive legal rights. The trend of the courts has been to construe liberally the terms of the contract in favor of the medical school. This approach is typical in educational contract cases. However, it is at variance from the more traditional viewpoint that a contract should be construed strictly with respect to the person drafting the contract, in this case the medical school.[19]

Handicapped students

The ADA, originally enacted by Congress in 1990, is changing how medical schools and all other schools approach handicapped students.[20] This act requires medical schools to make "reasonable accommodations" for students with certain physical and mental disabilities. Dyslexia, narcolepsy, drug and alcohol dependency, and mental disorders all fall within the scope of disabilities and certain protections of the law, along with the more traditional physical handicaps.[21] Little case law has as yet developed.

Substance of content of medical school education

Increasingly the demands to include new information in the medical school curriculum (e.g., courses on acquired immunodeficiency syndrome [AIDS]) have produced a problem of serious dimensions in medical school class scheduling. The phenomenon can be seen both within the medical school educational process and the process of health care law instruction within the legal community.[22]

The AIDS crisis exemplifies the difficulty of providing education and maintaining medical ethics within the medical school process. The medical student is presented with the dilemma when assigned to a rotation that requires treatment of AIDS patients. AIDS demonstrates the potential for new requirements of specific substantive courses within medical school education by state law, a step that would be historically unique within the medical school process.[23]

Substance of content requirements also have been increasingly dictated in a variety of other areas, on both a voluntary and an involuntary basis.[24] These trends point to the tendency toward further standardization of the medical school education process.

House officers

A medical school graduate is required to complete at least 1 year of postgraduate training in an internship, usually in a hospital. Many then go on to advanced training programs, residencies, and fellowships certified by a variety of organizations.

In the past, house officers were considered employees and were subject to the whim of the hospital administration. A recent California court decision, noting the impact of the arbitrary cancellation of a house officer's contract on his or her career, imposed the requirement of a due process hearing, with all its protections.[25]

Clinical training programs raise potential questions in the area of medical malpractice. There is considerable divergence among jurisdictions on the standard of care for residents in the academic medical context. Although *Rusk v. Akron General Hospital* represents the position that a special standard of care is applicable for interns and residents within the medical school and clinical context, more recent cases suggest that the standard of care to be applied should be the standard of a general physician or the standard of the specialty in which the resident is being trained.[26-28] Although there appear to be no reported cases covering the standard of care for medical students, the medical student, intern, or resident must be aware that he or she could be held to the standard of care applicable to the attending physician supervising his or her education and clinical process.[29]

In addition, the team-teaching approach presents informed consent issues. Consent is specific to the individual physician. Thus consent given by the patient to allow the attending physician to engage in a procedure does not automatically grant consent for the procedure to be performed by proxy (e.g., by a resident or intern), even if the procedure is done at the attending physician's or senior resident's request.[30] In the academic medical context several possibilities for liability arise that do not normally arise within the private practice setting. The attending physician and student must be aware of the potential for liability, take steps to ensure proper consent on the part of the patients, and maintain the highest possible standards of care.[31]

MEDICAL LICENSURE
Theory and requirements

Power of the state. To exclude any incompetent practitioners, the state may require that professionals obtain a license to practice medicine and perform surgery. The state has a right to continue to evaluate a physician's professional practice. "The right of a physician to toil in his profession . . . with all its sanctity and safeguards is not absolute. It must yield to the paramount right of government to protect the public health by any rational means."[32]

Licensing statutes are justified under a state's sovereign power to protect the health and welfare of its citizens. Medical practice acts create and define the composition of a state medical board, define the requirements for licensure, and vest the board with the authority to license candidates. The state medical board is mandated to regulate the practice of medicine in the public interest and to advance the medical profession. Establishing and vigilantly enforcing standards of conduct to ensure the competence and the scruples of physicians are the responsibilities of the board. This stewardship is viewed by courts as an entrustment by the state and is subject to judicial review.

Licensure statutes were originally designed to exclude the untutored, unskilled, and incompetent from the practice of medicine by certifying a minimally acceptable qualification of training, knowledge, and competence after evaluating and certifying submitted credentials. In a landmark case in 1898 the U.S. Supreme Court stated that licensure powers could be extended beyond credentialing to include standards of behavior and ethics. The case held that, in a physician, "character is as important a qualification as knowledge."[33] Sanctions may include denial of license, revocation of license, suspension of license, probation, oral or written reprimands, imposition of monetary fines, and censuring.

The authority of the courts to oversee the licensing of physicians also is mandated by statute. The courts, however, seldom intercede until the physician has completely exhausted his or her administrative remedies, unless the licensing board has acted wholly outside of its jurisdiction. At the conclusion of the administrative proceedings, the courts typically intervene only when the physician successfully argues that the licensing board violated the physician's constitutional rights, acted outside of its jurisdiction, or failed to follow its own rules and regulations.

Types of licensure. Virtually all state medical licenses are unlimited (i.e., unrestricted to any particular branch of medicine or surgery). Thus the holder of a medical license may take routine histories and do physical examinations or perform specialized neurosurgery under the same license.

Some states have a restricted license for postgraduate training, such as residency. In some cases the credentialing process is delegated de facto to the supervising institution. Physicians in state hospitals or correctional facilities sometimes hold licenses restricted to such institutional use. Again, the respective state legislature, medical board, or both sets forth the specific types of licensure available in that state.

As a sanction, some physicians may be restricted to institutional practice as a result of disciplinary proceedings in which supervision of practice is deemed appropriate. Such licensure curtailment is sometimes supplanted by other restrictive techniques, such as probation. Some states provide temporary licensure, allowing locum tenens work or allowing an expert visiting a medical school to engage in clinical activities.

Obtaining a license. As a necessary function of its duty to protect the public interest, a state board may require physicians and related practitioners to demonstrate a certain degree of skill and learning. It may also include conditions of licensure bearing a direct, substantial, and reasonable relationship to the practice of medicine, such as a statutorily specified amount of malpractice insurance coverage, before the licensee may practice medicine. In exercising its licensing authority the state has the inherent power to determine precisely the qualifications the applicant must possess. It may investigate educational credentials, professional competence, and moral character. The applicant bears the burden to prove his or her fulfillment of all requirements for licensure.

U.S. citizenship was once required for medical licensure, but that requirement was struck down by the U.S. Supreme Court in 1973 as unconstitutional discrimination. Another barrier to licensure was a residency requirement of a specific number of months. That requirement also was struck down as discrimination that only furthered the parochial interest of state physicians. Closely related to residency restrictions is reciprocity licensure. A state is not required to license a physician merely because he or she holds a license in another state; otherwise the state would be obligated to automatically grant a license to everyone who holds a license in every other state. Thus reciprocity is neither constitutionally discriminatory nor an infringement on a physician's rights and privilege of practice. Most states also have established a minimum age of 21 years for licensure.

Invariably, "good moral character" is required for licensure. A typical reason for denying a license on that ground is a prior criminal conviction, even if the crime on which the conviction was based has no obvious connection with the practice of medicine. Such candidates must be prepared to demonstrate total rehabilitation. The nature of the offense is a material consideration. For example, a licensing board should be prepared to differentiate between a trespass conviction arising out of a 1970s antiwar demonstration and the offense of grand larceny.

State requirements of educational achievement for licensure vary but have generally been upheld. Educational requirements cannot be arbitrary and must be rationally related to competence. Requirements of preprofessional education and professional education from "accredited schools" have been held reasonable and valid.[34] Experience requirements of postgraduate education are likewise considered to be rational, reasonable, and valid. If an individual's experience has provided comparable or superior education but licensure required a diploma, it has been held that the diploma requirement was not capricious or arbitrary and did not deprive one of a constitutional right of due process or equal protection.[35] Requiring malpractice insurance, a recent mandate in at least one state (Idaho), was upheld as reasonable because it bears a rational relationship to the welfare of citizens.

Supervision and disciplinary sanctions

Grounds for discipline. Until a few years ago, licensure sanctions against physicians resulting from inadequate patient care were few and far between, in large part because of the reluctance of physicians to report or take action against colleagues. In particular, physicians feared that their colleagues who were reported would sue them for libel, slander, or restraint of trade. In addition, the boards were nearly impotent, having more restricted investigative abilities and less sanctioning authority than they enjoy today.

Recently, however, courts have held hospitals and physicians liable for failure to "ferret out" bad physicians. Legislatures have given administrative agencies new power and have granted immunity to honorable informants and their authorized listeners. Licensing boards no longer have to wait for a formal report or complaint; they may now begin an inquiry and proceedings on their own initiative. Some courts have even allowed licensing board proceedings while a criminal proceeding is pending.

Grounds for discipline of the medical licensee are generally set forth in statute as "unprofessional conduct." A licensee may be disciplined for the following:

- Alcohol or drug dependency
- Fraudulent procurement of a license
- Failure to cooperate with a medical board investigation
- Participation or involvement in a criminal abortion
- Sexual advances toward or sexual involvement with patients
- Sales of medical licenses
- False or inaccurate patient records
- Misrepresentation of hospital status to patients
- Revocation or curtailment of hospital privileges
- Fraud involving reimbursement of patients' expenses by third parties
- Improperly prescribing, administering, or dispensing controlled substances
- Diverting or giving away controlled substances
- Transmission of disease by improper sterilization procedures
- Weight control therapy abuse
- Patient neglect (abandonment, real or constructive)
- Unprofessional or dishonorable conduct or gross misconduct
- Malpractice
- Communication of confidential patient information
- Failure to comply with legal requirements, such as reporting venereal disease, birth registration, and suspicious death or injury
- Permitting, aiding, or abetting unlicensed personnel to perform medical procedures normally restricted to a physician (When a physician's practice policies are challenged by the licensing board, the courts have held that the practices must be harmful or misleading and not merely generally unacceptable to the medical community.)
- Conviction of a crime, if the crime in question has been made a basis for a license revocation by statute
- Criminal activity, including fraud involving Medicare, Medicaid, the state insurance companies, and patient reimbursement; improperly prescribing, administering, or dispensing controlled dangerous substances; and conviction of a felony or misdemeanor (e.g., sexual assault, possession of an unlicensed firearm, or accepting a bribe in violation of either a state or federal law)

The least precise ground for disciplinary action is the allegation of unprofessional, immoral, dishonorable, or gross misconduct.[36-40] Such concepts are difficult to define. It is manifestly impossible to categorize all of the acts subject to discipline. Such unspecific and vague standards are enforceable because there is a common professional understanding of what the public interest requires. Precise definitions made by the state medical boards are usually left intact, but on occasion the courts reverse them and impose their own defini-

tions. As long as a board bases its finding of unprofessional conduct or gross misconduct on expert testimony (on the record) as to the proper standard of care, the board should be upheld.

Discipline on grounds of incompetence, negligence, or malpractice is also somewhat vague and difficult to define. Incompetence is not established by rare and isolated instances of inadequate performance; rather, repeated defects in the exercise of everyday skills are the gist of such complaints. In rare cases a single act of gross negligence is so wanton that it sufficiently demonstrates incompetence.

Fraud and deceit in the practice of medicine are grounds for discipline; most often fraud or deceit is alleged when a physician bills a third party (Medicare or an insurance company) for work he or she did not perform. Fraud or deceit in nonprofessional activities is an offense more often in the nature of moral turpitude or immoral conduct.

A felony conviction empowers the board in most states to revoke a license.[41] In some states, revocation cannot occur until all appeals have been exhausted. Misconduct in another state also may be grounds for revocation. Fraudulently obtaining a license and aiding and assisting an unlicensed practitioner in the practice of medicine also are grounds for revocation.

Discipline for failure to complete training and educational requirements, if mandated by a state statute, has been upheld as constitutional. Discipline for violation of medical board regulations is typically upheld, particularly if the legislative intent was to delegate to the state medical board the power to set standards of competence and conduct. Such regulations must be in the public interest and, although generally viewed favorably, are nevertheless subject to judicial review.

Medical boards have become increasingly active in dealing with physicians who practice while impaired by alcohol or controlled substances. Some states track these physicians through the traditional disciplinary route. Other states have formally established recovery programs that give physicians an opportunity to avoid formal disciplinary proceedings if they quickly agree to comprehensive treatment, supervision of their medical practice, and random testing.

Defenses to disciplinary charges. One of the most common practitioner defenses is that due process of law was denied by the board's commingling of investigative and adjudicatory functions within the same administrative agency. Courts have generally rejected this argument, stating that, absent a showing of bias, there was not sufficient risk of prejudice to taint the decision.[42]

At the initiation of disciplinary procedures, the practitioner may raise a number of specific defenses. These defenses include the statute of limitations, entrapment, unlawful search and seizure, double jeopardy, recovery from impairment (with or without impaired physician committee monitoring), and jurisdictional challenges to a medical board proceeding after voluntary surrender of a license.

Occasionally, disciplinary proceedings are brought years after the alleged improper conduct of the physician, most often because of the initial unwillingness of witnesses to come forward or because of the lengthy processes in state and federal courts. Generally a defense of inordinate delay in prosecution for an alleged offense from the too distant past, though valid in criminal and civil judicial proceedings, has been considered an invalid defense in administrative disciplinary proceedings.[43] However, some states specifically include a statute of limitations. Whether or not he or she practices in one of the few states with a statute of limitations on medical board disciplinary proceedings, the physician can defend by asserting the "equitable doctrine of laches." This doctrine protects defendants in cases of an unexcused delay in bringing a disciplinary procedure that is inequitably prejudicial to the defendant.

Entrapment is a defense that asserts that law enforcement agents coerced, tricked, induced, or persuaded the defendant physician to commit an offense that would not have been committed if not for the agents' conduct. Entrapment may be a valid defense, but in a few cases the defense has been rejected as being limited to criminal proceedings.[44]

Evidence gained by unlawful search and seizure may sometimes be suppressed and may constitute a successful defense. Courts typically explore the policies underlying the exclusionary rule before automatically applying it to professional licensure proceedings.[45] However, this evidence is not always subject to the usual prohibition because of the necessity of strict supervision in certain highly regulated business activities (e.g., firearms or narcotics).[46]

Double jeopardy (the risk of double punishment for a single offense), alleged in instances of multiple license revocations, has been held an invalid defense. In addition, a board may impose discipline even when the physician has prevailed in a related criminal proceeding and the principle of double jeopardy does not apply.[47]

A defense of recovery from an impairment (with or without monitoring from an impaired physician committee) or assertion of the right to resume practice after voluntary surrender of license is not in and of itself a defense in sanction proceedings. Typical board considerations when recovery is alleged include establishing that the impairment was the cause of misconduct, that the subject has indeed recovered, that the recovery has arrested the threat to public health and safety, and that relapse is unlikely.

Presentation by a convicted felon of a "certificate of rehabilitation" under a "Rehabilitated Convicted Offenders Act" is not a dispositive defense. Proof of a degree of rehabilitation does not preclude a license authority from disqualifying applicants.[48]

A jurisdictional challenge based on voluntary surrender of (or failure to renew) a license depends on whether the physician retains any remaining rights to revive the license. Furthermore, the state can assert an interest in going forward with its proof at a time when evidence and witnesses' memories are fresh.[49]

R.P. Reeves has described the defense of winning by "intimidation."[50] Such defenses include "tying up" board members or assistant attorneys general and staff with repeated requests for continuances, voluminous discovery requests, subpoenas for spurious documents or witnesses, floods of character witnesses, applications for stays, and collateral attacks in federal court.

Finally, physicians facing disciplinary charges have tried to bring federal civil rights actions under 42 U.S.C. § 1983. Because boards are sitting in both their prosecutorial and quasijudicial capacities when carrying out disciplinary functions, board members and their staffs are usually granted absolute immunity from such suits.[51] Physicians who bring such suits also may be ordered to pay the attorney fees of their successful opponents.

Commingling investigative and judicial functions. It is a common objection to disciplinary action that a fair hearing is denied when matters are judged by a board that is also investigating the charges. Commingling sometimes occurs because of practical limits of funds and personnel. Commingling has been recognized as prejudicial only when there was an actual showing of bias.[52] Thus a court found no denial of due process in a situation wherein the physician asserted

that the member of the Board who moved that the order to show cause be served upon him was thereafter appointed hearing officer and conducted the hearing, that complainant counsel was employed by the Board, and that before the hearing all the Board members, including the hearing officer, had access to the investigatory materials collected in the . . . complaint file. In addition, he [appeared] to assert that one or more of the Board members who participated in the decision to issue the order to show cause also participated in the ultimate decision to revoke his license.[53]

This finding is in contrast to a court finding of necessary bias in which two board members commenced an unauthorized investigation. After one posed as a patient, they filed formal charges and appeared as investigators and witnesses before their fellow board members, who voted to suspend an optometrist's license.[54]

Disciplinary proceedings before formal charges are filed. A physician can be brought to the board's attention by a variety of sources—professional colleagues, nurses and other health care professionals, anonymous written or oral communications, conversations overheard by board employees, news exposés, and so forth. Frivolous complaints are not pursued. Granting of public access to dismissed complaints varies from state to state. States must balance the danger of unjustified notoriety against the value of keeping boards accountable by allowing the public to scrutinize dismissed complaints. Formal complaints or reports filed by patients, hospitals, other physicians, insurance companies, courthouse clerks, state or federal agencies, and the Federation of State Medical Boards constitute major informational sources of disciplinary procedures.

Although it is usually not required, the board may notify the physician that a complaint has been received, thus providing the physician an opportunity to respond. Many complaints, however, can be dismissed without prior notice to the physician.

The investigative powers of boards vary. All boards, by statute, have subpoena powers. However, successful challenges limiting subpoena powers have been made. To protect confidentiality, some state and federal laws limit discovery of records from mental health or alcohol and drug treatment centers.

The accused physician does not have the right to subpoena board witnesses for deposition or to subpoena the board's investigative files. Civil trials typically have a wide-open discovery process that seeks to uncover all the opposition's facts. However, professional disciplinary discovery proceedings are much more limited, especially before formal charges are filed.

Disciplinary proceedings after formal charges are filed. The license to practice medicine and surgery is a right substantive enough to warrant compliance with all the requirements of due process (i.e., proper notice of charges, notice of the hearing before a properly constituted tribunal, the right to cross-examine and produce witnesses, and the right to a full consideration and fair determination based on the facts).

Proper notice need not be exact and formal, but it must be sufficient to permit a full opportunity to prepare an adequate defense.[55] Hearings, which are usually required by statute to be public, are typically held before a hearing officer or, because of financial constraints, the board en bloc without a hearing officer. The structure of the hearings is controlled by statute or agency rules. Some boards employ a hearing officer who reviews the records of the investigative officers and makes findings of fact, conclusions of law, and recommendations. Other boards employ a hearing officer to sit only as a judge who rules on motions and the admissibility of evidentiary documents while the board sits as a jury. Other board cases are tried by a subcommittee of the entire board, and the subcommittee then reports its findings and recommendations to the board en bloc.

In whatever process is devised under state law, full opportunity must be given to challenge the testimony of adverse witnesses and other evidence in a proceeding before the full board.[56] The right to appear with counsel is uniform. During the pendency of the formal adjudicatory hearing, the board, as the decision-maker, must be sufficiently separated from its own investigative agents so that it may be free from bias and prejudice.[57]

The rules of evidence in a board hearing are not identical to courthouse rules of evidence. Hearsay testimony, both written and oral, is commonly admissible as long as it goes to prove an issue and sustain a finding. The evidence must be substantive. Whether the evidence must be sufficient to establish a "preponderance," a "clear preponderance," "clear and satisfactory proof," or "clear and convincing proof" varies by state.

The final decision, rendered by a hearing officer or a board en bloc, must adopt specific findings of fact, which is a concise and explicit statement of the events supporting the decision. It also must contain conclusions of law in a form that permits judicial review. Appeals to the judicial process generally are limited to reviews, not retrials. Stays pending further appeal are within the discretion of the court. Courts are sometimes prohibited by statute from granting such stays, but even then a court can intervene with a stay if the physician successfully asserts that he or she is likely to prevail on a procedural due process claim. When a board has determined its sanction, courts are generally reluctant to interfere unless persuaded that there has been a clear abuse of discretion.

Discovery. Efforts to determine the nature and extent of witnesses against a defendant physician before the time of hearing are termed *discovery*. The administrative law process normally offers opportunity for full use of normal pretrial discovery. Depositions, interrogatories, requests to produce, requests for admission, and inspection of site can be used to determine the strength and intensity of the state board's case.

Because the administrative context is sometimes more informal, legal counsel or a defendant physician may in some jurisdictions merely request copies of evidentiary documents in an informal manner to shortcut the normal, formal discovery process. Diligent legal counsel should inquire with the board attorney about specific board rules or procedures related to expediting the pretrial discovery process.

Recusal of board members. Generally, state administrative law provides a mechanism to request the recusal of any board member who "cannot accord a fair and impartial hearing or consideration."[58] Usually that request must be accompanied by an affidavit and must be promptly filed upon discovery of the alleged disqualification, stating with particularity the grounds on which it is claimed that a fair and impartial hearing cannot be accorded. This threshold issue must be determined quickly by the board.

This pretrial remedy must be exercised with care. An unsuccessful or frivolous attempt to disqualify a board member may ignite other board members' passions against the defendant physician. Historically this remedy is rarely sought in the administrative law process and is rarely granted. There is a strong presumption that the administrative tribunal is unbiased.[59] However, if evaluation of the case and the board's process indicates substantial grounds that make recusal necessary, it should be strongly considered.

Attorney fees. Some states' statutes provide that, when an administrative proceeding is brought without reasonable basis or is frivolous, the board may become liable for the licensee's attorney fees.[60] This statute is powerful. Under the proper circumstances it can be an "equalizer" to help the defendant physician retain his or her rights. Making aggressive demands for attorney fees and putting the agency on notice may give a defendant physician leverage in settlement negotiations or may result in the dismissal of charges.

Sanctions. All state boards have laws authorizing sanctions, some more detailed than others. License revocation is the most severe sanction available because its term is indefinite, usually "forever placing the offender beyond the pale."[61] Other sanctions include suspension, probation, written or oral reprimand, censure, curtailment of professional activities, and monetary fines.

Restoration of a revoked license requires a petition and review process that could take years to complete. If the cause was physician impairment and if a board so chooses, a surrendered license may be restored without protracted and formalized procedures if and when demonstrated recovery can be established. Suspension of a license is similar to a revocation, except that it is for a limited period of time.

Probation is a formalized sanction in which a formal surveillance procedure is initiated, most often as a result of mental illness or alcohol and drug abuse. Terms and conditions of probation must be set forth in the board order. Systematic and periodic reviews are implemented, typically for years, because relapse remains a valid concern years later.[62]

Reprimand (a formal and sharp rebuke) and censure (a judgment of fault and blame) are intended to induce a mending of ways. They are lenient sanctions granted when probation is deemed too severe. In practice, such actions are more effective as a means of defining minimal acceptable levels of conduct than as a means of disciplinary enforcement. Licenses may be restricted to prohibit writing any prescriptions, to prohibit writing Schedule II controlled dangerous substance prescriptions, to limit hospital practice, or to limit all practice beyond supervised positions in state hospitals or teaching centers. In the past, restricted licensure has been used to provide supervision of the wayward, but this practice has fallen from favor because of an insufficient emphasis on the rehabilitation of restricted physicians.

Sanctions are generally imposed only after the physician has received notice and an opportunity to be heard in the adversary proceeding, with witnesses, cross-examination, and the like as set forth earlier. However, if a board determines that there is an imminent and material danger to patients or public health, safety, and welfare, a summary suspension, and later hearing, can be imposed. However, the physician is entitled to a prompt, postsuspension hearing that concludes without appreciable delay.[63] Summary suspension is the single exception to the rule that sanctions are imposed only after a full hearing.

Sanctions to protect the public are the primary responsibility of the medical board. Public opinion has become increasingly critical of the paucity of revocations, inadequate supervision, and investigative impotence.[64] A perception persists that professional compassion for a colleague can sacrifice public protection and that some sanctions are inconsistent, lenient, and seemingly ineffective. Contributing factors to the inadequacy of the boards include court-issued stay orders, injunctions, appeals, new trials granted on technical grounds, inadequate financing, and resistance by defense attorneys, hospital administrators, and district attorneys.

National collectors of disciplinary data. Two national clearinghouses currently collect disciplinary data on physicians. These data are retained and made available to other boards in states where a physician may hold a license, principally in response to reports of physicians "jumping jurisdictions" after disciplinary action is taken in one state of licensure.

The Federation of State Medical Boards in Fort Worth, Texas, has maintained a national clearinghouse on physician discipline for several years.[65] The federation collects information about disciplinary actions taken by the 65 member jurisdictions and then transmits a summary of those actions to each of the other jurisdictions on a monthly basis. State medical boards can then contact a sister state and obtain details of disciplinary action taken against a physician who is also licensed in their state.

A part of the 1986 Health Care Quality Improvement Act (Pub. L. 99-660) established the National Practitioner Data Bank.[66] Like many federal projects, the data bank was initially slow to receive adequate funding and slow to get under way. The legislation included a requirement that hospitals must query the data bank at least every 2 years about all physicians on their staff. Medical boards and certain others also may query the data bank. Federal law requires medical boards and hospital staffs that impose a curtailment on a license of more than 30 days to report that incident to the data bank.

Open Meeting Act and Open Record Act. There is a traditional perception in the medical profession that medical boards should regulate and discipline in private. This belief has aroused suspicion regarding conspiracies of silence. Exposés by the media and the increasing publicity of malpractice claims have created legislative pressure to revamp the traditional regulatory process of a medical board.

Most states have enacted "sunshine laws" that include an Opening Meetings Act and an Open Records Act.[67] States also have enacted "sunset laws," which require an administrative board to reprove periodically its reason for existence to a legislative body. The purpose of these laws is to require all government agencies, including medical boards, to give advance public notice of all activities, to carry these activities out in public view, and to provide access to the press. However, most do not require that frivolous complaints become public matters, and most do not allow public inspection of board investigative records before they are made public at a hearing.[68] Some boards distribute periodic newsletters listing regulations and specific sanctions imposed on physicians, including the practitioner's name, address, and listed infractions.

Such measures are taken to assure the public that regulation is active and vigorous.

Appeals. Judicial review of an administrative decision usually is limited to determining whether the administrative agency acted arbitrarily, capriciously, or fraudulently; whether the order was substantially supported by the evidence presented; or whether the administrative agency's actions were within the scope of its legal authority as created by the statute. Although courts review a decision of law made by the administrative agency, decisions regarding the credibility of evidence and witnesses ordinarily are a matter for the administrative agency itself and are overturned only if they are clearly contrary to the overwhelming weight of the evidence. Courts seldom intervene to substitute their judgment in determining a sanction or an assessment of mitigating circumstances.

Although there is no fundamental right to appeal an administrative decision, virtually all jurisdictions grant appeal by state statute. Licensees have fought any limitation of the appeals process by arguing that such limits would compromise access to the judicial process and limit board accountability.

Typically, courts restrict appeals to the appeals process specified by statute. This restriction could result in denying judicial access until the board has had a rehearing or the petitioner has exhausted all other administrative remedies. Some statutes typically limit judicial appeals to those approved by the board, known as *by leave appeals,* as opposed to those allowed by right. Courts typically limit their scope of review to the issues of law. Rarely, however, courts have granted a new trial as part of the appeals process, as if no administrative proceeding had occurred.

As a practical matter, some state courts may choose to review cases however they like, accepting limits that suit their convenience or needs. On one hand, they may choose to protect a licensee from administrative arbitrariness with strict scrutiny.[69] On the other hand, they may choose to accept virtually all board findings with routine affirmance.

Restoration of a license. Restoration of a license after revocation or suspension is a matter of serious concern for the public, the profession, and the physician. The odds of restoration are against the physician. And the physician clearly bears the burden of proof to demonstrate that there has been a substantial change of conditions in his or her qualifications, practice methods, or both since the discipline was originally imposed. The process of reinstatement has no due process entitlements, supposedly because reinstatement rights are not substantive enough property rights to warrant such protection.[70]

A surrendered license cannot be used to avoid a restoration process and consequent hearing and sanction. Licenses so surrendered are deemed final. In suspension, as compared with revocation, resumption of practice is automatic. There also is an early automatic reinstatement for a licensee who has failed to pay a routine renewal fee.

In the restoration process, a petition must be submitted (usually after at least 1 year) to initiate a preliminary investigative process. The investigation might involve an interview of the petitioner, review of character references, and contacts with other law enforcement agencies. The board might take steps to ensure that those providing character references are fully familiar with the facts the board found that led to the initial loss of license. Board concern focuses on rehabilitation and maintenance of skills, and it always keeps the public interest in mind. If a restoration petition is denied, reconsideration, future resubmission, or court challenges are available as alternative appeals. A court appeal of a denied reinstatement petition has virtually no chance of success because the decision is left to the board's discretion. A board may require a minimum waiting period before resubmission of a reinstatement petition.

CONCLUSION

Physicians and the medical services they provide greatly affect public health, safety, and welfare. Because of that impact and the historically high-profile nature of the medical profession, state government has the authority to regulate medical education and to erect a medical licensure process. The state also exercises a continuing jurisdiction over the professional activities of licensed and practicing physicians and may impose sanctions thereon. Currently the pendulum of public opinion is swinging to favor more oversight and accountability of physicians, rather than less.

ENDNBOTES

1. Shakespeare, *As You Like It,* Act 1, Scene 3.
2. *Steinberg v. Chicago Medical School,* 354 N.E. 2d 586 (Ill. App. 1976).
3. *DeMarco v. Chicago Medical School,* 352 N.E. 2d 356 (Ill. App. 1976); *In re Florida Board of Bar Examiners,* 339 So. 2d 637 (Fla. 1970).
4. *Cannon v. University of Chicago,* 559 F. 2d 1063 (7th Cir. 1977).
5. *Alevy v. Down State Medical Center,* 384 N.Y.S. 2d 82 (1976).
6. *University of California Regents v. Bakke,* 438 U.S. 265 (1978).
7. *Craig v. Boren,* 429 U.S. 190 (1976).
8. Smith, *A Third Rate Case Shouldn't Make Hard Law,* Jurisdoctor 31 (Feb. 1978).
9. *DeFunis v. Odegoard,* 416 U.S. 312, 94 S.Ct. 1704, 40 L.Ed. 2d 164 (1974).
10. *DeFunis v. Odegoard,* 529 P. 2d 438 (Wash. 1974).
11. Pub. L. 101-336, 104 Stat. 327 (codified at 42 U.S.C. § 12101 *et seq.*). An excellent discussion of the ADA is found at Jones, *Overview and Essential Requirements of the Americans with Disabilities Act,* 64 Temple L. R. 471 (Summer 1991).
12. 42 U.S.C. § 12181.
13. *Board of Curators of the University of Missouri v. Horowitz,* 96 S.Ct. 948 (1978).
14. *Sanders v. Ajir,* 555 F.Supp. 240 (W.D. Wis. 1983).
15. *Ross v. Pennsylvania State University,* 445 F.Supp. 147 (M.D. Penn. 1978).
16. *Goss v. Lopez,* 95 S.Ct. 729 (1975).
17. *Matthews v. Eldridge,* 424 U.S. 319 (1976).
18. *Ewing v. Board of Regents University of Michigan,* 742 F. 2d 913 (6th Cir. 1984), *cert. granted* 53 U.S.L.W. 3687 (U.S. Mar. 25, 1985).
19. *Lions v. Salva Regina College,* 568 F. 2d 200 (1st Cir. 1977).
20. 42 U.S.C. § 12101 *et seq.*

21. S. Rep. No. 116, 101st Cong., 1st Sess. 22 (1989); H.R. Rep. No. 485, 101st Cong., 2d Sess. 56 (1990).
22. *Teaching Health Law, A Symposium,* 38 J. Legal Educ. 489-497, 505-509, 545-554, 567-576 (Dec. 1988).
23. J.W. Burnside, *AIDS and Medical Education,* 10 J. Legal Med. 19 (Nov. 1, 1989).
24. Allen R. Felhous & Robert D. Miller, *Health Law and Mental Health Law Courses in U.S. Medical Schools,* 15 Bull. Am. Acad. Psychiatric Law 319 (Dec. 1987).
25. *Eneklal v. Winkler,* 20 Cal. 3d 267, 142 Cal. Rptr. 418, 572 P. 2d 32 (1977).
26. *Rusk v. Akron General Hospital,* 84 Ohio App. 2d 292, 171 N.E. 2d 378 (1987).
27. *McBride v. United States,* 462 F. 2d 72 (9th Cir. 1972).
28. *Pratt v. Stein,* 298 Pa. Super. 92, 444 A. 2d 674 (1982).
29. Ben A. Rich, *Malpractice Issues in the Academic Medical Center,* 36 Del. Law J. 641-646 (Dec. 1987).
30. *Id.* at 652.
31. Harold I. Hirsch, *The Evils of Admitting Private Patients to Hospitals with Teaching Programs: A View From Outside the Ivory Tower,* 16 Legal Aspects Med. Prac. (Nov. 1988).
32. *Lawrence v. Board of Registration in Medicine,* 239 Mass. 424, 428, 132 N.E. 174 (1921).
33. *Hawke v. New York,* 170 U.S. 189, 194 (1898).
34. *Dent v. West Virginia,* 129 U.S. 114, 123 (1888).
35. *In re Hansen,* 275 N.W. 2d 700 (Minn. 1978).
36. This includes false or deceptive advertising. Many states have specific statutes and regulations providing for discipline on this ground.
37. *Brun v. Lazzell,* 172 Md. 314, 191 A. 240 (1937) (revocation of license to practice dentistry based on guilty plea to criminal charges of indecent exposure).
38. *Raymond v. Board of Registration in Medicine,* 387 Mass. 708, 443 N.E. 2d 391-394 (1982) (where the board disciplined a physician upon his conviction for possession of unregistered submachine guns the court held that "lack of good moral character and conduct that undermines public confidence in the integrity of the medical profession are grounds for discipline.").
39. *Urick v. Comm. Board of Osteopath Examination,* 43 Pa. Commw. 248, 402 A. 2d 290 (1979) (court upheld licensure revocation for committing a crime of moral turpitude where the physician was convicted of conspiracy to use the mails to defraud and conspiracy to unlawfully distribute and possess Schedule II controlled substances).
40. *Lawrence v. Board of Registration in Medicine,* 239 Mass. 424, 428, 430, 132 N.E. 174 (1921) (gross misconduct in the practice of medicine is not too indefinite as a ground for discipline).
41. Includes felonies clearly unrelated to the practice of medicine, such as income tax evasion.
42. *Withrow v. Larkin,* 421 U.S. 35 (1975).
43. Note that a statute of limitations defense was not valid to block admission into evidence in a licensure proceeding, a felony conviction more than 3 years old was admissible, even where that state required that legal actions be commenced within 3 years. *Colorado State Board of Medical Examiners v. Jorganson,* 198 Colo. 275, 599 P. 2d 869 (1979).
44. *See generally* R.P. Reaves, *The Law of Professional Licensing and Certification* 255-257 (1st ed. 1984).
45. *See, e.g., Emslie v. State Bar of California,* 11 Cal. 3d 210, 520 P. 2d 991, 1000 (1974) (rule not applied to attorney disciplinary action); *Elder v. Board of Medical Examiners,* 241 Cal. App. 2d 246, 50 Cal. Rptr. 304 (1966), *cert. denied* 385 U.S. 1001 (1967) (rule applied in disciplinary action against physician).
46. *United States v. Biswell,* 406 U.S. 311 (1972).
47. *Arthurs v. Board of Registration in Medicine,* 383 Mass. 299, 418 N.E. 2d 1236 (1981).
48. *Hyland v. Kehayas,* 157 N.J. Super. 258, 384 A. 2d 902 (1978).
49. *See Cross v. Colo. State Bar of Dental Examiners,* 37 Colo. App. 504, 508, 552 P. 2d 38 (1976) ("It is logical and sensible that where such grave charges of . . . unprofessional or dishonorable conduct are alleged, the Board has the right to preserve (any) evidence . . . of these charges otherwise witnesses may disappear and the passage of time itself may well dim or even eradicate the memory of the witnesses and thus preclude the construction of an adequate record.").
50. R.P. Reeves, *The Law of Professional Licensing and Certification* 258 (1st ed. 1984).
51. *See, e.g., Horowitz v. State Board of Medical Examiners of Colorado* 822 F. 2d 1508 (10th Cir.) (members of state medical board absolutely immune for actions in connection with suspension of podiatrist's licensure), *cert. denied* 484 U.S. 964 (1987); *Vakas v. Rodriquez,* P. 2d 1293 (10th Cir.), *cert. denied* 469 U.S. 981 (1984); *see Batz v. Economou,* 438 U.S. 478, 508-517 (1978).
52. *See Withrow v. Larkin,* 421 U.S. 35 (1975).
53. *Raymond v. Board of Registration in Medicine,* 387 Mass. 708, 714-15 (1982).
54. *3600 I. Rogers v. Texas Optometry Board,* 609 S.W. 2d 248 (Tex.) (1980).
55. *Bloch v. Ambach,* 528 N.Y.S. 2d 204 (N.Y. App. Div. 1988).
56. *Physicians and Surgeons,* 61 Am. Jur. 2d § 105 (1981).
57. *Morrissey v. Brewer,* 408 U.S. 471, 92 S.Ct. 2593, 33 L.Ed. 2d 484 (1972).
58. *See, e.g.,* 75 O.S. 1991, § 316.
59. *Schneider v. McClure,* 456 U.S. 188, 102 S.Ct. 1665, 72 L.Ed. 2d 1 (1982); *National Labor Relations Board v. Ohio New & Rebuilt Parts, Inc.,* 760 F. 2d 1443 (6th Cir.), *cert. denied* 474 U.S. 1020 (1980).
60. *See, e.g.,* 12 O.S. 1991, § 941B.
61. Derbyshire, *Offenders and Offenses,* 19 Hosp. Prac. 981 (1984).
62. Shore, *The Impaired Physician, Four Years After,* J.A.M.A. 248:3127 (1982).
63. *See Barry v. Barchi,* 443 U.S. 55, 66 (1979); *Ampueto v. Department of Professional Regulation,* 410 So. 2d 213 (Fla. D.C. App. 1982) (6-month delay in postsuspension hearing found unreasonable).
64. *See* 18 Hosp. Prac. 251 (1983) (10-year saga of a license revocation).
65. Federation of State Medical Boards, 2630 West Freeway, Suite 138, Fort Worth, TX 76102-7199.
66. Codified at 42 U.S.C. § 11101 *et seq.*
67. *See, e.g.,* 25 O.S. 1991, § 301 *et seq.,* and 51 O.S. 1991, § 24A.1i.
68. *See, e.g.,* 51 O.S. 1991, § 24A 12 *et seq.*
69. R.P. Reeves, *supra* note 50, at 276.
70. *Hicks v. Georgia State Board of Pharmacy,* 553 F.Supp. 314 (Ga. 1982), *citing Meachum v. Fano,* 427 U.S. 215, 228 (1976).

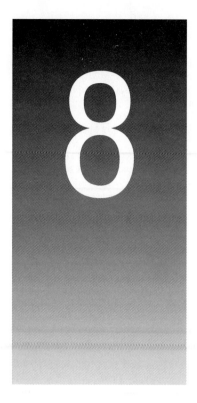

Medical staff peer review in the credentialing and privileging of physicians

MARVIN FIRESTONE, M.D., J.D.
ROBERT E. SCHUR, J.D.

MEDICAL STAFF PEER REVIEW
CREDENTIALING
PRIVILEGING
PROCTORING
DUE PROCESS
PHYSICIAN RIGHTS UNDER MANAGED CARE
APPLICATION OF DUE PROCESS PRINCIPLES
CONFIDENTIALITY AND PEER REVIEW PRIVILEGE
PEER REVIEW CORRECTIVE ACTION: AN UNFAIR PROCESS?

MEDICAL STAFF PEER REVIEW

The purpose of credentialing medical staff is to maintain quality patient care. This is an ongoing process during which the physician's training, skill, experience, and clinical competence are evaluated to ensure that the privileges granted match the physician's expertise.[1] The application of "corporate liability" concepts to hospital malpractice lawsuits after the landmark case of *Darling v. Charleston Community Memorial Hospital*[2] led to more aggressive physician peer review because hospitals could no longer deny responsibility for acts and omissions by their staff physicians. To encourage more aggressive peer review by the medical staffs, many states have enacted immunity statutes to protect hospitals' peer review committees.[3] In addition, federal law related to Medicare and Medicaid programs mandate some form of peer review if hospitals are to be compensated for services.[4] Therefore federal and state laws, regulations, and case law all emphasize a hospital's duty to monitor patient care and serve as the impetus for credentialing. The Joint Committee on Accreditation of Healthcare Organizations (JCAHO) also requires its member hospitals to have a credentialing process in place for accreditation and hold the hospital's governing board ultimately responsible for peer review by its medical staff.[5]

The Health Care Quality Improvement Act (HCQIA) of 1986 grants health care entities and peer review committees immunity from liability for credentialing and privileging activities as long as due process is afforded the affected physician. The HCQIA also established the National Practitioner

Data Bank (NPDB), an information clearinghouse regarding licensure actions, malpractice payments, and final adverse actions taken by hospitals and other health care entities that restrict physicians' practice privileges for more than 30 days. Hospitals and other health care entities must also query the NPDB when credentialing physicians for appointment and reappointment to the medical staff.

CREDENTIALING

Case law regarding credentialing generally supports the premise that a hospital could be held liable for a patient injured by a staff physician because the hospital should have known of the physician's poor performance or incompetence and failed to investigate or take reasonable corrective action. After the *Darling* case, the Wisconsin Supreme Court ruled in *Johnson v. Misericordia Community Hospital*[6] that the hospital had a duty to properly credential physicians on its staff even when the physician falsified his or her application for privileges. Similarly, in *Elam v. College Park Hospital*,[7] the court held that the hospital may be responsible for the conduct of its physicians under the doctrine of corporate negligence. These cases underscore the need for ongoing peer review to maintain quality care.

All credentialing criteria must be clearly stated in the medical staff bylaws and communicated to members of the medical staff and new applicants. Any changes adopted by the medical staff must be approved by the hospital's governing body. The medical staff bylaws should clearly identify the mechanisms and procedures to be used in the credentialing processes for appointment and reappointment. Standards for the evaluation and verification of applicant information, the delineation of privileges, and the procedures for appealing adverse decisions should also be clearly documented in the bylaws or rules and regulations of the medical staff. Applicants should not be asked for information related to gender, nationality, race, creed, sexual orientation, age, religion, ethnic origin, or any other data that can be viewed as having a discriminatory purpose. Likewise, provisions of the Americans with Disabilities Act (ADA) protect rehabilitated drug or alcohol abusers; therefore information requested of applicants should address *current* alcohol or drug abuse that has not been rehabilitated.

PRIVILEGING

The objective of the privileging decisions should be the delineation of the specific diagnostic and therapeutic procedures, whether medical or surgical, that may be performed in the hospital and the types of clinical situations to be managed by the physician. The JCAHO requires that privileges be granted before any care is provided to patients, noting that temporary privileges must be time limited. Physicians working in outpatient facilities owned or managed by JCAHO-approved health care entities are also subject to the credentialing and privileging process.

PROCTORING

For all new applicants for privileges (or additional privileges) and for physicians who may be returning to practice after a significant absence, proctoring is usually required for a time to ensure that the physician is competent to perform the procedures for which privileges are requested. Appropriate proctors should be selected and can include members of the medical staff who are noncompetitors, when possible, and senior active staff who have privileges in the same area of practice. The number of cases or length of proctoring and the method of proctoring (such as direct observation or prospective and retrospective review of cases) should be determined and communicated to the applicant in writing. The form of the proctor's report should be standardized and submitted to the department chair for periodic review. The physician being proctored should be apprised of his or her progress, including observed strengths and weaknesses, and should be given copies of any written evaluations submitted to the department chair. Final recommendations of the proctor should then be reviewed by the department chair and forwarded to the credentialing committee for final recommendation to the medical executive committee. Privileges approved by this committee should be formally granted by the governing board.

DUE PROCESS

In the context of medical staff peer review in credentialing and privileging, *due process* refers to the fair and consistent treatment of physicians who first apply for privileges or who reapply for privileges that were involuntarily restricted, suspended, or revoked. Clearly written due process procedures must be established, understood, and properly implemented by the hospital because physicians have legal rights to protect their careers. In government-owned hospitals, these rights may be found under the due process provisions of the United States and in state constitutions, but in privately operated hospitals, constitutional rights may not apply.[8]

Cases in which the power of the medical staff was abused for discriminatory or other improper motives have led some states' courts and legislatures to gradually extend legal protections to physicians whose staff privileges are attacked. Since the 1950s, the trend has been toward upholding the physician's right to fully practice his or her profession, a right that has in some states been considered "fundamental" for purposes of extending constitutional protections.[9] This view mandates fair procedures in disciplinary actions for medical staff.[10] Fair procedure includes, at a minimum, adequate notice of the charges on which the action is based and the opportunity to present evidence on one's own behalf to an unbiased decision-maker.[11] However, other protections usually found in civil and criminal actions, such as the right to cross-examine adverse witnesses and the right to be represented by counsel, have generally not been accorded in disciplinary hearings.

State laws provide for the right to legally challenge a decision restricting or terminating medical staff privileges, but judicial review may be limited by numerous factors, including the requirement that one must fully exhaust all available administrative remedies before seeking redress in the courts. Courts have traditionally shown a great deal of deference to the decisions of administrative bodies such as hospital boards and committees, even when due process may have been lacking at the administrative level, and are loathe to interfere in what is viewed as the exclusive bailiwick of hospitals and physicians.

Although many states have begun to address these issues, there is wide variance in the extent to which physicians' rights to practice in the hospital can be protected under the law. Most states, however, have done nothing to address similar problems created by managed care organizations, medical societies, and other entities that perform peer review and credentialing functions but that are not necessarily required by law to have an organized and independent medical staff.

PHYSICIAN RIGHTS UNDER MANAGED CARE

In California, the law applying to hospitals extends by statute to state medical societies, but only recently have the courts begun to extend the same protections in cases involving private insurers, health maintenance organizations, and managed care payors.[12] These cases hold that entities controlling "important economic interests" may not arbitrarily deprive a physician of privileges or contract rights without providing a fair hearing procedure, even if existing law requires that the action be reported to the state medical board or to the NPDB.[13]

In the seminal *Delta Dental* case, the court determined that the managed care organization had a duty to accord its member dentists the right to common law fair procedure in a dispute over a reduction in the payment rates because the plan was "the largest dental health plan in California, covering over 8 million individuals."[14] Thus the court apparently viewed the importance of the defendant's market power in general, rather than its impact on the plaintiff's business in particular, as controlling.

In the *Ambrosino* case that followed *Delta Dental,* the plaintiff podiatrist was terminated from participation in a managed care plan on the basis of "a short-term chemical dependency problem" that he claimed did not render him impaired to practice.[15] The plan refused to grant him a hearing because under its contract, any history of substance abuse was considered grounds for termination. The court first cited *Delta Dental* for the proposition that "[t]he common law right to fair procedures has recently been held to extend to health care providers' membership in provider networks such as that operated by defendant because managed care providers control substantial economic interests "[16] Then in determining that the *Delta Dental* criteria had been met, the court noted that approximately 15% of the plaintiff's patients were insured by defendant and concluded that therefore the plaintiff "had a common law right to fair procedures, including the right not to be expelled from membership for reasons which are arbitrary, capricious and/or contrary to public policy," notwithstanding the termination-at-will clause in the participation contract.[17]

These two cases were hailed by many as opening a new era in the law relating to managed care and physicians' rights. However, there was ample support for the *Ambrosino* decision in long-standing California case law, including the 1974 *Ascherman* case.[18] The true significance of the *Delta Dental* case seems to be that the common law right to fair procedure was accorded there despite the fact that no issue of the plaintiff's competence, fitness, or quality of care was raised; the decision to reduce payments under the plan was purely economic. The retroactive nature of the action, and consequently its effect on previously "vested" rights, also seems to have been an important factor. The California Supreme Court has recently extended the fair procedure doctrine to cases of "economic credentialing," wherein a hospital or managed care entity terminates participation on a physician plan for purely business reasons without according the affected physicians notice or a fair hearing.[19] Whether the courts will be willing to extend this doctrine to hospital privilege cases is uncertain.

APPLICATION OF DUE PROCESS PRINCIPLES

Due process requires that the right to practice medicine not be infringed on in an arbitrary or capricious manner.[20] The critical question concerns what procedures will suffice to satisfy due process requirements. Unfortunately there is no one answer to this query; due process varies according to the facts and circumstances of each case and according to the law of each jurisdiction where it is applied. The Supreme Court has stated that:

Due process is flexible and calls for such procedural protections as the particular situation demands. Consideration of what procedures due process may require under any given set of circumstances must begin with a determination of the precise nature of the government function involved as well as of the private interest that has been affected by governmental action.[20]

The nature and extent of the private interest involved are necessarily fact-based determinations based in most cases on the application of state law.

A flexible formula suggests that the type of hearing afforded may vary from case to case. Clearly, however, due process requires "some form of hearing" before an individual may be deprived of a protected interest.[21] Furthermore, it is generally accepted that "in a highly technical occupation (like the practice of medicine), the members of the profession should have the power to set their own standards. Due process requires that the evaluations of whether one gets along and meets the standards not be made in bad faith or arbitrarily and capriciously."[22] On the other hand, there is no constitutional requirement that physicians be given a formal adversarial hearing, nor even that the decision-makers be completely uninvolved in the underlying matter.[23] "The common law requirement of a fair procedure does not compel formal proceedings with all the embellishment of a court trial, nor adherence to a single mode of due process. It may be satisfied by any one of a variety of procedures which afford a fair opportunity for an applicant to present his position."[24] Under the HCQIA, peer review participants are immune from civil liability in connection with the peer review action if the affected physician is given a fair procedure under the terms outlined in the statute.[25]

Various elements constitute "fair procedure" or "due process" under the law, depending on the particular jurisdiction's legislative and judicial history of providing protection in this area. California offers what is probably the most comprehensive legislative scheme protecting the medical staff privileges of physicians (and similar property interests), as well as judicial interpretation and application of the law. For example, in California, the required hearing procedures include an unbiased hearing officer; an unbiased trier of fact, whether composed of a panel of peers or an arbitrator (or arbitrators); notice of the nature of the proposed action, the right to a hearing, and the time in which to request a hearing; notice of the reasons for the proposed action and of the fact that the action will be reported when final; and the right to inspect and copy documents to be used in support of the adverse action and to learn the identity of witnesses to be called by the representatives of the medical staff.[26] The precise methods to be followed may vary according to the rules and regulations of the institution.

Although medical staff bylaws vary from one institution to the next, most are similar in providing for an initial investigation by a credentials committee or similar body, during which the physician generally has few (if any) procedural rights but may be required to appear and answer questions in the matter; a hearing, including the basic elements previously discussed; and an appeal to the governing board of the hospital, medical society, or other institution. Medical societies have promulgated model medical staff bylaws prescribing procedures for each of these steps, and these models are generally geared toward ensuring a fair procedure for the physician whose privileges are under review.[27] Model bylaws are an excellent resource for attorneys and administrators involved in drafting and updating bylaws in any jurisdiction.

The final element of due process in adverse actions affecting staff privileges is that of judicial review. This right also varies considerably from one jurisdiction to another, again depending on each state's interpretation of *due process,* the property or liberty rights recognized, and the extent to which the courts have been willing to intervene in what have traditionally been considered private, or semi-public, concerns. Nevertheless, the majority of jurisdictions now recognize the right to obtain redress in the courts when due process is not provided by the institution with respect to medical staff privileges. Judicial review may be limited to a review of the written record of proceedings held by the peer review body or may encompass a full evidentiary hearing de novo, although the latter may be available only under limited circumstances.

CONFIDENTIALITY AND PEER REVIEW PRIVILEGE

Generally, records of peer review actions and proceedings are exempted from discovery and evidentiary use in civil actions. This may be expressed as an "immunity" from discovery, as an evidentiary "peer review privilege," or both. Exceptions may be found in cases in which a plaintiff has made a bona fide, prima facie case against the hospital for negligently credentialing the physician or in which the litigation concerns the physician's rights against the institution (as opposed to a malpractice claim). Some courts have upheld the protection against discovery in such actions, and some have not. There is also an open question as to whether, and in what circumstances, a peer review participant otherwise entitled to claim a privilege may waive it by voluntarily disclosing the records or facts pertaining to the peer review action; at least one court has held that a participant in the peer review process who may not be compelled to testify to the "privileged" matters may nevertheless do so of his own free will.[28]

Confidentiality may be ensured by means other than the law. Medical staff bylaws often require members involved in peer review proceedings to hold confidential all information and records relating to the proceedings or otherwise be subjected themselves to disciplinary action. The authors are unaware of any case challenging such a provision. However, it is important to keep in mind that in some states, the bylaws may be considered a binding contract, whereas in others the courts have not adopted that view.

Numerous instances continue to exist in which a physician's medical staff privileges may be revoked or withdrawn and due process protections cannot be invoked, such as when a hospital acts for purely business or economic reasons or some other cause that does not relate to the quality of care practiced by the physician or his or her fitness to practice. For example, courts have held that a hospital may close its staff or a particular service, such as radiology or anesthesiology, or award an exclusive contract to one physician or group while excluding all others (including those already on staff). Although such actions have occasionally been challenged on both due process and antitrust theories, these cases have failed to produce decisions limiting the hospital's discretion to make such decisions, even when the resulting effects on individual physicians are harmful or seemingly anticompetitive.[29]

PEER REVIEW CORRECTIVE ACTION: AN UNFAIR PROCESS?

Most physicians must carry hospital staff privileges in one or more facilities. The medical staff is self-policing and is independent of the hospital.[30] Its functions include reviewing the care provided by its physician members to patients and acting as a liaison between the hospital administration and individual physicians. As a peer review body, the medical staff is responsible for shielding patients from incompetent or unstable physicians; at the same time, by controlling physicians' access to both the patients and the facilities, the medical staff wields considerable power over physicians, and when that power is abused, the physician's professional reputation, standing, and license to practice may be disrupted and damaged.

Despite a growing trend toward protecting physicians' fundamental rights and interests in medical staff privileges, medical staffs continue to operate independently, without strict controls, when determining which physicians are granted credentials and which physicians should lose their credentials. At every stage of the disciplinary process, the affected physician is at a disadvantage. The disciplinary hearing under medical staff bylaws is like a malpractice action against the affected physician with one's own colleagues acting as witnesses, prosecutors, and judges. Dozens of charges involving the care of numerous patients may be leveled at one time. If the physician loses, he or she will probably have no insurance coverage against either the costs of defense or the economic impact on his or her medical practice.

There is little opportunity to obtain discovery of evidence before it is presented. The chairman of the medical executive committee usually selects the jury panel members and hearing officer (sometimes subject to the physician's challenges for bias, which may be overruled). There may be use of hearsay evidence, including medical opinions of experts who cannot be compelled to appear and be cross-examined. Frequently, the physician is denied the assistance of counsel in the hearing room and must represent himself or herself or depend on a medical colleague to act in a representative capacity. Other procedural protections, such as the right to subpoena witnesses or documents, are usually lacking, and witnesses in a peer review hearing may enjoy absolute immunity from civil suits for slander or malicious injury, even if their testimony is false.[31] The hospital and medical staff members are also immune from suit under federal law unless it is proved that they acted in bad faith when taking the peer review action.[32]

An adverse outcome for the physician may destroy his or her career. Actions adversely affecting medical staff privileges must be reported by the hospital to the state medical board, as well as the NPDB and the Healthcare Integrity and Protection Data Bank, nationwide data bases accessible to hospitals and managed care organizations.[33] The state Medical Board may then commence an investigation, finding the physician an easy target because damning evidence has already been compiled in the medical staff hearing. Although the state medical board may decide not to prosecute, in almost all cases it can do nothing to aid the physician to clear his or her name, regain staff privileges, or obtain redress for the economic, professional, and emotional injuries sustained. The physician's reputation and career may be ruined, and his or her legal recourse is extremely limited. Although physicians have sued for deprivation of hospital staff privileges on any number of legal theories, including breach of contract, various tort theories, and antitrust, these suits are difficult, costly, and rarely successful.

Although the objective of peer review is to ensure the quality of care and retention of competence of medical staff, peer review functions as performed by physician staff members who are uncompensated for their efforts retain the risk of being sued by the affected physician despite immunity statutes. In addition, peer review immunity may not necessarily be extended if a federal claim, such as antitrust or unlawful discrimination, is proved.

Clearly, there is a continuing need for improvement in the credentialing and peer review processes. Extension of procedural due process principles to all facets of peer review must be accomplished with due respect to the realities of the health care environment and marketplace. Although credentialing and peer review remain as important functions of the organized medical staff, the courts and legislatures are increasingly involved in the process. Physicians and hospitals alike should continuously assess their peer review processes in light of the evolution of the law.

ENDNOTES

1. *See generally,* F.A. Rozovsky, L.E. Rozovsky & L.M. Harpster, *Medical Staff Credentialing: A Practical Guide* (American Medical Association, Chicago, 1994).
2. *Darling v. Charleston Community Memorial Hospital,* 211 N.E. 2d 253, 260 (1965).
3. *See* Hammock, *The Antitrust Laws and the Medical Peer Review Process,* 9 J. Contemp. Health Law Policy 419 (1993).
4. Blum, *Medical Peer Review,* 38 J. Legal Educ. 525 at 531 (1988).
5. ECRI, *Medical Staff Credentialing, in Healthcare Risk Control. Risk Analysis: Medical Staff I,* Volume 3 (ECRI, Plymouth Meeting, Penn. Reissued January 1996).
6. *Johnson v. Misericordia Community Hospital,* 301 N.W. 2d 156 (Wis. 1981).
7. *Elam v. College Park Hospital,* 132 Cal.App. 3d 332, 183 Cal.Rptr. 2d 156 (1982).
8. Most states' laws still distinguish between public and private hospitals in determining whether, or to what extent, a physician is entitled to due process in respect to the termination or restriction of medical staff privileges. Others have largely eliminated this distinction, either by finding "state action" in the hospital's acceptance of federal funds, such as Hill-Burton Act payments, or by focusing on the quasipublic character of a hospital's business. *See, e.g., Ascherman v. San Francisco Medical Society,* 114 Cal.Rptr. 681 (Cal.App. 1974); *Silver v. Castle Memorial Hospital,* 497 P. 2d 564 (Hawaii 1972) (*cert. denied,* 409 U.S. 1048, *re-h'g denied* 409 U.S. 1131); *Peterson v. Tucson General Hospital, Inc.,* 559 P. 2d 186 (Ariz. Ct. App. 1976). In California the courts have expressly held that a common law doctrine of "common law fair procedure" exists and requires the same elements of fair procedure as would be required under a due process analysis. *Applebaum v. Board of Directors of Barton Memorial Hospital,* 104 Cal.App. 3d 648, 163 Cal.Rptr. 831 (1980).
9. *See, e.g., Ascherman v. San Francisco Medical Society, supra* note 8.
10. California's statutory scheme governing procedures in medical staff privileges disciplinary hearings may be found in Cal. Bus. Prof. Code, §§ 809, *et seq.*
11. *Applebaum, supra,* note 8.
12. *Potvin v. Met Life Insurance,* 22 Cal. 4th 1060, 997 P. 2d 1153, 95 Cal.Rptr. 2d 496 (2000); *Delta Dental Plan of California v. Banasky,* 33 Cal.Rptr. 2d 381 (Cal.App. 1994); *Ambrosino v. Metropolitan Life Insurance Company,* 899 F.Supp. 438 (N.D. Cal. 1995); *Hallis & Nopoletano v. CIGNA Health Care of Connecticut, Inc.* (1996), 680 A. 2d 127, *cert denied,* 137 LED 2d 308; *Paul J. Harper, MD v. Healthsource New Hampshire, Inc.,* 674 A. 2d 962 (1995).
13. *Supra* note 9.
14. *Ibid* note 12, 33 Cal.Rptr. 381, 385.
15. *Ibid* note 12, 899 F. Supp. 438, 440.
16. *Id.* note 12, 899 F. Supp. 445.
17. *Id.*
18. *Ibid,* note 12.
19. *Potvin v. Metropolitan Life Insurance Company (2000),* 22 Cal. 4th 1060, 997 P. 2d 1153, 95 Cal.Rptr. 2d 496 reaffirms *Ambrosino* by stating that the key issue in determining whether a payor entity must accord a fair procedure hearing to its members is the defendant's ability to control significant economic interests, following *Ascherman* and other existing case law.
20. *Anton v. San Antonio Community Hospital,* 19 Cal. 3d 802, 823, 567 P. 2d 1162, 140 Cal.Rptr. 442 (1977); *see also, Anton v. San Antonio Community Hospital,* 132 Cal.App. 3d 638, 183 Cal.Rptr. 423 (1982).
21. *Mathews v. Eldridge,* 424 U.S. 319, 335 96 S. Ct. 893, 963, 47 L.Ed. 2d 68 (1975).
22. *Stretten v. Wadsworth Veterans Hospital,* 537 F. 2d 361, 369, n.18 (9th Cir. 1976).
23. *Arnett v. Kennedy,* 416 U.S. 134, 94 S.Ct. 1633, 40 L. Ed. 2d 15.

24. *Pinsker v. Pacific Coast Society of Orthodontists,* 12 Cal. 3d 541, 555, 526 P. 2d 253, 116 Cal.Rptr. 245 (1974). *See also, Tiholiz v. Northridge Hospital Foundation,* 151 Cal.App. 3d 1197, 11203, 199 Cal.Rptr. 338 (1984) (procedures must ensure physician is "treated fairly"); *Cipriotti v. Board of Directors,* 147 Cal.App. 3d 144, 152, 196 Cal.Rptr. 367 (1983) (procedural protections are designed to give the physician "an opportunity to confront the witnesses and evidence against him and to present his defense").

25. 42 U.S.C. § 11112(b).

26. Cal. Bus. Prof. Code § 809, *et seq.*

27. *See, e.g.,* California Medical Association Model Medical Staff Bylaws.

28. *See, e.g., West Covina Hospital v. Superior Court (Tyus),* 226 Cal.Rptr. 132 (1986), a California Supreme Court decision narrowly holding that the state's evidence code prohibition against discovery of peer review proceedings was no bar to a participant's *voluntary* testimony (i.e., that the privilege to protect such information could be waived).

29. *See, e.g., Jefferson Parish v. Hyde,* 466 U.S. 2 (1984); *Eszpeleta v. Sisters of Mercy Health Corp.,* 800 F. 2d 119 (7th Circ. 1986); *Beard v. Parkview Hosp.,* 912 F. 2d 138 (6th Cir. 1990); *Capital Imaging Associates v. Mohawk Valley Medical Assn,* 791 F. Supp 956 (N.D.N.Y. 1992); *Anne Arundel Gen. Hosp. v. O'Brien,* 432 A.2d 183 (Md. App. 1981); *Holt v. Good Samaritan Hosp.,* 590 N.E. 2d 1318 (Ohio App. 1990); *Caine v. Hardy,* 943 F. 2d 1406 (5th Cir. 1991).

30. The Joint Commission on Accreditation of Healthcare Organizations is one source of the requirement that medical staffs be self-governing. State laws also may require that the hospital not only recognize but also require independent governance of its professional staff. *See, e.g.,* 22 Cal. Code Regs. § 70701.

31. California provides such an absolute immunity to witnesses in a peer review proceeding (Cal. Civil Code § 47(b)) and a qualified immunity to all participants who act without malice in the reasonable belief that the action is warranted by the facts (Cal. Civil Code § 43.7). Federal law extends essentially the same protections under the Health Care Quality Improvement Act, 42 U.S.C. § 11111, *et seq.*

32. Immunity is provided under the "safe harbor" provisions of the federal Health Care Quality Improvement Act of 1986 (42 U.S.C. § 11111, *et seq.*) when the peer review body observes certain minimal standards for fair procedure and acts in good faith for the purpose of furthering quality health care. 42 U.S.C. § 11112(a).

33. The NPDB was created by the Health Care Quality Improvement Act of 1986 (*supra* note 8). Hospitals and other entities responsible for credentialing physicians are required not only to report to the NPDB when taking peer review actions, 42 U.S.C. § 11132, but also to query the NPDB when granting or renewing a physician's privileges. 42 U.S.C. § 11133. The Healthcare Integrity and Protection Data Bank was recently established under the provisions of the Health Insurance Portability and Accountability Act of 1996. 45C.F.R. § 61.1.

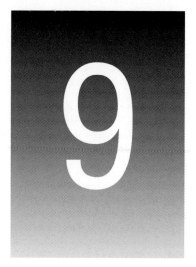

Physician as defendant in medical malpractice

PLAINTIFFS' THEORIES AGAINST PHYSICIANS
PHYSICIANS' DEFENSE THEORIES AGAINST PLAINTIFFS' CLAIMS OF NEGLIGENCE
AFFIRMATIVE DEFENSES
SETTLEMENT OF MALPRACTICE CLAIMS

The term *malpractice* refers to any professional misconduct that encompasses an unreasonable lack of skill or unfaithfulness in carrying out professional or fiduciary duties. Although the term *medical negligence* may be preferable to medical malpractice, the latter is used in this chapter because of the common and traditional usage of this term.

PLAINTIFFS' THEORIES AGAINST PHYSICIANS

Currently there are a number of legal theories or causes of action by which a patient as plaintiff may bring a lawsuit against a physician. Although negligence is the most common basis for a medical malpractice action imposing liability on a physician, physicians also may be involved in legal actions based on other legal theories. The physician must be aware that a suit often can be brought under several theories. If the plaintiff patient wins under any of these theories, recovery of a monetary award from the defendant physician may result. Alternative plaintiffs' theories against physicians are considered here after a discussion of the basic principles of medical negligence.

Medical negligence

Medical negligence is a breach of the physician's duty to behave reasonably and prudently under the circumstances that causes foreseeable harm to another. For a successful suit under a theory of negligence or in legal terms to present a cause of action for negligence, an injured patient (plaintiff) must prove each of the following four elements by the preponderance of evidence.

Duty. The first element of the negligence theory of liability is duty as created by the physician-patient relationship.

This duty requires that a physician possess and bring to bear on the patient's behalf that degree of knowledge, skill, and care that would be exercised by a reasonable and prudent physician under similar circumstances. In other words, a physician owes the patient a duty to act in accordance with the specific norms or standards established by the profession, commonly referred to as *standards of care,* to protect the patient against unreasonable risk.

A plaintiff may show that the defendant physician failed to exercise the required skill, care, or diligence by commission or omission (i.e., by doing something that should not have been done or by failing to do something that should have been done). It may not matter that the physician has performed at his or her full potential and in complete good faith. Instead the physician must have conformed to the standard of a "prudent physician" under similar circumstances.

There is no clear definition of the duty of a particular physician in a particular case. Because most medical malpractice cases are highly technical, witnesses with special medical qualifications must provide the judge or jury with the knowledge necessary to render a fair and just verdict. As a result, in nearly all cases the standard of medical care of a "prudent physician" must be determined based on expert testimony. In the case of a specialist the standard of care by which the defendant is judged is the care and skill commonly possessed and exercised by similar specialists under similar circumstances. The specialty standard of care may be higher than that required of general practitioners.

Although courts recognize that medical facts usually are not common knowledge and therefore require expert testimony, professional societies do not necessarily set the standard of care. The standard of care is an objective standard against which the conduct of a physician sued for malpractice may be measured, and it therefore does not depend on any individual physician's knowledge. In attempting to fix a stan-

The Editorial Committee updated this chapter. The committee gratefully acknowledges the past contribution of Martin B. Flamm, M.D., J.D., F.C.L.M.

dard by which the trier of fact may determine whether a physician has properly performed the requisite duty toward the patient, expert medical testimony from witnesses for both the prosecution and the defense is required. The trier of fact ultimately determines the standard of care, after listening to the testimony of all medical experts.

Breach of duty. The second element of medical negligence that must be proved by the plaintiff is that by failing to act in accordance with the applicable standard of care the defendant physician did not comply with the requisite duty, called *breach of duty.* The applicable standard of care must be proved before the plaintiff can prove that the physician breached that duty.

In most cases expert witnesses for the prosecution and the defense address the question of breach of duty while testifying as to the standard of care owed. Of course there are exceptions to every rule. Expert testimony may not be required if a plaintiff presents evidence showing that the defendant physician's substandard care is so obvious as to be within the comprehension of a layperson. Res ipsa loquitur, which literally means "the thing speaks for itself," is a legal doctrine that relieves the plaintiff from the requirement of proving duty and breach of duty through a physician expert witness. In other words, negligent care may be presumed. Res ipsa loquitur requires the plaintiff to show only that the outcome was caused by an instrumentality in the exclusive control of the defendant, that the plaintiff did not voluntarily contribute to the result, and that the injury was the type that normally does not occur in the absence of negligent care. After the plaintiff shows these elements, the burden of proof may shift to the defendant physician to prove otherwise. For example, the patient who discovers that a sponge or an instrument was left within his or her abdomen during surgery may have a res ipsa loquitur case. Causation and damages still may need to be proved by expert testimony, however.

Causation. The third element that must be proved by the plaintiff is causation. The plaintiff must show that a reasonably close and "causal connection" exists between the negligent act or omission and the resulting injury. In legal terms this relationship is commonly referred to as *legal cause* or *proximate cause.* The concept of causation differs markedly from that of medical etiology in that it refers to a single causative factor and not necessarily the major cause or even the most immediate cause of the injury, as is the case with medical causation or etiology. Although causation may seem to be an easy element for plaintiffs to prove, it is frequently the most difficult and elusive concept for the jury to understand because of the many complex issues.

Legal causation consists of two factual issues—causation in fact and foreseeability. Causation in fact may be stated as follows: An event A is the cause of another event B. If event B would not have occurred but for event A (known as the *but for test*), causation exists. This test is easily passed in some cases but not in others. Consider the following contrasting

examples. The patient with an intestinal perforation resulting from a surgeon's failure to remove an instrument from the abdominal cavity may suffer subsequent abdominal abscess, surgery, or death. But for the retained instrument, such a complication would not have occurred. In contrast, a physician's delay in the diagnosis of a highly aggressive malignant neoplasm might not necessarily affect the patient's chance of survival.

Foreseeability is the second causation issue. A patient's injuries and other damages must be the foreseeable result of a defendant physician's substandard practice. Generally the patient must prove only that his or her injuries were of a type that would have been foreseen by a reasonable physician as a likely result of the breach of the medical standard of care.

The law of causation varies widely from jurisdiction to jurisdiction, and its proof is currently in flux. In *Daubert v. Merrell Dow Pharmaceuticals* the U.S. Supreme Court addressed the admissibility of scientific evidence in a case involving expert testimony concerning causation.[1] This decision, which is followed in most jurisdictions, allows judges great discretion in deciding what scientific evidence is or is not admissible, especially as applied to the causation element.

Damages. The fourth element of the medical negligence suit is proof of damages. In general the concept of damages encompasses the actual loss or damage to the interests of the patient caused by the physician's breach of the standard of care. If the patient is not harmed, there can be no recovery. (The exception to this rule is "nominal damages," where a token sum, economically worthless, is awarded a plaintiff who has had his or her honesty, integrity, or virtue challenged and is vindicated by the satisfaction of having his or her claim honored. Although rare, the significance of an award of nominal damages is that it may serve as a prerequisite to the award of punitive damages.)

The purpose of awarding damages in a tort action is to ensure that the person who is harmed is made "whole" again or returned to the position or condition that existed before the tort. Because it is generally impossible to alleviate the effects of an injury resulting from medical malpractice, public policy demands redress through the award of monetary compensation to the plaintiff. The legal fiction is that money makes the damaged patient whole.

Damages may encompass compensation for a wide range of financial, physical, or emotional injury to the plaintiff patient. The law has recognized certain categories of damages, but categorization is often imprecise and inconsistent because some of these categories overlap and are not strictly adhered to by courts of all jurisdictions.

Compensatory damages are awarded to compensate the patient for losses. There are two types of compensatory damages—special and general. General damages are awarded for noneconomic losses, including pain and suffering, mental anguish, grief, and other related emotional complaints without any reference to the patient's specific physical injuries.

Special damages are those that are the actual but not necessarily the inevitable result of the injury caused by the defendant and that follow the injury as foreseeable and natural consequences. Typical items of special damages that are compensated by a monetary judgment include past and future medical, surgical, hospital, and other health care–related costs; past and future loss of income; funeral expenses in a case involving death; and unusual physical or medical consequences of the alleged injury, such as aggravation of a preexisting condition.

If a wrong was aggravated by special circumstances, punitive or exemplary damages, in addition to the injured patient's actual losses, may be awarded. Punitive damages, which are rarely awarded in medical negligence cases, are intended to make an example of the defendant physician or to punish his or her egregious behavior. Such damages generally are awarded when the defendant's conduct has been intentional, grossly negligent, malicious, violent, fraudulent, or with reckless disregard for the consequences of his or her conduct.

Other theories

Battery. In medical injury cases battery really is not a negligence action but an intentional tort. The law in general recognizes that an individual should be free from unwarranted and unwanted intrusion. In legal terms touching another person without that person's express or implied consent is a battery. The attempt to touch another person without consent is an assault. Assault can be considered an attempt at battery.

The law in all jurisdictions places considerable importance on this principle of personal autonomy, which traditionally has been reinforced by legislation dealing with patients' rights. In the medical setting, battery most often involves undesired medical treatment or nonconsensual sexual contact. To successfully prove a claim of medical assault or battery, the plaintiff must show that he or she was subjected to an examination or a treatment for which there was no express or implied consent. The treatment provided must be substantially different from that to which the patient agreed. There also must be proof that the departure was intentional on the part of the physician.

Unlike claims made under the negligence theory of consent, which is discussed later, there is no need to prove actual harm in battery cases, although harm may have occurred. The amount of damages of course relates directly to the amount of harm in most cases. For example, an operation that is not consented to but saves the patient's life likely will not result in damages, except in rare cases. However, if the patient suffers painful, crippling, or lingering effects, significant damages may be awarded.

Specific examples of medical battery include the performance of sexual "therapy" by a psychiatrist or other mental health care professional in the name of treatment, the unauthorized extension of a surgery to nonconsented bodily organs unjustified by the original procedure, and the nonconsensual treatment of Jehovah's Witnesses or others whose religious convictions limit therapeutic alternatives. Expert testimony regarding standard of care and breach of standard of care is not necessary in battery cases.

Although in some jurisdictions recovery still may be based on assault and battery theories, through legislation (sometimes as part of reform measures) most jurisdictions have removed the right to bring such an action because it is subsumed under other medical malpractice causes of action. This change is a result of the now nearly universal acceptance of the doctrine of informed consent. A physician may be negligent if he or she diagnoses or treats a patient without obtaining informed consent or an adequate informed consent for such a diagnostic or treatment procedure.

Informed consent. Patients must be capable of giving consent, must possess adequate information with which to reach a decision regarding a diagnostic procedure or treatment, and must be given ample opportunity to discuss alternatives with the physician. A failure to meet the requirements for an appropriate and adequate informed consent may be a departure from the recognized standard of care and may result in an action for failure to obtain "informed consent" against a health care provider.

Consent is a process, not a form. Physicians may fail in their duty to patients when they rely on a form or document for achieving "informed consent." Such a form can never replace the exchange of information between a patient and a health care provider, which is necessary to fulfill the requirements of an adequate informed consent. This topic is covered more thoroughly in Chapter 21.

Abandonment. Generally a physician has no duty to provide care to a person who desires treatment. However, a physician who agrees to treat a patient accepts the duty to provide continuity of care. Legal recognition of this duty follows from the reality that a sick or injured person is at risk until cured or stabilized. No physician can be available at all times and in all circumstances. Yet, physicians must provide an adequate surrogate when unavailable. Many physicians meet this obligation by making arrangements with a partner or nearby colleague in the same or similar field of practice. Backup may be provided by directing ambulatory patients to a nearby, physician-staffed hospital emergency department. Brief lapses of coverage are generally reasonable. For example, it is unlikely that a physician would be successfully sued for failure to attend simultaneous cardiac arrests for which no other physician was available. Physicians are sued when the unavailability of coverage for several hours harms a patient.

This duty to provide care is extinguished when the physician dies, when the patient no longer requires treatment for the illness under consideration, or when the physician gives reasonable notice to the patient of his or her intention to withdraw from the case. In the last case, however, the physician must give the patient time to arrange for care from another qualified physician or must arrange for a substitute physician who is acceptable to the patient. The original physician also must provide emergency care for the patient's condition and related medical problems until the patient has established a relationship with the new physician.

With the accelerated growth of managed health care plans, many physicians have become members of various health care networks. In some cases a physician may opt to leave a network to join another. Such an action per se does not necessarily end a physician-patient relationship, particularly if the patient opts to continue the relationship outside of the network payment scheme. Any physician who wishes to discontinue caring for patients previously seen in such a system may notify those patients of a change in managed care participation and arrange for appropriate transfer of care to a successor physician.

Breach of confidentiality. Physicians have a duty to respect the privacy interests of their patients. Generally, everything said by a patient or his or her family members to a physician in the context of medical diagnosis and treatment is confidential and may be revealed only under certain circumstances. In many states the physician-patient relationship is recognized by a statute that sets forth exceptions to the general rule of confidentiality. Some states rely on common law in this area. Each practitioner should know the rules that apply in his or her state and establish procedures for his or her employees to act accordingly.

In general, health care providers can safely release medical information to other treating physicians or consultants. In life-threatening emergencies, certain information pertinent to the patient's treatment also may be revealed to other medical personnel, even if the patient is unaware. The topic of patient confidentiality is dealt with in more detail in Chapter 22.

Breach of contract or warranty to cure. When a physician promises to effect a cure or to achieve a particular result and the patient submits himself or herself for treatment, the physician is generally liable if the treatment fails to achieve the promised result. The unhappy patient in such a situation can sue the physician in contract rather than in tort. This form of medical malpractice suit has become less common in recent decades. The major advantage for the plaintiff in a contract suit is that a medical standard of care need not be shown. The plaintiff must prove only that a promise was made and relied on, the promise was not kept, and damages resulted because of the broken promise.

The plaintiff in such a suit must prove how he or she was damaged by the physician's breach of promise. A successful plaintiff generally recovers an amount of money that would place him or her in a position comparable to the position he or she would be in had he or she not agreed to treatment. In many cases this amounts to a return of the surgeon's fees, plus a small sum for related expenses. Damages may be exceedingly high in some instances, however, such as when a professional performer is scarred or killed.

Most physicians at one time or another prognosticate for their patients. Courts understand this aspect of medical prac-

tice. Breach of contract or warranty actions usually arise when a physician sells a patient on a particular operation. To prevent a plethora of unwarranted suits, many states provide that no legal action may be taken for breach of a contract to cure unless the physician's promise is in writing.

Strict liability for drugs and medical devices. Strict liability (i.e., not negligence-based liability) is imposed on manufacturers, sellers, and distributors of unreasonably dangerous and defective products for injuries resulting from their use. Such liability is independent of negligence law, and a defendant's degree of care is irrelevant in lawsuits based on the concept of strict liability. However, the law recognizes that every drug and device used in medical practice is potentially hazardous. Therefore manufacturers, sellers, and distributors of such products are not liable for damages if they give adequate warnings about how to avoid the risks and make their products as safe as possible. These warnings must be given clearly, prominently, and in a timely manner, and they must be given to the proper person. Overpromotion of a product can negate the effect of otherwise adequate warnings.

Strict liability is dealt with in more detail in Chapter 12. Strict liability is mentioned here because many medical malpractice suits also include claims for harm caused by the physician's alleged failure to inform and adequately warn the patient of a dangerous or defective product in his or her role as "learned intermediary."

Strict liability reduces the plaintiff's burden of proof. It is much easier to prove that a product warning was not given or was inadequate than it is to show that a physician violated the standard of care. The plaintiff must show only that the product was defective or that the warning of its nondefective hazards was faulty and the deficiency of product or warning was a cause of the injury. Foreseeability is not required to make a case of strict liability against a defendant.

A strict liability case also can be brought when a defendant physician is uninsured or underinsured, and a solvent pharmaceutical house or device manufacturer may be found liable to pay a share of any judgment. Sometimes a defendant physician brings the drug manufacturer or device company into the suit as a "third-party defendant," requiring it to pay part or all of the plaintiff's damages, or the defendant treating physician also may be the seller of the drug or device.

Physician liability for the actions of other health care providers

Vicarious liability. Physicians usually employ or supervise other less qualified health care professionals. Physicians therefore owe their patients the duty to supervise nurses, technicians, and other subordinates properly. That duty may create vicarious liability, whereby one person may be liable for the wrongful acts or omissions of another. Several legal doctrines must be discussed in this context.

The simplest such doctrine is known as *respondeat superior* and states that an employer is liable for the negligence of his or her employees. For example, if a physician's office nurse injects a drug into a patient's sciatic nerve, causing injury, that patient may sue the physician for the nurse's negligence.

Physicians also may be held vicariously liable for the negligence of hospital employees they supervise under other legal doctrines. For example, surgeons have been sued for errors and omissions by operating room personnel under the "captain of the ship" doctrine. This doctrine holds a surgeon liable based on the legal action that he or she has absolute control, much like the captain of a ship at sea who is responsible for all the wrongs perpetrated by the crew. This doctrine was intended to offer a remedy to persons injured by negligent employees of charitable hospitals, which were otherwise legally immune from suit under the doctrine of charitable immunity.

The captain of the ship doctrine has been largely replaced by the "borrowed servant" doctrine in such situations. This latter doctrine holds surgeons responsible for hospital employees' negligent acts that are committed under their direct supervision and control.

Negligent referrals. Physicians today frequently request consultations from other physicians, especially regarding hospitalized patients. A referring physician usually is not liable for the negligence of the specialist. However, the referring physician may be liable for the specialist's misdeeds if each physician assumes the other will provide certain care that is omitted by both or if they neglect a common duty (e.g., postoperative care).

Physicians cannot attend or be available to all patients at all times. They have the duty to provide another physician to care for their patients when they cannot. Just as physicians generally are not liable for consultants' malpractice, they need not answer for care provided by other physicians who cover their practice. Exceptions include the use of covering physicians who are also partners and the negligent selection of covering physicians.

False imprisonment

False imprisonment is a tort that protects an individual from restraint of movement. False imprisonment may occur if an individual is restrained against his or her will in any confined space or area. The plaintiff is entitled to compensation for loss of time, for any inconvenience suffered, for physical or emotional harm, and for related expenses.

A physician holding a patient against his or her will, in absence of a court order, could be held liable for false imprisonment. Such situations arise in cases involving involuntary commitment of a patient with a mental disorder, where a patient is held without compliance with laws governing civil commitments.

Defamation

A statement is defamatory if it impeaches a person's integrity, virtue, human decency, respect for others, or reputation and lowers that person in the esteem of the community or deters third parties from dealing with that person. A defamatory statement can be made either in writing, which is called *libel,* or in verbal communication, which is called *slander.*

In general, truth is an absolute defense to defamation. Some jurisdictions have a rule that a statement that is substantially true, when published with good motives and justifiable ends, shall be a sufficient defense, even though it may not be literally true. For example, if a physician states publicly that a nursing home has 50 complaints against it and there were only 30, the statement likely would not be held defamatory.

Failure to warn and control

The failure of a physician to warn the patient or a third party of a foreseeable risk is a separate and distinct negligent act. A physician's duty of care includes the duty to identify reasonably foreseeable harm resulting from treatment and, if possible, to prevent it. It is increasingly recognized that a physician has the responsibility to warn patients of dangers involved in their care. Failure to advise the patient of known, reasonably foreseeable dangers leaves the physician open to liability for harm the patient suffers and injuries that patient may cause to third parties.

The courts have imposed the duty to warn on a physician when medications with potentially dangerous side effects are administered. If an administered drug might affect a patient's functional abilities (such as ambulation), the physician is obliged to explain the hazard to the patient or to someone who can control the patient's movements (e.g., family members or others who can reasonably be expected to have contact with the patient). The same duty is owed to patients engaged in any activity that may be hazardous, such as driving a car or operating machinery.

Similarly, when a physician learns that a patient has or may have a medical condition with dangerous propensities that may impair the patient's control of his or her activities, the physician has a duty to warn the proper persons, such as the patient's family members or others in contact with the patient. This duty to warn may apply whether the condition is completely diagnosed or is still under study.

In a number of cases physicians have been held liable to injured third parties for failure to warn them of the potentially dangerous mental condition of a patient. Similarly, patients' next of kin have successfully sued after the patients committed suicide, which could have been foreseen and potentially prevented by a physician.

Failure to report

Every jurisdiction has a list of diseases that must be reported to the authorities. The physician's failure to conform to the statutory requirement may make him or her liable for criminal penalties. Failure to report also has been held to be negligence per se (not requiring proof of negligence) in civil suits brought by injured patients or third parties.

Statutes in many states also require physicians to report battered children and abused elderly patients to the proper authorities. The physician is generally exempt from any civil or criminal liability for making a report pursuant to the terms of the statute. If the physician fails to report such abuse, he or she may be held liable to any individual who is damaged by this failure.

PHYSICIANS' DEFENSE THEORIES AGAINST PLAINTIFFS' CLAIMS OF NEGLIGENCE

A defendant physician can defeat a negligence claim by showing the absence of one or more of the requisite elements for the patient to prove medical negligence.

Absence of duty

The first defense to a negligence case is an attempt to show that there is no duty owed to the patient by the physician. If a physician can show that no physician-patient relationship exists, this "no duty" defense may suffice to defeat the plaintiff's action.

Physicians generally have no duty to treat new patients or patients of years past, with some exceptions. In some cases, even though a physician treats or diagnoses a condition, a duty exists only between the physician and the patient's employer (e.g., in certain occupational settings in which a physician, such as a plant physician, is employed).

In general, courts rarely hold that the "no duty" defense applies and have even held that a simple telephone consultation between a physician and emergency department personnel may be sufficient to create a professional relationship between the physician and patient, with the attendant requirements to comply with such duty.

A physician who wishes to withdraw from the care of certain patients, plans to relocate his or her practice, or simply retires must notify affected patients in a manner that an ordinary and reasonably prudent physician would do so in the same circumstances. Such notice is best made in writing and mailed postage paid to the patient's last known address. All patients receiving ongoing care for potentially serious ailments should be notified by certified mail, return receipt requested, at the last known address. Such patients should be informed that their physician will continue to see them for emergencies during a certain fixed and reasonable period of time. The physician may recommend a successor physician, provide a list of suitable physicians, or offer to forward records or copies of records (at reasonable or no cost) to another physician chosen by the patient.

In practice, when a physician retires or moves and sells his or her practice to a succeeding health care provider, patients' records are often sold as part of the transaction. However, physicians should be warned that many states have medical record retention acts, and these acts usually do not provide an exception for record-keeping requirements even in such a transfer. In such jurisdictions, physicians had best comply with statutory law and provide copies or keep copies of all pertinent records for the required statutory period. Although such medical retention statutes typically do not impose penalties for violation of the record-keeping act, physicians should follow such act or at an absolute minimum protect themselves by keeping such records for the minimum period of time for which they can be sued for medical negligence. Absent fraud, once the statutory period of limitations for filing a medical malpractice suit has passed or prescribed, physicians still may wish to check with their medical malpractice insurers concerning disposal of records to prevent waiver of any rights under the liability insurance carrier's rules.

No breach of duty (compliance with the standard of care)

A physician also must controvert the second element of the plaintiff's proof of negligence—breach of the standard of care. Because the plaintiff has the burden of proof, if all expert testimony and other evidence are equally balanced, the defendant physician will prevail.

Because rules of evidence generally prevent nonphysicians from testifying about the medical standard of care, the physician should attempt to prove compliance with the standard of care through the testimony of a credible medical expert. Because the trier of fact usually considers treating physicians (other than the defendant) credible, both the plaintiff patient and the defendant physician may seek to recruit one of the treating physicians to give supportive testimony. In practice, especially in past years, nondefendant treating physicians were often reluctant to appear, particularly if they received referrals from the defendant physician or were otherwise socially or professionally connected with him or her. For this reason, physicians engaged to testify for the plaintiff often are nontreating physicians who have no personal connection with the parties.

Because physicians are not insurers against harm or guarantors of a favorable outcome, defense to this element is that the defendant physician used the skill and knowledge common to other physicians in the specialty and applied such skills appropriately under the circumstances. Although there may have been a bad result, the bad result occurred in spite of the acceptable care being provided. Testimony that the defendant was available to the patient, interviewed and examined the patient appropriately, formed a reasonable differential diagnosis, performed the indicated tests to establish a diagnosis and rule out potentially more serious conditions, referred the patient for appropriate consultations in a timely manner, formed a reasonable diagnosis, treated the patient appropriately, adequately followed the case, and nevertheless made an error of judgment does not prove that he or she necessarily violated the standard of care, even though the patient may have been injured.

Other sources of evidence, in addition to expert testimony, include medical textbooks and other published medical data.

The admissibility of such evidence as proof of the standard of care varies among jurisdictions.

Medical texts or treatises may be effectively used to cross-examine the adverse medical expert; such cross-examination is accomplished by framing a proposition in the exact language used by the author of the medical text and asking if the witness agrees or disagrees. In such a situation of course the text must first be endorsed as being authoritative and relevant to the issue under consideration. Medical negligence cases tried in federal court, under the federal rules of evidence, allow statements from authoritative texts or medical journals to be read directly into evidence.

The defendant physician is not necessarily held to a standard of care advocated by the patient's medical experts. If there are alternative methods of diagnosis or treatment and a substantial minority of physicians agree with such alternatives, the physician may not be found negligent for using such alternatives, even though the majority of physicians do not adhere to such an alternative. In other words, employing a different method of diagnosis or treatment from that commonly used is not by itself evidence of a violation of the standard of care, especially if a "substantial minority" of "respected" physicians would have acted similarly under similar circumstances.

Lack of causation

The plaintiff cannot recover damages from a defendant physician unless the physician's malpractice caused the plaintiff's injuries. Under most theories of recovery, a plaintiff is required to prove that such malpractice was the actual cause-in-fact of injuries and that those damages were reasonably foreseeable. This element frequently affords an adequate defense for the physician, particularly in cases involving the misdiagnosis of cancer.

Traditionally the patient cannot be compensated for a delay in diagnosis and treatment if the delay did not materially affect the outcome of the disease. For example, a minimal delay in the diagnosis of a fatal high-grade malignancy may not have made a difference in the patient's outcome and therefore would not be compensable. In other words, death would have ensued despite earlier diagnosis and treatment. Jurisdictions following this traditional approach hold that in such a situation a plaintiff cannot recover any damages unless he or she can prove that there was a greater than 50% chance of survival if the diagnosis had been made earlier and treatment had been more timely.

Recently a growing trend has been to allow recovery "for loss of a chance" of a cure or improved outcome. Thus some jurisdictions allow a plaintiff's case to reach the jury even if the patient did not have a greater than 50% chance of survival or improved outcome in the absence of the physician's negligence. This loss of a chance doctrine, when applied by these courts using a "relaxed causation" or "substantial reduction" standard, focuses on the degree to which the defendant physician "cost" the plaintiff access to an improved chance of survival or recovery. The measure of damages is based on the portion of harm suffered by the patient as a result of the delay. The physician's defense is to controvert or minimize, through expert testimony, the percentage allocated to his or her delayed diagnosis.

Some jurisdictions no longer require plaintiffs to show that they have already suffered an actual loss because of a delay in diagnosis and treatment but require only some potential loss. In these jurisdictions the lost chance is viewed as a separate form of compensable injury. The focus is not on the ultimate physical harm but rather on the increased risk of harm because of the lost opportunity. In such "separate injury" jurisdictions the lower burden of proof allows the plaintiff recovery even if the plaintiff has been treated and is apparently healthy at the time of trial. Again, the physician's defense in these jurisdictions is to minimize or negate, through expert testimony, such risk of future problems.

No damages

The prevention or reduction of awarded damages is the defendant's primary goal in a lawsuit. To recover a monetary award, a plaintiff must introduce testimony and other evidence of damages, which often is difficult. In some cases the patient receives insurance or government benefits to cover expenses. In states that have eliminated the "collateral source" rule, evidence of such payment may reduce or obviate monetary damages.

AFFIRMATIVE DEFENSES
Contributory negligence, comparative negligence, and comparative fault

Under common law a patient's contributory negligence acted as a complete bar to any recovery for the negligent act of the defendant physician, no matter how slight the patient's negligence as compared with the physician's. This doctrine of contributory negligence was created to avoid "rewarding" persons for their own folly and to reduce the likelihood of collusion in suits between parties.

To avoid the potential for harsh results, however, contributory negligence as a concept has been largely replaced by the doctrine of comparative negligence. This innovation requires the trier of fact to determine the relative negligence of each party to a lawsuit and requires the judge or jury to assess monetary awards accordingly. Some states permit a plaintiff to recover only if the negligence of the plaintiff is less than that of the defendant.

A physician's duty to prevent harming the patient often is considered greater than any duty of the patient's. Only in limited circumstances can a physician escape liability as a result of a patient's negligence. For example, a diabetic patient who continues participation in a hazardous sport, despite a physician's clear warnings to cease participation, and suffers a secondary complication of the diabetes that results in injuries may pose such a case. However, defendant physicians have great difficulty proving negligence of the plaintiff. Rarely do the courts consider such socially destructive acts as smoking and drinking alcohol during pregnancy negligence on the part of the patient.

Comparative fault is a more recent legal doctrine designed by courts to allow apportionment of damages among negligent defendants. Some jurisdictions have experimented with various tests, including allocating damages based on a comparison of causation among all parties. In this case previous rules regarding contribution and indemnification among defendants have been rewritten. This area of the law currently is evolving.

Sovereign (government) immunity

In medieval times the concept that "the King can do no wrong" allowed the state to escape liability. As a consequence, if the state could do no wrong, its employed physicians and government hospitals could not be sued for malpractice. This was the law until relatively recently, when both federal and state governments passed tort claims acts that now allow suits against the sovereign and its representatives with some restrictions and limitations of damages. These statutes permit individuals who have been negligently injured by government workers, including government-employed physicians, to sue and recover from the government sometimes only after special notice or claim is first denied.

Statute of limitation

The idea that misdeeds must be litigated within a reasonable time is the basis for statutes of limitations. Plaintiffs are held to a duty to bring suit before the passage of time makes defense an unreasonable burden. The deadline for filing and serving certain legal claims varies from state to state, and different theories of recovery (i.e., felonies, breach of contract, torts, disputes over land ownership) may have different statutes of limitations.

The statute of limitation for medical negligence is generally the same as for other unintentional torts. If an injured patient sues a physician after the time set forth in the applicable statute of limitation has passed, the defendant may be entitled to dismissal.

The time allowed for filing suit is said to run from the date the negligence is discovered, which may present a special problem when the negligence was an omission or when injuries are apparent only after a long period. Most states stop or "toll" the running of time set forth in the statute during periods when the plaintiff would not be legally competent to commence the lawsuit without great difficulty. Examples include situations in which the plaintiff is a minor or is mentally incompetent. Other causes for such "tolling" include cases in which the physician fraudulently concealed the misdeed or continued to care for the patient beyond the limitation period.

Exculpatory agreements and indemnification contracts

Exculpatory agreements between physicians and patients appear to relieve the physician of liability for negligence. Although such contracts occasionally are upheld in other theories of liability, they are consistently struck down in the medical malpractice context. The rationale for not acknowledging such agreements is simply that they are contracts of adhesion. The fact that an ill patient is not in a position to negotiate terms or to reach a fair meeting of the minds, which is essential for a binding contract equity, dictates such an approach.

Contracts of indemnification usually arise between physicians and other individuals or institutions. For example, a hospital may agree to pay (indemnify) any damages incurred by the president of its medical staff for any liability resulting from carrying out the duties of that office. Conversely the chief of anesthesiology may agree to indemnify the hospital for any malpractice damages arising from the operation of the department, if no hospital employee is found to be negligent. Both types of contracts are generally upheld and effectively transfer enormous financial burdens from one party to another. Although such agreements often are represented as standard terms in an employment contract, they must be considered carefully.

SETTLEMENT OF MALPRACTICE CLAIMS

Practical aspects of defending any particular malpractice claim dictate the need for consultation with counsel and the malpractice insurer. In most cases a malpractice insurer provides counsel under the policy to defend the claim. Although a physician may believe that the best time to settle a malpractice claim (from his or her point of view) is at the time such claim occurs, procedural matters and substantive matters must be considered, and the physician's personal legal counsel may be able to give the best advice on this point.

The physician should contact his or her professional liability carrier as soon as there is even a suggestion of a potential claim and ask for a representative to handle the matter. The physician should always insist that an attorney rather than a claims adjuster handle the matter, even if the physician is willing to admit fault. Private counsel also should be retained to handle potential liability not covered by the policy or to advise the physician regarding negotiating a settlement in the course of the litigation. This advice is particularly important because the Health Care Quality Improvement Act of 1986 requires that the settlement of any medical malpractice claim for any amount in excess of $1 be reported.[2]

In practice, negotiation and settlement of a medical malpractice claim rarely occur before the phase of formal discovery procedures, which occur during the months between the filing of the suit and the scheduled trial. Discovery measures include interrogatories; requests for admissions; requests for production of documents or other items, such as x-ray films or fetal monitoring strips; and depositions of parties and witnesses. These measures are useful for ferreting out information; the prosecution and defense counsel use the same methods to determine the nature of the opposing party's case.

ENDNOTES

1. *Daubert v. Merrell Dow Pharmaceuticals,* 61 U.S. 6W 4805 (1993).
2. Health Care Quality Improvement Act, 42 U.S.C. §§ 11101 *et seq.* (1986).

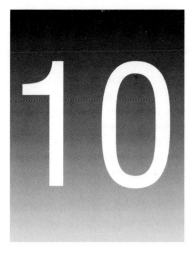

Medical testimony and the expert witness

JOSEPH D. PIORKOWSKI, Jr., D.O., J.D., M.P.H., F.C.P.M., F.C.L.M.

GENERAL RULES OF ADMISSIBILITY
SPECIAL CONSIDERATIONS
CONCLUSION

The use of medical experts in litigation has increased dramatically in recent years. In medical malpractice and product liability cases, expert testimony usually is necessary to establish one or more of the essential elements of a civil claim or defense. Similarly, in the criminal context, expert testimony generally is required to support claims of incompetency or insanity, and such testimony may be necessary to resolve issues about a defendant's potential for future dangerous behavior. Even when expert testimony is not required to prove an essential element of a claim or defense, medical experts increasingly are used to explain complex scientific concepts and aid the fact finders' understanding of the evidence.

Much of the popularity of using medical experts undoubtedly stems from the special status the law accords expert witnesses. "Unlike an ordinary witness, . . . an expert is permitted wide latitude to offer opinions, including those that are not based on first-hand knowledge or observation."[1] Because experts today can both offer opinions on ultimate questions of fact and explain fully the bases of their opinions, an expert witness provides a useful vehicle for a skilled trial lawyer to review the evidence on a particular issue and present it in a cogent and concise form for the jury.

At common law the presentation of expert testimony was rather cumbersome. Preliminarily the expert's background, training, and education were reviewed, and the court determined whether the witness was competent to render the proffered opinions. If the witness was found to be competent, the presentation of his or her direct testimony proceeded as a strictly regulated hypothetical question. A Florida court described the common law procedure for presenting an expert witness' direct testimony as follows:

When an expert is called upon to give an opinion as to past events which he did not witness, all facts related to the event which are essential to the formation of his opinion should be submitted to the expert in the form of a hypothetical question. No other facts related to the event should be taken into consideration by the expert as a foundation for his opinion. The facts submitted to the expert in the hypothetical question propounded on direct examination must be supported by competent substantial evidence in the record at the time the question is asked or by reasonable inferences from such evidence.[2]

The rationale for this procedure was that "[a]dherence to this form for the direct examination of an expert prevents the expert from expressing an opinion based on unstated and perhaps unwarranted factual assumptions concerning the event; facilitates cross-examination and rebuttal; and fosters an understanding of the opinion by the trier of fact."[3] In practice the use of hypothetical questions was tedious and came under harsh criticism. Wigmore's treatise on evidence contains the following sharp critique:

It is a strange irony that the hypothetical question, which is one of the few truly scientific features of the rules of evidence, should have become that feature which does most to disgust men of science with the law of evidence. The hypothetical question, misused by the clumsy and abused by the clever, has in practice led to intolerable obstruction of truth. In the first place, it has artificially clamped the mouth of the expert witness, so that his answer to a complex question may not express his actual opinion on the actual case. This is because the question may be so built up and contrived by counsel as to represent only a partisan conclusion. In the second place, it has tended to mislead the jury as to the purport of actual expert opinion. This is due to the same reason. In the third place, it has tended to confuse the jury, so that its employment becomes a mere waste of time and a futile obstruction.[4]

Rules 702 through 705 of the Federal Rules of Evidence (known as *the Rules*), enacted in 1975, simplify greatly the requirements for the admissibility of expert testimony. The Rules eliminate the requirement that evidence of the facts relied on by the expert be admitted into evidence; indeed the

Rules expressly permit an expert to rely on facts that are inadmissible. The Rules also obviate the necessity for using hypothetical questions, although hypothetical questions are still permissible. Most states eventually have followed the lead of the Rules as applied by the federal courts in eliminating at least some of the common law requirements. Although a great deal of variability still exists between states, the general trend since 1975 has been toward fewer procedural restrictions on the admissibility of expert testimony.

The first section of this chapter reviews the courts' approach to resolving frequently raised questions concerning the admissibility of medical or scientific expert testimony. Although this chapter focuses primarily on medical experts, cases interpreting the law dealing generally with expert testimony are discussed where useful. The major issues include (1) whether the subject matter of the expert's opinion is appropriate to the case, (2) whether the expert is sufficiently qualified to render the proffered opinion, (3) what types of information provide a proper basis for an expert witness' opinion, (4) the role of general consensus in the scientific community in evaluating the admissibility of expert testimony, and (5) other limitations that exist regarding the types of opinions experts can express. The second section of this chapter reviews some special considerations, including expert testimony in the form of medical literature, the "reasonable degree of medical certainty" standard, discovery of expert witnesses' opinions, and ethical considerations relating to the use of experts.

GENERAL RULES OF ADMISSIBILITY

The law governing the admissibility of expert testimony should be understood in light of two important background considerations. First, a constant tension exists in the law of evidence between two competency principles. One principle holds that deficient or problematic evidence should be inadmissible. Another principle holds that any problem or deficiency in evidence should affect only the weight given to that evidence rather than its admissibility. In no other area of the law of evidence is this tension so pronounced as in the area of expert testimony. Many of the rules reflect compromises between these two jurisprudential approaches.

Second, the trial judge is accorded broad discretion to determine whether expert testimony should be admitted or excluded in a given case. A trial court's decision of inadmissibility will be affirmed on review unless it is "manifestly erroneous."[6]

The subject matter of the expert's opinion

Under the common law, courts took a restrictive view of when expert testimony was appropriately admitted as evidence. The standard articulated in *Hagler v. Gilliland* represents the traditional test: "The admissibility of expert opinion evidence is governed by the rule that such evidence should not be admitted unless it is clear that the jurors themselves are not capable, from want of experience or knowledge of

the subject, to draw correct conclusions from the facts proved. It is not admissible on matters of common knowledge."[7,8] Stated somewhat differently, courts held that "the subject matter must be so distinctively related to some science, profession, business or occupation as to be beyond the ken of the average layperson."[9] If the subject matter was not beyond the ken of the average layperson, the opinion was deemed unnecessary and therefore inadmissible.

The standard articulated in the Rules, which has been adopted in form or in substance by most state courts, is much less hostile to expert testimony than the common law standard. Rule 702 provides, "If scientific, technical, or other specialized knowledge will assist the trier of fact to understand the evidence or to determine a fact in issue, a witness qualified as an expert by knowledge, skill, experience, training, or education, may testify thereto in the form of an opinion or otherwise."[10]

As interpreted by the courts, Rule 702 has three distinct requirements. First, the testimony must be composed of scientific, technical, or other specialized knowledge.[11] Second, the testimony must assist the fact finder in understanding the evidence or resolving a factual dispute in the case.[12] Third, the witness must be qualified to render the opinion. These three requirements are considered in greater detail in the following sections.

Requirement one: scientific knowledge. In *Daubert v. Merrell Dow Pharmaceuticals* the U.S. Supreme Court addressed the first of Rule 702's three prongs and noted that "[t]he subject of an expert's testimony must be scientific . . . knowledge."[13] The court explained that

The adjective "scientific" implies a grounding in the methods and procedures of science. Similarly, the word "knowledge" connotes more than subjective belief or unsupported speculation. The term "applies to any body of known facts or to any body of ideas inferred from such facts or accepted as truths on good grounds." Of course, it would be unreasonable to conclude that the subject of scientific testimony must be "known" to a certainty; arguably, there are no certainties in science. But, in order to qualify as "scientific knowledge," an inference or assertion must be derived by the scientific method. Proposed testimony must be supported by appropriate validation (i.e., "good grounds") based on what is known. In short, the requirement that an expert's testimony pertain to "scientific knowledge" establishes a standard of evidentiary reliability.[14]

The *Daubert* court emphasized that the approach to scientific knowledge is flexible.[15] "Its overarching subject is the scientific validity—and thus the evidentiary relevance and reliability—of the principles that underlie a proposed submission."[16] The court also noted that the inquiry must be directed to the principles and methodology used by the expert in reaching his or her conclusions and not to the conclusions themselves.[17]

To provide guidance to trial judges confronted with the question of whether proposed testimony constitutes scientific knowledge, *Daubert* identified four factors that bear on the inquiry but do not represent "a definitive checklist or test."[21] First, the court stated that "a key question to be answered in determining whether a theory or technique is scientific knowledge . . . will be whether it can be (and has been) tested."[22] The second factor is "whether the theory or technique has been subjected to peer review and publication."[23] Third, the known or potential rate of error for a particular scientific technique may be an appropriate consideration. Finally, the degree of acceptance of a theory or technique within the relevant scientific community may aid in determining whether expert testimony is admissible under Rule 702.

In *Kumho Tire Co. v. Carmichael* the U.S. Supreme Court clarified that the four factors articulated by the court in *Daubert* are neither exhaustive nor necessarily applicable in every case.[24] The list of factors set forth in *Daubert* "was meant to be helpful, not definitive."[25] The determination as to "whether *Daubert's* specific factors are, or are not, reasonable measures of reliability in a particular case is a matter that the law grants the trial judge broad latitude to determine."[26]

Requirement two: assisting the jury. The second prong of the subject matter inquiry is whether the expert's specialized knowledge will assist the jury in understanding the evidence or determining a fact in issue. The fact that expert testimony may not be necessary to prove an element of a claim or defense does not preclude its admissibility if the testimony is otherwise helpful to the trier of fact. "Helpfulness is the touchstone of Rule 702."[27]

Courts are divided on the question of whether expert testimony is admissible under Rule 702 when the subject matter of the testimony is within the knowledge or experience of laypersons. In *Ellis v. Miller Oil Purchasing Co.* the U.S. Court of Appeals for the Eighth Circuit reviewed a ruling in which the trial judge had excluded expert testimony by a qualified accident reconstruction expert.[28] The trial judge had determined "that the expert was in no better position than the jury to determine the answer."[29] In upholding the ruling the Eighth Circuit stated that "[w]here the subject matter is within the knowledge or experience of laypeople, expert testimony is superfluous."[30]

Other courts have reached the opposite conclusion. The U.S. Court of Appeals for the Third Circuit has stated that "there is no requirement that expert testimony be 'beyond the jury's sphere of knowledge.'"[31] In *Carroll v. Otis Elevator Co.* the U.S. Court of Appeals for the Seventh Circuit likewise upheld the admissibility of expert testimony on matters within the jury's ken.[32] The Seventh Circuit considered the admissibility of the testimony of an experimental psychologist with expertise in human behavior and perception. At trial the expert had testified that "brightly colored, red objects attract small children," that "[t]his elevator's red stop button was more brightly colored than others" and thus "was more attractive to small children than others," that "a covered stop button is less accessible to children than this uncovered one," and that "the more difficult a button is to push the less read-

ily it is actuated by a small child." In affirming the trial court's decision to admit this testimony, the Seventh Circuit stated that "[w]hile it is true that one needn't be B.F. Skinner to know that brightly colored objects are attractive to small children and that covered buttons or those with significant resistance are more difficult to actuate by little hands, given our liberal federal standard, the trial court was not 'manifestly erroneous' in admitting this testimony."[33]

The U.S. Supreme Court has declared that the requirement that expert testimony assist the trier of fact to understand the evidence or determine a fact in issue goes primarily to relevance. The court stated that "expert testimony which does not relate to any issue in the case is not relevant and, ergo, nonhelpful."[34]

Requirement three: the expert's qualifications. Rule 702 provides that a witness can be qualified by knowledge, skill, experience, training, or education. However, a witness need not demonstrate all of these bases to qualify as an expert.[35] In some cases practical experience alone has been held to be a sufficient basis for qualifying as an expert witness.[36] "Whether a witness is qualified as an expert can only be determined by comparing the area in which the witness has superior knowledge, skill, experience, or education with the subject matter of the witness' testimony."[37]

In the context of medical and scientific testimony, the court's approach to an expert's qualification often depends on the nature of the opinion at issue. In malpractice cases courts generally require that an expert witness rendering testimony on the medical standard of care be a physician, although courts have been less restrictive in permitting nonphysician witnesses to offer opinions on causation.[38]

[A] distinction must be made between testimony as to cause and testimony relative to the standard of care required of the physician. One need not necessarily be a medical doctor in order to testify as to causation. However, . . . [u]nless the conduct complained of is readily ascertainable by laymen, the standard of care must be established by medical testimony. Medical testimony means testimony by physicians.[39]

At common law, an expert testifying about the medical standard of care was required to demonstrate familiarity with the standard in the geographic location in which the defendant physician practiced. That requirement has been relaxed in numerous jurisdictions in cases in which the standard of care is the same throughout the United States.[40] Not all courts, however, follow the more liberal approach.[41]

A physician does not have to be board certified or even a specialist in a particular field of medicine to render an opinion about the standard of care applicable to that field.[42] "The training and specialization of the witness goes to the weight rather than admissibility of the evidence, generally speaking."[43]

An essential prerequisite to offering an opinion about the standard of care, however, is that the expert witness be familiar with the standard of care for the medical problem or procedure at issue.[44] "[M]ore than a casual familiarity with the specialty of the defendant physician is required. The witness must demonstrate a knowledge acquired from experience or study of the standards of the specialty of the defendant physician sufficient to enable him to give an expert opinion as to the conformity of the defendant's conduct to those particular standards."[45]

In *Hartke v. McKelway,* for example, the plaintiff, over the defendant's objection, was permitted to introduce the testimony of a physician regarding the standard of care for performing laparoscopic cauterization of the fallopian tubes.[46] Although the expert had performed several hundred tubal ligations, she had never performed a laparoscopic cauterization, had never assisted in the performance of such surgery, and had observed such an operation only twice. The appellate court noted that laparoscopic cauterization was a new procedure that was significantly different from the tubal ligation procedure. The court held that "[h]er reading of literature and conferring with other physicians on the eve of trial did not qualify her" and she "should not have been allowed to testify about the standard of care for laparoscopic cauterization."[47] The court concluded that "to give an opinion on whether the defendant complied with the applicable standard of care, the witness must be familiar with that standard."[48]

Similarly, in *Northern Trust Co. v. Upjohn Co.,* the court held that a specialist in emergency medicine and internal medicine was not competent to testify regarding the standard of care to be applied to a defendant, a specialist in obstetrics and gynecology.[49] The court did not make its decision, however, on the basis of the expert witness' field of specialization. Rather, the court examined the expert's knowledge, skill, experience, education, and training to determine whether he was adequately qualified to render an opinion on a pregnancy interruption procedure. The court stated:

He had never worked in an obstetrical or gynecological ward, had attended patients delivering babies "on occasion," but apparently had never been involved in pregnancy interruption procedures. He had never used the drug [that was administered to plaintiff], never seen it used and never observed the reactions of a patient receiving the drug. In fact, he had never had any experience with the drug in any manner and had not even read the insert and profile for the drug until he was asked to testify in [this] case.[50]

The court concluded that the expert "was not qualified to give an opinion . . . since he could not know what was customary practice for someone in [the defendant physician's] position."[51]

In *Smith v. Pearre* the Maryland Court of Special Appeals held that the trial court correctly excluded the testimony of a witness who was admittedly an expert in surgery.[52] The issue in the case involved the standard of care applicable to gastroenterologists. The expert witness was familiar with the standard of care for gastroenterologists at Yale University School of Medicine where he was a professor, but he was not familiar with the national standard of care for gastroenterologists.[53] The court stated that "[w]hile it is well established that a physician may render an opinion on a medical standard of care outside his own specialty, the witness must nevertheless possess the necessary qualifications and sufficient knowledge."[54]

In *Hedgecorth v. United States* the trial court considered whether two physicians—an ophthalmologist and an emergency medicine specialist—were qualified to give expert testimony regarding the standard of care for performing cardiac stress tests even though they were not cardiologists.[55] The court made a specific finding that both physicians "have demonstrated to this court that they are familiar with the appropriate standard of care with regard to stress tests. The fact that [these physicians] are not cardiologists does not render their testimony on stress testing inadmissible, but merely goes to the weight given it by . . . the trier of fact."[56]

The principle that emerges from these cases is that a physician's qualification to offer testimony on the standard of care in a particular case does not depend on the witness' title or field of specialization. Rather, it depends on whether the physician has sufficient familiarity with the standard of care applicable to the particular medical problem or procedure at issue to assist the trier of fact in determining the standard of care in the case.

Courts generally have been more receptive to receiving the testimony of nonphysician expert witnesses when the proffered testimony involves the issue of causation. In *Owens v. Concrete Pipe and Products Co.,* for example, the court determined that two experts in chemistry and pharmacology, both of whom had considerable experience in toxicology, should be permitted to testify "concerning topics such as the risks associated with varying degrees of exposure to certain chemicals."[57,58] The court stated that "[t]o the extent that their expert testimony is proffered for the purpose of establishing or rebutting causation, and is based on their knowledge of the chemicals rather than on a medical diagnosis of plaintiff's condition, their evidence is admissible."[59] Other courts have reached similar conclusions.[60]

In *Gideon v. Johns-Manville Sales Corp.,* the U.S. Court of Appeals for the Fifth Circuit considered whether the trial court properly admitted the testimony of the plaintiff's expert, "a biostatistician and epidemiologist specializing in the study of the causes of disease and its effects upon individuals and the public" in an asbestos case.[61] The defendants had objected that the nonphysician witness had given "medical testimony."[62] The court noted that the witness had not testified about the plaintiff's physical condition or prognosis. In affirming the trial judge's ruling admitting the testimony, the court concluded that the witness was qualified to render opinions about risk of cancer, decreased life expectancy associated with asbestosis, and the date when the toxic effects of inhaling asbestos were first known.[63]

Although courts generally have required that witnesses testifying about medical diagnoses must have medical training, they occasionally have permitted nonphysicians to offer opinions about a diagnosis when the witness' education, training, and experience demonstrate that the witness' opinion will assist the trier of fact. For example, in *Jackson v. Waller,* a case involving the contest of a will, the court permitted an optometrist to testify about the progressive nature of cataracts he observed while examining the testatrix's eyes for the purpose of fitting her for glasses.[64]

Jenkins v. United States involved an appeal of a criminal conviction in a case in which the defendant had relied solely on the defense of insanity.[65] The defendant had introduced the testimony of three psychologists, two of whom testified that the defendant's mental illness was related to his crime. The trial court instructed the jury that "[a] psychologist is not competent to give a medical opinion as to a mental disease or defect." The U.S. Court of Appeals for the District of Columbia Circuit reversed the defendant's conviction, stating "The determination of a psychologist's competence to render an expert opinion based on his findings as to the presence or absence of mental disease or defect must depend upon the nature and extent of his knowledge. It does not depend upon his claim to the title "psychologist."[66]

The court acknowledged that "[m]any psychologists may not qualify to testify concerning mental disease or defect. Their training and experience may not provide an adequate basis for their testimony."[67] Nonetheless, the court noted that "the lack of a medical degree, and the lesser degree of responsibility for patient care which mental hospitals usually assign to psychologists, are not automatic disqualifications."[68]

One common theme runs through all of these cases: "[T]he trial judge should not rely on labels, but must investigate the competence a particular proffered witness would bring to bear on the issues, and whether it would aid the trier of fact in reaching its decision."[69] When an expert is asked to render multiple opinions, the determination of whether the expert is qualified normally should not be made on an all-or-nothing basis. Rather, "expert opinion must be approached on an . . . opinion-by-opinion basis, and the court must . . . carefully examine each opinion offered by the expert to assess its helpfulness to the jury."[70] An expert may be qualified therefore to render some opinions but unqualified to render others.

In *Flanagan v. Lake,* for example, an appellate court considered whether a registered nurse was qualified to offer expert testimony on the issue of causation.[71] Although the court ultimately agreed with the trial court that the nurse was not qualified to offer such testimony, the court at the same time noted that the nurse would have been qualified to offer expert testimony concerning breaches of the standard of care allegedly committed by the nursing staff.[72]

Similarly, in *Perkins v. Volkswagen of America, Inc.,* a product liability case, the issue was the admissibility of testimony given by a specialist in mechanical engineering who had no experience in designing entire automobiles.[73] The U.S. Court of Appeals for the Fifth Circuit affirmed the trial court's decision to allow the expert to render opinions on general mechanical engineering principles but not to allow him to testify as an expert in automotive design.[74]

The foundation of the expert's opinion

At common law, ensuring that an expert's opinion had an adequate factual foundation presented little problem. Unless the expert was testifying on the basis of first-hand observation (as in the case of a treating physician testifying about his or her patient's diagnosis), the facts on which an expert's opinion was based generally had to be admitted into evidence before the expert could state an opinion. Thus the jury always had before it the expert's opinion, as well as all the testimony, records, and other evidence on which the expert's opinion was based.

The Rules relax the requirement that the underlying facts and data be admissible in evidence. Rule 703 provides that "the facts or data in the particular case upon which an expert bases an opinion or inference may be those perceived by or made known to the expert at or before the hearing. If of a type reasonably relied upon by experts in the particular field in forming opinions or inferences upon the subject, the facts or data need not be admissible in evidence."[75]

Rule 703 thus continues to permit experts to base their opinions on the traditional foundations (i.e., personal knowledge or facts made known to them at trial). However, Rule 703 expands the common law rule by permitting experts to base opinions on facts that have not been admitted into evidence and that are themselves inadmissible. The Advisory Committee explained the rationale behind this modification as follows:

[T]he rule is designed to broaden the basis for expert opinions beyond that current in many jurisdictions and to bring the judicial practice into line with the practice of the experts themselves when not in court. Thus a physician in his own practice bases his diagnosis on information from numerous sources and of considerable variety, including statements by patients and relatives, reports and opinions from nurses, technicians, and other doctors, hospital records, and X-rays. Most of them are admissible in evidence, but only with the expenditure of substantial time in producing and examining various authenticating witnesses. The physician makes life-and-death decisions in reliance upon them. His validation, expertly performed and subject to cross-examination, ought to suffice for judicial purposes.[76]

Rule 703 thus creates the anomalous situation of an expert being permitted to rely on inadmissible facts or data as the foundation for an admissible opinion. To ensure that the basis of the expert's opinion is reliable, the facts or data must be "of a type reasonably relied upon by experts in the particular field in forming opinions or inferences upon the subject."[77] Whether the facts or data are "of a type reasonably relied upon" is to be determined by the trial court. "Though courts have afforded experts a wide latitude in picking and choosing the sources on which to base opinions, Rule 703 nonetheless requires courts to examine the reliability of those sources."[78]

Before *Daubert,* federal courts were divided on the proper level of judicial scrutiny for evaluating whether an expert's opinion was based on facts or data of a type reasonably relied on by experts in the field. Judge Weinstein's decision in *In re "Agent Orange" Product Liability Litigation* summarizes the competing schools of thought:

Courts have adopted two judicial approaches to Rule 703: one restrictive, one liberal. The more restrictive view requires the trial court to determine not only whether the data are of a type reasonably relied upon by experts in the field, but also whether the underlying data are untrustworthy for hearsay or other reasons. The more liberal view . . . allows the expert to base an opinion on data of the type reasonably relied upon by experts in the field without separately determining the trustworthiness of the particular data involved.[79,80]

At issue in *Agent Orange* was whether expert witnesses proffered by the plaintiffs who were relying on symptomatology checklists completed by the plaintiffs and "prepared in gross for a complex litigation" were basing their opinions on facts or data of a type reasonably relied on by physicians.[81] The court found that such checklists "are not material that experts in this field would reasonably rely upon and so must be excluded under Rule 703."[82]

This court's reasoning reflected the restrictive approach.[83] In particular, the court did not defer to the expert on the question of whether the facts or data he relied on were of a type reasonably relied on by experts in the field. Rather, the discussion focused on the pivotal role of the trial judge in assessing the foundation of the expert's opinion. "[T]he court may not abdicate its independent responsibilities to decide if the bases meet minimum standards of reliability as a condition of admissibility. If the underlying data is so lacking in probative force and reliability that no reasonable expert could base an opinion on it, an opinion which rests entirely upon it must be excluded."[84]

Factual foundation. Regardless of the type of information on which an expert's opinion is based, courts generally require that an expert's opinion have an adequate factual foundation. "The trial court's examination of reasonable reliance by experts in the field requires at least that the expert base his or her opinion on sufficient factual data, not rely on hearsay deemed unreliable by other experts in the field, and assert conclusions with sufficient certainty to be useful given applicable burdens of proof."[85]

At common law the trial judge could easily enforce this foundation requirement. If factual assumptions were included in a hypothetical question but no evidence was contained in the record to support the existence of the assumed facts, an objection to the hypothetical question would be sustained and the expert's opinion would not be admitted.

Under the Rules, expert testimony lacking an adequate factual foundation usually has been excluded by Rule 703 (for reasons discussed previously), Rule 401, Rule 403, or some combination thereof.[86] Rule 403, which is discussed later in the section on Additional Limitations, permits the trial judge to balance the evidence's probative value against other concerns to determine the admissibility of the evidence. Obviously an expert's opinion that has no factual basis has little if any probative value and thus can properly be excluded. "[E]ven if a witness is eminently qualified, even if there is merit to his views, and even if [Rules] 702, 703, 704, and 705 are most liberally interpreted, there must be and ought to be some reliable factual basis on which the opinions are premised."[87] Although expert testimony that lacks a foundation should properly be excluded by the trial court, it is also generally accepted that "the relative weakness or strength of the factual underpinning of the expert's opinion goes to weight and credibility, rather than admissibility."[88]

The decision of the U.S. Court of Appeals for the District of Columbia Circuit in *Richardson v. Richardson-Merrell, Inc.* illustrates how courts assess whether an expert's opinion has an adequate factual foundation.[89] In *Richardson* the plaintiffs alleged that the administration of the antinausea drug doxylamine/pyridoxine (Bendectin) during pregnancy caused their child's birth defects. After a trial resulting in a jury verdict in favor of the plaintiffs, the trial judge granted judgment notwithstanding the verdict in favor of the defendant. The trial court concluded that the plaintiffs' expert's opinion lacked "a genuine basis, 'in or out of the record,'" and "that his 'theoretical speculations' could not sustain the [plaintiffs'] burden of proving causation."[90]

The Court of Appeals in *Richardson* agreed that the plaintiffs' expert's opinions did not have an adequate foundation. The court stated, "Whether an expert's opinion has an adequate basis, and whether without it an evidentiary burden has been met, are matters of law for the court to decide."[91] The court proceeded to analyze the adequacy of the foundation of the plaintiffs' expert's opinion. The court noted that the expert had "predicated his opinion upon four different factors: (1) chemical structure activity analysis, (2) in vitro (test tube) studies, (3) in vivo (animal) teratology studies, and (4) epidemiological studies."[92] The court determined that the first three types of studies "cannot furnish a sufficient foundation for a conclusion that Bendectin caused the birth defects at issue in this case."[93] The court then noted that "the drug has been extensively studied and a wealth of published epidemiological data has been amassed, none of which has concluded that the drug is teratogenic."[94] The plaintiffs' expert was able to establish a statistically significant association between Bendectin and the injury at issue only by "recalculating" epidemiological data previously published in peer-reviewed scientific journals.[95] Several other courts have reached conclusions similar to *Richardson.*[96]

Medical causation. Since *Daubert,* in cases involving medical causation issues courts seem to have changed the heading under which they perform their analyses; rather than considering whether an expert opinion has an adequate factual foundation under Rule 703, courts now appear to be considering whether the opinion is "derived from scientific knowledge" under Rule 702. Substantively, however, the analyses appear essentially identical with the critical focus being reliability of the expert's testimony.

In *Porter v. Whitehall Laboratories, Inc.,* for example, the Seventh Circuit considered a trial court's order granting summary judgment based on the need for the plaintiff to prove causation through expert testimony and the inadmissibility of the expert testimony proffered.[97] The case revolved around whether ibuprofen use could cause rapidly progressive glomerulonephritis (RPGN). One expert offered only a "curbside opinion" as opposed to "an analytical, scientific opinion." A second expert could not offer his opinion to a reasonable degree of medical certainty. The third expert "admitted that if his personal hypothesis turned out to be correct, it would be the first case in history in which ibuprofen caused RPGN." A fourth expert admitted that his proffered opinion was outside his area of expertise.[98] The trial court, in holding that the testimony of the proffered experts was inadmissible, had "posited that the expert must be able to compare the data at hand with a known scientific conclusion or relationship."[99] In affirming the ruling the Seventh Circuit stated: "If experts cannot tie their assessment of data to known scientific conclusions, based on research or studies, then there is no comparison for the jury to evaluate and the experts' testimony is not helpful to the jury."[100]

Similarly, in *Chikovsky v. Ortho Pharmaceutical Corp.* the Court considered the admissibility of an expert's opinion that the drug tretinoin (Retin-A) is a teratogen.[101] The court noted that the expert was not aware of any published study or treatise that found that tretinoin caused birth defects.[102] Although the expert testified that the dose is relevant in determining whether a substance can act as a teratogen, he knew of no studies that provided a basis for concluding that the plaintiff could have received a sufficient dose of tretinoin to cause such effects.[103] Finally, although the expert contended that vitamin A (a chemically related compound) could cause fetal harm when administered to pregnant women in some doses, he did not know at what level vitamin A became unsafe and he had "performed no comparisons between the dose of vitamin A in the study and that found in Retin-A."[104] The court concluded "as a matter of law that [the expert's] opinions are not based on scientifically valid principles and, therefore, do not meet the reliability requirements of Rule 702 as interpreted by the Supreme Court in *Daubert.*"[105]

The analysis of the adequacy of a scientific expert's factual foundation appears to reach the same conclusion regardless of whether the analysis is conducted under the rubric of Rule 702 or Rule 703.[106] Whether an expert witness' opinion has an adequate factual foundation is an issue that arises most often in the context of medical causation opinions. The issue also can arise, however, in other contexts, such as standard of care opinions.

In *Davis v. Virginian Railway Co.,* for example, the U.S. Supreme Court reversed a judgment in favor of the plaintiff arising from a medical malpractice claim.[107] The court held that "[n]o foundation was laid as to the recognized medical standard for the treatment [at issue]." The court held that the opinion of the plaintiff's expert that "he did not 'think that [the treatment] is proper'" did not provide an adequate foundation for a jury to determine the applicable standard of care.[108]

In *Stokes v. Children's Hospital, Inc.* the court granted judgment as a matter of law in favor of the defendant because the plaintiff's expert "was required to lay the foundation as to 'the recognized medical standard'" but failed to do so.[109,110] The court noted that "[I]n a case in which expert testimony is required, it is insufficient for the expert to state his opinion as to what he or she would have done under similar circumstances. . . . Rather, the jury must be informed of 'recognized standards requiring the proper . . . procedures under the circumstances.'"[111]

The role of "general acceptance" of scientific evidence. For the past several decades, many federal and state courts have held that before medical or scientific expert testimony can be admitted into evidence the principles from which the expert's opinions were derived must have attained general acceptance within the relevant scientific community. This standard was first articulated in *Frye v. United States,* an appellate decision from the District of Columbia Circuit, and has been referred to as the *Frye test.*[112] The Frye test has been applied to testimonial evidence and all forms of scientific evidence.

In *Frye* the court considered and rejected the admissibility of results of a systolic blood pressure deception test (a precursor of the polygraph). The court stated:

Just when a scientific principle or discovery crosses the line between the experimental and demonstrable stages is difficult to define. Somewhere in this twilight zone the evidential force of the principle must be recognized, and while courts will go a long way in admitting expert testimony deduced from a well-recognized scientific principle or discovery, the thing from which the deduction is made must be sufficiently established to have gained general acceptance in the particular field in which it belongs.[113]

The *Frye* court recognized that jurors can be unduly influenced by evidence that purports to be "scientific." Such evidence by its very nature carries with it an aura of accuracy and reliability. The Frye test was intended to protect jurors from placing excessive stock in scientific evidence until the principles from which the evidence was derived have gained general acceptance in the appropriate scientific community. "The requirement of general acceptance in the scientific community assures that those most qualified to assess the general validity of a scientific method will have the determinative voice."[114]

The Frye test, however, has encountered many difficulties in application.[115] Whether the evidence sought to be admitted has gained general acceptance in the appropriate field can depend on whether the "field" is defined broadly or narrowly. Also, courts have never adequately defined what constitutes "general acceptance." Although courts have recognized that *Frye* "does not require unanimity of view," no clear standard has emerged for measuring "general acceptance" among the relevant scientific community.[116]

The Rules, which were enacted more than half a century after the *Frye* decision, do not mention the Frye test or any need for scientific evidence to be generally accepted as a precondition to admissibility. Federal Courts of Appeal were sharply divided for years on the issue of whether the Frye test survived the enactment of the Rules. Some courts reasoned that no common law of evidence survived the enactment of the Rules and that the drafters of the Rules intended to abolish *Frye*. Other courts reasoned that the Rules were not intended to be an exhaustive codification of the law of evidence. These courts reasoned that the drafters would not have overruled such a well-accepted, long-standing standard without so much as a comment in the Advisory Committee Notes or a statement in the legislative history.

The U.S. Supreme Court finally resolved the question in *Daubert*.[117] The court held that the Frye test was superseded by the adoption of the Rules. The court made it clear, however, that the Frye "general acceptance" test was one of many factors bearing on the reliability of an expert's methodology. The court stated that "'general acceptance' can yet have a bearing" on the question of whether evidence is sufficiently reliable to justify its admission.[118] The court stated:

A "reliability assessment does not require, although it does permit, explicit identification of a relevant scientific community and an express determination of a particular degree of acceptance within that community." Widespread acceptance can be an important factor in ruling particular evidence admissible, and "a known technique which has been able to attract only minimal support within the community," may properly be viewed with skepticism.[119]

The Frye test continues to be important for another reason. State courts, which are not governed by the Rules, may still employ the Frye test. The Supreme Court of Florida, for example, in a post-*Daubert* decision asserted the continuing vitality of *Frye* as the standard for the admissibility of scientific evidence in Florida.[120]

Additional limitations

Three other limitations on the admissibility of expert testimony warrant brief mention. First, expert witnesses are not permitted to offer legal conclusions. Second, expert witnesses cannot express opinions about the credibility of other witnesses. Third, expert testimony, like all evidence, can be excluded if its probative value is substantially outweighed by other specific considerations.

At common law, expert witnesses were prohibited from giving opinions that embraced an ultimate issue; the rationale was that permitting experts to opine on an ultimate issue would invade the province of the jury. Rule 704 modified the common law rule, stating: "[t]estimony in the form of an opinion or inference otherwise admissible is not objectionable because it embraces an ultimate issue to be decided by the trier of fact." Thus under Rule 704 an expert is permitted to offer an opinion on an ultimate issue of fact.[121]

Rule 704 did not, however, open the door to experts opining on legal conclusions. As the U.S. Court of Appeals for the Fifth Circuit explained in *Owen v. Kerr-McGee Corp:*

Rule 704, however, does not open the door to all opinions. The Advisory Committee notes make it clear that questions which would merely allow the witness to tell the jury what result to reach are not permitted. Nor is the rule intended to allow a witness to give legal conclusions. [A]llowing an expert to give his opinion on the legal conclusions to be drawn from the evidence both invades the court's province and is irrelevant.[122]

Despite the seemingly simplistic distinction between permissible expert testimony on ultimate issues of fact and prohibited expert testimony on conclusions of law, courts have had great difficulty distinguishing between the two in practice. Moreover, courts have not been consistent in applying any set of standards to differentiate opinions of ultimate fact from legal conclusions.

The second limitation is that experts cannot express opinions about the credibility of other witnesses.[123] Evaluating the credibility of witnesses is exclusively the function of the jury. Several courts have excluded expert opinions that effectively tell the jury which witnesses to believe; such opinions are deemed both unhelpful and irrelevant.

In *State v. McCoy,* for example, the Supreme Court of Appeals of West Virginia reversed a defendant's rape conviction based in part on the testimony of a psychiatrist who stated that the alleged rape victim was "still traumatized by this experience."[124,125] The court stated that the psychiatrist's "testimony amounted to a statement that she believed the alleged victim and by virtue of her expert status she was in a position to help the jury determine the credibility of the most important witness in a rape prosecution."[126] The court determined that the psychiatrist's testimony encroached "too far upon the exclusive province of the jury to weigh the credibility of the witnesses and determine the truthfulness of their testimony."[127] The court concluded that "admission of her testimony was reversible error."[128]

Courts have held, however, that expert testimony is not inadmissible simply because it may have the indirect effect of bolstering another witness' credibility.[129] "Much expert testimony tends to show that another witness either is or is not telling the truth. That fact by itself does not render the testimony inadmissible."[130]

The third limitation is that, in addition to satisfying the standards on the admissibility of expert testimony imposed by Rules 702 though 705 of the Rules, expert testimony must not violate any of the other rules governing the admissibility of evidence at trial. A frequent obstacle to the admissibility of expert testimony is Rule 403, which provides: "Although relevant, evidence may be excluded if its probative value is substantially outweighed by the danger of unfair prejudice, confusion of the issues, or misleading the jury, or by considerations of undue delay, waste of time, or needless presentation of cumulative evidence."[131]

As the U.S. Supreme Court has noted: "Expert evidence can be both powerful and quite misleading because of the difficulty in evaluating it. Because of this risk, the judge in weighing possible prejudice against probative force under Rule 403 of the present rules exercises more control over experts than over lay witnesses."[132]

Thus even if an expert witness is qualified, the testimony would be helpful, and the basis is proper, the trial court has the discretion to exclude the witness' testimony if it would cause unfair prejudice, confuse the issues, mislead the jury, or waste time.

Preliminary questions of admissibility

An important practical issue with respect to the testimony of medical experts is how a litigant procedurally challenges the admissibility of expert testimony. Courts' practices vary greatly. Some courts require in limine motions concerning such matters to be filed well in advance of trial. Other courts permit challenges to an expert witness' qualifications to be raised for the first time when the witness takes the stand.

Some courts have held that before excluding expert testimony based on Rule 702, 703, or 403 the trial court must hold an in limine hearing to establish a sufficient factual record to support its decision. For example, in *In re Paoli R.R. Yard PCB Litigation* the U.S. Court of Appeals for the Third Circuit reversed a district court's original order granting summary judgment in favor of the defendants because the trial court's rulings excluding evidence pursuant to Rules 702 and 703 were not supported by a sufficiently detailed factual record.[133,134] The Third Circuit also "reversed the district court's Rule 403 determinations, holding that Rule 403 exclusions should not be granted pretrial absent a record which is 'a virtual surrogate for a trial record.'"[135]

On remand in *Paoli,* after a period of discovery, defendants again moved in limine to exclude the opinions of plaintiffs' experts and for summary judgment. The district court, pursuant to Rule 104(a) of the Rules, held 5 days of in limine hearings.[136] At the hearing, three of the plaintiffs' experts testified and 10 physicians and scientists testified for the defense as to the reliability of plaintiffs' experts' opinions.[137] The district

court "filed extensive opinions (totalling 330 pages) setting forth not only findings of fact but also its reasons for again excluding the vast bulk of plaintiffs' expert evidence."[138] In affirming in part and reversing in part the district court's rulings, the Third Circuit implicitly approved the manner in which the district court conducted the Rule 104 hearing.[139]

Similarly in *Hall v. Baxter Healthcare Corp.* the court held a hearing pursuant to Rule 104(a) that "spanned 4 intense days" at which "experts on both sides were questioned by counsel, the court, and the [court's] technical advisors."[140,141] (The court appointed as "technical advisors" experts in the fields of "epidemiology, rheumatology, immunology/toxicology, and polymer chemistry.") The issue in *Hall* involved the admissibility of the plaintiffs' experts' opinions that atypical connective tissue disease had been caused by the plaintiff's silicone gel breast implants. In addition to holding an evidentiary hearing, the parties provided the court with videotaped summations and proposed questions to guide the court's technical advisors in evaluating the experts' testimony.[142] The court's technical advisors then submitted reports, and both sides were provided with an opportunity to question them.

In *Kumho Tire,* the U.S. Supreme Court stated that the "abuse of discretion" standard of review applied both to the "trial court's decisions about how to determine reliability" and to "its ultimate conclusion."[143] The Supreme Court noted that "[o]therwise, the trial judge would lack the discretionary authority needed both to avoid unnecessary 'reliability' proceedings in ordinary cases where the reliability of an expert's methods is properly taken for granted and to require appropriate proceedings in the less usual or more complex cases where cause for questioning the expert's reliability arises."[144]

These decisions provide some guidance to trial courts grappling with the appropriate scope of a hearing to decide pretrial motions in limine in a complex case.

SPECIAL CONSIDERATIONS
Use of medical and scientific literature as evidence

All state and federal courts in the United States allow medical literature to be used for some purposes at trial. The traditional rule was that learned treatises and articles could be used during cross-examination to impeach or contradict the testimony of a testifying expert; such materials could not, however, be admitted as substantive evidence because of the prohibition against hearsay.

"Virtually all courts have, to some extent, permitted the use of learned materials in the cross-examination of an expert witness."[145] Courts vary greatly, however, on what threshold requirement must be met before such materials can be used for impeachment. Courts generally permit a treatise or article to be used for impeachment if the witness relied specifically on that treatise or article in forming his or her opinions.[146] Other courts permit a treatise or article to be used for impeachment in the absence of the witness' reliance if the witness acknowledges that the source is a recognized authority in the field. Still other courts permit such material to be used for impeachment even if the witness being impeached does not acknowledge the source as a recognized authority, if the authoritativeness of the source can be established through the testimony of other witnesses or by judicial notice.[147]

The admissibility of medical and scientific literature as substantive evidence has been the focus of heated debate. Opponents of admissibility argue that (1) the field of medicine changes so rapidly that treatises quickly become dated, (2) the trier of fact may be unable to understand complex technical passages that may be presented out of context, (3) the author is not available for cross-examination, and (4) medical literature is unnecessary as substantive evidence when live expert witnesses are available.[148]

On the other hand, proponents of the substantive admissibility of medical literature argue that (1) treatises generally are more up to date than live experts; (2) attorneys will be able to protect against confusion, the selective presentation of material, or passages being presented out of context; (3) cross-examination is not necessary when a live expert is available to explain the treatise or article; (4) the scrutiny of the peer review process lends a high degree of reliability to opinions or conclusions published in peer-reviewed scientific literature; and (5) the author of a treatise or medical article has no interest in the outcome of the particular case at issue.[149]

The proponents of admissibility succeeded in recent years in having the absolute prohibition against the substantive admissibility of medical literature replaced with a more liberal standard in the Rules in about half of the states. Rule 803(18) of the Rules is representative of the prevailing standard.

Although Rule 803(18) creates an exception to the hearsay rule for medical literature, it addresses the concerns of the opponents of admissibility and contains provisions to alleviate some of these concerns. For example, Rule 803(18) requires that the statements in the medical literature sought to be admitted either be "relied upon by the expert witness in direct examination" or "called to the attention of an expert witness upon cross-examination." This requirement ensures that an expert witness is available to explain the passage introduced into evidence, thereby diminishing the concern about the author's unavailability for cross-examination. Rule 803(18) also requires that the proponent of the evidence demonstrate that the source is "established as a reliable authority" through either the testimony of the witness on the stand, another expert witness, or judicial notice. Finally, Rule 803(18) provides that "the statements may be read into evidence but may not be received as exhibits."[150] This provision helps to ensure that the jury does not give undue weight to medical literature vis-á-vis the testimony of live expert witnesses. This requirement also ensures that the jury will not rely on any portion of the treatise or article other than the passages admitted by the court.

The "reasonable degree of medical certainty" standard

Some courts require that an expert hold opinions on causation and prognosis with "a degree of confidence in his conclusions sufficient to satisfy accepted standards of reliability."[151] "A doctor's testimony can only be considered evidence when he states that the conclusion he gives is based on reasonable medical certainty that a fact is true or untrue."[152]

Courts are in general agreement that expert testimony stating that a conclusion is "possible" does not meet the standard for admissibility with respect to the party who bears the burden of proof.[153] "A doctor's testimony that a certain thing is possible is no evidence at all. His opinion as to what is possible is no more valid than the jury's own speculation as to what is or is not possible."[154]

Courts differ, however, as to how much certainty is enough to constitute "a reasonable degree of medical certainty." Some courts have held that the standard requires only that the conclusion is more probably true than not; this formulation renders the phrase synonymous with "more probable than not." Such courts often permit experts to testify in terms of a "reasonable probability."[155] Other courts reject that standard. In *McMahon v. Young,* the court stated:

Here, the only evidence offered was that [plaintiff's condition] was "probably" caused [by defendant's conduct], and that is not enough. Physicians must understand that it is the intent of our law that if the plaintiff's medical expert cannot form an opinion with sufficient certainty so as to make a medical judgment, there is nothing on the record with which a jury can make a decision with sufficient certainty so as to make a legal judgment.[156,157]

Regardless of which standard they apply, courts generally look to the substance of an expert's testimony rather than the form in determining whether the witness has testified with the requisite degree of certainty. In *Matoff v. Ward* the Court of Appeals of New York stated:

Granted that "a reasonable degree of medical certainty" is one expression of . . . a standard [of a witness's degree of confidence in his or her conclusions] and is therefore commonly employed by sophisticates for that purpose, it is not, however, the only way in which a level of certainty that meets the rule may be stated. [T]he requirement is not to be satisfied by a single verbal straightjacket alone, but, rather, by any formulation from which it can be said that the witness' "whole opinion" reflects an acceptable degree of certainty. To be sure, this does not mean that the door is open to guess or surmise.[158,159]

Discovery of the expert witness' opinions

The Rules' elimination of many of the common law restrictions regarding the admissibility of expert testimony was premised on the belief that the adversarial system is capable of exposing the deficiencies in an expert's opinions. The drafters of the Rules recognized, however, that advance knowledge of the expert's opinions and the bases of the opinions is "essential for effective cross-examination."[160]

In civil cases, Rule 26 of the Rules "provides for substantial discovery in this area, obviating in large measure the obstacles which have been raised in some instances to discovery of findings, underlying data, and even the identity of the experts."[161] The majority of states also provide for ample discovery of the opinions of testifying experts. However, a few states, such as New York and Oregon, severely restrict pretrial discovery of the identities and opinions of testifying experts.

The law regarding discovery of testifying expert witnesses in civil cases currently is quite varied. The Federal Rules of Civil Procedure (FRCP) were amended December 1, 1993. The Rules as amended (called *the new Rules*) have not been adopted by all U.S. district courts; some federal courts continue to follow the rules that were in effect before December 1, 1993 (called *the old Rules*). Some federal courts permit the attorneys by agreement to opt out of the new Rules and continue to use the old Rules. Most state courts continue to use discovery provisions that closely parallel the old Rules.

Although a detailed review of the law regarding discovery of expert witnesses is beyond the scope of this chapter, a brief review of the applicable provisions of Rule 26 of the old Rules and the new Rules is useful. Under the old Rules, discovery pertaining to experts who were expected to testify at trial is governed by Rule 26(b)(4)(A). Rule 26(b)(4)(A)(i) allowed a party, through interrogatories, to require any other party to provide the following four categories of information concerning each expert witness who was expected to testify at trial: (1) the expert's identity, (2) the subject matter of the expert's expected testimony, (3) the substance of the facts and opinions to which the expert is expected to testify, and (4) a summary of the grounds for each opinion.[162] In practice, at a scheduling conference early in a case, many courts routinely set a date by which each party is required to file a "Rule 26(b)(4) Statement." Typically the Rule 26(b)(4) Statement is required to set forth the information discoverable under Rule 26(b)(4)(A)(i).

The old Rules also provide that "[u]pon motion, the court may order further discovery by other means, subject to the restrictions as to scope and such provision . . . concerning fees and expenses as the court may deem appropriate."[163] The old Rules do not permit a party to depose another party's testifying expert without first obtaining leave of court. In most jurisdictions, however, it is customary for parties by agreement to take the depositions of each other's experts without obtaining leave of court.

Under the new Rules, discovery of expert testimony is governed by Rule 26(a)(2) and Rule 26(b)(4). Rule 26(a)(2)(A) requires a party to disclose to other parties "the identity of any person who may be used at trial to present evidence under Rules 702, 703, or 705 of the Federal Rules of Evidence."[164] Rule 26(a)(2)(B) then requires a more extensive disclosure than that required under the old Rules:

[T]his disclosure shall, with respect to a witness who is retained or specially employed to provide expert testimony in the case or whose duties as an employee of the party regularly involve giving expert testimony, be accompanied by a written report prepared and signed by the witness. The report shall contain a complete statement of all opinions to be expressed and the basis and reasons therefor; the data or other information considered by the witness in forming the opinions; any exhibits to be used as a summary of or support for the opinions; the qualifications of the witness, including a list of all publications authored by the witness within the preceding 10 years; the compensation to be paid for the study and testimony; and a listing of any other cases in which the witness has testified as an expert at trial or by deposition within the preceding 4 years.[165]

Thus the new Rules place an affirmative disclosure obligation on the party who intends to call the expert as a witness at trial; it is no longer incumbent on other parties to obtain such information through interrogatories.

In *Sylla-Sawdon v. Uniroyal Goodrich Tire Co.,* for example, the Eighth Circuit affirmed the district court's decision to limit an expert's testimony where, instead of submitting a report that complied with the court's scheduling order (which was quite similar to the new Rules), the expert submitted an affidavit that lacked the specificity mandated by the court's scheduling order and a curriculum vitae (CV).[166] The district court had limited the expert's testimony to matters set forth in his affidavit and his CV.[167] The court held that "[t]he failure to comply with the Scheduling Order is not excused because [the opposing party] elected to depose [the expert]."[168]

Rule 26(b)(4)(A) expressly authorizes a party to depose "any person who has been identified as an expert whose opinions may be presented at trial," thereby harmonizing the rule with what has been the customary practice under the old Rules.[169] Both the old Rules and the new Rules provide that "the court shall require that the party seeking discovery pay the expert a reasonable fee for time spent in responding to discovery."[170]

The old Rules and the new Rules both also contain a provision governing discovery of nontestifying retained experts. Rule 26(b)(4)(B) provides that "opinions held by an expert who has been retained or specially employed by another party in anticipation of litigation or preparation for trial and who is not expected to be called as a witness at trial" can be discovered only "upon a showing of exceptional circumstances under which it is impracticable for the party seeking discovery to obtain facts or opinions on the same subject by other means."[171]

In criminal cases, Rule 16 of the Federal Rules of Criminal Procedure contains the major provisions governing the discovery of an expert witness' opinions. Rule 16(a)(1)(E) provides:

At the defendant's request, the government shall disclose to the defendant a written summary of testimony the government intends to use under Rules 702, 703, or 705 of the Federal Rules of Evidence during its case-in-chief at trial . . . The summary provided under this subdivision shall describe the witnesses' opinions, the bases and the reasons for those opinions, and the witnesses' qualifications.[172]

Rule 16(b)(1)(C) requires the defendant to make a similar disclosure at the government's request "[i]f the defendant requests disclosure under subdivision (a)(1)(E) of this rule and the government complies."[173] These subdivisions of Rule 16 were added as part of the 1993 amendments; they represent a major expansion of federal criminal discovery. The Advisory Committee explained that "[t]he amendment is intended to minimize surprise that often results from unexpected expert testimony, reduce the need for continuances, and to provide the opponent with a fair opportunity to test the merit of the expert's testimony through focused cross-examination."[174]

Rule 16 also contains provisions governing discovery of reports of examinations and tests. Rule 16(a)(1)(D) provides:

Upon request of a defendant the government shall permit the defendant to inspect and copy or photograph any results or reports of physical or mental examinations, and of scientific tests or experiments, or copies thereof, which are within the possession, custody, or control of the government, the existence of which is known, or by the exercise of due diligence may become known, to the attorney for the government, and which are material to the preparation of the defense or are intended for use by the government as evidence in chief at the trial.[175]

Rule 16(b)(1)(B) imposes a similar, although somewhat different, disclosure requirement on the defendant "[i]f the defendant requests disclosure under subdivision (a)(1)(C) or (D) of this rule, upon compliance with such request by the government." The defendant's disclosure requirement includes only "results or reports of physical or mental examinations and of scientific tests or experiments made in connection with the particular case."[176] The defendant is required to produce only materials "which the defendant intends to introduce as evidence in chief at the trial or which were prepared by a witness whom the defendant intends to call at the trial when the results or reports relate to that witness' testimony."[177]

Rule 12.2 imposes a notification requirement on a criminal defendant if the defendant "intends to rely upon the defense of insanity at the time of the alleged offense," or "[i]f a defendant intends to introduce expert testimony relating to a mental disease or defect or any other mental condition of the defendant bearing upon the issue of guilt."[178,179]

Ethical considerations

Two ethical considerations relating to the use of expert witnesses warrant mention. First, paying a contingent fee to an expert witness is not permitted in most jurisdictions. The American Bar Association (ABA) Model Code of Professional Responsibility includes a disciplinary rule that states: "[A] lawyer shall not pay, offer to pay, or acquiesce in the payment of compensation to a witness contingent upon the content of his testimony or the outcome of the case."[180] The ABA Model Rules of Professional Conduct do not expressly prohibit the payment of a contingent fee to an expert witness, but Model Rule 3.4 prohibits offering "an inducement to a witness that is prohibited by law."[181] The Comment to Rule 3.4 also notes that "the common law rule in most jurisdictions is that . . . it is improper to pay an expert witness a contingent fee."[182]

The second ethical consideration relates to ex parte contacts with expert witnesses in civil proceedings. ABA Formal Opinion 93-378, which was issued in November 1993, concluded:

[A]lthough the Model Rules do not specifically prohibit a lawyer in a civil matter from making ex parte contact with the opposing party's expert witness, such contacts would probably constitute a violation of Rule 3.4(c) if the matter is pending in federal court or in a jurisdiction that has adopted an expert-discovery rule patterned after Federal Rule 26(b)(4)(A). Conversely, if the matter is not pending in such a jurisdiction, there would be no violation.[183]

The Committee noted that neither the Model Rules nor the Model Code contains "an automatic bar to lawyers initiating contact with the opposing parties' experts."[184] The Committee characterized Rule 26(b)(4)(A) of the new Rules and similar state provisions as the "exclusive procedures for obtaining the opinions, and the bases therefor, of the experts who may testify for the opposing party."[185] Because Rule 26(b)(4) and similar state rules make no provision for informal discovery of expert witnesses' opinions, the Committee concluded that "in those jurisdictions a lawyer who engages in such ex parte contacts would violate Rule 3.4(c)'s prohibition against knowingly disobey[ing] an obligation under the rules of a tribunal."[186]

CONCLUSION

The next decade promises to be a dynamic period with respect to the law governing medical testimony and expert witnesses. The U.S. Supreme Court's decisions in *Daubert* and *Kumho Tire* provide general guidance regarding the proper role of the trial court in ensuring the reliability of expert testimony. The full impact of those landmark decisions and their practical effect on the practice of litigation involving medical experts, however, remain to be determined.

ENDNOTES

1. *Daubert v. Merrell Dow Pharms.*, 509 U.S. 579, 592 (1993).
2. *Nat Harrison Assoc's., Inc. v. Byrd,* 256 So. 2d 50, 53 (Fla. Dist. Ct. App. 1971).
3. *Id.*
4. 2 J. Wigmore, *Evidence* § 686, at 962 (Chadbourn rev. 1979) (footnote omitted).

5. The American Bar Association Section of Litigation published an excellent treatise entitled *Expert Witnesses,* which was written in part and edited by Professor Faust F. Rossi. The treatise includes three parts—a careful review of the relevant law of evidence, a section that provides general guidance for the litigator on the practical aspects of working with experts, and a section that provides practical guidance on specific types of experts.

6. *Salem v. United States,* 370 U.S. 31, 35 (1962). In *General Electric Co. v. Joiner,* 522 U.S. 136, 118 S.Ct. 512, 515 (1997) the United States Supreme Court clarified that "abuse of discretion" is the appropriate standard that an appellate court should apply in reviewing a trial court's decision to admit or exclude expert testimony under *Daubert.*

7. *Hagler v. Gilliland,* 292 So. 2d 647, 648 (Ala. 1974).

8. *Id.*

9. *Dyas v. United States,* 376 A. 2d 827, 832 (D.C.) (quotation omitted), *cert. denied,* 434 U.S. 973 (1977).

10. Fed. R. Evid. 702.

11. *Supra,* note 1 at 579, 600.

12. *Breidor v. Sears, Roebuck & Co.,* 722 F. 2d 1134, 1139 (3d Cir. 1983).

13. *Supra,* note 1 at 589-590.

14. *Id.* (quotation and citations omitted).

15. *See Id.* at 594 595.

16. *Id.* at 594-595.

17. *Id.*

18. Reference deleted in proofs.

19. Reference deleted in proofs.

20. Reference deleted in proofs.

21. *Supra,* note 1 at 594-595.

22. *Id.*

23. *Id.*

24. *Kumho Tire Co. v. Carmichael,* 526 U.S. 137, 119 S.Ct. 1167, 1175-1176 (1999).

25. *Id.* at 1175.

26. *Id.* at 1176.

27. *Supra,* note 12 (emphasis added).

28. *Ellis v. Miller Oil Purchasing Co.,* 738 F. 2d 269, 270 (8th Cir. 1984).

29. *Id.* at 270.

30. *Id.* at 270.

31. *Linkstrom v. Golden T. Farms,* 883 F. 2d 269, 270 (3d Cir. 1989) (quoting *In re Japanese Elec. Prods.,* 723 F. 2d 238, 279 (3d Cir. 1983), *rev'd on other grounds,* 475 U.S. 574 (1986).

32. *Carroll v. Otis Elevator Co.,* 896 F. 2d 210, 212 (7th Cir. 1990).

33. *Id.* at 212.

34. *Supra,* note 1 (quoting 3 J. Weinstein & M. Berger, *Weinstein's Evidence* ¶ 702[02], at 702-18[1988]).

35. *See American Tech. Resources v. United States,* 893 F. 2d 651, 656 (3d Cir.), *cert. denied,* 495 U.S. 933 (1990).

36. *Federal Crop Ins. Corp. v. Hester,* 765 F. 2d 723, 728 (8th Cir. 1985).

37. *Supra,* note 32.

38. *Shea v. Phillips,* 98 S.E. 2d 552 (Ga. 1957).

39. *Rodriguez v. Jackson,* 574 P. 2d 481, 485 (Ariz. Ct. App. 1977) (emphasis original and citation omitted); *but see Harris v. Robert C. Groth, M.D., Inc.,* 663 P. 2d 113 (Wash. 1983).

40. *See McNeill v. United States,* 519 F.Supp. 283, 287 (D.S.C. 1981).

41. *In Falcon v. Cheung,* 848 P. 2d 1050, 1054 (Mont. 1993), for example. The court disqualified an expert who had never practiced medicine in Montana, had never practiced at a rural hospital in another state, and therefore was unfamiliar with the standard of practice in rural Montana.

42. *Frost v. Mayo Clinic,* 304 F.Supp. 285, 288 (D. Minn. 1969).

43. *Baerman v. Reisinger,* 363 F. 2d 309, 310 (D.C. Cir. 1966).

44. *Swanson v. Chatterton,* 160 N.W. 2d 662 (Minn. 1968); *Hartke v. McKelway,* 526 F.Supp. 97, 101 (D.D.C. 1981), *aff'd,* 707 F. 2d 1544 (D.C. Cir.), *cert. denied,* 464 U.S. 983 (1983).

45. *Fitzmaurice v. Flynn,* 356 A. 2d 887, 892 (Conn. 1975).

46. *Supra,* note 44 *Hartke.*

47. *Id.* at 101.

48. *Id.*

49. *Northern Trust Co. v. Upjohn Co.,* 572 N.E. 2d 1030, 1041 (Ill. App. Ct.), *appeal denied,* 580 N.E. 2d 119 (1991), *cert. denied,* 502 U.S. 1095 (1992).

50. *Id.* (citation omitted).

51. *Id.*

52. *Smith v. Pearre,* 625 A. 2d 349, 359 (Md. Ct. App.), *cert. denied,* 632 A. 2d 151 (Md. 1993).

53. *Id.*

54. *Id.*

55. *Hedgecorth v. United States,* 618 F.Supp. 627, 631 (E.D. Mo. 1985).

56. *Id.*

57. *Owens v. Concrete Pipe and Prods. Co.,* 125 F.R.D. 113, 115 (E.D. Pa. 1989).

58. *Id.*

59. *Id.*

60. *See Backes v. Valspar Corp.,* 783 F.2d 77, 79 (7th Cir. 1986); *Roberts v. United States,* 316 F. 2d 489, 492-493 (3d Cir. 1963).

61. *Gideon v. Johns-Manville Sales Corp.,* 761 F. 2d 1129, 1136 (5th Cir. 1985).

62. *Id.*

63. *Id.*

64. *Jackson v. Waller,* 10 A. 2d 763, 769 (Conn. 1940).

65. *Jenkins v. United States,* 307 F. 2d 637, 643-644 (D.C. Cir. 1962).

66. *Id.* at 643, 645.

67. *Id.* at 644.

68. *Id.* at 646.

69. *Mannino v. International Mfg. Co.,* 650 F. 2d 846, 850 (6th Cir. 1981).

70. *Zenith Radio Corp. v. Matsushita Elec. Indus. Co.,* 505 F.Supp. 1313, 1333 (E.D. Pa. 1980), *aff'd in part and rev'd in part,* 723 F. 2d 238 (3d Cir. 1983), *rev'd on other grounds,* 475 U.S. 574 (1986).

71. *Flanagan v. Lake,* 666 A. 2d 333 (Pa. Super. Ct. 1995).

72. *Id.* at 335.

73. *Perkins v. Volkswagen of Am., Inc.,* 596 F. 2d 681, 682 (5th Cir. 1979).

74. *Rimer v. Rockwell Int'l. Corp.,* 641 F. 2d 450, 456 (6th Cir. 1981) (permitting a pilot to testify about experiences as a pilot, experiences of other pilots, and a forced landing that he made as a result of a fuel siphoning problem in a plane similar to that at issue in the case, but excluding pilot's opinion that the plane's fuel system had been defectively designed).

75. Fed. R. Evid. 703.

76. Notes of Advisory Committee on 1972 Proposed Rules, Fed. R. Evid. 703.

77. *Supra,* note 75.

78. *Soden v. Freightliner Corp.,* 714 F. 2d 498, 505 (5th Cir. 1983).

79. *In re "Agent Orange" Prod. Liab. Litig.,* 611 F.Supp. 1223, 1244 (E.D.N.Y. 1985), *aff'd,* 818 F.2d 187 (2d Cir. 1987), *cert. denied,* 487 U.S. 1234 (1988).

80. *Id.* at 1243-1244 (citations omitted).

81. *Id.* at 1247.

82. *Id.* at 1246.

83. The U.S. Court of Appeals for the Third Circuit, for example, adopted the liberal approach to Rule 703 in *DeLuca v. Merrell Dow Pharmaceuticals, Inc.,* 911 F.2d 941, 952 (3d Cir. 1990). In that case the court determined that an expert who had relied on his own reanalysis of published epidemiological data was basing his opinions on the same epidemiological data that the defendant's expert used in formulating her opinions. *Id.* at 953. The court held that Rule 703 did not require the plaintiff's expert to accept the conclusions of the authors of the studies upon whose data he relied. The court concluded that there was no basis for excluding the plaintiff's expert's opinion under Rule 703. In *In re Paoli R.R. Yard PCB Litigation,* 35 F. 3d 717, 747-749 (3d Cir. 1994), *cert. denied,* 115 S.Ct. 1253 (1995), however, the Third Circuit

III Professional Medical Liability

overruled *DeLuca* and its liberal approach to Rule 703. The court stated, "Judge Weinstein's view is extremely persuasive, and we are free to express our agreement with it because we think that our former view is no longer tenable in light of *Daubert*." *Id.* at 748. Although the Supreme Court's holding in *Daubert* was based on Rule 702 and not Rule 703, the Third Circuit nonetheless held that "[i]t makes sense that the standards are the same, because there will often be times when both Rule 702 and Rule 703 apply." *Id.* Thus after *Paoli*, U.S. Courts of Appeals are in agreement that "it is the judge who makes the determination of reasonable reliance." *Id.*

84. *Supra*, note 79.

85. *Id.*

86. *Lynch v. Merrell-National Lab.*, 830 F. 2d 1190, 1196-97 (1st Cir. 1987).

87. *Johnston v. United States*, 597 F.Supp. 374, 401 (D. Kan. 1984) (quoted in *In re Agent Orange*, 611 F.Supp. at 1250).

88. *Taenzler v. Burlington N.*, 608 F. 2d 796, 798 n.3 (8th Cir. 1979).

89. *Richardson v. Richardson-Merrell, Inc.*, 857 F. 2d 823 (D.C. Cir. 1988), *cert. denied*, 493 U.S. 882 (1989).

90. *Id.* at 829.

91. *Id.*

92. *Id.*

93. *Id.* at 830.

94. *Id.* at 832.

95. *Id.* at 831.

96. *See Brock v. Merrell Dow Pharms., Inc.*, 874 F. 2d 307, 313 (5th Cir. 1989), *modified on reh'g*, 884 F. 2d 166 (5th Cir. 1989), *cert. denied*, 494 U.S. 1046 (1990); *supra*, note 86.

97. *Porter v. Whitehall Labs., Inc.*, 9 F. 3d 607 (7th Cir. 1993).

98. *Id.* at 614-615.

99. *Id.* at 614.

100. *Id.*

101. *Chikovsky v. Ortho Pharm. Corp.*, 832 F.Supp. 341 (S.D. Fla. 1993).

102. *Id.* at 345.

103. *Id.*

104. *Id.* at 346.

105. *Id.*

106. *See Glaser v. Thompson Med. Co.*, 32 F. 3d 969, 975 (6th Cir. 1994) (reversing lower court's decision to exclude expert testimony based on studies that had undergone peer review, were published in reputable medical journals, and had "clearly explained, solid scientific methodologies"); *Sorensen v. Shaklee Corp.*, 31 F. 3d 638, 649 (8th Cir. 1994) (affirming lower court decision excluding expert opinion where "the experts . . . reasoned from an end result in order to hypothesize what needed to be known but what was not"; no reliable evidence that alfalfa tablets contained ethylene oxide or that ethylene oxide causes mental retardation); *see also Wheat v. Pfizer, Inc.*, 31 F. 3d 340, 343 (5th Cir. 1994) (in affirming summary judgment, court stated that proffered testimony was a hypothesis that lacked an empirical foundation and had not been subjected to peer review and publication and was therefore inadmissible).

107. *Davis v. Virginian Ry., Co.*, 361 U.S. 354, 357-358 (1960).

108. *Id.*

109. *Stokes v. Children's Hosp., Inc.*, 805 F.Supp. 79, 82-83 (D.D.C. 1992), *aff'd without op.*, 36 F. 3d 127 (D.C. Cir. 1994).

110. *Id.* at 82 (quoting, *supra*, note 107).

111. *Id.* (omissions in original) (quoting *Levy v. Schnabel Found. Co.*, 584 A. 2d 1251, 1255 [D.C. 1991] [citation omitted]).

112. *Frye v. United States*, 293 F. 1013 (D.C. Cir. 1923).

113. *Id.* at 1014.

114. *United States v. Addison*, 498 F. 2d 741, 743-744 (D.C. Cir. 1974).

115. *See* Gianelli, *The Admissibility of Novel Scientific Evidence: Frye v. United States, a Half Century Later*, 80 Colum. L. Rev. 1197, 1208 (1980).

116. *Massachusetts v. Lykus*, 327 N.E. 2d 671, 678 (Mass. 1975).

117. *Supra*, note 1.

118. *Id.* at 594.

119. *Id.* (citations omitted).

120. *Flanagan v. Florida*, 625 So. 2d 827 (Fla. 1993). *See California v. Leahy*, 882 P. 2d 321 (Cal. 1994) (reaffirming use of general acceptance test of admissibility of scientific evidence in California); *Nebraska v. Carter*, 524 N.W. 2d 763 (Neb. 1994) (affirming continuing vitality of "general acceptance test" of admissibility in Nebraska); *Arizona v. Bible*, 858 P. 2d 1152, 1183 (Ariz. 1993) (continuing to apply general acceptance test in Arizona "notwithstanding legitimate criticism of *Frye*"), *cert. denied*, 114 S.Ct. 1578 (1994); *Washington v. Cissne*, 865 P. 2d 564, 569 (Wash. Ct. App. 1994) (acknowledging that Washington courts continue to employ *Frye* when determining admissibility of evidence based on novel scientific procedures), *review denied*, 877 P. 2d 1288 (Wash. 1994).

121. Rule 704(b) includes a specific limitation that is applicable only to cases in which an expert witness is testifying with respect to "the mental state or condition of a defendant in a criminal case." This rule precludes an expert witness from stating "an opinion or inference as to whether the defendant did or did not have the mental state or condition constituting an element of the crime charged or of a defense thereto." Fed. R. Evid. 704(b).

122. *Owen v. Kerr-McGee Corp.*, 698 F. 2d 236, 240 (5th Cir. 1983).

123. *Henson v. Indiana*, 535 N.E. 2d 1189, 1192 (Ind. 1989).

124. *West Virginia v. McCoy*, 366 S.E. 2d 731 (W. Va. 1988).

125. *Id.* at 737.

126. *Id.*

127. *Id.* (quoting *Kansas v. McQuillen*, 689 P. 2d 822 [Kan. 1984] [C.J. Schroeder, dissenting]).

128. *Id.*

129. *Minnesota v. Meyers*, 359 N.W. 2d 604 (Minn. 1984).

130. *Id.* at 609.

131. Fed. R. Evid. 403.

132. *Supra*, note 1 at 579, 595 (quoting Weinstein, *Rule 702 of the Federal Rules of Evidence is Sound: It Should Not be Amended*, 138 F.R.D. 631, 632 [1991]).

133. *In re Paoli R.R. Yard PCB Litig.* ("Paoli I"), 916 F. 2d 829 (3d Cir.), *cert. denied*, 499 U.S. 961 (1991).

134. *Id.* at 855-859.

135. *In re Paoli R.R. Yard PCB Litig.*, 35 F. 3d 717, 735 (3d Cir. 1994) (quoting Paoli I, 916 F. 2d at 859-860).

136. *Id.* at 736.

137. *Id.*

138. *Id.* at 732.

139. *Id.* at 738-741.

140. *Hall v. Baxter Healthcare Corp.*, 947 F.Supp. 1387 (D. Or. 1996).

141. *Id.*

142. *Id.*

143. *Supra*, note 18 at 1167, 1176.

144. *Id.*

145. McCormick, *Evidence* § 321, at 900 (3d ed. 1984).

146. *Id.*

147. *Id.*

148. *See* 6 J. Wigmore, *Evidence* § 1690 (1979); J. King, *The Law of Medical Malpractice in a Nutshell* 100-103 (1977); F. Rossi, *Expert Witnesses* 135-136 (1991).

149. *Id.*

150. Fed. R. Evid. 803(18).

151. *Matott v. Ward*, 399 N.E. 2d 532, 534 (N.Y. 1979).

152. *Palace Bar, Inc. v. Fearnot*, 381 N.E. 2d 858, 864 (Ind. 1978).

153. *See Cohen v. Albert Einstein Med. Ctr.*, 592 A. 2d 720 724 (Pa. Super. Ct. 1991), *appeal denied*, 602 A. 2d 855 (Pa. 1992).

154. *Supra*, note 152 (emphasis in original).

155. *See Parker v. Employees Mut. Liab. Ins. Co.*, 440 S.W. 2d 43, 46 (Tex. 1969).

156. *McMahon v. Young*, 276 A. 2d 534, 535 (Pa. 1971).

157. *Id.* (citation omitted).
158. *Supra,* note 151.
159. *Id.* (citation omitted).
160. Notes of Advisory Committee on 1972 Proposed Rules, Fed. R. Evid. 705.
161. *Id.*
162. Fed. R. Civ. P. 26(b)(4)(A).
163. *Id.*
164. Fed. R. Civ. P. 26(a)(2)(A).
165. Fed. R. Civ. P. 26(a)(2)(B).
166. *Sylla-Sawdon v. Uniroyal Goodrich Tire Co.,* 47 F. 3d 277 (8th Cir. 1995), *cert. denied,* 116 S.Ct. 84 (1995).
167. *Id.* at 284.
168. *Id.*
169. *Supra,* note 162.
170. Fed. R. Civ. P. 26(b)(4)(C).
171. Fed. R. Civ. P. 26(b)(4)(B).
172. Fed. R. Crim. P. 16(b)(1)(C).
173. Fed. R. Crim. P. 16(b)(1)(E).
174. Notes of Advisory Committee on 1993 Amendment, Fed R. Crim. P. 16.
175. Fed. R. Crim. P. 16(a)(1)(D).
176. Fed. R. Crim. P. 16(b)(1)(B) (emphasis added).
177. *Id.*
178. Fed. R. Crim. P. 12.2(a).
179. Fed. R. Crim. P. 12.2(b).
180. ABA Model Code DR 7-109(C).
181. ABA Model Rule 3.4(b).
182. Comment 3 to ABA Model Rule 3.4.
183. ABA Formal Opinion 93-378 (Nov. 8, 1993) (emphasis in original).
184. *Id.*
185. *Id.* (brackets in original).
186. *Id.*

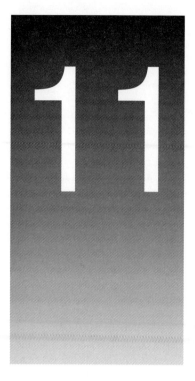

Liability of health care entities for negligent care

JOHN R. FEEGEL, M.D., J.D., M.P.H., F.C.L.M.

Corporate liability for negligent care and treatment on the part of health care providers was historically limited so that the corporation was responsible only for its employees, acting within the scope of their duties; for the hazardous conditions of its physical plant; and for the equipment it provided. The hospital was considered a facility where physicians, usually contracted privately by patients before their arrival, could practice medicine restricted only by the state regulatory boards. It was the physician rather than the hospital who was licensed to practice medicine. Under these circumstances the physician was considered an independent contractor from whom the patient could seek compensation in case of injury caused by professional negligence.

When the health care provider was a direct employee of the hospital, however, the hospital also could be held liable for injuries to the patient under the doctrine of respondeat superior. In this regard the hospital was treated similarly to other corporate entities whose employees offered services to the public. Where the employee acted within the scope of his or her duties, the employer was held responsible for the outcome. In earlier times some hospitals were run as charitable institutions (eleemosynary), and as such either they were held immune from liability or their damages as a result of liability were greatly reduced on the theory that the charitable contributions were not intended to be used by the donors as compensation for fault. Later, as health care institutions became insured and began accepting other sources of income, the rationale for these exemptions or restrictions dissolved. Other institutions, such as government-run hospitals, escaped liability under the sovereign immunity doctrine. No lawsuit could be brought against the state unless the state gave its permission. With growing recognition of the unfairness of the exemption, local, state, and federal legislation allowed claims to be brought for the negligent acts of its employees, albeit with numerous and varied restrictions, conditions, and caps on selected damages.

In the modern era the law is no longer simply concerned with the corporate responsibility of hospitals. It also must deal with the rapidly emerging variants and mutations of organized health care providers. These additional corporate entities now include managed care organizations (MCOs), health maintenance organizations (HMOs), preferred provider organizations (PPOs), independent practice associations (IPAs), permutations of all of these types based on their internal organizations, and the increasingly popular professional associations (PAs) or professional corporations (PCs) under which one or more physicians can own and be employed by a self-owned third party.

Statements and citations that hereinafter mention "the hospital" as the corporate entity also apply to the newer varieties of health care organizations. (Those statements that are not perfectly applicable should at least be considered as a potential bellwether of things to come.)

Under the theory of corporate negligence the hospital may be held responsible for the acts and omissions of its apparent (ostensible) agents under certain circumstances, even when they were thought to be nonemployees or independent contractors. This theory recognizes that the hospital has a nondelegable duty to provide reasonable and safe health care to its patients and that direct liability can arise for negligent care. Liability for employees may additionally arise out of the doctrine of vicarious liability, in which one may be responsible for the actions of others whom he or she controls.

Hence the responsibility of the health care institution for proper selection, retention, and supervision of professionals on its staff has assumed newer and more hazardous proportions for the corporation. No longer can the hospital simply delegate to a volunteer staff committee the responsibility to examine a staff applicant's credentials and history of prior performance before granting full or restricted staff privileges. Nor can the physician on staff be allowed to practice negligently without some form of reasonable and prudent supervision or review of continued performance. Under the newer doctrine of corporate negligence the hospital or other health care organization may share responsibility with the negligent physician for the consequences of his or her acts or omissions.

LEGAL BASIS FOR THE HOSPITAL'S DUTY TO PATIENTS

Case law has expanded the scope of the hospital's independent duty of care to its patients. The law may now impose on the hospital the responsibility for monitoring the activities of its independent medical staff and supervising the quality of medical care provided within it. Where the negligence of its health care personnel is imputed to the hospital under legal theories, such as respondeat superior and ostensible agency, the hospital may be held liable along with the individual whose negligence gave rise to the cause of action.

Under the legal doctrine of corporate liability a hospital may have a duty to properly select and credential its staff physicians for clinical privileges and a duty to monitor its staff physicians as part of the implied contract between the patient and the hospital.[1] The hospital may even have a duty to intervene actively and affirmatively when a physician is negligent and a duty to prevent the errant staff physician from endangering hospitalized patients. Mere documentation of the problem with the physician may not be enough.

Traditionally the determination of a hospital's liability for negligent acts of members of its medical staff depended on the legal relationship between the hospital and the physician. At one end of the legal continuum was the salaried physician, who was a hospital employee. Under the doctrine of respondeat superior the hospital would be jointly liable for the physician's negligence.[2,3] At the other end of the continuum was the independent contractor staff physician, who admitted patients under his or her care to the hospital. In the past the hospital was seldom liable for an independent contractor staff physician's negligence, even if the negligent actions occurred within the hospital.[4,5] Whether a physician is considered an employee may depend less on the written contract between the institution and the physician than on the actions and appearances. Thus if the hospital provides supplies, equipment,

uniforms, meals, parking spaces, billing services, and ancillary personnel, a physician who claims to be an independent contractor may be held to be a de facto employee, particularly if the physician does not maintain an office elsewhere. The conditions set by the Internal Revenue Service may have significance here and should be considered.[6] If a patient seeks treatment directly from the hospital rather than from the physician who negligently caused the injury or if the hospital provides the patient no choice as to which physician provides a particular service as part of treatment, courts may view that physician as an employee and apply the doctrine of respondeat superior, even if the treating physician is considered an independent contractor for other purposes. If a hospital represents to the patient that a physician is a hospital employee but the doctor actually is an independent contractor, a court may still hold the hospital vicariously liable for the physician's acts. This legal theory of liability is called *ostensible* or *apparent agency.*

To hold a hospital liable on a corporate liability theory, a plaintiff must show that the hospital staff knew or should have known that the physician whose negligence caused the plaintiff's injury was providing substandard care. A plaintiff relying on an ostensible agency theory need show only that he or she looked to the hospital for treatment and that the assigned attending physician negligently injured the patient in the provision of the treatment sought.

The hospital's liability for the negligence of a physician whose practice is hospital based, such as an anesthesiologist or pathologist, was previously determined by the contractual arrangements between the physician and the hospital. These arrangements were referred to in determining whether the physician was more like an employee or an independent contractor, ordinarily a question of fact for the jury to decide.[7-9] Under the ostensible agency doctrine the contract issue is moot. The theory of apparent agency is applicable where a hospital holds out a physician as its agent or employee, and a patient accepts treatments from that physician in the reasonable belief that it is being rendered on behalf of the hospital.[10-12]

In *Pederson v. Dumouchel* the court recognized the need for a hospital to adhere to its own rules and regulations designed to control and regulate a staff physician's conduct.[13] In this case an injured child was examined by a physician, who diagnosed a fractured jaw. A dentist was called in to perform oral surgery, and the physician who diagnosed the fracture left the hospital. The operation was performed without the diagnosing physician in the operating room. The child suffered intraoperative cerebral anoxia and sustained permanent brain damage. The hospital was found to be negligent because it had not enforced its own rules, which provided that no surgery was to be performed without a physician present.

However, the case most often cited as extending and expanding hospital responsibility to include a direct duty to patients is *Darling v. Charleston Memorial Hospital.*[14] In this Illinois case a general practitioner who had not treated a leg fracture in several years set and cast a patient's fractured leg. As a result of negligence, the leg had to be amputated. The physician settled with the plaintiff. The hospital was found liable for failing to require the physician to obtain a consultation. *Darling* came to engender the concept that a patient is entitled to expect that the hospital will provide reasonable care and that the hospital has a duty to monitor and oversee the treatment provided by physicians practicing in the hospital.

In *Fiorentino v. Wenger* the court held that a hospital may be found liable if it allows a physician to provide services to hospital patients when those in charge of granting hospital privileges know or should know through reasonable inquiry that the physician is likely to commit malpractice.[15] This knowledge may consist of notice that the physician's staff privileges were rescinded at another hospital because the physician had conducted improper and radical surgery.

Mduba v. Benedictine Hospital held that a nonsalaried physician, despite his contract to the hospital to operate the emergency room, was an employee of the hospital.[16] The reasoning was based on the court's observation that the physician's fees were based on rates guaranteed by the hospital and that he was subject to the rules and regulations of the hospital's governing board.

In *Corleto v. Shore Memorial Hospital* the court held that a hospital could be found liable for permitting a known incompetent physician to perform an operation negligently and for failing to remove him from the case after his incompetence became obvious to the hospital.[17] The court held that the hospital was ultimately responsible for the care of its patients, and therefore it had a duty to act when it had reason to know that malpractice would probably occur.

Under the corporate negligence theory a hospital may be liable for negligently failing to establish adequate procedures to ensure the safety and welfare of patients, including cases in which the hospital knew or should have known that the physician who caused injury to the patient was not qualified to practice in the hospital but nevertheless granted or renewed the physician's hospital privileges. Earlier, some courts limited the hospital's duty to supervise staff physicians to situations involving only employee physicians or to situations of gross negligence by the hospital. Apparently these courts were concerned that the imposition of a broad duty of hospitals to supervise care would impair independent physicians' discretion in purely medical decisions. Other jurisdictions have imposed a duty on hospitals to use reasonable care in the selection of staff physicians if detectable information exists about a physician's incompetence or lack of qualifications. Such notice can be inferred from records related to denying or restricting privileges at other hospitals or the existence of prior malpractice claims against the physician. If there is no notice of a physician's incompetence and no apparent reason to rescind or deny privileges, a hospital may escape liability. A physician's membership on the medical staff does not by itself create corporate liability for the hospital or health care organization.

NONDELEGABLE DUTY

One of the landmark decisions in the emergence of hospital liability through the theory of nondelegable duty for the acts of a nonemployee, independent contractor emergency room (ER) physician is *Jackson v. Power.*[18] Jackson fell from a cliff and was airlifted to Fairbanks Memorial Hospital (FMH) where he was examined by Dr. Power, an independent contractor. Severe internal injuries allegedly went untreated as a result of Power's negligence. The court's discussion of ostensible agency centered on whether Jackson or other patients so transported to FMH without their specific request for a designated physician created the requisite appearance of the ER physician as an ostensible agent of the hospital or whether such a patient should have known the treating physician was not an employee of the hospital. The court said that it was a question for the jury. However, in considering the theory of nondelegable duty the court made an historic decision: A general acute care hospital has a nondelegable duty to provide nonnegligent physician care in its ER. As an acute care facility FMH was mandated by statute to provide a physician in the ER at all times and that FMH was accredited by the Joint Commission on Accreditation of Hospitals (JCAH, now the Joint Commission on Accreditation of Healthcare Organizations [JCAHO]), which imposed standards for operation of the emergency department. In these statutes and standards, as well as the hospital's own bylaws, the court found a duty on the part of FMH to provide physician care in its ER. Next, the court sought to answer the single question of whether that duty could be delegated. Seeking guidance, the court turned to an airplane crash case in which Alaska Airlines contended that responsibility had been delegated by subcontract to Chitina Air Service.[19] Looking to the principles governing safety of passengers on common carriers, the Alaska Supreme Court held that the principal carrier would not be allowed to avoid liability by engaging in separate subcontracts to provide food, perform maintenance, or even supply crews. In *Jackson* therefore the same court saw clear similarities in the responsibility of hospitals in supplying various services to patients and held that the duty to provide physicians and nonnegligent care for patients in its ER was nondelegable. Such a duty does not extend, however, to situations in which a patient is negligently treated in the ER by a physician of the patient's own choice.

In recognizing the doctrine of corporate negligence the Florida Supreme Court held that a hospital has a duty to select and retain competent physicians who, even though they are independent practitioners, would be providing in-house patient care through their hospital staff privileges. In *Insinga v. LaBella* the court added that the hospital's responsibility for the physician's acts does not extend to acts outside the hospital.[20] This concept probably is not applicable where hospitals enter into direct associations with the physician or purchase the staff physician's private practice and continue to refer patients to him or her. Under those limited circumstances the court may see an inducement of the patient to visit the physician's "private" office because of the referral or the endorsement of the care by the hospital.

STANDARDS TO MEASURE HOSPITAL CONDUCT

Many courts have distinguished the facts involved in determining the standard of care required of a hospital from those of *Darling,* thereby blunting the impact of that case on the hospital's requisite standard of care. Some courts have held that a hospital will not be held liable for an act of malpractice performed by an independently retained physician unless it had reason to anticipate that the act of malpractice would take place. *Lundahl v. Rockford Memorial Hospital* distinguished the facts of Darling on the grounds that the physician in *Lundahl* had been an employee of the hospital and assigned to the ER.[21] In *Lundahl* a boy was taken to a hospital where he was examined by a physician employed by the hospital. The patient was then referred to a staff orthopedist who was not an employee of the hospital. After the orthopedist replaced a moleskin traction strip with a floating splint, a blood clot formed, eventually requiring an amputation. The boy claimed that the hospital had a duty to review the medical care being given to him by the orthopedist. In *Lundahl* the appellate court ruled that the decision to treat a patient in a particular manner was a medical question to be made solely by the treating physician not by the hospital, thus refusing to extend the holding in *Darling.*

Other courts have held that the only way a hospital could be liable for negligent performance of professional services by a member of its staff would be if the plaintiff proved that the hospital had been negligent in its original selection of an unskilled physician.[22] However, in *Pogue v. Hospital Authority of DeKalb County* a partnership was under contract to staff an ER.[23] Although the contract provided that the services performed would be "subject to surveillance by the medical staff of the hospital" and had to be performed in keeping with "good medical practice," the contract also specifically provided that the partners were "independent contractors." In finding that the hospital was not liable for negligence of one of the partnership's members, the court held that the hospital had no right to direct specific medical techniques employed by the physicians. The hospital was not liable when the physician's negligence related to a matter of professional judgment as long as the hospital did not have the right to control the physician's diagnosis and treatment of the patient.

In *Vanaman v. Milford Memorial Hospital,* a case with facts similar to those in *Darling,* a 1970 court came to an opposite conclusion.[24] A mother brought her child to the ER with a fractured leg. Her own physician could not be located, so she asked to see the on-call physician, who set the leg, applied the cast, and treated the child in his office after her release from the hospital. The on-call physician, not the hospital, billed for his services. When permanent disability of the

leg resulted, the parents sued both the physician and the hospital. In finding that the hospital was not liable, the court said that the medical staff was an organized body with qualifications and privileges approved by the governing board of the hospital for patient care. The court held that the hospital had functioned only as a referral service and had not practiced medicine itself. This view probably is outdated.

However, some courts have recognized and reaffirmed the concept enunciated in *Darling.* In *Ohligschlager v. Proctor Community Hospital* a patient experienced severe pain and swelling in her arm near the point of insertion for intravenous infusion.[25] The patient informed a nurse's aide of the pain, but the aide allegedly did nothing. The patient suffered skin necrosis, requiring skin grafting, as a result of infiltration of the intravenous medication, which the physician had ordered in an incorrect concentration. The patient brought a malpractice suit, charging that the hospital's negligence was the proximate cause of her injuries. The court said that there was sufficient evidence to require submission to the jury of the issues of whether the hospital had failed to heed the patient's complaints and whether it failed to properly supervise the injection ordered by the physician. Citing *Darling,* the court said that the hospital was under the duty to "conform to the legal standard of reasonable conduct in the light of the apparent risk."

In *Tucson Medical Center v. Misevch* the court restated the duty of the hospital, acting through appropriate committees, to ensure the competence of members of its medical staff.[26] The decision stated that the hospital was responsible to a patient if failure to properly supervise an incompetent physician results in the patient being injured. In this case the plaintiff contended that a physician staff member was negligent in administering anesthesia to the plaintiff's wife during disk surgery, and as a result of this negligence, she suffered cardiac arrest and died. The key contention against the hospital was that the anesthesiologist was under the influence of alcohol at the time of the operation and that the hospital was negligent in retaining him on its medical staff.

The court pointed out that among the duties a hospital owes to patients with respect to competence of its medical staff is supervision of the physicians on its staff. The court stated that through the concept of "corporate liability" a hospital and its governing body may be held liable for injuries resulting from negligent supervision of members of its medical staff. The court reasoned that a hospital assumed certain responsibilities for the care of its patients and thus was required to meet the standards of responsibility commensurate with that trust. If the medical staff were negligent in the exercise of its duty to supervise its members or in failing to recommend action by the hospital's governing body before a patient's injury, the hospital would be negligent. The court specifically stated that when the hospital's alleged negligence is predicated on an omission to act, the hospital will not be held responsible unless it had reason to know that it should have acted within its duty to the patient. Therefore knowledge (actual or constructive) is an essential factor in determining whether the hospital exercised reasonable care under the circumstances. The court buttressed this argument by quoting the standards of the JCAH, which stated that "In a hospital accredited by the JCAH, the medical staff is responsible to the governing body of the hospital for the quality of hospital patient care. It therefore evaluates the qualifications of applicants and members to hold staff privileges and recommends curtailment and exclusion when necessary."

A hospital's lack of knowledge of a physician's incompetence also can result in liability if the hospital, through the exercise of due diligence, could have acquired such knowledge and acted so as to prevent the plaintiff's injury and failed to do so. In the Memorandum of Decision in *Gonzales v. Nork* the court held that a hospital had a duty to its patients to protect them from the malpractice of an independently retained surgeon who was a member of the hospital's staff if the hospital knew, had reason to know, or should have known that the negligent acts were likely to occur.[27] In this case a private physician member of the medical staff had admitted to performing unnecessary and negligent spinal surgery on a hospital patient, a 27-year-old man who had suffered from back pain after being injured in an automobile accident. Three years after this operation the hospital administrator heard a rumor that the surgeon's malpractice insurance had been canceled. Because the hospital required staff physicians to have such insurance, it investigated and found that the rumor was true. The hospital promptly placed the surgeon in a monitoring program under which he was forbidden to operate without another qualified surgeon present.

During the trial, the surgeon admitted to performing at least 26 other unnecessary operations over 9 years. The court indicated that the hospital's liability was based on its duty to protect its patients from malpractice by members of its medical staff. Although the hospital had no knowledge of the surgeon's propensity to commit malpractice, it was negligent because it had failed to investigate an earlier malpractice case in which the surgeon had been sued. The court concluded that mere compliance with the prevailing JCAH standards did not discharge the hospital from its duty to its patients because those standards furnished no effective means of detecting a fraudulent physician. The court also concluded that the hospital's system of peer review of the quality of patient care was random, casual, subjective, and uncritical. Therefore at the time of the patient's surgery the hospital had no actual knowledge of the surgeon's fraud and incompetence. The judge in essence said that the hospital had a duty to protect its patients from malpractice by members of its medical staff, and therefore the hospital governing board was "corporately responsible for the conduct of its medical staff."

The standard of care that the hospital must use to discharge the duty enunciated in Nork was detailed and illustrated in *Johnson v. Misericordia Community Hospital,* a case involving the credentialing of a physician member of the medical staff.[28] The court stated that a hospital owes a duty to its patients in selecting medical staff and granting surgical privileges. In this case a patient contended that the hospital was negligent in appointing the surgeon to the medical staff and in granting him surgical privileges.

Testimony established the surgeon's negligence; this fact was not challenged on appeal. It also established that the surgeon misrepresented the truth on his application and authorized the hospital to verify all information given. The hospital's administrative records were devoid of any procedures used in the appointment of the surgeon to the medical staff organization. The court concluded that these procedures would have uncovered inter alia that at two hospitals the surgeon's privileges were revoked, at another hospital he was denied privileges, he was neither board certified nor board eligible, and 10 malpractice suits had been filed against him.

The appellate court held that a hospital had a duty to exercise reasonable care to permit only competent physicians and surgeons the privilege of using its facilities. It concluded that had the hospital exercised ordinary care in the staff selection process, it would not have appointed the surgeon to its medical staff, and thus the patient in the case would not have been negligently injured. The court enunciated the theory that a hospital owes a duty of care of its patients to refrain from any act that will cause foreseeable harm or an unreasonable risk of danger. The concept of institutional responsibility is interwoven with foreseeability.

Once the duty is established, the standard of care is the degree of care ordinarily exercised by the average hospital in granting staff privileges. Although a hospital is not the ensurer of competence of its medical staff, it will be charged with gauging and evaluating the knowledge that would have been acquired had it exercised ordinary care in investigating its medical staff applicants. In addition to judicial recognition of the direct duty of a hospital to exercise reasonable care in selecting and retaining staff physicians, some courts have enunciated a duty to supervise the health care provided by physician staff members. The hospital's duty to promulgate regulations to oversee the clinical performance of physicians was enunciated in *Bost v. Riley,* which adopted the concept of corporate negligence for failure to supervise medical treatment.[29] The plaintiff contended that inadequate physician progress notes were evidence of negligent care that resulted in the patient's death. In determining the hospital's liability the court held that hospitals have a duty to make a reasonable effort to monitor and oversee the treatment prescribed and administered by physicians practicing in the hospital. The court noted that the hospital may have breached its duty to the patient by failing to enforce its own internal rule requiring the keeping of accurate progress notes.

Other legal decisions have tended to limit the hospital's duty to supervise medical treatment. In *Cox v. Haworth* the patient was hospitalized so that his privately retained physician could perform a myelogram.[30] During the course of treatment, the patient sustained permanent injury to the spinal cord. The patient alleged that the hospital was negligent in not obtaining informed consent before the medical procedure was performed. No negligence by the hospital personnel during performance of the myelogram was alleged. The court refused to interpret the doctrine of corporate liability as imposing a duty on a hospital to inform and advise the patient of the nature of medical procedures to be privately performed.

The limitations placed on the expansion of the doctrine of corporate liability probably represent judicial recognition that hospitals are not well equipped to supervise patient care actively and concurrently. The personal nature of the physician-patient relationship requires that the physician exercise necessary discretion. Moreover, it is impractical for the hospital to stand over a physician and personally supervise the quality of medical care rendered.

Overseeing the quality of physician performance is a different matter. Review of medical staff clinical performance is a retrospective process because hospitals must ordinarily delegate the review function to a number of medical staff committees (such as quality assurance, risk management, and credentials). The procedure for selection and retention of medical staff members is essentially a retrospective process. To project future performance, the committees use a historical data base describing the physician's training, experience, and prior performance. Some courts have conditioned a hospital's duty to supervise the quality of care or competence of its staff on the hospital's knowledge, either actual or constructive, and awareness of a physician's incompetent acts. This approach uses the agency law principle that a corporation is bound by the knowledge acquired by or by the notice given to its agents or officers, who are within the scope of its authority in reference to matters to which its authority extends. In *Fridena v. Evans* the court held that the negligent physician was an officer of the hospital who held a medical administrative position as chief of the medical staff.[31] This relationship became the linchpin for imputing knowledge of the physician's incompetence to the hospital. In holding that the hospital had "actual notice" of the physician's incompetence, the court concluded that the hospital had been negligent in failing to supervise the incompetent physician's performance.

Insight into the law's reluctance to create the unusually difficult task of supervising physicians as a responsibility of hospital staffs was provided in *Elam v. College Park Hospital.*[32] The court indicated that the hospital had a duty of "continuing evaluation" of the staff physicians' clinical performance, apparently a less onerous and more achievable modification of the requirement that a hospital supervise the actual medical care. Such a requirement did not necessarily require concurrent supervision and on-line intervention.

Additional modifications of the duty to supervise physicians were expressed in *Pickle v. Curns.*[33] The court rejected the contention that a hospital has a duty to ensure that physicians practicing on its premises never commit negligent acts. Instead the court formulated the hospital's duty as one to prevent injuries resulting from negligent acts of its staff physicians when it knew or should have known that the physician would perform a negligent clinical task.

The trend evinced by these cases is to impose a duty on the hospital to supervise medical treatment only when the hospital has been put on notice by past negligent acts. Thus the law does not impose on hospitals a duty to concurrently supervise the administration of medical care but rather to monitor a physician's provision of medical services through patient care assessment committees.

In addition to responsibilities to patients regarding medical staff conduct, hospitals must have adequate policies to protect the welfare of patients receiving care in their institutions and must establish an organizational structure to carry out those policies. A violation of this duty is illustrated in *Polischeck v. United States,* a case in which a hospital was held liable for failing to have the patient examined or her chart reviewed by a licensed physician before her discharge.[34] The hospital permitted ER patients to be admitted and discharged by physician assistants, who under state law were not considered qualified to make such determinations.

In *Ravenis v. Detroit General Hospital* a court imposed direct liability on the hospital for failing to have appropriate standards of care related to handling tissues to be transplanted from donor cadavers.[35] Several patients were injured as a result of contaminated cornea transplants because the hospital had no policy that required the performance of necessary tests on the donor or the donor tissue.

MEDICAL STAFF SELECTION, MONITORING, AND SUPERVISION

Courts have recognized the hospital's duty to select, monitor, and supervise independent contractor members of the medical staff. Although a hospital's overall monitoring system is closely examined when a hospital is named in a suit, the hospital is not considered to be guarantor of the adequacy of medical care rendered in its facility. Isolated negligent acts of an otherwise competent independent contractor physician generally are not evidence of negligence on the part of the hospital.

The hospital is responsible for obtaining reasonably available information on prospective staff members regarding their credentials and any prior negligent conduct. In *Joiner v. Mitchell County Hospital Authority* a patient complaining of chest pain was examined at the hospital by an independent contractor member of the medical staff.[36] The physician advised the patient that the condition was not serious and sent the patient home. Shortly after he returned home, the patient's condition worsened and he died. The patient's estate sued the hospital directly for its negligence in permitting an allegedly known incompetent physician to continue to serve on its medical staff. The court rejected the hospital's contention that it was relieved of liability by delegating its authority to screen medical staff applicants to the members of the existing staff, reasoning that the medical staff simply acted as an agent for the hospital in screening applicants. The court held that because the hospital knew or because, based on information in the hospital's possession, it was apparent that the physician was incompetent, the hospital did not act with reasonable care in permitting the physician to remain a member of the staff.

A hospital also may incur liability if it has implemented a data system for evaluating the qualifications of its staff members but has failed to use this system to restrict the clinical privileges of a physician who has demonstrated incompetence. In *Purcell v. Zimbelman* the court ruled that the hospital had "notice" of the surgeon's incompetence, based on evidence that prior similar operations performed by the surgeon had resulted in lawsuits against him and other hospitals.[37] Significantly the court concluded that the failure of the hospital surgical department, which had reviewed the surgeon's various mishaps in the operating room, to take any corrective action against the surgeon did not relieve the hospital of its duty to protect the patient.

If a hospital has not implemented review procedures to properly credential and appraise staff physicians' clinical performance, plaintiffs must demonstrate review procedures that would have placed the hospital on notice. *Reynolds v. Mennonite Hospital* involved a negligence lawsuit against several hospitals for damages caused by allegedly unnecessary surgery.[38] The plaintiffs claimed that the hospital failed to comply with certification and review procedures. The court said, however, that such failure, even if the surgeries were unnecessary, was not necessarily sufficient to prove that the hospital was directly negligent. The hospitals had no notice of any flaw in the qualifications or background of the surgeons or of any circumstances existing before this plaintiff's surgery that would have caused the hospital to limit or revoke the physicians' privileges to operate. The court pointed out that a hospital is not an ensurer of a patient's safety; therefore because nothing in the record indicated that an evaluation of the surgeons' capabilities would have disclosed substandard practices, the hospital was not negligent.

In *Braden v. St. Francis Hospital* the plaintiff alleged that an unnecessary amputation was performed by a staff surgeon, that the hospital had a duty to exercise proper supervision to prevent unnecessary and wrongful surgery, and that it breached this duty.[39] In support of these allegations the plaintiff offered inter alia statistics showing that the allegedly negligent staff surgeon had performed significantly more amputations than the average number of amputations performed by other surgeons on the hospital staff. The plaintiff also referred to the hospital's bylaws, which documented an elaborate administrative structure of supervision and monitoring to ensure quality care. The court held that a hospital does not generally expose itself to liability for negligence unless it

knows or should know of a propensity on the physician's part to commit negligent acts. The court pointed out that statistics themselves do not indicate a proclivity on the part of the staff surgeon to perform unnecessary amputations because multiple surgeries do not necessarily support a reasonable inference that any one procedure, including the procedure in this case, was unnecessary or negligently performed.

EXPANDING HOSPITAL LEGAL DUTIES

Kirk v. Michael Reese Hospital expanded a hospital's liability beyond its patients to individuals affected by the actions of patients.[40] In this case the hospital discharged a patient on medication that should not be combined with alcohol, especially if the patient intends to drive. The patient consumed alcohol and subsequently was involved in a car accident in which an injured third party sued both the patient and the hospital. The court ruled that the hospital had an obligation to that third party, an individual who had not been admitted or treated in the hospital.

In general, hospitals do not have a duty to ensure that its staff physicians render medical care competently outside the hospital setting. In *Pedroza v. Bryant* the court held that a hospital is not liable for injuries resulting from malpractice committed in the private office of a nonemployee physician before the patient was admitted to the hospital.[41] The plaintiff charged that the hospital was negligent in not ensuring that its staff physician, the patient's private physician, was competent. Noting that the physician's negligent acts had occurred entirely outside the hospital, the court stated that for the plaintiff to prevail, the court would have to extend the hospital's duty of care under the corporate liability doctrine to patients treated by staff members in their private offices, where the hospital is not involved. The court declined to do so. The court pointed out that acts of malpractice committed by staff physicians outside the hospital are relevant only if the hospital has actual or constructive notice of them and negligently fails to take some action. The court stated that the hospital is not an inspector or ensurer of the private office practices of its staff members. Within the hospital, the delineation of staff privileges may reasonably affect the procedures used by staff members.

The doctrine of corporate liability may encompass a duty for the hospital to inform the patient or the patient's survivors when it is aware of a deviation from the standard of care that has caused an injury. The rationale for the duty is that when a hospital knows that a deviation from the standard of care has caused an injury, the failure to inform the patient or the patient's survivors may constitute fraudulent concealment. In *Kruegar v. St. Joseph's Hospital* the court held that whether fraudulent concealment was present was a question of fact for the jury to determine.[42] In this case the plaintiff was advised by her husband's physicians that he had died of heart failure during an operation. Nearly 3 years later, it was anonymously disclosed to the survivor that malfunction of the respiratory machine used during the operation had contributed to the cause of death. The plaintiff filed suit and alleged that the hospital had a duty to inform her of this fact and was therefore precluded from asserting the statute of limitations as a defense. The court noted that fraud can exist even when no false statement is made and stated that the suppression of a material fact, which a party is bound in good faith to disclose, is equivalent to a false representation.

A hospital must be sensitive to emerging areas of liability for failure to warn, particularly in areas involving the adverse side effects of radiation therapy and other types of advanced medical treatment and the possibility of contact with communicable diseases. Case law principles governing a hospital's duty to warn in these instances are still developing. *Knier v. Albany Medical Center Hospital* dealt with the hospital's duty to warn the general public that one of its employees had come in contact with a patient who had a communicable disease.[43] A nurse's family sued the hospital for failing to warn them that the nurse had been exposed to a contagious disease. The court ruled that it did not have an obligation to warn her family, friends, or the public at large that she had been exposed to scabies.

Far more dangerous than scabies is the threat of acquired immunodeficiency syndrome (AIDS). The hospital's duty to warn patients that a surgeon was infected with the human immunodeficiency virus was explored in a 1991 New Jersey case, when the hospital restricted the surgeon's privileges until he provided proof of informed consent from his patients. At odds here were the duty of confidentiality to the surgeon as patient and the duty of the hospital to protect other patients from "risk of harm." The superior court held that the restriction and temporary suspension of surgical privileges did not violate the New Jersey law against discrimination.[44] This area of the law is obviously unsettled, and further developments in many jurisdictions should be researched before a health care professional or the health care corporation acts. AIDS is considered a handicap in many states, is protected by special laws of confidentiality in others, and is a reportable disease (although not with disclosure of the patient's name) everywhere. How these competing issues will play out remains to be seen. A full discussion is provided in *Dellinger.*[45]

MANAGED CARE ORGANIZATIONS

An MCO is designed to facilitate the management and financing of health care while delivering services to its enrolled members. The most common type is the HMO, which in turn may consist of groups of physicians under contract to an employer or an insurer, independent practice networks, staff model organizations with direct employment of physicians, and open-ended networks that allow enrollees to seek services from within and from outside the organization. Regardless of the variant, MCOs share a common goal to provide health care services at reduced costs through consumer competition.

Cost containment measures may include direct incentive payments to physicians to decrease patient-initiated use of services, reduction of physician involvement where overuse can be demonstrated, fixed fees for identified procedures, and predetermined annual payments for comprehensive care (the so-called capitation payment). These cost containment measures may require the physician to restrict or deny some health care measures requested by the patient. The physician under these conditions becomes the "gatekeeper." Conflicts may arise when the patient feels harm has resulted from the restriction or denial of care. Indeed the physician may concur that the restrictions are contrary to his or her own medical judgment.

The MCO may face liability for the improper selection and retention of the physicians or other professionals with whom it contracts to provide services to enrollees. This area of liability is similar to that of corporate liability for a hospital's negligence in providing hospital staff privileges, and cases cited elsewhere in this chapter should be reviewed. Because the MCO may function as the provider, the payor, and the quality reviewer, it may be exposed to liability for alleged breaches in each of these areas.

In *Harrell v. Total Health Care, Inc.* the appellate court found that an HMO had failed in its duty to properly select the physician with whom it contracted to care for the plaintiff, noting a history of malpractice and incompetence.[46] The Missouri Supreme Court found the HMO free of liability on statutory grounds but did not reject the theory of corporate liability.

In *McClellan v. Health Maintenance Organization of Pennsylvania,* the court found the doctrine of nondelegable duty nonapplicable to this HMO because the HMO did not provide on-site health care services.[47] The court, however, apparently recognized the theory of corporate liability for negligent staff selection and retention.

Because MCOs also are employers, the theory of respondeat superior is applicable to hold the HMO liable for the negligence of its employees and agents acting within the scope of their duties. A staff model HMO was held liable for acts of its physicians in *Robbins v. HIP of New Jersey.*[48] In *Sloan v. Metropolitan Health Council, Inc.* the HMO exercised control over the physician.[49] In *Schleier v. Kaiser Foundation Health Plan of Mid-Atlantic States* the physician was a consultant rather than an employee, yet the HMO was held liable for his acts after the appellate court determined that the HMO "controlled" him through its medical director.[50]

Where the physicians were found to be independent contractors and the HMO did not directly treat patients, negligence was not imputed to the organization *(Mitts v. HIP of Greater New York).*[51] A similar conclusion was reached in a case in which an HMO contracted with an IPA and had no direct control over medical decisions. In this case the court refused to apply respondeat superior *(Chase v. Independent Practice Association).*[52]

Under the theory of apparent or ostensible agency, HMOs have been held liable for negligent acts of affiliated physicians who were not directly employed. Courts have considered whether the HMO "held out" the physician as an agent, whether the patient looked to the HMO rather than the designated physician for care, whether the physician was chosen from lists supplied by the HMO, and whether the HMO restricted the patient's choice of physician.[53] However, HMOs were not held liable when the HMO had exercised no professional control over the physician, such as in *Raglin v. HMO Illinois, Inc.,* or where the state law prohibits the HMO from practicing medicine *(Williams v. Good Health Plus, Inc.).*[54,55] If an HMO physician specifically promised a given result and the patient relied on that promise, the HMO could be held liable for breach of contract when the result was not forthcoming from the treatment *(Depenbrok v. Kaiser Foundation Health Plan, Inc.).*[56]

In *Wickline v. State of California* a patient alleged that her premature discharge from hospital care, based on the utilization review decision to deny additional hospitalization, led to the amputation of her leg.[57] She sued the California Medicaid program (Medi-Cal) for its interference with her physician's judgment to keep her hospitalized. The California appellate court held that only the physician could be held responsible for the premature discharge but allowed that the program could be held liable if there were a defect in its cost containment measures that caused harm. In *Wilson v. Blue Cross of So. California* the utilization review organization of a private insurer refused extension of a patient's hospitalization for depression.[58] The patient committed suicide after discharge. The court said the utilization review organization, the insurer, and the utilization review physician could be held liable. Unlike in *Wickline,* in *Wilson* there was inter alia no clear public policy expressed in the statute that required a cost containment utilization review process. The private insurance provisions requiring cost containment review and restriction of services were not public policy.

DIRECT LIABILITY OF MANAGED CARE ORGANIZATIONS

MCOs also are subject to direct liability for organizational or corporate negligence. These cases usually revolve around the negligent selection and retention of incompetent physicians. The theory applied is essentially the same as that of corporate liability of the hospital.[59] The more recent application of these well-tested decisions to an HMO is evident in *Harrell v. Total Health Care Inc.,* where a Missouri court of appeals upheld a decision against a nonprofit HMO for negligent selection of a physician who was held out to subscribers on its list of specialists.[60]

As courts continue to consider MCOs "health care providers," particularly staff model HMOs in which care and treatment are dispensed instead of merely financed, it is anticipated that direct liability for negligent supervision and control of its physicians will increase. Establishing a coherent and consistent appropriate standard of care in this area for MCOs may be difficult and as yet remains unclear.[61] The federal government's efforts to reform health care nationwide may attempt to set practice parameters that some courts may interpret as "standards."

CONTRACT AND WARRANTY THEORIES

Dissatisfied subscribers may seek relief in the courts via legal theories other than negligence. These theories include breach of contract or warranty or misrepresentation by the MCO. *Williams v. Health America* and *Boyd v. Albert Einstein Medical Center* provide examples, albeit unsuccessful at the time, of these theories.[62,63] The more the MCO becomes a "provider" of health care for its subscribers, the more the court can be expected to find contractual or fiduciary relationships between it and the patient.

ERISA

Some claims of malpractice by MCOs may be preempted under the Employee Retirement Income Security Act of 1974 (ERISA).[64] A complete discussion of ERISA is neither possible nor appropriate here. Suffice it to mention that where an MCO, HMO, or PPO plan is offered to an employee as part of a benefit package, it may be qualified as an ERISA program and thus subject to federal regulation. If so qualified, the preempted claims in malpractice usually are those resulting from defective design or implementation of cost containment or claims handling systems or those resulting from vicarious or direct liability for negligence by the provider. At present there does not seem to be any sense of urgency by state or federal courts to preempt medical malpractice claims against MCO providers *(DeGenova v. Ansel).*[65] However, the issue has not quietly faded away. It may become more popular with further federal involvement in health care and attempts to correct so-called malpractice crises.[66]

PROFESSIONAL SERVICE CORPORATIONS

Professional service corporations, variously known as a *PC* or *PA,* are products of state legislatures. Specific regulations, restrictions, limitations, and liabilities for these corporations and their shareholders, agents, and employees should therefore be researched in the applicable state statutes.

If Florida can be used as an example, professionals, such as physicians, lawyers, accountants, and many others, may incorporate for the sole and specific purpose of rendering professional services, provided that the shareholders are duly licensed individually to render the same service.[67] Motivation for incorporation by professionals includes tax benefits, pension plans, group ownership of property or contracts, and escape of the more open liability for the acts of others in a partnership. The corporation cannot legally provide professional medical services, but it can be owned by the individual licensed professionals, contract with others as a provider of health care services, own and convey property, employ persons (who need not be licensed) for managerial purposes, employ licensed professionals who need not be shareholders, sue, and be sued.

Under these professional service corporation arrangements the individual professionals do not escape liability and responsibility for their own acts. The professional corporation assumes liability and responsibility for the professional acts of its employees, including the individual licensed professional, "up to the full value of its property."[68]

The PA may purchase professional liability insurance to cover all of its professional employees and others acting within the scope of their duties, and each licensed professional may purchase individual liability coverage. Strict attention should be paid to these variables by all seeking to purchase coverage for the corporation, its shareholders, or both and for the employees, as well as by all those to whom professional employment is offered. The terms may vary significantly from state to state.

Conversely the liability of individual shareholders for the nonmalpractice liability of the professional corporation has been held in some jurisdictions to be limited to an extent similar to that of shareholders of nonprofessional corporations. For example, for ordinary business debts or nonprofessional contracts entered into solely in the name of the corporation, the assets of the individual shareholders should be exempt. Compare *We're Associates Co. v. Cohen et al.,* where individual shareholders of a professional corporation of attorneys were not held responsible for the corporation's default on its lease, with *South High Dev. Ltd. v. Weiner et al.,* where the bar rules made the individual lawyers guarantors for the acts of their professional corporation when professional duties were concerned.[69,70]

In the sale or lease of a piece of expensive medical equipment, such as a computed tomography machine, the prudent vendor may require that the individual professionals as shareholders cosign along with the corporation itself. Notification of the professional corporation at the time of notice to one of its shareholders in an action for malpractice is customary or required in many states, but failure to do so is not necessarily fatal because the intent of the state legislature allowing professional corporations was not to provide an escape mechanism for the errant individual.

CONCLUSION

The role of the hospital and other corporations providing patient care has significantly changed in recent years. No longer is the hospital simply a physician's workplace that merely furnishes room, board, operating rooms, sophisticated equipment, nurses, attendants, and other personnel. Today, physicians and the health care corporation both play integral roles in the treatment of the patient. The hospital has assumed the role of a health care center and is ultimately responsible for the health care provided within its walls. The public expec-

tation is that the hospital will act to ensure the overall quality of care rendered. The doctrine of corporate liability is an attempt to pragmatically focus the law on the modern relationships between legal doctrine and social and economic reality. The courts are moving away from an overly strict application of traditional but archaic doctrinal rules and guidelines in recognition of these changing relationships among the hospital, health care corporation, patients, subscribers or enrollees, and physicians.

The corporate nature of the modern hospital has demanded recognition of the corporate negligence theory. A common thread running through those legal cases that have applied the corporate negligence theory is the court's role in identifying and analyzing the organizational structure of the hospital. This approach recognizes that hospitals have assumed the dual role of delivering services and reviewing and monitoring the physicians it appoints to its staff. The duty, however, does not automatically render the hospital liable for all malpractice committed by physicians if the hospital has been reasonable in its procedures and has carefully selected and monitored its medical staff. The movement to assign responsibility for all types of professional malpractice, including acts of independently practicing physicians, to the hospital corporation itself has been slow to develop in the medical care field, although it has become the most common form of legal responsibility in nearly all other aspects of "enterprise liability" in American law during this century.

ENDNOTES

1. *Insinga v. LaBella,* 543 So. 2d 209 (1989) (Fla.).
2. *Bing v. Thunig,* 143 N.E. 2d 3 (1957) (N.Y.).
3. *Sepaugh v. Methodist Hospital,* 202 S.W. 2d 985 (1946) (Tenn.).
4. *Byrd v. Marion General Hospital,* 162 S.E. 738 (1932) (N.C.).
5. *Moon v. Mercy Hospital,* 373 P. 2d 944 (1962) (Colo.).
6. 1992-22 I.R.B. 59.
7. *Carroll v. Richardson,* 110 S.E. 2d 193 (1959) (Va.).
8. *Seneris v. Haas,* 291 P. 2d 915 (1957) (Cal.).
9. *Brown v. Moore,* 247 F. 2d 711 (1957) (Pa.).
10. *Cuker v. Hillsborough County Hospital Authority,* 605 So. 2d 998 (1992) (Fla.).
11. *Orlando Regional Medical Center v. Chmielewski,* 573 So. 2d 876 (1990) (Fla.).
12. *Arthur v. St. Peter's Hospital,* 405 A. 2d 443 (1979) (N.J.).
13. *Pederson v. Dumouchel,* 431 P. 2d 973 (1967) (Wash.).
14. *Darling v. Charleston Memorial Hospital,* 211 N.E. 2d 253 (1965) (Ill.).
15. *Fiorentino v. Wenger,* 227 N.E. 2d 296 (1967) (N.Y.).
16. *Mduba v. Benedictine Hospital,* 384 N.Y.S. 2d 527 (1976) (N.Y.).
17. *Corleto v. Shore Memorial Hospital,* 350 A. 2d 534 (1975) (N.J.).
18. *Jackson v. Power,* 743 P. 2d 1376 (1987) (Ala.).
19. *Alaska Airlines v. Sweat,* 568 P. 2d 916 (1977) (Ala.).
20. *Supra* note 1.
21. *Lundahl v. Rockford Memorial Hospital,* 235 N.E. 2d 671 (1968) (Ill.).
22. *Clary v. The Hospital Authority of the City of Marietta,* 126 S.E. 2d 470 (1962) (Ga.).
23. *Pogue v. Hospital Authority of DeKalb County,* 170 S.E. 2d 53 (1969) (Ga.).
24. *Vanaman v. Milford Memorial Hospital,* 262 A. 2d 263 (1970) (Del.).
25. *Ohligschlager v. Proctor Community Hospital,* 303 N.E. 2d 392 (1973) (Ill.).

26. *Tucson Medical Center v. Misevch,* 545 P. 2d 958 (1976) (Ariz.).
27. *Gonzales v. Nork,* No. 228566 (Cal. Sup. Ct., Sacramento Co.) (1974) (Cal.).
28. *Johnson v. Misericordia Community Hospital,* 301 N.W. 2d 156 (1980) (Wis.).
29. *Bost v. Riley,* 262 S.E. 2d 391 (1980) (N.C.).
30. *Cox v. Haworth,* 283 S.E. 392 (1981) (N.C.).
31. *Fridena v. Evans,* 622 P. 2d 463 (1981) (Ariz.).
32. *Elam v. College Park Hospital,* 183 Cal. Rptr. 156 (1982) (Cal.).
33. *Pickle v. Curns,* 435 N.E. 2d 877 (1982) (Ill.).
34. *Polischeck v. United States,* 535 F.Supp. 1261 (1982) (Pa.).
35. *Ravenis v. Detroit General Hospital,* 234 N.W. 2d 411 (1976) (Mich.).
36. *Joiner v. Mitchell County Hospital Authority,* 189 S.E. 2d 412 (1972) (Ga.).
37. *Purcell v. Zimbelman,* 500 P. 2d. 335 (1972) (Ariz.).
38. *Reynolds v. Mennonite Hospital,* 522 N.E. 2d 827 (1988) (Ill.).
39. *Braden v. St. Francis Hospital,* 714 P. 2d. 505 (1985) (Colo.).
40. *Kirk v. Michael Reese Hospital,* 513 N.E. 2d 387 (1987) (Ill.).
41. *Pedroza v. Bryant,* 677 P. 2d, 166 (1984) (Wash.).
42. *Kruegar v. St. Joseph's Hospital,* 305 N.W. 2d 18 (1981) (N.D.).
43. *Knier v. Albany Medical Center Hospital,* 500 N.Y.S. 2d 490 (1986) (N.Y.).
44. *Estate of William Behringer, M.D. v. The Medical Center at Princeton, et al.,* 592 A. 2d 1251 (1991) (N.J.).
45. G.A. Reed & S.W. Malone, *Acquired Immunodeficiency Syndrome,* Ch. 13 in *Healthcare Facilities Law* (A.M. Dellinger ed., Little Brown and Company, Boston, 1991).
46. *Harrell v. Total Health Care, Inc.,* 781 S.W. 2d 58 (1989) (Mo.).
47. *McClellan v. Health Maintenance Organization of Pennsylvania,* 604 A. 2d 1053 (1992) (Pa.).
48. *Robbins v. HIP of New Jersey,* 625 A. 2d 45 (1993) (N.J.).
49. *Sloan v. Metropolitan Health Council, Inc.,* 516 N.E. 2d 1104 (1987) (Ind.).
50. *Schleier v. Kaiser Foundation Health Plan of Mid-Atlantic States,* 876 F. 2d 174 (1989) D.C.
51. *Mitts v. HIP of Greater New York,* 478 N.Y.S. 2d 910 (1984) (N.Y.).
52. *Chase v. Independent Practice Association,* 583 N.E. 2d 251 (1991) (Mass.).
53. *See Boyd v. Albert Einstein Medical Center,* 547 A. 2d 1229 (1988) (Pa.); *Dunn v. Praiss,* 606 A. 2d 862 (1992) (N.J.); *Decker v. Saini,* 88-361768 NH (1991) (Mich.).
54. *Raglin v. HMO Illinois, Inc.,* 595 N.E. 2d 153 (1992) (Ill.).
55. *Williams v. Good Health Plus, Inc.,* 743 S.W. 373 (1987) (Tex.).
56. *Depenbrok v. Kaiser Foundation Health Plan, Inc.,* 144 Cal.Rptr. 724 (1978) (Cal.).
57. *Wickline v. State of California,* 239 Cal.Rptr. 810 (1986) (Cal.).
58. *Wilson v. Blue Cross of So. California,* 271 Cal.Rptr. 876 (1990) (Cal.).
59. *See Darling v. Charleston Community Hospital,* 211 NE 2d 253 (1965) (Ill.); *Purcell v. Zembelman,* 500 P. 2d 335 (1992) (Ariz.); *Corleto v. Shore Memorial Hospital,* 350 A. 2d 534 (1975) (N.J.); *Elam v. College Park Hospital,* 183 Cal.Rptr. 156 (1982) (Cal.); *Blanton v. Moses Cone Memorial Hospital,* 354 S.E. 2d 455 (1987) (N.C.).
60. *Harrell v. Total Health Care Inc.,* 781 S.W. 2d 58 (1989) (Mo.).
61. *See* D. Kinney & M. Wilder, *Medical Standard Setting in the Current Malpractice Environment: Problems and Possibilities,* 22 U.C. Davis L. Rev. 421 (1989).
62. *Williams v. Health America,* 535 N.E. 2d 717 (1987) (Ohio).
63. *Boyd v. Albert Einstein Medical Center,* 547 A. 2d 1229 (1987) (Pa.).
64. 29 U.S.C.A. § 1001-1461.
65. *DeGenova v. Ansel,* 555 A. 2d 147 (1988) (Pa.).
66. W.A. Chittenden III, *Malpractice Liability and Managed Health Care: History and Prognosis,* Tort & Ins. L. J. 451-496 (Sp. 1991).
67. Ch. 621 Florida Stat. (1991).
68. Ch. 621.07 Florida Stat. (1991).
69. *We're Associates Co. v. Cohen et al.,* 480 N.E. 2d 357 (1985) (N.Y.).
70. *South High Dev. Ltd. v. Weiner et al.,* 445 N.E. 2d 1106 (1983) (Ohio).

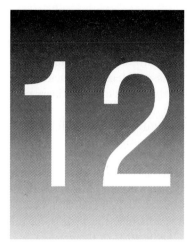

Medical product liability

PHARMACEUTICAL BACKGROUND
GOVERNMENT REGULATION OF THE PHARMACEUTICAL INDUSTRY
STRICT LIABILITY AND PHARMACEUTICALS
RECENT CASES
CONCLUSION

The concept of strict liability eliminates the need to prove negligence for an injury caused by a defective product.[1] However, policy interests have shaped the unique nature of pharmaceutical case law to provide multiple exceptions to the standard rules of strict liability. Some of the exceptions favor plaintiffs.[2] In such cases manufacturer liability is easier to prove and is often decided with minimal evidence.[3] Other exceptions favor the defendants in drug-related litigation. The most notable exception is comment k to Section 402A of the Restatement (Second) of Torts.[4] Comment k distinguishes some pharmaceuticals from most other manufactured products by stating that the manufacturer is not held liable for injury resulting from consumption of drugs that are seen as unavoidably unsafe. Use of these drugs is justified in spite of the apparent medical risks. Certain products are unavoidably dangerous and are incapable of being made safe when manufactured properly. Currently a majority of courts agree with the Restatement's view and find some drugs dangerous by nature, but it is unclear which drugs are unavoidably unsafe.[5]

The courts treat pharmaceuticals differently than other manufactured products. One reason for this different treatment is the interaction between the patient's body and the drug's chemical compound. When a drug is ingested, the response of an individual patient is difficult to predict. Every effect and each adverse reaction is unique. Frequently the response to the chemical depends more on the individual's physiology than on the product design. Therefore a safely designed drug for every situation or every individual may be illusory. Some commentators consider the pharmaceutical industry sufficiently unique to be categorized separately from all other forms of product liability.[6] Others believe the drug manufacturer should be held to the same form of strict liability as other industries.[7] Still others contend that the pharmaceutical companies should be strictly liable for their products but define the role of liability differently, usually holding manufacturers to a lesser standard.[8]

PHARMACEUTICAL BACKGROUND
Drug industry

The drug industry in America has changed dramatically since the 1930s and 1940s. Early pharmaceutical companies generally produced a complete line of medication to serve pharmacists' needs.[9] These companies spent little money on research, development, and advertising. Customarily the basic drug ingredients constituted 75% of corporate expenditures.[10]

The impetus for change was the increasing efficacy of drugs.[11] In the early part of the century, even with hundreds of compounds on the market, few "cures" could be credited to pharmaceuticals.[12] Most drugs sold were used for supportive care and did little to affect the course of illness directly. However, by the late 1940s and early 1950s drugs took the offensive against disease.[13] Penicillin and other broad-spectrum antibiotics heralded a new age in which medicine could directly attack foreign cells without harming the host. Because most drugs are effective against only one or two conditions, hundreds of drugs are sold. In the United States, more than 1000 physiologically active compounds are available.[14] These compounds in turn are mixed with other compounds that produce hundreds of thousands of products.[15]

Adverse reactions are unwanted interactions between a drug and a recipient's physiology. Multiple forms of adverse reactions are possible with any drug. Hypersensitivity or allergic reactions, drug interactions, excessive amounts of the desired effect, unavoidable side effects, and activation of physical illness are a few of the adverse reactions possible. Wherever possible, a manufacturer should seek to discover and eliminate these unwanted side effects. Adverse reactions to drugs remain one of the major causes of hospitalization,

The Editorial Committee updated this chapter. The committee gratefully acknowledges the past contributions of Martin J. MacNeill, D.O., J.D., F.C.L.M., and Sandy Sanbar, M.D., Ph.D, J.D., F.C.L.M.

illness, and death in the nation. Some authors believe that more than 140,000 deaths per year are caused by adverse drug reactions in the United States.[16] A product, however, that is highly beneficial to millions of patients may be deadly to a few. Most commentators agree that a prescription drug should not be considered defective because an unusually sensitive user develops an adverse reaction.[17]

Known adverse reactions

Pharmaceutical manufacturers are required to warn adequately of known dangers in the administration of their product.[18]

Unknown adverse reactions

Possibly more serious than known side effects are those that remain undiscovered until an adverse reaction occurs in the ultimate consumer. Although no national consensus exists, some courts consider an undiscovered side effect a defect and impose the same strict liability as with other defects.[19] Others look to comment k of Section 402A and insulate drugs from standard product liability.[20]

GOVERNMENT REGULATION OF THE PHARMACEUTICAL INDUSTRY

Government regulation of the pharmaceutical industry is discussed in detail in Chapter 48.

STRICT LIABILITY AND PHARMACEUTICALS
Strict liability as applied to pharmaceuticals

Most courts categorize rules of liability that apply to prescription drugs differently than rules for other products. Some courts have held that the rules of strict liability should not apply to some drugs.[21] Other courts apply a limited form of strict liability with less stringent rules for drugs. Still other courts do not differentiate between drugs and other manufactured products.[22]

The Restatement (Second) of Torts, Section 402A, comment k, describes some drugs as "incapable of being made safe." For example, "the vaccine for the Pasteur treatment of rabies" often "leads to very serious and damaging consequences when it is injected." Such a drug is "properly prepared, and accompanied by proper directions and warning, is not defective, nor is it unreasonably dangerous."[23] Comment k does not seek to prevent all suits against drug manufacturers. Although it protects drug manufacturers against liability for design defects, it does not immunize them against suits for manufacturing defects or inadequate warnings.

Multiple policy considerations are behind the adoption of strict liability in torts. Some of these considerations include compensation or spreading of the loss between all consumers of a product, deterrence, encouraging useful conduct by both parties to an action, protecting consumer expectations, and improving the allocation of resources.[24] Multiple approaches have been used by the courts in the development of the concept of defectiveness. One approach is the consumer expectation test, which weighs whether a product is unreasonably dangerous beyond the danger contemplated by the ordinary consumer.[25] This test has fallen from favor in a majority of courts because it relies on the term unreasonable as a requirement of defectiveness. Reasonableness is a negligence concept.[26] If a danger generally is known to the ordinary consumer, the product is not per se defective.[27]

Another approach is the risk/utility test,[28] which balances the risk of danger associated with a product and the utility of the product to the consumer. This test is the approach used most often to determine defectiveness.[29] The emphasis is on the safety of the product rather than the reasonable or unreasonable action of the manufacturer. Some of the factors considered in a risk/utility analysis include the severity of the risk, the likelihood of harm, the benefits of the product, and the feasibility of an alternative design.[30] Once a product is determined to be dangerous, the court then must balance the product's utility against its dangers. Many courts refuse to classify a drug as unreasonably dangerous if the drug's utility to mankind is considered greater than the potential for injury to an individual.[31]

Last, some jurisdictions offer an alternative test that uses a bifurcated standard—either consumer expectation or risk/utility.[32] Use of the disjunctive expands recovery potential for plaintiffs.

Types of defects

First, a manufacturing defect might cause one "batch" of the drug to deviate from the norm. Second, a design defect, such as a basic intrinsic flaw in the chemical design, could exist.

Manufacturing defects. Manufacturing defects are those that deviate from the manufacturer's design or specifications and thus are different than the usual product that "comes off the assembly line."[33] Manufacturing defects typically are easy to identify because the products are flawed. Even though the cause of the manufacturing defect usually is negligence, difficulty in proof requires a strict liability standard, without regard to the manufacturer's reasonableness in protecting its process from error. The consumer expectation test is used because the consumer expects a product to be free of defects.

As an industry, pharmaceutical manufacturers have maintained a good record, keeping manufacturing defects to a minimum. From 1966 to 1971 the U.S. Food and Drug Administration (FDA) ordered 1935 drug recalls for mistaken labeling, contamination, adulteration, or incorrect dosage.[34] Apart from the sulfanilamide disaster, few episodes of death or disability have been caused by manufacturing defects.[35] Recent cases are discussed later in this chapter.

Design defects. Whereas a manufacturing defect involves an isolated deviation from the norm, a design defect involves the entire line of products. Such a product is manufactured according to specifications but remains unreasonably dangerous for its intended use.[36] Difficulty in determining a design defect situation arises when the courts attempt to define "reasonable danger."[37]

If a design is defective, all of the products manufactured using that design are defective. The evaluation of design defect by the jury is based on a four-prong test involving (1) feasibility of an alternative design (2) at the time of the manufacture that was (3) commercially available and (4) would not destroy the product's productivity.[38] Some courts hold that the "FDA's decision of product marketability disposes of the defect issue."[39] These courts conclude that, if the FDA does not approve a product, "the product must be considered unavoidably unsafe as a matter of law and thus outside the parameters of strict liability for defective design."

Occasionally the government accepts responsibility for drug defects. In 1976 the government statutorily accepted liability for any adverse reactions to the swine flu immunization,[40] The government took the position of the manufacturer for the purpose of liability.[41] This legislation was repealed in 1978.[42] A similar program of "no-fault compensation" was created by the National Childhood Vaccine Injury Act.[43] This legislation has a dual purpose. First, it allows easier access to compensation for those children who have suffered hypersensitivity reactions to vaccines.[44] Second, it provides liability protection for manufacturers of the vaccine, allowing them to continue their production.[45]

Warning

Manufacturer's duty to warn. Products that are both properly designed and correctly manufactured may still be dangerous and will be considered defective if not accompanied by a proper warning.[46] The supplier of any product, including the manufacturer of pharmaceuticals, is under a duty to use reasonable care to warn adequately about the risks associated with the use of its product.[47] This duty extends to the risks about which the manufacturer knows and to those about which, through reasonable care, it should have known.[48]

The duty of a pharmaceutical manufacturer to warn arises when the product is known to cause a particular side effect. The manufacturer is not responsible for unforeseeable or unknown dangers it is unable to discover with reasonable care.[49] Nor is the company a guarantor of the safety of a product that causes an unusual hypersensitivity reaction if that reaction was not a known side effect of the product.[50]

The "unavoidably dangerous" protection afforded prescription drugs under the Restatement (Second) of Torts, Section 402A, comment k, applies unless the manufacturer has provided an adequate warning of potential adverse reactions.[51] The protection does not extend to those manufacturers who have failed to follow FDA guidelines for testing and marketing of their product.[52]

Drugs are an exception to the rule requiring a warning of danger to the ultimate consumer.[53] The drug manufacturer's duty to warn includes a warning to physicians of the special risks that accompany normal use.[54] In the majority of cases there is no duty to warn the patient directly.[55] For the sake of pharmaceutical warnings the physician is considered the "learned intermediary," and as such in most instances the duty to warn ends when an adequate effort is made by the company to instruct physicians of the drug's potential side effects.[56,57] The pharmaceutical manufacturer has no obligation to warn the ultimate user of danger propensities "where there is an intermediary who is not a mere conduit of the product, but rather administers it on an individual basis."[58] After the manufacturer has given the physician the necessary information, it is then the physician's duty to warn the patient.[59]

The manufacturer's duty to warn does not end with the purchase of the drug by the patient. Postsale warnings also are required. The manufacturer is considered an expert with regard to its product.[60] As an expert, the manufacturer has the duty to stay abreast of the scientific data in the field and the further duty to warn physicians of potential harm caused by the product.[61]

If an unknown hazard is discovered after the drug has been sold, the manufacturer is required to make reasonable efforts to inform the consumer.[62] This requirement usually is satisfied with warnings to physicians in the form of "Dear Doctor" letters or via detail persons. One court has said that "[a]lthough a product may be reasonably safe when manufactured . . . risks thereafter revealed by user operation and brought to the attention of the manufacturer or vendor may impose upon one or both a duty to warn."[63,64]

The manufacturer is responsible for performing studies of its product when adverse reactions are reported. The results of these studies, if adverse to the product, must be reported to the public (i.e., physicians).[65] This duty to report new adverse findings extends to more than the research of the manufacturer and includes all industry knowledge (i.e., state of the art). Constructive knowledge of potential side effects is presumed with the publication of articles in scientific journals that relate to the product.[66]

Although the duty of drug manufacturers to provide warnings usually extends only to the physician, in cases in which the manufacturer knows that the product will reach the public without individualized medical intervention the drug manufacturer also must warn the public at large.[67,68] Such an example is immunizations; everyone is given a standardized dose of the vaccine without individualized dosing by the physician.[69] Likewise, birth control pills are given out without much individual attention. Therefore no protection exists for the drug producer under the learned intermediary rule in situations in which the manufacturer had actual or constructive knowledge of the potential for the public to acquire the product without significant physician intervention.[70]

Adequacy. Adequacy of the warning is a major issue in determining reasonableness. If the warning is adequate, the defendant drug producer will usually prevail, even if the product is unavoidably unsafe.[71] The warning is adequate when it is obviously displayed, when it gives a fair appraisal of the extent of the danger, and when it properly instructs the user in how to use the product.[72] Likewise, a warning is adequate when it "warns with the degree of intensity demanded by the nature of the risk."[73] A warning, however, may be inadequate if it is "unduly delayed, reluctant in tone or lacking in a sense of urgency."[73]

Even if an adequate warning of the risk is given, it will not insulate the manufacturer from liability when a cure for the defect could have been accomplished with little effort. Moreover, statements that lead the user to minimize the importance of the warning may diminish the value of an adequate warning. For example, one manufacturer's warning concerning birth control pills contained studies showing an increased incidence of thrombosis in British women taking the pill. The court held that having a study dealing with British women did little to amplify concern of thrombosis in American women and therefore did not adequately warn this group.[74]

In addition, most courts require warnings to be given if an allergic reaction may affect a substantial number of people.[75] Some courts have imposed a duty to warn of rare adverse reactions if the end result would be exceedingly serious.[76] The Restatement (Second) of Torts states that "[w]here . . . the product contains an ingredient to which a substantial number of the population are allergic . . . the seller is required to give warning . . . and a product bearing such a warning, which is safe for use if it is followed, is not in defective condition, nor is it unreasonably dangerous."[77]

Methods. Warnings may be satisfied in a number of ways. Labeling package inserts, advertising, and interaction with drug company detail persons all may act as adequate warnings to decrease liability.

LABELING. The FDA has numerous requirements for the labeling of pharmaceuticals.[78] These are minimum requirements only and do not relieve the manufacturer of its duty to fully warn of dangers of which it has actual or constructive knowledge.[79] The basic labeling regulation as promulgated by the FDA is that all material facts relating to the drug are to be presented on the package.[80]

PACKAGE INSERTS. The package insert is the method developed by the FDA for instructing physicians and patients about the makeup, side effects, indications, and dosing of a product.[81] The most important feature of the package insert is the requirement that the information contained therein be completely based on substantial evidence. No "hype" or promotion is permitted to be included. Because physicians have almost unlimited access to drug information through a variety of sources, the package insert is not intended to be the most current repository of information concerning the benefits of a drug. Instead, its purpose is to inform the physician of any substantial evidence relating to the drug's benefits or side effects.

The package insert contains information based on data submitted to the FDA by the manufacturer dealing with the safety and efficacy of the drug.[82] A physician is not required to follow the instructions on the package insert. However, if the physician chooses not to follow the instructions, he or she may be concerned about increased liability.[83] This fear leads many physicians to practice "cookbook medicine" (i.e., following the product insert instructions implicitly without regard to the patient's individual reactions). However, in general most physicians do not dispense drugs; thus they do not see the product inserts, which can be problematic. Likewise, although pharmacists have access to inserts, they usually rely on computer data for the majority of their product information.

Some courts construe a manufacturer's failure to comply with rules requiring package inserts as constituting negligence per se.[84] Other courts have held that failure to follow statutory regulation concerning inserts is not a controlling issue.[85]

ADVERTISING. Emphasis on product promotion is one of the more controversial actions of the pharmaceutical industry. Manufacturers spend more than one fourth of their gross income from drug sales on marketing.[86] The majority of this money is spent on advertising and detail persons. The Pharmaceutical Manufacturers Association, realizing the importance of this issue, has promulgated the Code of Fair Practices in the Promotion of Drug Products. But, as with many such professional ethical codes, the written word is often overlooked for an improved bottom line.

For most prescribing physicians, drug manufacturers are the dominant if not the only source of information regarding drug risks and benefits. Other independent sources of information, such as medical journals, may be reluctant to publish research that is critical of drug manufacturers' products because drug advertising accounts for the largest share of medical journals' revenue.[87]

Courts have held drug manufacturers liable for advertisements that dilute proper warnings or reduce the physician's reliance on a package insert.[88] Courts have held that a company incurs liability if it causes a prescribing physician to disregard the warnings mandated by the FDA.[89] Some courts have held the manufacturer liable, even when the physician acted in a negligent manner, if the physician's actions were induced through overpromotion.[90]

Drug manufacturers may be held to a warranty standard based on advertising. Drug manufacturers rarely expose themselves to liability by expressly warranting their products.[91] Instead, exposure to breach of warranty liability most often arises through implied warranty and misrepresentation.

DETAIL PERSONS. Detail persons—the sales representatives of ethical drugs—occupy a position different from those of other salespersons. Their potential misrepresentation of the product, rather than being harmless fluff, may lead to death or disfigurement of the ultimate consumer. Detail persons, acting as the liaison between physicians and the manufacturer, are the most common transmitters of new information concerning pharmaceuticals. The pharmaceutical industry employs almost 40,000 detail persons.[92]

Detail persons are frequently torn between a desire to increase the substantial profits of the drug manufacturer and a duty to inform the physician of product side effects and possible contraindications.[93] There is great potential for detail persons to mislead physicians in an attempt to increase sales. Manufacturers are vicariously liable for the actions of the detail persons who are within the scope of their employment.[94] Some courts have held that the liability extends even beyond the scope of employment.[95] An otherwise adequate warning provided by the company can be nullified by an overzealous detail person. High-pressure sales by intense, occasionally knowledgeable detail persons often determine physician use patterns. Even though the oral communications of detail persons are difficult to monitor as to completeness or accuracy, drug companies cannot escape liability for the improper overpromotion of safety by detail persons.

If a detail person convinces the physician to disregard warnings provided by the manufacturer, the company may be held liable with regard to the cause of the injury.[96] At least one court has held that detail persons have a duty to warn of potential adverse reactions.[97] Liability is possible because the physician might otherwise have been aware of the risks that were involved had the detail person given adequate warnings.[98]

Causation

As in negligence actions, causation must be proved in strict tort liability. Professor Prosser states that "[s]trict liability eliminates both privity and negligence; but it still does not prove the plaintiff's case."[99] The standard elements of proof, as enumerated in Section 402A of the Restatement (Second) of Torts, are (1) proof that the product was defective, (2) proof that the defect existed at the time it left the control of the defendant, (3) proof that the defect created a product that was unreasonably dangerous for the intended or foreseeable use, and (4) proof that the defect caused the injury.[100] Within the pharmaceutical industry, causation is most commonly proved through epidemiological and statistical studies, expert testimony, direct or circumstantial evidence, or a combination of these methods.[101]

In situations in which the plaintiff is unable to identify the defective product's specific manufacturer, an industry-wide liability has been devised.[102] Liability may be imposed on every manufacturer of a generic product. It is then the responsibility of the various defendants to prove that they did not supply the defective product.[103]

On the other hand, a design defect is easier to prove because all of the same types of drugs are equally defective and available for testing. In a failure to warn case the plaintiff must prove that lack of proper warning was the proximate cause of the injury. The failure to warn must be the direct link between the product and the injury. The plaintiff must further show that the manufacturer either knew or should have known about the danger of harm from the drug.[104] Defendant liability may be severed by the introduction of an intervening cause. In strict liability litigation, courts are willing to view intervening causes as unforeseeable.[105]

Most courts view the terms *user* and *consumer* liberally. Historically, privity was required before permitting recovery. Today, a user may be far removed from the initial privity of contract.[106] If it is foreseeable that an individual will be a user, that individual is a potential plaintiff.[107] If, for example, the patient were to ingest multiple drugs, each drug might be viewed as a cause-in-fact of the subsequent harm. At least one court has held a manufacturer of one defective drug liable for the entire injury sustained by the ingestion of multiple drugs.[108]

The foreseeability of the harm caused by a product is an issue in many courts.[109] Some courts now reject the foreseeability of the harm approach and instead look to the foreseeability of the use.[110]

Physician and pharmacist liability

Many physicians and pharmacists are not fully informed of the potential side effects associated with the drugs they prescribe. One study revealed that less than 13% of drug use was evaluated as rational, 21.5% was considered questionable, and amazingly more than 65% was judged irrational.[111] Because of the prevalence of drug use in the treatment of patients, many malpractice cases could have pharmaceutical components.

The application of traditional liability rules to pharmaceutical manufacturers is problematic. For example, the defined consumer of prescription drugs is the physician, not the patient. The patient has little input into the drug selected by the physician. The physician holds a position as a "learned intermediary" and as such takes on some of the manufacturer's liability even in the case of product defect.[112]

Physicians and pharmacists who find themselves in a suit resulting from a defective product have some recourse.[113] There is a potential tort action against the manufacturers of the defective products both for the injury to the patient and for damage to reputation and earnings.[114] In many circumstances this action leads to plaintiffs playing one potential defendant against another.[115]

Defenses

Defenses to strict product liability differ from one jurisdiction to the next as discussed in the following sections.

Assumption of the risk. The Restatement (Second) of Torts describes assumption of the risk as "the form of contributory negligence which consists of voluntary and unreasonable encounter of a known danger."[116] If the consumer knew of the product's defect but disregarded the danger and used the product, he or she is barred from seeking to recover against the defendant. The defendant must prove that the plaintiff knew and understood the danger and "voluntarily and unreasonably" consented to being exposed to it.[117]

Assumption of the risk is an essential concept in pharmaceutical litigation defense. If adequate warning is given to the physician and the physician disregards these dangers, then the physician and patient have assumed some of the risk for potential adverse reactions.

Comparative fault. Comparative fault measures the plaintiff's fault in comparison to the manufacturer's fault and places a percentage value on each. Most states with comparative negligence systems have applied a comparative fault scheme to strict tort liability litigation.[118] In a pure system a plaintiff may recover the percentage of damage caused by the defendant, regardless of the fault attributable to the plaintiff.[119]

The goal of strict tort liability is to avoid making the manufacturer an insurer for product-induced injuries. Comparative fault provides more equity in allocating risks and preventing manufacturers and other consumers from sharing in the costs attributable to those who fail to use products carefully. Most courts that have permitted a comparative fault defense also have permitted defenses of assumption of the risk and misuse.[120] The jury usually is instructed to combine the percentage from each of these defenses and award the percentage of fault as the sum of the three.[121]

Product misuse. The defense of product misuse is permitted when the plaintiff has used a product for a purpose not reasonably foreseeable to the manufacturer.[122] The Restatement (Second) of Torts recognizes the defense of product misuse. Comment h of Section 402A provides that "if the injury results from abnormal handling, . . . the seller is not liable."[123] The defense of misuse may be used if the plaintiff's misuse of the product was a contributing cause of the injury.[124] To assert this defense, the plaintiff's misuse of the product must be unforeseeable. The definition of the term *unforeseeable* is the important issue. Taking four times the standard dose of a medication may be foreseeable but taking five times may be unforeseeable. There is no standard, fixed, arbitrary cutoff. The fact-finder must determine foreseeability on a case-by-case basis.

Damages

Similar to negligence litigation, strict liability provides for property and personal damage recovery.[125] With both negligence and strict liability, damage is part of a prima facie case.[126] Commentators differ in their views regarding punitive damage awards in strict liability litigation. Some assert that punitive damage awards should be granted as punishment for wanton, willful, reckless, malicious, or outrageous conduct.[127] Other jurisdictions grant punitive damage awards to deter others who might commit the same outrageous conduct.[128] Most jurisdictions use punitive damages for any combination of the preceding reasons.[129]

Punitive damage awards are common in strict liability litigation involving pharmaceutical products.[130] The plaintiff has the burden of proving the defendant's outrageous conduct by presenting clear and convincing evidence.[131] Punitive damage awards punish inappropriate manufacturing practices and stop product suppliers from making economic decisions but do not remedy the product's defects.[132] The most common type of drug cases in which punitive damages are granted are those in which the manufacturer had knowledge of adverse reactions but failed to properly warn of the danger.[133]

RECENT CASES

In 1993 the California Supreme Court held generally in *Anderson v. Owens-Corning Fiberglass* that a manufacturer was strictly liable for injuries caused by its failure to warn of dangers known to the scientific community at the time the product was manufactured and distributed.[134] In 1988 the court applied this rule to manufacturers of prescription drugs in *Brown v. Superior Ct.*[135]

In 1996 the California Supreme Court held in *Carlin v. Sutter County Superior Ct.* that prescription drug manufacturers may be strictly liable under state law for failure to warn, so long as the risk of injury is either actually known or scientifically ascertainable at the time of the drug's distribution.[136] The court was not persuaded to adopt a standard of simple negligence for only that industry. The court also found that FDA regulations do not preempt common law tort remedies for failure to warn and that FDA action or inaction may be admissible to show whether a risk was known or scientifically ascertainable.

In 1996 in *Wagner v. Roche Laboratories* the Ohio Supreme Court held that expert testimony that a drug manufacturer knew or should have known of synergistic side effects of its drug and certain antibiotics was specific enough and of sufficient probative value to create under state product liability law a question of fact as to the adequacy of warnings contained in an FDA-approved package insert.[137]

Silicone breast implants

In 1997 Dr. Jack Snyder published an exhaustive law review article on the subject of silicone breast implants in which he noted that breast implant litigation had reshaped the concept of compensable "soft tissue injury" in the 1990s.[138] Snyder noted that between 1977 and 1992 breast implant product liability cases were primarily resolved on evidentiary or procedural grounds. Plaintiffs alleged negligence, strict liability, fraudulent misrepresentation, and breach of express and implied warranty. His analysis of past, present, and future breast implant lawsuits included the potential defendants, causes of action and defenses, causation hurdle, case management (including the traditional case-by-case method), consolidation, bifurcation, multidistrict litigation, class actions, dormant dockets, future injuries, and federal-state coordination.

In 1988 the FDA reclassified breast implants in the category of the most strictly regulated medical products.[139] In 1991 the FDA learned that Dow Corning Corporation had not disclosed evidence suggesting it had safety concerns about breast implants. In 1993 the commissioner of the FDA, D. David Kessler, announced that the availability of silicone breast implants would be severely limited. What followed was a flood of litigation resulting in billions of dollars in judgments and settlements. The breast implant cases are cited, reviewed, and superbly discussed by Snyder.

Statutory compliance and tort liability

Professor Michael D. Green discussed the topic of statutory compliance and tort liability in 1996 at a product liability symposium.[140] In discussing the proper balance between the tort system and regulation in the context of prescription drugs and the FDA's vigorous oversight of the industry, Green articulated his reasons that a regulatory compliance defense, in which tort law would defer to FDA regulation, is quite attractive. However, he concluded by suggesting that a regulatory compliance defense may impact the types of drug litigation that occur but drug litigation would not disappear.

Preemption in medical device cases

The verdict in *Medtronic Inc. v. Lohr* was handed down by a sharply divided U.S. Supreme Court in June 1996.[141] *Lohr* raises significant questions about whether preemption is still a viable defense in medical device cases. Lohr filed suit in Florida state court against Medtronic based on the failure of a pacemaker lead. The case was removed to federal court, then the district court granted Medtronic's summary judgment on the grounds that Lohr's claims were preempted by the Medical Device Amendments to the Federal Food Drug and Cosmetic Act of 1938.[142] The U.S. Supreme Court held in a five-to-four decision that none of Lohr's claims were preempted. For a thorough discussion of *Lohr,* see the excellent article by Quenton F. Urquhart Jr. and Robert E. Durgin.[143]

CONCLUSION

The public should be free to purchase goods without fear of defect. Strict tort liability is a valid means to ensure that products function without causing injury. On the other hand, it is unreasonable to expect all products to be totally safe and risk free for consumers. A knife with a dull blade might be safer than one with a sharp blade, but part of the sharp knife's efficacy is due to the cause of its dangerous propensity, namely, its sharpened edge. Ice cream would be safer without the heavy cholesterol content, but the joy of eating it comes from its richness, which clogs our arteries. Medication is unique because it is ingested into the body with the knowledge that in a certain number of individuals there will be serious side effects.

It is true that drugs can be made safer, but even so certain idiosyncratic reactions will occur and cause a few to suffer. The answer might be for the government or the manufacturer to set up a trust fund for those few individuals who experience such reactions. Rather than hamper the medical establishment with increased liability, the courts should take the forefront in the fight to provide a strong defense for drug manufacturers.

ENDNOTES

1. *Greenman v. Yuba Power Prod.,* 59 Cal. 2d 57, 377 P. 2d 897, 27 Cal. Rptr. 697 (1963); Restatement (Second) of Torts § 402A (1) (1965).
2. *See* Comment, *DES and a Proposed Theory of Enterprise Liability,* 46 Fordham L. Rev. 963 (1978).
3. *See Wells v. Ortho Pharmaceutical Corp.,* 788 F. 2d 741 (11th Cir. 1986), cert. denied, 479 U.S. 950 (1986).
4. Restatement (Second) of Torts § 402A cmt. k (1965).
5. *See, e.g., McElhaney v. Eli Lilly & Co.,* 575 F.Supp. 228 (D.S.D. 1983).
6. *See, e.g.,* Scott, *Medical Product and Drug Causation: How to Prove It and Defend Against It,* 56 Def. Couns. J. 270 (1989); Leighton, *Introduction to the Symposium on Chemical and Food Product Liability,* 41 Food Drug Cosm. L. J. 385 (1986); Schwartz, *Unavoidably Unsafe Products,* 42 Wash. & Lee L. Rev. 1139 (1985).
7. McClellan, *Drug Induced Injury,* 25 Wayne L. Rev. 1 (1978); Maldonado, *Strict Liability and Informed Consent: 'Don't Say I Didn't Tell You So,'* 9 Akron L. Rev. 609 (1976); Merrill, *Compensation for Prescription Drug Injuries,* 59 Va. L. Rev. 1 (1973); Keeton, *Product Liability: Drugs and Cosmetics,* 25 Vand. L. Rev. 131 (1972).
8. Britain, *Product Honesty Is the Best Policy: A Comparison of Doctor's and Manufacturer's Duty to Disclose Drug Risks and the Importance of Consumer Expectations in Determining Product Defect,* 79 N.W. U.L. Rev. 342 (1984); Fink, *Education in Pharmacy and Law,* 26 J. Legal Educ. 528, 538 (1974).
9. *See* Staudt, *Determining and Evaluating the Promotional Mix,* Modern Medicine Topics 8 (July 1957).
10. *See* E. Ackerknecht, *Therapeutics from the Primitives to the 20th Century* (Hafner Press, New York 1973).
11. *Id.* at 144-145.
12. *Id.* at 145.
13. *Id.* at 30.
14. U.N. Industrial Development Organization, *The Growth of the Pharmaceutical Industry in Developing Countries: Problems and Prospects,* at 23, U.N. Doc. ID/204, U.N. Sales No. E.78.II.B.4 (1978).
15. Halberstrom, *Too Many Drugs?* F. on Med. 3 (Mar. 1979).
16. Tally & Laventurier, *Drug-Induced Illness,* 229 J.A.M.A. 1043 (1974).
17. *See, e.g.,* Restatement (Second) of Torts § 402A, cmt. c (1965).
18. *See Id.* at cmt. j (1965).
19. *See, e.g., Brochu v. Ortho Pharmaceutical Corp.,* 642 F. 2d 652 (1st Cir. 1981).
20. *See, e.g., Johnson v. American Cyanamid Co.,* 239 Kan. 279, 285, 718 P. 2d 1318, 1323 (1986).
21. *See, e.g., Id.* (quoting Restatement (Second) of Torts § 402A cmt. k [1965]).
22. *Supra,* note 19.
23. Restatement (Second) of Torts § 402A cmt. k (1965) (emphasis in original).
24. D. Fisher & W. Powers Jr., *Products Liability: Cases and Materials* 50-51 (1988).
25. Restatement (Second) of Torts § 402A cmt. g (1965).
26. *Id.* at § 395 (1965).
27. *Id.* at § 402A cmt. i (1965).
28. *See, e.g., Boutland of Houston, Inc. v. Bailey,* 609 S.W. 2d 743, 746 (Tex. 1980.)
29. *See, e.g., Phillips v. Kimwood Mach. Co.,* 269 Or. 485, 525 P. 2d 1033 (1974); *Dosier v. Wilcox-Crittendon, Co.,* 45 Cal. App. 3d 74, 119 Cal. Rptr. 135 (1975).
30. Wade, *On the Nature of Strict Tort Liability for Products,* 44 Miss. L. J. 825, 829 (1973).
31. *See contra, supra,* note 19.
32. *Barker v. Lull Engineering Co.,* 20 Cal. 3d 413, 573, P. 2d 443, 143 Cal. Rptr. 225 (1978) (permitting the use of either the consumer expectation test or the risk/utility test).

33. *Id.* at 225, 241.

34. M. Silverman & P. Lee, *Pills, Profits and Politics* 333 (University of California Press, Berkeley 1974).

35. A batch of sulfanilamide was improperly mixed with a lethal solvent causing the death of many patients during the 1950s. J. Schnze, *Governmental Control of Therapeutic Drugs: Intent, Impact, and Issues, in The Pharmaceutical Industry* 9-10 (C. Lindsay ed. 1978). For a competent evaluation of the history of the drug industry, *see* G. Porter & H. Livesay, *Merchants and Manufacturer: Studies in the Changing Structure of the Nineteenth Century Marketing* (1971).

36. Comment, *Can a Prescription Drug be Defectively Designed?: Brochu v. Ortho Pharmaceutical Corp.,* 31 De Paul L. Rev. 247 (1981).

37. Birnbaum, *Unmasking the Test for Design Defect: From Negligence to Strict Liability to Negligence,* 33 Vand L. Rev. 593 (1980).

38. Isaacs, *Drug Regulation, Product Liability, and the Contraceptive Crunch: Choices Are Dwindling,* 8 J. Leg. Med. 533 (1987) (strict liability and duty to warn).

39. *See, e.g., Collins v. Ortho Pharmaceutical Corp.,* 195 Cal. App. 3d 1539, 231 Cal. Rptr. 396 (1986).

40. National Swine Flu Immunization Program of 1976, Pub. L. No. 94-380, 90 Stat. 1113; *see also Ducharme v. Merrill-Nat'l Labs.,* 574 F. 2d. 1307 (5th Cir.), *cert. denied,* 439 U.S. 1002 (1978).

41. 90 Stat. 1116.

42. Health and Services Amendments of 1978, Pub. L. 95-626, 92 Stat. 3551.

43. Pub. L. 99-660, 100 Stat. 3755 (codified at 42 U.S.C. §§ 300aa-1 to -33 [1986]).

44. 100 Stat. 3758 (codified at 42 U.S.C. § 300aa-10 (1988)).

45. 100 Stat. 3758-59 (codified at 42 U.S.C. § 300aa-11 (1988)).

46. *See, e.g., Basko v. Sterling Drug,* 416 F. 2d 417, 426 (2d Cir. 1969); *see also Jacobson v. Colorado Fuel & Iron Corp.,* 409 F. 2d 1263, 1271 (9th Cir. 1969).

47. Restatement (Second) of Torts § 12 (1965).

48. *See, e.g., Lindsay v. Ortho Pharmaceutical Corp.,* 637 F. 2d 87 (2d Cir. 1980); *Sterling Drug, Inc., v. Cornish,* 370 F. 2d 82 (8th Cir. 1966); *Incollingo v. Ewing,* 444 Pa. 263, 282 A. 2d 206 (1971), *rev'd on other grounds,* 491 Pa. 561, 421 A. 2d 79 (1977).

49. *Griggs v. Combe, Inc.,* 456 So. 2d 790 (Ala. 1984); *Freeman v. United States,* 704 F. 2d 154 (5th Cir. 1983).

50. *Gravis v. Parke, Davis & Co.,* 502 S.W. 2d 863 (Tex. Civ. App. 1973).

51. *Davila v. Bodelson,* 103 N.M. 243, 704 P. 2d 1119 (App. 1985).

52. *Id.*

53. *See, e.g., Buckner v. Allergan Pharmaceuticals,* 400 So. 2d 820 (Fla. Dist. Ct. App. 1981); *supra,* note 48, *Lindsay; Id.* at 91.

54. *See, e.g., Fellows v. USV Pharmaceutical Corp.,* 502 F.Supp. 297 (D. Md. 1980) (the manufacturer has a duty to provide warnings to physician, but the duty does not extend to the patient); *Ezagui v. Dow Chemical Corp.,* 598 F. 2d 727 (2d Cir. 1979).

55. *Id.*

56. *Reyes v. Wyeth Laboratories,* 498 F. 2d 1264 (5th Cir.), *cert. denied,* 419 U.S. 1096 (1974).

57. *See Leesley v. West,* 165 Ill. App. 3d 135, 518 N.E. 2d 758 (App. Ct.), *appeal denied,* 119 Ill. 2d 558, 522 N.E. 2d 1246 (1988); *Stone v. Smith, Kline & French Laboratories,* 447 So. 2d 1301 (Ala. 1984); *Mauldin v. Upjohn Co.,* 697 F. 2d 644 (5th Cir. 1983).

58. *Bacardi v. Holzman,* 182 N.J. Super. 422, 424, 442 A. 2d 617, 618 (1981).

59. *See Crain v. Allison,* 443 A. 2d 558, 562 (D.C. App. 1982); *Salis v. United States,* 522 F.Supp. 989, 1000 (M.D. Pa. 1981).

60. *Barson v. E.R. Squibb & Sons,* 682 P. 2d 832 (Utah 1984).

61. *Id.* at 834 (citing *McEwan v. Ortho Pharmaceutical Corp.,* 270 Or. 375, 528 P. 2d 522 (1974)).

62. *Schenebeck v. Sterling Drug,* 423 F.2d 919 (8th Cir. 1970).

63. *Id.*

64. *Cover v. Cohen,* 61 N.Y. 2d 261, 268, 461 N.E. 2d 864, 871, 473 N.Y.S. 2d 378, 385 (1984) (citations omitted).

65. *See supra,* note 62; *O'Hare v. Merck & Co.,* 381 F. 2d 286 (8th Cir. 1967).

66. *Feldman v. Lederle Laboratories,* 97 N.J. 429, 479 A.2d 374 (1984); *see also* Gilhooley, *Learned Intermediaries, Prescription Drugs, and Patient Information,* 30 St. Louis L. J. 633 (1986).

67. *See supra,* note 19; *Dyer v. Best Pharmacal,* 118 Ariz. 465, 577 P. 2d 1084 (Ct. App. 1978).

68. *See supra,* note 56; *Davis v. Wyeth Laboratories,* 399 F. 2d 121 (9th Cir. 1968).

69. *Brazzell v. United States,* 788 F. 2d 1352 (8th Cir. 1986).

70. *Williams v. Lederle Laboratories,* 591 F.Supp. 381 (S.D. Ohio 1984).

71. *Formella v. Ciba-Geigy Corp.,* 100 Mich. App. 649, 300 N.W. 2d 356 (1980).

72. Madden, *The Duty to Warn in Products Liability: Contours and Criticism,* 89 W. Va. L. Rev. 221, 310-20 (1987); *Richards v. Upjohn Co.,* 95 N.M. 675, 679, 625 P. 2d 1192, 1196 (Ct. App. 1980).

73. *Seley v. G.D. Searle & Co.,* 67 Ohio St. 2d 192, 198, 423 N.E. 2d 831, 837 (1981).

74. *McEwan v. Ortho Pharmaceutical Corp.,* 570 Or. 375, 528 P. 2d 522 (1974).

75. *Kaempfe v. Lehn & Fink Prods. Corp.,* 21 A.D. 2d 197, 249 N.Y.S. 2d 840 (App. Div. 1964), *aff'd,* 20 N.Y. 2d 818, 231 N.E. 2d 294, 284 N.Y.S. 2d 818 (1967).

76. *Tomer v. American Home Prod. Corp.,* 170 Conn. 681, 368 A. 2d 35 (1976); *Crocker v. Winthrop Laboratories,* 514 S.W. 2d 429 (Tex. 1974).

77. Restatement (Second) of Torts § 402A (1965).

78. 21 C.F.R. § 201 (1990).

79. *Supra,* note 66, *Feldman.*

80. 21 C.F.R. § 201.5 .10 (1990).

81. *Pharmaceutical Mfr. Ass'n. v. Food & Drug Admin.,* 484 F.Supp. 1179 (D. Del. 1980).

82. 21 C.F.R. § 201.5 (1990).

83. *Ohligschlager v. Proctor Community Hosp.,* 55 Ill. 2d 411, 303 N.E. 2d 392 (1973).

84. *Lukaszewicz v. Ortho Pharmaceutical Corp.,* 510 F.Supp. 961, *amended,* 532 F.Supp. 211 (E.D. Wis. 1981).

85. *See MacDonald v. Ortho Pharmaceutical Corp.,* 394 Mass. 131, 475 N.E. 2d 65 (1985), *cert. denied,* 474 U.S. 920 (1985).

86. Harrell, *Pharmaceutical Marketing, in The Pharmaceutical Industry* 80 (C. Lindsay ed. 1978).

87. *See* S. Greenberg, *The Quality of Mercy* 267-283 (Atheneum, New York 1971).

88. *Love v. Wolf,* 226 Cal. App. 2d 378, 38 Cal. Rptr. 183 (1964). Wolf, 226 Cal. App. at 399-400, 38 Cal. Rptr. at 196 (citation omitted).

89. *See Toole v. Richardson-Merrell, Inc.,* 251 Cal. App. 2d 689, 60 Cal. Rptr. 398 (1967).

90. *See, e.g., Stevens v. Parke, Davis & Co.,* 9 Cal. 3d. 51, 507 P. 2d 653, 107 Cal. Rptr. 45 (1973).

91. *But see Spiegel v. Saks 34th Street,* 43 Misc. 2d 1065, 252 N.Y.S. 2d 852 (Sup.Ct. 1964), *aff'd,* 26 A.D. 2d 660, 272 N.Y.S. 972 (1966).

92. Pharmaceutical Manufacturers Association, *Prescription Drug Industry Fact Book* 56 (Washington, D.C. 1986).

93. *See generally* J. Lidstone, *Marketing Planning for the Pharmaceutical Industry* (1987); R. Norris, *Pills, Pesticides and Profits* (1982).

94. Restatement (Second) of Agency § 229 (1958).

95. *See, e.g., Schering Corp. v. Cotlow,* 94 Ariz. 365, 385 P. 2d 234 (1963).

96. *Supra,* note 90.

97. *Supra,* note 48, *Incollingo.*

98. *See, e.g., supra,* note 62; *Krug v. Sterling Drug, Inc.,* 416 S.W. 2d 143 (Mo. 1967).

99. Prosser, *The Fall of the Citadel (Strict Liability to the Consumer),* 50 Minn L. Rev. 791, 840 (1966).

100. Restatement (Second) of Torts § 402A (1965).

101. Middlekauff, *The Current Law Regarding Toxic Torts: Implications for the Food Industry,* 41 Food Drug Cosm. L. J. 387, 404-05 (1986).

102. Comment, *Industry Wide Liability,* 13 Suffolk U. L. Rev. 980 (1979); *Mulcahy v. Eli Lilly & Co.,* 386 N.W. 2d 67 (Iowa 1986) (DES market share liability).

103. Comment, *The Market Share Theory: Sindell's Contribution to Industry Wide Liability,* 19 Hou. L. Rev. 107 (1982).

104. Restatement (Second) of Torts § 402A.

105. *See generally* D. Fischer & W. Powers Jr., *supra,* note 89, at 409-411.

106. Restatement (Second) of Torts § 402A cmt. l (1965).

107. *Winnett v. Winnett,* 57 Ill. 2d 7, 310 N.E. 2d 1 (1974).

108. *Supra,* note 46, *Basko.*

109. *Helene Curtis Indus. v. Pruitt,* 385 F. 2d 841, 859-864 (5th Cir. 1967); Bigbee v. Pacific Tel. & Tel. Co., 34 Cal. 3d 49, 665 P. 2d 947, 192 Cal. Rptr. 857 (1983).

110. *See, e.g., Baker v. International Harvester Co.,* 660 S.W. 2d 21 (Mo. Ct. App. 1983).

111. M. Silverman & P. Lee, *supra,* note 103, at 289-290.

112. Comment, *Strict Tort Liability/Negligence/Prescription Drugs: A Pharmaceutical Company Owes No Duty to a Non-Patient Third Party to Warn Doctors or Hospitals of the Side Effects of a Drug and a Hospital or Doctor Owes No Duty to a Non-Patient Third Party to Warn a Patient of the Effects of a Prescription Drug,* 77 Ill. B. J. 227 (1988); Comment, *Torts: Duty to Warn—Incorrect Prescription of Unavoidably Unsafe Drugs,* 22 Kan. L. Rev. 281 (1984).

113. *See* Merrill, *Compensation for Prescription Drug Injuries,* 59 Va. L. Rev. 1, 50-68 (1973).

114. *See, e.g., Oksenholt v. Lederle Laboratories,* 294 Or. 213, 656 P. 2d 293 (1982); Mobilia, *Allergic Reactions to Prescription Drugs: A Proposal for Compensation,* 48 Alb. L. Rev. 343, 364-365 (1984).

115. *See* Willig, *Physicians, Pharmacists, Pharmaceutical Manufacturers: Partners in Patient Care, Partners in Litigation?* 37 Mercer L. Rev. 755 (1986).

116. Restatement (Second) of Torts § 402A cmt. n (1965).

117. *Smith v. Clayton & Lambert Mfg. Co.,* 488 F. 2d 1345, 1349 (10th Cir. 1973).

118. *Daly v. General Motors Corp.,* 20 Cal. 3d 725, 575 P. 2d 1162, 144 Cal. Rptr. 380 (1978).

119. *Mulherin v. Ingersoll-Rand Co.,* 628 P. 2d 1301, 1303-1304 (Utah 1981).

120. *See generally,* Fischer, *Products Liability: Applicability of Comparative Negligence to Misuse and Assumption of the Risk,* 43 Mo. L. Rev. 643 (1978).

121. *See, e.g., Duncan v. Cessna Aircraft Co.,* 665 S.W. 2d 414 (Tex. 1984).

122. *Perfection Paint & Color Co. v. Konduris,* 147 Ind. App. 106, 107, 258 N.E. 2d 681, 682 (1970).

123. Restatement (Second) of Torts § 402A cmt. h (1965).

124. *Supra,* note 119.

125. *See* Restatement (Second) of Torts § 402A (1965).

126. *See generally,* W. Prosser, *Law of Torts* § 96 (4th ed. 1971).

127. *See* Restatement (Second) of Torts § 908(2) (1965).

128. *See, e.g., Malcolm v. Little,* 295 A. 2d 711 (Del. 1972).

129. *See, e.g., Miller v. Watkins,* 200 Mont. 455, 653 P. 2d 126 (1982); *Newton v. Standard Fire Ins. Co.,* 291 N.C. 105, 229 S.E. 2d 297 (1976); *see also,* W. Keeton et al., *Prosser and Keeton on Torts,* § 2, at 9 (5th ed. 1984).

130. *See Hoffman v. Sterling Drug,* 485 F. 2d 132, 144-147 (3d Cir. 1973).

131. *Acosta v. Honda Motor Co.,* 717 F. 2d 828, 833 (3d Cir. 1983).

132. *Neal v. Carey Canadian Mines,* 548 F.Supp. 357 (E.D. Pa. 1982), *aff'd, Van Buskirk v. Carey Canadian Mines,* 791 F. 2d 30 (3rd Cir. 1986).

133. *See G.D. Searle & Co. v. Superior Court,* 49 Cal. App. 3d 22, 122 Cal. Rptr. 218 (1975); *Roginsky v. Richardson-Merrell, Inc.,* 378 F. 2d 832 (2d Cir. 1967); *supra,* note 89.

134. *Anderson v. Owens-Corning Fiberglass,* 810 P. 2d 549.

135. *Brown v. Superior Ct.* 751 P. 2d 470.

136. *Carlin v. Sutter Court Superior Ct.* (No. S045912, 8/30/96).

137. *Wagner v. Roche Laboratories* (No. 95-1209, 11/13/96).

138. J.W. Snyder, *Silicone Breast Implants. Can Emerging Medical, Legal, and Scientific Concepts be Reconciled?* 18 J. Legal Med.133-220 (1997).

139. C.F.R. § 878.3540 (1990).

140. Products Liability Symposium, *Statutory Compliance and Tort Liability: Examining the Strongest Case,* 30 U. Mich. J.L. Ref 461 (Spring 1997).

141. *Medtronic Inc. v. Lohr* 116 S. Ct. 2240 (1996).

142. Medical Device Amendments to the Federal Food Drug and Cosmetic Act of 1938 (21 U.S.C. § 360 c et seq. (West Supp. 1996).

143. Q.E. Urquhart, Jr. & R.E. Durgin, *Medtronic v. Lohr: Is There a Future for Preemption in Medical Device Cases?* 64 Def. Couns. J. 45 (January 1977).

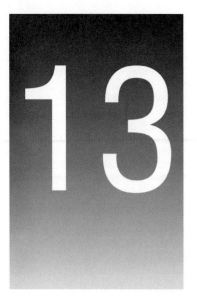

Nursing and the law

JUDITH A. GIC, R.N., J.D.

MEDICAL MALPRACTICE
EMPLOYER'S DIRECT NEGLIGENCE
WORKPLACE TORTS OTHER THAN MALPRACTICE
GOOD SAMARITAN LAWS
PROBLEMS ASSOCIATED WITH NONTRADITIONAL WORKPLACES
NURSES AND THE FAIR LABOR STANDARDS ACT
NURSES AND UNIONS
NURSING LICENSURE

MEDICAL MALPRACTICE

Many state laws governing claims for medical malpractice specify that the actions or inactions of nurses may be the basis for a malpractice lawsuit.[1,2] Even when state law does not consider negligence on the part of a nurse to be malpractice, the nurse can still be held liable for negligence. Either way—malpractice or negligence—nurses can be sued for their mistakes.

Nurses, unlike physicians, are frequently sued because they are usually employed by the hospitals where they work. (Of course, many nurses work outside hospitals, but the majority is still employed there.) The employment relationship may allow the plaintiff to add the employer hospital as a defendant and to make its assets (or those of its insurer) vulnerable to a judgment. This incentive is not always present, but generally, the more solvent defendants there are in a case, the more money the plaintiff may ultimately recover.

Standards of care in nursing

Generally applicable standards. *Malpractice* is usually defined simply as conduct that fails to meet an appropriate standard of care—the care that a reasonably prudent nurse would provide—and that causes an adverse result. Every adverse result is not the consequence of malpractice, however. Some adverse results may be unavoidable even with the best care. Malpractice occurs only when the adverse result could have been avoided through reasonably prudent care. In *Lenger v. Physician's General Hospital, Inc.,*[3] for example, a patient sued for complications that arose after a nurse breached the standard of care by not following the physician's feeding instructions. However, there was no malpractice because there was no evidence that the misfeeding caused the complications. In other words, the

adverse result had nothing to do with the misfeeding and could not have been avoided even if the nurse had not erred.

Defining what the nurse should have done—the standard of reasonably prudent care—is often the critical issue in a malpractice case. At the most general level, the nurse's care should be consistent with generally accepted knowledge and practice. As one court stated (with respect to a specialist nurse)[4]:

A nurse who practices her profession in a particular specialty owes to her patients the duty of *possessing the degree of knowledge or skill* ordinarily possessed by members of her profession actively practicing in such a specialty under similar circumstances. It is the nurse's duty to exercise the degree of skill ordinarily employed, under similar circumstances, by members of the nursing profession in good standing who practice their profession in the same specialty and to use reasonable care and diligence, along with his/her best judgment, in the application of his/her skill to the case.

However, this level of generality is not always helpful, given the highly technical and fact-dependent nature of malpractice cases. The facts of a case help the court define a more specific standard of care for determining liability in that case. Even then, a range of complementary (and occasionally conflicting) choices may still remain because there are so many potential sources of nursing standards.

For example, a patient's injury may arise from something as basic as a nurse's failure to chart the administration of medication, causing another nurse to repeat the dose. Fundamental nursing education may define the appropriate standard of care concerning patient charts. Hospital policy and general standards issued by the American Nurses Association and the Joint Commission on Accreditation of Healthcare Organizations may also address the issue. In such cases, the court may rely on one of the available standards or on some combination of standards that complement one another in directing how a reasonably prudent nurse should act.

In another situation, an injury may result from a highly technical failure involving anesthesia. In deciding whether the nurse was negligent, the court would need to compare the nurse's behavior with that of a reasonably prudent nurse. Its first question might be whether the nurse was a nurse anesthetist or a general registered nurse specially tasked to work with anesthesia.[5] A nurse anesthetist would probably be held to a higher standard. Nurse anesthetists are organized into a professional association (the American Association of Nurse Anesthetists) that has issued protocols for patient treatment. A nurse anesthetist would be expected to satisfy those standards, whereas a general registered nurse might not. Many other nurse specialties are organized similarly (e.g., Association of Women's Health, Obstetrical and Gynecological Nurses; Emergency Nurses Association; American Association of Operating Room Nurses; American Subacute Care Association). A court may agree that these specialist associations help define the appropriate standard of care for nurses regularly practicing within that specialty.[6]

In both of these scenarios, the standard is implicitly national in application. In some malpractice cases, such as those relating to treatment options or decisions relating in turn to the size or wealth of the health care institution and its surrounding community, the standard of care is local. The local standard generally does not apply when as in the example scenarios, either a specialist standard applies or the conduct involves basic nursing skills. In *Ross v. Chatham County Hospital Authority,*[7] an issue in the lawsuit that resulted from leaving a surgical instrument in the patient was whether, and how, application of a local standard might affect a finding of liability. The court concluded that the hospital's location would not matter because "the ability of an operating room employee to count the surgical instruments present at the beginning and end of an operation obviously would not be affected by the size or location of the hospital."[8]

Courts themselves are also extremely important sources for standards of care because they interpret and apply the complementary and sometimes conflicting standards of the various professional organizations. To the extent that a court relies on a particular standard to decide a case, that standard actually becomes the law.

Duty to follow physician's instructions. Whatever local or national standard applies, a physician's orders supplement the standard and in some cases override it. If a physician instructs a nurse to perform a certain action and the nurse fails to do it, resulting damages will be charged to the nurse's negligence.

This obligation is the nurse's shield when the nurse performs as instructed but the result is bad. In *Moore v. Carrington,*[9] an emergency department physician and nurse failed to resuscitate a child. The hospital could not be held liable for any fault of the physician because he was an independent contractor, not an employee. Neither the nurse nor her employer, the hospital, could be held liable because she had done as the physician instructed. Consequently, it was legally possible for only the physician to be held liable (although the jury, after looking at the facts, decided that the physician had not committed malpractice).

Liability for breaches of the standard

Liability for nurse malpractice always falls on the responsible nurse and may also fall on the nurse's employer or supervising physician (or both). The employer and the supervising physician may be the same, as in an office-based practice; however, the employer and the supervising physician are often not the same, as in hospital-based practice, in which the physician is rarely the nurse's employer.

The law assigns shared responsibility for the nurse's malpractice to the employer, the physician, or both parties based on a standard that, like much else in the law, is much easier to state than to apply with consistency. When the malpractice arises out of work that the nonemployer physician supervises and controls, the physician is considered to have "borrowed" the nurse for purposes of that work, so the nurse's actual employer is not liable. When the malpractice arises out of any other work of the nurse, then the nurse's employer is liable. Both results are rooted in the ancient doctrine of respondeat superior, which makes superiors in all lines of work responsible for the negligent (and in some cases, even the intentional) misdeeds of their employees when they act in the course and scope of their employment.

The responsibility is said to be "shared" by the nurse and the other party because the nurse remains liable. Shared liability, also known as *solidary liability* or *joint and several liability,* means that both the nurse and the respondeat superior codefendant are each liable for the full judgment, giving the plaintiff the option of seeking the full judgment against the nurse from either the nurse (in all probability, the nurse's insurer), the nurse's co-defendant employer (again, probably the insurer), or any other co-defendant or seeking some portion from any of these parties. However, some state laws may limit the responsibility of a co-defendant to an amount no greater than that co-defendant's share of the fault, as determined by the jury.[10]

Although a physician or a hospital may have to share a nurse's liability for the nurse's malpractice, a nurse should never have to share a physician's or a hospital's liability for their malpractice. Legal responsibility runs up, not down, the chain of command; that is why it is called *respondeat superior.*

It may seem obvious, but the first questions to ask in a malpractice case concern who committed malpractice, who breached the standard of care, and who is liable. Unfortunately, every party may have a different answer to those questions, for at least two reasons. First, the parties may disagree about the facts: about who did what, when, where, and why. Second, they may disagree about the legal effect of the facts, in particular about who (e.g., the physician, the nurse, or someone else) had a legal duty of care under one or another version of the facts. In some cases, the law forecloses disagreement over who had the duty of care. In *Ravi v. Williams,*[11] for example, it was determined that Alabama law holds surgeons, not nurses, responsible for removing all sponges from the patient before closing an abdominal incision. In thousands of other fact patterns and jurisdictions, the answer may not be so clear-cut.

Although the parties may disagree about who breached the standard, the only answer that really counts is the judge's or jury's. In a real case, the plaintiff generally sues as many people as reasonably possible and lets the lawsuit's fact-finding process zero in on the culpable parties. Early predictions about whose fault it was may be wrong. In *Mosey v. Mueller,*[12] the jury found the hospital liable under respondeat superior for a nurse's negligence in leaving a surgical instrument inside a patient. The appeals court reversed the finding of the nurse's negligence. It concluded, "Evidence established that the surgical nurses had no responsibility to count or account for surgical instruments during a surgical procedure and that such accountability was the sole responsibility of the surgeon."[13] As a result, the nurse was exonerated.

Nurse's own liability. A nurse who has committed malpractice is liable primarily for the damages. The mere fact that the plaintiff may focus collection efforts against a wealthier co-defendant, such as the nurse's employer, does not eliminate the nurse's liability (or the possibility that the nurse's employer will take some adverse job action, such as discipline or termination, or that the state licensing board will suspend or revoke the nurse's license). A nurse must be satisfied that he or she has malpractice insurance, provided by either the self or the employer. In selecting the amount of coverage, the nurse should be aware of any caps or limits on damages that exist under state law.

Physician liability. A physician may incur respondeat superior liability for a nurse's negligence if the physician was either the nurse's actual employer or, during the procedure in question, exercised such supervision and control that a court would *treat* the physician as *if* he or she had been the actual employer. In the second case, the nurse is said to be the physician's "borrowed servant."

In *Hunnicut v. Wright,*[14] the plaintiff sued for injuries caused by a screw and washer that fell off a medical instrument and stayed in his body. The evidence showed that a hospital-employed "scrub tech" failed to tighten the screw after sterilizing it and that if he had done so, the screw and washer would not have fallen off. The surgeon was not the technician's actual employer, so the plaintiff argued that the surgeon should be *treated as* the actual employer. However, the court concluded that the surgeon did not have sufficient supervision or control over the scrub nurse's sterilization and reassembly of the instrument to be treated as the nurse's actual employer and held liable for the negligence. As the court determined in this case[15]:

> The routine acts of treatment which an attending physician may reasonably assume may be performed in his absence by nurses of a modern hospital as part of their usual and customary duties, and execution of which does not require specialized medical knowledge, are merely administrative acts for which negligence in their performance is imputable to the hospital.

On the other hand, the necessary degree of supervision and control was present in *Hudmon v. Martin*[16] for a nurse to be a physician's borrowed servant. In that case, the surgeon and scrub nurse were working together to prepare a patient for surgery, and the surgeon directed the scrub nurse to fill a syringe with a certain fluid. The nurse filled it with the wrong fluid, which injured the patient when the surgeon injected it.

Hospital liability. A hospital may incur respondeat superior liability for an employee nurse's negligence when the nurse is not acting under the supervision and control of a physician; in other words, the nurse has not been "borrowed" and remains an employee of the hospital (or another nonphysician employer). Most nursing occurs outside of a physician's direct supervision and control, with the nurse relying on education, training, and common sense. In these cases, the plaintiff cannot blame the physician for the nurse's negligence.[17] The negligence remains with the nurse, and the nurse's employer will probably share it.

The hospital may also incur respondeat superior liability even when the negligent nurse was acting under a physician's supervision and control but only when the hospital employs both the nurse and the physician. In that case, the supervising physician cannot borrow the nurse from the hospital because the physician works for the same hospital.[18]

General areas in which nurses may be found in breach of standard

How a nurse may breach the appropriate standard of care is a question with innumerable answers. Injury-causing errors can occur in countless ways, and this chapter does not attempt to catalog them. The result would quickly become outdated because new technologies and treatments constantly offer new pitfalls for malpractice. Also, the new (and the old) pitfalls are often practice specific; some types of errors that can occur in a gerontology practice are not likely to occur in a neonatal practice, for example.

Considering nurses' significant role in administering medications to patients, it is not surprising that this is one of the largest areas for negligence actions against nurses. The negligence may take many forms because there are many facets to this nursing activity. A nurse may accidentally give the wrong medicine or the wrong dose, may give the medication to the wrong patient, may administer it incorrectly (e.g., by mouth instead of by injection), or may make another mistake.

The error may not cause physical consequences in the patient for some time. Other circumstances may make it initially difficult to determine that a patient received something in error and may delay the necessary backtracking to define the error. For that reason, some cases of negligent administration are resolved by applying the evidentiary principle of res ipsa loquitur. This principle is founded on the idea that the patient could not have suffered the medical result in question without there having been some negligence. It relieves the plaintiff of proving what may be unprovable: the exact nature of the care provider's mistake. On the other hand, the mistake becomes apparent immediately as when in *Loveland v. Nelson,*[19] a dentist injected a patient's gum with Lysol instead of anesthetic.

A related mistake is giving a patient the wrong type of blood. A nurse may mix up two patients' different blood types,[20] type the blood incorrectly,[21] retrieve the wrong type of blood from the blood bank,[22] think the physician ordered one type when in fact another was ordered, or make some other mistake. Whatever the cause of the mistake, its consequences can be severe and include death.[23]

Other key roles of nurses (and therefore prime areas for malpractice suits) are monitoring patients, documenting patients' conditions and treatments, and taking appropriate responsive actions, including keeping physicians up to date on patients' conditions. In *Louie v. Chinese Hospital Association,*[24] a nurse neglected to tell a physician that a patient appeared to grow restless and confused. The patient was suffering from a neurological disorder and had been sedated. Later, the patient fell while trying to get out of bed. The physician testified that he might have changed the patient's medicine if he had been told about the patient's mental state.

Finally, suspecting or knowing that a physician has failed to treat the patient adequately or has discharged a patient prematurely requires the nurse to take appropriate steps to remedy the problem. This should not include the nurse undertaking to treat the patient—such an action might violate important restrictions on the practice of medicine by nonphysicians—but must include bringing the concerns to an appropriate person. The policies of hospitals and other large-scale health care providers should address this issue and tell nurses where to report such concerns. Smaller facilities may not have instituted such policies, but nurses who work there must nonetheless not neglect this important duty. They should raise their concerns with their nursing superiors and if necessary the physician's partners or colleagues.

A nurse may have some concern about losing his or her job because of questioning a physician's treatment decisions. In many states, it is illegal to fire anyone who opposed conduct that he or she reasonably believed was illegal. This principle should protect a nurse who opposes the reasonably believed illegality of malpractice.

Criminal liability for medical malpractice

In rare but well-publicized instances, medical malpractice has been so extreme that criminal charges have resulted. Perhaps the most publicized was the case of Dr. Wolfgang Schug, who was accused of second-degree murder, involuntary manslaughter, and willful injury to a child after he discharged the child from a rural northern California hospital so that his parents could drive him to a distant pediatrics-equipped hospital. The child died on the road. The state alleged that Dr. Schug should have arranged for transport by ambulance or helicopter. The charges were eventually dismissed,[25] but other health care providers have been convicted in connection with malpractice.[26]

Physicians have not been prosecutors' only target. In *State v. Winter,*[27] a registered nurse was convicted of simple manslaughter and sentenced to 5 years in prison after she mistakenly transfused the wrong blood into a patient and then intentionally took several steps to conceal the error, "including failing to inform the patient's physician of her error, secreting and disposing of the remainder of the blood on realizing her mistake, and changing notations on . . . [the patient's] chart to mask the effects of the transfusion reaction."[28]

The nurse's intentional and deceptive misconduct may have made *Winter* a strong case for punishment, but prosecutors have tried nurses on weaker facts. Just because the nurses in the two cases discussed next were acquitted does not detract from the basic point: nurses face the possibility of criminal prosecution for malpractice.

In the first case, a Denver-area grand jury indicted three nurses on charges of criminally negligent homicide in the death of a day-old baby. The baby's physician wrote a prescription for penicillin to be injected in the baby's hip muscle. A hospital pharmacist misinterpreted the prescription and filled it at 10 times the prescribed dosage but correctly showed that it was to be given in the hip muscle. When one of the three nurses received the medication from the pharmacy, she consulted a neonatal nurse practitioner who told the nurse to give the medicine intravenously instead of in the hip muscle. The homicide charges that followed this mistake carried a maximum jail term of 6 years and a maximum fine of $100,000.

Two of the nurses eventually pled guilty under an arrangement that called, in part, for each to perform 24 hours of public service and to satisfy other conditions set by the Colorado Nursing Board, which suspended each for 1 year with subsequent 2-year probationary periods. The third nurse was acquitted at trial. The pharmacist who misfilled the prescription received a letter of admonition from the Colorado Board of Pharmacy but was not charged because according to published reports, prosecutors believed that the much higher dosage would not have killed the baby if it had been administered through the hip muscle as prescribed and as the pharmacist correctly indicated.[29]

In the second case, *Caretenders, Inc., v. Kentucky,*[30] the state tried two registered nurses, one licensed practical nurse, and their employer (a home health agency) for knowing and willful neglect of a patient. When admitted to a hospital, the patient was dirty and covered with extensive bedsores. Evidence showed that agency employees did not turn the patient as ordered, did not keep her clean, and kept bad records of their patient care activities, and it also showed that the agency failed to train and supervise its employees properly. The nurses were acquitted, but the agency was convicted and fined $8333.

EMPLOYER'S DIRECT NEGLIGENCE

The negligence discussed so far has been the nurse's own negligence and the liability for that negligence as shared under the doctrine of respondeat superior. In some instances, a nurse's employer may be negligent with respect to nursing services without regard for whether the nurse is negligent. In this situation, the negligence is the employer's *own,* instead of shared. This can happen when, for example, the employer fails to maintain an adequate nursing staff. In such a situation, a nurse may do everything that is reasonably prudent under the circumstances, but the circumstances (created by the nurse's employer) are so bad that a mistake by the nurse is a reasonably foreseeable result. In this situation, the negligence should be the employer's alone, not the nurse's.

When the nurse is negligent, the employer may be negligent too. Although the nurse's negligence arises out of failure to satisfy the standard of care, the employer's negligence arises out of some failure that contributes to the nurse's failure.

In *Perez v. Mercy Hospital of Laredo,*[31] the co-defendant hospital settled for $15 million in a case alleging that an overworked nurse mistakenly injected paralysis-inducing vecuronium bromide (Norcuron) into a patient in the intensive care unit (ICU); the medication stopped his breathing and caused brain damage. The evidence showed that the nurse had been working 72-hour weeks in the ICU and was finishing an 18-hour shift when the alleged mistake occurred. However, the evidence also showed that the nurse had failed a placement agency test that covered administration of medication and that the hospital fired the nurse 2 days after the patient's brain damage was discovered. In addition to the money payment, the hospital also agreed to institute a policy limiting ICU nurses to working only 60 hours a week. Because the case was settled before trial, there was no final determination that the nurse, the hospital, both, or neither was negligent. However, the allegation was that the hospital failed to exercise reasonable care in scheduling such long shifts for the ICU nurses and that this failure contributed to the medication error.

An employer may contribute to a nurse's mistake in other ways. For example, a nurse may harm a patient by neglecting to monitor vital signs regularly. If a reasonable check of the employment history would have shown that the nurse had been fired from an earlier job for the same mistake, then the hospital may have been negligent for failing to perform such a reasonable check. If there had been similar complaints against the nurse during the nurse's current employment but no one had documented them or if the documents had been simply placed in a personnel file with no action taken, the employer may have been negligent for retaining a nurse whom it would have been reasonable to fire. Finally, if the employer acquired new monitoring equipment but failed to train nurses on its use, the employer may have been negligent for failing to train.

WORKPLACE TORTS OTHER THAN MALPRACTICE
Patient battery by nurses

Nurses and their employers may be held liable for torts other than negligent errors that constitute malpractice. Intentional misconduct toward patients is an unfortunate but prime example, especially in nursing homes and other facilities for patients with long-term, subacute conditions. Such employers must be particularly careful in screening, retaining, and training employees. An Oklahoma jury awarded $1.25 million in damages against a nursing home because a drunk aide harshly slapped a patient while trying to bathe him.[32]

Obligation to preserve patient privacy and confidentiality

Privacy is a broad right that everyone enjoys with respect to personal information, and invasion of privacy is a widely recognized basis for filing a lawsuit. Confidentiality is a somewhat narrower right, since it is rooted specifically in a patient's medical records. Together, the rights of privacy and confidentiality preserve the nondisclosure of patients' medical records as well as other private information regardless of whether it has been documented in a medical record.

Although nurses must be careful to preserve the confidentiality of both records and other private information, they should be particularly on guard concerning the latter. Nurses' jobs, especially in institutional or home health settings, often bring them into relatively informal contact with patients' visiting family and friends. These contacts present a dangerous opportunity for a nurse to reveal confidential patient information to a person not entitled to receive it.

Such inadvertent disclosures should ordinarily be considered within the course and scope of the nurse's employment, with the result that the nurse's employer should have to share any civil liability under the principles of respondeat superior. However, a nurse may have to bear alone the liability for a purposeful breach. In *Jones v. Baisch,*[33] the nurse's employer was dismissed as a defendant in a case based on a nurse's breach of confidentiality. The nurse had told friends about a specific, named patient who had herpes. The court ruled that the nurse was not acting in the course and scope of employment when she made the disclosure.

Violence against nurses in the workplace

Spectacular incidents of crime in the workplace have focused attention on the risks that Americans face as employees. Nurses are certainly not immune from these risks, since their jobs bring them in contact with patients, families, and co-workers who may be under significant stress.

Employers of nurses may be liable for violence against them, just as they may be liable for the workplace injuries of other employees. Depending on the applicable state law and the facts of the case, an injured nurse's sole avenue of recovery against the employer may be through worker's compensation (plus whatever insurance and disability benefits may be available). For injuries caused by an act that was unintentional, regardless of whether it was the act of a co-worker or a nonemployee, the compensation due to the injured nurse is usually limited to only worker's compensation. Worker's compensation would probably also be the only compensation for intentional injuries caused by a nonemployee. However, for intentional injuries caused by a co-worker, the nurse may be able to hold the employer responsible in tort for much greater damages.

GOOD SAMARITAN LAWS

With few exceptions, no one has a duty to go out of the way to render aid to anyone in need. The main exception is health care providers at work: they have duties to their patients (including those they have had to accept as patients in their emergency departments). However, even a highly trained nurse generally has no duty to cross the street and give cardiopulmonary resuscitation to a nonpatient suffering a heart attack. Any nurse who did so could be held liable for an injury resulting from lack of reasonably prudent care under the circumstances.

Good Samaritan laws encourage emergency caregiving by reducing the possibility of liability; they alter the ordinary rules that govern actions based on negligent conduct. As already seen, *malpractice* can be simply defined as failure to satisfy an appropriate standard of care, which is what a reasonably prudent health care provider would do in the same circumstances. These laws tell courts to ignore reasonable prudence and instead ask whether a caregiver acting gratuitously at the scene of an emergency met the relatively lower standard of providing care in good faith.[34] Some state laws also grant Good Samaritan status to someone gratuitously providing services on behalf of organizations such as the American Red Cross.[35] Some states' Good Samaritan laws not only encourage emergency caregiving but actually require it.[36] Because coverage and the standard of care applied to those covered may vary from state to state, nurses should be familiar with the laws in their jurisdiction. Cases interpreting Good Samaritan laws generally hold that they do not excuse negligence in actual emergency departments, physicians' offices, or other places where the caregiver has the equipment and resources to act in a reasonably prudent manner.[37]

PROBLEMS ASSOCIATED WITH NONTRADITIONAL WORKPLACES

Nursing practice is not limited to hospitals and medical offices. With the increase in the number of senior citizens in America, nurses more often work outside of the traditional, highly supervised venues and visit their patients in places such as their home, assisted-living facilities, and hospices.

One of the primary challenges of this kind of nursing practice is maintaining good communication with patients' physicians. It is well known that nurses and their employers may be held liable for nurses' failure to communicate promptly and accurately with physicians.[38] Obviously, the possibility of miscommunication or of a communications breakdown is much greater when the nurse and physician do not work side by side and may in fact have very limited one-to-one contact.

Communication is just one concern, however. Before assigning nurses to relatively unsupervised duties, their employers must be certain of their overall competence and judgment. Employers who fail to do so may be held liable, not just under respondeat superior for the nurses' malpractice, but also for their own negligence in hiring, retention, or training.

Nontraditional nursing also increases the possibility of liability for torts indirectly related to patient treatment. For example, nurses who make house calls are probably more likely to be involved in traffic accidents within the course and scope of their employment than nurses who generally work at one fixed location. Applicable state law may allow injured persons to hold nurses' employers liable for such accidents.

NURSES AND THE FAIR LABOR STANDARDS ACT

The Fair Labor Standards Act (FLSA) requires most employers[39] to pay all their employees the minimum wage plus overtime wages for each hour over 40 in a work week unless an exemption applies.[40] There are three major exemptions: salaried workers who actually perform the duties of a bona fide executive, administrative employees, and professional employees (the "white collar" exemptions).[41] A nurse could fall into any one of these three categories, depending on his or her duties. Each exemption has detailed standards for the type of duties that qualify the employer to claim the exemption.

One of the standards for the executive exemption is having the primary duty of managing a department that includes at least two other employees; for example, a director of nursing could be an exempt executive employee. One of the standards for the administrative exemption is having the primary duty of nonmanual work directly related to the employer's management policies or general business operations; a nurse might be exempt under this standard if, for example, he or she manages only one assistant but has overall responsibility for the employer's program on improving patients' quality of life. One of the standards for the professional exemption is having knowledge acquired through specialized instruction and study; at least every registered nurse whose job is nursing (as opposed to managing or administering) might be exempt under this standard.[42]

Despite their variations, each white-collar exemption requires duties for which the exempt employee exercises independent judgment and discretion.[43] Any nurse who does not have this freedom to act should receive overtime pay.

In addition to actually performing the duties of a bona fide exempt employee, the nurse must also be paid on a salaried basis (or on a fee basis, if the exemption is administrative or professional[44]). *Salaried* generally means that the employee gets the same amount per pay period with no variation for the quantity or quality of work (except in weeks when the employee performs no work at all). *Fee basis* generally means the employee receives a fixed amount of money per "unique" job or project.[45]

The uniqueness requirement may be a problem for some employers. For example, a home health agency might agree to pay its nurses a fixed fee per patient visit with no overtime. On each visit, the nurse encounters a different health problem and exercises independent judgment and discretion to address it. The nurse's duties fully meet the duties standard for the professional exemption. However, is this a proper case for fee-basis payment? It probably is not because even though each visit is different, considered together, they may not meet the regulation's strict standard for "unique."[46] Consequently, the nurse cannot be paid on a fee basis, so the employer must, to preserve the overtime exemption, pay him or her on a salary basis.

An employer who merely pays a nurse on an hourly basis has no ground for claiming an exemption, as the court held in *Brock v. Superior Care.*[47] In this case, the employer treated its nurses as independent contractors instead of employees. It paid them on an hourly basis with no overtime. This would be permissible if the nurses really were not employees, since the FLSA covers only employment relationships, not independent contractor relationships. The court, however, concluded that the nurses were employees and that they should have been paid overtime because, even if they performed duties that qualified for the exemption, they were not paid on a salary or fee basis.

For nurses who are nonexempt (entitled to receive overtime pay), employers have several options. The most familiar is to pay overtime at 1 1/2 times the employee's regular hourly rate for each hour over 40 in a 7-day work week. Another involves modifying the normal 40-hour overtime standard. The FLSA provides that a hospital or other establishment primarily engaged in the business of providing in-residence care to the ill or elderly may use a 14-day work week if it pays overtime for each hour that an employee works over 8 hours in a single day and for each hour over 80 in the 14-day period, as long as the employee agrees to the arrangement.[48]

There are some other possible arrangements, such as an agreement to pay a fixed sum (e.g., a salary) for either regular hours or for a combination of regular and overtime hours plus an additional overtime premium[49] as well as an agreement to pay a fixed sum plus overtime for widely fluctuating hours (a Belo contract).[50] Also, public hospitals can, to a limited degree, pay overtime in the form of compensatory time off instead of in cash wages.[51]

A significant question for on-call nurses, regardless of which option the employer uses, is whether to count time as time *worked.* The general test is whether the "time is spent predominantly for the employer's benefit or for the employee's."[52] If during on-call time a nurse has no obligation to the employer but to respond to a call if it comes, the time is probably not compensable. If, on the other hand, the nurse must remain within, say, a 5-mile radius of the hospital, then the time probably is compensable.

NURSES AND UNIONS

Within limits, nurses have the legal right to unionize and to require their employers to bargain with them through their unions. The most significant limit is that federal labor law concerning unions does not cover an employer if it is "any . . . political subdivision" of a state.[53] Such an employer is not covered if it is either "(1) created directly by the state, so as to constitute departments or administrative arms of the government, or (2) administered by individuals who are responsible to public officials or to the general electorate."[54] Employees of such employers can certainly unionize, but they have no federal right to do so and no federal remedy if their employer takes steps to prevent unionization. Even though employees of a "political subdivision" of a state have no union rights under federal law, they may under state law.

Another limit—one that applies to nurses with union rights under federal law—pertains to acute care hospitals. The National Labor Relations Board (NLRB), which plays a large role in enforcing federal labor laws, ruled in 1989 that in ordinary circumstances, there can be only eight "bargaining units" in acute care hospitals (as defined in the NLRB's rule).[55] A bargaining unit is a group of workers whose interests are similar enough that one representative can speak fairly for all of them. One of these eight designated units is made up of all *registered* nurses at the hospital. Licensed practical nurses and other nurses would have to be in a separate bargaining unit, one that comprises "[a]ll professionals except for registered nurses and physicians." Two exceptions to this rule are when the circumstances are not ordinary (such as when one of the rule-mandated bargaining units contains a very small number of workers) and when a labor organization seeks certification of a bargaining unit that combines two or more of the rule-mandated units.

In all other circumstances, the NLRB determines the appropriateness of a proposed bargaining unit of nurses on a case-by-case basis, as it does for all other types of bargaining units.[56] In making this determination, the NLRB presumes that a single-facility bargaining unit of certain employees (such as registered nurses) is more appropriate than a multifacility unit. For example, if a hospital corporation owns five hospitals within a single metropolitan area, the employer may prefer that all its registered nurses at all five hospitals be organized into one bargaining unit; that way, the corporation will bargain with only one representative over the terms and conditions of employment for all registered nurses at all five hospitals. However, the NLRB's presumption—it is a rebuttable presumption, so it can be disproved—is that there should be a separate bargaining unit for the registered nurses at each hospital.[57] The representative need not be the same for all five units, and the bargained-for terms and conditions may also differ from unit to unit.

Finally, nurses who qualify as "supervisors" have no federally protected union rights; all such employees (not just nurses) are by definition members of management rather than labor. A supervisor is[58]:

[A]ny individual having authority, in the interest of the employer, to hire, transfer, suspend, lay off, recall, promote, discharge, assign, reward, or discipline other employees, or responsibly to direct them, or to adjust their grievances, or effectively to recommend such action, if in connection with the foregoing the exercise of such authority is not of a merely routine or clerical nature, but requires the use of independent judgment.

Supervisor status exists when all three of the following critical questions have an affirmative answer[59]:
1. Can the employee perform even 1 of the 13 items just listed?
2. Does performing the job require the employee's independent judgment?
3. Is the performance is in the interest of the employer?

With respect to nurses, the Supreme Court has held that nurses who direct other employees (including other nurses) on matters of patient care do so in the interest of their employer.[60] Such a nurse *may* be supervisor; the other two questions must be answered before this conclusion can be reached.

Although the Supreme Court has laid to rest (for now, at least) the meaning of *in the interest of the employer,* there is currently a controversy over the term *independent judgment,* especially as it pertains to licensed practical nurses employed as charge nurses at nursing homes.[61] At most, it can be said that resolving whether a nurse exercises "independent judgment" with respect to 1 of the 13 listed items depends on the facts of the case and the legal precedents from the federal appellate court that will decide the case.

NURSING LICENSURE

States have the authority to regulate nurses and other health care practitioners by legislating the requirements for getting and keeping a license to practice.[62] These regulations vary from state to state, so a nurse must be familiar with the requirements in the state or states where he or she practices.

License requirements cannot violate state and federal constitutional requirements. For example, a state probably could not make getting a nursing license significantly harder for out-of-state nurses solely for the purpose of preserving nursing jobs for current state residents. A state also probably could not

enact a license-revocation procedure that did not provide any procedural standards or any opportunity for appeal.

In the absence of such constitutional problems, federal law has very little to say about nursing licensure. However, federal law may affect a nurse's employability with an employer that receives federal funds. For example, federal law requires that nursing care in a skilled nursing facility "must meet professional standards of quality."[63] It also provides that home health agencies must employ only those who meet competency standards established by the federal Department of Health and Human Services and who are actually competent to serve patients.[64]

Federal courts provide an unlikely forum for seeking damages when a nurse believes that a state wrongly revoked his or her license. In *O'Neal v. Mississippi Board of Nursing,*[65] two Mississippi nurses unsuccessfully sued state board members under federal law for wrongly revoking their licenses. The board revoked their licenses for false or negligent record-keeping. Mississippi state law allowed the nurses to appeal the board's decision to the state courts. The first-level state court affirmed the board's revocation, but the second-level state court reversed and restored the nurses' licenses.

With their licenses restored, the nurses then sued in federal court, alleging that the board's mistake in revoking their licenses amounted to a violation of constitutional rights. They sued both the board itself and individual board members. The district court dismissed the claims against all defendants, and the Fifth Circuit affirmed. It concluded that suing the board itself was equivalent to suing the state in federal court, which the eleventh amendment to the Constitution prohibits. It also concluded that board members could not be held liable because of the doctrine of absolute quasijudicial immunity. This doctrine provides immunity to public officials when they act in the role of judges or prosecutors; the court held that this document provided immunity to the board members when they decided the evidence warranted revocation of the nurses' licenses (even though the decision was ultimately found to be wrong).[66]

ENDNOTES

1. An excellent book-length treatment of legal issues facing nurses is Marcia Andrews, Kathy Goldberg & Howard Kaplan, eds., *Nurse's Legal Handbook* (3d ed., Springhouse, Springhouse, Pa. 1996).
2. *See* George L. Blum, Annotation, *Medical Malpractice: Who Are "Health Care Providers," or the Like, Whose Actions Fall within Statutes Specifically Governing Actions and Damages for Medical Malpractice,* 12 A.L.R. 5th 1 § 15 (1993).
3. *Lenger v. Physician's General Hospital, Inc.,* 455 S.W. 2d 703 (Tex. 1970).
4. *King v. Dep't of Health & Hospitals,* 728 So. 2d 1027, 1030 (La. Ct. App.) (emphases added), *writ denied,* 741 So. 2d 656 (La. 1999).
5. Tasking a general registered nurse to function as a nurse anesthetist might itself be negligence, but it would be chargeable to the person responsible for not having a certified registered nurse anesthetist available, not to the nurse.
6. *See, e.g.,* 1 Steve E. Pegalis & Harvey F. Wachsman, *American Law of Medical Malpractice* (2d ed., Clark Boardman Callaghan, Deerfield, Ill. 1992).
7. *Ross v. Chatham County Hospital Authority,* 408 S.E. 2d 490 (Ga. App. 1991).

8. *Id.* at 493.

9. *Moore v. Carrington,* 270 S.E. 2d 222 (Ga. 1980).

10. *See, e.g.,* La. Civ. Code Ann. art. 2324(B) (West 1999).

11. *Ravi v. Williams,* 536 So. 2d 1374, 1376 (Ala. 1988).

12. *Mosey v. Mueller,* 218 N.W. 2d 514 (Wis. 1974).

13. Id. at 519.

14. *Hunnicut v. Wright,* 986 F. 2d 119 (5th Cir. 1993).

15. *Id.* at 123.

16. *Hudmon v. Martin,* 315 So. 2d 516 (Fla. Dist. Ct. App. 1975).

17. *Striano v. Deepdale Gen. Hosp.,* 387 N.Y.S. 2d 678 (N.Y. App. Div. 1976).

18. In some cases even a nonemployee physician (such as a contract physician in an emergency department) is regarded as a hospital employee. *Ryan v. N.Y.C. Health & Hospitals Corp.,* 633 N.Y.S. 2d 500, 501 (N.Y. App. Div. 1995).

19. *Loveland v. Nelson,* 209 N.W. 835 (Mich. 1926).

20. *Parker v. Port Huron Hosp.,* 105 N.W. 2d 1 (Mich. 1960).

21. *Redding v. United States,* 196 F.Supp. 871 (W.D. Ark. 1961); *Berg v. New York Soc. for Relief of the Ruptured and Crippled,* 136 N.E. 2d 523 (N.Y. 1956) (medical technician's error).

22. *Parker v. St. Paul Fire & Marine Ins. Co.,* 335 So. 2d 725 (La. Ct. App.), *writ denied,* 338 So. 2d 700 (La. 1976); *Kyte v. McMillion,* 259 A. 2d 532 (Md. 1969).

23. *National Homeopathic Hosp. v. Phillips,* 181 F. 2d 293 (D.C. Cir. 1950); *Ward v. Orange Mem. Hosp. Ass'n, Inc.,* 193 So. 2d 492 (Fla. Dist. Ct. App. 1966).

24. *Louie v. Chinese Hospital Association,* 57 Cal.Rptr. 906 (Cal. Dist. Ct. App. 1967).

25. Maura Dolan, *Judge Acquits Rural Doctor of Murder of Infant Patient,* Los Angeles Times (Feb 21, 1998); Maura Dolan, *Doctor's Trial Begins in Baby's Death,* Los Angeles Times (Feb 4, 1998); Maura Dolan, *A Medical Mistake or Murder?* Los Angeles Times (Jan 7, 1998).

26. *See, e.g.,* Lynette Holloway, *Abortion Doctor Guilty of Murder,* New York Times (Aug 9, 1995); *Samitier v. State,* 654 So. 2d 308 (Fla. Dist. Ct. App. 1995) *(per curiam).*

27. *State v. Winter,* 477 A. 2d 323 (N.J. 1984).

28. *Id.* at 324.

29. Keith Coffman, *Nurse Acquitted in Death; Improper Injection was Fatal to Newborn,* The Denver Post (Jan 31, 1998); Kieran Nicholson & Marilyn Robinson, *2 Nurses Plead Guilty in Death of Newborn; Deferred Judgment, Public Service Ordered,* The Denver Post (Jan 23, 1998); Ann Schrader & Marilyn Robinson, *Baby's Nurses Face Homicide Charges,* The Denver Post (April 29, 1997).

30. *Caretenders, Inc., v. Kentucky,* 821 S.W. 2d 83 (Ky. 1991).

31. *Perez v. Mercy Hospital of Laredo,* No. 98-CVQ-492-D3 (341st J.D.C., Webb County, Texas), as reported in Rebecca Conklin, *Hospital Changes Work Hours Policy as Part of $15 Million Med Mal Settlement,* Lawyer's Weekly USA (Nov 29, 1999).

32. *Rodebush v. Oklahoma Nursing Homes, Ltd.,* 867 P. 2d 1241 (Okla. 1993).

33. *Jones v. Baisch,* 40 F. 3d 252 (8th Cir. 1994).

34. *See, e.g.,* La. Rev. Stat. Ann. § 9:2793(A). (West 1999).

35. *See, e.g.,* La. Rev. Stat. Ann. § 9:2793.2 (West 1999).

36. *See* Minn. Stat. Ann. § 604A. 01(1) (West 1988 & Supp. 2000); Vt. Stat. Ann. tit. 12, § 519(a) (1973).

37. *Colby v. Schwartz,* 78 Cal. App. 3d 885, 891-92, 144 Cal.Rptr. 624, 627 (Cal. Dist. Ct. App. 1978); *Guerrero v. Copper Queen Hosp.,* 537 P. 2d 1329 (Ariz. 1975).

38. *See, e.g.,* Helen Creighton, *Law Every Nurse Should Know* (4th ed., WB Saunders, Philadelphia 1981).

39. The Fair Labor Standards Act does not cover employees of a state. *Kimel v. Florida Bd. of Regents,* No. 98-791 (U.S. Jan 11, 2000). The interpretation of *state* is much narrower than the public employee exclusion discussed later in the section on nurses and unions.

40. 29 U.S.C.A. §§ 206-07 (West 1998).

41. 29 U.S.C.A. § 213(a)(1) (West 1998). Among other exemptions is one for employees providing companionship services, such as some employees of home health agencies. The exemption should not cover any nurses who provide skilled services to home health patients. 29 U.S.C.A. § 213(a)(15) (West 1998); 29 C.F.R. § 552.6 (1999); Office of Enforcement Policy Priv. Ltr. Rul. (May 15, 1998), *reprinted in* 6A Lab. Rel. Rep. (BNA) § 99:2157, 2158.

42. Department of Labor regulations recognize that nursing meets the basic definition of a profession on grounds it requires a course of specialized instruction and study. 29 C.F.R. 541.301(e)(1) (1999).

43. *Id.* at §§ 541.1 - 541.3.

44. *Id.* at § 541.313(a).

45. *Id.* at § 541.313(b).

46. *See* Office of Enforcement Policy Priv. Ltr. Rul. (April 27, 1998), *reprinted in* 6A Lab. Rel. Rep. (BNA) § 99:8152.

47. *Brock v. Superior Care,* 840 F. 2d 1054 (2nd Cir.), *modified on other grounds,* 28 Wage & Hour Cas. (BNA) 1016 (2nd Cir. 1988).

48. 29 U.S.C.A. § 207(j) (West 1998).

49. 29 C.F.R. §§ 778.113 and 778.114 (1999); Office of Enforcement Policy Priv. Ltr. Rul. (Oct 31, 1997), *reprinted in* 6A Lab. Rel. Rep. (BNA) § 99:8101.

50. 29 U.S.C.A. § 207(f) (West 1998); *Walling v. A.H. Belo Corp.,* 316 U.S. 624 (1942); 29 C.F.R. §§ 778.402-778.414 (1999); Office of Enforcement Policy Priv. Ltr. Rul. (Sept 15, 1997), *reprinted in* 6A Lab. Rel. Rep. (BNA) § 99:8103.

51. 29 U.S.C. § 207(o) (West 1999).

52. *Armour & Co. v. Wantock,* 323 U.S. 126, 133 (1944).

53. 29 U.S.C.A. § 152(2) (West 1998).

54. *N.L.R.B. v. Natural Gas Utility District,* 402 U.S. 600, 604-605 (1971) (internal quotation omitted).

55. 29 C.F.R. § 103.30 (1999). The Supreme Court approved the NLRB's authority to issue the rule in *American Hosp. Ass'n v. N.L.R.B.,* 499 U.S. 606 (1991).

56. 29 U.S.C.A. § 159(b) (West 1998).

57. Visiting Nurses Ass'n, 324 N.L.R.B. 55 (1997); Manor Health Care Corp., 285 N.L.R.B. 224 (1987).

58. 29 U.S.C.A. § 152(11) (West 1998).

59. *N.L.R.B. v. Health Care & Retirement Corp. of America,* 511 U.S. 571, 573-574 (1994).

60. *Id.* at 577.

61. In *N.L.R.B. v. Attleboro Associates,* 176 F. 3d 154 (3rd Cir. 1999), the Third Circuit held that licensed practical nurses employed as charge nurses, with respect to certified nursing assistants, exercised independent judgment in recommending discipline, adjusting grievances, and assigning and responsibly directing nurses and were thus supervisors, since the other two critical questions were not in dispute. Under similar circumstances, the Sixth Circuit also held that such nurses at a nursing home were supervisors in *Beverly Enterprises v. N.L.R.B.,* 165 F. 3d 290 (4th Cir. 1999) *(en banc).* However, in *Beverly Enterprises v. N.L.R.B.,* 165 F. 3d 960 (D.C. Cir. 1999), the District of Columbia Circuit held that charge-nurse license practical nurses in a bargaining unit that also included registered nurses were not supervisors and thus entitled to protection under federal labor law.

62. *Semler v. Oregon State Bd. of Dental Examiners,* 294 U.S. 608, 611 (1935).

63. 42 U.S.C.A. § 1395i-3(b)(4)(A) (West 1992 & Supp. 1999).

64. 42 U.S.C.A. § 1395bbb(a)(3)(A) (West 1992 & Supp. 1999).

65. *O'Neal v. Mississippi Board of Nursing,* 113 F. 3d 62 (5th Cir. 1997).

66. Absolute quasijudicial immunity also protected medical board members in *Watts v. Burkhart,* 978 F. 2d 269 (6th Cir. 1992); *Bettencourt v. Bd. of Registration in Medicine of the Commonwealth of Massachusetts,* 904 F. 2d 772 (1st Cir. 1990); and *Horwitz v. State Bd. of Medical Examiners of the State of Colorado,* 822 F. 2d 1508 (10th Cir.), *cert. denied,* 484 U.S. 964 (1987).

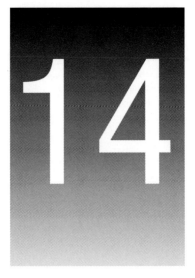

Dental litigation: triad of concerns

BRUCE H. SEIDBERG, D.D.S., M.SC.D., J.D., D.A.B.E., F.P.F.A., F.A.A.H.D., F.C.L.M.

LEGAL CONSIDERATIONS
STANDARD OF CARE
COMMON LITIGATION AREAS
TRIAD OF CONCERN
EMERGENCY CARE
ADDITIONAL AREAS OF CONCERN
CONCLUSION

The health care profession has been deluged with peaks and valleys of malpractice cases alleging various degrees of negligence, including incompetence, departure from the standard of care, failure to diagnose, failure to obtain consent, performing unnecessary treatment (practicing defensive dentistry), and providing poor treatment. Although most litigation literature refers to medicine, dentistry also has been burdened with its own set of frivolous and meritorious cases. Local dental societies, dental districts, and dental peer review committees have seen an increase in the number of complaints about dentists.[1] The current litigious and consumer-oriented society at times considers the treatment performed by dentists and the work done by automobile mechanics on equal terms.[2]

Society has become litigious for many reasons; economic factors and the belief that dentists might be an easy target to satisfy the patient's greed encourage these suits. In reviewing the literature and litigated cases and consulting with attorneys throughout the country, the author has categorized dental litigation into three major areas of concerns, referred to as the *triad of dental litigation,* each with a series of related subcategories. The triad consists of the *physician-patient relationship* (PPR), *informed consent,* and *documentation.* Although the three areas share equal importance, the base of the triangle is the PPR, in which communication skills prevail. In his risk-prevention skills manual, Tennenhouse[3] presents a series of 22 categories containing 119 recommendations for avoiding dental litigation.

Dentists are rapidly realizing that any patient may resort to litigation. Cautionary measures help dentists avoid legal involvement.[4] To reduce potential malpractice actions, each practitioner must have a risk-prevention skill (RPS) program in force. RPS programs, clinical and nonclinical, are designed to help health care practitioners incorporate management methods into their private practices that alleviate and control patient injury and liability problems, act to detect failure on the part of systems or persons, and prevent bad things from happening. They are developed to provide solutions for the entity's protection, relying more on process improvement than simple risk transfer.[5] The goals of a health facility risk manager are to design programs that keep patients free from insults and injuries and protect the practitioners' licenses. Each dentist is the risk manager for his or her own office: The level of risk that each dentist wants to assume is an individual choice. Every dentist must decide what level of risk he or she is comfortable with because there are various degrees of consequences. An action arising from risks can lead to no action, mediation, peer review, or formal adjudication. Each action carries its own set of consequences, from monetary penalties to adverse effects on licensure or practice.

The primary cause of malpractice litigation in dentistry is patient injury or perceived injury. The primary reason for submission of a complaint to a mediation committee is lack of proper communication with the patient or perceived excessive fees. The National Society of Dental Practitioners[6] has identified 12 ways that a dentist can get sued (Box 14-1). Recommended ways to avoid problems are listed in Box 14-2. Zinman's[7] criteria for dealing with a potential lawsuit are outlined in Box 14-3. To minimize the liability risk, dentists must avoid causing patients to seek legal counsel by communicating properly and must not create damaging record-keeping evidence. Dentists must improve the cooperation amongst members of the dental team, generalists and specialists, and improve the trust and satisfaction of patients and their families. Satisfied patients usually do not pursue lawsuits.

In a litigation-prone society, in addition to those dentists who allegedly provide treatment of an inferior quality, dentists whose treatment merely does not bring about the desired results could be the targets of lawsuits. Special types of negligence relating to dentistry and the principal legal duties of the dental health care provider are listed in Boxes 14-4 and 14-5.

137

BOX 14-1. TWELVE WAYS TO GET SUED

1. Neglect to pay a fee.
2. Refuse to negotiate the return of a fee.
3. Guarantee or promise a result.
4. Exceed your level of competencies.
5. Fail to obtain informed consent.
6. Be inaccessible to a patient with complaints.
7. Be unavailable, or fail to provide coverage for patients of record.
8. Fail to refer.
9. Fail to diagnose or treat a pathological condition.
10. Fail to prescribe or prescribe incorrect medications.
11. Fail to meet a reasonable standard of care.
12. Make treatment errors (e.g., treat the wrong tooth).

From National Society of Dental Practitioners, 12; 4; 97.

BOX 14-2. HOW TO AVOID LAWSUITS

Be professional and courteous.
Keep good, accurate records.
Communicate with patients and colleagues, especially those who are confused or unsure.
Obtain adequate informed consent.
Predict an appropriate prognosis.
Do not be egotistical about second opinion diagnoses.
Do not be greedy (i.e., do not overbill).

BOX 14-3. HOW TO APPROACH A DENTAL MALPRACTICE CASE

Do not try to settle the matter on your own.
Do not discuss the case with colleagues.
Do not be short-changed by your defense counsel.
Do not be your own private detective.
Do not rely on hold-harmless agreements.
Do not alter records.
Treat patients who have a need; do not treat patients to satisfy greed.
Learn from the experience.

Modified from Edwin Zinman, *What to Do When a Patient Plans to Sue,* Dent. Mgm't. 32-35 (March 1986).

BOX 14-4. SPECIAL TYPES OF DENTAL NEGLIGENCE

Abandonment
Failure to refer
Failure to obtain informed consent
Failure to warn
Failure to follow a manufacturer's directions

BOX 14-5. PRINCIPAL LEGAL DUTIES OF DENTISTS

Duty to care
Duty to inform
Duty to maintain confidentiality
Duty to maintain accurate records

The duty of care exists and persists for as long as there is a PPR, whether active or passive, unless there is some express or clearly implied effort to terminate the relationship.

LEGAL CONSIDERATIONS

The legal theories and principles of malpractice and the elements of negligence that apply to medicine, which are outlined in many of the chapters of this text, apply to dentistry as well but are not repeated here. All dentists should be familiar with the elements of negligence and the generalities and with the reasons that patients bring litigatory actions. As Former President George Bush[8] said when he made reference to the liability system, " . . . the simple truth [is that] not every unfortunate medical [dental] outcome is a result of poor medicine [dentistry]; . . . you cannot make life risk free." However, dentists can try to practice risk free.

Black letter law is made by legislative bodies creating statutes and can lead to loss of licensure; civil law cases are decided in the courts, based on English common law, and can lead to a monetary fine and a tarnished reputation. There are shades of gray in the law, and it is the attorney's responsibility to learn the case details and defend it appropriately; courts and juries make the final decisions regarding the dentist, who makes the diagnosis and decides to treat or refer.

STANDARD OF CARE

All dentists are expected to conduct their practices within a certain standard of care, which is the benchmark against which a dentist's conduct is measured.[9] The law recognizes that there are differences in dentists' abilities just as there are differences in the abilities of people engaged in other activities. To practice dentistry, a dentist is not required to have the extraordinary knowledge and ability that belongs to a few dentists of exceptional ability. However, every dentist is required to remain reasonably informed regarding new developments in his or her field and to practice dentistry in accordance with approved methods and means of treatment in general use.

Standard of care is defined as the reasonable care and diligence ordinarily exercised by similar members of the profession in similar cases and like conditions, given due regard for the state of the art. Initially an analysis of local community standards was implied. A dentist was held liable only for the level of competence, concern, and compassion that society would expect of the average dentist in the community in which that dentist practiced. James and co-workers[10] defined the legal concept of standard of care from a community standard to a national standard. Curley[11] also addressed the definitions of standard of care. Today the dentist must meet the national standard because several courts have found that the conduct of a specialist should be measured against national standards of care.[12]

The ethical basis of standard of care is beneficence (i.e., to recommend the best therapy while minimizing potential harm and to avoid placing a patient in a situation in which there is an unreasonable risk of harm).[13] General practitioners are required to exercise the same degree of care and skill as a specialist acting in the same or similar circumstances, locality not withstanding. In *Taylor v. Robbins*[14] the dentist failed to use accepted treatment techniques, and in *Perry*[15] the locality rule was nullified when sufficient foundation was recognized that the local and national standards did not differ.

COMMON LITIGATION AREAS

The scope of dental litigation touches every phase of dentistry, some more than others (Table 14-1). Common reasons for litigation include failure to refer; failure to diagnosis and treat periodontal disease; dissatisfaction with prosthetics; endodontic failures and mishaps; extraction errors, including the extraction of the wrong tooth; implant failure; adverse consequences, such as paresthesia; temporomandibular dysfunction; poor crown margins; failure to pretreat the patient with subacute bacterial endocarditis by giving antibiotics; failure to obtain the patient's medical history; writing an im-

proper prescription; child abuse; sexual harassment; and inappropriate use of intravenous sedation. The allegations in the preceding list usually include a form and a degree of negligence, incompetence, or gross negligence. In negligence cases the allegation is that the practitioner knew what to do and did not do it, in incompetence cases the assertion is that the practitioner never knew what to do, and in gross negligence cases the accusation is that the practitioner knowingly put a patient at risk.

Patients seek legal advice when they think that negligence has occurred. In a 1994 study by Beckman,[16] 54% of plaintiffs who settled malpractice suits filed between 1985 and 1987 indicated that another health care provider suggested maloccurrence. In addition, 71% identified problematic PPRs. A poor interpersonal relationship with a patient usually is the result of communication barriers set up by the dentist's staff or by office policy. When a dissatisfied patient is unable to discuss his or her problems with the dentist, he or she becomes frustrated. When a patient is unhappy with the care provided yet owes a fee and the dentist pursues or sues to recover the fee, the patient becomes irate. If a patient changes dental providers and has to pay a second time to receive the same treatment within a short period, he or she becomes suspicious. If a dental provider does not communicate potential problems to a patient and misleads him or her relative to treatment, the patient becomes upset. Individually or in combination the aforementioned problems lead to conflicts that may direct patients to an attorney's office. Markus[17] and Dorn[18] address methods of dealing with patient conflict. Both suggest that conflict must be understood, escalation checked, and resolution skills developed.

In a "failure to diagnose" case the injury on which the suit is premised is not the patient's original detrimental condition. Rather, the injury occurs later, as a result of the misdiagnosis and failure to treat, after the problem develops into a more serious condition that poses greater danger or requires more extensive treatment.[19]

TABLE 14-1 Claim data from various insurance sources

Procedure	Claims (%)
Endodontics	15-25
Extraction, simple	12-15
Crown/bridge work	15-20
Fixed partial denture	8-15
Routine dental care	8-17
Extraction, surgical	8-12
Removable partial dentures	3-8
Comprehensive orthodontics	3-8
Complete dentures	3-8
Periodontics	5-12
Paresthesia	8-12
Other (e.g., failure to refer, failure to diagnose, implant failures, temporomandibular joint pain, failure to give a patient with subacute bacterial endocarditis antibiotics)	3-15

TRIAD OF CONCERN
Physician-patient relationship

The PPR is a fiduciary relationship in which mutual trust and confidence are essential.[20] Any time a professional gives advice or expresses an opinion to a patient in a professional manner, regardless of location, and there is actual and significant contact between the two, duties are incurred. When there is no contact and the involvement is limited to a simple observation regarding the patient, with limited suggestions being offered, no direct duty to the patient is assumed.[21] The relationship is based on contract law, with rights and obligations affecting all concerned. The fiduciary principle relates to the fact that the dentist has knowledge and skill based on which the patient entrusts his or her care. It promotes open disclosure of all specifics and encourages the free flow of information between the individuals. The mutuality of contract principle originates when a patient requests services and the dentist agrees to render the services. Consideration, usually in the form of a professional fee, binds the contract. In most cases gratuitous treatment and advice establish a relationship and invoke all the duties of that relationship. No money has to change hands. Once the relationship begins, the patient is endowed with various rights that include but are not limited to freedom from bodily harm, the right to choose and consent to treatment, the right to refuse treatment, and the right to privacy and confidentiality. To reduce the liability risk, the dentist must strive to improve cooperation between members of the health care team, which includes staff and prior and subsequent caregivers. The dentist also must endeavor to improve the trust and satisfaction of their patients and their families. Once the relationship begins, a series of communication skills must be practiced: A proper history is taken, the case is presented, informed consent is obtained, referrals are made if necessary, and the patient is given a strict understanding of what to expect.

The relationship can be terminated without incurring liability for abandonment only if the patient withdraws from treatment voluntarily, the patient no longer requires care, or the provider is unable or unwilling to provide continued care and gives reasonable notice to the patient. Failure to terminate the professional relationship in an appropriate manner can lead to an action of abandonment. Improper unilateral termination of the PPR by the practitioner at a time when there is a need for continuing care constitutes causation of concern for the patient and possible breach of duty. Before suggesting the termination of care for a patient, a dentist must ensure that the patient is whole and not in the middle of a procedure. Whatever treatment has been started must be completed. A short, kind, and to-the-point letter must be sent to the patient. See Figs. 14-1 and 14-2 for sample letters. Emergent care must be provided for a reasonable time, usually 30 days. A letter must be sent via certified mail, with return receipt requested.

Good communication with a patient usually ensures a relationship without conflict. Staff members must be taught how to communicate with a patient without suggesting that any previous treatments were questionable, poor, or improper. Emanuel and Emanuel[22] identify and discuss four models of PPRs—paternalistic, informative, interpretive, and deliberative.

Informed consent

The doctrine of informed consent is based on a special fiduciary relationship between the dentist and the patient, a relation of trust, confidence, and responsibility. The approach to obtaining informed consent used to be maternalistic/paternalistic in that the patient listened to the practitioner with respect and trust. Smith[23] reviewed current literature from various sources to develop a general sense and understanding of informed consent. He found that the doctrine of informed

consent had significantly influenced relationships among health care practitioners and their patients in the last 25 years. He also identified an erosion of the paternalistic approach leading to an increase in patient sovereignty and decision-making. Now, in the litigious society that exists, the approach must be the sharing of information.

Date
Patient's Name
Address

Dear_____,
I will no longer be able to provide dental care to (you/your children). If (you/your children) require dental care within the next_____days, I will be available, but in no event will I be available after _____, 2001.

To assist (you/your children) in continuing to receive dental care, I will make records available as soon as you authorize me to send them to another dentist.

Sincerely,

Dentist's Name

Fig. 14-1. Sample letter of withdrawal.

Date
Patient's Name
Address

Dear_____,
This letter will confirm our conversation of today in which you discharged me as your dentist. In my opinion your condition requires continued dental care. If you have not already done so, I suggest that you employ another dentist without delay.

You can be assured that, at your request, I will furnish the dentist you select with information or copies of your records regarding the diagnosis and treatment that you have received from me.

Very truly yours,

Dentist's Name

Fig. 14-2. Sample letter confirming patient termination of relationship.

Some negligence lawsuits have been related to lack of informed consent; the elements of such suits are listed in Box 14-6. Informed consent is discussed in detail in Chapter 21. The concepts and details apply equally to medicine and dentistry and therefore are not be repeated in this chapter.

Documentation

"From the facts, the issues arise. Without the facts, there are no issues." This maxim essentially states that, if nothing has been written, there are no facts, and therefore it is considered that nothing has been done. It easily can be restated to read, "If there are issues, there must be facts. Without the facts, there will be issues," probably legal in nature. Patient records are considered legal documents, as well as business records. It is the presumption in law that all entries are accurate, are truthful, and were entered in a reasonable time frame. What is written around the time of the event is less likely to be biased or inaccurate. The longer the dentist or staff member waits to write about the event, the less credible the entries are.

A dentist's written records can be his or her best friend or worst enemy. If subpoenaed, the records continue to testify long after the dentist has gone. The records end up in the jury room, where the jurors can review them more carefully than the testimony heard on the stand. Records are put into evidence because of relevancy, materiality, and competency. They serve to record prior history, diagnosis, and therapies rendered. They provide continuity between providers, partners in group practices, and interested third parties. They also allow transfer between dental providers.

There are many facets of a dental record.[24,25] Aside from containing the patient's personal identification information, the record should include a current and thorough medical questionnaire. There also must be a current dental history; notations of a complete oral, head, and neck examination; documentation of diagnostic tests and results; a copy of the memorialization document of informed consent; and notes regarding any changes in the treatment plan. In addition, copies of letters, laboratory reports, and termination of care documents and notes regarding telephone calls, questions,

complaints, pharmacy prescriptions and refills, and canceled or missed appointments are part of the documentation. Diagnostic evidence, such as radiographs, photographs, and study models, is another integral part of a dental record. Records must follow the universally accepted SOAP format of record-keeping (Box 14-7).

Reviewing the medical history with the patient is just as important as disclosing information during the informed consent dialogue. At this point in the examination or consultation the dentist can determine whether any of the patient's medical conditions would interfere with or impact dental care. In the event that there is a question about an entry on the medical record or a medication the patient is taking, the dentist is obligated to consult the patient's physician before commencing with treatment.[26]

Records should be well written, legible, and accurate. There should be no words scratched out, no words covered with correction fluid or tape, and absolutely no alteration in any form. Any alteration or spoilation is frowned upon and is detrimental to the dentist's credibility. Spoilation[27] is the destruction or loss of records and in court can destroy or impair the patient's ability to prove negligence or other tortuous conduct in a malpractice lawsuit against the provider.

BOX 14-6. ELEMENTS OF AN INFORMED CONSENT LAWSUIT THAT COULD CONSTITUTE NEGLIGENCE

1. A patient-physician relationship is proved to have existed.
2. The provider had a duty to disclose information.
3. There was a failure to provide information.
4. If the information had been supplied, the patient would not have consented to treatment.
5. Failure to disclose was the proximal cause of the plaintiff's injury and damages claimed.

BOX 14-7. UNIVERSALLY ACCEPTED RECORD-KEEPING FORMAT: SOAP

Subjective data

This section of the record contains the patient's chief complaint or complaints. It should state how the patient says he or she feels, what his or her symptoms are, and what specifically has resulted in this visit to the dental office.

Objective findings

What does the dentist observe, see, or find in examination of a patient? This area involves the critical clinical examination and all of the diagnostic tests and results.

Assessment

Taking into consideration all of the comments made by the patient and all that he or she has observed, the dentist makes an assessment of the patient. The subjective and objective data guide the provider's diagnostic and treatment thought process.

Plans

The thought process materializes in this section, and a treatment plan is determined. When presentation of this plan is prepared for the patient, there should be an ideal treatment plan and a secondary treatment plan that would work well for the patient. Often, secondary plans are chosen because of economic issues. Patients also prefer to make choices.

The dentist has custodial rights to record ownership. The patient has proprietary rights. Records cannot be withheld from patients for any reason when they are requested in writing; however, only copies should be provided. The dentist should receive a proper authorization before releasing copies of records. The dentist must never part with the original dental records or any of the original components. In the event that there is a monetary refund to the patient for nonconfrontational purposes, a general release should be signed by the patient.

Records should be retained for a minimum of 6 years for adults and 6 years plus 1 year after the age of majority for minors, but it is preferable to keep records forever and store them someplace safe. Without the defense of records, a dentist will have difficulty winning a case. Usually, tolling time of law begins at the time of the alleged negligence, when treatment ends for normal care, or when the patient recognizes a problem. When a foreign object is the subject of the lawsuit, the statute could change in time to 1 year from the date of discovery. Continuation of treatment also affects the statute of limitations, which differs with each jurisdiction. Therefore the onus is on the practitioner to know how long the statute is, to understand the ramifications or exceptions, and to keep records for at least 5 years longer than required by law.

EMERGENCY CARE

Every office must establish a policy for handling emergency calls during and after office hours. When a patient or potential patient telephones the office and speaks with the dentist or a staff member, certain information, such as the medical history, premedical requirements, and nature of the complaint, must be gathered. When the dentist speaks with a patient and provides any information, a PPR begins. The conversation must be well documented, and follow-up policies must be in place. Emergency services, specifically for patients of record, are the responsibility of the dental practitioner, and thus the office must have a policy. Every dentist must have at least an answering service, answering machine, a mechanism of reachability, or some type of available coverage. Every dental practitioner must be available for and must respond to the emergent needs of patients of record in a timely manner. Before prescribing any medication, over the counter or prescription, the dentist must be familiar with the patient and his or her medical history.

ADDITIONAL AREAS OF CONCERN

Life is becoming more legally complex, and as a result many dentists will see the inside of a courtroom at some point in their careers. Some will called as expert witnesses; others will serve as jurors. Unfortunately, some will be defendants in malpractice actions. In addition to the dentists who allegedly provide treatment of an inferior quality, any dentist whose treatment does not bring about the desired result could be the target of a lawsuit in a litigation-prone society.

False claim acts (fraud)

False claim acts involve the knowledge that a claim is false, deliberate ignorance, or reckless disregard for the truth. The areas of concern for false claims are improper coding or upcoding, double billing, billing for services not yet rendered, unbundling or bundling of services, waiver of deductibles and co-insurance, and alteration and destruction of records. These areas also constitute insurance fraud.

Dental areas of consideration

General dentistry. Every patient has specific expectations for the outcome of dental care, and for whatever reason the dentist may not be able to satisfy that expectation. Unless the patient knows and is prepared for a lesser result, the patient may be dissatisfied. Finances may drive a treatment plan that could alter expectations. If the patient needs specialty procedures, the general dentist should not succumb to pressure to perform procedures that he or she is not comfortable with. Similarly a general dentist should not succumb to the directives of a managed care organization to perform a lesser procedure when he or she knows that the proposed procedure is necessary for appropriate patient care.

The dentist should provide the patient with treatment options and should not try to "sell" a specific treatment plan; he or she should explain the plan in layman's terms so that the patient comprehends the proposal. Consent should be obtained for every procedure to be done but is specifically important for invasive procedures. During efforts at restoration, the dentist must be observant to avoid overhanging margins, poor reconstruction, an overbite or underbite, and improper post insertions. Another litigation concern for general dentists is the failure to diagnose periodontal disease, endodontic problems, or cancerous and other medical conditions. Failure to refer to a specialist when necessary also is actionable.

Periodontics. Gingival health and cosmetics are a big part of periodontal care. Retaining the dentition also is important. There are periodontal procedures that will alter the gingival appearance, hence lengthening teeth and affecting cosmetics and function. If such alterations become a necessity, the patient must be informed before treatment. The patient must participate in the treatment plan, clearly understand the periodontist's goal, and recognize that he or she must comply with good oral hygiene or the goal cannot be accomplished. At times periodontal care involves the cooperation of other dental specialists, as well as the general dentist. Paresthesia is a concern but not as much as in other phases of dentistry. Periodontists are now included in the team of specialists who place implants and must specifically describe all aspects of implantology to the patient.

Oral and maxillofacial surgery. Some of the components of a lawsuit regarding surgery pertain to the extraction of the wrong tooth. Although the oral surgeon receives a prescription for a service to be rendered, the onus is on the oral surgeon to ensure that the diagnosis is correct and that the patient understands which tooth will be extracted before performing the procedure. After an extraction, unforeseen circumstances, such as dry sockets or sinus involvement, could present. Root tips can be left behind, jaws fractured, and foreign bodies aspirated. Although these events are unforeseen, they are possibilities and should be discussed as potential risks before the procedure is performed. Paresthesia is a common subject of litigation because many patients are unaware of nerve patterns and what could happen when an invasive procedure is performed. Some procedures are more difficult than others and can place stress on the jaw structures, causing trismus, temporomandibular joint dysfunction, or both.

Implantology. Patient selection, implant selection, and implant team member selection are of utmost importance in this area of dentistry. Expectations should be discussed and no guarantees made. Strict informed consent procedures must be adhered to so that all of the known risks are outlined for the patient, and team records must be accurate and consistent. Patients must comply with all instructions given by the implant team. Possible concerns include sinus perforations, mandibular canal perforations, and paresthesia. The patient should be told how much time and commitment are involved with this procedure, the potential longevity of the effect, and the prognosis.

Endodontics. Endodontic procedures can be successful in more than 98% of cases when the condition is properly treated, the restoration of the tooth is appropriate, and the tooth is periodontally sound. Yet, problems and mishaps occur in endodontic therapy, and not necessarily all of them can be considered negligence. The root canal system anatomy varies from tooth to tooth and patient to patient. Many patients' root canal systems are tortuous, narrow, and constricted or calcified. With newer techniques including microscopes, enhanced vision aids, light sources, and instrumentation, the ease of endodontic therapy has increased. However, difficulties (usually related to the anatomy and chronological age of the teeth and the more heavily restored and involved teeth) remain in many cases. Perforations of tooth structure in the chamber or root surfaces, the sinus, and the mandibular canal are not uncommon. It is best for an endodontist to prepare a post space within the anatomy of a canal. When the restorative dentist does not follow the path of canal anatomy in preparation for the post placement, failure can easily follow. Other concerns in endodontic care are crown and bridge fractures occurring during access preparations, paresthesia, instrument breakage, and the swallowing of instruments if the proper rubber shield is not used.

Fixed prosthetics. Fixed prosthetics are more commonly referred to as *crowns* and *bridges*. Considerations in this area of dentistry include improper margin adaptation, unrealistic cosmetic expectations, occlusal problems, and retention problems. Before preparing and treating teeth by applying fixed prosthetics, the practitioner should perform a complete endodontic and periodontal examination. Litigation has resulted from cases in which teeth with evidence of existing periapical pathology have been restored. Once crowns and bridges have been permanently cemented, endodontic therapy and periodontal therapy are possible but much more difficult. After the recent cementation of crowns, periodontal treatment risks the exposure of root structure. In addition, endodontic treatment performed after a final cementation can cause alteration or breakage of the crown, the bridge, or even the abutment.

Removable prosthetics. The most common concern among patients with removable or partially removable prosthetics (dentures) is a poor fit, which usually results from loss of bony ridge structure and poor impression techniques. In patients with removable partial dentures, poor fit can be a result of poorly designed rest areas and clasps. Improper stress on abutments can cause endodontic and periodontic pathology. Additional concerns in this area of dentistry are the mobility of abutments, failure to meet the cosmetic expectations of a patient, temporomandibular joint involvement, and defects of various products.

Orthodontics. Orthodontics used to be for the young, but now increased attention is paid to adult orthodontics aimed at correcting patients' cosmetic defects. Orthodontics deals with improving jaw development and ensuring appropriate occlusal contact. Some of the problems in this area are failure to meet the patient's cosmetic expectations, external apical root resorption, internal resorption, root canal system calcifications, temporomandibular joint problems, injury associated with the appliances, and untoward facial changes.

Pedodontics. Children are sometimes difficult to treat. Some methods of physical restraint can be construed as child abuse. Problems arise because of the patient's age, behavioral problems, and the interpretive abuse situations. Additional difficulties involve improper parental consent to various treatments and the tendency for young patients to neglect oral hygiene.

Paresthesia. Paresthesia is in a category of its own because it can result from any invasive procedure in oral surgery, endodontics, periodontics, or implantation. It can result from a poorly directed mandibular inferior alveolar nerve injection, improper surgical flapping of tissue in the mandible, involvement of the mental nerve, third molar extraction, or recklessness of care. Nerves commonly involved are the inferior alveolar nerve, lingual nerve, chorda tympani nerve, and mental nerve, as well as the peripheral sensory branch nerves. Paresthesia can involve the lower lip, a portion of the tongue, and the chin. It also can cause diminished taste and slurred speech. The dentist should be acutely aware of this possibility because paresthesia can be a temporary and transient situation or a permanent situation. The practitioner should discuss this risk with the patient before discussing the invasiveness of a procedure. Corrective treatment should be recommended when necessary. The patient should be afforded all means of communication, and all conversations and recommendations should be accurately recorded in the dental record.

Additional issues. Failure to recognize medical problems; improper use of nitrous oxide; failure to diagnose[28] and refer; complications with anesthesia; failure to recognize the depressed patient's normal functions during treatment; and improperly monitoring and charting bodily functions, such as blood pressure, cardiac function, and respiration, also can lead to lawsuits.

CONCLUSION

When all risks are considered in dentistry, most are rare and are not causation for negligence. There are defenses that can help each dentist prevent litigation. The primary line of defense is to avoid encouraging the patient to seek legal counsel by communicating properly. A second line of defense is to obtain appropriate consent for treatment. The final line of defense is to avoid creating damaging evidence by keeping accurate and appropriate dental records. Defenses exist for the action of negligence. Contributory negligence is the conduct on the part of the plaintiff that contributes to his or her own injury. Comparative negligence compares the negligence of the plaintiff and defendant solely in terms of blameworthiness and apportions the damages accordingly. Assumption of the risk is when the plaintiff assumes the risk because he or she has the knowledge, comprehension, and appreciation of a procedure and voluntarily chooses to encounter it.

This chapter includes a synopsis of risks and thoughts pertaining to risk management in dentistry. The entire textbook includes all of the elements of malpractice and negligence and should be read and understood by every dental practitioner. The dentist chooses the level of risk that he or she works with, and his or her license to practice dentistry will come under scrutiny in the event that he or she strays from the standard of care. Included is a list of suggested reading references and case history summations that support this thesis.

ENDNOTES

1. New York State Education Department, *Disciplinary Cases for Dentistry from 1994-1997* (New York State Education Department, Albany, NY).
2. Robert Nora, *Dental Malpractice: Its Causes and Cures,* 17 Quintessence International (1986).
3. Daniel Tennenhouse, *Dental Risk Prevention Manual* (Tennenhouse Publications, Calif.).
4. Norman Ascherman, *How to Spot the Malpractice-Minded Patient,* Dental Management (Oct 1985).
5. AHA Insurance Resource Inc, *Market Monitor,* No. 8 (Fall 1999).
6. Burton Pollack, *Risk Management Newsletter* (National Society of Dental Practitioners 1999-2000).
7. Edwin Zinman, *What to Do When a Patient Plans to Sue,* Dent. Mgmt. 32-35 (Mar 1986).
8. George Bush, *New York Times* (Feb 23, 1990).
9. Kevin Ricotta, Personal communication (Buffalo, NY).
10. A.E. James, S. Perry, R.M. Zaner, J.E. Chapman, & T. Calvani, *The Changing Concept of Standard of Care and the Development of Medical Imaging Technology,* 7 Humane Medicine (Oct 1991).
11. Arthur Curley, *Standard of Care Definition Varies,* 53 J. Am. Coll. Dent. (Fall 1986).
12. R. Shandell & P. Smith, *Standard of Care: The Preparation and Trial of Medical Malpractice Cases,* 1.01 Law J. Press (2000); *Advincula v. United Blood Services,* 176 Ill. 2d 1, 678 N.E. 2d 1009, 1018 (1996).
13. Bruce Weinstein, *Ethics and Its Role in Dentistry,* Gen. Dentistry (Sept/Oct 1992).
14. *Taylor v. Robbins* Tex., Harris County 281st Judicial District, No. 85-28095 (May 4, 1988).
15. *Perry v. Magic Valley Regional Medical Center,* Idaho Supreme Court, opinion No. 13 (Feb 28, 2000).
16. Beckman, *Doctor-Patient Relationship and Malpractice,* 154 Arch. Med. 1365 (1994).
17. L. Markus, AMA News (March 2, 1992).
18. B. Dorn, AMA News (March 2, 1992).
19. *Burlingham v. Mintz,* 891 P. 2d 527, 529 (Mont. 1995).
20. F. Buckner, *The Physician-Patient Relationship,* Med. Pract. Mgmt. (Sept/Oct 1994).
21. ACLM, *Liability Arising from Consultation,* 8 Med. Leg. Lessons (June 2000).
22. E.J. Emanuel & L.L. Emanuel, *Four Models of the Physician-Patient Relationship,* 267 J.A.M.A. (1992).
23. T.J. Smith, *Informed Consent Doctrine in Dental Practice: A Current Case Review,* 1 J. Law and Ethics in Dent. (1988).
24. *Morgan v. Olds,* 417 N.W. 2d 232, 235 (Iowa 1987).
25. P.J. Oberbreckling, *The Components of Quality Dental Records,* Dent. Econ. (May 1993).
26. P.G. Stimson & L.A. George, *How to Practice Defensive Dentistry,* 61 J. Greater Houston Dent. Soc. (March 1990).
27. F. Buckner, *Spoilation of Evidence: The Destruction, Alteration, or Loss of Medical Records,* Med. Pract. Mgmt. (Sept/Oct 1993).
28. R. Shandell & P. Smith, *Failure to Diagnose: The Preparation and Trial of Medical Malpractice Cases,* 1.01 Law J. Press (2000), *St. George v. Pariser,* 253 Va. 329, 484 S.E. 2d 888, 891 (1997).

RELATED CASE CITATIONS

ATLA, *Case Summary Survey 1986-1991,* Professional Negligence Law Reporter.

Brimm v. Malloy, Mich., Oakland County Circuit Court, No. 85 298 750 NO (Aug 5, 1987) (orthodontics, improper use of dental appliances).

Campbell v. Virginia Park Dental Ctr., Mich., Wayne County Circuit Court, No. 90-004143-NH (Aug 1, 1991) (wrongful death).

Canterbury v. Spence, 464 F. 2d 722 (D.C. Cir., 1972), *cert. denied,* 409 U.S. 1064 (1974).

Chang v. Frigeri, 76 A.D. 2d 643.

Coert v. Ryan, Wis., Milwaukee County Circuit Court, No. 657-296 (July 1, 1987) (informed consent, failure to consider alternatives).

D'Amour v. Board of Registration in Dentistry, 567 N.E. 2d 1226 (Mass. Sup. Jud. Ct., March 19, 1991). Dentist's license was suspended for gross misconduct (taking nude photographs of a patient in the name of science); the decision was remanded for reconsideration. The dentist contended that there was a relationship between temporomandibular joint pain and scoliosis.

Dillard v. MacGregor Dental Centers, Inc., Tex., Harris County 127th Judicial District Court, No. 85-50994 (July 14, 1987) (paresthesia, general dentistry, wisdom teeth extraction).

German v. Nichopoulos, 577 S.W. 2d 197 (Tenn. Ct. of App.) (requires disclosure to patient regarding the risks incident to a proposed diagnosis for treatment).

Ginsburg v. Golden, Md., Health Cl. Arbitration, No. 93-107 (Feb 25, 1994) (orthodontics, failure to diagnose root resorption).

Graddy v. New York Medical College, 19 A.D. 2d 426.

Harrison v. Bradley, Md., Health Claims Arbitration No. 84-498 (Mar 13, 1986) (orthodontics, failure to x-ray).

Isaksen v. Protopappas, Cal., Orange County Superior Court, No. 40-28-06 (June 20, 1986) (medical history, wrongful death).

Johnson v. International Dental, Ariz., Pima County Superior Court, No. 227157 (Apr 10, 1987) (paresthesia, wisdom tooth removal).

Kavanaugh v. Nussbaum, 71 N.Y. 2d 535.

Koslowski v. Sanchez, La., East Baton Rouge Parish District Court, No. 313, 459, Div. "B" (Nov 11, 1988) (paresthesia, Sargenti paste).

James Lantier, *Vicarious Responsibility,* personal correspondence.

Limongelli v. State Board of Dentistry, 616 A. 2d 945 (N.J. Superior Ct., Dec 1, 1992).

McCormack v. Gerren, N.Y., Albany County Supreme Court, No. 1454-86 (Apr 13, 1988) (improperly fitting dentures).

McGrath v. State Board of Dentistry, No. 25 C.D. 1993, Pennsylvania Commonwealth Court (Oct 19, 1993). Pennsylvania appeals court upholds license suspension of dentist convicted of Medicaid fraud.

Moore v. Curry, 577 So. 2d 824 (La. Ct. of App., April 3, 1991). Dentist found not negligent in failing to diagnose ameloblastoma.

Morgan v. MacPhail, Pa. Lexis 2739 (Dec 24, 1997). Informed consent doctrine applies to surgical procedures alone; courts maintain the surgical/nonsurgical distinction for informed consent.

Nathanson v. Kline, 186 Kan. 393, 350 P. 2d 1093 (1960).

Ong v. Department of Professional Regulation, 565 So. 2d 1384 (Fla. Dist. Ct. of App., Aug 23, 1990). Dentist reprimanded, fined, and given a 90-day license suspension for negligent treatment of a patient's chronic periodontitis.

Pasquale v. Siegel, N.Y., Queens County Supreme Court, No. 15103/86 (Mar 19, 1990) (failure to give antibiotics, subacute bacterial endocarditis).

Pastorelli v. Saltzman, N.Y., Queens County Supreme Court, No. 14620/80 (June 27, 1991) (delayed diagnosis of cancer).

Pelnar v. Neumeier, Mich., Menominee County Circuit Court, No. 86 4472 CZ (Nov 13, 1989) (failure to diagnose, periodontics).

Puglissi v. Klein, U.S. District Court, D. Del, No. 88-481-JJF (Sept 19, 1989) (failure to diagnose: decay).

Schloendorff v. Society of New York Hospital, 105 N.E. 92 (N.Y. 1914).

Bruce H. Seidberg, *Case Summaries* (personal files of dental-legal consultant), Mediation Committee, Onondaga County Dental Society.

Simpson v. Davis, Kansas Supreme Court, 549 P. 2d 950 (endodontics, swallowed instrument, deviation of standard of care).

St. Paul Fire & Marine Ins. Co. v. Shernow, 610 A. 2d 1281 (Conn. 1992) (sexual abuse).

VanTreese v. Whitcomb, U.S. District Court, E. D. Mich., No. G88-629-CA7 (Oct 22, 1990) (failure to refer).

Walter v. Smith, Mo., Jackson County Circuit Court, No. CV-89-23467 (Oct 26, 1992) (fraud to patient).

Woitalewicz v. Wyatt, Neb., Hall County District Court, No. 86-152 (Sept 13, 1986) (oral surgery, osteomyelitis).

REFERENCES

A. Bernstein, *Avoiding Medical Malpractice* (Pluribus Press, Chicago 1991).

W. Harold Bigham, *A Lawyer's View of the Legal Implications of Periodontal Disease Recognition,* J. Tenn. Dent. Assoc. (Apr 1985).

Sherry Case, *Terminating the Doctor-Patient Relationship,* N.Y. State Dent. J. 18-19 (Apr 1993).

Bruce R. Donoff, *Dentists as Physicians of the Mouth,* 125 J.A.D.A. 20-25 (Jan 1994).

F. Edwards, *Medical Malpractice* (Henry Holt, New York 1989).

W.W. Feuer, *Medical Malpractice Law* (Lawprep, Irvine, Calif. 1990).

R.M. Fish, M.E. Ehrhardt & B. Fish, *Malpractice Managing Your Defense* (Medical Economics, Oradel, N.J. 1990).

D. Foreman, *Dental Law* (Directed Media 1990).

D. Foreman, *How to Become an Expert Witness* (Directed Media, 1989).

B. Friedland, *Physician-Patient Confidentiality,* 15 J. Legal Med. 249-277.

Paul Gerber, *Can Your Records Withstand the Malpractice Test?* Dent. Mgmt. (Apr 1985).

Albert Good, *Statute of Limitations in Dental Malpractice Actions,* LIX W. Va. Dent. J. (Jan 1985) (limitation period does not begin to run until the patient knows or has reason to know of the malpractice).

H.B. Jacobs, *The Spectre of Malpractice* (Medical Quality Foundation 1988).

H.B. Jacobs, *Understanding Medical Malpractice and Maximizing Recovery in all Medical Malpractice and Personal Injury Cases* (Medical Quality Foundation 1988).

J.H. King, *The Law of Medical Malpractice in a Nutshell* (West Publishing, St Paul, Minn. 1986).

M.D. McCafferty & S.M. Meyer, *Medical Malpractice: Bases of Liability* (Shepard's/McGraw-Hill, Colorado Springs, Colo. 1987).

W.O. Morris, *A Lawyer's View as to How A Dentist Can Keep His House in Order,* 72 N.W. Dent. 45-48 (Sept/Oct 1993).

Elliott B. Oppenheim, *Presenting an Objective Standard of Care in Med-Mal Litigation,* Med. Malp. Law & Strategy 4-6 (Feb 1998).

B.R. Pollack, *Handbook of Dental Jurisprudence and Risk Management* (PSG Publishing, Littleton, Mass. 1987).

D. Poynter, *The Expert Witness Handbook* (Para Publishing 1987).

Prosser, *The Law of Torts* §§ 18, 32 (5th ed. 1984).

F. Rozovsky, *Consent to Treatment* (Little Brown, Boston 1990).

N. Schafler, *Medical Malpractice Handling of Dental Cases* (Shepard's/McGraw-Hill, Colorado Springs, Colo. 1991).

Julian Steiner, *The Dental Malpractice Crisis: What It Means for the Dental Assistant,* 55 Dent. Assist. (Mar/Apr 1986) (record-keeping accuracy and confidentiality, physician-patient relationship, vicarious decisions and treatment recommendations by the dental assistant).

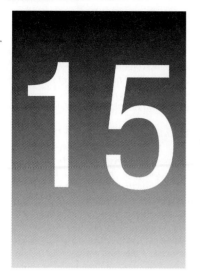

Antitrust

DAVID P. CLUCHEY, M.A., J.D.
EDWARD DAVID, M.D., J.D., F.C.L.M.

HISTORY AND INTRODUCTION
CONDUCT VIOLATIONS
ENFORCEMENT
DEFENSES
ROBINSON-PATMAN ACT
RECENT DEVELOPMENTS IN ANTITRUST AND HEALTH CARE REFORM

HISTORY AND INTRODUCTION

The principal objective of antitrust laws is the prohibition of practices that interfere with free competition in the marketplace. Business enterprises are expected to compete on the basis of price, quality, and service. The underlying assumption of the antitrust laws is that "the unrestrained interaction of competitive forces will yield the best allocation of our economic resources, the lowest price, the highest quality, and the [greatest consumer satisfaction.]"[1]

The U.S. economy underwent far-reaching and significant change after the Civil War. Technological development and rapid industrialization led to the emergence of a complex economic system. The laissez-faire policy of government during this time led to the amassing of vast economic power by individuals and certain large firms. Often this power was used to destroy smaller rivals with the goal of achieving and maintaining market control.

The public response to this economic system was colored by the changing social conditions of urbanization and immigration. Many felt that business firms should not be permitted to accumulate such wealth and exercise such great control over economic conditions. Discontent was particularly prominent among farmers and laborers. The specific targets of their outrage were the giant combinations that came to be called trusts. Chief among these was Standard Oil, apparently the first to use the trust device as a vehicle for merging numerous enterprises into a cohesive entity.[2] Various other trusts followed. The trust device was largely replaced after the turn of the century by the holding company, but the name *trust* remained.[3]

The last two decades of the nineteenth century saw the legal authorities in some states moving to break up business trusts. By 1890, 14 states had constitutional provisions prohibiting monopolies, and 13 had antitrust statutes.[4] These statutes commonly outlawed any contract, agreement, or combination to fix a common price. They also prohibited activity that tended to limit the quantity of a product sold or manufactured. Although some success was realized, the state constitutional provisions and statutes were for the most part ineffective in controlling or breaking up the large business combinations of the day.[5] This failure was due in part to the limit of each state's jurisdiction. The business enterprise could reincorporate in another state or otherwise change its practices to avoid specific restrictions. This perception of business' abuse of power led to public demand that Congress deal with trusts on a national basis.[6]

The congressional response to public outrage about monopoly and predatory business practices was the Sherman Antitrust Act of 1890. Because of opposition to the trusts from both political parties, passage of the Sherman Act took several years. Senator Sherman's proposals were strenuously attacked despite the nearly unanimous desire to enact antitrust legislation. The debates focused on the limits of the commerce power as the constitutional basis for such legislation and the definition of common law restrictions on monopolies and predatory business practices.

The Sherman Act as finally enacted has been described as being "as good an antitrust law as the Congress of 1890 could have devised."[7] It was a compromise that restated common law principles prohibiting restraints of trade and monopolization. However, the Sherman Act went beyond common law in several respects. Unlike common law prohibitions that were entirely civil in nature, the Sherman Act provided for criminal prosecution and penalties.[8] The Sherman Act also expressly provided the United States the authority to bring civil actions to enjoin violations of the act and authorized private citizens damaged by violations to seek injunctive relief and treble damages. The nationwide effect of the act and access to the federal courts resolved the most serious problems of limited jurisdiction under state law.

Indifference and failure characterized early antitrust policy under the Sherman Act.[9] The drafters of the Sherman Act had intended to curb both the power and monopolistic abuses of the great trusts. It had been assumed that the Sherman Act would be self-enforcing because the business community would follow its prohibitions. Assumptions of voluntary compliance proved incorrect. The Trans-Missouri Freight Association case was the government's first major antitrust victory.[10] The Supreme Court overturned a lower court determination that the prohibitions of the Sherman Act did not apply to price-fixing agreements between members of a railroad association. This decision was quickly followed by successful prosecutions in *United States v. Joint Traffic Association* and *United States v. Addyston Pipe & Steel Co.*[11,12] Overall, however, results were not impressive, and one senator was able to compile a list of 628 trusts formed between 1898 and 1908.[13]

After the enactment of the Sherman Act, there was substantial concern about its general language. In 1911 the Supreme Court decided the Standard Oil case.[14] In *Standard Oil* the court interpreted Section 1 of the Sherman Act as a prohibition on "unreasonable restraints of trade" and left to the courts the task of applying this "rule of reason."[15] Some concluded that the ambiguity of the statutory language and the new rule of reason gave excessive discretion to the courts. A movement for explicit prohibition of practices inimical to free competition gained momentum, and in 1914 Congress passed the Clayton Act.[16]

In 1914 Congress also passed the Federal Trade Commission (FTC) Act.[17] The FTC was modeled on the Interstate Commerce Commission, and it was anticipated that the commission would notify businesses of conduct that violated the FTC Act by issuing cease-and-desist orders without initial penalty. The FTC Act was another attempt to alleviate the uncertainty caused by the general language of the Sherman Act. The language of these three basic antitrust laws has been changed little since 1914.[18]

Before 1975, it generally was believed that the antitrust laws did not apply to the health care industry. In 1975, however, the Supreme Court held in *Goldfarb v. Virginia State Bar* that "learned professions" were not exempt from the antitrust laws.[19] Consequently the court has applied the antitrust laws to the activities of both individual health care providers and institutional health care providers, finding that the provision of medical service, as a "trade or commerce," is within the scope of the antitrust laws.[20,21] Especially since the 1980s, with the health care industry undergoing substantial restructuring in response to pressure to reduce costs and governmental regulatory changes, the industry has experienced an increasing number of antitrust actions.[22]

CONDUCT VIOLATIONS

Section 1 of the Sherman Act prohibits combinations, contracts, and conspiracies in restraint of trade among the states or with foreign nations.[23] To violate this section, an individual must engage in some type of concerted action that restrains trade in interstate commerce or with foreign countries. One of the issues concerning this concerted action requirement is whether joint action by two subsidiaries of the same parent corporation can lead to antitrust liability. In *Copperweld Corp. v. Independent Tube Corp.*, the Supreme Court held that a parent corporation and its wholly owned subsidiary are legally incapable of conspiring in violation of Section 1 of the Sherman Act.[24] Further extending the court's reasoning in *Copperweld* that an agreement between two subdivisions of a single corporation was not likely to be anticompetitive, courts have generally determined that two subsidiaries wholly owned by the same parent corporation are legally incapable of conspiring with one another for purposes of the Sherman Act.[25,26] Similarly, when an acute care hospital was alleged to conspire with its corporate affiliate, the court found no concerted action under the Sherman Act.[27] The same reasoning has been applied in concluding that a hospital and its medical staff—a creature of the hospital—do not engage in concerted action for the purposes of the antitrust laws.[28]

The interstate commerce requirement is a prerequisite to the jurisdiction of the federal courts over alleged antitrust violations. The conduct in question must have an appreciable impact on interstate commerce.[29]

In the health care field the Supreme Court has found that a particular hospital was not strictly a local, intrastate business because of the impact that it exerted on the purchases of drugs and supplies from out-of-state sources, as well as the revenues derived from out-of-state insurance companies.[30] Denial of staff privileges may satisfy an "effects" test by showing that commerce in the form of medical insurance from out-of-state sources, supplies from out-of-state sources, and interstate patients using a hospital was affected.[31] On the other hand, a number of courts have not found the interstate commerce requirement satisfied in cases involving denial of hospital privileges.[32] Almost all business can be found to have some connection with interstate commerce. This connection, no matter how tenuous, may serve to bring the conduct of a health care provider within the scope of the relevant antitrust statutes. Note, however, that the Clayton Act requires that the prescribed activity be in commerce. This requirement limits jurisdiction to persons or activities within the flow of interstate commerce, and incidental effects on interstate transactions are insufficient to confer jurisdiction.[33] This provides little solace to potential defendants because the Sherman Act provisions are broad enough to reach most anticompetitive conduct prohibited by the Clayton Act.

Rule of reason

Section 1 of the Sherman Act prohibits restraints of trade but contains no explicit limiting language. In interpreting this language, the courts initially struggled with the question of whether Congress intended to prohibit all restraints of trade. In 1911 the Supreme Court decided *Standard Oil Co. of New*

Jersey v. United States, which held that Section 1 of the Sherman Act was intended to prohibit only unreasonable restraints of trade.[34] What constitutes an unreasonable restraint of trade remains somewhat ambiguous, but since *Standard Oil,* the general approach to allegations of illegal restraints of trade has been to evaluate the alleged restraints under the rule of reason. The rule of reason requires a court applying Section 1 of the Sherman Act to evaluate whether a restraint of trade is an unreasonable restraint on competition. If it is found to be unreasonable, it is in violation of the statute. The rule of reason was described by Justice Brandeis in *Chicago Board of Trade v. United States* as follows:

Every agreement concerning trade, every regulation of trade, restrains. To bind, to restrain, is of their very essence. The true test of legality is whether the restraint imposed is such as merely regulates and perhaps thereby promotes competition or whether it is such as may suppress or even destroy competition. To determine that question the court must ordinarily consider the restraint as applied; the nature of the restraint and its effect, actual or probable. The history of the restraint, the evil believed to exist, the reason for adopting the particular remedy, the purpose or end sought to be attained are all relevant facts.[35]

Substantial debate has revolved around what courts may consider in evaluating the reasonableness of a restraint. The current view is that courts are limited to considering impacts on competition and may not consider social policy or some worthy purpose allegedly furthered by the restraint. In the application of antitrust principles to the conduct of health care providers, this issue is confronted when a restraint is defended on the grounds that it advances quality of care, access to care, or some other laudable public purpose.

A good example of the Supreme Court's approach to this issue is found in the discussion of the ban on competitive bidding by professional engineers considered by the court in *National Society of Professional Engineers v. United States.*[36] The society defended the ban as a means of minimizing the risk that competition would produce inferior engineering work, thereby endangering public safety. Noting that the Sherman Act does not require competitive bidding but prohibits unreasonable restraints on competition, the court pointed out that:

Petitioners' ban on competitive bidding prevents all customers from making the price comparisons in the initial selection of an engineer, and imposes the Society's view of the costs and benefits of competition on the entire marketplace. It is this restraint that must be justified under the Rule of Reason, and petitioner's attempt to do so on the basis of the potential threat that competition poses to the public safety and the ethics of its profession is nothing less than a frontal assault on the basic policy of the Sherman Act.[37]

Despite this rather strong statement about the scope of the rule of reason, some lower courts have been willing to consider issues other than the impact on competition in applying the rule of reason in cases involving the health care industry. In *Wilk v. American Medical Association, Inc.* the Court of Appeals for the Seventh Circuit indicated that it would allow a jury to consider issues of patient care in evaluating a prohibition on dealing with chiropractors as a restraint on trade under the rule of reason.[38] The court held that once the plaintiffs had established that the defendants' conduct had restricted competition, the burden shifted to the defendants to show that they had a genuine and objectively reasonable concern for patient care, that this concern had motivated the conduct in question, and that the concern would not have been satisfied with a less restrictive alternative.[39] The court was careful to distinguish this approach from a general consideration of the public interest served by the restraint, which would have put its approach in direct conflict with the Supreme Court decisions noted earlier.[40]

In *Hospital Building Co. v. Trustees of Rex Hospital* the Court of Appeals for the Fourth Circuit used a narrow rule of reason to permit a nonprofit hospital to defend against charges of market allocation and a concerted refusal to deal on the grounds that the planning activities in which the hospital participated were undertaken in good faith and their actual and intended effects were contemplated by federal health planning legislation.[41] This special rule of reason was described by the court as follows:

Because on this view the relevant federal health care legislation is in limited derogation of the normal operation of the antitrust laws, we further think that the burden of proof to show reasonableness of challenged planning and activities under this special rule of reason should be allocated as an affirmative defense to defendants seeking on this ground to avoid antitrust liability. On this basis a claimant, such as plaintiff here, makes out a prima facie case by showing acts that, but for the health care planning legislation, would constitute a per se violation of § 1 under traditional antitrust principles. This establishes liability for appropriate damages unless the defendants then persuade the trier of fact by a preponderance of the evidence that their planning activities had the purpose (and effect if plaintiff proves anticompetitive effects) only of avoiding a needless duplication of health care resources under the objective standard of need above defined.[42]

It remains to be seen whether the Supreme Court will be willing to accept considerations of patient care in rule of reason analysis in the health care industry.[43] In *FTC v. Indiana Federation of Dentists* the court rejected the patient care argument when the restraint did not produce any procompetitive benefits.[44] The court, however, left open the possibility that if concerns for the quality of patient care lead to the adoption of restraints that have procompetitive effects, the patient care concerns may be considered to balance against the anticompetitive effects of the restraints.[45]

Rule of reason analysis, even if limited to issues of competition, can be extremely complex, and the burden of litigating a rule of reason case is substantial. This factor was recognized by the courts, and a presumption of unreasonableness was established quite early for certain specific categories of anticompetitive conduct.[46] This presumption is known as the per se rule.[47]

Per se rule

In contrast to the rule of reason, the courts will apply a per se rule of illegality to practices that generally have been shown to have anticompetitive effects on competition. These practices are presumed to be illegal without inquiry into specific anticompetitive effects.

There are certain agreements or practices which because of their pernicious effect on competition and lack of any redeeming virtue are conclusively presumed to be unreasonable and therefore illegal without elaborate inquiry as to the precise harm they have caused. . . . Among the practices which courts have deemed to be per se unlawful are price-fixing . . . ; division of markets . . . ; group boycotts . . . ; and tying arrangements.[48]

Because application of the per se rule forecloses an in-depth analysis of the alleged restraint and its market effect and risks, sweeping potentially procompetitive activity within a categorical condemnation, the Supreme Court has cautioned that "[i]t is only after considerable experience with certain business relationships that courts classify them as per se violations of the Sherman Act."[49] Therefore when the case involves a professional association or an industry in which certain restraints on competition may be essential to its product, the Supreme Court has declined to invoke the per se rule, even though it is apparent on their face that the restraints in question will increase price or constitute a refusal to deal.[50,51] Instead the court undertakes a "quick-look" analysis under the rule of reason to ascertain the likelihood of anticompetitive effects, reasoning that an observer with even a rudimentary understanding of economics could conclude that the restraints would have an anticompetitive effect on customers and markets.[52]

The use of such a "quick-look" analysis, however, is not unlimited. In a recent case, *California Dental Association v. FTC,* the Supreme Court stated that, where the anticompetitive effects of given restraints are comparably obvious, the rule of reason demands a more thorough inquiry into the consequences of those restraints than the quick-look analysis.[53] In this case, California Dental Association (CDA), a voluntary nonprofit association of local dental societies, required its dentist members to refrain from advertising falsely or misleadingly under its Code of Ethics.[54] To help members comply with the code, CDA issued a number of advisory opinions and disclosure rules, which cautioned that price advertising must be based on verifiable data substantiating any comparison or statement of relativity and suggested that quality advertising is likely to be false or misleading because it cannot be measured or verified. The FTC brought action against CDA for unreasonably restricting truthful, nondeceptive discount or quality advertising in violation of Section 5 of the FTC Act.[55] The Court of Appeals for the Ninth

Circuit found the restrictions on across-the-board discount advertising to be a naked restraint on price competition and the nonprice advertising restrictions to be a form of output limitation. Accordingly the court held that these restrictions were sufficiently anticompetitive on their face to constitute unreasonable restraints of trade under a quick-look analysis.[56] The Supreme Court, however, found that the obvious anticompetitive effect that triggers the quick-look analysis had not been proved with respect to both the restraints on discount advertising and the restraints on nonprice advertising. According to the court, even assuming that the CDA disclosure rules essentially bar advertisement of across-the-board discounts, it does not obviously follow that such a ban would have anticompetitive effects. As a matter of economics, it is possible that "any costs to competition associated with the elimination of across-the-board advertising will be outweighed by gains to consumer information (and hence competition) created by discount advertising that is exact, accurate, and easily verifiable (at least by regulators)."[57]

In a similar vein the court found that restricting quality or patient comfort advertising may have a procompetitive effect by preventing false or misleading claims that distort the market. Based on the foregoing analysis, the court held that an extended examination of the possible factual underpinnings should be conducted so as to determine whether the advertising restraints violate the relevant antitrust law. Although the court did not elaborate on the scope of such an extended examination, its aversion to the quick-look analysis in *California Dental Association* may signal the court's inclination to adopt a heightened rule-of-reason analysis when the restraints in question arise in a professional context.[58]

Specific violations

Price-fixing. The courts have found certain types of conduct to have so pernicious an effect on competition and to be so lacking in any redeeming virtue that they are accorded per se illegal status.[59] One such type of conduct is price-fixing. As the Supreme Court noted in *United States v. Trenton Potteries Co.,* "the aim and result of every price-fixing agreement, if effective, is the elimination of one form of competition."[60] The economic power to fix a price reflects control of a market. It does not matter whether or not the fixing of prices is exercised in a reasonable or unreasonable manner. An agreement that creates such power "may well be held to be . . . unreasonable . . . without the necessity of minute inquiry whether a particular price is reasonable or unreasonable . . . and without placing on the government . . . the burden of ascertaining . . . whether it has become unreasonable through the mere variation of economic conditions."[61]

The agreement to fix prices need not be formal. The agreement itself can be demonstrated by circumstantial evidence.[62] An agreement that tampers with price (whether it raises, lowers, or stabilizes prices) is a per se violation.[63] Even agreements that affect price indirectly often are prohibited.[64] Once a practice is characterized as price-fixing, it is per se illegal. Making that characterization, however, can be difficult.

The leading price-fixing decision in the health care field is *Arizona v. Maricopa County Medical Society.*[65] There the Supreme Court applied the per se rule to an agreement among physicians to set maximum fees pursuant to a foundation program established by the county society. Approximately 70% of the physicians in Maricopa County were involved in the Maricopa plan. These physicians agreed not to charge more than the maximum agreed price for specified services and agreed with insurance companies to provide care to insured patients on that basis. The society defended the foundation plan on the grounds that it fixed only maximum prices, that it was an agreement among members of a profession, that it had procompetitive justifications, and that the courts should further investigate the health care industry before applying a per se rule to the conduct of health care providers. The majority in *Maricopa* rejected each of these arguments and held that the setting of maximum prices constituted per se illegal price-fixing.[66] The majority was unwilling to assign any weight to the unique characteristics of the market for physician services or to the plan's purported cost containment purposes.[67]

Reimbursement policies of health insurance companies have been challenged as illegal price-fixing agreements.[68] Courts have shown interest in such claims when evidence of provider control over reimbursement rates may exist.[69] When the evidence shows unilateral action with an effect on prices, courts have not been receptive to claims of price-fixing.[70]

Agreements or approaches resulting in the stabilization of prices generally are considered per se violations. Relative value scales have been challenged as price-fixing mechanisms because they allegedly tend to standardize charges for professional services. The FTC entered into multiple consent orders barring the use of relative value scales in the late 1970s.[71]

The critical issue of rising health care costs has led the purchasers of health care services to take various actions in an effort to stabilize or reduce their costs. Individual action rarely poses antitrust concerns. Collective action, including the joint buying of services through preferred provider organizations (PPOs), however, may trigger antitrust price-fixing concerns.[72] An agreement among buyers not to compete on price in the purchase of goods or services is just as much unlawful price-fixing as is a similar agreement among sellers not to compete on price.[73]

However, joint purchasing of health care can be procompetitive by allowing individual purchasers to share information and develop skills in negotiating and contracting collectively with health care providers.[74] Therefore, absent significant market power, such joint purchasing programs should be able to pass muster under the Sherman Act. When joint purchasers possess some market power, the purpose of the joint purchase must be scrutinized more closely and the

probable procompetitive effects of the arrangement must be weighed against possible anticompetitive harm.[75]

By the same token, hospitals can typically purchase supplies and services jointly without antitrust concerns. The Supreme Court has implicitly sanctioned wholesale purchasing cooperatives as arrangements seemingly designed to increase economic efficiency and render markets more rather than less competitive.[76] The Department of Justice (DOJ) and the FTC, in the 1996 Statements of Antitrust Enforcement Policy in Health Care (Health Care Statements) also emphasize that most joint purchasing arrangements among hospitals or other health care providers increase efficiencies and do not raise antitrust concerns.[77] The Statements provide a safety zone for any joint purchasing arrangement among hospitals and other health care providers if (1) the purchases account for less than 35% of the total sales of the purchased product or service in the relevant market and (2) the cost of the products and services purchased jointly accounts for less than 20% of the total revenues from all products or services sold by each competing participant in the joint purchasing arrangement. Beyond the safety zone, the law is not clear. Some suggest that the procompetitive effect inherent in joint purchasing arrangements dictates that a flexible per se standard should be applied.[78] Under this standard, horizontal pricing agreements among joint purchasers would be per se unlawful unless the purchasers could make an argument that the joint purchasing resulted in productive efficiencies and these efficiencies could be achieved only through an agreement designed to force prices below competitive levels.[79] Whether the courts will accept such a standard is difficult to predict.

Some large purchasers of health care services have sought to lower costs by insisting that health care providers include a so-called most favored nation clause in the agreement for the purchase of services. The purpose of such clauses is to ensure that the purchaser receives the lowest price given to any other purchaser. Although, in the usual case the antitrust law would support efforts to lower prices, when the purchaser has market power, a most favored nation clause could bring the price-cutting process to a halt because any additional price cut would have to be shared with the large purchaser.[80]

The development of new vehicles for the delivery of health care services has led to creative approaches to limiting prices paid for those services. This action in turn has sometimes resulted in allegations of price-fixing being put forward by private parties. In one such instance the Eleventh Circuit upheld a conclusion that there was no price-fixing involved in the negotiation of a reimbursement schedule by a PPO, in which the payers decided the maximum amount they were willing to pay providers for medical services and the providers decided whether they were willing to accept the limitation on reimbursement.[81]

Physicians seeking to avoid price-fixing problems should not agree with competing physicians on any term of price, quantity, or quality. Agreement on fee schedules and relative value scales is prohibited.[82] Although there may be exceptions to this relatively simple statement, the purported exceptions should be carefully examined with the assistance of competent and experienced antitrust counsel.

Tying and exclusive dealing. Tying may be defined as the sale or lease of a product or service conditioned on the buyer taking a second product or service. Tying arrangements may be attacked as unreasonable restraints of trade under Section 1 of the Sherman Act.[83] Anticompetitive tying arrangements are specifically prohibited by Section 3 of the Clayton Act and are deemed illegal under Section 5 of the FTC Act.[84,85] The Clayton Act is rarely encountered in suits against physicians and other health care providers because it applies only to the sales of commodities.[86]

The legal standard employed in evaluating tying arrangements may be viewed as a modified per se rule. This standard was discussed by the Supreme Court in the health care context in *Jefferson Parish Hospital District No. 2 v. Hyde.*[87] In *Jefferson Parish* the East Jefferson Hospital had entered into an exclusive agreement with Roux and Associates for the provision of anesthesiology services at the hospital. Dr. Edwin Hyde, a board-certified anesthesiologist, had applied for admission to the hospital's medical staff, and because of the exclusive contract the hospital's board had denied his application. Hyde sued the hospital and others, alleging that East Jefferson Hospital had engaged in tying by mandating that any person using services of the hospital requiring anesthesia also use the services of anesthesiologists employed by Roux and Associates. In *Jefferson Parish* the Supreme Court described an illegal tying agreement as follows: "[T]he essential characteristic of an invalid tying arrangement lies in the seller's exploitation of its control over the tying product to force the buyer into the purchase of a tied product that the buyer either did not want at all, or might have preferred to purchase elsewhere on different terms."[88] The court concluded that tying should be subject to per se condemnation when the probability of anticompetitive forcing is high.[89]

In general, to invoke the per se rule against a tying arrangement, the plaintiff must establish the existence of two separate products. In addition, the plaintiff must show that the party accused of tying has sufficient market power in the tying product to force acceptance of an unwanted tied product and that it has used that power to tie the products.[90]

In applying this analysis to the facts of *Jefferson Parish* the court concluded that East Jefferson Hospital had no significant power in the market for hospital services—the alleged tying product.[91] Absent this condition, the court was unwilling to apply the per se rule against the arrangement. In evaluating the arrangement under the rule of reason, the court concluded that there was insufficient evidence in the record to support a finding that the arrangement unreasonably restrained competition.[92]

Before the court's decision in *Jefferson Parish* there was substantial debate about whether inpatient hospital care could be divided into a number of different products for purposes of a tying analysis. In *Jefferson Parish* the court had no difficulty determining that the evidence amply supported the treatment of anesthesiology services as a separate product for purposes of the tying analysis.[93] The mere fact that services, such as anesthesia and surgery, are functionally linked does not foreclose treating the services as separate products.[94] This determination depends on a realistic appraisal of whether the products are distinct in the view of the purchasers and whether there is a distinct demand for each product.[95]

The utility of *Jefferson Parish* in evaluating the antitrust risks in other factual contexts is limited. The decision in the case turned entirely on an analysis of the market power of East Jefferson Hospital with regard to in-patient services. The court has, however, once again made it clear that no special consideration will be given to the fact that an alleged antitrust violation occurs in a health care context.[96]

Illegal tying issues also may arise when a health maintenance organization (HMO) conditions membership in the HMO network of medical prescription providers on a pharmacy's agreement to give its third-party administrator business to a subsidiary of the HMO. In *Brokerage Concepts, Inc. v. U.S. Healthcare, Inc.,* U.S. Healthcare refused to approve the application of a small Pennsylvania pharmacy chain for participation in its medical prescription network until it transferred its third-party administrator business to Corporate Health Administrators, a U.S. Healthcare subsidiary.[97] The Third Circuit Court of Appeals found no illegal tying, reasoning that U.S. Healthcare did not exercise appreciable market power in a properly defined tying market and that the alleged tying posed no harm to competition in the market for the tied product.[98]

An exclusive dealing arrangement involves an agreement by one party to buy particular products exclusively from another party. This arrangement has the effect of foreclosing to competitors of the seller the opportunity to compete for the purchases of buyers who are parties to exclusive dealing agreements. Exclusive dealing arrangements have been challenged under Section 1 of the Sherman Act, Section 3 of the Clayton Act, and Section 5 of the FTC Act.[99-101] Generally, exclusive dealing is regarded as a vertical restraint, which is evaluated under the rule of reason.[102] In evaluating exclusive dealing arrangements under Section 3 of the Clayton Act, the Supreme Court has found a violation where the arrangement foreclosed competition in a substantial share of the line of commerce affected.[103] In a more recent case the court used the same test but conducted a rigorous structural analysis and considered a number of unique characteristics of the market in concluding that a substantial share of the market was not foreclosed by the arrangement.[104]

Exclusive dealing agreements are common in the health care industry. A typical example is a contract between a physician or a group of physicians and a hospital to provide exclusive services to that hospital in a particular medical specialty, such as pathology, radiology, anesthesiology, or emergency medicine. In *Jefferson Parish* the arrangement between Roux and Associates and East Jefferson Hospital is properly characterized as an exclusive dealing arrangement. The court did not find sufficient evidence of anticompetitive impact on competition among anesthesiologists as a result of the arrangement to find it unreasonable and noted that Hyde did not undertake to prove unreasonable foreclosure of the market for anesthesiological services.[105] Nevertheless, Justice O'Connor, representing the view of four justices, noted:

Exclusive dealing is an unreasonable restraint on trade only when a significant fraction of buyers or sellers are frozen out of a market by the exclusive deal. . . . When the sellers of services are numerous and mobile, and the number of buyers is large, exclusive dealing arrangements of narrow scope pose no threat of adverse economic consequences. To the contrary, they may be substantially pro-competitive by ensuring stable markets and encouraging long-term, mutually advantageous business relationships.[106]

In evaluating the facts of *Jefferson Parish* as exclusive dealing, Justice O'Connor readily concluded that there was no potential for an unreasonable impact on competition as a result of the arrangement between Roux and Associates and the hospital.[107]

Before the decision in *Jefferson Parish,* a number of lower courts had upheld exclusive dealing arrangements between physicians and hospitals. *Harron v. United Hospital Center, Inc.* dealt with a radiologist's suit brought after he lost an exclusive contract because of a hospital merger.[108] The merged entity had contracted with a second physician to operate its radiology department. The Fourth Circuit Court of Appeals upheld the right of the new hospital to contract on an exclusive basis with another physician, stating that it was "frivolous to urge that the employment of a single physician to operate the radiology department of a hospital invokes the Sherman Act."[109]

The exclusion of an anesthesiologist from a hospital because that hospital had awarded an exclusive contract to the physician group with which the plaintiff had formerly been associated was the focus of concern in *Dos Santos v. Columbus-Cuneo-Cabrini Medical Center.*[110] The plaintiff anesthesiologist sued the hospital and the anesthesiology group under Sections 1 and 2 of the Sherman Act and under the Illinois Antitrust Act. The Seventh Circuit Court of Appeals vacated a preliminary injunction against the exclusive arrangement and remanded the case back to the District Court, noting that in its opinion the district court had improperly limited the relevant geographic market solely to the hospital from which the plaintiff was excluded. The Court of Appeals suggested, "should the instant case proceed to trial, the district court should reconsider on the basis of more complete evidence its preliminary finding regarding the relevant market."[111] The

court also suggested that the District Court "reexamine the basis of its conclusion that there is no effective competition among hospitals."[112] Although the Court of Appeals disposed of the case on a finding that the plaintiff had not satisfied other necessary prerequisites for the issuance of a preliminary injunction, it also expressed doubt that the plaintiff would succeed on the merits.[113]

Allegations of exclusive dealing also have been brought against a variety of exclusive contracting arrangements in the managed care context. In *U.S. Healthcare, Inc. v. Healthsource, Inc.,* Healthsource, a New Hampshire HMO, offered its panel physicians greater compensation if they agreed to a clause that precluded them from serving as participating physicians for any other HMO plan.[114] The First Circuit Court of Appeals held that the exclusive clause in question did not constitute an illegal restraint on competition. Absent a compelling showing of foreclosure of substantial dimension, the court saw no need to pursue any further inquiry into Healthsource's motive, the balance between harms and benefits, or the possible existence and relevance of any less restrictive means of achieving the benefits. It emphasized that proof of substantial foreclosure and "of probable immediate and future effects" in the market are the essential basis for an attack on an exclusivity clause.[115]

An exclusive dealing allegation is unlikely to prevail absent a convincing showing that a substantial portion of a rigorously defined relevant market is foreclosed by the arrangement. It also may be assumed that a court will consider seriously and weigh in the balance of a rule of reason analysis any legitimate procompetitive aspects of the arrangement.[116]

Concerted refusals to deal (boycotts). A concerted refusal to deal occurs when a group of competitors or a competitor and others through collective action exclude or otherwise interfere with the legitimate business activities of one or more other competitors. Courts use the terms *boycott* and *concerted refusal to deal* interchangeably when referring to the exclusion of a competitor by collective action. Boycotts involve concerted action and are challenged under Section 1 of the Sherman Act.[117] In general, boycotts have been held to be per se violations of the antitrust laws.[118] More recently, however, the Supreme Court has taken a more flexible approach, insisting that the potential for anticompetitive impact be established before the per se rule will be applied.[119]

In *Northwest Wholesale Stationers, Inc. v. Pacific Stationery and Printing Co.* the Supreme Court concluded that the exclusion of a retail office supply store from a nonprofit cooperative buying association was not a per se violation of the antitrust laws. The court noted that the per se rule generally has been applied in those cases where "the boycott . . . cut off access to a supply, facility, or market necessary to enable the boycotted firm to compete, . . . and frequently the boycotting firms possessed a dominant position in the relevant market."[120] The court held that:

A plaintiff seeking application of the per se rule must present a threshold case that the challenged activity falls into a category likely to have predominantly anticompetitive effects. . . . When the plaintiff challenges expulsion from a joint buying cooperative, some showing must be made that the cooperative possesses market power or unique access to a business element necessary for effective competition.[121]

Because such showing had not been made in *Northwest Stationers,* the court remanded the case for a review of the rule of reason analysis undertaken by the district court.

Although myriad opportunities exist within the health care arena for boycott activity, the issue has arisen most commonly in cases involving the refusal of medical staff privileges at a hospital. Existing members of a medical staff, who would be in direct competition with an applicant for staff privileges, often have significant influence, if not control, over the determination of whether or not to grant privileges. In some circumstances a denial of privileges may constitute an effective bar to competition (e.g., denial of privileges to a new physician at the only hospital in a community). The privileges issue is complicated by the fact that the training, professional competence, and need for a new physician may be relevant and legitimate issues for the hospital considering an application for privileges, and physicians currently active in the applicant's specialty will have substantial expertise and information to contribute regarding these questions.

The lower courts that have examined boycott allegations in the context of disputes over privileges have adopted a variety of approaches. In *Weiss v. York Hospital* the Court of Appeals for the Third Circuit concluded that the conduct of members of a hospital medical staff in opposing the granting of hospital privileges to a class of osteopathic physicians was the equivalent of a concerted refusal to deal.[122] Ultimately the court determined that the per se rule should be applied to this conduct.[123] It suggested, however, that rule of reason analysis would be appropriate if questions of professional competence or unprofessional conduct were at issue or the exclusion was otherwise based on public service or ethical norms.[124]

In *Wilk v. American Medical Association, Inc.* the plaintiff chiropractor sued a number of medical organizations under the Sherman Act for an alleged conspiracy to induce individual medical physicians and hospitals to refuse to deal with the plaintiff and other chiropractors.[125] Although the trial court instructed the jury on the per se rule, the Court of Appeals for the Seventh Circuit concluded that in the context of these facts "the nature and extent of [the] anticompetitive effect are too uncertain to be amenable to per se treatment."[126] Moreover, the court determined that the existence of substantial evidence of a patient care motive for the conduct of the organizations made application of the per se rule inappropriate.[127] Other courts have adopted a similar approach.[128]

In *Patrick v. Burget* the U.S. Supreme Court reinstated a treble damages verdict in excess of $2 million against three Oregon physicians because of their participation in a peer review process that recommended that the plaintiff surgeon's hospital privileges be revoked.[129] Although the reason given for revocation was substandard care, the evidence strongly supported the conclusion that the true motivation was anticompetitive bias. Although there is some protection for peer review activities under the state action exemption and the Health Care Quality Improvement Act of 1986, peer review activity stemming from anticompetitive motivation that results in the denial or revocation of hospital privileges may be held to be illegal group boycott activity.[130,131]

In addition, the issue of concerted refusal to deal has been raised when a PPO denied a physician's application for provider membership. In *Levine v. Central Florida Medical Affiliates, Inc.* the plaintiff internist sought physician provider membership with Healthchoice, a PPO in which physicians agreed to accept no more than a maximum allowable fee for services rendered to plan enrollees in exchange for a potentially higher volume of patients. Healthchoice denied Levine's request on the ground that it did not need any more internists in his geographic area.[132] The Court of Appeals for the Eleventh Circuit determined that the per se rule was not warranted in analyzing the alleged boycott because the plaintiff failed to prove that Healthchoice had market power and because selective contracting may be a method through which Healthchoice limited its provider panels in an effort to achieve quality and cost containment goals, thereby enhancing its ability to compete against other networks.[133] Applying a rule-of-reason analysis, the court found that Levine's illegal boycott claim could not succeed because he failed to define the relevant product and geographic markets and failed to prove that Healthchoice had sufficient market power to affect competition.[134] The Levine court's decision and in particular its unwillingness to adopt a per se analysis indicate that, absent necessary market power, a multiprovider network, such as a PPO, would have ample leeway in selecting its preferred providers without incurring antitrust liability.[135]

Market allocation. Another type of conduct that raises serious questions of restraint of trade is market allocation. Competitors, by agreeing to divide geographic markets or customers, can achieve the benefits of monopoly as to their exclusive market share. In general the Supreme Court has regarded market allocation agreements among competitors as per se illegal under Section 1 of the Sherman Act.[136] There are, however, substantial questions of characterization that qualify that statement. For example, territorial or customer restraints that are insisted on by a party operating at a different level of production, such as restraints imposed by a manufacturer on wholesalers, will be evaluated under the rule of reason.[137] There may be a substantial question whether the market allocation scheme is the primary objective of an agreement among competitors or merely ancillary to an otherwise legitimate joint venture. If the latter is the case, the court may well evaluate the entire venture under the rule of reason.[138]

Market allocation agreements among hospitals or physicians could take the form of agreements on geographic placement of institutions or offices. This type of arrangement could be characterized as a geographic market division. Agreements allocating the provision of certain services exclusively to particular hospitals or physicians would be another approach to market division. Evaluation of such agreements is likely to raise complex questions of motivation and anticompetitive effect. For example, some such arrangements may be dictated or at least approved by a state agency under applicable health planning statutes. The significance of such approval by a state agency is discussed in the section on defenses. Joint ventures among hospitals generally have not been challenged by federal antitrust enforcement agencies.[139]

Market allocation issues also arise in the context of managed care. In *Blue Cross & Blue Shield United of Wisconsin v. Marshfield Clinic,* the Court of Appeals for the Seventh Circuit affirmed a jury verdict upholding the plaintiff's market allocation claim under Section 1 of the Sherman Act.[140] The evidence in this case showed that Marshfield Clinic and North Central Health Protection Plan (North Central), an HMO, established "free flow" arrangements that allowed the physicians of North Central, a subsidiary of Marshfield Clinic, to refer patients to each other without getting each HMO's approval. The plan of the physician who rendered the service would bill the other plan for its cost. As part of the arrangements, the parties involved purposely chose not to place in writing clear descriptions of their respective service areas so as to minimize any risks of antitrust violations, but their understanding was to discourage the physician providers of one plan from establishing practices in the service area of the other plan. Based on these findings, the Court of Appeals for the Seventh Circuit upheld the jury's determination that the defendants had engaged in a market allocation.[141]

Monopolization. Section 2 of the Sherman Act prohibits monopolization, attempts to monopolize, and conspiracies to monopolize.[142] Section 2, by its terms, does not prohibit monopoly. The antitrust laws promote competition. As a result of competition a successful competitor may achieve a monopoly in a particular market. To declare such a result illegal seems unfair and illogical.[143]

The Supreme Court has suggested that a monopolization offense has two elements: "(1) the possession of monopoly power in the relevant market and (2) the willful acquisition or maintenance of that power as distinguished from growth or development as a consequence of a superior product, business acumen, or historic accident."[144]

Determination of the existence of the first element may be complicated. Monopoly power has been defined by the courts as the "power to control prices or exclude competition."[145] Although the Supreme Court has suggested that monopoly power may be inferred from a predominant share of the relevant market, substantial question remains as to what constitutes a "predominant share" and how the "relevant market"

should be defined.[146,147] Over time, the calculation of market share and the definition of the relevant market have become much more sophisticated.[148]

The second element of monopolization—the willful acquisition or maintenance of monopoly power—may be similarly elusive. In *United States v. Aluminum Co. of America* the court suggested that by embracing new opportunities and anticipating the need for new capacity Alcoa had monopolized the market for aluminum ingot.[149] More recently the courts appear to require something more than behavior motivated by legitimate business purposes to support a charge of monopolization.[150]

The offense of attempt to monopolize generally requires the proof of three elements: (1) specific intent to control prices or to exclude competitors, (2) predatory conduct directed to accomplishing this purpose, and (3) a dangerous probability of success.[151] Precise definition of conduct that satisfies these elements has proven to be controversial.[152]

In a recent example of an attempted monopolization case in the health care field, *Delaware Health Care, Inc. v. MCD Holding Co.,* Delaware Health Care (DHC), a provider of home care, brought an antitrust action against MCD Foundation and its subsidiaries, asserting that before the formation of Infusion Services of Delaware (ISD), a subsidiary of MCD Foundation, discharge planners of MCD's subsidiary hospitals recommended home care providers to patients on an informal rotating basis.[153] When ISD was formed, however, this informal rotation process was dismantled, and the defendant hospitals issued a directive to channel patients only to ISD. In addition, ISD was given exclusive access to patients in defendant hospitals' rooms to solicit business. As a result, ISD quickly gained a substantial share of the home infusion therapy market in the county where DHC and 13 other home care providers operated. DHC alleged two specific methods by which defendants had attempted monopolization. First, MCD Foundation "leveraged" its monopoly in the hospital market to extend its monopoly into the home health care market. Second, defendant hospitals denied DHC access to an "essential facility," the home care patients already discharged or about to be discharged from the defendant hospitals, and those patients' records. In response, MCD Foundation and the other defendants moved for summary judgment.[154]

With respect to the "leveraging" claim, the District Court for the District of Delaware started by analyzing the defendants' monopoly power in the "upstream" hospital market. Without monopoly power in the hospital market, there could be no illegal leveraging of the downstream home care market. Because the parties agreed that the relevant upstream product market was inpatient hospital services, the court turned its attention to the determination of the proper geographic market, noting that "[t]he geographic market must be broad enough that consumers would be unable to switch to alternative sellers in sufficient numbers to defeat an exercise of market power."[155]

Rejecting the defendants' argument that DHC failed to define the relevant market according to the "standard methodology" of the DOJ Merger Guidelines by considering the crucial forward-looking component that asks what patients would do in the event of a price increase, the court found that the Elzinga-Hogarty (E-H) test analyzing the flow of consumers in and out of the proposed market may be proper because a reasonable juror could conclude that consumers of health care would not choose to leave their local hospital market as a result of a price increase.[156] Moreover, the court held that MCD Foundation and its subsidiary hospitals' 62% share of the market, together with other evidence, could prove that the defendants possessed monopoly power in the particular geographic market. However, to succeed on the leveraging claim, DHC also had to prove that the use of the defendants' monopoly power in in-patient hospital services had resulted in "actual or threatened" monopoly power in the home infusion therapy market. It was this element that the court held DHC had failed to establish. According to the court, the information that 75.9% of ISD's patients are residents of the county does not by itself define the county as the geographic market. To define that market, DHC must consider all home infusion therapy services produced in the county. Moreover, the court opined that the home therapy market could not be properly analyzed using the E-H test. The prong of the E-H test that measures the percentage of the goods or services produced outside the market that were purchased by consumers within the market does not aid the analysis of the geographic market because the home care services are always produced in the consumer's residence. Consequently the court granted the defendants' motion for summary judgment on the illegal leveraging claim.[157]

With respect to the "essential facility" claim, the court found that, even accepting DHC's alleged inability to gain referrals for the defendant hospitals' patients as true, other sources of business for DHC existed in a sufficient amount that the patient discharge and referral process at defendant hospitals could not be considered an "essential facility." Given the availability of these other sources of business within DHC's service area, the access to the defendant hospitals' patient discharge process could not be deemed vital to DHC's competitive viability, and the denial of such access would not necessarily inflict a severe handicap that threatened to eliminate competition in the market. Accordingly the court held that DHC's evidence was insufficient to survive summary judgment on its essential facility claim.[158]

In the context of health care the most common instance of alleged monopolization is the situation in which a hospital with monopoly power is acting to maintain that power and to avoid competition.[159] Similarly an association of all or most physicians of a given specialty in a relevant market could support a finding of monopoly power in support of an allegation of monopolization.[160] In particular contexts an HMO, PPO, or other provider organization could face monopolization allegations.

Mergers. Mergers between business entities are generally evaluated under Section 7 of the Clayton Act.[161] Section 7 prohibits mergers in which the effect may be "substantially to lessen competition, or to tend to create a monopoly" in an activity "affecting commerce in any section of the country."[162] The purpose of Section 7 is to reach incipient problems of monopoly, and hence the rather broad language noted previously.

Section 7 applies to the acquisition of stock or assets of any person by any other person. It is clear that the term *person* includes corporations and unincorporated business enterprises and that the section applies to partial acquisitions of assets.[163,164] Section 7 may apply to joint ventures, as well as to more complete integration of business resources.[165]

The determination of whether an acquisition or merger substantially lessens competition or tends to create a monopoly has generated enormous controversy. In applying Section 7, the Supreme Court has engaged in increasingly rigorous structural analyses of the effect of the transaction on competition.[166] This trend also has been true of merger analysis undertaken by the FTC.[167]

The merger guidelines issued by the DOJ in 1968 and substantially revised in 1982, 1984, and 1992 have been exceptionally useful and influential in advancing the analysis of the competitive effect of mergers. The merger guidelines provide a structured approach to defining relevant product and geographic markets.[168,169] The merger guidelines use the Herfindahl-Hirschman index to measure market concentration and provide an outline of enforcement policy for different levels of and increases in market concentration.[170]

Merger cases brought in the health care context generally have involved for-profit hospitals.[171] Hospitals represent one of the largest economic entities engaged in the provision of health care services, and the expansionary activities of for-profit hospital chains have elicited the interest of antitrust enforcement authorities. Whether the developing merger activities of other types of health care providers will elicit the same interest remains to be seen.

When a merger involves nonprofit hospitals, the initial dispute may concern the threshold issue of whether the FTC has authority to challenge the merger under Section 7 of the Clayton Act.[172] Section 7 provides in relevant part: "[N]o person subject to the jurisdiction of the Federal Trade Commission shall acquire the whole or any part of the assets of any other person . . . where in any line of commerce . . . in any section of the country, the effect of such acquisition may be substantially to lessen competition."[173]

Some courts have held that to determine those persons "subject to the jurisdiction of the Federal Trade Commission" a court must turn to the FTC Act, which excludes nonprofit institutions from the jurisdiction of the FTC.[174] Other courts and the government, however, have taken the view that the

FTC's jurisdiction to enforce the Clayton Act is determined by Section 11 of the same act, which provides no exemption for nonprofit hospitals.[175]

The Statements of Antitrust Enforcement Policy in Health Care, revised and reissued by the DOJ and the FTC in 1996, address the issue of mergers among hospitals.[176] Statement 1 provides a safety zone for mergers "between two general acute care hospitals where one of the hospitals (1) has an average of fewer than 100 licensed beds over the three most recent years, and (2) has an average daily inpatient census of fewer than 40 patients over the three most recent years," and the hospital has been in operation for longer than 5 years.[177] The DOJ and FTC recognize that a hospital qualified for safety zone protection is often the only hospital in a relevant market and is unlikely to achieve the efficiencies that larger hospitals enjoy. A merger involving such a hospital is unlikely to have a substantial anticompetitive effect.[178]

Outside of the safety zone, hospital mergers are evaluated under the 1992 Merger Guidelines. The Statements do recognize that "[m]ost hospital mergers and acquisitions do not present competitive concerns."[179] This statement suggests that the government enforcement agencies might take a less strict approach in analyzing hospital mergers than mergers in other industries. For example, approximately 229 hospital mergers occurred between 1987 and 1991, and the federal antitrust enforcement authorities investigated only 27 and challenged only 5.[180]

ENFORCEMENT

The federal antitrust laws are enforced by the DOJ, the FTC, and private persons. In addition, state attorneys general have authority under Section 4C of the Clayton Act to bring federal antitrust actions as parens patriae on behalf of the citizens of the state.[181] They also enforce antitrust laws enacted by their state legislatures.

On the federal level, the Antitrust Division of the DOJ is responsible for enforcing the Sherman Act and the Clayton Act through either civil or criminal prosecutions. The FTC is mainly charged with the enforcement of the FTC Act and has concurrent jurisdiction with the Antitrust Division over some sections of the Clayton Act.

Any person or entity that has been injured by conduct in violation of the antitrust laws may bring a lawsuit under Section 4 of the Clayton Act for treble damages, costs of suit, and attorney's fees. To maintain such a private antitrust cause of action, a plaintiff must demonstrate (1) that it has suffered an injury (2) to business or property by (3) the violation of an antitrust law.[182] Over the years, the Supreme Court has required that the injury suffered by a private party be an "antitrust injury." That is, the injury suffered by a private person must be a type of injury that "the antitrust laws were intended to prevent and that flows from that which makes the defendants' acts unlawful."[183] Only after establishing an "antitrust

injury" may a plaintiff proceed to the liability and damage issues in a private lawsuit.

DEFENSES
State action exemption

There are a number of defenses or exemptions from liability under the antitrust laws. Although some of these exemptions are the result of action by Congress creating a specific statutory exception to the application of the antitrust laws, perhaps the most important—the state action exemption—was created by judicial decision.

The state action exemption is grounded on the principle of federalism. A state may choose to displace competition in the provision of certain goods or services within its borders and to replace market control with state regulation. As long as this action by the state qualifies under the state action exemption, private parties are protected from liability under the federal antitrust laws for acting in compliance with this state mandate.

The state action exemption was initially articulated by the Supreme Court in *Parker v. Brown.*[184] At issue in *Parker* was whether a raisin marketing program that had the effect of restricting production and maintaining prices but was created by state legislation was in violation of federal antitrust laws. In refusing to rule against the state program, the Supreme Court noted:

> We find nothing in the language of the Sherman Act or in its history which suggests that its purpose was to restrain a state or its officers or agents from activities directed by its legislature. In a dual system of government in which under the Constitution, the states are sovereign, save only as Congress may constitutionally subtract from their authority, an unexpressed purpose to nullify a state's control over its officers and agents is not lightly to be attributed to Congress.[185]

In a number of cases decided since *Parker v. Brown,* the Supreme Court has elaborated on the state action exemption.[186] In *California Liquor Dealers v. Midcal Aluminum Inc.* the Supreme Court suggested a two-pronged test for determining whether a state regulatory scheme is exempted from the federal antitrust laws.[187] First, the restraint must be clearly articulated and affirmatively expressed as state policy.[188] Second, the anticompetitive conduct must be actively supervised by the state.[189]

Most recently the Supreme Court has reaffirmed the two-prong Midcal test as the appropriate analytical approach for evaluating anticompetitive conduct by private parties acting pursuant to state statute.[190] The court also has made clear that the second prong of the Midcal test is not applicable to municipalities.[191]

The state action exemption has been raised as a defense by defendants in a variety of health care–related antitrust suits. A number of state statutes have been suggested as a basis for the state action exemption, including state certificate of need statutes, state statutes mandating physician peer review, and state authorization of municipal- and county-owned hospitals to grant or deny physician privileges.[192-194] The lower courts have engaged in substantial debate as to whether a state statute constitutes a clearly articulated and affirmatively expressed state policy to displace competition and whether there is adequate state supervision to satisfy the Midcal test.

In several cases in which municipalities have been sued for allegedly anticompetitive conduct in contracting for ambulance services, the lower courts have applied only the first prong of the Midcal test.[195] Requiring an explicit state policy to displace competition, these courts successfully anticipated the Supreme Court's decision in *Town of Hallie v. City of Eau Claire,* holding that the second requirement of *Midcal*—active state supervision—was not required when a municipality was following an expressed state policy.[196] Liability of municipalities and other political subdivisions for damages under the antitrust laws has now been clarified by statute.[197]

The Supreme Court has recently clarified the active supervision prong of the state action exemption. The clarification was made in the 1992 case *FTC v. Ticor Insurance Co.*[198] In the Ticor decision the court described state action immunity as "disfavored" and explained that active supervision means more than endowing a state agency with the duty to regulate.[199]

Explicit and implied exemption

Of course the antitrust statutes are subject to any limits and exemptions that Congress chooses to place on them. Over the years, Congress has enacted a number of specific exemptions for labor organizations, the business of insurance (to the extent regulated by state law), agricultural cooperatives, fishery associations, joint newspaper operating agreements, intrabrand territorial restrictions on franchisees of soft drink companies, joint small business programs for research and development, agreements between businesses necessary for the national defense, and joint exporting companies.[200-208]

Partially in response to the decision in *Patrick v. Burget,* Congress enacted the Health Care Quality Improvement Act of 1986.[209,210] This statute provides a general immunity from damages under the antitrust laws for physicians engaging in professional peer review.[211] In addition, any person providing information to a professional review body regarding the competence or professional conduct of a physician is given immunity from damages under state or federal law.[212,213] In the event that a suit is brought against a person engaging in professional peer review and is unsuccessful, the statute imposes liability on the person bringing the suit for the costs of suit, including a reasonable attorney's fee, if the claim of the person bringing suit was frivolous, unreasonable, without foundation, or in bad faith.[214]

In addition to the exemptions noted, there are express exemptions to aspects of the antitrust laws in the statutes establishing federal regulatory schemes for particular industries. These exemptions are generally specific and limited in scope.[215]

A more difficult question is generated when Congress has not enacted a specific statutory exemption to the antitrust laws but has entrusted authority over certain matters in an industry to a regulatory agency. The question becomes whether Congress has by implication created an exemption from the antitrust laws. In general, implied exemptions from the antitrust laws are disfavored by the courts and are found only when there is a clear conflict between the antitrust laws and other federal statutes.[216]

In the context of health care the Supreme Court has refused to find an implied exemption from the antitrust laws in federal health planning legislation.[217] In *National Gerimedical Hospital,* Blue Cross defended against a charge of anticompetitive conspiracy as a result of denying a hospital participating status by arguing that it was acting pursuant to the local Health System Agency (HSA) plan and furthering the purposes of the National Health Planning and Resources Development Act (NHPRDA) of 1974.[218] The Supreme Court concluded that in light of the strict approach taken in evaluating the claims of implied exemption to the antitrust laws Blue Cross would remain subject to the antitrust laws in this case. The court was not persuaded that there was a clear repugnancy between the NHPRDA and the antitrust laws, at least not on the facts of this case.[219] The court left open the possibility that an implied exemption from the antitrust laws might be found in other factual contexts in the health care industry, specifically for activities necessary to make the federal health planning legislation work.[220]

Noerr-Pennington doctrine

The courts have created an exemption from the antitrust laws for conduct by private parties intended to influence governmental action by the legislative, judicial, or executive branches. This exemption is known as the *Noerr-Pennington doctrine,* drawing its name from two U.S. Supreme Court cases wherein the court discussed the defense.[221] The underlying purpose of the Noerr-Pennington doctrine is to protect the right of citizens to petition government and to ensure that government's access to information about the desires of citizens remains unimpaired by the threat of liability under the antitrust laws.[222] Although the Noerr-Pennington doctrine is available to protect persons genuinely undertaking to influence governmental action, it is not available where the conduct is "a mere sham to cover what is actually nothing more than an attempt to interfere directly with the business relationships of a competitor."[223]

Appeals to certificate of need agencies and to physician licensing boards are types of conduct that may be subject to Noerr-Pennington protection unless subject to the sham exception just noted.[224] Hospital peer review committees have not been recognized as governmental agencies for purposes of the Noerr-Pennington doctrine.[225] Unilateral or joint action that does not take the form of an appeal to a governmental decision-maker is not accorded protection under Noerr-Pennington.[226]

ROBINSON-PATMAN ACT

In light of the recent practice of physicians dispensing medications and the joint venture movement, the Robinson-Patman Act is pertinent.[227] The act prohibits vendors from selling and customers from buying supplies at discriminatorily low prices (i.e., prices not generally available to other customers). The statute forbids price discrimination by vendors among their purchasers so as to lessen competition. However, an amendment to the Non-Profit Institutions Act exempts nonprofit hospitals but only on supplies purchased for the facility's "own use."[228] The exemption allows nonprofit purchasers to receive discounts on supplies for their own use. Customarily, nonprofit hospitals have paid less for drugs than the corner pharmacy, with the buyer and seller being protected by the statutory exemption.

In *Abbott Laboratories v. Portland Retail Druggists Association,* "for their own use" was interpreted as applying to hospital purchases of drugs dispensed for admitted patients, emergency department clientele, patients about to be discharged, some patients receiving out-patient treatment, and for personal use of employees, students, and physicians but not for walk-in customers.[229] "Own use" also has been defined as referring to treatment of hospital emergency department patients, patients receiving out-patient treatment on hospital premises, and immediate take-home use by discharged patients. These hospitals also may resell products to the medical staff for the personal use of physicians and their dependents. Although the potential liability in damages for defendants in antitrust actions should not be taken lightly, in the health care field it appears that these suits are more likely to be pursued as a threat to alter the defendants' conduct than with the expectation of recovering a judgment. Thus far, recoveries have been uncommon among reported cases.

RECENT DEVELOPMENTS IN ANTITRUST AND HEALTH CARE REFORM

In recognition of the substantial structural change occurring in the health care industry in recent years, the DOJ and the FTC issued Statements of Antitrust Enforcement Policy in Health Policy, regarding mergers and joint activities in the health care arena.[230] The first of these statements was issued on September 15, 1993. These statements were expanded and revised in September 1994 and further revised and reissued in August 1996. The most recent version of the statements addresses the following nine specific topics:

1. Hospital mergers
2. Hospital joint ventures involving expensive medical equipment
3. Hospital joint ventures involving specialized clinical or other expensive health care services
4. Providers' collaboration to provide non-fee–related information to purchasers of health care services
5. Providers' collaboration to provide fee-related information to purchasers of health care services
6. Provider exchanges of price and cost information
7. Joint purchasing arrangements among health care providers
8. Physician network joint ventures
9. Multiprovider networks

The statements issued by the federal antitrust enforcement agencies include antitrust safety zones in seven of the nine areas discussed. Conduct will not be challenged absent extraordinary circumstances when it falls within one of these zones. Analytical principles and illustrations are included for activity falling outside of the safety zones. The statements also commit the agencies to an expedited review process on antitrust issues in health care. The agencies will respond to requests for an opinion on enforcement intentions within 90 days after all necessary information is received regarding matters addressed in the statements, except nonsafety zone merger requests and requests regarding multiprovider networks. The agencies will respond within 120 days to requests on all other nonmerger health care matters.

Several of the statements of antitrust enforcement policy rely on a four-step rule of reason analysis for health care joint ventures that fall outside the safety zones defined by the agencies. The first step in this process is to define the relevant market. Typically, doing so involves the identification of the service being produced by the joint venture. The second step is to evaluate the competitive effects of the venture. This step begins with an examination of the structure of the relevant market and continues with an analysis of whether the joint venture restricts competitive activity among health care providers participating in the venture. In the event that it is determined that the venture has anticompetitive effects, it will be necessary to undertake the third step in the process and evaluate the impact of procompetitive efficiencies likely to be generated by the venture. This step includes the balancing of procompetitive efficiencies against the anticompetitive effects of the venture. Any venture in which the anticompetitive effects predominate will not survive this step of the analysis. The fourth step is the evaluation of collateral agreements that are likely to restrict competition to ensure that these collateral agreements are reasonably necessary to achieve the procompetitive efficiencies to be generated by the venture. This description of the rule of reason analytical approach reflects a refinement of judicial approaches and is likely to be drawn on by judges and attorneys faced with making such an analysis.

The statements of antitrust enforcement policy are an extraordinary and unprecedented effort by antitrust enforcement agencies to provide guidance to participants in the health care industry. The statements were motivated by the uncertainty generated by the antitrust laws at a time of fundamental change in the health care industry. Consolidations, mergers, and restructuring continue in the health care industry, driven primarily by market forces. These changes in the health care industry will generate significant antitrust questions for many years to come.

ENDNOTES

1. *Northern Pacific Railway v. United States,* 356 U.S. 1, 4-5 (1958).
2. Standard Oil adopted the trust format in 1879, and this action was followed by the rapid development of trusts in other industries. The trust as a vehicle for combining economic power commonly involved a trust agreement among the shareholders of the corporations involved. This agreement gave control over the stock in the corporations to the trustees, in return for which the shareholders received trust certificates evidencing their interest in the property controlled by the trust.
3. *See generally,* E. Kinter, *Federal Antitrust Law* (1980).
4. *Id.* at 130.
5. *Id.* at 128, 130.
6. *See generally,* E. Letwin, *Law and Economic Policy in America,* 53-99 (1965); *Kinter, supra* at 125-129.
7. Letwin, *supra* at 95.
8. Initially a violation of the act was a misdemeanor punishable by a fine of up to $5000 and by imprisonment of up to 1 year. The maximum fine was increased in 1955. In 1974 a violation of the act was made a felony, and penalties were substantially increased. A corporation may now be fined up to $10 million and any other person, $350,000. The maximum term of imprisonment is now 3 years. The Sherman Act is codified at 15 U.S.C. § 1-7.
9. *See generally,* Letwin, *supra* at 106-142.
10. *United States v. Trans-Missouri Freight Association,* 166 U.S. 290 (1897).
11. *United States v. Joint Traffic Association,* 171 U.S. 505 (1898).
12. *United States v. Addyston Pipe & Steel Co.,* 175 U.S. 211 (1899).
13. 51 Cong. Rec. 14218 21 (1914).
14. *Standard Oil Co. of New Jersey v. United States,* 221 U.S. 1 (1911).
15. *Id.* at 138.
16. Act of October 15, 1914, ch. 322, 38 Stat. 730, 15 U.S.C. §§ 12-27. The Clayton Act deals specifically with tying, exclusive dealing, price discrimination, and mergers.
17. Act of September 26, 1914, ch. 11, 38 Stat. 717, 15 U.S.C. §§ 41-51.
18. The most significant change was the amendment of the law of price discrimination by the Robinson-Patman Act in 1936. Act of June 19, 1936, ch. 592, 49 Stat. 1526.
19. *Goldfarb v. Virginia State Bar,* 421 U.S. 73 (1975).
20. *E.g., Summit Health, Ltd. v. Pinhas,* 500 U.S. 322 (1991).
21. *E.g., Hospital Building Co. v. Trustees of Rex Hospital,* 425 U.S. 738 (1976)
22. *See* Phillip A. Proger, *Application of the Sherman Act to Health Care: New Developments and New Directions,* 59 Antitrust L.J. 173 (1990).
23. 15 U.S.C. § 1.
24. *Copperweld Corp. v. Independent Tube Corp.,* 467 U.S. 752 (1984).
25. *Id.* at 772.
26. *See, e.g., Directory Sales Management Corp. v. Ohio Bell Tel. Co.,* 883 F. 2d 606, 611 (6th Cir. 1987); *Hood v. Tenneco Texas Life Ins. Co.,* 739 F. 2d 1012, 1015 (5th Cor. 1984). *But see In re Ray Dobbins Lincoln-Mercury v. Ford Motor Co.,* 671 F. Supp. 1525, 1544 (W.D.Va. 1984) (*Copperweld* does not apply to an allegation of conspiracy between two subsidiaries of the same parent corporation), *affir'd on other issues in an unpublished opinion,* 813 F. 2d 402 (4th Cir. 1985).
27. *Advanced Health-Care Serv. v. Radford Community Hosp.* 910 F. 2d 139, 143, 146 (4th Cir. 1990).
28. *See Weiss,* 745 F. 2d at 814-817, *cert. denied,* 470 U.S. 1060 (1985); *Feldman v. Jackson Memorial Hospital,* 571 F.Supp. 1000 (S.D. Fla. 1983), *aff'd,* 752 F. 2d 647 (11th Cir. 1985); *Cooper v. Forsyth County Hospital Authority,* 604 F.Supp. 685 (M.D. N.C. 1985). *But see Nurse Midwifery Associates v. Hibbett,* 918 F. 2d 605 (1990), *cert. denied,* 112 S.Ct. 406 (1991). It is, of course, clear that a medical staff is composed of individual physicians, and the conduct of physicians within a medical staff or as individual competitors in the market for physician services is not protected by the *Copperweld* doctrine. *See* discussion of this point in Weiss, 745 F. 2d at 815-816; *see also Nurse Midwifery Associates,* 918 F. 2d 605 (1990), *cert. denied,* 112 S.Ct. 406 (1991).
29. *See Summit Health, Ltd. v. Pinhas,* 500 U.S. 322 (1991); *McLain v. Real Estate Board of New Orleans,* 444 U.S. 232 (1980).
30. *Hospital Building Co.,* 425 U.S. 738, 744 (1976).
31. *Summit Health,* 500 U.S. 322 (1991); *Everhart v. Jane C. Stormont Hospital and Training School for Nurses,* 1982-1 Trade Cas. (CCH) 164, 703 (D. Kan. 1982).
32. *See, e.g., Cardio-Medical Associates v. Crozer-Chester Medical Center,* 536 F.Supp. 1065, 1073-1074 (E.D. Penn. 1982), *rev'd,* 721 F. 2d 68 (3d Cir. 1983); *Riggall v. Washington County Medical Society,* 249 F. 2d 266, 269 (8th Cir. 1957), *cert. denied,* 55 U.S. 954 (1958); *Nankin Hospital v. Michigan Hospital Service,* 361 F.Supp. 1199, 1210 (E.D. Mich. 1973).
33. *See Gulf Oil Corp. v. Coff Paving Co.,* 419 U.S. 186, 194 (1974).
34. *Standard Oil,* 221 U.S. 1 (1911).
35. *Chicago Board of Trade v. United States,* 246 U.S. 231, 238 (1918).
36. *National Society of Professional Engineers v. United States,* 435 U.S. 679 (1978).
37. *Id.* at 695. *See also Fashion Originator's Guild of America v. Federal Trade Commission,* 312 U.S. 457 (1941).
38. *Wilk v. American Medical Ass'n, Inc.,* 719 F. 2d 207, 227 (7th Cir. 1983), *cert. denied,* 467 U.S. 1210 (1984).
39. *Id.* at 227.
40. *Id.* at 226.
41. *Hospital Building Co.,* 691 F. 2d 678, 685 (4th Cir. 1982), *cert. denied,* 464 U.S. 890 (1983).
42. *Id.* at 686.
43. *See Arizona v. Maricopa County Medical Society,* 457 U.S. 332 (1982) (health care industry entitled to no unique treatment).
44. *FTC v. Indiana Federation of Dentists,* 476 U.S. 447, 459 (1986).
45. *See Id.* at 464.
46. The development of this presumption in the area of price-fixing began with *United States v. Joint Traffic Ass'n,* 171 U.S. 505, 568 (1897), continued in *United States v. Trenton Potteries Co.,* 273 U.S. 392, 397 (1927), and reached its high point in *United States v. Socony-Vacuum Oil Co.,* 310 U.S. 150, 221-223, 224 n. 59 (1940).
47. The term *per se* was first used in *Socony-Vacuum,* 310 U.S. at 223.
48. *Northern Pacific Railway,* 356 U.S. at 5.
49. *United States v. Topco,* 405 U.S. 596, 607-07 (1972).
50. *See National Society of Professional Engineers,* 435 U.S. 679 (1978); *Indiana Federation of Dentists,* 476 U.S. at 458.
51. *See NCAA v. Board of Regents,* 468 U.S. 85, 100 (1984).
52. *California Dental Association v. FTC,* 526 U.S. 756, 770 (1999).
53. *See Id.* at 770-778.
54. *Id.* at 760.
55. 15 U.S.C.S. 45.
56. *California Dental Association,* 526 U.S. at 763.
57. *Id.* at 775.
58. The court in *California Dental Association* seemed to suggest that a detailed market analysis might not be necessary in that case. It was, however, not entirely clear how extensive the examination needed to be to satisfy the rule of reason analysis. As the court stated, "[T]here is generally no categorical line to be drawn between restraints that give rise to an intuitively obvious inference of anticompetitive effect and those that call for more detailed treatment. What is required, rather, is an enquiry meet for the case, looking to the circumstances, details, and logic of a restraint. *Id.* at 780-781.
59. *Northern Pacific Railway,* 356 U.S. 1 (1958).
60. *Trenton Potteries Co.,* 273 U.S. at 397.
61. *Id.* at 397-398.
62. *Eastern States Lumber Association v. United States,* 234 U.S. 600, 612 (1914).
63. *Socony-Vacuum,* 310 U.S. at 221.
64. *But see Broadcast Music Inc. v. Columbia Broadcasting System, Inc.,* 441 U.S. 1, 23 (1979).
65. *Maricopa County Medical Society,* 457 U.S. 332 (1982).
66. *Id.* at 357.

67. *Id.* at 351. *Maricopa* was decided by a vote of four to three, two justices not participating. The dissent criticized the failure of the majority to recognize the uniqueness of the market for medical services. *Id.* at 366 n. 13.

68. *See, e.g., Glen Eden Hospital v. Blue Cross & Blue Shield of Michigan,* 740 F. 2d 423 (6th Cir. 1984).

69. *Id.* at 430.

70. *See, e.g., Kartell v. Blue Shield of Massachusetts, Inc.,* 749 F. 2d 922 (1st Cir. 1984).

71. The American College of Radiology, 3 Trade Reg. Rep. (CCH) 121, 236; Minnesota State Medical Association, 3 Trade Reg. Rep. (CCH) 121, 293; the American College of Obstetricians and Gynecologists, 3 Trade Reg. Rep. (CCH) I21, 171; the American Academy of Orthopedic Surgeons, 3 Trade Reg. Rep. (CCH) 121, 171.

72. *See* Clark C. Havighurst, *Antitrust Issues in the Joint Purchasing of Health Care,* Utah L. Rev. 409, 417 (1995).

73. *Mandeville Island Farms, Inc. v. American Crystal Sugar Co.,* 334 U.S. 219, 235 (1948).

74. Havighurst, *supra,* at 422.

75. *Id.* at 428

76. *Northwest Wholesale Stationers, Inc. v. Pacific Stationery and Printing Co.,* 472 U.S. 284, 295 (1985) (quoting from *Broadcast Music,* 441 U.S. at 20).

77. Department of Justice and Federal Trade Commission Statements of Antitrust Enforcement Policy in Health Care, 1996-4 Trade Reg. Rep. (CCH), s. 13,153.

78. *See* Roger D. Blair & Jeffrey L. Harrison, *Cooperative Buying, Monopoly, Power, and Antitrust Policy,* 86 Nw. U. L. Rev. 331, 366 (1992).

79. *Id.* at 366-367.

80. *Cf. Blue Cross & Blue Shield United of Wisconsin v. Marshfield Clinic,* 65 F.3d 1406,1415 (7th Cir. 1995), *cert. denied,* 516 U.S. 1184 (1996).

81. *Levine v. Central Florida Medical Affiliates, Inc.,* 72 F. 3d 1538, 1548 (11th Cir. 1996).

82. *See* "Remarks of Charles F. Rule Before the Interim Meeting of the American Medical Association House of Delegates," Dallas, Texas, December 6, 1988.

83. 15 U.S.C. § 1.

84. 15 U.S.C. § 14.

85. 15 U.S.C. § 45.

86. 15 U.S.C. § 14.

87. *Jefferson Parish Hospital District No. 2 v. Hyde,* 466 U.S. 2 (1984).

88. *Id.* at 12.

89. *Id.* at 15-16.

90. *Id.* at 17. Justice O'Connor, in an opinion concurring with the judgment in *Jefferson Parish,* which three other justices joined, suggests three prerequisites to an illegal tie: (1) The seller must have power in the tying product market; (2) there must be a substantial threat that the seller will acquire market power in the tied product; and (3) there must be a coherent economic basis for treating the tied products as distinct products. *Id.* at 1571. She also rejected per se treatment of tying arrangements even if these conditions are met. *Id.* at 37-40.

91. *Id.* at 26-27.

92. *Id.* at 29.

93. *Id.* at 21.

94. *Id.* at 22-24.

95. *Id.* at 23.

96. *Id.* at 25-26, n. 42 (citing *Maricopa County Medical Society,* 457 U.S. 332 [1982]); *National Gerimedical Hospital v. Blue Cross,* 452 U.S. 378 (1981); *American Medical Ass'n v. United States,* 317 U.S. 519 (1943).

97. *Brokerage Concepts, Inc. v. U.S. Healthcare, Inc.,* 140 F. 3d 494, 501 (3d Cir. 1998).

98. *Id.* at 519.

99. 5 U.S.C. § 1.

100. 15 U.S.C. § 14.

101. 15 U.S.C. § 45.

102. *Continental T.V., Inc., v. GTE Sylvania, Inc.,* 433 U.S. 36 (1977). *See also Jefferson Parish Hospital,* 466 U.S. at 45 (J. O'Connor, concurring).

103. *Standard Oil Co. v. United States,* 337 U.S. 293, 314 (1949).

104. *Tampa Electric Co. v. Nashville Coal Co.,* 365 U.S. 320 (1961).

105. *Jefferson Parish Hospital,* 466 U.S. at 30 n. 51 (1984).

106. *Id.* at 45 (J. O'Connor, concurring).

107. *Id.*

108. *Harron v. United Hospital Center, Inc.,* 522 F. 2d 1133 (4th Cir. 1975), *cert. denied,* 424 U.S. 916 (1976).

109. *Id.* at 1134.

110. *Dos Santos v. Columbus-Cuneo-Cabrini Medical Center,* 684 F. 2d 1346 (7th Cir. 1982).

111. *Id.* at 1354.

112. *Id.* at 1355.

113. *Id.* at 1352.

114. *U.S. Healthcare, Inc. v. Healthsource, Inc.,* 986 F.2d 589, 592 (1st Cir. 1993).

115. *Id.* at 596-597.

116. *See, e.g., Jefferson Parish Hospital,* 466 U.S. at 45 (J. O'Connor, concurring); *U.S. Healthcare, Inc. v. Healthsource, Inc.,* 986 F. 2d 589 (1st Cir. 1993).

117. 15 U.S.C. § 1. Section 1, by its terms, requires some contract, combination, or conspiracy for a violation of the section to occur. Unilateral action by a businessman has long been recognized as legitimate conduct unrestrained by the antitrust laws. *United States v. Colgate Co.,* 250 U.S. 300 (1919). One significant exception to this proposition would be unilateral action, which could be characterized as monopolization or as an attempt to monopolize.

118. *See Klor's, Inc. v. Broadway-Hale Stores, Inc.* 359 U.S. 207 (1959); *United States v. General Motors Corp.,* 384 U.S. 127 (1966).

119. *Northwest Wholesale Stationers,* 472 U.S. 284 (1985).

120. *Id.* at 294 (citations omitted).

121. *Id.* at 2621.

122. *Weiss v. York Hospital,* 745 F. 2d 786, 818 (3d Cir. 1984), *cert. denied,* 470 U.S. 1060 (1985).

123. *Id.* at 820.

124. *Id.* at 820. The court drew on language from *Arizona v. Maricopa County Medical Society,* 457 U.S. 332, 348-349 (1982), recognizing some limited vitality for a learned professions exemption from the operation of the antitrust laws.

125. *Wilk,* 719 F. 2d 207 (7th Cir. 1983), *cert. denied,* 467 U.S. 1210 (1984).

126. *Id.* at 221.

127. *Id.* at 221. *See* discussion of the rule of reason approach in *Wilk* at 182.

128. *See, e.g., Pontious v. Children's Hospital,* 552 F.Supp. 1352 (W.D. Pa. 1982); *Chiropractic Cooperative Association of Michigan v. American Medical Ass'n.,* 617 F.Supp. 264 (E.D. Mich. 1985).

129. Patrick, 486 U.S. 94 (1988).

130. *See* discussion at 174-175.

131. 42 U.S.C. §§ 11101-11152. This statute was, in part, in response to the verdict in the trial court in *Patrick v. Burget.*

132. *Levine v. Central Florida Medical Affiliates, Inc.,* 72 F. 3d 1538, 1542-1543 (11th Cir. 1996).

133. *Id.* at 1550.

134. *Id.* at 1552.

135. *See, e.g., Doctor's Hospital v. Southeast Medical Alliance,* 123 F.3d 301 (5th Cir. 1997). In this case a PPO controlled by local hospitals terminated the defendant hospital's membership, and accepted a rival hospital in the area as a new member instead. The court applied the rule of reason and found insufficient evidence of injury, noting that the plaintiff was affiliated with several other PPOs in the area and that the plaintiff failed to show that its exclusion from the defendant PPO would lead to increased prices under managed care plans, diminished consumer choice, or an impact on its long-term ability to compete. 15 U.S.C. § 1.

136. *United States v. Topco Associates, Inc.,* 405 U.S. 596 (1972).

137. *Continental T.V. v. G.T.E. Sylvania,* 433 U.S. 36 (1977).

138. *Cf. Broadcast Music,* 441 U.S. 1 (1979).

139. *See, e.g., Department of Justice and Federal Trade Commission Statements of Antitrust Enforcement Policy in Health Care,* 1996-4 Trade Reg. Rep. (CCH), section 13,153.

140. *Blue Cross & Blue Shield United of Wisconsin v. Marshfield Clinic,* 65 F.3d 1406, 1416 (7th Cir. 1995).

141. *Id.*

142. 15 U.S.C.A. § 2.

143. *United States v. Aluminum Co. of America,* 148 F. 2d 416, 430 (2d Cir. 1945) ("The successful competitor, having been urged to compete, must not be turned upon when he wins.")

144. *United States v. Grinnell Corp.,* 384 U.S. 563, 571 (1966).

145. *United States v. duPont & Co.,* 351 U.S. 377, 391 (1956); *accord Grinnel Corp.,* 384 U.S. at 571.

146. *Grinnell Corp.,* 384 U.S. at 571.

147. *In Aluminum Co. of America,* 148 F. 2d at 424, Judge Learned Hand noted that "The percentage we have already mentioned—over 90—results only if we both include all 'Alcoa's' production and exclude 'secondary.' That percentage is enough to constitute a monopoly; it is doubtful whether 60% or 64% would be enough; and certainly 33% is not."

148. *See* in this regard the revised merger guidelines issued by the United States Department of Justice in 1992; § 2.1 Product Market Definition; § 2.3 Geographic Market Definition; § 2.4 Calculating Market Shares.

149. *Aluminum Co. of America,* 148 F. 2d at 431.

150. *Aspen Skiing Co. v. Aspen Highlands Skiing Co.,* 472 U.S. 585, 603-605 (1985); *Berkey Photo Inc. v. Eastman Kodak Co.,* 603 F. 2d 263, 274 (2d Cir. 1979), *cert. denied,* 444 U.S. 1093 (1980).

151. *See William Inglis & Sons v. ITT Continental Baking Co.,* 668 F. 2d 1014, 1027 (9th Cir. 1981), *cert. denied,* 459 U.S. 825 (1982).

152. *See, e.g.,* Cartensen, *Reflections on Hay, Clark and the Relationship of Economic Analysis to Rules of Antitrust Law,* 83 Wis. L. Rev. 953 (1983); Cooper, *Attempts and Monopolization: A Mildly Expansionary Answer to the Prophylactic Riddle of Section Two,* 72 Mich. L. Rev. 373 (1974).

153. *Delaware Health Care, Inc. v. MCD Holding Co.,* 957 F. Supp. 535 (D.Del. 1997), *aff'd,* 141 F. 3d 1153 (3d Cir. 1998).

154. *See Id.* at 538-539.

155. *Id.* at 541 (citation omitted).

156. *Id.* at 541-543.

157. *Id.* at 544-546.

158. *Id.* at 547-548.

159. *See, e.g.,* Weiss, 745 F. 2d at 825, *cert. denied,* 470 U.S. 1060 (1985) (§ 2 violation reversed because no showing of willful conduct on part of hospital); *Robinson v. Magovern,* 621 F.Supp. at 887 (30% market share does not constitute monopoly power).

160. Allegations of monopolization, inter alia, by the attorney general of the State of Maine against an association of anesthesiologists in Portland, Maine, resulted in a consent decree restricting the practices of that association. *State of Maine v. Anesthesia Professional Ass'n,* Maine Superior Court, Consent Decree, June 12, 1984. In *Bhan v. NME Hospitals, Inc.,* 772 F. 2d 1467 (9th Cir. 1985) a nurse anesthetist alleged violations of §§ 1 and 2 of the Sherman Act by anesthesiologists and a hospital acting in combination to deny access to the hospital to nurse anesthetists.

161. 15 U.S.C. § 18. The FTC may review a merger pursuant to 15 U.S.C. § 45, which incorporates the provisions of Section 7. *Stanley Works v. FTC,* 469 F. 2d 498, 499 n. 2 (2d Cir. 1972), *cert. denied,* 412 U.S. 28 (1973).

162. 15 U.S.C. § 18.

163. 15 U.S.C. § 12. In regard to asset acquisitions, the acquiring party must be subject to the jurisdiction of the FTC. For discussion of this point, *see* Miles and Philip, *Hospitals Caught in the Antitrust Net: An Overview,* 24 Duquesne L. Rev. 489, 664 (1985), *and see FTC v. University Health Inc.,* 938 F. 2d 1206 (11th Cir. 1991) and *U.S. v. Rockford Memorial Hospital,* 898 F. 2d 1278 (7th Cir. 1990).

164. 5 U.S.C. § 18.

165. *United States v. Penn-Olin Chemical Co.,* 378 U.S. 158 (1964).

166. *Cf. United States v. Von's Grocery Co.,* 384 U.S. 270 (1966), with *United States v. General Dynamics Corp.,* 415 U.S. 486 (1974) and *United States v. Marine Bancorporation,* 418 U.S. 602 (1974).

167. *See, e.g., Hospital Corporation of America,* 3 Trade Reg. Rep. (CCH) I22, 301 (FTC Oct. 25, 1985); American Medical International, 3 Trade Reg. Rep. (CCH) I22, 170 (FTC July 2, 1984).

168. 1992 Merger Guidelines, § 2.1.

169. *Id.* at § 2.3.

170. The Herfindahl-Hirschman index (HHI) is the sum of the squares of the individual market shares of all the firms judged to be appropriately included in the market. An HHI of below 1000 in a postmerger market generally is considered unconcentrated, whereas an HHI above 1800 generally is considered highly concentrated. An HHI between 1000 and 1800 will be reviewed with emphasis on the increase in the HHI caused by the merger and other factors. This statement is a summary explanation of the process followed under the Merger Guidelines and reference to the Merger Guidelines is strongly recommended.

171. *See Hospital Corporation of America v. FTC,* 807 F. 2d 1381 (7th Cir. 1986), *cert. denied,* 481 U.S. 1038 (1987); American Medical International, 3 Trade Reg. Rep. (CCH) 122,170 (FTC July 2, 1984); *United States v. Hospital Affiliates International, Inc.,* 1980-1981 Trade Cases (CCH) 163, 721 (E.D. La. 1980); *American Medicorp, Inc. v. Humana, Inc.,* 445 F.Supp. 589 (E.D. Pa. 1977).

172. *See, e.g., FTC v. Freeman Hospital,* 69 F.3d 260 (8th Cir. 1995).

173. 15 U.S.C. s. 18.

174. *See, e.g., United States v. Carilion Health Service, Inc.,* 707 F. Supp. 840 (W.D. Va. 1988), *aff'd without opinion,* 892 F.2d 1042 (4th Cir. 1989).

175. *See, e.g., FTC v. University Health, Inc.,* 938 F.2d 1206, 1214-1215 (11th Cir. 1991); *United States v. Rockford Memorial Corp.,* 898 F.2d 1278 (7th Cir. 1990), *cert. denied,* 498 U.S. 920 (1990).

176. 4 Trade Reg. Rep. (CCH) s. 13,153, Statement 1.

177. *Id.*

178. *Id.*

179. *Id.*

180. *See* Statement of Charles A. James, Acting Assistant Attorney General, Antitrust Division, to the Joint Economic Committee of the House-Senate Subcommittee on Investment, Jobs and Prices, June 24, 1992.

181. 15 U.S.C. s. 15c.

182. *See Brunswick Corp. v. Pueblo Bowl-O-Mat, Inc.,* 429 U.S. 477 (1977).

183. *Id.* at 489.

184. *Parker v. Brown,* 317 U.S. 341 (1943).

185. *Id.* at 350.

186. *See, e.g., Goldfarb v. Virginia State Bar,* 421 U.S. 773 (1975); *Cantor v. Detroit Edison Co.,* 428 U.S. 579 (1976); *Bates v. State Bar of Arizona,* 433 U.S. 350 (1977).

187. *California Liquor Dealers v. Midcal Aluminum Inc.,* 445 U.S. 97 (1980).

188. *Id.* at 105.

189. *Id.*

190. *See Patrick v. Burget,* 486 U.S. 94 (1988); *see also Southern Motor Carriers Rate Conference v. United States,* 471 U.S. 48 (1985). In *Southern Motor Carriers* the court rejected the contention that to gain the benefit of the state action exemption the anticompetitive conduct of the private party must be compelled by the state statute.

191. *Town of Hallie v. City of Eau Claire,* 471 U.S. 34 (1985).

192. *See, e.g., State of North Carolina ex rel. Edmisten v. P.I.A. Asheville, Inc.,* 740 F. 2d 274 (4th Cir. 1984), *cert. denied,* 469 U.S. 1070 (1985).

193. *See, e.g., Marrese v. Interequal, Inc.,* 748 F.2d 373 (7th Cir. 1984), *cert. denied,* 472 U.S. 1027 (1985); *Quinn v. Kent General Hospital, Inc.,* 617 F.Supp. 1226 (D.C. Del. 1985).

194. *See, e.g., Coastal Neuro-Psychiatric Associates v. Onslow County Hospital Authority,* 607 F.Supp. 49 (D.C.N.C. 1985).

195. *Springs Ambulance Service v. City of Rancho Mirage,* 745 F.2d 1270 (9th Cir. 1984); *Gold Cross Ambulance and Transfer v. City of Kansas City,* 705 F.2d 1005 (8th Cir. 1983), *cert. denied,* 469 U.S. 538 (1985). Both cases involved exclusive contracts for the provision of ambulance services to the citizens of the municipalities.

196. *Town of Hallie,* 471 U.S. at 47.

197. Local Government Antitrust Act of 1984, Pub. L. 98-544, October 24, 1984, 15 U.S.C. §§ 34-36.

198. 112 S.Ct. 2169 (1992).

199. *Id.* at 2178.

200. 15 U.S.C. § 17.

201. 15 U.S.C. §§ 1011-1015 (McCarran-Ferguson Act). *See Union Life Insurance Co. v. Pireno,* 458 U.S. 119 (1982); *Group Life & Health Ins. Co. v. Royal Drug Co.,* 440 U.S. 205 (1979); *St. Paul Fire & Marine Ins. Co. v. Barry,* 438 U.S. 531 (1978).

202. 15 U.S.C. § 17; 7 U.S.C. §§ 291-292 (Capper-Volstead Act).

203. 15 U.S.C. § 521 (The Fisheries Cooperative Marketing Act).

204. 15 U.S.C. § 1801-1804 (The Newspaper Preservation Act).

205. 15 U.S.C. §§ 3501-3503 (The Soft Drink Interbrand Competition Act of 1980).

206. 15 U.S.C. § 638(d)(1), (2).

207. 15 U.S.C. §§ 640, 2158.

208. 15 U.S.C. §§62, 4001-4021 (Webb-Pomerene Act, Export Trading Company Act of 1982).

209. *Patrick,* 486 U.S. 94 (1988).

210. 42 U.S.C. §§ 11101-11152.

211. The professional review action must meet the standards set forth in 42 U.S.C. § 11112(a). This immunity may be lost if a health care entity fails to report information as required by the statute. 42 U.S.C. § 11111(b).

212. Professional review body is defined at 42 U.S.C. § 11151 (11). It includes a health care entity conducting professional review and any committee of a health care entity or of a medical staff of such an entity conducting such review when assisting the governing body of the institution.

213. Immunity is not provided if the information is false and the person providing it knew it was false. 42 U.S.C. § 11111(a)(2).

214. 42 U.S.C. §11113.

215. *See, e.g.,* The Reed-Bullwinkle Act, 49 U.S.C. § 10706 (joint rate filings with ICC by carriers); the Shipping Act of 1916, 46 U.S.C. § 813a, 814 (rate agreements between maritime carriers).

216. *See, e.g., United States v. National Association of Securities Dealers,* 422 U.S. 694 (1975); *United States v. Philadelphia National Bank,* 374 U.S. 321 (1963); *Silver v. New York Stock Exchange,* 373 U.S. 341 (1963).

217. *See National Gerimedical Hospital v. Blue Cross,* 452 U.S. 378 (1981).

218. 42 U.S.C. § 3001 (National Health Planning and Development Act of 1974).

219. 452 U.S. at 391.

220. *Id.* at 393 n. 18.

221. *Eastern Railroad Presidents Conference v. Noerr Motor Freight, Inc.* 365 U.S. 127 (1961); *United Mine Workers v. Pennington,* 381 U.S. 657 (1965).

222. *Noerr Motor Freight,* 365 U.S. at 137.

223. *Id.* at 144; *see also Professional Real Estate Investors Inc. v. Columbia Pictures Industries, Inc.,* 113 S.Ct. 1920 (1993); *City of Columbia v. Omni Outdoor Advertising, Inc.,* 111 S.Ct. 1344 (1991); *California Motor Transport Co. v. Trucking Unlimited,* 404 U.S. 508, 513 (1972).

224. *See,* e.g., *Hospital Building Co.,* 692 F. 2d at 687-688; *Feminist Women's Health Center v. Mohammad,* 586 F. 2d 530, 442-447 (5th Cir. 1978).

225. *Feminist Women's Health Center,* 586 F.2d at 454.

226. *Virginia Academy of Clinical Psychologists v. Blue Shield of Virginia,* 624 F. 2d 476, 482 (4th Cir. 1980), *cert. denied,* 450 U.S. 916 (1981).

227. Robinson-Patman Antidiscrimination Act, ch. 592, § 1-4, 49 Stat 1526, 15 U.S.C. 13, 13a, 13b, 21a, 13c (1936).

228. Non-Profit Institutions Act, ch. 283, 52 Stat. 446, 15 U.S.C. 13c (1938).

229. *Abbott Laboratories v. Portland Retail Druggists Ass'n,* 425 U.S. 1 (1976).

230. 1996-4 Trade Reg. Rep. (CCH), § 13,153. In the 1996 revised statements the agencies elaborated on their discussion in two critical areas—physician and multiprovider networks.

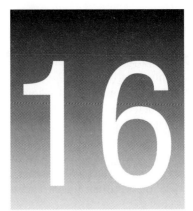

Crimes by health care providers

STAN TWARDY, J.D., LL.M.

CRIMES BY HEALTH CARE PROVIDERS
CRIMES AGAINST THE PERSON
CRIMINAL PROCEDURE

CRIMES BY HEALTH CARE PROVIDERS

The twenty-first century had barely dawned when the magnitude of medical care fraud was highlighted by a record $745 million in criminal and civil penalties that Columbia/HCA Healthcare Corp. agreed to pay for Medicare frauds, including mishandling of home health care, billing, and laboratory claims.[1] Several Columbia executives have already been convicted. Also in the beginning of the new century, in the second highest combination of criminal and civil fines, Fresenius Medical Care of North America of Lexington, Mass., agreed to pay $486 million to the U.S. government for fraud involving medically unnecessary kidney dialysis, deliberate duplicate billings, "nutrition therapy," and kickbacks to nephrologists.[2] Two vice presidents of its subsidiary companies also pleaded guilty, and three others were indicted in an ongoing investigation of the company's 800 dialysis facilities by the Federal Bureau of Investigation (FBI). FBI officials described the schemes as a "corporate strategy of criminal behavior." This single fine exceeded the total of $480 million netted by the federal government in 1998 from all health care frauds combined, according to the Justice Department.

Although the United States spends approximately $1 trillion a year on health care, estimates of the amount of money actually lost to health care frauds vary greatly, but both the government and private health care providers calculate losses in billions of dollars. The closest approximation made by the Office of Inspector General of the Department of Health and Human Services was $13.4 billion in 1999. In its report to Congress, the General Accounting Office reported that $19.1 billion in government money was wasted during the fiscal year 1998 and that overpayments were made in 14 federal programs administered by nine federal agencies, including Medicare. The largest waste was by Medicare, which paid $12.6 billion in fraudulent and improper payments to the fee-for-service sector. The General Accounting Office described the figures as "the tip of the iceberg." The Inspector General also estimates that more than half of the $1.4 billion spent on infusion therapy from 1995 through 1998 represented fraudulent claims and

that overpayments to Medicare managed care organizations (MCOs) could cost $34 billion by the year 2010.

The FBI has described health care frauds as its highest-priority white-collar crimes. Some 500 agents work almost exclusively on health care frauds in close cooperation with the Inspector General of the Department of Health and Human Services, states' attorneys general, and district attorneys throughout the United States. As a result, hundreds of physicians, nurses, hospital administrators, accountants, and even billing clerks have received long-term prison sentences. At the end of 1999, there were some 4000 cases pending. The FBI claims that the fraudulent providers of medical care are frequently the most incompetent physicians, nurses, and home care operators.

Prosecution criteria

The U.S. Department of Justice issued prosecution criteria for health care frauds that are especially applicable to corporations. Among others, these criteria include the following:

1. The nature and seriousness of the wrongdoing
2. The pervasiveness of the misconduct
3. The individual's or organization's history of similar wrongdoing
4. Voluntary disclosure or a willingness to cooperate in the investigation
5. The existence or inadequacy of corporate compliance programs
6. The corrective actions taken
7. The collateral consequences of the lawbreaking
8. The sufficiency of noncriminal sanctions

The directive points out that even minimal wrongdoing may justify criminal prosecution if the misbehavior was pervasive, was carried out by employees, and was known by the company's top managers. Conversely, the document states that single acts by a rogue employee may not be sufficient justification for criminally charging the employer.

In addition to other criminal statutes, the FBI relies increasingly on antikickback (1) false claims; (2) and false statements laws; (3) mail, wire and Internet frauds, and (4) the Racketeer Influenced and Corrupt Organizations (RICO) Act, and money laundering. The Works Incentives Improvement Act, signed into law in December 1999, now allows state units that control Medicaid fraud to also tackle certain Medicare frauds when they also involve Medicaid recipients.

According to the Health Care Financing Administration (HCFA), the newer target areas of more aggressive criminal investigation and prosecution include, among others, patient referrals to entities in which the physician has a financial interest, patient dumping regulations, nursing home oversight, quality care issues, substandard care in managed care plans, and pharmaceutical and billing frauds. Prosecutors who in the past have been reluctant to get caught in the battle of experts over quality care are increasingly finding academic and other expert witnesses willing to testify. In nursing home cases, in which witnesses are often feeble minded and inarticulate, disgruntled employees often act as whistle-blowers and make excellent witnesses. Juries are also increasingly inclined to punish nursing homes for abuse of patients. Intensified prosecutions are also directed at individual physicians because of inadequate involvement in patient care, especially in nursing homes.

Numerous physicians are regularly being convicted for submitting improper claims and short-changing patients on medical examinations and treatment. The FBI receives hundreds of tips from patients who suspect, or have detected, possible fraud by their health care providers. The Department of Defense has also announced that it will intensify assistance to U.S. attorneys in conducting aggressive prosecutions of individuals and institutions who short-change patients in providing care under the Department's guidelines.

Understanding criminal law

The purpose of criminal law is to define socially intolerable conduct and to make specific prohibitions punishable by law. Criminal procedure deals with constitutional safeguards and the working mechanism of American courts to ensure justice and fairness. A health care provider who runs afoul of criminal law may be consoled by the array of constitutional safeguards that ensure a fair trial. The Anglo-American system of justice provides more safeguards for the criminal defendant than any other system in the world. In this system the criminal accused is deemed innocent until proved guilty. In other judicial systems the criminal defendant must prove innocence.

In a civil case the facts at issue must be proved by a "preponderance of the evidence." In a criminal case the state or federal government must prove its case "beyond a reasonable doubt." Some legal scholars define *preponderance of the evidence* as being merely more likely than not, something more than a 50% probability; this is the standard for civil litigation, which includes most malpractice cases. In contrast, when a criminal defendant is tried, the prosecution must prove beyond a reasonable doubt that a crime was committed and that the defendant committed the crime. This means that a rational and fair juror would be convinced of the defendant's guilt and would not reasonably hesitate to vote for the conviction. In criminal cases, this usually means that a jury must be unanimous or that at least two thirds of the jurors approve the conviction. A conviction of a felony in any state or foreign country, even if unrelated to medical practice (e.g., tax evasion, possession of an unlicensed machine gun, intimidation of expert witnesses in a malpractice action, conspiracy to murder a spouse, sexual misconduct with a minor), often carries a mandatory revocation or suspension of license and hospital privileges.

Physicians who are not U.S. citizens, aside from criminal penalties on conviction and the possible revocation or suspension of license, may lose their resident alien status and be deported. Deportation often can be forestalled when the physician's wife, husband, or children are American citizens. Unlike the federal government, which has only delegated powers to enact and enforce substantive criminal laws, every state has inherent authority by virtue of its police powers granted by the Constitution to regulate internal affairs for the protection or promotion of the health, safety, welfare, and morals of its residents. This is why most states have their own, often dissimilar, criminal codes.

Modern criminal law recognizes two major classes of crimes and a number of miscellaneous offenses and violations. By definition a *felony* is a crime punishable by imprisonment for 1 year or more. Felonies include crimes such as murder (e.g., withdrawal of a comatose patient's life support), manslaughter, rape, robbery, larceny, kidnaping, arson, burglary, most narcotics and insurance frauds, and sex with a minor.[3] Misdemeanors are crimes that are punished with imprisonment of no more than 1 year. The term *misdemeanor* is applied to the widest range of criminal activity and includes the broadest gradation of offenses and degrees of unpermitted activity (e.g., failure to report child abuse, refusal to allow patients to examine and copy their medical records, willful disclosure of health care information to unauthorized people).

Another category of criminal and quasicriminal offenses—both felonies and misdemeanors—are the so-called strict liability offenses. The major significance of such offenses is that certain defenses, such as mistakes, are generally unavailable. These are usually offenses that are part of regulatory schemes (e.g., practicing medicine or nursing without a license, writing prescriptions without a valid registration from the Drug Enforcement Agency [DEA] or narcotics license from the state).

In the health care field, federal and state agencies, under delegation from Congress or state legislatures, have created a multitude of rules and regulations, the violation of which may be punishable as a crime. These rules and regulations include the DEA's wide-ranging regulations on the licensing and the supervision of prescribing, storing, and dispensing controlled substances; the regulations of the Internal Revenue Service; and various regulations from the health department, including reporting requirements of certain contagious diseases. Violations of these regulations may be enforced either criminally or administratively by revocation of licenses and heavy fines. In most states there is a third category of offenses and violations, or *prohibited acts,* as they are sometimes called. These acts, although technically crimes, are so minor in nature that the law refuses to classify them as misdemeanors. These include a host of activities such as violating minor traffic laws, allowing dogs to be unleashed, spitting in public, and littering.

After being apprehended, the accused may be held pending a preliminary hearing that will in turn determine whether there are sufficient grounds to hold the accused for trial or for presentation to a grand jury; the case may also be taken directly before a grand jury. The preliminary hearing magistrate also may release the accused on bond or may hold the accused for a grand jury hearing or trial. The grand jury and the magistrate may reject the allegations and free the suspect. Also, the prosecuting attorney may refuse to proceed, which is known as a case of *nolle prosse.*

The defendant is found guilty when each and every element of the crime prescribed by the legislature and the culpability of the suspect must be proved beyond a reasonable doubt to the trier of facts: a jury, judge, or both. In prosecuting a crime the government provides the forum, courtroom, judge, jury, and other necessary functions and functionaries. If the criminal defendant cannot afford a defense attorney or other necessary defense materials, the state provides them within reason. The accused must be afforded his or her constitutional rights, both federal and state (if appropriate), of due process and equal protection under the law. At trial the accused may (1) plead guilty, thus obviating the need for an actual trial; (2) plead not guilty and be tried; or (3) plead nolo contendere (meaning, "I will not contest the charges"), which although not a guilty plea, is a tacit confession of guilt. After conviction or plea, the judge determines the penalty, if any. Frequently, pleading guilty or nolo contendere is based on plea bargaining between the state's and defendant's attorneys. If the defendant is convicted, the government exacts a penalty: fine, imprisonment, or probation. The victim may also sue the criminal in tort, or the victim may apply to the government for victim compensation. Both the federal government and many states have such programs.

Elements of a crime

The essential elements of a crime are (1) intent (mens rea) and (2) the act (actus reus). To constitute a crime, the act must be volitional, and the intent must be to accomplish the criminal purpose. In the case of misdemeanor offenses and violations the law does not always inquire whether the criminal intent was present. (For example, the traffic court judge does not inquire into the intent of a person who went through a red light, failed to stop at a stop sign, or made a left turn without signaling.) However, "pulling the plug" on a patient presupposes the intent to kill combined with an act to further that purpose. For misdemeanors and petty offenses the element of intent is not normally a consideration. Lack of intent is not a defense for the category of crimes committed while the defendant was intoxicated or under the influence of drugs. The law takes the position that such acts are voluntary and that a misconduct in such a state is predictable; therefore criminal liability should be attached.

Lesser included offenses

Another concept that underlies criminal law in American jurisprudence is the theory of "lesser included offenses." For example, murder usually includes such lesser offenses as manslaughter and battery, robbery usually includes larceny with the added element of force or threat of force against a person, and burglary includes an unlawful trespass into a dwelling with the intent to commit a larceny or another crime. A person cannot, by definition, commit a burglary unless trespassing has been committed; a person cannot be guilty of robbery unless that person is also guilty of larceny. The significance of lesser included offenses comes into play when a jury cannot agree on a major crime or when because of extenuating circumstances the jury decides to punish the wrongdoer for a lesser included offense. Although pulling the plug may be premeditated murder, if there are extenuating circumstances, the jury may convict the defendant only of a lesser included offense of manslaughter.

Vicarious culpability

Modern American jurisprudence also tends to disregard distinctions between principals and accessories to a criminal act. The streamlined approach tends to regard an accessory before the fact (one who supplies a weapon but does not participate in the murder) not as some quasiinnocent bystander but as an actual participant in the crime. Under this theory, drivers of getaway cars are responsible for murders committed by bank robbers almost to the same extent as if they themselves had pulled the trigger. The accessory after the fact is treated differently and is not liable for acts performed before his or her involvement. Modern jurisprudence is also abandoning the designation of participants in the crime as accessories; instead, they are regarded as accomplices who are liable for all the foreseeable consequences of the criminal act they that intended to aid or in which they participated. The physician may be vicariously liable for the acts of his or her employees when allowing them unsupervised access to controlled substances, when allowing them to call in prescriptions without consulting him or her, or when inducing, encouraging, or ordering them to fill out fraudulent insurance claims or commit other criminal acts.

Under the theory of accomplices, the test of criminal activity is the foreseeability that the crime will be committed and the weight the law attaches to the acts done to further the conspiracies or crimes. Of special interest to physicians are acts that cannot be committed alone or acts committed by a perpetrator who is legally considered incapable of committing the crime directly because of his or her special status.

In the case of accomplices, not all accomplices to the crime are convicted. If one escapes, is acquitted, or is not caught, another may nevertheless be convicted as if he or she alone had committed the crime. Secretaries and bookkeepers often have been prosecuted as accomplices for helping falsify billing records or as accessories after the fact for helping cover up Medicare frauds. However, when threatened with criminal prosecution, office workers almost invariably make deals with prosecutors. They are not prosecuted in exchange for providing testimony against the physician. Such former employees are often the most devastating witnesses against physicians.

Accessory after the fact

An accessory after the fact is anyone who renders assistance to a felon after an offense has been committed, even though the accessory had no prior knowledge of the commission of the crime. The assistance may involve harboring a fugitive, providing funds for escape, or hindering the prosecution by delaying the discovery of the crime or apprehension of the felon. In Medicare and insurance fraud cases, this often involves helping falsify medical records. In modern American jurisprudence, failure to report a felony generally no longer makes one an accessory after the fact.

Conspiracies

Conspiracy is a separate and distinct crime from the substantive criminal acts committed pursuant to the plan. Conspiracy consists merely of an agreement or plan by two or more people who have the specific intent to commit a crime or engage in dishonest, fraudulent, or immoral conduct that is injurious to public health and morals. Previously, in addition to intent, it was required that some overt act in furtherance of the conspiracy must have been committed. This requirement has been virtually abandoned in American jurisprudence. For instance, if a hospital administrator and a physician agree to fill hospital beds with nursing home patients (who do not require hospitalization) to create revenue for the hospital, the administrator may be convicted of conspiracy even though his or her acts in furtherance of the conspiracy consisted only of a telephone call or no act at all. It may be sufficient that the administrator and the physician tacitly agreed to defraud Medicare or an insurance carrier. In most states, proof of the agreement would have been sufficient even if it had not been made in person and there had been no act such as the telephone call. Manufacturers, sellers, and prescribers of unapproved drugs have been convicted of conspiracies (e.g., the amygdalin or vitamin B_{17} [Laetrile] cases).[4]

In Boston, Margaret S. Telgeheder, a former marketing executive for National Medical Care's medical products division, pleaded guilty to arranging "hundreds of thousands of unnecessary tests" while serving as the company's vice president of marketing and manager of Lifechem, a clinical blood laboratory for a subsidiary company.[5] Several other executives were also convicted for conspiracy to pay kickbacks to obtain referrals for the laboratory business, fraudulent Medicare billing, and numerous counts of mail fraud and conspiracy to defraud Medicare of millions of dollars.

A factual impossibility to commit a crime (e.g., when conspirators agree to kill somebody who is already dead) is no defense. However, there can be no conspiracy when the objective of the conspiracy is not illegal. The concept of conspiracy involves the accomplishment of an objective prohibited by law. Conspiracies may be punished as criminal and civil acts. Thus a conspiracy to destroy a physician's practice by excluding that physician from hospitals or otherwise defaming or disgracing him or her may be punishable as a crime, even though the mere denial of privileges would not have been a criminal offense. The physician may concurrently seek civil remedies in a lawsuit for damages. In practice, however, unless the circumstances of the case involving civil wrongs are particularly outrageous, the district attorney usually refrains from prosecution, letting the victim seek remedy in civil law.

Defenses to crimes

The substance of the criminal laws and procedures involving criminal trials and convictions is governed by the strict application of the constitutional standards of due process and equal protection. These concepts are constantly redefined by the courts in a tug-of-war between liberal, socially oriented standards and more conservative approaches that balance the rights of the accused against the more important rights of society and victims of crime. The defense of entrapment is being raised frequently in prosecutions resulting from the crackdown on physicians who overprescribe drugs to "professional patients" and undercover agents, prescribe drugs in the absence of adequate need or examination, or prescribe drugs in return for sexual favors.

In addition to allowing admission of office charts, the courts allow virtually unlimited production of records kept by accountants, attorneys, and others. This virtually eliminates the defense of self-incrimination from records held by a third party (e.g., hospital, insurance company, or even the physician's professional corporation). The courts also extend virtually unlimited access to bank records when requested under grand jury subpoenas. The courts hold that such compulsion, even though incriminating, is not within the privilege against self-incrimination. The Fifth Amendment privilege against self-incrimination does not protect against compulsion to furnish specimens of body fluids, pubic hair, or head hair; to provide a handwriting sample or a voice exemplar; to stand in a lineup; to wear particular clothing; or to provide a hair exemplar.[6,7] The courts allow physicians great latitude to conduct physical examinations and tests. These procedures may include involuntary minor surgery to remove bullets that may be evidence, rectal and vaginal examinations, penis scraping to reveal menstrual blood that may be a rape victim's type, fingernail scraping, and blood tests, provided they are done in a medically acceptable manner.[8] Because taking x-ray films is potentially harmful and more invasive, the courts are more hesitant to allow them.[9] Forcibly taken impressions of a defendant's teeth for comparison with bite marks on the body of a homicide victim have been permitted by the court.[10] Procedures requiring general anesthesia and potentially risky procedures generally are not permitted.[11] Statements by criminal suspects can be used against them if they had been warned about self-incrimination (see the section on Miranda rights). Statements made to a psychiatrist generally may not be used because they may constitute self-incrimination.[12]

The court decided that it was self-defense when a physician shot and wounded a patient with acquired immunodeficiency syndrome (AIDS) who threatened to bite him. Similarly a psychiatric nurse claimed self-defense after using a fatal chokehold on a threatening patient. The defense of faith healing and the freedom to choose or refuse medical treatment continue to be litigated. Parents are usually found criminally liable for failing to provide medical care to a minor child when, if medical care had been provided, the child almost certainly would have survived. Under the guise of protecting the rights of the unborn child, a case went all the way to the U.S. Supreme Court, which held that a woman could not be compelled to have a cesarean delivery against her religious beliefs because a physician feared that a vaginal delivery could be harmful to the infant. Many states expressly protect patients who in good faith rely on spiritual means or prayer for healing, although the question of how far such laws may be extended to parents caring for minor children is unclear. The U.S. Supreme Court has also held that states have the responsibility to provide court-appointed psychiatrists to indigents charged with capital crimes.

Causation

Before a criminal defendant can be convicted, it must be shown that his or her act was indeed the cause of the criminal result or was a substantial contributing factor in causing the criminal result. Whereas the mind may get lost in the labyrinth of contributory factors to the crime, modern jurisprudence focuses on the sine qua non, or the so-called but-for test. This test determines whether without such an act the crime would not have happened. For example, if the defendant had not fired the shot, the deceased would still be alive. In applying the second criterion of a substantial factor, a crime is recognized even though the but-for test was failed. Such an example occurs when the deceased receives two in-

juries from separate and independent sources (e.g., he or she is kicked to the ground by one person and run over by an oncoming car). Another example occurs when three people play Russian roulette, and one is killed. The conduct of the survivors may be deemed a substantial factor, and they may be charged with manslaughter based on their reckless endangerment of the life of the deceased.

Criminal law recognizes both acts of commission and acts of omission as causes of crime. The gravity of the crime varies if the physician or nurse who had the duty to care for a patient failed negligently or intentionally to provide life-sustaining medications or deliberately provided an overdose, causing that patient's death. For purposes of criminal law, a victim's preexisting conditions do not release the defendant from liability. For instance, victimizing a person who has the unusual and unknown fragility of hemophilia or heart disease is a risk that the wrongdoer takes, even though the same act might not have caused death or serious injury to a healthy individual.

With regard to causation the law also distinguishes between intervening and superseding causes. Other legally recognized multiple causations include concurrent, independently sufficient causes; foreseeable intervening forces that do not break the causation chain; and foreseeable dependent causes for which more than one culprit may be held liable. An intervening cause is a cause that occurs after the act of the defendant but before the occurrence of the result. When the intervening cause is sufficient to absolve the defendant from responsibility, it is a superseding cause. An example involves medical complications in which the foreseeable causes may be dependent. An individual stabbed in the arm is hospitalized and contracts blood poisoning from the use of improperly sterilized instruments. The patient dies. The intervening blood poisoning flowed from the stabbing injury and was foreseeable. Most cases hold that medical complications, medical malpractice, and even the victim's refusal to undergo surgery or other treatment are foreseeable dependent causes. Whatever the defenses, excuses, or justifications, a fundamental principle of criminal law is that these defenses must be asserted to cast a reasonable doubt on the culpability of the defendant. Whereas the burden of proof in a civil case is a mere preponderance of the evidence (variously expressed as 51% or more), the standard in criminal cases is beyond a reasonable doubt.

Excuses

Among the most frequently invoked defenses excusing criminal culpability are infancy, mental illness, intoxication, mistake, entrapment, and duress. With regard to infancy, most American jurisdictions hold that children under the age of 7 years are conclusively presumed to be incapable of committing a crime. This may be a legal fiction, but it is sustained by the courts as being essential to protect children. Children between the ages of 7 and 14 years are presumed to be incapable of criminal responsibility, but this presumption may be rebutted by evidence of maturity and understanding of the moral and legal consequences of their behavior. Such adolescents are frequently used by "pushers" to transport and deliver narcotics or to steal. When it comes to crimes committed by people older than 14 years, criminal responsibility attaches, but there is a large body of juvenile law that tempers punishment and provides for rehabilitation. Some states provide that youths younger than 16 years must be tried in special family courts and that juvenile convictions be expunged on attainment of legal maturity at age 18. In some cases the law provides that juveniles may be tried as adults on determination of mental age as opposed to chronological age.

Mental illness. Theoretically, mental illness presumes an incapacity to hold the defendant morally responsible for his or her conduct. It is usually defined in law as "insanity." However, *insanity* is not a medical term, and it is beyond the scope of this chapter to discuss beyond explaining some definitions the medical and legal quagmires and controversies surrounding the defense of insanity. *Insanity,* as defined by the traditional M'Naghten rule, postulates that a person is not guilty by reason of insanity if the following four conditions are met: (1) at the time of the criminal act, (2) the person was laboring under a mental disease or defect (3) that prevented him or her from knowing (4) either the nature and quality of the act or that the act was wrong.

Whereas the M'Naghten rule focuses on capacity for blameworthiness, the "irresistible impulse" test focuses on volitional controls. It extends the insanity defense to a myriad of situations in which the accused may have known that his or her conduct was wrong and criminal but was supposedly incapable of controlling the conduct. However, the question of what constitutes an "impulse" remains unanswered. Some courts hold that even if the accused spent a lot of time brooding and reflecting, the acts may still be the result of an impulse. Although the M'Naghten rule is still widely used, one of the newer variations is the American Law Institute's Model Penal Code formulation of a "substantial capacity" test, which is a merger of the older M'Naghten rule and the "irresistible impulse." The result is a test that absolves criminal defendants of criminal responsibility if the following three conditions are met: (1) as a result of the mental disease or defect, (2) the defendant lacks substantial capacity (3) to either appreciate the criminality of his or her conduct or to conform it to the requirements of law.

There are virtually hundreds of variations of what constitutes mental disease or defect, including organic brain damage, mental retardation, psychosis, addiction to alcohol that produces significant permanent mental defects (temporary disorientation or emotional frenzy are not sufficient), and various degrees of psychopathic personality. In the case of retarded people or others suffering from mental illness short of insanity, a "diminished responsibility" defense may be asserted to mitigate the culpability and reduce the charge. Although traditionally the accused was presumed to be sane and

it was the burden of the defendant to plead and prove the defense of insanity, there is a growing trend to shift this burden to the prosecution to prove beyond a reasonable doubt that the accused was sane at the time of the crime after the issue of insanity has been raised by the defendant. About half of the states and the federal criminal code have shifted this burden to the prosecution. There is also a growing trend to determine the issue of insanity separately from guilt. When a defendant is found to be insane, he or she would not be acquitted by reason of insanity, but the issue of insanity would be considered in the determination of punishment. In practice a successful assertion of the insanity defense usually means that the defendant is committed to a mental hospital and kept there until a psychiatrist or judge is convinced that he or she is no longer dangerous.

Drunkenness. Intoxication caused by alcohol or drugs may impair the individual's ability to appreciate the significance of his or her criminal conduct and under certain circumstances may negate culpability. However, voluntary intoxication is increasingly held to be an invalid excuse for general intent crimes such as rape, battery, and trespass. Voluntary intoxication is not a defense to strict liability offenses such as statutory rape, mishandling of drugs, or serving liquor to minors. Performing surgery while under the influence of alcohol or drugs is almost invariably prosecuted as criminal negligence. Intoxication may serve as a defense to such subjective intent crimes as larceny in which an honest mistake, which negates the mental state, may operate as a defense.

Mistakes of law. The following are a few exceptions to the rule that ignorance of the law is no excuse:

1. When the government has not made information about the law reasonably available to all those who may be affected. This exception usually applies to situations in which the laws punish inaction or omission, such as failure to obtain a license or permit or failure to file certain information with appropriate governmental agencies (e.g., if reporting venereal diseases, AIDS, or certain birth defects is mandatory).
2. When there is reasonable reliance on an official government pronouncement and the defendant has made reasonable efforts to find out about such a law and reasonably believes that his or her conduct is not criminal.
3. When the defendant reasonably relies on erroneous official interpretation of the law by a public officer or agency responsible for the interpretation and enforcement of the law, such as an erroneous interpretation of controlled substance laws by ranking officials of the DEA.

Entrapment. The defense of entrapment excuses the commission of a crime if a law enforcement officer, federal or state, actually instigates or induces an otherwise innocent person to commit the crime. The test of entrapment is the subjective disposition of the defendant before police involvement. This is often the case when undercover agents prevail on gullible physicians to prescribe pain medication without proper examination or need. The defense of entrapment is not available in cases involving personal violence.

Duress. The defense of duress or compulsion is available when a person commits a criminal act under a threat by another, thus causing the accused to reasonably believe that he or she is in danger of imminent death or great bodily harm unless the criminal act is committed. The threat must be present and imminent and may not involve economic circumstances in which the person is unable to resist the threat. However, no coercion or threat excuses an infliction of serious physical violence on another.

Privileged conduct

Criminal conduct involving the killing or injuring of another person is justified in cases of self-defense, defense of others, crime prevention, defense of property, and necessity. Use of reasonable force and self-defense are permissible when an individual reasonably believes that he or she is in imminent danger of impermissible aggression. The individual may use such force as is necessary to avoid being injured, but the use of excessive force may result in criminal liability. Normally, being pushed, shoved, grabbed, or hit with bare hands does not justify shooting the aggressor. The use of deadly force in self-defense is permitted only in response to deadly force or a reasonably perceived threat of deadly force. Courts are divided as to whether a person must retreat from the aggressor before using deadly force in self-defense. Some jurisdictions require what is called *retreat to the wall* before permitting deadly force in self-defense. Such retreat is required only if it is completely safe and makes it possible to avoid the aggressor. The duty to retreat does not apply if the aggressor enters the home or in some states the office of the attacked individual. The rights of self-defense and the privilege of using physical force are permissible only to prevent physical bodily harm. The rights do not apply in the case of insults. Self-defense is more liberally interpreted in the western and southern states, and the use of deadly force in self-defense is most severely circumscribed in states that have rigid retreat requirements, such as New York and New Jersey. The right of defense of others varies with the circumstances, but generally the defender of others is protected only if the person he or she helped was truly acting in self-defense or acted to protect their lives or that of others.

Prevention of crimes

Private citizens and police officers have the right to use whatever nondeadly force is reasonably required to prevent the commission of a crime or the immediate escape of a perpetrator from the scene of either a misdemeanor or a felony. Deadly force may be used only when such force is reasonably believed to be necessary to prevent the commission or completion of crimes such as homicide, violent assault, kidnaping, robbery, rape and other forcible sex offenses, burglary, and arson. The private citizen who uses force to prevent a crime may be criminally prosecuted if the person killed or injured did not actually commit or attempt to commit a serious or, as the law calls it, an "atrocious" felony. Police officers may use deadly force when they believe it is necessary to prevent the commission or consummation of what they reasonably believe to be an atrocious felony.

Defense of property

The law allows only the moderate use of nondeadly force in the defense of property. Whereas deadly force may not be used to protect property, it may be used when the person defending the property acts in self-defense, such as in robbery and arson situations.

Necessity

The destruction of private or public property may be justified in reasonable attempts to extinguish a fire or prevent it from spreading, if the harm that may have been caused by the fire is greater than the harm caused by the attempts to avoid it.

Justified killings

The law accepts as a defense the justified killings by public servants such as police officers, soldiers, or executioners in the performance of their duty.

Inchoate crimes

Mere preparation to commit a crime without actually committing the crime falls into the category of anticipatory, preparatory, or unsuccessful criminal acts in which the actual intended harm did not develop but the accused did manifest a willingness to cause such harm.

Attempts

Attempted crimes are criminal offenses if some significant act with the intent to commit a criminal act is established. Mere preparation to commit a crime is not enough. A person can be convicted of attempted murder for pulling the plug, even when the plug was reinserted and the patient did not die.

Impossible crimes

A person may be criminally liable if he or she attempts to commit a crime that is physically impossible but that would have been committed had the facts been true as the accused believed them to be. Examples include an attempt to kill someone with an unloaded gun or a gun that jammed, a rape attempt precluded by the attacker's impotency, and an attempt to steal a wallet from an empty pocket. In some instances, renunciation of a crime acts as a defense when the attempt to commit the crime is voluntarily abandoned, the withdrawal occurs before the attempted offense is completed, or the defendant makes a substantial effort to prevent the attempted crime by either dissuading accomplices or calling the police.

Prestigious defendants

Although it was no surprise that many Columbia/HCA executives went to jail and many others remain under investigation and are awaiting trial, it was a surprise and a shock to many that some of the nation's leading medical institutions have been caught in allegations of Medicare and Medicaid fraud. In the case of *United States v. University of Chicago*,[14] some 40% of all the highest-coded Medicare claims submitted for outpatient physician services were upcoded from one to four levels. The University faces penalties that could exceed $100 million. Also, in 1999, Georgetown University Medical Center agreed to pay the federal government $5.3 million to settle allegations of fraudulent billing by its University Faculty Practice Group, which billed Medicare for Part B medical services performed by residents and interns.[15]

Donald J. Kirks, the former chief of radiology at Children's Hospital in Boston, was sentenced to 2 years' probation for embezzling health care funds from the Children's Hospital Radiology Foundation, a not-for-profit group.[16] Dr. Kirks was chairman and president of the foundation, which also trained and supervised radiology residents at the hospital and at the Harvard Medical School. He was regarded as a world-renowned expert in pediatric radiology and traveled widely while double-dipping into travel expenses to the tune of some $60,000.

Blue Cross and Blue Shield of Massachusetts has agreed to reimburse $4.75 million to the Federal Government for falsely billing for claims that the Blue Cross, not Medicare, should have paid as a primary payor; Medicare paid many claims that should have been paid by the private insurance company.[17] Humana Co., Inc., of Louisville agreed to pay the Department of Justice $15 million for managed care premium overpayments, whereas Nova Southeastern University in Tampa agreed to pay $4.2 million to children and elderly patients recipients of Medicaid and Medicare for improper mental health care.[18] The University of Vermont Fletcher Allen Health Center agreed to reimburse the government $3 million for anesthesia overbillings.[19]

The Mount Sinai School of Medicine in New York City agreed to pay $2.3 million to resolve charges that it fraudulently obtained Medicare funds.[20] The former administrator of the school's psychiatry department agreed to pay $339,300 for submitting claims for certain services that the medical schools said were "personally and identifiably provided by its faculty physicians." The University of San Diego Medical Center agreed to pay $8.3 million to settle false claims to Medicare and Tricare, the military health care program, and The University of Washington Medical Center agreed to pay $3.6 million for billing for hundreds of unauthorized procedures.[21] These included "investigational" devices not approved for marketing by the Food and Drug Administration,

including electronic heart devices such as pacemakers and automatic defibrillators; the university also provided services and other procedures for which improper reimbursements were sought. Staten Island University Hospital in New York agreed to pay a record $45 million to settle overbilling cases and to provide $39 million in uncompensated or free services to indigent patients over 20 years.[22] The company also agreed to retain an independent review organization to monitor its billing compliance over a 5-year period and to report results to the New York attorney general.

Rocky Mountain Hospital and Medical Service, d/b/a Blue Cross and Blue Shield of Colorado, and New Mexico BCBS, Inc., agreed to pay $1.5 million in criminal fines and $12 million in civil settlements for conspiring to obstruct federal audits to conceal evidence of poor performance by destroying and altering documents to claim inappropriate costs.[23] Olsten Corp. of Melville, N.Y., a leading provider of home health care, agreed to pay $51 million in a settlement with the U.S. Department of Justice, and its subsidiary Kimberly Health Care, Inc., will pay $10 million in criminal fines arising from a great variety of Medicare fraud charges. Olsten and its subsidiaries operate management and staffing services for home health agencies in Florida, Georgia, and several other states. As part of the plea agreement, Olsten agreed to assist the FBI in its investigation of Columbia/HCA, which acted with Olsten to receive illegal reimbursements for costs Columbia incurred in buying home health agencies from Olsten and other providers. Columbia was also charged with having illegally billed Medicare for its sales and marketing activities and using employees as so-called community educators and home care coordinators to arrange for referrals from physicians and search hospital files to find beneficiaries about to be discharged and needing home care.[24]

The U.S. Department of Justice announced that Walgreen Company paid $7.6 million in a case brought under the False Claims Act alleging that Walgreen only partially filled prescriptions but billed Medicaid, Tricare, and the Federal Employees Health Benefits Program for the full amount. The agreement settles allegations against Walgreen in 25 states and Puerto Rico. Whistle-blower pharmacist Louis Mueller will receive $678,000, or 15%, of the amount recovered by the government.[25] Pharmacist Mueller also reported similar practices at Eckerd stores, which is also being pursued by the government.[26]

To combat such frauds, both the federal government and the states have created new units specializing in health care fraud and have embarked on vigorous programs of criminal prosecutions, example setting, and fraud prevention.[27] The most notable of such new units are within the FBI and state attorneys general's Medical Fraud Control Units (MFCUs). Local and state prosecutors also are increasingly deputized as special assistant U.S. attorneys, enabling them to more fully enlist the aid of federal law enforcement and to prosecute their cases in federal courts. In addition to health care frauds, these prosecutorial activities also focus heavily on many aspects of drug abuse. Boards licensing health care professionals also are allowing many of these special prosecutors to press for suspensions and revocations of physicians', nurses', and pharmacists' licenses in conjunction with criminal proceedings. When criminal convictions are difficult to obtain, prosecutors usually succeed in getting professional license revocations or at least suspensions or revocations of narcotic licenses. Such proceedings, although not criminal in nature, can be professionally devastating and require a much lesser burden of proof than criminal prosecutions.

The Office of the Inspector General of the Department of Health and Human Services is now actively pursuing health care frauds by focusing mostly on revocations and suspensions of federal reimbursements. Because these revocations and disqualifications from federal reimbursements range in the hundreds of millions of dollars and can last for years, they are a strong deterrent to both institutions and individual practitioners.

Billing frauds

One of the more vigorously prosecuted areas is submission by health care providers of false and fraudulent claims under the Medicaid and Medicare programs. It is a felony to knowingly make false and material statements in the processing of Medicare claims.[28-31] Furthermore, physicians who defraud the government or private insurance companies and use the U.S. Postal Service to do so face additional penalties for mail and wire fraud.[32] A physician who is prosecuted in a criminal case may subsequently be left defenseless in a civil action[33] because factual matters litigated in the criminal action will act as a bar to their relitigation in civil action through collateral estoppel.[34,35]

In most instances, criminal prosecutions for health care fraud usually involve the federal government. Physicians also should be aware that criminal responsibility may arise from any material false statements made to the federal or state governments and to private insurance companies. Conviction for such frauds generally also results in suspension or revocation of a medical license. Medical fraud also may involve misrepresentations of certain therapies, other treatments, or untested remedies that allegedly produce miraculous cures for ailments. Criminal prosecutions are often carried out against physicians who offer these false cures to patients either verbally or through the mail, and severe penalties are often invoked. In *People v. Privitera,*[36] several groups challenged California's prohibition on using amygdalin or vitamin B_{17} (Laetrile) to treat cancer. The constitutional challenge raised the issues that the statute was vague, was overly broad, and violated equal-protection concepts. The vagueness charge regarding that portion of the law prohibiting the "prescribing, selling, or administering of any unapproved drug, medicine, compound, or device to be used in the diagnosis, treatment, or alleviation of cancer" was not supported by evidence.

Cases regarding billing errors usually center on massive, flagrant, and pervasive general fraudulent billing and mail and wire fraud. These frauds are usually perpetrated on numerous patients, insurers, and the government with the clear intent to rip off the health care system through "creative billing" over an extended time. These billing error cases primarily include charges for services that were never performed; repetitive patterns of unnecessary procedures, hospitalizations, or both; giving and receiving of kickbacks, bribes, or rebates; and false representations for certification of hospitals, nursing homes, intermediate care facilities for the mentally retarded, and home health agencies. Most frequently, individual physicians are charged with fraud for using higher billing codes or for "unbundling" Current Procedural Terminology (CPT) codes. Each CPT code specifically describes the procedure performed. When a physician uses a higher code (called *upcoding*), he or she is misrepresenting what was actually done and is billing and getting paid for services that were not performed. Patient visits under the coding system are categorized as brief, limited, intermediate, comprehensive, and extended. These categories are based on the amount of time spent and the services performed. If a physician charges for 30 minutes for writing a prescription and designates it as an "extensive" consultation instead of a "minimal" consultation, the jury will recognize it as fraud. The hospital records or office notes also would indicate what else the physician did. If he or she consistently used the highest codes, the criminal modus operandi will be obvious to the jury. Testimony that each case was very complex and required the physician to spend an inordinate amount of time with patients is easily refuted. When a physician is "unbundling" codes, he or she is double-billing for services performed. The physician is paid once for the whole job (called a *global fee,* which includes all the services rendered) and a second time for the specific things the physician did. The defense of making "mistakes" in using the incorrect codes is not very credible when it can be shown that the same mistakes were made over and over again on numerous patients and always in favor of the physician. Billing for treatment given to dead patients is increasingly picked up by computers that record the date and time of death.

Other fraudulent transactions have included double-billing for fees as attending physician and as a consultant on the same patient at the same time. This is double-billing for the same service by any name. Another fraud involves billing separately for different medications prescribed to the same patient because the physician was already paid for his diagnosis and treatment, which includes prescribing. In virtually all cases of Medicare and Medicaid fraud the courts have ordered full restitution.

In addition, heavy fines were imposed in conjunction with jail terms or probation. Federal sentences are based on mandatory guidelines, which leave little discretion to judges.

Medaphis Corp., an Atlanta company that provides business management services to physicians, agreed to pay the United States a total of $50 million to settle allegations of submitting false claims for emergency physicians to various federal health care programs.[37] The company typically upcoded services rendered as having been more acute then actually provided by physicians. Medical Pathology Laboratory, Ltd., and its owner, Dr. Charles Wilkinson of Meridian, Miss., agreed to pay $1.2 million for fraudulent Medicare billing for some 15,000 tests.[38] The U.S. attorney prosecuting the case pointed out that under the federal False Claims Act, prosecution is a allowed if the fraudulent billing was done knowingly or through deliberate ignorance or reckless disregard. The $1.2 million recovery includes treble damages and investigative costs.

Ventura County in California, agreed to pay the federal government $15 million to settle claims for submitting false bills to Medicare for outpatient psychiatric services.[39] The county attempted to develop the team approach to mental health, which included psychiatrist, social workers, welfare department personnel, and others. Eventually, the social plan replaced psychiatric treatment, and there was no psychiatrist left on the team. Instead the county randomly selected a staff psychiatrist's Medicare provider numbers and included them on bills submitted to Medicare.

A joint operation by FBI agents and U.S. postal inspectors led to the arrests and conviction of six Los Angeles telemarketers for Data-Med and its owner Bryan D'Antonio, who defrauded more than 12,000 individuals of some $4.4 million in the Los Angeles area; this scam involved setting up businesses doing medical billing for physicians who purportedly expressed interest in instructions on how to over-bill.[40] In another case, after paying a $495,000 fine for submitting false claims through the Bradford Regional Medical Center, the hospital's consultants, Metzinger Associates, who were co-defendants in the case for advising hospitals on how to "maximize" reimbursements, were ordered to pay a $60,000 fine and to give the U.S. attorney for the eastern district of Pennsylvania 250 hours of consulting time to help unravel complex fraud cases.[41] The consultants previously advised the hospitals on how to unbundle, double-bill, and bill for medically unnecessary laboratory services. In California, Dr. Santiago Cadag was sentenced to 3 years in prison and ordered to pay restitution of $290,000 for submitting fraudulent bills to Medi-Cal for ghost patients, submitting fictitious treatments, and allowing unlicensed physician's assistants to practice medicine and charge for unneeded injections.[42]

Intentional and negligent conduct

The health care provider may become a criminal defendant in many ways, sometimes even inadvertently. Most often, prosecutions result from multifaceted problems, such as kickbacks from referrals of phantom patients to specialists, physical ther-

apy, and laboratories for tests; billing frauds, including oft-repeated "mistakes" or visits; use, dispensing, and theft of medications; writing of false or fictitious prescriptions; Medicare and Medicaid frauds; rape; homicide (death resulting from surgery, administration of medications, abandonment, improper care, improper prescription or injection of medications, or drug or alcohol intoxication during surgery); death or injuries resulting from refusal or failure to provide medical or surgical treatment; reckless nursing or pharmaceutical errors; excessive restraints; abuse of children or the elderly; criminal malpractice; income tax fraud; "rebates" from pharmacies; conspiracies; practicing without a license or with a suspended or revoked license; intimacy with minors or psychiatric patients; assault and battery during examination or treatment of a female patient; abortion and fertility problems; and most recently the wide-ranging debate about assisted suicide and euthanasia.

The criminal liability of physicians, dentists, nurses, and pharmacists frequently results from a high degree of reckless and negligent conduct. What the law calls *criminal negligence* is largely a matter of degree, incapable of a precise definition. Whether or not criminal negligence exists is a question for the jury. The law requires a showing of "gross lack of competency or gross inattention, or wanton indifference to the patient's safety, which may arise from gross ignorance of the science of medicine and surgery or through gross negligence, either in the application and selection of remedies, lack of proper skills in the use of instruments, and failure to give proper attention to the patient" (e.g., "practicing fraudulently with gross incompetence and gross negligence" by failing to take and record vital signs of a patient to whom the physician administered anesthesia, using investigational and non–FDA approved substances).[43] The fact that the patient consented to a specific treatment or operation is no defense to the criminal action against the physician.

The courts have been very careful not to hold physicians criminally responsible for patient deaths resulting from a "mere mistake of judgment" in the selection and application of remedies or for inadvertent deaths.[44] However, willful and wanton conduct is clearly criminal. For example, Dr. Nancy Lynn Moyer was sentenced to 70 months of imprisonment for stealing morphine from her critically ill and dying patients in the intensive care unit.[45] Dr. Moyer inserted the hypodermic needle and syringe into her patients' morphine-delivery device and removed some of the morphine and replaced the stolen morphine with saline solution. The court described her conduct as "reckless disregard" and "extreme indifference." Expert witnesses at the trial testified that Dr. Moyer's action created patient risks of increased pain, agitation, infection, and air embolism. Dr. Moyer was also sentenced to an additional 48 months for obtaining controlled substances through fraud by using forged prescriptions. In addition, a Harvard-educated physician and husband-and-wife owners of a "hole in the wall" pharmacy in rural Northern California were charged with defrauding Medi-Cal of approximately $3 million in narcotic prescription schemes that also left at least three people dead of overdoses.[46] Dr. Frank Fisher and pharmacy owners Stephen and Madeline Miller were charged with 3 counts of murder, 10 counts of unlawfully prescribing controlled substances, 7 counts of prescribing to addicts or habitual users, grand theft, submission of false claims, and aggravated white-collar crimes. Elsie Arrington Monroe, a certified nurses aide, and the Shawnee Care Center in Shawnee, Okla., were charged with first-degree manslaughter for pushing and shoving Lina Jones, an elderly, decrepit, and somewhat mentally incapacitated resident of the center, causing Jones to break a hip. The injury resulted in Jones' death from an acute pulmonary embolism as a complication of the broken hip.[48]

The ongoing unprecedented scrutiny, aided by a high level of computerization and widespread use of undercover agents, has brought to light a variety of crimes committed by physicians, nurses, pharmacists, hospitals, clinics, nursing homes, and other health care practitioners and facilities. Even though small in number, these pill pushers, quacks, and welfare cheats can give the medical profession a "black eye." Their creativity in stealing appears to be unlimited in both scope and ingenuity. An overview of some of these schemes in the 1999 and prior Reports by the National Association of Attorneys General (NAAG) lists the following examples of fraud in fee-for-service health care:

1. Overutilization: using treatments, including office visits, laboratory tests, therapy, and prescriptions, that are not required.
2. Pharmacy fraud: billing for prescriptions and supplies not delivered or providing lower-priced or generic products and billing for higher-priced medications or supplies.
3. Billing fraud: billing for services not needed or not performed, billing for nonexistent patients, or billing for products not needed or not supplied. Another form of billing fraud is the "intentional mistake." Hospitals are frequently caught in this web of billing fraud. The use of cumbersome billing procedures providing incredible detail, covering everything from the room charge to aspirin tablets, can conceal charges of intentional mistakes that frequently escape payor scrutiny.
4. Marketing and enrollment frauds: enrolling ineligible or nonexistent individuals or misrepresenting the availability of medical equipment and rehabilitative procedures.
5. Frauds in the procurement of Medicaid contracts: falsifying financial solvency and misrepresenting staffing or assisted daily living activities such as eating, bathing, toileting, turning, and positioning.
6. Durable equipment or supplies fraud: selling and purchasing (by the payor for the patient) of long-use or durable medical equipment (DME), such as a wheelchair or another device, that is not needed or is of a lesser quality than that for which billed. The sale of DME is a source of regular and heavy abuse.
7. Supplies fraud: billing the patient for nondurable items, such as dressings not delivered or not used by the patient, or billing for supplies not needed but delivered and charged nonetheless. The provider may be the direct victim of supplies fraud (such as when a supplier delivers a lesser quantity or lesser quality than that for which the payor is billed). Whatever costs the hospital may incur in the area of supplies, it will pass on—together with the fraud—to the patient and the ultimate payor.
8. Unbundling: charging separately for procedures that are usually combined or "bundled" into a single charge (diagnosis-related group) in which the single charge is less than the sum of the separate charges.
9. Upcoding: billing for a more expensive procedure than the one used or using a more expensive procedure when a less costly one could have been used. This is a type of billing fraud.
10. Legal scams: engaging in worker's compensation fraud and filing false injury claims, such as faked accidents. The success of such scams requires that the "victim" and his or her lawyers work with physicians, therapists, and other health care providers to secure compensation for false accident or injury claims. Lawyers have also created fictitious companies and instigated or covered up fraudulent billing, sometimes for nonexistent services and facilities.
11. Kickbacks: receiving payments in the form of rebates and referral fees used as business inducements. Most are illegal under the antikickback statues adopted by the federal government and many state governments.

Perhaps the best example, which illustrates virtually all these frauds, is the case of Parkshore Adult Care Centers and its owner Lawrence Friedman. In this $62 million fraud, Parkshore brought its clients, mostly older Russian immigrants, to the centers in ambulettes, and virtually all the care it provided was Russian-language television and food specifically chosen to attract Russians, which included herring, gefilte fish, and borscht. The company provided minimal, if any, health care services, but virtually all billing was based on supposed Medicaid and Medicare claims. The operation was actually little more than glorified revolving-door, three-shifts-a-day centers for the elderly. In another case, a day-care center in Brooklyn apparently even had a beauty parlor.[49]

Massive and typical frauds

In Oklahoma, which has one of the most aggressive health care fraud investigative programs in the country, FBI agents, aside from arresting the acting commissioner of health and several of his associates, are investigating dozens of nursing home operators and others involved in kickbacks, false claims, and failure to provide necessities to patients. The officials were charged with bribes to give advance notice of "surprise" inspections, overlook massive fraud, not enforce regulations, and harass competitors. PacifiCare of Oklahoma, Inc., agreed to pay $9 million to settle allegations that it violated the False Claims Act by overcharging the Federal Employees Health Benefits Programs in Oklahoma City and Tulsa, after having guaranteed that the government would pay the same price as commercial entities for a given package of health benefits.[50] An Oklahoma-based physician billing company and its founder, Dr. J.D. McKean, Jr., have agreed to pay the United States and 28 states $15 million in to settle a case alleging fraudulent billing, upcoding of claims, and billing for services more extensive than those actually provided by physicians.[51] Recently a physician staffing company, EmCare, Inc., of Dallas, settled Medicare, Medicaid, and other federal medical programs fraud claims for $7,750,000 in an Oklahoma City case. ACR New York, Liberty Testing Laboratories and its President Albert Huerta, and Columbia/ HCA Healthcare Corp. paid the State of Oklahoma $107,031 for "billing irregularities" in Medicaid fraud reimbursements. Agents swooped down on Qualicare, Inc., a local health care company, and arrested its owners on charges of conspiring to defraud Medicare of more than $1.5 million. They had set up a phony management company, Monarch Management, to draw illegal Medicare fees. All have now pleaded guilty and are awaiting sentencing. Oklahoma FBI chief Richard Marquise says that the FBI will show "zero tolerance," in investigating health care frauds, either large or small, and no matter how convoluted and complex, and will devote the necessary resources to track the culprits.

Elsewhere, bogus claims ranged from a psychiatrist who provided psychotherapy to a 98-year-old nursing home resident who was in a coma[52] to a chiropractor who billed for spine adjustments for a 33-day-old infant. The chiropractor, Dr. Robert Guzek, had his license suspended for 100 years, was fined $1 million, and is now facing charges of defrauding Medicaid of $4.7 million. The Indiana attorney general said, "Guzek used his license to heal as a license to steal." In Arkansas, Dr. Robert E. Blackwell, a preacher who conducted his dental practice next to his church and engaged in massive fraudulent billing, was sentenced to 60 months in prison, fined $666,000, and ordered to pay restitution of $21,000 in a Medicaid fraud scheme.[53] A University of California professor, Dr. Sergio Stone, was convicted of federal mail fraud in connection with fraudulent billing and is currently under investigation after patients said that their eggs or embryos were taken without their consent and implanted in other women, resulting in 15 babies of uncertain parentage.[54] The professor was fired and the university's Center for Reproductive Health closed. The University paid $17 million to settle lawsuits by former patients.

The continuing parade of Columbia/HCA Healthcare Corp. executives included the conviction of Jay A. Jarrell, former chief executive officer (CEO) of Columbia/HCA in southern Florida, to 33 months of imprisonment and restitution of $1.6 million for Medicare, Medicaid, and 10 civilian health and medical programs of the uniformed military services and Champus frauds at Fawcet MRI of Hospital in Tampa.[55] Louisiana attorney Gary Wayne Sheffield, who operated Sheffield's Neighborhood Kid Medical Clinic in New Orleans, was charged with Medicare fraud for routinely billing "face-to-face physician office visits," when he only printed medical information from the Internet and placed the printouts in patients' charts. Sheffield also submitted hundreds of false billings for what he referred to as *staffings,* when the clinic's nutritionist, social worker, and physician supposedly met with the patients to discuss care. No such meetings took place. Witnesses informed investigators that Sheffield pulled random patient files, looking for the last date the patient visited the office to determine when to submit the fraudulent bills. Sheffield faces up to 5 years in prison and a $20,000 fine for each false billing.

Two brothers who were also practicing osteopathic physicians, Robert LaHue and Ronald LaHue, and Dan Anderson, former Chief Executive Officer of Baptist Medical Center in Kansas City, Mo., were sentenced to a total of more than 13 years in prison and 9 years of supervised release for conspiracy to solicit, receive, and pay bribes in schemes from which the hospital also received $59.8 million in Medicare reimbursement for treating nursing home patients referred by the LaHue brothers.[56] They were also ordered to pay $317,000 in fines and restitution.

Psychiatric frauds

Including billing fraud, psychiatric and psychological services are reportedly among those most frequently prosecuted. Criminal responsibility for physical measures and involuntary administration of medications to mentally disordered patients is very broad, especially if the patient does not present an imminent danger to self or others. There have been numerous cases of psychiatrists who billed individually for group therapy sessions in which they did not provide individual medical services to patients. In some instances, psychiatrists have not provided any care but have hired "therapists" and counselors without degrees and billed for fictitious care and nonexisting patients. One psychiatrist practiced "wave therapy." He billed heftily for individual care, which involved merely waving a hand at children who were drawing cartoons under the supervision of an unlicensed counselor. Atlanta psychiatrist James E. McClendon was convicted in one of the largest psychiatric scams in the United States. He was jailed for 78 months for fraudulently billing Medicaid $8.6 million. Dr. McClendon submitted more than 77,000 false claims in which he falsely claimed to have provided psychotherapy to after-school and summer programs for children.[57] Ohio psychiatrist

Dr. Sammy I. Michael was convicted on 7 counts of mail fraud and 35 counts of making false statements for billing Medicare, Medicaid, and private insurance programs for group psychotherapy services when in fact Dr. Michael entertained patients by showing them movies such as *Lethal Weapon, Tootsie, Ghostbusters,* and *Batman.*

Dr. Walter O. Anderson and his son Walter O. Anderson, Jr., were indicted on 43 counts of Medicare fraud and 1 count of conspiracy for falsely billing Medicaid more than $3.7 million in false claims of psychiatric care to schoolchildren in their clinics in Meridian and Laurel, Miss.[58] According to officials, the Andersons did not provide any psychiatric care to the children. The Jewish Memorial Hospital and Rehabilitation Center in Boston was fined $261,100 and ordered to perform $24,000 worth of community service for falsifying records by ordering employees to "white out" nonreimbursable codes for mental disorders and replace them with medical diagnoses.[59] A Boston area psychiatrist, Dr. Richard Skodnek, vainly tried an insanity plea, claiming he suffered "a psychotic delusion that caused him to overbill." He was sentenced to 46 months in prison and more than $1.3 million in restitution and fines for submitting hundreds of false insurance claims to Medicare, Blue Cross and Blue Shield, Bay State Health Care, and Tufft's Associated Health Plans. In San Antonio, children were kidnaped and brought to a psychiatric hospital for a 30-day stay, the maximum length of time before insurance benefits are exhausted. At the end of the 30 days, all such children were miraculously cured; no child was released before the exhaustion of insurance benefits. Another instance of "individual" treatment billed at a maximum rate involved a provider who took five children to McDonald's, where, as "special therapy," the children ordered their own hamburgers. In Somerset, Penn., Dr. Jopinder Harika explained to the judge that he billed 1000 hours of fictitious psychiatric care at $85 per hour because, "I could use the money and it was good for the hospital which otherwise might not have been able to provide good psychiatric care."

Nursing home scams and mistreatment of residents

In what was described as one the most outrageous examples of patient abuse in a nursing home, a Massachusetts judge sentenced nurse's aide Stacy H. Arruda to 5 years of imprisonment for force feeding one patient her own feces and slapping, kicking, and spitting on other patients who lived at the Wilmington Woods Nursing Center.[60] Witnesses testified that Arruda assaulted five patients, all of whom were over 80 years of age, on several occasions; they also said she beat the patients and pulled their hair. Judge Sandra Hamlin of Middlesex Superior Court, who sentenced Arruda, described it as the most disturbing example of elder abuse and, according to experts, the most egregious incident anywhere in the country. Six patients at three facilities owned by Guardian Post Acute Services, Inc., of Corte Madeira, Calif., were left un-

attended for days, were forced to lie in their own feces and urine, and developed bedsores, which often became infected.[61] In addition to allegations of three deaths, prosecutors charged that one elderly patient was sexually assaulted. Criminal charges were brought not only against individual attendants but also against the company, which had previously been cited for more than 60 compliance violations in the previous 3 years. New York nurse Laura Stiggins, who also served as a town justice, was convicted of assaulting her elderly patient in a nursing home by striking her so forcefully that the resident had several broken ribs.[62] In San Francisco, Beverly Enterprises, Inc., the nation's largest nursing home chain, agreed to pay $175 million and relinquish 10 of its nursing homes for defrauding Medicare.[63] The company submitted phony nurse sign-in sheets and fabricated documents to support its bills; the homes were in California, Georgia, Kansas, South Carolina, and Washington.

Indicative of a growing trend to find and prosecute nursing home administrators and staff members who criminally mistreat patients is the zeal of Oklahoma Medical Fraud Unit Director Tully McCoy, recipient of the 1999 Inspector General's Award. His unit was cited as a model for Medicaid fraud investigative work. Several dozen successful Oklahoma prosecutions included, among others, conviction of rape by instrumentation at the Waleetka Care Center, where attendant Adam Wesley Bishop was sentenced to 7 years of imprisonment for using his fingers to penetrate the vagina of a female resident and touching the breasts of other residents.[64] In Arizona a Pima County jury found two licensed practical nurses guilty of abusing a 67-year-old woman in a nursing home by subjecting her to at least 10 enemas in a 2-hour period. In Melbourne, Fla., a 53-year-old nursing home aide fled the country after being released on bail for physically abusing three elderly residents; she sprayed cleaning fluid into their faces and placed a metal clip on one victim's tongue. Richard H. Johnson, a certified nursing assistant at the Wesley Health Care Center in King County, Washington, pleaded guilty to two counts of indecent liberties with a paralyzed 79-year-old nursing home resident; he admitted to sexually touching her breasts and vaginal area.

Sanctions of up to $10,000 for each incident of physical harm to nursing home residents will become immediately collectible from the nation's 17,000 nursing homes if the facilities are found to have harmed residents in two consecutive state surveys, according to the HCFA. The agency received $50 million from Congress in 1999 to do more frequent surveys and to promptly investigate abuse allegations.

Hospitals and clinics

Nine leading hospitals agreed to pay fines in lieu of facing criminal charges for illegally dumping patients from their emergency departments. The hospitals included Kaiser Foundation Hospital in Los Angeles; Iowa Lutheran Hospital in Des Moines, Iowa; St. John's Episcopal Hospital in Smithtown,

N.Y.; Martin Luther and Hospital Medical Center in Anaheim, Calif.; Charter South Bend Health System in Granger, Ind.; Olean General Hospital in Olean, N.Y.; Doctors Hospital of Wentzville, Mo.; Atlantic General Hospital of Berlin, Md.; and Joaquin Community Hospital of Bakersfield, Calif. In addition to possible criminal prosecutions, hospitals with emergency departments that participate in Medicare are subject to civil fines under the Emergency Medical Treatment and Active Labor Act. In California, operators of Clinica Santa Maria and Clinica San Jose in Long Beach were jailed for 1 year each for billing for fictitious patients under five false provider numbers and for paying drivers to bring in patients with Medi-Cal cards.[65] Two Philadelphia area hospitals, the Lankenau Hospital and Methodist Hospital, were fined $303,684 and $103,432, respectively, under the False Claims Act for submitting false Medicare claims with the principal diagnoses of more complex illnesses than supported by the medical records and for misusing pneumonia diagnoses codes.[66]

Frauds and abuse in dentistry

San Diego dentist Farzan Alami-Rad and 13 other individuals were convicted in California in a $1 million fraud scheme of paying $20 to $100 for each Medi-Cal beneficiary whom they brought to Dr. Alami's three clinics.[67] The dentist conspired with "enrollers," who went door-to-door in low-income areas and offered inducement such as cash and gifts to card-holders to go to the Alami clinics. Dr. Alami's office managers also allowed unlicensed individuals to perform dental procedures. Frank William Meyer, a pediatric dentist in Kansas City, Mo., was sentenced to 29 months in prison for scheming to defraud the Medicare program of $64,000.[68] He also lost his medical license and was ordered to pay $75,000 in restitution to the Medicaid program and $125,000 to the U.S. government. Dr. Meyer submitted more than $178,000 in false and fraudulent claims for services not rendered, and he padded bills. Dentist Lewis M. Irving, Jr., owner of Gentle Dental Care in Bridgeton, N.J., was sentenced to 4 years in prison, fined $40,658, and ordered to pay restitution of $175,342 for fraudulently billing Medicaid for full noble metal crowns when he installed only temporary crowns; the attorney general reported that there were more than 1600 false entries on Dr. Irving's claim forms. David W. Young, an Oregon dentist, went to jail for perjury after lying about his criminal background and licensing histories in other states. In Miami, dentists Nicholas Michael Murado and Christopher Paul Lodenquai were indicted on 107 counts of organized fraud and Medicaid provider fraud for upcoding chair-side denture relines and billing them as laboratory relines when no relines of any type were performed on nursing home residents.

Managed care fraud

Fraud in managed care differs primarily in the incentive for underutilization, which is fraudulent when used to deny patients access to contracted services merely to line the pockets of providers. Managed care frauds also include, among others, submission of false cost data to justify higher capitation payments, registration of fictitious enrollees or those who have left the area, payment of kickbacks for referral of healthy patients, avoidance of unhealthy and high-risk groups, and denial of necessary contracted services.[70] In addition, numerous MCOs have been convicted of the following types of fraud: falsifying or misrepresenting professional credentials, providing "quack" treatments, overenrolling patients, charging a single patient to more than one MCO, failing to remove deceased patients from capitation lists, paying kickbacks for referrals, and giving referrals to laboratories and specialized services in which the provider has a financial interest.

Medical equipment frauds

Medical equipment is one of the most fertile fields for medical frauds. Richard Pregler, a Chicago-area supplier of diapers, defrauded Medicare of more than $7 million by obtaining reimbursement for processing urinary devices when he actually supplied adult diapers, which are not covered.[71] He was sentenced to 40 months imprisonment and ordered to pay $4.8 million in restitution; the court also ordered his home, several cars, and $641,000 in cash forfeited to the United States. Alan Cone, president of Health Care One and World, was found guilty on 58 counts of conspiracy to defraud the United States of some $186,000 as well as wire and mail fraud in seeking reimbursement for orthotic knee braces when he was actually supplying nonelastic compression garments and leggings.[72] New York Health Plan, Inc., and its president and CEO, Jay Fabrikant, pleaded guilty to charges of illegally billing Medicaid for some 6700 patients that the state claims were intentionally deleted from physicians' rosters after the company learned that its managed care contract with the state would be terminated.[73] Oklahoma obtained guilty pleas from two men who started a DME company and billed Medicaid for more than 50 oxygen concentrators for nursing home patients when none was used. Blanca Valle, president of B & V Medical Equipment in Miami, was charged with 39 counts of Medicaid provider fraud and one count of organized fraud for receiving $206,069 by forging physicians' signatures on certificates of medical necessity. The Florida attorney general also reported the indictment of Angelica Posada, owner of A & A Family Medical Equipment, Inc., for billing Medicaid $209,000 for oxygen concentrators, which were never received by Medicaid recipients. In Hialeah, Fla., Nelson DeLaCerda, president of Flamingo Medical Equipment Co., was indicted on 61 counts of Medicaid provider fraud for receiving $654,194 obtained by submitting 1503 forged physicians' signatures on certificates of medical necessity.

Fictitious clinics

A Texas health care attorney, Waylon E. McMullen, was convicted in Tennessee on three criminal counts of participating in a conspiracy to defraud Medicare by filing false claims and creating shell companies as vehicles for diverting reimbursements as management fees.[74] He used the fraudulently obtained funds to purchase the Gulf Coast Healthcare Corp. By using the provider numbers of two Miami physicians who had no knowledge of his scheme, Edgar Hernandez, owner of BBC Medical Center, created a fictitious medical clinic that filed electronically for claims in excess of $63,000.

Sightseeing ambulances

"An ambulance company isn't a taxi," Maryland Attorney General J. Joseph Curran, Jr., said after Gary Jefferson, owner of Care Plus and Ambulance Service, Inc., of Baltimore, was sentenced to 10 years of imprisonment for stealing more than $440,000 through Medicare and Medicaid frauds. "Mr. Jefferson took the government for an expensive ride that he will now have to fund out of his own pocket," Curran said. Jefferson was ordered to pay restitution of over $166,000 to Medicaid and almost $389,000 to Medicare. Georgia Freitag, a Chicago Company ambulance owner, was convicted on 16 counts of mail fraud, making false claims, and health care fraud in a scheme that bilked Medicare of more than $500,000.[75] The allegations involved transport of patients by ambulance when the service was not medically necessary, destruction of records, excessive mileage for trips, and trips that never occurred.

Racketeer-influenced and corrupt organizations

Criminal prosecutions for medical fraud also may involve multiple violations, which in turn may lead to violations of the RICO Act. Such prosecutions involve jail penalties and stiff fines and permit the government to trace assets and forfeit other private property allegedly purchased with the illicitly obtained funds. The Florida attorney general filed a racketeering lawsuit against Rite Aid Corp. in Tampa, for defrauding some 29,000 uninsured customers for pain and other prescription medications, supposedly to compensate for revenues lost in meeting competition.[76] The company specifically targeted uninsured patients coming from emergency departments because they would be unlikely to shop around for the best price for pain-relieving medicines, the attorney general said.

Home health care

A federal judge in Miami sentenced Susan Regueiro, a registered nurse, to 12 years in prison and $15.2 million in restitution for masterminding one of the largest health care fraud schemes by using a "large network of bogus nursing groups" to submit false Medicare billings for people not qualified to receive home health services under Medicare and for others to whom little or no services were provided.[77] Best Nursing Care, Inc., of Miami was charged with bilking Medicaid programs of more than $1 million for bogus home health visits to the elderly.[78] Among those arrested were several registered nurses who worked for the agency, including a lieutenant with the Hialeah Fire Department. The nurses allegedly were paid $20 for each set of false nursing notes they wrote for phony home visits, and clerical workers allegedly created fraudulent client files using boilerplate medical language. Many of the elderly clients knowingly participated in this scan, signing fraudulent home nursing visit forms in return for light housekeeping and neighborhood errands by the staff of Best Nursing Care. Several physicians were paid cash for elderly clients they referred to the home health care agency, according to the attorney general. Ramon Dominguez, owner of the now-defunct St. John's Home Health Agency, Inc., of Miami, was sentenced to almost 6 years in prison and ordered to pay $12.9 million in restitution in a $10 million Medicare billing fraud and money-laundering and nursing home kickbacks.[79]

Pharmacies

In Kansas City, Mo., $10 million of bulk quantities of pharmaceuticals were purchased at deeply discounted prices for a nursing home, but the drugs were instead resold to various pharmaceutical wholesalers in California, Florida, Kentucky, Nevada, Ohio, and Oregon.[80] A Springfield, Ill., pharmacy repackaged unused portions of medications from nursing home patients and long-term care clients and resold them; the pharmacy was fined $1 million for fraudulently billing Medicare for both the original prescriptions and the resold ones, without giving any credit to Medicare for the unused portions of the prescriptions.[81] State and local authorities in Tampa arrested some 60 individuals who participated in a black-market scheme in which medications were purchased at discount from Medicaid recipients and sold to 11 South Florida pharmacies to be mixed with other orders; several Miami physicians allegedly wrote the prescriptions.[82]

Knoll Pharmaceutical Co. and its parent company, BASF Corp., agreed to pay $41.8 million to 37 states for fraudulently marketing levothyroxine sodium drug products used to treat hypothyroidism, a product used by some 8 million people in the United States.[83] The company also tried to prevent publication of a study showing that Synthroid, a competing product, and some lower-priced generic thyroid medicines were bioequivalent in strength, potency, and effectiveness.

In Brooklyn, Ricci Pharmacy owner Joseph F. Pappalardo and a pharmacy employee, Phyllis Fitton, were indicted for stealing approximately $1.4 million by falsifying prescription records of Medicaid recipients and submitting phony claims. Baltimore pharmacist Yasin M. Husain and his wife Tahir were prosecuted for theft and Medicaid fraud for billing for unusually expensive prescriptions that were not dispensed. New Jersey pharmacist Kanu Raval was convicted for adding to the number of refills allowed by otherwise-valid prescriptions and for adding refills to prescriptions that should have had none. He then billed for the refills without dispensing any additional drugs.

Footloose podiatrists

Citywide Foot Care clinics, operating a chain of New York City podiatry facilities, and 13 podiatrists and administrative staff members were indicted on charges of Medicare fraud for falsely billing Medicare and private insurance carriers for higher-price services, such as foot surgeries, x-ray studies, and neuromuscular tests when lower-cost routine foot care treatment, such as toe nail clipping and foot washing, was what was medically necessary.[85] In addition, the defendants charged for services never rendered; double-billed patients, insurance plans, and Medicare for the same procedures; created false and fraudulent medical notes to deceive Medicare about its practices; and lured Medicare beneficiaries with promises of "free foot exams" to obtain the patients' Medicare billing numbers and then using these numbers for fraudulent billing. After pleading guilty in Albany, N.Y., to a podiatric scam in which he billed Medicaid for foot molds he never provided to patients, Dr. Charles DeCiutiis went to jail for 3 years; he also was ordered to make restitution totaling $134,366. Dr. Douglas Hamilton was indicted in Las Vegas for setting up the Nail Clinic, from where he billed Medicare $132,000 for treating patients suffering from toenail and fingernail fungus. The indictment charges that Hamilton filed claims for follow-up patient evaluations and whirlpool treatments that never occurred, fungal cultures that were never analyzed, and specimen removal since scrapings were not performed.[87]

Kickbacks

The legal definition of *kickbacks* is extremely broad. The federal antikickback statute makes it a felony for any person (or organization) to offer or pay "remuneration" (bribe or rebate) to any person or induce the person either to purchase a product or to refer a patient for whose care the government would be ultimately responsible. Thus a physician, a pharmacist, or a physical therapist receiving a referral from anyone who may gain from it is subject to prosecution. "Safe harbor" exceptions include employees, certain consultants, investments, and equipment rentals; these are strictly construed, and legal advice should be sought in almost all cases. A New Jersey physician, Dr. Joseph Piccotti, pleaded guilty to a kickback scheme involving Medicare fraud for ordering DME and supplies from a supply company that he partially owned; Dr. Piccoti also pleaded guilty to filing false certificates of medical necessity, claiming that patients had lymphedema when they did not to obtain reimbursement for the pumps his company sold.[89] Elsa Hernandez, a former director of St. John's Home Health Agency, Inc., in Miami, was sentenced to 63 months in prison for conspiring with 13 other individuals and paying kickbacks in a $42 million scheme of filing false Medicare claims and awarding contracts to outside groups in assisting them in filing false claims.[90]

Assisted suicide

With Dr. Jack Kevorkian safely behind bars, assisted suicide has faded from headlines, but the issue remains very much alive in American medical jurisprudence. Some states have enacted separate statutes that make it, or that do not make it, a crime to knowingly assist or encourage a suicide.

Other punitive actions

Allegations of criminality, even when there are no convictions, are almost invariably followed by separate investigations. There is often drastic disciplinary action by state licensing boards, the DEA, and state narcotic-control authorities, as well as the barring of reimbursements from Medicare, Medicaid, other federally funded and supported programs, and insurance plans for federal employees. Many contracts for health maintenance organizations and preferred provider organizations provide for the dismissal of physicians tainted by criminality. Theoretically, all such actions should find their way into the National Practitioner Data Bank, resulting in denials of licenses and hospital privileges to errant physicians. Prosecution of nurses is rather infrequent. It primarily involves the use, theft, and distribution of drugs. In a few rare cases, nurses have been charged with murder or manslaughter for pulling the plug on patients, recklessly ignoring patients' symptoms and problems, allowing patients to die by not calling physicians in a timely fashion, abandoning patients, and practicing with revoked or suspended licenses. Nurses also have been accused of racial bias, as in one case in which a nurse used a racial epithet toward an unruly patient and removed him from a dialysis machine, leaving dialysis needles in his arm.[91]

CRIMES AGAINST THE PERSON
Homicide

Homicide is the killing of a human being by another human being. As far as the law is concerned, a homicide may be criminal or innocent. It may be caused by an act of commission (the actual killing) or omission (when one has a duty to take life-saving action but does not do so). The criminal act constitutes an act causing the death of another human that must be committed with criminal intent and without lawful excuse or justification. The law divides criminal homicides into three main categories, as follows: (1) murder, (2) voluntary manslaughter, and (3) involuntary manslaughter. Within these categories the law recognizes various types of crimes and degrees of culpability. With murder, voluntary manslaughter, or involuntary manslaughter, the victim does not have to die immediately. Traditionally, if the victim died within 1 year of the shooting, stabbing, or poisoning, the perpetrator could be charged with murder. However, modern American jurisprudence embraces any unlawful causation of death and extends the period to as long as 3 years. Deaths resulting from negligent medical treatment, failure to provide treatment, or provision of improper or inadequate treatment are seldom treated as murder despite pressure from distraught family members. Absent outrageous or severely aggravating circumstances, even grossly negligent physicians usually are charged with only involuntary homicides.

To sustain a conviction of criminal homicide, the prosecution must establish that the victim was alive at the time of the death-causing act by another person. These thorny questions of when life begins and ends are largely a matter of expert medical testimony and state law, and they carry with them a Pandora's box of medical and legal problems that will continue to be hotly debated within both professions for some time.

Infanticide

From the standpoint of medical law, one of the most frequently encountered types of homicide is infanticide. Most states still adhere to the rule that there is no homicide unless the child has been born alive. The traditional determination of a live birth for purposes of a homicide conviction requires that the child must be physically separated from the mother and must give clear signs of independent viability, such as breathing or crying. This definition has been repeatedly challenged by prosecutors with the help of medical testimony that seeks to establish that a living fetus is indeed a human being. This has resulted in a number of convictions in which some courts have found individuals guilty of murdering both the mother and the unborn child after they shot or stabbed a pregnant woman. Some states, led by California, have even modified the homicide laws to include in the definition the unlawful killing of a human being or a fetus with malice aforethought. However, such laws expressly exclude abortion procured with the consent of the mother. Efforts to change laws to include abortions under homicide definitions have so far been unsuccessful. Allegations of criminality for failure to treat infants with spina bifida have been dismissed. A physician may encounter infanticide under a great variety of circumstances. Sometimes, he or she may be deemed to have caused the death of the child, and if the death was the result of neglect or willful misconduct, the physician may be found guilty.

In other cases, suffocation of infants may be disguised as "crib death." Infant deaths also may have been caused by parents through acts of abuse, such as drowning, scalding, or starving. Prenatal injuries to the infant resulting from drug abuse by the mother during pregnancy have also led to criminal prosecution in several states. If the physician is aware or suspects such infanticides, he or she is legally obligated to report them. Unfortunately, in the majority of cases, physicians are unwilling to become involved, and most infanticides are allowed to pass as "accidents."

Euthanasia

There are two types of euthanasia. The first type, called *active euthanasia* or *mercy killing,* is a crime in every state. In such cases the physician takes an active role in the death of a patient by disconnecting a life-support system or administering a lethal dose of a medication. In the second type, called *passive euthanasia,* a crime may not have been committed, particularly in jurisdictions in which the concept of a "living will" has been approved by the state legislature. *Passive euthanasia* simply means no further measures (e.g., therapy) are taken against the patient's wishes. Instead, the patient is kept merely as comfortable as possible, and nature is allowed to take its course. In California, two respected practitioners faced murder charges, which were later dismissed on technical grounds, for disconnecting the life-support system of an allegedly terminally ill patient.[92] At the Kaiser Foundation Hospital in Harbor City, Calif., a patient suffered cardiopulmonary arrest in the recovery room, and although he was successfully resuscitated, he remained in a coma. It was alleged that there may have been insufficient staff present in the postoperative area (one nurse for five patients). Without the consent of the family, the attending physicians terminated the patient's comatose state after 11 days. The attending physicians disconnected the respirator; ordered the nurses not to use endotracheal mist to assist the patient's breathing, allowing the patient to suffocate; and removed the patient's intravenous line. To the attending physicians, the proper choice in this medical situation was to permit the patient to die. From the prosecutors' viewpoint, removal of the respirator and intravenous line amounted to murder. They argued that any shortening of life is a homicide, and if it is intentional, it should be construed as murder.[93] The prosecutors alleged the following[94]:

1. That the physicians lied to the family about the patient's condition
2. That the physicians stated the patient had reached a state of "brain death," when in fact they were not certain at all of the actual state of the patient
3. That the physicians withheld information about a problem in the recovery room, where there was insufficient nursing supervision and inadequate response
4. That a physician's order not to treat cardiac dysrhythmias (an alteration in the pacing rhythm of the heart) was out of the ordinary, if not conspiratorial, in nature
5. That the physicians committed murder because the patient had been taken off the intravenous line, dehydrated, and starved to death.

Most important, the prosecutors stated that these actions prevented the patient from ever having a chance to recover. Even those sympathetic to the physicians who pulled the plug felt that a physician should never take such an abrupt step as pulling an intravenous line. Expert witnesses on the subject of coma and chances for survival described the incident as a medical embarrassment. One of the defendant physicians was quoted as saying, "I will fight to the death to keep bureaucracy and lawyers out of our medical group." By his actions, it appears that this physician achieved just the opposite.

Forcible feeding

In another case a California district attorney refused to press criminal charges of battery against physicians and nurses who forcibly fed a suicidal quadriplegic. As a result, the patient sought a civil injunction to stop the feedings. The patient claimed a right to starve herself to death and achieve a death with dignity while in the confines of the hospital. Although the patient failed in her civil suit, it was still possible that the physicians and nurses involved could have been found criminally liable for battery in the unauthorized forced feeding if the patient was not found to be incompetent.

"Innocent" crimes

A physician is also capable of imparting an element of criminality to an otherwise lawful act. This is particularly true in cases in which a physician attempts to spare a family's feelings but causes further hardship and suffering by issuing an incorrect death certificate or failing to report deaths under suspicious or unusual circumstances to the medical examiner or coroner. Such crimes arise many times in the cases of "overdoses." In most states it is a misdemeanor to fail to report death under unnatural circumstances to the coroner or medical examiner. In many states, there are also misdemeanor charges for failure to report (1) all manner of violent deaths, including those caused by thermal, chemical, electrical, or radiation injuries; (2) deaths caused by criminal abortion, whether apparently self-induced or not; (3) deaths occurring without a physician in attendance; (4) deaths of people after unexplained comas; (5) medically unexpected deaths during the course of a therapeutic procedure; (6) deaths of prisoners at penal institutions; and (7) deaths of those whose bodies are to be cremated, buried at sea, transported out of state, or otherwise made unavailable for pathological study. Civil and criminal penalties also may be imposed for failure to report diseases that constitute a threat to public health.

Abusive therapy

The illegality of beatings as therapy is still an unclear area of legal medicine. If the physician makes outrageous claims about the success of such therapies, the criminal responsibilities are much clearer, even if the defendant is released on a technicality.[95] However, in *State v. Killory*[96] a psychologist was convicted of administering "therapy" under the guise of beating his naked 15-year-old niece with paddles; the "patient" was also whipped with a leather belt. Although this therapy appears to be of dubious value at best, it can be debated whether the issue is the age of the patient or the therapy used. Such matters are further complicated by the fact that

many patients who allege abuse—physical, sexual, or otherwise—are currently or were past psychiatric patients whose testimony will be regarded dubiously by any judge or jury. Without corroborating evidence, the statements of mental patients often make it difficult to separate fabrications and exaggeration from the truth.

Intimate therapy

Improper or immoral conduct by physicians or dentists toward patients may result in criminal prosecution for rape or child molestation. Such crimes also may lead to disciplinary measures, including loss of licensure to practice.[97] The courts have repeatedly stated that offenses relating to moral turpitude are not relegated only to actions in the lines of professional practice.[98] Again, however, because most alleged rape cases against physicians involve psychiatric patients, they are difficult to prosecute. Psychiatric patients have little credibility with a jury.

Another obstacle to criminal prosecution is the embarrassment and unwillingness of the witnesses to testify. Unless the suit involves minors or other unusual circumstances, the defense to such charges is usually that the acts alleged were between consenting adults. An example of one of the more bizarre criminal prosecutions in this area involved a Chicago dentist. Apparently a patient emerged from anesthesia to find the dentist in a rather compromising position on top of her. The patient's screams brought the receptionist running into the room, and she saw enough of the dentist's activities to help convict her employer of rape. The defendant further compounded his problems by attempting to bribe his receptionist into repudiating the statements she had made to police. In *Roy v. Hartogs*[99,100] a New York court described criminal prosecutions in sexual abuse cases as functioning to protect "patients from deliberate and malicious abuse of power and breach of trust by psychiatrists, where the patient entrusts her body and mind in the hope that the psychiatrist will use his best efforts to effect a cure."

Numerous cases involve psychiatrists and other physicians accused of having sexual intercourse with their patients. Although most of these actions are civil suits, rape and elements of fraud may be found in cases in which large sums of money were obtained by physicians from their patients under false pretenses. In such cases criminal charges may ensue.

CRIMINAL PROCEDURE
Burden of proof

In a criminal case the prosecution must prove beyond a reasonable doubt that a crime was committed and that the defendant committed the crime. This means that a rational and fair juror would be convinced of the defendant's guilt and would have no reasonable hesitation to vote for the conviction. In criminal cases this usually means that a jury must be unanimous or that the conviction must be approved by at least two thirds of the jurors.

Constitutional safeguards

What makes a criminal case different is that the defendant can invoke a broad array of constitutional safeguards that are not generally applicable in civil litigation. Some of these safeguards include the following:

1. The Fourth Amendment, which provides protection against unreasonable arrests, searches, and seizures
2. The Fifth Amendment, which provides for a grand jury indictment, includes prohibitions against double jeopardy and compelled self-incrimination, guarantees due process of law, and in practice, translates into the application of much more rigid standards than those used in civil trials
3. The Sixth Amendment, which includes the right to a speedy trial, the right to a public trial by a jury of peers, the right to confront and cross-examine adversarial witnesses, the right to subpoena favorable witnesses, and the right to be represented by a lawyer
4. The Eighth Amendment, which prohibits excessive bail and any form of cruel and unusual punishment

The U.S. Supreme Court has interpreted these constitutional safeguards and thus provided definitions of how they should be applied. Thus denial of due process may include almost any allegation that law enforcement authorities have engaged in improper behavior. (For example, one court held that due process was violated when a defendant's stomach was forcibly pumped by police officers to extract two morphine capsules. The court ruled that such evidence was not admissible at trial because "it shocked the conscience of the court.")

Legal technicalities

Prosecutors are often frustrated by the legal technicalities that are imposed by courts in the strict interests of constitutional due process and that allow criminals to escape convictions. The foremost of these is the "exclusionary rule," which prohibits the use of illegally obtained evidence no matter how strongly it proves the defendant's guilt. Such cases include finding victims' bodies, murder weapons, or large quantities of narcotics in areas that were searched without a properly executed search warrant (e.g., trunk of a car, a shed behind the house). Incriminating evidence against criminal defendants may also be suppressed when the court finds that the defendant's right to privacy was violated. The exclusionary rule also prohibits the use of any information or investigative leads that prove the culpability of the defendant when such information was obtained as a result of illegal conduct on the part of the investigating officers. This is known as the *doctrine of fruits of the poisonous tree*. The gathering of evidence against an accused person is also severely limited by court rulings circumscribing electronic surveillance. Thus in cases in which wiretapping was not properly authorized, the defendant was not advised subsequently that his or her telephone was "bugged," or the defendant was not provided transcripts of the taped conversation, the intercepted conversation may be excluded from use as evidence against the criminal defendant.

Warrants and searches. The validity of a search, even where the incriminating evidence is discovered, can be challenged on the basis that the issuing judge was not neutral, that the warrant did not exactly describe the things to be seized or the place or person to be searched, or that the warrant was not based on a sworn affidavit of a trustworthy or reliable informant establishing probable cause to justify the search. More recently, some commonsense rules liberalizing the requirements for warrants and searches under exigent circumstances have been enacted. These exceptions grant police the right to stop and search moving vehicles in which they have probable cause to believe that contraband will be found. Even then, most courts continue to hold that once the vehicle is stopped and passengers arrested, a warrant may still be needed to search the immobilized vehicle, open the trunk, or open bags or suitcases in the vehicle.

Other instances in which search without a warrant is permissible include hot pursuit and searches incident to an arrest, in which the arrested individual may be searched for any weapons on his or her person and within the area of his or her immediate control. This area does not include the trunk of an automobile or adjoining rooms. When police officers assert that the arrestee assented to the search, they must prove by clear and positive testimony that there was no actual or implied duress or coercion. People entering the United States by land, sea, or air are subject to border searches without a warrant. Courts also generally have upheld searches of airline passengers before boarding by holding that passengers may avoid such searches by agreeing not to board the aircraft. Subjecting luggage and mail suspected to contain narcotics to a "sniff test" by trained narcotic-detection dogs does not constitute a "search." Also, the "open fields" doctrine allows searches of land outside the dwelling house and outbuildings, where evidence may be in plain view, as in the case of marijuana plants.

Administrative searches of medical offices, pharmacies, pharmaceutical plants, and storage facilities are often allowed without warrants under narcotics laws on the theory that license to handle controlled substances allows governmental agencies to inspect and verify the appropriate storage and dispensation of controlled substances. Such searches also are permitted for the seizure of spoiled or contaminated food, in the storage and selling of highly toxic chemicals, and in the sale of guns.

Detentions and arrests. A police officer may arrest a person without a warrant when the officer has reasonable grounds to believe that a felony has been committed and that the person committed it. An arrest without a warrant also can be made for misdemeanors committed in the presence of police officers. However, nonemergency arrests cannot be made in a private home without a warrant. In the absence of exigent circumstances, all arrests without warrants made in homes are presumed to be unreasonable and illegal. The only exception is the detention of occupants of a house or apartment during the execution of a valid warrant for narcotics or contraband. A police officer may stop a person without probable cause for arrest if the officer has a reasonable suspicion of criminal activity or that person's involvement in a crime. However, the police officer may frisk such a person only if the officer has a reasonable belief that the person may be armed and dangerous. Police officers also must have full probable cause to bring a suspect to a police station for questioning.

Miranda warnings. A major safeguard against self-incrimination is the requirement that the criminal defendant be given the Miranda warnings, which inform the criminal defendant of (1) the right to remain silent and not to answer any questions asked by the police, (2) the possibility that any statement made may be used as evidence, (3) the right to have an attorney present during the questioning, and (4) the possibility that an attorney will be appointed if the accused cannot afford one. Based on the Miranda doctrine, thousands of confessions by criminals have been declared inadmissible because the arresting officer did not adequately provide this warning before questioning the suspect. The question of whether the confessions were tainted, coerced, or illegal is one of the most common grounds for appeal by convicted criminals. A suspect may waive his or her Miranda rights, provided that the waiver is done knowingly, voluntarily, and intelligently. This is done most commonly in cases in which a suspect wishes to present exculpatory evidence to the police. However, once the suspect starts talking voluntarily, anything the suspect says may be used against him or her.

Right to counsel

The most pervasive right of a criminal defendant is the right to be assisted by an attorney in all criminal proceedings. The courts have defined *criminal proceedings* as events "where substantial rights" of a criminal accused may be affected. The test is always whether the attorney's presence would safeguard against any inherent danger of unfairness. The accused always has the right to be represented by an attorney at a preliminary hearing in which a judge determines whether there is probable cause to prosecute. No such right exists when the accused appears before a federal grand jury, which determines whether there is probable cause to prosecute. A person subpoenaed before a grand jury does not have the right to receive Miranda warnings and may be convicted of additional charges of perjury if he or she testifies falsely. Although a grand jury witness does not have the right to an attorney in the grand jury room, he or she may interrupt the testimony to step outside the grand jury room and consult with an attorney. The grand jury system is also used in a number of states east of the Mississippi.

The accused does not have a right to an attorney when blood samples or handwriting exemplars are taken, when hair samples are taken, or when photographs are shown to potential witnesses. Criminal defendants frequently allege that although they were represented by a retained or appointed counsel, their constitutional right to effective assistance to counsel was violated or denied because the attorney was "incompetent." Such allegations are made against even the most highly experienced and competent attorneys after the criminal defendants are convicted.

Starting criminal prosecution

The Fifth Amendment constitutional requirement that the criminal suspect be indicted by a grand jury does not apply to the states. However, it does require judicial determination of probable cause before anyone is deprived of his or her liberty for an extended time. Thus criminal proceedings frequently are started by arrest warrants, probable cause hearings, or grand jury indictments. In some instances, filing of information by the prosecutor is authorized in lieu of a grand jury hearing. In all instances the accused must be apprised of the nature of all elements of the offense so that the defense can be prepared. The initiation of a criminal prosecution is strictly a matter of prosecutorial discretion, and prosecutors have extremely broad discretion regarding whom to prosecute and what crimes to charge. It is also a matter of prosecutorial discretion not to prosecute certain individuals or certain crimes as long as no individuals are singled out for prosecution or are not selectively prosecuted. In most cases the courts have no power to interfere with a decision not to prosecute, but if the courts find abuse of discretion in cases of selective prosecution, they will dismiss the case.

The law is very strict in that a prosecutor must disclose to the accused any exculpatory information derived from the investigation of the case. This is known as the *Brady doctrine,* and failure to adhere to it constitutes a denial of due process. This information must be disclosed even if the defendant does not ask for it.

The Sixth Amendment guarantee of a speedy trial has been variously interpreted by the courts as prejudicing the defendant by possible loss of defense witnesses, resulting in greater likelihood of conviction. The speedy trial provisions come into play only after the charges have been filed. The period during which charges may be filed is determined by the applicable statutes of limitations. These statutes vary with the specific charges and are governed by federal and state law.

Plea bargaining

A plea bargain is an agreement between the prosecutor and the defendant that allows the defendant to plead guilty to a lesser charge in return for a lesser sentence. The courts require that such pleas must be made knowingly and voluntarily. There is no violation of due process if the prosecutors charge the accused with more serious crimes when plea bargaining negotiations break down. However, the courts are usually liberal in allowing an accused to withdraw a guilty plea and stand trial. In virtually all cases the courts refuse to accept plea bargains unless the defendant is represented by an attorney and thoroughly understands the nature of the plea bargaining agreement.

Right to jury trial

The Sixth Amendment right to jury trial has been held by the U.S. Supreme Court to apply to the states. Exceptions to the right to jury trial are petty offenses that carry penalties of no more than 6 months' imprisonment and that do not involve serious offenses. Criminal contempt proceedings provide for a jury trial only if the punishment is more than 6 months in jail. The traditional doctrine that the jury must be composed of 12 jurors has been ruled not to be a constitutional requirement. Juries of 6 members are increasingly allowed in criminal cases on the basis that they provide sufficient group deliberation. Many defendants prefer 12-person juries because there are greater possibilities of disagreements resulting in acquittals and hung juries. Although in the cases of 6-person juries, unanimity is required, the Supreme Court has upheld noncapital felony convictions based on 10-to-2 and 9-to-3 jury votes for conviction.

The Fourteenth Amendment prohibits racial discrimination in the selection of petit and grand juries. Whereas systematic discrimination in the selection of juries results in reversal and remand for a new trial, the Supreme Court does not require proportional representation of all the component ethnic groups of the community in every jury. In selecting jurors, the prosecution and the defense attorneys each have the right to dismiss a certain number of prospective jurors on peremptory challenges without giving any reason for doing so. Both the prosecutor and the defense attorney may dismiss any number of jurors challenged for cause. These are jurors who indicate that they would not impose the death sentence; would not follow the law; are friends or relatives of the plaintiff, the defendant, or their attorneys; or because of a degree of bias and prejudice, would be unable to judge the case based solely on the evidence presented in court.

The Sixth and Fourteenth Amendments guarantee the right to a public trial. The press cannot be excluded from trials, and state laws vary regarding whether criminal proceedings can be televised, regardless of the defendant's objections.

Witnesses

No witness may testify anonymously; the law requires that each person who testifies in a criminal proceeding must give his or her name, address, and other information that would enable the defendant to determine any possibility of bias and allow the defense to impeach such a witness. *Impeachment* means discrediting a witness by showing prior inconsistent statements, previous convictions, or untruthfulness.

Medical expert witnesses play a key role in many criminal trials. Most frequently, forensic pathologists testify to the causes of death, the time of death, or the instruments used to commit the crime. Psychiatrists are frequently called to testify when the issue of insanity is raised. When medical expert witnesses give conflicting opinions, the juries are free to accord whatever weight they choose to whichever expert seems more credible.

Protection against self-incrimination

The Fifth Amendment, which protects against self-incrimination, provides that no person shall be compelled in any criminal case to be a witness against himself or herself. Both defendants and witnesses have the right in a legal proceeding to refuse to answer any incriminating questions. Whereas the defendant's right to remain silent may not be challenged, the court may offer immunity to witnesses, thereby forcing them to testify under penalty of being held in contempt.

The trial

Constitutional safeguards of due process require that the accused be presumed innocent and that the prosecution have the burden of proving all of the elements of the criminal offense beyond a reasonable doubt. Before anyone can be convicted of a crime, the prosecution must prove the corpus delicti (the body of the crime), or simply that a crime has been committed. A defendant's confession to a crime without any corroboration is insufficient to satisfy this requirement. Individuals have been known to confess to crimes that they never committed for a variety of reasons ranging from insanity to a desire for notoriety. In some states, there can be no conviction for homicide unless the body of the victim is found; however, in other states, there can be a conviction but no sentence of death in a case in which the body has not been recovered.

Although not expressly written in the Constitution, the most fundamental ingredient of a fair trial in Anglo-American jurisprudence is that the accused is presumed to be innocent until proved guilty and that the prosecution must prove every element of the crime beyond a reasonable doubt. Although the courts have refused to put a percentage figure on "beyond a reasonable doubt," the U.S. Supreme Court has ruled that due process is violated if, viewing all the evidence in the light most favorable to the prosecution, no rational judge or jury would have found the defendant guilty of the crime of which he or she was accused.

A guilty plea is a voluntary renunciation of the Sixth Amendment right to jury trial. It is estimated that up to 95% of all criminal cases are settled by guilty pleas. To ensure that guilty pleas are voluntary, judges use long questionnaires to ascertain that there was no coercion or promises of a more lenient sentence offered in return for the guilty plea. Theoretically an accused may not be punished more severely for pleading innocent and asserting his or her right to a jury trial than by pleading guilty. In practice, however, it is often alleged that people who plead guilty receive lesser sentences.

Double jeopardy

One of the foremost constitutional safeguards is the right against double jeopardy. The Fifth Amendment provides that "no person shall be subject for the same offense to be twice put in jeopardy of life or limb." This provision is intended to protect individuals from harassment, to achieve certainty and finality in criminal proceedings, and to reduce the chances of convicting an innocent person. The states and the federal government can reprosecute an individual if jeopardy has not yet attached. In a jury case, jeopardy attaches when the jury is impaneled and sworn. In a bench trial, jeopardy attaches only when the prosecution has started the presentation of the evidence. The exceptions to these rules include cases in which a mistrial is caused by the misconduct of the defendant or the defendant's defense counsel, the jury is unable to reach a verdict, the judge dies or becomes ill, or it is discovered that a juror should be dismissed for cause after the jury has been impaneled. The courts have broad discretion to declare a mistrial if it is found that a trial cannot be fairly continued. Although this is sometimes perceived as double jeopardy, the same crime may be prosecuted separately by both the state and the federal government based on the doctrine of separate sovereignties. The Supreme Court has upheld the right of a state to convict a bank robber who was tried and acquitted in federal court for the same crime. The defendant was retried by the state when the FBI found considerable additional evidence after the acquittal on federal charges and turned it over to the state prosecutor.

Double jeopardy does not apply to separate offenses based on the same crime. Timothy McVeigh was sentenced to death for blowing up the Murrah Federal Building in Oklahoma City and killing eight federal law enforcement agents, which are federal crimes. Without putting him in double jeopardy, the State of Oklahoma could also prosecute him for the same explosion and killing 160 other individuals, for which he was not prosecuted because murder is a state crime. This is exactly what Oklahoma is doing to Terry Nichols, an accomplice who did not receive the death penalty. This is being litigated under the doctrine of separate sovereignties.

Criminal and civil trials did not put O.J. Simpson in double jeopardy. In the criminal case the state prosecuted Simpson for the crime of double murder. In the civil case, although the evidence was virtually identical, the families of the victims sued for compensation. In an Illinois case the defendant was charged with the murder of his wife and three children. The prosecution tried him first for the murder of the wife and one child, and after he received 20-year and 45-year sentences, the prosecution tried him for the murder of the second child, for which the court imposed the death penalty. The prosecution could have tried the defendant a fourth time for the death of the third child to maximize the penalty if the death sentence had not been imposed.

Exceptions to double jeopardy

As a general rule, if a defendant appeals his or her conviction, the right against double jeopardy is waived. This is usually the case when an appellate court remands the case for a new trial. An exception occurs when the appellate courts hold that the evidence on which the conviction was based was legally insufficient and the defendant should have been acquitted. Another exception is that a defendant may not be retried for a greater offense of which he or she was found innocent when the conviction is appealed on a lesser included offense. Although technically a defendant who won a reversal and new trial may be given a more severe sentence after reconviction, this is viewed with great disfavor by the appellate courts; such sentences are usually reduced to the original sentence. It is the courts' way of saying that the defendant should not be punished for exercising the right to appeal. Time served on the original conviction is also credited against the sentence after a retrial.

ENDNOTES

1. Wall Street Journal (May 19, 2000).
2. False Claims Act & *United States ex rel West v. Biotrax Int.*, E.D. Pa. 99-CIV-3223; *United States ex rel Strelov v. National Medical Care, Inc.*, E.D. Pa. 96-CIV-7423; *United States ex rel Piacentile v. Diagnostic Services, Inc.*, E.D. Pa. 97-CIV-4071.
3. 47 A.L.R. 4th 18.
4. *People v. Privitera*, 591 P. 2d 919, *cert. denied*, 444 U.S. 949.
5. Health Care Fraud Report (June 30, 1999 & Oct 6, 1999).
6. *Walters v. Secretary of Defense*, 725 F. 2d 107.
7. *United States v. Dougall*, 919 F. 2d 932.
8. *Brent v. White*, 398 F. 2d 503, *cert. denied*, 393 U.S. 1123.
9. *United States v. Ek*, 676 F. 2d 379.
10. *Wade v. State*, 490 N.E. 2d 1097.
11. *Winston v. Lee*, 470 U.S. 753.
12. *United States v. Leonard*, 609 F. 2d 1163.
13. Endnote deleted in pages.
14. *United States v. University of Chicago*, N.D. Ill. 96-C-8273.
15. Health Care Fraud Report (May 19, 1999).
16. *United States v. Kirks*, D. Mass. 99-10058.
17. Health Care Fraud Report (Jan 27, 1999).
18. Health Care Fraud Report (Feb 24, 1999).
19. *United States v. Poulton*, D. Vt. 99-CIV-269.
20. Health Care Fraud Report (Oct 6, 1999).
21. *United States ex rel Seal*, W.D. Wash 94-747D, *settled* Sept 15, 1999.
22. Health Care Fraud Report (Oct 6, 1999).
23. *United States v. Blue Cross Blue Shield of Colorado*, D.N.M. 960650 CS.
24. Health Care Fraud Report (July 8, 1999).
25. *United States v. Walgreen*, M.D. Fla. 96-84.
26. *United States ex rel Mueller v. Eckerd Corp.*, M.D. Fla. 95-2030, *complaint unsealed* Feb 4, 1998.
27. *Health Care Fraud in a Managed Care Environment*, Report by the National Association of Attorneys General (April 1996).
28. *State of Wisconsin v. Kennedy*, 314 N.W. 2d 884 (Wis. Ct. App. 1981).
29. *United States v. Matank*, 482 F. 2d 1319 (9th Cir. 1973).
30. *People of the State of New York v. Montesano*, 459 N.Y.S. 2d 21, 445 N.E. 2d 197 (1982).
31. *People of the State of New York v. Chaitin*, 462 N.Y.S. 2d 61 (1983).
32. *United States v. Perkal*, 530 F. 2d 604 (4th Cir. 1976).
33. *See, e.g.*, under 31 U.S.C.A., § 231, 323[a].
34. *United States v. Zulli*, 418 F. Supp. 252 (1975).
35. *Id.*
36. *People v. Privitera*, 55 Cal. App. 3d Supp. 39, 128 Cal.Rptr. 151 (1976).
37. *United States v. Medaphis*, W.D. Mich., 95-857, *settlement announced* July 12, 1999.

38. *United States v. Medical Pathology Laboratory,* S.D. Miss. 98-578 BN.
39. *United States v. Ventura County,* 98-7734 J. S.L.
40. *United States v. D'Antonio,* C.D. Calif. CR-99-158.
41. *United States v. Metzinger,* E.D. Pa. 94-7520.
42. *California v. Cadag,* BA109552, *sentenced* March 4, 1999.
43. *State v. Lester,* 149 N.W. 297.
44. *Cole v. New York State Dept. of Education,* 465 N.Y.S. 2d 637.
45. *United States v. Moyer,* 8th Cir. No. 98-1981.
46. *California v. Fisher,* F-99-1134.
47. Endnote deleted in pages.
48. NAAG (May/June 1999).
49. Dan Barry & Katherine E. Finkelstein: *Golden Opportunity: A Special Report—Brooklyn Boom in Elderly Care Is Laid to Fraud,* New York Times (Feb 7, 2000).
50. Health Care Fraud Report (June 2, 1999).
51. *United States ex rel Semtner v. Emergency Physician's Billing Services,* W.D., Okla. CIV-94-617, *settled* Oct. 13, 1999.
52. Health Care Fraud Report (Dec 1, 2000).
53. *Blackwell v. Arkansas,* CR-98-456.
54. *Fertility Clinic Scandal Costs Professor His Job,* New York Times (March 17, 2000).
55. *United States v. Jarell,* M.D. Fla. 97-52 CR-FTM 25.
56. *United States v. Anderson,* D. Kansas, 98-20030 JWL.
57. *United States v. McClendon,* 11th Cir. No. 98-9557.
58. *Mississippi v. Anderson,* Cir. Ct. 99-562.
59. Health Care Fraud Report (Jan 12, 2000).
60. NAAG (July 1999).
61. Health Care Fraud Report (June 16, 1999).
62. Medicaid Fraud Report (April 1999).
63. *Nursing Home Company to Pay for Fraud,* New York Times (Feb 4, 2000).
64. Medicaid Fraud Report (April 1999).
65. NAAG (April 1999).
66. Lankenau, Health Care Report (Jan 12, 2000).
67. *California v. Alami-Rad,* CD 144620, (June 1, 1999).
68. *United States v. Meyer,* W.D. Mo. 98-00077-01-CR.
69. Endnote deleted in pages.
70. *Id.*
71. *United States v. Pregler,* N.D. Ill. 98-CR- 469.
72. *United States v. Cone,* S.D. Cal. 98-1828.
73. *New York v. Fabrikant,* Sup. Ct. No. 7055/98.
74. *United States v. Sailors,* M.D. Ten 96-00131.
75. *United States v. Freitag,* N.D. Ill., 99-CR 218.
76. *Florida v. Rite Aid Corp.,* 99-5200.
77. *United States v. Regueiro,* S.D. Fla. 97-574.
78. *Fla. v. Mares,* F. 99-12386.
79. *United States v. Dominguez,* S.D. Fla. 98-CR-777.
80. *United States v. Ferro,* W.D. Mo. 99-00180.
81. *United States v. LTC Pharmacy, Inc.,* C.D. Ill. 99-100072.
82. *Florida v. Fraga,* 99-29753.
83. Health Care Fraud Report (Aug 11, 1999).
84. Endnote deleted in pages.
85. *United States v. Bell,* S.D. N.Y. 99-1553 MAG.
86. Endnote deleted in pages.
87. *United States v. Hamilton,* D. Nev. CRS-99415 HDM.
88. Endnote deleted in pages.
89. *United States v. Piccoti,* D. N.J. 97-432.
90. *United States v. Hernandez,* S.D. Fla. 98-963-CR.
91. *Hall v. Biomedical,* 671 F. 2d 300.
92. American Medical News (Sept 16, 1983).
93. *Id.*
94. *Id.*
95. *Hammer v. Rosen,* 181 N.Y.S. 2d 805, *modified on other grounds,* 198 N.Y.S. 2d 65, 165 N.E. 2d 756.
96. *State v. Killory,* 243 N.W. 2d 475.
97. *Cadilla v. Board of Medical Examiners,* 103 Cal.Rptr. 455.
98. *Barski v. Board of Regents,* 111 N.E. 2d, *aff'd,* 347 U.S. 442.
99. *Roy v. Hartogs,* 366 N.Y.S. 2d 297.
100. *Id.*

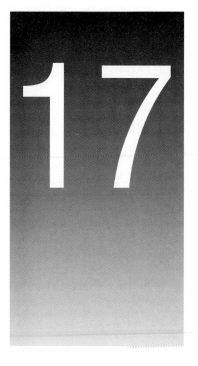

Countersuits by health care providers

BRADFORD H. LEE, M.D., J.D., M.B.A., F.A.C.E.P., F.C.L.M.

Recent years have seen a precipitous increase in the incidence of medical malpractice litigation. This increase has taken the form of a dramatic rise in the number of suits filed and in the size of judgments and settlements. Although many of the suits filed have some legitimate basis, physicians and their insurance carriers have noted a rise in the number of actions filed that lack substantial merit. To counteract these nonmeritorious claims, physicians have sought recourse through countersuits.

Physician countersuits have been conspicuously, although not uniformly, unsuccessful. Countersuits for abuse of process, malicious prosecution, intentional infliction of emotional distress, defamation, barratry, and negligence have been consistently rejected by the courts for numerous reasons.

POLICY CONSIDERATIONS

State and federal courts must weigh a number of opposing public policy issues when deciding whether to permit countersuits. On one hand, courts have recognized a policy favoring protection of individuals from unjustified and oppressive litigation. On the other hand, courts have sought to protect the public interest by providing injured parties with free and open access to the courts. Countersuits exert a chilling effect on injured persons who would seek legal redress.

When an individual with a meritorious claim is faced with the possibility of a countersuit, many legal scholars and members of the judiciary believe that the potential plaintiff's right of access to the courts is threatened. In this situation the nation's legal system for redress of wrongs would be threatened with failing to protect the rights of the individual, and many meritorious claims for damages would not be pursued. The end result could well be to leave the injured party without adequate remedy. On the whole, courts have given far greater weight to preserving the peace by favoring free access to the courts. This policy choice renders it extremely difficult for wrongfully sued physicians and others to seek an effective remedy via countersuits.

Most physician countersuits are brought against the physician's former patient (plaintiff in the original medical malpractice action) and the patient's attorney. As the countersuit litigation progresses, the focus usually shifts from the former patient to the attorney. This shift occurs because the patient frequently raises the defense that he or she relied on legal advice from the attorney regarding the merits of the case. As a practical matter, because most unsuccessful medical malpractice plaintiffs have limited resources, a judgment against a former patient is rarely collectible. The patient's attorney, however, is frequently covered by a legal malpractice liability policy; thus a judgment against a defendant attorney, if covered in the policy, usually is paid. The attorney's insurance carrier may be more willing and able to settle than the insured. The attorney's defense is weaker than that of the former client. The attorney usually can claim only that, before initiating the medical malpractice action, he or she relied on information from the client. The attorney will then claim that such information was inaccurate and led to an unjustified

The author gratefully acknowledges the assistance of law student Catherine "Kate" Duval in updating this chapter. Her superb research skills, persnickety nature, and drive for perfection helped immensely.

medical malpractice action. Another defense is that the attorney acted reasonably, obtained the advice of medical experts, and relied on their advice before filing suit.

MALICIOUS PROSECUTION

The tort of malicious prosecution has its origin in English common law. It developed as a remedy against persons who unjustifiably initiated a criminal proceeding. Modern English law has not extended this tort to allow redress against persons wrongfully instituting a civil action. A minority of jurisdictions in the United States follow that conservative approach. However, the majority of jurisdictions in the United States currently permit suits based on malicious prosecution if someone wrongfully initiated a civil lawsuit.

The moving party in a malicious prosecution suit must prove facts that satisfy the four elements of the cause of action: (1) Initial suit was terminated in favor of the plaintiff, (2) it was brought without reasonable or probable cause, (3) it was actuated by malice, and (4) the counterclaimant suffered a "special grievance." A physician countersuit based on malicious prosecution can be instituted only after the medical malpractice action has been terminated; it cannot be instituted while the medical malpractice action is still pending. A formal, favorable determination of the malpractice suit for the physician defendant must come first. That favorable determination generally need not be a jury verdict for the physician but may be a voluntary dismissal by the patient or an involuntary dismissal by the court.[1] To serve as a basis for a malicious prosecution action, the malpractice action must not have been terminated solely on procedural grounds.

The mere fact that the party complained against has prevailed in underlying action [sic] does not itself constitute favorable termination, though such fact is ingredient [sic] of favorable termination, but such termination must further reflect on his innocence of alleged wrongful conduct; if termination does not relate to merits, reflecting on neither innocence of nor responsibility for alleged misconduct, termination is not favorable in the sense it would support a subsequent action for malicious prosecution.[2]

The most difficult element for a physician to establish in a malicious prosecution action is lack of probable cause. Mere failure of a patient to prevail in a medical malpractice action does not by itself indicate lack of probable cause. Courts realize that the complex legal issues and fact patterns surrounding medical malpractice litigation contain substantial uncertainties. In many such cases questions of liability and damages are not resolved until the trial. Therefore a physician must show that the former patient's attorney had no reasonable basis for an ordinarily prudent person to believe that there was merit to the case. It is usually difficult to prove this element because courts give attorneys a great degree of latitude in pursuing malpractice actions. Courts are even more understanding concerning the early stages of litigation before discovery has progressed. Some courts have liberalized this element by holding that an attorney's failure to investigate and conduct reasonable discovery supports a finding of lack of probable cause.

Malice traditionally implies a motive of ill will. As with the element of lack of probable cause, a showing of malice on the part of the patient or attorney may prove to be an insurmountable barrier. Because of this extreme difficulty, some courts have liberalized the malice requirement. These courts will find that malice is present if there is a lack of a reasonable belief in the likelihood that the malpractice action will be successful. Where that suit was begun primarily for a purpose other than adjudication of a reasonably valid claim, malice may be inferred.

The states are divided concerning the damage element. In the majority of jurisdictions that recognize the tort of malicious prosecution, only proving "special injury" can satisfy the damage element. This requirement is based on the historical origin of malicious prosecution suits. They arose as a redress for the initiation and prosecution of an unwarranted criminal action. Those jurisdictions recognizing the special injury rule require a showing of (1) arrest or imprisonment of the physician, (2) seizure of property, or (3) injury different from that ordinarily sustained by malpractice defendants. Special damages do not include the costs of the physician's defense, increased liability insurance premiums, or injury to the physician's standing in the community. Rather, special damages are those in the nature of business losses. If the physician cannot prove that he or she has lost patients, for example, as a direct result of the groundless malpractice suit, the special damages requirement is not met. The occurrence of one or more of the three types of special injuries is quite rare. To date, no special damages have been awarded in a malicious prosecution suit based on a prior medical malpractice suit in such a jurisdiction. As a result, there has been a complete lack of success in prosecuting the tort of malicious prosecution in those states requiring a showing of special damages.

A number of states that recognize the tort of malicious prosecution, however, require only that the physician demonstrate some injury to establish the damage element. This element may include the attorney's fees incurred to defend the prior medical malpractice action. Other possible damages include the physician's mental anguish, loss of reputation in the community, decreased patient flow, and loss of income. Even an increase in liability insurance premiums caused by the prior medical malpractice claim could be sufficient to meet the damage requirement.

At least two malicious prosecution judgments for physicians have been upheld on appeal. In 1980 an intermediate appellate court in Tennessee allowed a malicious prosecution judgment.[3] During prosecution of the medical malpractice action, it was determined that the attorney continued to press the case without his client's consent.

The patient's attorney also made allegations in his original complaint that were not predicated on information provided by the client; they were fabricated by the attorney. Finally, the plaintiff lost the case and the plaintiff's attorney filed a groundless appeal—again without his client's consent. The key finding was that continued prosecution of a medical malpractice suit, without the plaintiff's authorization, constituted clear-cut evidence of lack of probable cause.

The Kentucky Supreme Court decided a second malicious prosecution action in favor of a physician in 1981.[4] In that case the patient plaintiff had sustained an orthopedic injury before being diagnosed and treated by the defendant physicians. The element of lack of probable cause was established by the fact that the attorney filed a malpractice suit with full knowledge that the plaintiff had suffered the injury before the defendants assumed the plaintiff's care.

In summary, these two cases indicate that the difficult burden of establishing lack of probable cause can be met. These courts upheld judgments for physicians in situations in which an attorney prosecuted a suit without the client's consent and in which an attorney recklessly or knowingly maintained suit against a wholly blameless physician.

Since 1981, continuing inroads have been made by appellate courts in furthering the liability of the tort of malicious prosecution. In 1982 the Kentucky Supreme Court reversed a directed verdict for the defendant and returned the case to the trial court level for rehearing.[5] In 1983 the Kansas Supreme Court reversed a summary judgment for the defendant and returned the case to the state court level for retrial.[6] In 1985 a California intermediate appellate court partially sustained a physician's victory on appeal but remanded the case to the trial court for a new trial.[7] Finally, in 1986 a California intermediate appellate court reversed a summary judgment for the defendant and returned the case to the state court level for retrial on its merits.[8] Although none of these state appellate court decisions represents a complete victory on the merits by the physician plaintiff, each certainly indicates a recognition on the part of the appellate courts that malicious prosecution is a viable tort and should be afforded respect at both the trial and the appellate court levels.

An opinion in a California Supreme Court case rendered in 1989 dramatically increased the burden of proving a malicious prosecution action.[9] Before this ruling, the attorney who filed the prior medical malpractice action had to fulfill a two-part test to establish that the action was brought with probable cause. First, he or she had to have a subjective belief that the claim merited litigation; second, that belief had to be satisfied by an objective standard of legal tenability.

The California Supreme Court, in a unanimous decision, ruled that the two-part test was invalid. The court stated that the only standard to be applied was that of objectivity, and if the prior attorney could show that objective tenable evidence supported the prior malpractice claim, his or her subjective beliefs at that time were unimportant in establishing a basis for proper probable cause.

Also, in the same case the court indicated that the party bringing the action for malicious prosecution could not introduce into evidence opinion testimony of expert witnesses as to whether a reasonable attorney could conclude that the claims advanced in the prior action were tenable. The Supreme Court felt that the objective tenability of the prior action was a matter to be determined solely by the present trial judge.

In essence this important California case greatly increased the burden of a physician wishing to prove lack of probable cause in a prior medical malpractice action. It also greatly reduced the defensive burden of the prior attorney in establishing that he or she brought the prior action with necessary probable cause.

Since 1985 a rather interesting development has occurred at the trial court level involving a variation of the tort of malicious prosecution. As previously discussed, the typical defendants in a physician countersuit based on this theory of liability are the original patient plaintiff in the prior medical malpractice action and his or her attorney. Several recent trial court cases, which have not reached the appellate level, have named the prior plaintiff's expert medical witness as a co-defendant in the physician's subsequent suit for malicious prosecution, based on a conspiracy theory of liability.

Conspiracy is a legal theory of liability usually applicable in criminal actions. A conspiracy occurs when two or more individuals agree to carry out an illegal act. Many jurisdictions permit a conspiracy theory of liability to be pleaded in a civil action. The theory of liability for including the expert medical witness in the malicious prosecution lawsuit is that he or she participated in the prior medical malpractice action by providing expert medical witness advice while knowing that the medical malpractice suit had no merit. In many jurisdictions a co-conspirator, such as a participating expert medical witness, would be jointly and severally liable for all damages along with the other co-conspirators (the former patient and his or her attorney).

This new basis of liability for nonmeritorious expert medical witness participation in medical malpractice suits is likely to make physicians much more cautious to avoid participating in obviously nonmeritorious litigation. Cases of this type should deter many medical expert "hired guns" from participating in those cases in which there is no reasonable basis for believing that medical errors were committed by the treating defendant physician.

ABUSE OF PROCESS

Abuse of process is a cause of action frequently employed by physicians after what is perceived as an unjustified medical malpractice action. The elements of this cause of action include unauthorized use of an otherwise legal process, existence of an ulterior purpose in bringing the original malpractice suit, and damages sustained by the physician defendant as a result of the abuse of process.

Unlike the tort of malicious prosecution, abuse of process does not require proof of prior favorable determination or lack of probable cause. The principal difficulty faced when prosecuting this cause of action is proof of an ulterior purpose. To establish this element, the physician must demonstrate that the original use of legal process in bringing the medical malpractice action, although justified initially, was later perverted and that the process itself was employed for a purpose not contemplated by the law.

Note that institution of a meritless lawsuit is not sufficient by itself to state a cause of action for abuse of process. Physicians sometimes allege that the original, groundless medical malpractice suit was brought merely to coerce a nuisance settlement. However, a majority of courts have rejected this argument as insufficient to fulfill the requirement of an improper ulterior purpose.

In 1980 the Nevada Supreme Court upheld a countersuit based on an abuse of process.[10] In that case the defendant physician was alleged to have been negligent in the treatment of bed sores that the patient developed while under the physician's care. A thorough review of the facts indicated that there was absolutely no basis for initiating or prosecuting the medical malpractice action. Shortly before trial, the patient's attorney attempted to settle for the nominal sum of $750. The physician refused to settle. The case was tried without the plaintiff's attorney having retained an expert witness, and the plaintiff lost the malpractice case.

The Nevada Supreme Court found that the plaintiff's attorney had used an alleged claim of malpractice solely for the ulterior purpose of coercing a nuisance settlement. His offer to settle for $750, his failure to investigate the facts properly before filing suit, and the absence of essential expert testimony at trial supported a case for abuse of process. Although this court recognized the threat of litigation to coerce a settlement as satisfying the ulterior purpose element, it is unlikely that other jurisdictions will expand on this holding because of the great weight that courts place on the public policy of providing injured parties free and open access to the courts.

DEFAMATION

The tort of defamation can be committed when an oral or written false statement is made to a third party about another person and is damaging to that person's reputation and good name. Countersuits based on the tort of defamation rely on the principle that an unfounded suit attacks the professional reputation of the defendant physician.

Defamation has not proven effective as a cause of action on which to base a countersuit because of an underlying privilege covering oral and written statements made in the course of judicial proceedings. That privilege immunizes patients and their attorneys from liability for any reasonable communication made in the course of a lawsuit. The purpose of this privilege is to permit the free expression of facts and opinions necessary to decide the merits of a lawsuit. The threat of defamation lawsuits would have a chilling effect on access to the courts and on honest testimony and would be contrary to the public interest in the free and independent operation of the courts.

However, in a 1963 countersuit based on defamation, a California intermediate appellate court ruled in favor of the physician.[11] On the other hand, the fact pattern in this case was unusual *and subsequent decisions have criticized the court's ruling.* In the original medical malpractice action the defendant physician was charged with negligent diagnosis and treatment of a child, resulting in the child's death. A local reporter contacted the office of the plaintiff's attorney for information. That attorney reiterated his formal allegations and added additional, unsubstantiated charges. Those charges were incorporated into a subsequent newspaper article. The defendant physician read that article and contacted the newspaper, demanding that the false allegations be formally retracted in a subsequent article. A newspaper official contacted the attorney who had made the original allegations and asked if the facts set forth in the article were true. The attorney assured the newspaper official that they were true and later supported his claims with formal, written correspondence with the newspaper.

The physician sued for defamation and prevailed at trial. The judgment was upheld on appeal because the attorney's statements to the newspaper were not made in pursuit of the underlying malpractice litigation. The wrongfulness of the attorney's false statements was compounded by his failure to retract them when the newspaper contacted him to substantiate his allegations. Defamation may be a viable form of action in countersuits in which erroneous statements are made outside of usual judicial proceedings. In such circumstances the privilege covering judicial proceedings will not protect an attorney or a patient who makes false statements that are injurious to a physician.

NEGLIGENCE

The law of negligence requires that individuals do not subject other persons to unreasonable risks of harm. A countersuit based on negligence alleges that the patient's attorney was negligent in unreasonably bringing an unfounded lawsuit against the physician. However, under negligence law the plaintiff must prove that the defendant owed him or her a duty. No physician has succeeded with a countersuit based on negligence and prevailed at the appellate level.

Courts have consistently held that an attorney owes no duty to a party, other than his or her client, unless that party was intended to benefit from the attorney's actions. In the usual medical malpractice action an attorney owes a duty to the client (the patient) to zealously represent him or her and to prosecute the claim. Requiring a concurrent duty to a physician not to file an unjustified suit would create a conflict of interest between attorney and client, denying the latter a right to effective counsel and free access to the courts.

INTENTIONAL TORTS

Intentional torts alleged by physicians in their countersuits against plaintiffs and their attorneys from a prior medical malpractice action include invasion of privacy, intentional infliction of emotional distress, and barratry (persistent incitement of lawsuits). Although the courts have, in dictum, lauded the application of these causes of actions as being novel and innovative, they have consistently rejected them.

CONSTITUTIONAL MANDATE

Some jurisdictions do not recognize the common law countersuits. Innovative attorneys in those states have attempted to create new theories of liability to permit physicians to bring successful countersuits. In other states in which there are major stumbling blocks to countersuits, attorneys have sought to establish such novel theories.

For example, Illinois courts require proof of a "special injury" to prove malicious prosecution. This requirement effectively prevents physicians from winning a countersuit of this nature. However, the Illinois Constitution specifically provides that "every person shall find a certain remedy in the laws for all injuries and wrongs which he receives to his person, privacy, property, or reputation. He shall obtain justice by law, freely, completely, and promptly."

An attorney representing a radiologist who was sued unsuccessfully seized on this wording and attempted to fashion a new cause of action based on constitutional mandate. He argued that, because Illinois case law required a showing of special injury, physicians were precluded from successfully bringing a malicious prosecution action. Therefore any wrongs suffered from unjustified malpractice suits had no remedy. This attorney argued that the Illinois Constitution gives a broad remedial right to such plaintiffs who are unable to obtain remedies by more conventional common law causes of action.

An intermediate appellate court in Illinois found that the pertinent section of the Illinois Constitution was merely a philosophical expression and not a mandate for a legal remedy.[12] The court ruled that, as long as some remedy for the alleged wrong exists, this constitutional section does not mandate recognition of any new remedy. It so held in spite of the fact that a physician wrongfully sued is effectively precluded from countersuing. Because the common law remedy of malicious prosecution technically is available to him or her, the courts will not create a new cause of action based on constitutional mandate.

PRIMA FACIE TORT

A form of countersuit recently relied on by creative attorneys attempting to carve out a new countersuit cause of action is the prima facie tort. The elements of this tort are intentional infliction of harm, without excuse or justification, by an otherwise lawful act, causing special damages to the physician.

Innovative attorneys had to resort to this cause of action because of the clear failure of the more conventional causes of action. Charges that the patient's attorney was negligent in failing to ascertain the merits of the case before filing suit have been summarily dismissed because the patient's attorney is not considered to have a duty of care to an adverse party—the physician. As for claims based on the attorney's breach of the attorney's oath not to bring frivolous suits, courts generally consider that private citizens are not proper parties to enforce such oaths and that any disciplinary action must come from the organized bar. Charges of barratry (i.e., the practice by an attorney of habitually pursuing groundless judicial proceedings) have been dismissed on the ground that barratry is a criminal offense with only a public remedy, not a private one.[13] Casting about for some means of avoiding the strictures of these closely defined causes of action, attorneys in three recent malpractice countersuits have laid before the courts a more novel form of action—the prima facie tort. Although in all three instances the physicians ultimately lost, the cases point the way for possible future physician countersuits.

Prima facie tort is a remedy of fairly recent origin; it grew out of an opinion delivered in 1904 by Supreme Court Justice Oliver Wendell Holmes in a case involving a conspiracy among several Wisconsin newspapers to draw away the advertising customers of a rival paper. In appealing their conviction the defendants pointed out that their stratagems had been, strictly speaking, perfectly legal and that they were really being tried for their motives. They argued that motive alone is not a proper line of inquiry for the court. Justice Holmes disagreed, holding that even lawful conduct can become unlawful when done maliciously and that such conduct becomes actionable even when it does not fit into the mold of an existing cause of action.[14]

Out of these general principles there eventually grew the specific cause of action known as *prima facie tort*. Unlike malicious prosecution, abuse of process, or the other torts described earlier, prima facie tort has not been accepted or even introduced in all jurisdictions. Ohio, New York, Georgia, Missouri, and Minnesota have recognized the tort by name, whereas Massachusetts recognizes the principle without the label. Oregon, on the other hand, once enforced the action but has since discarded it.

No appellate court has thus far upheld a countersuit judgment based on a prima facie tort theory. The reason generally stated is that prima facie tort should not be used to circumvent the requirements of a traditional tort remedy, such as malicious prosecution. The courts stress the need for open access to the judicial system and state that the prima facie tort should not become a catch-all alternative for every countersuit that cannot stand on its own. Appellate courts have refused to accept prima facie tort when relief technically is available under traditional theories of liability.

APPEALS RESULTS

Approximately 30 physician countersuits have been decided by appellate courts in recent years. In nearly all of these suits the courts have ruled against countersuing physicians and in favor of medical malpractice plaintiffs and their attorneys. At least four appellate decisions have favored physicians who brought countersuits. Specifically there have been at least two successful appeals of malicious prosecution actions, one successful appeal of an abuse of process action, and one successful appeal of a defamation action.

CONCLUSION

Although the absolute number of medical malpractice claims has increased dramatically in recent years, there has been no concomitant increase in the number of successful physician countersuits. Because the courts recognize the strong public policy interest in ensuring that injured parties have free and open access to the judicial system, they are extremely reluctant to allow countersuits because it is believed that countersuits would have a chilling effect on a party's ability to seek legal redress. Despite the application of many innovative and novel causes of action, physician countersuits have been and will probably continue to be conspicuously, although not uniformly, unsuccessful.

ENDNOTES

1. *Raine v. Drasin,* 621 S.W. 2d 895 (Ky. 1981).
2. *Lackner v. La Croix,* 25 Cal. 3d 747, 159 Cal.Rptr. 693, 602 P. 2d 393 (1979).
3. *Peerman v. Sidicaine,* 605 S.W. 2d 242 (Tenn. App. 1980).
4. *Supra* note 1.
5. *Mahaffey v. McMahon,* 630 S.W. 2d 68 (Ky. 1982).
6. *Nelson v. Miller,* 233 Kan. 122, 660 P. 2d 1361 (1983).
7. *Etheredge v. Emmons,* no. A014929 (Cal.App. 1985).
8. *Williams v. Coombs,* 179 Cal.App. 3d 626 (1986).
9. *Sheldon Appel Co. v. Albert & Oliker,* 47 Cal. 3d 863 (765 P. 2d 498) (1989).
10. *Bull v. McCuskey,* 615 P. 2d 957 (Nev. 1980).
11. *Hanley v. Lund,* 32 Cal.Rptr. 733 (1963).
12. *Berlin v. Nathan,* 381 N.E. 2d 1367 (1978).
13. *Moiel v. Sandlin,* 571 S.W. 2d 567 (Tex. Civ. App. 1978).
14. *Aikins v. Wisconsin,* 195 U.S. 194 (1904).

GENERAL REFERENCES

Logan, *Physician Countersuits,* 32 Med. Trial Tech. Q. 153 (1985-1986).

M.D. McCafferty & S.M. Meyer, *Medical Malpractice Bases of Liability* (Shepard's/McGraw-Hill, Colorado Springs, Colo. 1985)

S.R. Reuter, *Physician Countersuits: A Catch-22,* 14 U. of San Francisco L. Rev. 203 (1980).

W.E. Shipley, *Medical Malpractice Countersuits,* 84 A.L.R. 3d 555.

Linda A. Sharpe, *Medical Malpractice Countersuits,* 61 A.L.R. 3d 555 (supersedes the previous ALR citation).

M.J. Yardley, *Malicious Prosecution: A Physician's Need for Reassessment,* 60 Chi. Kent L. Rev. 317 (1984).

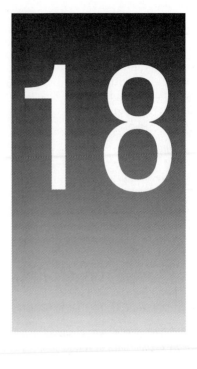

18 Health insurance and professional liability insurance

JAMES G. ZIMMERLY, M.D., J.D., M.P.H., L.L.D. (Hon)
JAMES R. HUBLER, M.D., J.D.

HEALTH INSURANCE AND PROFESSIONAL LIABILITY INSURANCE
INSURANCE CONTRACTS AND INTERPRETATION
INSURANCE RATES AND REGULATION
ACCOUNTING REPORTS
POLICY PROVISIONS AND CLAIMS
NATIONAL PRACTITIONER DATA BANK
RISK RETENTION GROUPS
ADDITIONAL PREDICTIONS

Insurance is a system that protects against the risk of individual loss by distributing, according to the law of averages, the burden of losses over a large number of individuals. Payment of the premium serves to contribute to the coverage fund and provide compensation for any members of the group who may suffer from a defined loss. There are numerous types of insurance coverage available, including life insurance, health and disability insurance, fire and casualty insurance, title insurance, and liability insurance.

HEALTH INSURANCE AND PROFESSIONAL LIABILITY INSURANCE

Ordinarily, health insurance is discussed within the framework of health and disability insurance. Typically, other forms of employment-related benefits and medical malpractice insurance are discussed within the context of liability insurance. In this section these two subjects are best served if discussed in conjunction with one another because both areas inevitably intersect in practice. Basically, in medical malpractice the insureds are physicians and other health care providers. They in turn add their insurance costs into their fees. For all intents and purposes, patients are self-insured through a variety of health care plans. Both areas of coverage for medical and health-related purposes are increasingly the subjects of legislative debates, complex litigation matters, federal and state regulatory schemes, media attention, and public concern. Be-

The authors gratefully acknowledge the past contributions of Richard F. Gibbs, M.D., J.D., L.L.D., F.C.L.M.; Richard W. Moore, Jr., J.D., C.P.C.U.; and Erica F. Cohen, J.D.

cause change is occurring so rapidly, these debates promise to expose many interesting legal issues in the coming years.

Health insurance

Health insurance is a fairly modern construct and differs from other types of coverage in that it is a entirely a voluntary system, unlike liability insurance, which is required. In addition, unlike other forms of personal protection coverage, most employers provide heath insurance coverage. Although formulated to indemnify the insured for cost of care and treatment, coverage for health care is sometimes provided alternatively through worker's compensation insurance (for those injured within the scope of employment) and by general liability policies, such as the personal injury protection coverage mandated by statute in most states as part of standard automobile insurance contracts. Much has changed within the past decade with respect to health insurance, and thus heath insurance is often the target of both state and federal regulation. These changes are largely in reaction to the nation's health care crisis and concerns of affordability, access to care, and quality of care. Though numerous factors have contributed to this phenomenon, the high cost of medical liability insurance for practitioners, rapid increases in technology, and aging of America are often cited as significant complexities. In efforts to balance the often competing needs of the public, health care insurance is offered in a variety of forms, including the traditional service-benefit plan, such as Blue Cross Blue Shield; health maintenance organizations (HMOs); and hybrid plans, such as preferred provider organizations (PPOs) and exclusive provider organizations (EPOs).

A service-benefit plan generally involves the payment of a premium and then the additional requirements of a deductible and co-payments. Generally these policies directly reimburse the participating provider of heath services, limit coverage, and often exclude services such as routine checkups and other health maintenance protection. These policies differ from the more common indemnity insurance, which does not limit the insured to a pool of participating providers but limits its recovery to what is deemed to be "usual and customary" and a number of other specifically listed exceptions. Interestingly, recent studies, including that by the Dartmouth Atlas of Health Care, suggest that "geography is destiny," meaning treatments and costs largely depend on locality.[1]

A current and increasingly more common approach to health care is the HMO. These plans, which are forms of independent or self-insured policies, are subject to federal regulation under the Federal Health Maintenance Act of 1988. Basically the HMO does not require extensive copayments or deductibles, but after payment of a premium it provides members service through a network of contracted providers. HMOs quite often compensate providers through a general scheme of periodic payment without respect to specific treatments, unlike service-benefit plans, which reimburse providers on a case-by-case, visit-by-visit payment scheme for costs incurred. Hybrid plans, such as PPOs and EPOs, combine various characteristics of the service-benefit plan with the HMO. Participants therefore are permitted to choose from a list of specifically contracted providers or go outside the system, although reimbursement is limited if they choose the latter option.

Recently, health insurance has been the center of public and legislative debate. Each issue exposes several of the complexities unique to health insurance. In 1997 the debate focused on coverage for mammographies to facilitate the early detection of breast cancer in women. This debate over coverage also involved medical experts' genuine disagreement with respect to the effectiveness and utility of the technology involved and providers' attempts to contain health care costs. Similarly, media attention has focused on issues such as statutorily mandated minimum-required hospital stays for maternity patients.[2] Additional regulation of the private health care industry included an extension of coverage for treatment of mental illness, an area that previously was a common exclusion to coverage. These statutory changes illustrate the difficult task of balancing expert opinions, health care costs, the health and safety of the public, and the traditional notions of free trade and contractual freedoms.

Professional liability insurance

Professional liability coverage is best discussed in conjunction with health care coverage because it is often cited as one of the reasons for the high cost of health care in the United States. The advent and growth of HMOs and related programs have created many new issues with respect to the lia-

bility of the health care industry. Some experts argue that HMOs, in the aggregate, are increasing health care costs as a result of numerous factors, including the rising number of misdiagnoses and litigation over limited access to specialists' care. In addition, public debate often targets the increased number of malpractice claims as the cause of limited access to and affordability of medical liability coverage and thus the reason physicians practice defensive medicine to insulate themselves.

Overall, in medical practice, insurance is a contract in which, in consideration of a certain payment or premium paid by the insured physician, the insurance company or carrier agrees (in the case of an injury or harm caused by negligence) to pay to the aggrieved party a sum of money agreed on or determined by a trier of fact—judge, jury, or arbitration panel—to compensate for the losses resulting from the injury. Similar to other insurance providers, medical liability carriers are bound by the duty to act in good faith, which includes the duty to defend the insured through litigation, indemnification, or settlement.

Recent developments in the field of medical liability insurance include extension of federal liability protection to medical volunteers under the Federal Tort Claims Act. This Medical Volunteer Act allows those who volunteer their efforts to do so without fear of being personally liable for medical malpractice actions that may arise in the course of their duty.[3] In addition, many states, including California, have imposed statutory caps on punitive damage awards to limit recovery in medical malpractice actions. Although the constitutionality of such schemes often has been challenged, they have been upheld. However, other statutory provisions have been repealed, including a 2-year statute of limitations on the filing of a malpractice claim. The legislative intent of these medical liability statutes overall is to contain health care costs by reducing the number of suits, limiting the dollar amounts of damage awards, and thereby alleviating some of the unpredictable financial and administrative burdens on the insurance industry. Similarly, within the context of medical liability suits, in addition to naming the treating physician, it is common today to extend liability to residents, referring physicians, nurses, hospitals, HMOs, and volunteer health care workers.

In a California case, *Commissioner of Corporations v. Take Care Health Plan,* the court levied a $500,000 civil fine against the HMO for failing to authorize an experienced pediatric surgeon to surgically remove a child's Wilms' tumor.[4] The statutory violation for which the HMO was fined involved California's Knox-Knee Health Care Service Plan Act, which requires health care providers to provide appropriate service to its members without hindrance by "fiscal and administrative motives." In a more recent case, *Petrovich v. Share Health Plan of Illinois, Inc.,*[5] a patient who was a member of an HMO sued the HMO for medical malpractice, alleging that the HMO was vicariously liable for the conduct of the participating physician who treated her. The treating physician failed to order a follow-up magnetic resonance image to rule out an oral malignancy (the patient was later diagnosed with squamous cell carcinoma) because he felt that the HMO would not pay for the test. The Illinois Supreme Court held that (1) an HMO may be held vicariously liable for the negligence of its independent-contractor physicians under the doctrine of apparent authority and (2) such liability also may be imposed under the doctrine of implied authority. Several other states have recognized the rights of patients to bring claims against their managed care organizations (MCOs) for delays in treatment, testing, or transfer.[6] In addition, many jurisdictions allow HMO patients to sue on breach of fiduciary duty grounds for denial of medical treatment when such denials would pass on savings to physicians and administrators in the form of bonuses.[7] These cases represent a trend toward increased liability and expanded theories of recovery against HMOs for the actions of physicians.

On the opposite end of the spectrum many managed care plans require physicians to agree to indemnify the MCO for any claims made against the company for the physicians' negligence. The physicians may be liable for the full cost of the claim, as well as attorneys' fees and expenses. To avoid large out-of-pocket expenses, physicians must be certain that their insurance policy does not limit or exclude contractual liability coverage.

INSURANCE CONTRACTS AND INTERPRETATION

In modern society perhaps no written contract is entered into more frequently and read less often than the insurance contract. Even when the purchaser reads the contract, he or she typically does not read it at the time of purchase but only after a loss has occurred. The insured usually does not read the contract to determine what it says so much as to determine whether a particular incident is covered.

The primary purpose of any insurance contract is to indemnify the policyholder against certain losses. This absence of any potential gain generally distinguishes insurance contracts from wagering and is the core theme behind many of the limitations within the contract.

The essential concept of the insurance contract is the attempt to define those losses that are covered by the insuring agreement and those that are not. As a result, certain conditions, limitations, and exceptions are used to limit the general promise to cover losses. Because of the virtually limitless number of factual situations to which an insurance contract may conceivably apply, definitional problems and attempts to make comprehensible contracts have represented considerable challenges to the legal and insurance communities. Attempts to address all foreseeable factual situations have resulted in the complexity of insurance language and its interpretation by the courts. In a study by the Pennsylvania Insurance Department, based on the FLESCH readability scale (a method of testing the readability of documents by as-

signing point values for length and complexity), the Bible received a readability score of 66.97 out of a perfect readability score of 100, Einstein's theory of relativity scored 17.72, and the standard automobile insurance policy scored 10.31.[8]

Interestingly, state statutory requirements often attempt to eliminate these problems of readability by imposing their own standards on the formation of contracts. Massachusetts, for example, requires that before delivery of the policy can take place, the contract must achieve a score of 50 on the FLESCH scale.[9] Not unlike other states' laws, the Massachusetts law also sets forth specific requirements as to size, typeface, and color of the print, as well as other mandatory requirements for the actual printing, organization, and order of the policy.

Aspects

An insurance contract is characterized by the following five basic elements: (1) an insurable interest who is subject to loss, (2) an insurer who assumes risk of the defined loss, (3) the use of a general scheme to indemnify this loss, and (4) a group made of substantial membership to contribute to the coverage fund, (5) each with their own insurable interest.[10] Although most contracts involve the exchange of goods for money, the insurance contract is an agreement to provide protection or indemnity upon the occurrence of some future event. Because its performance depends on an event that may or may not occur, the insurance contract is referred to as an *aleatory contract.* The essential purpose of insurance is to distribute the individual uncertain losses to the group and, by spreading the risk of loss, increase the certainty of the cost of the loss in the form of the insurance premium.[11] Another aspect of the insurance contract that is important for modern court interpretations is that it is a contract of adhesion. With the exception of large commercial ventures, the insurer typically draws the contract. The purchaser has the option of purchasing the contract or not purchasing it. In recent years a rule of strict construction has evolved in interpreting insurance contracts. Under this judicial concept, any doubt or ambiguity in the contract is construed against the insurer because the insurer prepared the contract.[12] Courts will often apply this approach regardless of the strength of the bargaining power of the two parties. As a practical matter, many court decisions regarding contracts based on seemingly clear language have determined that the contract is ambiguous when applied to specific facts because not all contingencies can be anticipated by the drafter of the document. In this particular area the courts have vastly expanded the extent of contractual liability in recent years.[13]

Another aspect of the concept of the aleatory contract is that in some jurisdictions courts have been willing to recognize the reasonable expectations of the policyholder, even if he or she failed to read the policy. This theory has allowed courts to go beyond the clear and unambiguous language of the policy and determine in equitable situations that the policyholder is entitled to recovery despite the specific wording of the contract purchased. The reasonable expectations approach assumes unequal bargaining power between the drafter and draftee and attempts to resolve this inequity. The reasonable expectations approach, although applied in a wide variety of situations, often is used in resolution of disputes over heath insurance coverage. In *Ponder v. Blue Cross of Southern California* the policy explicitly listed "temporomandibular joint syndrome" within a section of general limitations and exceptions to coverage for a "high option performance plan." The court, however, held in favor of the insured and allowed recovery for this specifically listed exception to coverage, reasoning that the contract language must be plain and conspicuous and must not "disappoint the reasonable expectations of the purchaser."[14]

Some courts have been willing to take this duty to protect the insured even further and as a result have adopted the "wayfaring fool" doctrine. This doctrine requires the insurer to use language that is plain and clear enough that the average person, even if he or she is a fool, could interpret it correctly. This approach allows courts to interpret policies in favor of the insured without regard to what is reasonable and based almost entirely on the subjective understanding of the particular injured party. Because of the severity of this approach against the interests of the insurer and the hesitancy of courts to "rewrite" contracts, it is rarely used.[15] Because insurance is an essential element of most commercial and financial transactions of everyday life, courts and legislatures have a much different attitude toward insurance transactions than toward ordinary commercial transactions. Courts have recognized that a contract of insurance requires the highest degree of good faith between the parties; therefore the failure to disclose vital information, dishonesty, or fraud on the part of either party results in the declaration of the contract as voidable at the option of the innocent party.

As an executory contract, insurance contracts will not be performed by the insurer until some future point in time. This factor has formed the historical basis of the strict regulation of insurance contracts and the insurance industry. Starting in the 1920s, states took an active role in regulating the insolvency of insurance companies to ensure that they had the financial stability to meet their future obligations. This basic goal of insurance regulation has been expanded significantly in the last 10 to 15 years to include many aspects of consumer protection, such as limitations on the company's right to cancel agents and insurance policies and regulations on unfair claim settlement practices. Many states also strictly regulate insurance rates.

Formation

As with any contract, the insurance contract must have a lawful object, must be entered into by competent parties evidencing genuine assent, and must be supported by sufficient consideration. However, in many insurance contracts these elements are present as a matter of routine commercial transactions. Typically the first contact made when purchasing insurance is with an insurance agent. As a general rule, the efforts of an agent are viewed as merely soliciting offers for insurance. However, a person described as an agent may not be an agent on behalf of the insurance company at all. Similarly a differentiation must be made between a general or managing agent and a soliciting agent because their duties and powers to bind the company differ. A soliciting agent is hired by the managing agent, whose powers are clearly broader, and he or she may be either independent or exclusive to that particular company. A clear distinction is also made in insurance law between an agent for an insurance company and a broker, who is an agent for the insured.[16] An agent for the company typically has authority under the American Agency System to bind the company to policies, accept payments on behalf of the company, and represent the interests of the company in other authorized ways when dealing with the insured. A broker represents the insured in the procurement of insurance. Because a broker does not represent the insurance company, he or she does not have the authority to bind the company or accept premiums on its behalf but operates as the agent of the applicant for purposes of seeking coverage. This fact is of particular importance in cases involving the defalcation of an agent and whether coverage is in effect.

In property-casualty contracts the insurance company typically does not accept risk until its office has received the application and reviewed it. The exact date and time that coverage became effective are of critical importance because it is essential for coverage that the loss occurred within the coverage period. In many typical business transactions the time required for this procedure is too long, and the company gives the agent authority to bind coverage on the occurrence of certain events. The issuance of such an immediate binder represents a binding contract to purchase the policy and provides immediate short-term coverage pending the execution of the completed policy. Although a binder is a brief document, it must contain the basic information needed to reach an agreement and indicate the type of coverage purchased. As a practical point, when insurance contracts are entered into, the distinction between a true company agent and a broker must be recognized and the extent of the agent's authority to bind the company must be determined.[17]

Many courts continue to adhere to the general rule that acceptance of the application by the insurance company cannot be inferred from mere silence or delay. However, the majority of courts now hold that the insurer is liable under the contract if it was negligent in not acting on the application in a reasonable time.

Fraud

If one party to a contract has been guilty of fraud, the contract is voidable at the election of the innocent party.[18] In this sense the law distinguishes between fraud and mere folly or carelessness. In most cases courts require the first four of the following five elements for a contract to be rescinded on the basis of fraud. The fifth element is necessary to show damage.[19]

1. False representation: The falsity is of a past or existing fact.
2. Material fact: The materiality is determined by whether the fact influenced or induced the party to enter the contract.
3. Intent to deceive: The party must have intended to deceive or at least have been recklessly indifferent to the truth or falsity of the statement.
4. Reasonable reliance: The innocent party must have been justified in relying on the statement.
5. Injury or loss must be shown before damages can be recovered.

False statements of opinions generally do not constitute fraud. An individual who knows that another is merely stating an opinion relies on that opinion at his or her own peril.[20] An exception to this rule involves statements of an opinion by a person who claims to be an expert with particular knowledge of the subject matter. In such cases false opinions by an expert constitute misrepresentation when dealing with a layperson. By the same token, a statement by a layperson concerning the law is considered a statement of opinion. A statement made by an attorney, who is presumed to be an expert, can be reasonably relied on by a layperson.

For fraud to be found, the party must establish either an intent to deceive or reckless indifference to the truth. Because it is frequently difficult to establish the subjective intent, the surrounding circumstances typically are shown in each case to establish the intent.[21] The requirements of a material fact and reasonable reliance are closely related. Typically a material fact is one that would influence or cause a party to enter into a contract. It is difficult to see how a person could reasonably rely on a fact that was not material to the contract, but typically in these cases, if the fact is relied on by the party claiming the fraud, chances are that materiality will be found.[22] The key question is whether the fact would have influenced the insurer's decision to accept the application. This question relates to whether the concealed facts indicate an increased risk to the insurer, such as the failure to reveal prior losses.

A number of particular types of fraud are found in insurance contracts. A common type of fraud is a situation in which an individual impersonates the applicant when taking a medical examination in connection with life or health insurance. In some fraudulent situations there is collusion between the agent and the third party to defraud the insurance company in a certain way, such as withholding adverse information on the application.[23] Closely related to this type of fraud is that of concealment, in which a material fact of importance to the contract is withheld. Although courts generally have not imposed the duty to reveal prior losses or claims, the presence of a specific question regarding loss history may result in a claim of concealment.[24] Most courts

agree that an applicant for insurance must be reasonably diligent in notifying the insurer of material facts that come to his or her knowledge even after making the application. However, the person owes no allegiance to disclose facts learned after the insurance contract has been entered into, even though delivery occurs at a later time.

Incontestability clause

Common to life and health insurance contracts is a clause wherein the parties agree that the validity of the contract cannot be contested after the policy has been in effect for a certain period. This clause is obviously contrary to the basic aspect of contract law that fraud negates consent. The presence of this clause in life insurance contracts is a result of their long-term nature. It is believed unfair for the company to receive premiums over an extended period only to declare the contract invalid at the time of death because of some earlier misrepresentation. The incontestability clause does not extend coverage or preclude a showing that the person had no insurable interest.[25] For example, in the 1973 Illinois case *Crawford v. Equitable Life Assurance Society of United States,* recovery under a group life insurance contract was denied despite the incontestability clause, where the decedent and her husband falsely listed her occupation as "company treasurer." The policy was for the insurance of only those employees working more than 32 hours per week, and thus the subject of the policy was not even a member of the class intended to be covered by the policy.[26] The reach of the clause, however, though generally otherwise applying to fraud in the application, makes an additional exception where it is part of a scheme for profit, such as an attempt to murder the insured or substitute a person to take the insured's medical examination.[27]

Waiver, estoppel, and election

An insurer may deny liability based on one of the reasons previously discussed. However, the insurer may be unable to assert one of its defenses because the insurer has waived the defense, has been estopped from asserting the defense, or has elected not to take advantage of the defense.[28] Although these three concepts are closely related, they have clearly distinctive characteristics. A waiver is an intentional relinquishment of a known right. As such, it is a contractual right, typically contained in the policy, that requires no proof of materiality. An example of a contractual waiver is a life insurance policy in which the company agrees to pay premiums during a period of the insured's total disability. An example of a waiver outside the policy is where the company declares a life insurance policy void when the insured enters the military service. If the insured is killed as a result of military service, a representative of the company may notify the beneficiary that the company will waive the defense because the insured died in the service of his or her country. Even a subsequent letter stating that the company has changed its position will not invalidate the express waiver. One primary difference in insurance law is that some waivers are binding even in the absence of consideration.[29]

On the other hand, estoppel in insurance law is a representation of fact relied on by one party that makes it unfair for the other party to refuse later to be bound by the representation.[30] A typical example occurs when an agent of the company assures the insured that he or she is covered for a certain event that is not covered by the language of the policy. Of course, in these situations it is necessary that the reliance on the representation was reasonable, the insured was prejudiced as a result, and the fact was material. As distinguished from waiver, estoppel is tortious in nature and relies on a false representation. By comparison, election is simply the choosing between two available rights that relinquishes the right not chosen. A typical example of an election is when an insurer must decide whether to accept a premium and afford coverage or reject a tender of premium. If the insurer elects to accept the premium, it should be bound by that choice and not permitted to reserve its position.

Reservation of rights

One area of insurance law where the concepts of waiver, estoppel, and election come into play is when a claim is made against the insured for which the insurer may not be liable because of a valid contractual defense. If the insurer elects to defend the insured, as obligated under the contract, there is no problem. However, many instances in which the insurer needs to take action could be interpreted as defending the insured, even before its obligation to defend is determined. A typical example is when the company needs to undertake further investigation to determine whether the facts of the incident fall within the coverage provided in the contract.[31] Because this could be interpreted as a waiver of the right to decline coverage, a company typically notifies the insured by using a reservation-of-rights notice.

The reservation-of-rights notice states that, although the company is proceeding with a certain action, it is for the purpose of determining whether there is coverage under the policy and does not represent a waiver of any future rights of the company to decline coverage. Although this notification clearly should prevent the insured from relying on the activities of the insurance company to create estoppel because it is a unilateral action, it may not always be effective. To be fully protected, the insurer may seek a nonwaiver agreement. This contractual agreement between the insured and the insurance company indicates that neither party will waive any of its rights under the policy as a result of the investigation or initial defense of the action. Typically, both of these procedures are limited in time and scope of information necessary to determine whether there is coverage under the policy.[32]

Bad faith

Regardless of how courts interpreted the provisions of the policy, despite construing the contractual ambiguities against the drafter or using the reasonable expectations of the insured, in the past it was at least certain that a recovery was limited to the coverage limits of the policy. Recently, however, a number of jurisdictions, led by California, have accepted the rationale that in addition to a contractual remedy for breach of a contract some types of breach can also result in a tort remedy.[33] These courts have determined that in every contract there is an implied covenant of good faith and fair dealing, which essentially means that neither party can do anything that will injure the right of the other to receive the benefits under the agreement.[34] These so-called bad faith actions have developed during the last 25 years in the wake of the landmark California case, *Communale v. Traders and General Insurance Company.*[35] In this case the court held that the insurance company that defends an insured against liability to a third person must compensate the insured for the full judgment if the insured is held liable beyond the policy limits because of the insurer's bad faith in refusing a settlement offer. The result of such cases has been that companies must be careful in dealing with claims that could potentially exceed the limits of the particular insurance policy involved.[36] Typically the insured is notified of this possibility and informed that he or she may wish to retain an independent counsel. As a result, the insurance company is pressured by the plaintiff and by its own insured to settle the case, when possible, within the policy limits.

In addition, the implication of good faith extends to all dealings between the insurer and the insured. Typical examples include the application of contractual defenses to the insured and the obligation to make first-party payments directly to the insured, such as with life and health contracts. The adverse consequences of these types of cases arise because damages may be awarded in excess of the policy limits and in some states, such as California, punitive damages may be based on a bad faith case. In the case of *Frazier v. Metropolitan Life Insurance Company* the company failed to pay $12,000 in death benefits under a life insurance policy on the grounds that the insured had committed suicide.[37] The jury found that the refusal was improper and awarded the $12,000 under the contract, as well as $150,000 for emotional distress and $8 million in punitive damages. Although this award was subsequently reduced and reversed in part on statute of limitation grounds, it illustrates the potential impact on actuarially determined rates that do not anticipate judgments over the policy limits.

Bad faith claims often arise in the context of a company's breach of its contractual duties and a failure to defend or a failure to settle. The insurance industry's relationship to its insured is often understood to be a fiduciary relationship requiring the highest of standards of good faith and fair dealings. The company is required to protect the interests of its insured without hindrance by pecuniary or administrative motives. One of the most extreme examples of an insurer's failure to act in good faith and breach of its duty to defend is the California case of

Betts v. Allstate Insurance Company. In *Betts* the insurer refused to accept a settlement offer within the policy limits and thus exposed an insolvent teenager to extensive personal liability to such an extent that the actions of the carrier and the legal counsel (provided by the insurer) amounted to what the court considered "willful manipulation" with "the intent to vex, injure, and annoy."[38] As a result of this breach of duty on the part of the insurer, Betts was awarded substantial recovery in the form of punitive and exemplary damages.

Recent expansion of the legal concept of bad faith includes recognition by the courts of an action for reverse bad faith. Ordinarily the duty to act in good faith is recognized as a responsibility on the part of the insurer; however, it is also binding on the insured. This action may arise in situations in which the insured refuses to cooperate in an investigation, often because the investigation may implicate a family member. This concept of reverse bad faith has limited applicability in that it is mainly a defense strategy used to defeat coverage rather than a source of potential damage recovery.[39]

INSURANCE RATES AND REGULATION

Historically the insurance business can be described as being highly competitive. In many cases a large number of sellers provide policies of insurance that are fairly uniform, encouraging price competition.[40] This aspect of the industry helps distinguish it from the public utility area in which a monopoly or semimonopoly has been granted by the state with the addition of rate regulation, which as a practical matter frequently guarantees a rate of return. In contrast, over the years a number of insurance companies have become insolvent and therefore unable to meet their obligations.

Despite the advantages of allowing open market competition to regulate business conduct under the rubric of the antitrust laws, two specific distinctions have created the need for some regulation by governmental agencies. Because insurance is essentially an exchange of a premium for a future promise to perform, the executory nature of these contracts makes the insolvency of an insurance company particularly damaging to the purchasers of insurance. At the same time, the pricing of insurance is based on the gathering of statistical evidence and the use of actuarial science to determine, based on past experience, what levels of future losses and expenses are likely.

Companies have historically combined data because of the limitations on an individual company in gathering statistical information in any one geographical area and for any one class of risks. By applying the law of large numbers these combined data more accurately predict future losses than the data from any individual company. Therefore both the need to regulate companies' solvency to ensure their ability to pay claims and the need to share loss data between companies have placed them outside the conceptual framework of the antitrust laws and required more direct government regulation.

Role of rating bureaus

Particularly before World War II, rating bureaus were used by the property-casualty insurance industry to gather actuarial data. These bureaus were composed of insurance company members and had the clear purpose of securing uniformity in premium rates, coverage design, and other matters related to the business of insurance. Many state laws authorized rating bureaus to act in concert with insurance companies in setting rates. Although some of these organizations were limited to the function of collecting and disseminating statistical data and other information (the statistical agent function), other types were allowed specifically to recommend rates or make rate filings.[41] Before World War II these organizations were exempt from the antitrust laws by court interpretation because they were not deemed to be in commerce.[42]

The U.S. Supreme Court in *Southeastern Underwriters Association v. U.S.* held that bureau activity was subject to the federal antitrust laws, based on an expanded definition of what constituted commerce.[43] However, in response to the Southeastern Underwriters case and the fear that without the ability to share loss data it would simply be impossible to set accurate rates, the U.S. Congress passed Public Law 15, the McCarran-Ferguson Act.[44] This act reaffirmed the desirability of state insurance regulation and the principle that federal statutes should have no application to the "business of insurance" where specifically regulated by the state, except for those federal statutes that dealt specifically with insurance. The McCarran-Ferguson Act also had an exception for boycotts, coercion, or intimidation subject to federal law.

Subsequent to this congressional action, all states specifically authorized rating bureau activity in most lines of property-casualty insurance. Before that decision, the practical activities of the states in regulating rates were somewhat limited and focused primarily on ensuring that all rates were sufficiently high to guarantee the continued solvency of companies. In an effort to preempt federal regulation by specifically showing that the states were affirmatively engaged in regulating insurance, a number of states passed fairly specific laws establishing statutory standards for the determination of insurance rates. These laws were fairly uniform because language recommended by the National Association of Insurance Commissioners was adopted by many states, and the laws centered on three statutory criteria that rates not be "excessive, inadequate, or unfairly discriminatory."[45] Many of these laws required the "prior approval" of rates before they could be charged. Despite the continued existence of the prior approval laws, a number of important states, including Illinois and California, persist in allowing competition rather than direct state regulation as the method of ensuring fair rates. Even in these states, however, significant regulation of insurance company activities occurs.

Direct regulation

The degree of regulation of rates in the insurance business outside of property-casualty lines has been more limited. Typically, no portion of the insurance code provides for direct state regulation of rates for life insurance or most types of health insurance. Part of the reason for this differentiation results from the fact that these lines of insurance have remained independent and there is no equivalent to the types of rating bureaus that once dominated rate-making in property-casualty lines. Some specific lines, such as credit life insurance and credit accident and health insurance, have been regulated indirectly by the states through the use of their Unfair Trade Practice Acts and the requirement that policy forms be approved.[46]

In part because of the advantages given to Blue Cross Blue Shield over commercial insurance by virtue of their tax-exempt status, some states have taken a strong position regarding the regulation of their risk classifications. In *Blue Cross v. Insurance Department* the court allowed a rate to be disapproved because it did not include a community rating factor that would reduce the rate differential between those policies issued to elderly individuals and those issued to others, primarily employer groups.[47]

Today, most property-casualty rate regulatory laws place the rate-making initiative with the individual insurance company or rating bureau, and approval or disapproval power rests with the state. In addition to having the authority to determine overall rate levels, most of these laws have been interpreted to include authority over risk classification systems.[48] In most areas of insurance the risk potentials of individuals fall within certain broad classifications. In automobile insurance, for instance, it has been documented that young men have increased losses as compared with either young women or all adult drivers. It is also clear that drivers operating in congested urban areas have higher loss exposure than operators in rural areas. Therefore insurance companies have sought to divide the risks they insure into broad classifications that allow the rates for these classifications to more closely match the risk potential of the members of the group.[49] This method has resulted, for instance, in the rating of groups and individuals differently for purposes of accident and health insurance and in charging different premiums for medical malpractice coverage based on the type of practice and in some cases geographical considerations. Particularly in recent years these rate regulatory laws have been used in some jurisdictions to form a basis for the regulation of the solvency of insurance companies and to address issues of affordability.

The actuarial method of determining rates is not overly complicated from a mathematics standpoint; it generally involves arithmetic and simple algebra. However, because this method requires predicting future events based on past experience, it is subject to many of the same shortcomings as any economic projection. In the short run the degree of estimation necessary in this process makes it unlikely that premiums will be exactly right for any given policyholder during that time because of errors in both overestimating and underestimating. In the long run this process results in a fairly accurate approximation of future losses over a number of years. However, this degree of uncertainty allows some states to exercise their judgment concerning socially and politically acceptable rates for various classes of insured. Particularly in times of increasing costs it is tempting for a regulator to determine that physicians cannot pay for the increased cost of medical malpractice insurance or that the elderly cannot afford the cost of Medicare supplemental insurance.[50] Without a statutory requirement that insurance companies provide this coverage, they will not continue to write coverage for which the approved premium does not cover the cost.

Thus companies have withdrawn from offering coverage in some states for such lines as medical malpractice and automobile insurance. In response to these situations during the last 10 years, a number of states have mandated participation of property-casualty companies in various residual market mechanisms. These are basically pooling arrangements that provide coverage the free market economy cannot provide under these circumstances. Some type of pooling or assignment of risks has been established for so-called uninsurable automobile risks in every state of the country.[51] In addition a number of states have established joint underwriting associations to deal with unavailable coverage, such as medical malpractice and liquor liability insurance. Although frequently intended merely to cover high-risk applicants who cannot otherwise be insured in the voluntary market, a number of these arrangements have grown to become a major, if not the only, source of coverage within a state.[52] Currently in Massachusetts, more than half the drivers, as well as virtually all the physicians and hospitals, are insured through such industry-sponsored joint underwriting associations.

State regulation

In addition to regulating the rates that insurance companies charge, the states have taken action to regulate insurance companies in other aspects of their operations. Because of some past abuses, many states have regulations involving the handling of claims. These regulations typically set standards for dealing with policyholders who have claims, create administrative procedures to ensure fair treatment, and establish periodic audits by the insurance departments to ensure compliance.

Despite the best efforts of insurance departments to ensure that companies are solvent, insolvencies continue to occur. Therefore states have established guarantee funds to ensure that claims will be paid even after an insolvency. All states currently have property-casualty guarantee funds, and many states have life and health funds. When a company becomes insolvent, these guarantee funds require that the rest of the industry step in to ensure that claims will be paid.[53]

A number of states have passed regulations that limit a company's right to cancel or not renew existing policies. In many cases these regulations establish notice requirements for cancellation so that substitute coverage can be purchased, and in some cases they limit the right to cancel a policyholder so that person will not need to be treated as a high risk and insured through a residual market mechanism.[54]

Further state regulation includes a statute of limitations on the filing of actions for recovery. This effort is obviously an attempt to minimize the court's already overburdened dockets, to further discourage frivolous or meritless suits, to narrow the scope and increase the accuracy of discovery, and to help alleviate the burdens on the insured and insurer by reducing the difficulties in establishing reserves for long-tailed losses and other such administrative tasks complexified by delayed action. In addition, state regulation has taken the form of caps on recovery, such as in the case of tort recovery; attempts to mandate arbitration; and mandatory plans for no-fault recovery. This no-fault recovery is most common within the framework of automobile liability coverage and worker's compensation coverage and is an attempt to use the insurance industry to reduce tort liability by limiting recovery to the limits of the policy and foreclosing opportunities for additional compensation through the courts. Therefore recovery in a worker's compensation action would preempt tort action against the employer and compensate for medical expenses and disability coverage without looking toward the individual's primary insurance for contribution. New Jersey represents an extreme example of no-fault coverage in both industries and the overall trend toward alternative systems of coverage.

State versus federal regulation

As discussed previously, insurance is one of the few highly regulated aspects of our economy that has been left to the states to regulate. Under earlier interpretations of the Constitution, antitrust laws were not applicable to insurance because insurance was not considered commerce. When this belief changed in 1944 with *Southeastern Underwriters,* Congress stepped in quickly to ensure state regulation of insurance by passing the McCarran-Ferguson Act.[55] At the same time, states regulated insurance with renewed vigor, using the McCarran-Ferguson Act exception to prevent federal preemption.

More recently, a line of cases has construed the McCarran-Ferguson Act exception narrowly and has opened the door for increased antitrust scrutiny of insurance practices. Even under McCarran-Ferguson the federal government is always free to regulate insurance by any statute passed that specifically deals with insurance. In 1979 the landmark case, *Group Life and Health Insurance Company v. Royal Drug Company,* interpreted what constitutes the "business of insurance."[56] This case determined that the business of insurance is "the contract between the insurer and the insured" or the "underwrit[ing] and spreading of the risk." Therefore the exemption did not extend to contracts between insurance companies and drugstores to provide low-cost prescriptions

to group insured. Whereas it may constitute the business of insurance companies, it does not constitute the business of insurance. In another leading case, *Barry v. St. Paul Fire and Marine,* the court expanded the definition of what constituted a boycott within the boycott exception to McCarran-Ferguson.[57] Thus under present law, unless the activity is core to the concept of insuring a risk, it is subject to antitrust action.

In addition to this indirect regulation through the antitrust laws, the federal government has taken a direct hand in some aspects of insurance that are of national concern. Within the federal government, the Federal Insurance Administration has been involved with a number of federal insurance programs. These programs are limited to crime coverage and flood insurance. Additional federal regulation of the insurance industry includes the extension of the Employee Retirement Income Security Act of 1974 (ERISA) to include employment-provided health care plans. ERISA was enacted to protect the rights of employees, their dependents, and their beneficiaries with respect to benefit pension-type plans. Benefit plans covered by ERISA include those that provide medical, surgical, or hospital care. Overall, ERISA preempts state laws and provides for exclusivity of federal regulation over employment-provided pension and welfare plans. The statute continues to be a frequently litigated issue in lawsuits within the insurance industry.

Coverage of patients with HIV or AIDS

Average lifetime health care costs for acquired immunodeficiency syndrome (AIDS)–related illnesses have grown from initial low-cost estimates of $55,000 to more than $155,000.[58] The development of expensive new medications, which extend the life expectancy of patients infected with human immunodeficiency virus (HIV), is increasing the cost of insuring such individuals. The rising costs have received attention from self-insured employers, as well as insurers in general. Approximately one half of the American workforce now receives employee health benefits through employer "self-insured" plans.[59]

Self-insured plans are regulated exclusively by federal law, whereas insured plans are regulated at the state and federal levels. As mentioned earlier, ERISA[60] is a federal law that protects employees covered by employer-sponsored health insurance plans. State insurance laws prevent insurers from reducing health insurance benefits after a disease is diagnosed, but ERISA has a loophole for self-insured employers. Self-insured employers can reduce or eliminate coverage for a particular illness after a sick employee submits a claim. These self-insured employers are not currently subject to state health insurance regulations.[61] States may regulate certain aspects of a plan; however, they cannot regulate the content of self-insured plans.

Many state regulations that apply to insurers do not apply to self-insured employers. Many states have prohibited exclusions of AIDS coverage in insurance policies.[62] As many as two thirds of the states have legislative guidelines regarding AIDS that prohibit distinctions based on disability.[63] The loophole allowed by ERISA does not prevent employers from avoiding state insurance regulation by self-insuring. Courts have upheld the self-insured company's right to limit benefits for employees who contract HIV or AIDS, despite state laws that would have prohibited similar modification of coverage if not "self-insured."[64] However, many of these cases were tried before the Americans with Disabilities Act (ADA) was enacted.

The ADA[65] may provide protection to sick employees of self-insured companies. The U.S. Supreme Court expanded the federal disabilities law and ruled that asymptomatic HIV is a disability under the ADA.[66] The ADA prohibits its employers from discriminating on the basis of disability but permits ERISA self-insureds to continue to underwrite, classify, and administer risks, as long as the plans are carried out according to accepted principles of insurance risk classification.[67]

The Equal Employment Opportunity Commission (EEOC) interprets the ADA and guides employers in its implementation. The EEOC recognizes that a cap on lifetime benefits for those with AIDS would be considered a disability-based distinction because it "singles out a particular disability."[68] However, the EEOC allows employers to show that a disability-based distinction is not disparate treatment and is justified by the risks or costs associated with the disability. Employers may show this in several ways, including similar treatment of like illnesses, actuarial data, and a necessity to preserve the finances of the plan, or they can attempt to prove that the limitation is required to provide affordable heath coverage for employees.[69]

Courts vary in their decisions regarding whether postclaim cutoffs for AIDS patients are protected under the ADA.[70] Section 302(a) of Title III provides, "No individual shall be discriminated against on the basis of disability in the full and equal enjoyment of the goods, services, facilities, privileges, advantages, or accommodations of any place of public accommodation."[71] Much of the debate in these cases revolves around whether Section 302(a) of Title III applies to goods and services provided by insurers. The central issue has not addressed whether such claims are considered discrimination.[72]

Self-insured employers may cap benefits unless a preexisting contractual agreement limits such amendments. Currently, under ERISA and the ADA, to cap benefits to AIDS patients, self-insured employers must show classification and unequal treatment based on sound actuarial principles and experience.[73] The financial protection of the self-insured and the plan participants may require such postclaim reductions. However, the ADA may be found to limit the loophole created by ERISA for self-insured employers in limiting coverage for certain diseases.

ACCOUNTING REPORTS

The purpose of insurance accounting is to provide information regarding the financial status of the ongoing business operation to interested parties. It is critical that information be provided to the management of the insurance company for use in making both day-to-day and long-term decisions. This information should be both reasonably accurate and contemporary.[74]

In addition, a number of individuals outside the corporation require current information. For stock insurance companies the Securities and Exchange Commission imposes requirements concerning annual statements that aid those contemplating investment in the company. In addition, state insurance departments, which are responsible for overseeing insurance company operations within their boundaries, need accounting information to protect consumers. In this latter role the states are assisted by the National Association of Insurance Commissioners (NAIC). The NAIC has established uniform accounting standards for use by all insurance companies when filing statements in the various states in which they do business.

In addition to this financial information, there is a parallel system for gathering rate-making information to be used by the insurance companies and departments in setting rates. Although these systems collect similar information, the purpose of the information requires different forms of data. Therefore the accounting data that appear in the annual statement cannot serve as a basis for establishing rates because the primary purpose of such data is company solvency. Although the ultimate goals of insurance accounting are similar to those of any other business entity, the usual aspects of the insurance industry result in substantial differences in the accounting rules and practices employed.

Insurance problems

In all lines of insurance, particularly in long-tail lines, such as medical malpractice, product liability, and hazardous waste, this matching of revenues and expenses is much more difficult. In medical malpractice, for instance, the insurance policy is typically sold for a 1-year term based on a fixed premium. Because claims arising out of incidents occurring during the policy period often are not reported until 5 or even 10 years after the term has ended, only a small fraction of the claims to be paid out of that premium will have been reported by the end of the accounting period. Once reported, another 3 to 5 years may transpire before the disposition of the claim. In some states, such as New York, an individual claim may remain unsettled for as long as 25 years after the policy period has closed.[75] Under these circumstances, it is readily apparent that, although the revenue is known at the end of the accounting period, the great bulk of the cost in terms of the payment of losses and accompanying attorneys' fees will remain substantially unknown for a number of years. These facts, however, are of little consolation to the executive planning the company's future or to the shareholder determining whether to hold or sell stock.

Loss reserves

Because claims may not be reported, investigated, and settled for a number of years, the actual paid loss and associated loss adjustment expenses cannot be determined in a timely manner. Therefore estimates are made of the ultimate value of the claims that have been and will be filed. These estimates give the insurer an indication of the size of future claims to be paid from present premiums and future investment income. Although this method suffers from problems inherent in making any economic prediction, steps are taken to ensure its accuracy.

There are a number of ways to determine the ultimate value of the claims that have been filed; however, the method typically used in medical malpractice insurance and other "large claim" lines is the individual estimate method. When a loss is reported to the insurer, a reserve is established by the field or home office claims staff. The reserve equals the estimated amount necessary to ultimately settle the claim. The company then aggregates the individual estimates on all of the claim files in statistical records. This method works best when claims are definite and the number of claims is too small for the application of reliable averages, particularly because the claims vary greatly in their severity.

For lines involving smaller claims that arise frequently, it is possible to base the reserves on the average value of claims of various types. A third method sometimes used is the loss ratio method in which the ultimate losses in a particular line of insurance are estimated by applying an assumed loss ratio to the premiums earned during the period. This method merely establishes a theoretical reserve and is required in some lines of insurance to establish the minimum statutory loss reserves. This formula approach is not widely used because of its arbitrary nature, yet adjustment of this reserve for actual results in subsequent periods improves the accuracy with time.

Naturally, when a case is first reported to an insurance company, little is known concerning the facts of the case, statements by witnesses, or other information from which the degree of liability or amount of damage can be estimated. However, over a period of time the claims staff develops information on the amount of damages involved, such as lost wages, health costs incurred, or the repair of specific damage. Staff members also take statements, talk to expert witnesses, and receive reports from defense counsel. When a claim is initially reported, a reserve is established based on currently available information. As the investigation of the file develops, this reserve is changed to reflect the best estimate of ultimate liability at that time. Thus, on an individual case basis, the reserves that are established for losses change from the time the file is opened until the ultimate disposition is made. When these files are aggregated, they produce a statistical loss development pattern that can be used by the actuary to produce a historical record of how reserves tend to change with the age of a case.

Obviously the establishment of reserves on individual cases is subjective and requires a great deal of practical experience in handling similar cases. To improve uniformity,

more senior levels of company staff or committees typically set reserves on larger cases. An individual adjuster handling a claim will have a relatively low level of reserve authority and must go to a supervisor or manager to establish higher levels of reserves. Even the local office does not have authority to establish reserves at the highest claim levels, and usually a committee of senior claims staff at the home office has the ultimate responsibility on large cases. Despite the active and high level of consultation that goes into establishing these reserves, some offices and companies may have a bias toward setting reserves higher or lower than necessary in the aggregate.

Aggregate case reserves are not used directly in a financial statement; rather, the information is turned over to an actuary for certain critical adjustments. One of the important functions of the actuary is to analyze in an historical perspective the accuracy with which loss reserves have been established. The actuary compares the record of loss reserves established over time on cases in which the ultimate payments have actually been made. This method enables the actuary to establish statistically the tendency of claims personnel to either overestimate or underestimate the amount necessary to ultimately settle the case. Therefore from an actuarial perspective the critical element is not whether reserve estimates are too high or too low but whether the methods used to establish these reserves result in a uniform approach. This analysis by the actuary produces factors that, when multiplied by the case reserves, produce an adjusted aggregate reserve that eliminates any historical bias.

Incurred but not reported

The methods discussed previously establish reserves on known cases. However, at any time there are potential claims from incidents that occurred during the policy period but are as yet unreported. A good example of this is medical malpractice, in which fewer than 10% of claims are reported during the policy year and almost none of those will result in a final payment. Therefore at any given time an insurance company is responsible for incurred losses on incidents that have occurred but have not yet been reported. Although case reserves cannot be established for claims not filed, to ignore them simply because the company has not received a report would be to significantly understate liabilities and thus substantially overstate income. To accurately view a company's financial position, these future claims must be taken into account. Again, the actuary can make an historical analysis based on past reporting patterns in determining what percentage of claims will be reported at a given point in time after the close of a particular policy year. This produces a statistical estimate of the dollar value of those incurred claims that will be reported in the future. Thus a company's loss costs during a particular year are made up of the adjusted reserves on reported cases and the reserves for incurred but unreported claims.

Insurance statutory accounting

The NAIC blank. Annual statements must be filed with the insurance department or other agency within each state in which a company is doing business. These forms are required by statute in all states and are both open for public inspection and used by financial data services, such as Bests Insurance Reports: Property-Liability.

The NAIC was formed in 1871 to establish, among other things, uniform financial blanks for insurance companies. The association also establishes rules governing the preparation of the annual statement to ensure uniformity among the states. In effect these instructions, along with the examiner's manual, provide the source for statutory insurance accounting principles. Currently the annual statement blank is an oversized booklet containing more than 60 pages of financial statements and exhibits. However, these statements are filed with regulators for solvency purposes and do not form the basis for rate-setting activities.

During the 1920s and 1930s general accounting changed. It became oriented less toward informing management and more toward providing information for potential investors. Statutory insurance accounting did not follow this trend but continued to emphasize solvency considerations. Rather than focusing on accurate measurement of current income, statutory accounting assesses the company's ability to pay all of its liability if it were to go out of business. For this regulatory purpose the rules concerning statutory accounting are conservative.

Major differences between statutory accounting and generally accepted accounting practices

ADMITTED AND NONADMITTED ASSETS. For federal income tax accounting and generally accepted accounting practices (GAAP) purposes, no distinction is made between assets and nonadmitted assets. Nonadmitted assets in statutory accounting represent types of assets that, though generally considered to have value for noninsurance purposes, are not admitted to an insurance company's statutory balance sheet. Items such as investments not specifically authorized by statute, premiums due over 90 days, prepaid expenses, and office furniture are not included in statutory accounting assets because they are either not legally authorized or not sufficiently liquid. The focus is on whether these assets are liquid enough to satisfy the company's obligations.

Bonds are generally the largest single category of admitted assets of an insurance company and frequently represent more than half the total admitted assets. Typically, many states have statutory rules that limit stock to a prescribed percentage of the insurance company's admitted assets. In addition, property-liability insurance companies normally do not make substantial investments in mortgages because they may be difficult to convert to cash. Reinsurance placed with a company that is not authorized to transact business in the state also is not recognized under statutory rules. Because

bond values are sensitive to interest rate changes as the maturity of the bond increases, in the annual statement bonds are shown at an amortized cost that does not usually represent the true market value of the bonds. This avoids fluctuation in the price of bonds and shields policyholders' surplus from unnecessary fluctuations as long as the company has cash flow sufficient to cover operating expenses without liquidating its investments. Stocks are usually valued at the closing price quotation on the final day of the year.

PREPAID EXPENSES. The expenses attributed to the acquisition of new business, such as agents' commissions, are treated as expenses during the accounting period in which they were incurred. However, the corresponding premium revenue is treated as income over the entire contractual period. In GAAP accounting, acquisition expenses are capitalized and spread over the same period during which the revenues are earned. The insurance approach is conservative because it recognizes that a policy may be canceled at any time and thus may require a premium refund. However, this conservative approach creates an anomalous situation in insurance accounting. An expanding firm that is rapidly writing new business may find itself in solvency difficulties on its annual statement not because of an inability to make economic income but because the acquisition expenses appear on the income statement immediately, whereas the income is reported only over time as it is earned.

TIME VALUE OF MONEY. As previously discussed, the insurance company's liability for claims that have been incurred but not yet paid is accounted for by the various elements of reserves. Reserves are, in essence, the best estimate as to the ultimate settlement value of these incurred losses. As such, however, these liabilities actually will be satisfied in future years out of the assets represented by the premiums that have been earned, as well as the investment income on those assets held between the time of premium payment and claim settlement. Thus the assets include only the investment income earned to date, whereas the liabilities include the final settlement amount of cases. Because the future expenditure for claims is therefore not matched with the future flow of investment income, the liabilities, particularly in long-tail lines, such as medical malpractice, are overstated in relationship to the assets. Of course theoretically this difficulty could be rectified by simply taking the future claims and discounting them using some assumed interest rate and the time periods indicated by historic loss payment patterns. However, a number of subjective judgments must be made before these calculations can be made. Because companies could overstate their profitability by simply overdiscounting their liabilities, insurance departments have resisted attempts to include discounted liabilities in financial statements for most lines of insurance. Ironically, however, companies are frequently criticized by those outside the industry for overstating their losses as a result of statutory accounting.

Balance sheet

ASSETS. The major division of the annual statement shows various kinds of invested assets. These assets primarily include bonds, common stock, cash, and other invested assets. Another important category consists of noninvested assets, primarily agents' balances. These balances are insurance premiums due on insurance policies written within 90 days before the statement date. As discussed earlier, nonadmitted assets may be excluded entirely from the balance sheet or may have a portion of their values eliminated as being nonadmitted. For instance, agents' balances are considered overdue and nonadmissible after 90 days.

LIABILITIES. Obligations resulting from past or current transactions are liabilities. Historically, property-casualty insurance accounting has used the word reserves to describe those liabilities involving money for settling claims. This use should be compared with the use of the term reserve pertaining to life insurance, in which case it represents a segregation of retained earnings for specific purposes. This distinction is unfortunate because it causes considerable confusion when discussing an insurer's financial condition. An insolvent company has large reserves but insufficient assets to pay for them.

Reserves take into account losses, loss-related adjustment expenses, and unearned premiums. They typically equal approximately two thirds of a company's net admitted assets. As previously mentioned, the reserves for unpaid losses (established in the claim department as the best estimate of the ultimate cost of disposing of cases) include the actuarial adjustment to correct for overestimates and underestimates.

In addition to loss reserves on known cases currently being adjusted, there are also the reserves for incurred but not yet reported claims, which represent losses that have already been incurred in the sense that the incident leading to liability has already taken place. However, the losses are as yet unknown because the report of claim has not been made. Particularly in lines of insurance in which there is a large time lag between the incident and claim report, such as with medical malpractice, product liability, or hazardous waste, a substantial portion of the total reserves may be included in this category. The fact that these claims have not yet been reported makes them no less real, although they are actuarial estimates of the total value of these claims. To ignore them would be to substantially overstate the financial soundness of the company.

In addition to these reserves for unpaid losses, there is also a reserve for loss adjustment expense. This reserve is made up of two categories—allocated loss adjustment expense and unallocated loss adjustment expense. The unallocated loss adjustment expenses are the general overhead and costs of running a claims operation, which cannot be easily assigned to an individual claim file. On the other hand, as the name implies, allocated loss adjustment expenses are expenses directly attributable to a particular claim. As a practical matter, although some witness fees and other incidental expenses are included in allocated loss adjustment expenses, the great bulk of this expense represents defense counsel fees.

Because of the conservative nature of statutory accounting, a reserve also must be established for that portion of the paid premium that has not been earned during the accounting period. A policyholder can cancel the policy and receive a refund of premium; thus it is necessary to establish a liability for such contingency. Whereas the loss reserves show the company's liability for losses occurring during the period, the unearned premium reserves show the insurer's liability for providing coverage under continuing policies.

Capital and surplus.

The admitted assets minus the liabilities equals the "policyholders'" surplus. Initial capitalization provides the resources needed by the insurer to begin business. During continuing operations the policyholder surplus represents the financial protection that guards against insolvency created by fluctuating investment values or underwriting results.

Income statement.

The annual statement also includes a summary of operating results entitled, "Underwriting and Investment Exhibit Statement of Income." This statement shows the excess of premiums earned over any underwriting losses and expenses that are incurred during the period. The losses and loss adjustment expenses paid during the year in addition to the new reserves for unpaid losses and loss adjustment expenses are allocated against the period's revenues. Added to this gain from the insurance operations is the net investment income, including realized capital gains and losses. Finally, additional revenues and expenses from sources other than the insurance operation are added.

POLICY PROVISIONS AND CLAIMS
Occurrence vs. claims-made policy

Occurrence policies cover incidents occurring during the policy period without regard to when the claims are reported. The policy in effect at the time a service is performed covers a claim based on that service and reported in the future. Claims-made policies cover claims reported during the policy period, regardless of when a service is rendered, with some exceptions that are discussed later. Thus claims reported this year are covered by this year's policy; claims reported next year are covered by next year's policy, and so on.

If a policy is maintained with the same company during a person's entire professional life, there is little difference in actual coverage between the occurrence form and most claims-made policies being offered today. However, they are different products with different problems and advantages in specific situations, such as changing policies, changing type of practice, and retirement. They also can result in different comparative costs over a period of years. The average medical malpractice claim is made several years after the incident, and an additional 2 to 3 years are allowed for investigation and settlement. At the outside, a claim could be reported much later, and if a jury trial is necessary, the claim may not be closed for 20 years or more after the incident. In these long-tail lines of insurance it is equally important under either form of coverage that the insurer have the financial stability and backing to remain solvent for at least the period of time it takes for all claims to be closed. Obviously, because the occurrence form covers all future claims whenever reported, the company must be around to pay the claim. A typical claims-made policy covers an act or omission, provided the claim is first made against the insured and reported to the company during the policy period.

Requirements or limitations

Additional requirements or limitations to coverage are as follows:

- The insured has no prior knowledge of the claim at the time the policy went into effect.
- A retroactive exclusion limits covered claims to those that occur during the policy period or after a retroactive date (normally the date of the first claims-made policy with that company).
- Prior coverage of the claim for incidents occurring before the commencement of the policy is required, sometimes with the same company.

Prior knowledge of a claim. A claim does not require that suit actually be brought but only that there be a demand for something as the result of a covered activity. It includes the statement that the claimant intends to hold the insured responsible for the cost incurred in correcting a defect or the demand that the insured correct the problem without charge.[76] The idea behind a clause excluding prior claims that the applicant knows about is to permit the company to avoid assuming a known risk. The question that generally must be answered is whether a reasonable professional in similar circumstances would have known of the claim. Most policies require that the insured provide notice of the claim to the company within the policy period. However, some courts have allowed the notice to be made in a reasonable time where there is "excusable delay," and others have read the clear language of the policy strictly. Some courts have been accused of converting a claims-made policy into an occurrence policy by failing to strictly enforce the notice requirement.[77] Certainly it is in the best interest of the policyholder to inform the company of any incident that he or she has some reason to believe may give rise to a claim.

Retroactive exclusion clause. Most present claims-made policies exclude coverage for any incident that occurred before the date on which the policyholder first took out a claims-made policy with the company. This provision has no practical impact where the young physician takes out his or her first policy (with no prior incidents to cover) or where the policyholder is switching from an occurrence policy (prior incidents will be covered under the first policy). There can be

severe consequences, however, for others who are not sufficiently informed on how to avoid a gap in coverage.

An unfortunate example of the potential problems created by coverage gaps is presented in the case of *Gereboff v. Home Indemnity Company.*[78] This accounting firm had continuous policies with three companies. Home Indemnity covered the period in 1968 when the alleged malpractice occurred. St. Paul Fire and Marine covered the period in 1971 when the malpractice was first discovered by the insureds, and American Home had the coverage in 1973 when the suit was filed. Home Indemnity did not provide coverage because the claim was not reported during the period of its policy; St. Paul did not cover the claim because there was no claim made during the policy period; and American Home did not provide coverage because it had an exclusion for acts that occurred before the retroactive date when its first policy was written. Therefore, despite the significant premium that was paid, the accounting firm had no coverage for this claim.

As graphically illustrated by this case, gaps in coverage can easily occur in claims-made policies. Although they do not occur when switching from an occurrence to a claims-made policy, gaps can occur when switching from one claims-made policy carrier to another or when the insured ceases to purchase claims-made policies. If the claims-made policy terminates, for whatever reason, the insured has no coverage for claims arising from incidents before the termination date but reported after that date. Similarly the subsequent carrier would not provide coverage because of the prior act's exclusion. This problem can be remedied by purchasing a "reporting endorsement" to the policy.

To avoid a gap in coverage when a claim is made after the policy ended, many claims-made policies include a "discovery clause." The concept is as follows: if during the term of a claims-made policy the insured shall become aware of circumstances that may give rise to a claim or if the insured has notice of a possible claim and a claim is asserted after the policy expires, the claim relates back to the time that notice was given to the insurer and is deemed to be a claim made during the policy period. Despite the fear of nonrenewal or increased premiums, notification to the carrier immediately upon learning of any negligence or possible claim is strongly suggested.[79]

Reporting endorsements. The reporting endorsement is an amendment to a policy that provides that all claims arising from actions that occurred during the term of prior claims-made policies are covered regardless of when they are reported (assuming they are otherwise covered under the terms and conditions of those policies). In effect this amendment puts these claims on the occurrence basis.

Typically the reporting endorsement is purchased from the first company to cover these late reported claims. However, that company may not guarantee the purchase of the full reporting endorsement. To be fully covered, at some point the claims-made insured must purchase the reporting endorsement. The endorsement will be priced as of the year of its purchase, so it will be subject to all the accuracy considerations already discussed. Therefore, during periods of rapid cost increases, the reporting endorsement cost could be much higher than the amount saved in the first 4 claims-made years even when interest is earned on the savings.

Because these endorsements are typically rather expensive, some companies build the cost of limited reporting endorsements into the basic policy for insureds who have been with the company for some period of time. Usually the policyholder is entitled to this so-called free tail on death or disability. In addition, a physician may earn a portion or all of the free tail for retirement at a certain age by continuing with that same company for a period of years before retirement. These provisions, however, generally do not help the physician who is leaving the coverage area, changing companies, or changing practice.

Because medical malpractice coverage is rated based on whether the physician is in a high- or low-risk specialty, the reporting endorsement is rated on a similar basis. To prevent a physician in a high-risk specialty from changing to a low-risk one just before retirement simply to get the benefit of a lower-cost reporting endorsement that would still cover earlier high-risk claims, the company requires the physician to purchase a reporting endorsement any time there is a change to a lower-risk specialty. The cost of that endorsement is simply the difference between the cost of the endorsement in the higher-rated class and in the lower-rated one. This cost reflects the fact that the company will continue to cover subsequently reported high-risk losses. When the physician retires or otherwise changes status, he or she will pay only the reporting endorsement for the lower-rated class.

It is frequently asked whether, rather than purchase the unlimited reporting endorsement, the policyholder should just keep the claims-made policy in effect for the period of the statute of limitations for the type of exposure involved. This is a dangerous practice because of the many exceptions to the absolute statute of limitations in many jurisdictions. In medical malpractice most jurisdictions recognize some exceptions based on the "discovery rule." Under the variations of this rule the statute of limitations does not begin to run until the patient discovers the malpractice or reasonably should have discovered it.[85] In some cases this discovery includes the facts of the injury, whether the injury was caused by malpractice, and whether it resulted in irreparable harm. In addition, many statutes are extended for minors and have exceptions for continued treatment or allegations of concealment. Because of these exceptions to the general rule, in many cases the claim will not be barred no matter how late it is made.

Pricing

Although over years of continuous coverage there is no essential difference as to the totality of claims covered under either type of coverage, their total cost may be quite different. In the first year of coverage with an occurrence policy 100% of all the claims that arise from the first year of treatment are covered. By comparison, in the first year of coverage with a new claims-made policy only about 30% of the claims from the first year of treatment are covered. As the policy continues in effect, the claims-made policy covers larger and larger numbers of potential losses because the cumulative years of past treatment may produce reported and hence covered claims in any policy year. This gradual increase in the number of potentially covered claims results in a gradual increase in the premium for the claims-made policyholder until the fifth year of coverage, when the policyholder is paying the maximum, or mature, claims-made rate. This rate may be higher or lower than the occurrence rate but probably will be in the same range. The factors affecting the relative costs of the occurrence policy and the mature claims-made rate are discussed later.

It is frequently said that the fundamental difference between these two types of policies is that the claims-made policy eliminates the tail because it covers only reported claims. Although this is an important aspect of the policy, it is not technically true. The tail of a claim is the time between the incident giving rise to the claim and its ultimate disposition. As such, it is made up of the time lag in the claim being made and its report to the company, as well as the time required to investigate, settle, or litigate the claim. Only the delay in the report of the claim is eliminated in the claims-made policy.

If the average time between the incident and the report to the company is about 4 years and if it typically takes an average of 2 to 3 years to dispose of the claim, the average lag on an occurrence policy would be around 6 to 7 years as compared with 2 to 3 years for the claims-made policy. The significance for rating purposes is that a 1990 occurrence policy covering 1990 claims must estimate the number of claims and their cost on average through 1996 and for a few claims as far as the year 2010. On the other hand, that same incident in 1990 would be covered by some later years' claims-made policy, on average around 1994. Obviously, considering the difficulties in projecting future claims from 1990 incidents, the estimate made in 1994 (which would be made in pieces between 1990 and 2000 as the reported claims arising from 1990 incidents are reported to the company) will be considerably more accurate than those made in 1990 covering 20 years' worth of claim settlement activity.

Theoretically, if the exact changes in claim cost were known into the future, both of these rates would be equally accurate regardless of the rate of change from year to year. However, the volatility of these losses in the real world causes problems. If in predicting the ultimate cost of 1990 incidents for occurrence policies the cost has been underestimated, the claims-made policy (because its rates are set later in time and hence are more accurate) will appear higher over the course of time. By the same token, if the cost of future reported occurrence claims has been overestimated, the accuracy of a claims-made policy results in a lower cost over time. Over the last 20 years in medical malpractice there have been periods of overestimating and periods of underestimating. However, because of the rapid and generally underestimated increases in the underlying cost of medical malpractice during much of that time, the cost comparison has favored the occurrence policy.

The volatility in claims expense itself also has impacted on the overall cost of these coverages. An objective insurer should receive a higher premium for allocating its scarce resources to a risky line, such as medical malpractice. The absence of the risk premium as a result of strict rate regulation has caused commercial insurers to abandon this market in many states and leave it to the physician companies and residual markets, such as joint underwriting associations (which are required by statute to provide this coverage). Because the volatility of claims-made rates is less than that of occurrence rates, an insurer could write that claims-made policy for less, all things being equal.

Another factor results from the differences between claims-made and occurrence policies and has a bearing on their relative cost. All insurers take into account the future investment income that they will earn on their premium receipts when they set their rates. They do this by determining the future loss payment pattern for the policy and then discounting these values back to the policy year using an assumed investment yield. The insurer holds the premiums from occurrence policies for a longer period of time (from the payment of the premium by the insured until the payment of the claim). Thus in periods of high interest rates and particularly where the tail is long the relative cost of occurrence policies would decrease. However, these same factors also tend to make the premium savings to the insured in the first 4 claims-made years more valuable because the insured could invest the savings at higher rates of interest. Also the long payment pattern lowers the cost of the first 4 years because few claims would be reported in that year.

It may be difficult for physicians to change insurance companies. In a claims-reporting policy, a covered reported claim is only a claim in which a lawsuit has already been filed. For example, if a patient notifies a physician that he or she intends to sue, the policy coverage will not be triggered until the court documents are filed. A claims-reporting policy makes it difficult for a physician to change insurers because a new insurer does not want to take on a new insured who will generate immediate claims.[81] Some insurance companies offer physicians a retroactive effective date on the new policy, eliminating the need for tail coverage. They do so to encourage a change of carriers, and this type of insurance is known as *nose coverage.*

NATIONAL PRACTITIONER DATA BANK

Before the creation of the National Practitioner Data Bank, which lists malpractice actions against all physicians, settlement gave physicians closure and peace of mind regarding malpractice claims. Today, in addition to concerns over coverage limits and liability, physicians need to reserve the right to defend appropriate cases. The selection of an insurance company with a reputation for not settling claims too quickly is of utmost importance. Physicians should be wary of companies concerned more with protecting themselves than the insured physician.

Hammer clauses are provisions that shift the decision of whether to defend or settle to the insured physician. Hammer clauses typically place burdens on physicians who do not wish to settle. The most common condition is that the failure to settle will reduce the limits of coverage available to the sum for which a case could have been settled. This financial burden to the physician usually is too great to withstand the pressure to settle. Thus an insurance company with a strong defense history is preferable.

The National Practitioner Data Bank was created as part of the Heath Care Quality Improvement Act,[82] The act was passed to facilitate state and hospital awareness of physicians who have been disciplined in one state and move to another and become licensed. The reported physician cannot sue those who report in good faith. Malpractice payments by insurance companies must be reported. Use of an offshore malpractice insurer or self insurance does not preclude reporting.[83] Medical malpractice insurers may not obtain information from the National Practitioner Data Bank. The information is not subject to disclosure under the federal Freedom of Information Act.[84] Hospitals are expected to query the Data Bank during credentialing and re-credentialing of physicians.

RISK RETENTION GROUPS

During the ninety-ninth Congressional session, the United States was shaken by a crisis in the availability and affordability of commercial liability insurance. Congress was besieged with complaints regarding huge rate increases, mass cancellations of coverage, and entire lines of insurance virtually unavailable at any price. Crucial activities and services were hard hit. Such activities included those of municipalities, universities, child day-care centers, health care providers, corporate directors and officers, hazardous waste disposal firms, small businesses generally, and many others.

To some extent, the "insurance crisis" may be viewed as a repetition of a prior experience. The liability insurance business is cyclical, with alternating periods of expansion and contraction. The Product Liability Risk Retention Act of 1981 was in large part the result of concerns arising from the last contraction of insurance markets.[85] However, the current insurance problem is far more severe than those previously experienced. Different observers have attributed the high cost and limited availability of insurance to a wide variety of causes. Many observers contend that a multifaceted approach is required to deal with the insurance crisis.

The Federal Interagency Task Force on Product Liability premised the act on an 18-month study. It was believed that the proposed risk retention legislation would help address the fact that many rates appeared to be based on subjective underwriting judgments rather than actuarial techniques.[86] Because a risk retention group is simply a group of businesses or others who join together to set up their own insurance company and issue insurance policies to themselves, it was believed that encouraging such groups could reduce the subjective element in underwriting. The risk retention group would know its own loss experience and could adhere closely to it in setting rates. It was also believed that by providing alternatives to traditional insurance the 1981 act would promote greater competition among insurers to "encourage private insurers to set rates to reflect experience as accurately as possible."[87] These considerations remain valid and justify expansion of the scope of the 1981 act to include other lines of liability insurance. Congressional hearings indicated the existence of a multibillion-dollar insurance capacity shortage, and the creation of self-insurance groups was thought to provide a much-needed new capacity. Additionally, according to the Department of Commerce, "the knowledge that substantial insurance buyers can create their own alternative insurance mechanisms is incentive to commercial insurers to avoid sharp peaks and valleys in their costs."[88]

With respect to purchasing groups, risk retention group regulation seeks to enable insurance markets to translate into lower rates and better terms the efficiencies gained from the better loss and expense experience that might arise from the collective purchase of insurance. Federal legislation alleviated the problems of certain aspects of state laws. Some states have created capital and other requirements that make it difficult for risk retention groups to form or to operate on a multistate basis. Many states prevent insurance purchasing groups from achieving the advantages in rates and terms derived from the economic efficiency of collective purchasing that could contribute to resolving affordability and availability problems, or they prohibit purchasing groups altogether. Risk retention and purchasing groups were exempted from state law to allow them to achieve their beneficial effects.

The Federal Liability Risk Retention Act of 1986 changed existing law to permit risk retention groups in virtually every line of commercial insurance except worker's compensation.[89] The act preempts state law regulating insurance wherever the federal law applies. Where the federal act is silent, state law remains effective. Cases interpreting the act upheld a number of state requirements on insurers.[90]

Risk retention group enabling legislation is one of many initiatives to address the serious financial and operational problems in the liability insurance industry. Tort reform measures have proliferated and continue to be tested in the courts, legislatures, and marketplace. Most "tort reform" efforts are aimed more at claims limitation and less at liability factors or insurance regulation. However, as a major player in liability disputes, insurers have been intensely interested in such activities.[91]

ADDITIONAL PREDICTIONS

In addition to expansion of liability in the field of medical malpractice and health care insurance, rapidly advancing technology promises to expose many other interesting conflicts for the insurance industry as a whole. The mass marketing and boilerplate contracts that traditionally have characterized the insurance industry open the industry up to numerous types of liability because of the assumption of unequal bargaining power and advantage to the drafter of such policies. Increasing popularity of the Internet and other electronic interfacing systems has already been the subject of intense public debate. Offers to contract are currently being made over the Internet, and it is now possible to purchase insurance coverage virtually without any personal contact or hard copies of receipts or policies. This area of law has not yet fully developed and undoubtedly will require a new understanding of general principles of insurance contract law, as well as the expansion of state and federal regulation over such arrangements.

ENDNOTES

1. Robert Kazel, Almost Entirely on Location, *Business Insurance* (Feb 26, 1996).
2. Robert A. Rosenblatt, Federal Mandates in Health Insurance Alarm Providers Benefits, *Los Angeles Times* (Oct 3, 1996).
3. *Senate Votes for Liability Coverage to Medical Volunteers*, 10 Liability Week 15 (Apr 22, 1996).
4. David R. Olmos & Barbara Marsh, $500,000 Fine Against HMO Upheld: Health Case Involved Care Denied a Cancer Patient, *Los Angeles Times* (Oct 30, 1996).
5. *Petrovich v. Share Health Plan of Illinois, Inc.*, 241 Ill. Dec. 627 1999.
6. *Nealy v. U.S. Healthcare HMO, NY*, 93 N.Y. 2d 209, 711 N.E. 2d 621, (N.Y. 1999) and *Pappas v. Asbel*, 724 A. 2d 889 (Pa. 1998).
7. *Herdrich v. Pegram*, 154 F. 3d 362 (7th Circ. 1998); *see also Neade v. Portes*, 710 N.E. 2d 418 (Ill. App. Ct. 1999).
8. Pennsylvania State Insurance Department, Press Release (Feb 23, 1973).
9. Massachusetts General Laws Annotated, Chapter 175, § 2B, "Readability of Policy Form."
10. Vance, *The Law of Insurance* § 1 (3d ed. 1951).
11. R. Keeton, *Insurance Law* § 1.2, 2 (1971).
12. W. Shernoff et al., *Insurance Bad Faith Litigation* § 1.03 (1986).
13. G. Couche, *Couche on Insurance* § 15.83-86 (rev. ed. 1985).
14. *Ponder v. Blue Cross of Southern California*, 145 Cal. App. 3d 709, 193 Cal. Rptr. 632 (1983).
15. *Insurance Lawyers View "Wayfaring Fool" Doctrine*, Insurance Advocate (July 24, 1971).
16. *Pieri v. John Hancock Mutual Life Insurance Co.*, 92 R.I. 303, 168 A. 2d 277 (1961); *Furlong v. Donhals, Inc.*, 87 R.I. 46, 137 A. 2d 734 (1958); *Washington National Insurance Company v. Strickland*, 491 So. 2d 872 (S.Ct. Al. 1985).
17. *Belanger v. Silva*, 114 R.I. 266, 331 A. 2d 403 (1975); *Hancock v. State Farm Mutual Insurance Co.*, 403 F. 2d 375 (6th Cir. 1968).
18. *Eisenberg v. Continental Casualty Co.*, 48 Wis. 2d 637, 180 N.W. 2d 726 (1970); *Namco, Inc. v. American Employers Insurance Co.*, 736 F. 2d 187 (5th Cir. 1984).
19. Couche, *supra* note 13, § 35, at 1093; *Carpenter v. Sun Indemnity Co.*, 138 Neb. 552, 293 N.W. 400 (1940).
20. *Vackiner v. Mutual of Omaha Insurance Co.*, 179 Neb. 300, 137 N.W. 2d 859 (1965).
21. *Glickman v. Prudential Insurance Co.*, 151 Pa. Super. 52, 29 A. 2d 224 (1942).

22. *Burns v. Prudential Insurance Co.,* 201 Cal. App. 2d 868, 20 Cal. Rptr. 535 (1962).
23. *Fisher v. Prudential Insurance Co.,* 107 N.H. 101, 218 A. 2d 62 (1966).
24. *Shelter Insurance Co. v. Cruse,* 446 So. 2d 893 (La. App. 1984).
25. *Crawford v. Equitable Life Assurance Society of United States,* 56 Ill. 2d 41, 305 N.E. 2d 144 (1973).
26. Couche, *supra* note 13, § 72, at 2.
27. *Ludwinska v. John Hancock Mutual Life Insurance Co.,* 317 Pa. 577, 178 A. 28, *rev'd.* 115 Pa. Sup. 228, 175 A. 283 (1935).
28. *Clemmons v. Nationwide Mutual Insurance Co.,* 267 N.C. 495, 148 S.E. 2d 640 (1966); 1 A.L.R. 3d 1139.
29. *Therrien v. Maryland Casualty Co.,* 97 N.H. 180, 84 A. 2d 179 (1951); *Salloum Foods & Liquor, Inc. v. Parliament Insurance Co.,* 69 Ill. App. 3d 422, 388 N.E. 23, 27-28 (1979).
30. *St. Paul Fire and Marine Insurance Co. v. Molloy,* 46 Md. App. 520, 420 A. 2d 994 (1980), *rev'd on other grounds,* 291 Md. 139, 433 A. 2d 1135 (1981); *Sahlen v. American Casualty Co.,* 103 Ariz. 57, 436 P. 2d 606 (1968).
31. J. Moore, *Insurers' Preservation of Rights,* 26 For the Defense 23 (1984).
32. D. Wall, *Litigation and Prevention of Insurer Bad Faith* § 3.04 (1985).
33. *Id.,* at § 1.01.
34. Shernoff, *supra* note 12, at § 1.07.
35. *Communale v. Traders and General Insurance Co.,* 328 P. 2d 198 (Cal. 1958).
36. *Egan v. Mutual of Omaha Insurance Co.,* 24 Cal. 3d 809, 157 Cal. Rptr. 482, 598 P. 2d 452 (1979); *cert. denied,* 445 U.S. 912, 100 S.Ct. 1271, 63 L.Ed. 2d 597 (1980).
37. *Frazier v. Metropolitan Life Insurance Co.,* 169 Cal. App. 3d 90, 214 Cal. Rptr. 883 (1985).
38. *Betts v. Allstate Insurance Company,* 154 Cal. App. 3d 688, 201 Cal. Rptr. 528 (1984).
39. *California Casualty General Ins. Co. v. Superior Ct.,* 173 Cal. App. 3d 274, 218 Cal. Rptr. 817 (1987).
40. Comments on the NAIC Program to Monitor Competition, Patricia Danzon (Munch) (1979).
41. P. Danzon (Munch), *The Role of Rating Bureaus in Property-Liability Insurance Markets* (1980).
42. *Paul v. Virginia,* 75 U.S. (8 Wall.) 168 (1868).
43. *Southeastern Underwriters Ass'n v. U.S.,* 322 U.S. 533, 88 L.Ed. 1440, 64 S.Ct. 1162 (1944).
44. McCarran-Ferguson Act, Pub. L. No. 15 U.S.C. § 1011 (1945).
45. J. Mintel, *Insurance Rate Litigation,* 4 (1983).
46. *Id.,* at 5.
47. *Blue Cross v. Insurance Dept.,* 34 Pa. Commw. 585, 383. A. 2d 1306 (1975).
48. Mintel, *supra* note 45, at 113.
49. R. Holton, *Restraints on Underwriting* (1979).
50. *Medical Malpractice JUA v. Comm'r of Insurance,* 478 N.E. 2d 936 (Mass. 1985).
51. F. Lee, *A Profile of the Automobile Shared Market* (1979).
52. L. Soular, *Subsidization of Insurance: A Study of Residual Markets and Their Impact on Property-Casualty Insurers* (1980).
53. R. Marcus, *Directory and Chart of State Laws* (1985).
54. Holton, *supra* note 49.
55. McCarran-Ferguson Act, *supra* note 44, at § 1011-1015.
56. *Group Life and Health Insurance Co. v. Royal Drug Co.,* 435 U.S. 903, 98 S.Ct. 1448, 47 L.W. 4203 (1979).
57. *Barry v. St. Paul Fire and Marine,* 438 U.S. 531, 57 L.Ed. 2d 932, 98 S.Ct. 2923 (1978).
58. David R. Holtgrave & Steven D. Pinkerton, *Updates of Cost of Illness and Quality of Life Estimates for Use in Economic Evaluations of HIV Prevention Programs,* 16 J. Acquired Immune Deficiency Syndrome and Hum. Retrovirology 54 (1997). *See also* Fred Hellinger, *The Lifetime Cost of Treating a Person with HIV,* 270 J.A.M.A. 474 (1993).
59. Craig Copeland & Bill Pierron, *Implications of ERISA for Health Benefits and the Number of Self-Funded ERISA Plans,* EBRI Issue Brief No. 193, at 71 (Employee Benefits Research Inst., 1998).
60. 29 U.S.C. §§ 101-1461 (1994).
61. N. Mansfield, *Evolving Limitations on Coverage for AIDS: Implications for Health Insurers and Employers Under the ADA and ERISA,* 35 Tort & Insurance L.J. 1 (Fall 1999).
62. Arthur S. Leonard, *AIDS: Employment and Unemployment,* 49 Ohio St. L.J. 929, 960 (1989).
63. *See* Mansfield, *supra* note 61, at 122.
64. *Mcgann v. H&H Music Co.,* 946 F.2d 401 (5th Cir. 1991), *cert. denied,* 506 U.S. 981 (1992). *Owens v. Storehouse, Inc.,* 773 F.Supp. 416 (N.D. Ga. 1991).
65. 42 U.S.C. 12101-12117 (1994).
66. 18 S. Ct. 2196 (1998).
67. *See* Mansfield, *supra* note 61, at 119. Section 501 specifically provides that the ADA does not affect preexisting condition clauses included in insurance policies issued by employers.
68. *EEOC Interim Guidance on Application of ADA to Health Insurance,* 20 Pens. & Ben. Rep. 1303 (1993).
69. *See* Mansfield, *supra* note 61, at 125-126.
70. *Carparts Distribution Center v. Automotive Wholesalers Ass'n of New England, Inc.,* 37 F. 3d 12 (1st Cir. 1994) (the first federal appellate court to issue an affirmative ruling suggesting that the ADA will protect AIDS-related health care benefits from postclaim cutoffs).
71. 42 U.S.C. 12182(a) (1994).
72. *Doukas v. Metropolitan Life Ins. Co.,* 950 F.Supp. 422 (D.N.H. 1996). *See also Baker v. Hartford Life Ins. Co.,* 1995 WL 573430 at 3 (N.D. Ill., Sept 28, 1995). *See also Winslow v. IDS Life Ins. Co.,* 1998 WL 852876 (D. Minn., Sept 30, 1998). *Doe & Smith v. Mutual of Omaha,* 139 F. 3d 895 (7th Cir. 1999).
73. S. Flannery, *Employer Health-Care Plans: The Feasibility of Disability-Based Distinctions Under ERISA and the Americans with Disabilities Act,* 12 Hofstra Lab. L.J. 211 (1995).
74. C. Galloway & J. Galloway, *Handbook of Accounting for Insurance Companies* (1986); T. Troxel & C. Breslin, *Property-Liability Insurance Accounting and Finance* (2d ed. 1983); R. Strain, *Property and Liability Insurance Accounting* (3d ed. 1986).
75. J. Macginnitie, *Malpractice: Where We've Been and Where We May be Going,* National Medical Malpractice J.U.A. Seminar (1984).
76. *Williamson & Vollmer Eng'g, Inc. v. Sequoia Insurance Co.,* 64 Cal. App. 3d 261, 134 Cal. Rptr. 427 (1976); *Continental Casualty Co. v. Enco Ass'n. Inc.* 238 N.W. 2d 198 (Mich. App. 1976).
77. *Stine v. Continental Casualty Co.,* 315 N.W. 2d 887 (Mich. App. 1982); Windt, *Insurance Claims & Disputes,* § 12.02, at 12(1983).
78. *Gereboff v. Home Indemnity Co.,* 383 A. 2d 1024 (R.I. 1978).
79. F. Huszagh & K. Sorenson, *Professional Liability Insurance Issues,* in *Liability Insurance* 21 (Illinois Institute for Continuing Legal Education).
80. Long, *The Law of Liability Insurance,* § 12.02, at 12 (1983).
81. I. Tietelbaum, *Practice in Transition,* 11-14 (Summer 1996).
82. Title IV of Public Law 99-960, as amended (codified at 42 U.S.C. 11001). *See also* 45 C.F.R. Part 60.
83. David Freedman, *What's Reportable and Who Has Access to the Information,* 10 E.D. Legal Letter 63.
84. *Id.,* at 66.
85. Product Liability Risk Retention Act of 1981.
86. House report 97-190, p. 23.
87. House report 97-190, p. 4.
88. Congressional Record, S9229-S9230 (July 17, 1986).
89. Liability Risk Retention Act of 1986.
90. *Frontier Insurance v. Hager,* S. Dist. Iowa No. 87-645 (1988); *Pennsylvania Insurance Co. v. Corcoran,* Cir. No. 87-7858 (1988).

91. For discussion of such issues, *see* L.S. Maarema, *Public Regulation of Insurance Law: Annual Survey,* XXIV Tort and Insurance Law J. 472 (Winter 1989); S. Conley & L.H. Vitlin, *The Duties of Good Faith Owed by a Primary Insured to the Carriers Providing Excess Coverage,* 369 Practicing Law Institute Lit. 337 (Jan 1 1989), PLI Order No.

H4. 5062; P.B. Weiss, *Comments Reforming Tort Reform,* 38 Catholic Univ. L. Rev. 737 (April 1 1989); M. Hager, *Civil Compensation and Its Discontents: A Response to Huber,* 42 Stanford L. Rev. 539 (Jan 1 1990); P.W. Huber, *Liability: The Legal Revolution and its Consequences* (Basic Books 1988).

APPENDIX 18-1   Insurance glossary

ALE   Allocated loss expense. See *expenses.*

amortized value   See *investments.*

claim   A demand to pay. A claim is a demand against a physician or hospital. It may or may not be insured under a policy, depending on the coverage afforded and the nature of the offense.

claims frequency   The number of claims reported during a period of time, such as a year, expressed as a ratio to the number of physicians insured, for example, per 100 physicians.

class   Short for classification. A class is a subdivision of a "universe." To lump all insureds into the same rate grouping would be to overcharge one subgroup (or class) and to undercharge another. In medical malpractice insurance approximately 100 classes are based mostly on medical specialties. However, an insurer may have only seven rate groups, so each rate group contains several classes.

combined loss ratio   The sum of (a) the ratio of losses and loss adjustment expenses incurred to earning premiums and (b) the ratio of all other underwriting expenses incurred to written premiums.

coverage   The insurance afforded by the policy and the endorsements or riders attached to it.
  I. Claims-made coverage—The claims-made policy covers only those claims that are reported during the term of the (annual) policy, regardless of when the incident occurred.
  II. Occurrence coverage—The occurrence policy insures against all incidents that occurred during the term of the (annual) policy, regardless of how many years later they are first reported.

EPO   Exclusive provider organization.

expenses
  I. Loss expense
    A. ALE—Allocated loss expense. That claim expense that can be allocated to a specific claim. This type of expense is almost 100% loss legal (i.e., outside of defense attorneys' and expert witnesses' fees).
    B. ULE—Unallocated loss expense. The inside cost of running a claim department, including costs of employing supervisors and claim examiners, share of executive, heat, light, rent, and so forth.
  II. Commissions—Percentage of premiums paid to brokers.
  III. Taxes—Percentage of written premium paid to the state.
  IV. Administration and overhead—Includes actuarial, legal, accounting, and investment service fees, and so forth.

expenses incurred   The expenses paid during a period of time, such as a year, plus the change in expense reserves. Equal to paid expenses less outstanding expenses at the beginning of the period plus the outstanding expenses at the end of the year.

experience   A matching of premiums, losses, and expenses. May or may not include investment earnings, net profit, or both.
  I. Calendar year experience—Combines the premiums earned in a year and the losses incurred in the year.

  II. Accident year experience—Combines the losses incurred in a year and the premiums earned on policies in effect during that year. Changes over time. See separate definitions of *premium* and *expenses incurred.*

HMO   Health maintenance organization.

IBNR   Losses incurred but not reported. See *losses.*

investments
  I. Interest—The interest received on bonds in the portfolio.
  II. Maturity—Unlike stocks, bonds are debts that become due and payable at some time in the future, at which time they are said to mature.
  III. Portfolio valuations
    A. Market value—The value at which a bond could be sold today. Fluctuates widely, inversely with general interest rates, and directly with quality and other factors.
    B. Par value—The face amount (maturing amount) of each and all of the bonds.
    C. Price or purchase amount—The cost of the bonds; what was paid for them when they were purchased.
    D. Amortized value—A straight line indicating the trend from the date and amount of purchase to maturity at par. If a bond maturing in 10 years is bought at 90, its amortized value is 91 at the end of the first year, 92 at the end of the second year, and so on, regardless of the market values of the bonds at those times. Bonds of insurance companies are valued this way. If they were not, there would be a good many technical insolvencies when market values become abnormally depressed.
  IV. Realized capital gain (loss)—The difference between the purchase price of a bond and the amount for which it was sold. By selling the bond or letting it mature at par, a gain or a loss is realized, which is measured in dollars.
  V. Unrealized capital gain (loss)—The difference between the purchase price of a bond and what it's worth now at market. The bond has not been sold or has not matured, so the gain or loss is unrealized.

ISO   Insurance services office. A large organization located in New York City that gathers and processes the statistics of most insurance companies (not life) in the United States. ISO also publishes rate manuals for most lines of insurance (see *line*) in each of the states.

line   A line is a general kind of insurance, such as fire, automobile, or worker's compensation. The Annual Statement blank provides for 29 lines of insurance and leaves a line blank for some specialty lines. It separates malpractice liability from other types of liability.

losses   The most important statistic.
  I. Losses paid—The losses actually paid on a body of policies. Calendar year losses paid (see *experience—Calendar year*) are the losses paid out in a given period, for example, during 1982, on claims whenever occurred or reported but do not include loss adjustment expenses, which are separate. After a claim is paid, it is usually but not always closed. There are partial payments on claims that remain open. Indemnity payments are those made to claimants and do not include payments to defense attorneys (ALEs). Losses paid are indemnity payments only.

For a more comprehensive glossary of medicolegal terms, see the glossary at the back of the book.

II. Losses outstanding—The losses that are unpaid and are represented by loss reserves.
   A. Case reserves—*Case* is a claims department term meaning "claim" or "file." Technically it is accompanied by a claim number. When a claim is reported and set up, it gets a claim number and a "case estimate." That is, the claims department estimates the final liability of the claim, that amount goes into reserve, and liability is set up for its ultimate cost. The total of such estimates minus any amount paid thereon becomes the losses outstanding reserve for known cases.
   B. IBNR—Losses incurred but not reported. Some claims are not reported promptly; others are reported late because the injury takes a long time to become manifest. In any event, provision must be made for such claims, which are often reported 10 or more years after the event or injury. IBNR reserves, particularly for medical malpractice liability, are substantial and often exceed the reserves for known cases. They are calculated by the actuary and are based on past patterns of claims emergence, trended to the future.
   C. Loss adjustment expenses—See *expenses*.
III. Losses incurred—The sum of losses paid and losses outstanding, with reserves for both case estimates and losses IBNR. The estimated ultimate cost of a body of claims.

maturity   See *investments*.

no-pay claims   Claims closed without indemnity payment. Also known as *closed without payment* (CWOP). There may be some loss adjustment expense paid.

par value   See *investments*.

PPO   Preferred provider organization.

premium   The money a policyholder pays for the policy.
   I. Written premium—The sum total of all the premiums for all the policies written for a period (e.g., during 1990).
   II. Earned premium—That part of the premium for a policy that represents the expired part of the policy. If a policy has already run for 4 months, one third of its premium is earned and belongs to the company and two thirds is unearned and refundable to the policyholder if he or she cancels. A proper matching of premiums, losses, and expenses to determine profit includes earned premiums, losses incurred, and expenses incurred.
   III. Unearned premium—The premium representing the unexpired part of a policy. Equals the written premium minus the earned premium. Can become a substantial item on the balance sheet of an insurance company, and is carried as a liability because it is theoretically refundable.

reserve   A liability on the balance sheet for future payments. See *losses*. There are reserves for unearned premiums, for losses and loss expenses unpaid, and for other expenses unpaid. The solvency of a company can be determined only after all reserves and other liabilities have been taken into account.

statutory accounting   The system under which insurance companies must report to the state. Many businesses use generally accepted accounting principles (GAAP). Two major differences for joint underwriting associations (JUAs) are as follows: (1) under statutory accounting the JUA may not "discount" its reserves to take into account the investment income they will earn before they are paid out, and (2) the JUA may not be given credit for its "equity" in the unearned premium reserve. This is the prepaid acquisition expense, or commission paid to brokers. The unearned premium reserve, which is a liability, may not be reduced to reflect this prepaid expense.

ULE   Unallocated loss expense. See *expenses*.

underwriting profit (loss)   The amount left after subtracting from earned premiums in a period the sum of losses and loss expenses incurred in the same period. Investment income is not taken into account; when it is, the result is called *operating profit* or *loss*.

unrealized capital gains   See *investments*.

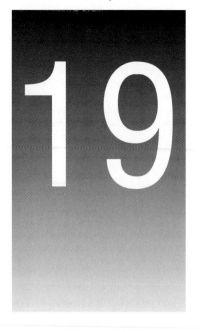

Risk management

RICHARD R. BALSAMO, M.D., J.D., F.C.L.M.
MAX DOUGLAS BROWN, J.D.

ORIGIN AND SCOPE
RISK IDENTIFICATION
RISK PRIORITIZATION
RISK CONTROL
RECENT DEVELOPMENT: USE OF ALTERNATIVE DISPUTE RESOLUTION
RISK PREVENTION
RISK FINANCING
EXTERNAL REQUIREMENTS
CONCLUSION

ORIGIN AND SCOPE

Risk management programs began in the 1970s as a response to increasing numbers of medical malpractice claims of hospitals, and they have since been adopted by other types of health care organizations. Risk management is the process of protecting an organization's financial assets against losses from legal liability. It is defined by the Joint Commission on Accreditation of Healthcare Organizations (JCAHO) as "clinical and administrative activities that [health care organizations] undertake to identify, evaluate, and reduce the risk of injury and loss to patients, personnel, visitors, and [the organization] itself."[1]

Comprehensive risk management is both reactive in its response to events that have already occurred and proactive in its prevention of further occurrences. The primary responsibilities of a comprehensive risk management program are identification of legal risk, prioritization of identified risk, determination of proper organizational response to risk, management of recognized risk cases with the goal of minimizing loss (risk control), establishment of effective risk prevention, and maintenance of adequate risk financing. Risk management in a health care organization requires knowledge of the law and of the legal process, an understanding of clinical medicine, and familiarity with the organization's administrative structure and operational realities.

The full scope of risk management encompasses all organizational activity—operational and clinical—because liability may originate in either area. This purview includes proper building maintenance and food preparation as well as adverse outcomes of medical care and accurate medical record keeping. This chapter, however, focuses on risk management as it relates to the medical care that is provided by a health care organization, called *"clinical" risk management.* Clinical risk management requires close cooperation between the legal department and the clinical administrators responsible for quality assessment and improvement and for clinical functional units (e.g., a hospital patient care unit, a medical office, or the physical therapy department).

Risk management is usually the prime responsibility of either a risk management department or the legal department, which in carrying out this function typically establishes a close working relationship with the clinical administrative staff. Nevertheless, important risk management functions, such as risk identification, clinical case review, and clinical risk prevention, are the direct responsibility of the clinical staff. Many organizations employ specialized staff, commonly called *risk managers,* who often have training and experience in a clinical field, such as nursing, to work with the legal staff and take day-to-day responsibility for some specified risk management functions, such as the management of recognized risk cases (risk control) and the coordination of overall risk management activity. In this chapter the term *risk administrators* refers to those individuals in an organization with formal, organization-wide risk management responsibility, most notably the legal staff and risk managers. In the context of clinical duties, the term's meaning incorporates clinical administrators such as the director of quality assessment and improvement (quality management) and the chief medical staff officer.

Role

The escalating frequency of litigation and the decreasing affordability of liability insurance have generated the demand for increased sophistication in the identification, control, prevention, and financing of medical risk. For example, the trust fund of a self-insured hospital represents a sizable and important asset of that hospital. A highly synergistic commonality of purpose exists between financial management and risk management. A risk administrator seeks to manage what is substantially a financial risk—the loss of financial assets. This loss occurs through the payment of claims for damages and expenses arising from untoward events that become potentially compensable through judgments or settlements and that may erode the hospital's assets and increase the cost of providing health care.[2]

Although the basic purpose of a risk management program is to minimize the cost of loss, there is a tendency to evaluate a risk management program solely from a financial standpoint with regard to current cases and claims. Most administrators of successful risk management programs agree that such a "bottom line" view misses the overriding purpose of a clinical risk management program. Risk management in a health care institutional setting should be considered first and foremost a means of improving and maintaining quality patient care—the cornerstone of risk prevention.[3]

In pursuing this goal, risk administrators must have a close, trusting relationship with the clinical administrators who have direct responsibility for many risk management functions. Effective risk management depends on their active participation. Moreover, formal organizational quality assessment and improvement functions should be operationally linked to the risk management program. This linkage should include the exchange of all relevant information and the sharing of formal risk management responsibilities to maximize the understanding of all risk management issues, specific cases, and organizational data. Nonclinical risk administrators must have quick, thorough, and reliable access to medical consultation about clinical issues, specific cases, and organization performance data. The proper relationship avoids duplication of effort, the potential for misunderstanding between the clinical and legal staffs, and the potential to work at cross-purposes in carrying out specific risk management functions.

Risk administrators and quality managers in turn must be operationally linked to and influential in the overall management of the organization. For example, tragic consequences can befall the health maintenance organization (HMO) whose risk and quality administrators' efforts to reverse increasing risk exposure resulting from poor after-hours access to care are ignored and defeated by a financially driven, organization-wide effort to reduce emergency room use.

Despite the necessity of a close working relationship, risk management and quality management are not ideally combined in one department. Risk management is an extension of the legal responsibilities of an organization. Thus an attorney ultimately should direct risk management activity. Fulfillment of quality management responsibilities requires detailed medical knowledge and the trust, respect, and attention of the medical staff. Thus quality management activity is best led and directed by a physician.

An effective risk management program begins with its system for identifying the specific events likely to result in loss and the general clinical areas of risk exposure. This system should be predicated on a current, thorough understanding of the varied sources of legal risk faced by a health care organization. Risk management then proceeds to risk prioritization, risk control, risk prevention, and risk financing.

Sources of legal risk: new developments and recent trends

Detailed discussion of the varied sources of legal risk that confront health care providers is covered elsewhere in this text and is beyond the scope of this chapter. However, it may be useful here to point out some recent data and trends that indicate the developing legal risks that are especially problematic for health care providers.[4]

The legal risk most commonly associated with the health care organization is medical malpractice. One of the more recent reports to provide detailed data on the clinical and operational sources of malpractice risk is that provided by St. Paul Fire and Marine Insurance Company in its 1999 year-end report. In this report, St. Paul offered its policyholders an analysis of claims of physicians and surgeons for the period between July 1997 and June 1999. Appendixes 19-1 through 19-3 demonstrate, respectively, St. Paul's findings as to the top 10 malpractice allegations by average cost, the top 10 malpractice allegations by frequency, and all malpractice allegations by location.

The growing use of clinical practice guidelines may develop as a cause of increased medical malpractice risk.[5] When followed, practice guidelines are widely viewed as means to improve the quality and appropriateness of care and as shields against liability. Unquestionably they provide great benefits to the extent that they improve the quality and efficiency of care. Unfortunately, they also have the potential to stultify and codify the practice of medicine by establishing innumerable sets of microstandards useful to plaintiffs in proving a departure from the standard of care. In the absence of legal protection accompanying their adoption, fear of deviating from guidelines and the difficulty of remembering their many details may bedevil physicians in years to come.

Another developing contributor to medical malpractice risk is the sometimes inordinate deference given to the principle of patient control over treatment choices. Obstetrical care may be the most problematic area. Today, many patients demand home deliveries, impose restrictions on care given to infants, and even refuse cesarean sections, all of which may pose a grave danger to an infant's health and increase the likelihood of an adverse outcome. Courts have generally been tolerant of patients' asserting their right to pick and choose how obstetrical care will be provided. At the same time, this attitude causes great unease among risk administrators, who note that the single-most costly source of risk to a health care organization is birth-related infant trauma, which usually can be avoided by cesarean section. In the absence of reasonable limitations on patient choices, it is fully expected that childbirth-related trauma and other adverse outcomes stemming from increasing patient control over care will grow even more costly to both physicians and their health care organizations.

Failure to obtain informed consent is another important source of risk. It may give rise to an intentional tort or may be a secondary count in a medical malpractice action. States are divided in their approach to determining what information must be provided to patients to enable them to decide whether to accept the risks of proposed treatment. Some states require the disclosure of information that a reasonable physician would disclose to that patient, whereas others require the disclosure of information that a reasonable patient would feel was material to his or her decision of whether to accept the risks of treatment. As more clinical outcomes performance data become available, those data may play an increasingly important role in determining the content of disclosure. Risk administrators must be aware of and educate their physicians about the need to meet the legal standard of disclosure, particularly if their organizations are located in states applying the "reasonable patient" standard. For example, a patient preparing to undergo heart bypass surgery at a hospital that is a high mortality outlier for this surgery might expect such information to be disclosed when the risks of surgery are discussed. In a cogent essay, physicians Topol and Califf argue for more extensive disclosure to patients of institution- and physician-specific outcomes data. Using coronary artery bypass surgery as an example, they suggest the following:

In the future, an ideal approach would be to shift "full disclosure" to inform patients. On the consent forms that patients sign before the procedure, the cardiologist and cardiac surgeon could include their actual risk and success rates, when appropriate, for the past several years, the cumulative number of procedures the physician has done, and the site's overall rate of complications for the procedure. This up-front disclosure to patients would be revolutionary because it is rarely practiced today. Without furnishing such data up front, we are not truly providing informed consent.[6]

Within the context of a patient's right to consent to or refuse treatment, an important question is whether care or treatment may be withheld or withdrawn from certain patients. The law in this area remains in a rather formative stage and varies from jurisdiction to jurisdiction. Generally speaking, care may be withheld if such care or treatment would be futile or would only delay the certainty of death. Withdrawal of care that has already been initiated is more problematic. In the absence of death, reliance may be given to living wills and durable powers of attorney for health care that under certain circumstances allow for care to be withdrawn. One or the other of these two types of advance directives is recognized by most states. In addition, some states have enacted health care surrogacy acts, which permit individuals other than the patient (usually the next of kin) in the absence of an advance directive to consent to or refuse medical care on behalf of a patient who lacks decisional capacity and may be terminally ill, in a persistent vegetative state, or suffering from an incurable or irreversible condition that will ultimately cause death. On the condition that they follow in detail the requirements set forth, these acts generally provide immunity from suit for health care providers who withdraw care from patients. In the absence of the death of a patient and in the absence of an executed advance directive, withdrawal of care may still be permissible on the order of a court of competent jurisdiction. Although resorting to courts may be costly and time-consuming and may generate media exposure, recourse to a court of law in an area that has not been previously clarified in a particular jurisdiction will provide the greatest amount of protection to the hospital, patient, family members, and other health care providers.

Another developing area of medical care–associated risk is maintenance of confidentiality. Examination of state law reveals an array of privacy protections, frequently with gaps and areas of uncertainty. Often, paper records are presumed, so the status of electronic data is unclear. Consequently a developing area of risk is the release of electronic, patient-level data to government regulators, business coalitions, insurers, and quality monitoring projects. A health care organization's marketing, information systems, and quality management staff may be insufficiently aware of confidentiality issues and therefore may release data with patient identifiers, such as name, address, and social security number, linked with personal information, such as diagnoses and procedures. All staff should be educated about the importance of maintaining patient confidentiality and should ensure that any electronic patient information released from their organization without specific patient consent is stripped of externally recognizable unique patient identifiers and is allowable under law.

Increasingly, health care institutions will be held accountable for the actions of providers on their staffs through the expansion of the corporate negligence theory, in which institutions have been held to have duties to properly maintain their facilities, to have available the necessary equipment, to hire, supervise, and retain competent and adequate provider staff, and to develop and implement policies and procedures that promote quality care. More recently, many courts have enhanced the corporate responsibility of health care institutions through the use of agency theory and a more expansive concept of corporate negligence, incorporating the duty to protect patients from medical staff negligence through the assumption of more control over the quality of care delivered within its facility and the duty to properly credential medical staff members.[7] The federal Health Care Quality Improvement Act of 1986 extended the corporate responsibility of health care organizations by requiring them to make reports to and check with the National Practitioner Data Bank maintained by the Department of Health and Human Services. Failure to check the data bank may subject an organization to the burden of being constructively informed of (i.e., deemed to have knowledge of) the information it would have received had it done so, with this information being admissible in medical malpractice actions.

Finally, important developing sources of medical liability risk for both managed care insurers and managed care providers are found in the areas of utilization review, benefit determination, and capitation reimbursement. The line between insuring care and directing care is rapidly evaporating. Insurers have exerted leverage through a variety of maneuvers, such as requiring second opinions, denying claims, and canceling provider agreements. In the trade-off of discounted fees for patient referrals, the best interests of patients may not always be given sufficient consideration. It is likely that this will be an area of increasing controversy between patients and health care organizations. Although verdicts against managed care organizations (MCOs) may serve as a wake-up call to insurers (e.g., *Fox v. Health Net of California*), hospitals and physicians have no immunity from being equally culpable if medical decisions are made on financial grounds.[8] Risk administrators of MCOs should be vigilant in searching for inappropriate financial incentives to limit benefit coverage and utilization of services.

RISK IDENTIFICATION
Importance of early risk identification

Risk of financial loss through legal liability presents itself to an organization in one of two ways. It can appear in the form of an individual patient event that, on inspection, carries with it a significant risk of liability. The actions that may result in liability in a specific case could be unique to that case or could be part of a general pattern of problem care or activity that can be referred to as *risk exposure*. Risk exposure can be identified even in the absence of a specific risk case related to it because a pattern of activity may be "risky" in terms of liability even though no specific patient injury related to that activity has yet occurred. The earliest recognition of both types of risk is crucial to a health care organization and as such is a fundamental risk management activity.[9]

The benefit of early risk detection is that it enables risk administrators to conduct the earliest possible investigation of any identified risk cases and to intervene against risk exposure with prevention strategies before any, or at least further, risk cases develop. Successful risk management departments do not wait to be sued before undertaking an investigation of a case and establishing a defense or settlement posture. Within a 2-year time (the period for most statutes of limitations pertaining to medical malpractice), valuable testimony and evidence about a risk case may be lost. All health care organizations should have a set of methods in place to obtain the earliest possible notice or warning of a specific risk case or risk exposure. Quick recognition of a risk case can enable attorneys and risk managers to record the facts of the case when the events are fresh in the minds of the participants and to counsel members of the organization on how to respond to the event. A particular opportunity exists to ensure that the organization delivers subsequent care and administrative services in an expedited and satisfactory way to minimize any patient and family anger over the incident. With proper methods in place, a risk management program should have knowledge of most risk cases long before service of process is made. More sophisticated risk management programs should have notice of 75% or more of the incidents that eventually result in lawsuits filed against the organization.

Methods

Most health care organizations use a variety of means to identify risk cases and risk exposure. In reactive case identification an organization assesses for risk in cases identified external to the organization as being problematic. In proactive case identification an organization initiates the identification of cases that are more likely than others to contain risk. Finally, in data-based performance monitoring an organization moves beyond the individual case as the basis of risk identification and focuses on performance monitoring as the means to uncover risk exposure. Risk administrators should use each of these three general approaches in their identification of risk cases and risk exposure. These approaches are complementary, for risk detected by one may be entirely missed by the others. Risk management programs that rely on only one or two of the approaches run the great danger of failing to recognize all identifiable risk cases and areas of risk exposure. However, some methods within each approach are more likely than others to detect risk, so risk administrators with limited resources should select those methods that are most cost-effective in their organizations. Once a case has been identified as a risk case it is managed according to the principles discussed in later sections on risk prioritization and risk control.

External case identification

Legal actions. The easiest and most instinctive approach to the identification of risk is the assessment of clinical events that come to an organization's attention in the ordinary conduct of its business. The clearest example of this is a lawsuit. Every organization is compelled to assess and respond to legal actions against it. Such an assessment usually entails a careful examination of the specific circumstances of the clinical case, including a peer review of the medical record. By definition, a lawsuit establishes a case as a risk case because even if an organization feels that the likelihood of loss from liability is small, the cost of preparing for litigation and the cost of the litigation itself amount to a significant financial loss even without the finding of liability.

Medical record requests. The review of medical records requested by attorneys is another method by which risk can be identified. The fact that an attorney is requesting the records indicates that the case is involved in some legal activity, and some organizations routinely review all such cases. However, reviewing all attorney-requested records, no matter how natural it may seem as a response, can be problematic. First, medical records may be requested for reasons other than suspicion of wrongdoing by providers or institution (e.g., disputes involving payment of claims or worker's compensation). In the absence of knowledge about the reason for the record request, detailed review of every requested record can be an unfocused activity that may produce a low yield of findings and hence may not be cost-effective. At the same time, a cursory review of requested records might produce reliable identification of those cases deserving more detailed review.

Patient complaints. Review of patient complaints is a good way to detect cases with risk and poor quality. Many organizations have a formalized mechanism for handling patient complaints. Often, descriptive statistics of patient complaints are generated routinely, such as a monthly compilation of all complaints by type, clinical/administrative area, and involved providers. A focused review of complaints that on their face suggest risk or poor quality can be a reasonably productive undertaking when attempting to discover problematic cases.

Billing disputes. Often, patients refuse to pay bills because they believe that the care received was substandard and therefore not deserving of payment. As a result, like patient complaints, review of billing disputes is an excellent method of identifying risk and quality deficiencies. However, the cost-effectiveness of reviewing billing disputes is compromised because some patients make accusations of poor quality simply to justify their refusal to pay for care. Even reviewing the records of only those billing disputes in which there is an accusation of poor quality would result in the review of many cases in which the accusation was knowingly unfounded. Detailed clinical review of all cases resulting in a billing dispute should probably be reserved for cases involving either large sums of money or significant accusations of substandard quality.

Internal case identification

Occurrence (incident) reporting. Rather than wait for a legal action, a record request, a patient complaint, or a billing dispute to initiate the process of risk identification, most organizations ask their staff to notify the risk management or legal department whenever an untoward or unusual incident occurs. This process is often referred to as *occurrence reporting.* Often a special form, commonly referred to as an *incident report form,* is provided for this purpose. This form indicates the minimum, specific information that must be provided about the incident (Appendix 19-4 is an exam-

ple). Although the information contained in incident reports is commonly protected from legal discovery by state law, some institutions request that reports of patient harm resulting from medical misdiagnoses, therapies, and procedures be reported verbally rather than in writing.

Incident reporting can be useful in identifying areas of risk exposure. Its usefulness as a method of identifying specific risk cases is limited, however, by a number of factors. The reliability of incident reporting can be compromised by the clinical staff's failure to appreciate a risk case or an area of risk exposure, uncertainty about what events to report, fear of getting involved, ignorance of how to file a report, and apathy. Risk administrators must recognize these barriers to reliable incident reporting and take active steps to eliminate them. Risk administrators should work hard to establish a trusting relationship with all physicians, who often see incident reporting as a nursing function and are wary of admitting the occurrence of adverse clinical outcomes. Physicians should be continually reassured that their communications will be held in the strictest confidence and that their statements will be protected from legal discovery. Physicians should be allowed to report incidents verbally, which should make reporting easier and somewhat alleviate their fear of reporting.

Progressive organizations actively cultivate a network of risk-sensitive and risk-educated clinical and administrative staff to facilitate incident reporting—a matrix of what can be called *risk management champions.* This effort is especially directed at having risk management champions in important areas of patient care and patient interaction. The theory underlying this matrix approach to information gathering is that within an organizational infrastructure (departments, units, sections, and ancillary services) there are certain essential intersections through which potential plaintiffs are likely to pass. Important intersections include a hospital's surgical recovery room, emergency room, intensive care unit, and patient relations department. In addition, the utilization management department, given its expanding role both in hospitals and in MCOs and the detailed data bases used, can be one of the best and most reliable sources of information about potential risk cases. Furthermore, the clinical departments of radiology and perhaps even more importantly pathology often are recipients of crucial information that medical malfeasance has occurred. Progressive risk administrators aggressively solicit and maintain a network of risk management champions located in important areas of patient contact.

A refinement of incident reporting is specified occurrence reporting. With this method, risk administrators specify a set of events that must be reported by staff. This approach takes incident reporting a step further to educate the staff about what specific events must be reported. Staffs are nonetheless still encouraged to report any unspecified event or possible area of risk exposure. Specified occurrences can be significant adverse outcomes of medical care (such as significant postoperative complications), accidents or mishaps in the provision of ancillary medical services (such as needle stick injuries), and non–medical-care-related accidents that occur in the institution (such as slip and fall injuries). Many of the specified occurrences are organization-specific based on the particular risk exposure history.

Random medical record review. Random medical record review was one of the first proactive approaches taken to uncover problem cases. It consisted of unfocused peer review of randomly selected medical records and for a time was a widespread "quality assurance" activity. However, because of its low yield of positive findings, it has now fallen into disfavor as a method of case identification in quality management. It never found use in risk management because the less frequent occurrence of risk, compared with quality deficiency, made this method cost-ineffective for risk identification. Nevertheless a program of random medical record review by providers can be beneficial in educating them about the wide variety of practice styles and approaches present among the staff and over time may lead to a group consensus on the identity of relatively weak performers.

Occurrence screening. In an effort to avoid the potential unreliability of occurrence reporting, many risk administrators identify groups of cases for screening review without depending on reporting from the staff. This method identifies groups of cases in which the yield of detailed review is likely to be higher than with routine review of cases identified through incident reporting (or its variant of specified occurrence reporting). The criteria used to identify cases for review are event based (e.g., all emergency room deaths) and can be specified as the result of a known institutional area of concern about clinical quality or risk (e.g., all coronary care unit deaths from cardiac dysrhythmias). The event that flags a case for review can on its face represent a quality problem (e.g., all medication errors), which may or may not create risk depending on the specific facts of the case, or can be nonspecific (generic). The latter events are generic in the sense that they are not particular to a certain type of case or a certain field of medical practice. Commonly used generic screening events, often called *generic indicators,* include unexpected in-patient death, unplanned postoperative return to the operating room during the same admission, and unplanned postdischarge readmission to the hospital within a specified time period (such as 14 days). The occurrence of a generic event does not imply a quality deficiency or the presence of risk in that case. That is, the fact that a patient recently discharged from the hospital needed to be readmitted within 14 days of discharge does not imply a quality or risk problem. Each case identified by a generic occurrence indicator must be carefully reviewed to determine whether any quality deficiency or risk is present.

Occurrence screening has found wider use in quality management than in risk management, where the approach to case evaluation is still based primarily on external case identification and occurrence reporting. Even in quality management, though, occurrence screening has met with mixed results as a method for uncovering quality deficiencies. Most cases that meet a criterion are not found by detailed peer review to have a quality deficiency, leading many to conclude that the expense involved in identifying the cases and then having them all reviewed by busy professionals is not justified by the relatively low yield of findings. The growing consensus is that most cases with quality problems and risk are not detected by the widely used generic screening criteria, and that of the cases that do meet screening criteria, after careful and time-consuming review most do not contain risk or a quality deficiency.

Case evaluation

Once a case has been identified as a possible risk case through one of the methods just discussed, the medical record is reviewed clinically. A physician who is an experienced reviewer of cases and who has an understanding of the potential sources of liability should first review the case. This physician should recognize the need to be completely objective in assessing for quality of care deficiencies, a risk event, and risk exposure. This physician may have a formal administrative role in the organization, such as the medical director overseeing the quality management activity. If the care is squarely within the field of the experienced physician reviewer, that review may be the only one necessary, especially if the physician finds no arguable evidence of quality deficiency or risk. In any cases of doubt the physician reviewer should refer the case to another physician for a second review. Risk administrators should realize that complex cases often involve care in more than one clinical field. Therefore it is imperative that all aspects of the patient's care be carefully reviewed. This may require a review by an internist or pediatrician (general or subspecialized) of surgical cases because all surgical cases involve at least some "medical" care.

Evaluation of clinical care by peer review usually includes determination of any culpability of the involved providers and institution. The results of case review can help assess the risk in that specific case, as well as identify organizational risk exposure or substandard providers. Unfortunately, peer case review as a method of identification of risk and quality deficiency is compromised by the understandable reluctance of clinicians conducting the review to criticize the care provided by colleagues with whom they may practice and socialize. This reluctance is magnified by the frequent defensive posture of clinicians regarding clinical care in general and the widespread fear that an adverse assessment will create interpersonal conflicts and be returned in kind when the roles of reviewer and reviewee are reversed in a future case. Moreover, clinicians often differ in the issues that they think are of paramount importance in a specific type of clinical case, which occasionally results in multiple reviewers of the same case focusing on different events and different aspects of care.[10] These factors create a bias against the recognition of poor quality and risk. This bias may be less problematic in a provider's assessment of system deficiencies, as opposed to provider-related deficiencies, but still could be considerable. Risk administrators must recognize the potential for this bias in provider assessments of individual cases and take decided action to minimize it. Initial review by a trained reviewer and the subsequent use of multiple reviewers can reduce the effects of this bias.

Many experienced risk administrators and clinical managers have had the experience of seeing two physicians come to dramatically different conclusions after reviewing the same case record.[11] Sometimes this discordance stems from a genuine disagreement over the proper clinical care for a specific problem. Occasionally, however, in complex cases two physicians (or other clinical providers) may focus on entirely different sequences of care and come to different conclusions about the case in question. Informed only that a suit has been filed by the family of a hospital patient who died unexpectedly as a result of postoperative sepsis, one reviewer may concentrate on postoperative wound care, whereas another may direct most attention to the question of whether the proper prophylactic antibiotics were given.

A second problem with peer review is that, even when practitioners agree on the specific care to be examined, they may not agree on the appropriate standard of care against which to judge the actual care provided. Indeed, some reviewers have difficulty articulating a standard of care at all and may appear to regard all but the most egregious care as acceptable.

A third problem with peer review is that often it is not thorough. Many practitioners, especially physicians, feel overwhelmed by the time demands of clinical practice and are unwilling to devote much energy to ancillary responsibilities like peer review. Moreover, physicians in particular are often hostile toward the legal process and may have a tendency to diminish the legitimacy of clinical issues identified through it. At times, physicians charged with conducting a case review only cursorily review the record, skimming physician notes and ignoring nonphysician notes all together. (Nonphysician notes are often of crucial importance in understanding the care in a case.) Laboratory data, radiology reports, and pathology data may receive only brief attention.

Risk administrators can use a number of approaches to increase the usefulness and reliability of peer review. One approach is to cultivate a network of willing, fair, and thorough case reviewers on which to rely. Risk administrators should continually reinforce the need for thoroughness and fairness in the evaluation of care by peers. Risk administrators should foster the development of this group with informal training and should demonstrate appreciation for the reviewers' efforts.

Another approach is to adopt a structured, explicit method of case review. Structured, explicit case review is designed to reduce the unreliability of case review through explicit identification of questionably problematic sequences of related care and the corresponding standards of care. Case review begins with a "foundation review" by an experienced case reviewer, preferably with a background in quality and risk management, who identifies the major processes of care and any issues associated with them. For each issue identified a written form is prepared that asks subsequent reviewers to explicitly state in writing the standard of care for all aspects of related care in which a problem was spotted and to assess the care against that standard. Reviewers can be asked to reference applicable published or organizational practice guidelines. Reviewers are given space to identify and comment on issues not identified during the foundation review.

A final technique is to ask more than one reviewer to perform a structured, explicit review. As stated earlier, it is often useful to have reviewers of different specialties assess a case, particularly if it is a surgical one.

Routine structured, explicit peer review of all cases identified as possible risk cases is too costly and is unnecessary. Although they are an important and indispensable source of information, most cases identified either internally or externally, with the exception of lawsuits, ultimately are not found to contain either risk or a quality deficiency. Therefore an experienced reviewer who can create a structured, explicit case review form if necessary should screen all identified cases first. Structured, explicit case review should be reserved for those cases that appear on initial screening review to have resulted in a serious adverse outcome and a measurable risk of liability.

Strengths and limitations of case identification methods

Although all case identification methods can reveal cases with a risk of loss, some are more useful than others in identifying cases with probable losses. For example, informal studies by hospitals indicate that incident reports are generally poor predictors of lawsuits, which perhaps is not surprising given the large number that are filed in organizations with aggressive risk management programs. However, incident reports remain useful sources of information that can reveal potential risk cases and areas of risk exposure. On the other hand, attorneys' requests for medical records, patient complaints, and billing disputes are factors associated with a higher probability that a lawsuit will follow.

However, case-by-case evaluation does not provide the entire picture of organization-wide clinical risk exposure and quality of care. It paints a picture only of those cases that were identified and is not a complete sample of all cases with risk, risk exposure, and quality problems. In particular, cases that result in a patient complaint are a biased sample of patients from which to make inferences about overall organizational clinical risk because not all patients are equally likely to register a complaint given the same care. Inferences about the general state of clinical risk exposure and quality of care should not be made solely from a review of cases flagged through external identification methods and by occurrence reporting.

Despite various strengths and limitations, all of the aforementioned methods for case identification should be used by a health care organization. Because no method is perfect, a case overlooked by one method may be detected by another. The use of a wide variety of case-specific risk identification methods can be enhanced but not replaced as a method of identifying risk exposure by data-based performance monitoring.

Data-based performance monitoring

Data-based performance monitoring is a method for assessing organizational quality of care and risk exposure that has developed recently and is growing in importance. It is a method for identifying areas of quality deficiency and risk exposure as opposed to specific risk cases. Its premise is that an indispensable way to assess organization-wide clinical risk exposure and quality of care is to monitor everyday activity, which has the benefit of avoiding the reporting bias encountered with many of the already discussed methods of risk identification. Data derived from continuous monitoring are used to either identify quality deficiencies and risk exposure or monitor an organization's response to corrective action taken to remedy previously identified quality and risk problems.

The initial purpose of data-based performance monitoring was the assessment of quality of care. Interinstitutional public release of data-based assessments of clinical performance began in earnest with the Health Care Financing Administration's report on hospital mortality rates in the care of selected Medicare patients. Subsequently, various projects have begun ongoing compilation and reporting of comparative hospital performance. Some are sponsored by state agencies and some by voluntary coalitions. Private comparative data are also available. A primary goal of these programs is to stimulate internal quality improvement through comparative performance assessments. Many organizations also gather clinical outcomes data internally and compare their results with published benchmarks or information obtained from outside data bases.

Risk administrators should be aware of all comparative performance data available on their organizations. Proper interpretation of comparative performance data requires a working familiarity with the strengths and limitations of clinical outcomes monitoring and provider performance profiling.[12,13] Heretofore, analysis of clinical outcomes data has been the province of clinical quality management staff, in no small part because of its substantial clinical and statistical content. However, comparative clinical outcomes data should be of great interest to risk administrators because they may point out areas of substandard hospital performance and consequently risk exposure. Hospitals with high adverse outcome rates (e.g., mortality) in specific areas of care should aggressively analyze their processes of care in an effort to reduce the rate of adverse outcomes to the lowest achievable levels. High adverse outcomes in specific clinical areas may indicate unusually high-risk exposure in those areas. Although performance data aggregated over hundreds and thousands of cases do not give information about a specific case, a pattern of persistently high severity-adjusted adverse outcomes in a specific clinical area may signal a deficiency in the quality of care, which may have already and could in the future lead to liability in specific cases. For example, a hospital with a high surgical mortality rate, after adjustment for the severity of illness of its patients before surgery, may have clinical problems that result in greater risk exposure than hospitals with lower rates. Comparative performance data afford risk administrators an excellent means of risk identification.

Performance data have a second important use. They are indispensable as a tool used inside an organization to continually assess its success in eliminating areas of known risk exposure. This process entails the design and continual measurement of risk indicators and is discussed later in the section on risk prevention.

RISK PRIORITIZATION

Risk administrators must prioritize identified risks to expend organizational resources in the most cost-effective way. Organizations usually have limited resources of personnel time and attention. Most risk administrators concentrate risk prevention efforts on events that are infrequent but of great consequence, on the one hand, and events that are of lesser import but of frequent occurrence.

A rare event of relatively minor consequence often can be handled directly without assembling a quality improvement team. Sometimes the source of risk exposure is suggested by a pattern of events or by data, and the challenge is first to discover the source of the problem. At times the cause of risk exposure is obvious, such as a physician office's failure to have all routine screening mammogram reports reviewed by a physician or nurse, and so preventive efforts can be focused immediately on faulty clinical or operational processes. The intensity of administrative risk prevention efforts should be tailored to the complexity of each individual risk. Clinical problems will usually require a multidisciplinary team, including physicians, with familiarity in all involved clinical and operational areas.

Risk prioritization is important in both assessing the proper response to a recognized risk case (risk control) and in allocating resources for risk prevention. For example, medication errors frequently occur in hospitals. These errors generally include delays in providing patients with prescribed doses of medicine. Identification of such delays is most frequently accomplished through incident reports but also may be identified through occurrence screening, random medical record review, or patient complaints. The total number of medication delays may then be divided between those delays that actually injured patients and those that had the potential to injure patients. Obviously, risk management personnel must give immediate attention to an error that has resulted in an injury to a patient. In determining the proper response to a medication delay, risk administrators should seek to answer the following questions: Did the error result in an injury to the patient? How significant was the injury? Was the injury of a temporary nature or of a more permanent nature? Has it compromised the care of the patient? Will the adverse effect on the patient extend beyond the current hospitalization? What was the reason for the delay? Was the delay the result of an individual error or a larger institutional problem? Is this an error that has occurred before, on a particular unit, or during a specific shift? Did a specific health care provider cause the error?

The differences between iatrogenic and custodial injuries serve as an illustration of the kind of considerations important in risk prioritization. The distinction between iatrogenic and custodial injuries is relevant when assessing these two types of injuries in terms of frequency and severity—the two major considerations in prioritizing the organization's response to specific risks. Frequency refers to how often the type of injury occurs, and severity refers to how likely it is that the type of injury will result in financial loss. Custodial injuries are estimated to account for as much as 75% to 85% of all patient injuries in hospitals and ambulatory care areas. However, measured in terms of financial loss, custodial injuries account for less than 25% of aggregate losses. Iatrogenic injuries, on the other hand, although less frequent than custodial injuries, account for approximately 75% to 85% of hospital losses.[14] The lesson to be learned from the distribution of risk between iatrogenic and custodial injuries is not that a concentrated effort should be directed only toward the prevention or management of iatrogenic claims; hospital risk management programs obviously must address both types of injuries. The lesson, rather, is that their relative risks must be carefully evaluated to achieve a balanced approach in preventing and managing both types of injuries.

Identification of major risks

What risks should be considered major risks? For most organizations a list of major risks can be found in their reporting requirements under excess liability policies. For hospitals, such mandatory reporting is typically required in the event of the following injuries to a patient: unexpected death; brain damage; neurological deficit, nerve damage, or paralysis; loss of limb; or failure to diagnose a condition that results in a continuous course of treatment. In addition to the aforementioned events, a catch-all provision is often included that requires reporting of any claim or medical incident the value of which is equivalent to a certain percentage (e.g., 50%) of the self-insured retention limits. This list is not exhaustive, but if a hospital risk management program is constrained because of financial or staffing limitations, it can serve as a priority list that fulfills most needs.

Key specific risks

Risk management programs of large health care organizations may find it necessary to use a more detailed list of key specific risks. Such a list may be compiled based on the individual ex-

perience of that organization. Using a hospital as an example, a typical list includes the following major headings: medication error, patient fall, equipment related, security related, blood related, surgery related, anesthesia related, food related, patient induced, policy related, radiology related, medical record related, laboratory related, intravenous line related, newborn related, maternal related, and physician related. Box 19-1 contains a representative sample of subcategories for each of the aforementioned key specific risks. The categorization of risks associated with a specific hospital will, of course, vary depending on the risk experience of that hospital.

RISK CONTROL

Risk control is the process of managing a recognized risk case to minimize the potential for loss. Most risk administrators find their time primarily directed toward risk control, rather than risk prevention, for an obvious reason: A lawsuit represents an actual loss. Even if successfully defended, a lawsuit will result in expenditures for its defense, primarily in terms of fees for legal counsel and expert witnesses. Tangentially there also may be an increase in insurance premiums or in the organization's deductible. Consequently, risk administrators find a greater part of their time allocated to risk control than to risk prevention.

Completing the initial investigation

On identification of a risk case an initial investigation is undertaken. This investigation has two purposes—the early assessment of probability and value of loss and the identification of relevant sources of information. The essential steps necessary to complete these objectives are (1) review of the medical record; (2) interview of the potential defendants for whom the organization provides insurance coverage; (3) identification, cataloging, and collection of physical evidence that may be relevant and could otherwise be lost or misplaced (e.g., monitor tracings, temporary logs, and policy and procedures); (4) identification of witnesses who may have information concerning the incident and who might have to be interviewed at a later time because of time constraints; and (5) collection of medical bills. This five-step initial investigation is not intended to serve as an extensive investigation or to replace the more thorough investigation conducted upon service of process. It is only a preliminary action to determine the essential facts of the case and to identify which personnel have personal information about the incident.

With this information in hand, risk managers and attorneys select and prioritize those incidents that warrant further investigation. This process fulfills the essential risk control functions of gathering and assessing information about potential losses and prioritizing time and efforts toward investigation of probable losses.

Predicting the potential plaintiff

An important part of identifying those risk cases likely to result in loss is predicting which patients will bring a lawsuit.

BOX 19-1. OPERATIONAL SUBCATEGORIES OF KEY HOSPITAL RISKS

Medication error

Adverse reaction
Wrong route
Wrong patient
Pharmacy error
Medication not given
Wrong medication given
Medication duplicated
Medication not ordered
Medication not given at correct
    time
Transcription error
Medication given despite hold
    order
Wrong dosage

Patient falls

Caused by a liquid or substance on
    floor
Fall from bed (siderails up? siderails
    down? position of siderails
    unknown?)
Fall in bathroom
Fall in room
Fall outside of room
Fall off table or equipment
Fall in elevator
Fall from crutches or walker
Fall outside of building
Fall from chair or wheelchair
Near fall with assistance

Equipment related

Failure of life support or monitor
Equipment missing or unavailable
Injury related to medical device

Security related

Personal property damage
Personal property disappeared
Injury resulting from conduct of
    another patient

Blood related

Wrong blood
Transfusion reaction
Delay in transfusion

Surgery related

Incorrect sponge count
Incorrect surgical instrument
    count
Surgical instrument broken
Loss of pathology specimen
Unplanned return to surgery
Removal of retained foreign
    body
Unplanned return after
    readmission

Anesthesia related

Respiratory distress reaction
Related to intubation or related to
    extubation

Food related

Poisoning
Foreign body
Improper diet
NPO order violated
Burns from foods or liquids

Patient induced

Attempted suicide
Self-mutilation
Refusal to consent to treatment
Returned late from approved pass
Discharge against medical
    advice
In possession of drugs, alcohol,
    or weapon

Policy related

Procedural error
Violation of physician order
Performance of wrong procedure
Autopsy signed with no autopsy
    performed

Laboratory related

Transport delay
Identification problem
Loss or damage of laboratory
    specimen
Incorrect reading

Intravenous line related

Infiltration
Wrong solution
Contaminated or expired solution
Line disconnected
Incorrect timing
Pump malfunction
Incorrect rate
Central line complication

Newborn related

Apgar scores of less than 3 at
    1 minute
Apgar scores of less than 7 at
    7 minutes
Skull fracture
Resuscitation
Transfer from in-house nursery to
    special-care nursery
Meconium aspiration

Maternal related

Maternal injury from obstetrical
    treatment
Blood loss

Physician related

Failure to diagnose
Unexpected death
Brain damage resulting from treat-
    ment
Neurological deficit or nerve injury
    resulting from treatment
Injury relating to resident supervision
Adverse reaction
Delay in response

Radiology related

Reaction to contrast dye
Unmonitored cardiac or respiratory
    arrest
Disappearance of films

Medical records related

Orders not charted
Consent not signed
Disappearance of record

As varied as plaintiffs may be, many of them share certain common characteristics. The following factors often determine which patients are most likely to sue a health care organization.

Poor or unexpected results. The most reliable identifying characteristic of the potential plaintiff is that he or she has suffered an unsatisfactory outcome as a result of or despite medical care. The outcome may be direct harm (e.g., a postsurgical complication) or a result that, although not harmful per se, is less than that expected after the care (e.g., unsatisfactory outcome of cosmetic surgery). A poor or unexpected result from medical care does not mean, of course, that any medical malfeasance has occurred.

Seriousness of injury. Another characteristic of the potential plaintiff is that the injury sustained is permanent and serious, involving death, disability, or disfigurement. Disability may be manifested in various ways; at a minimum, it usually must be sufficient to have resulted in lost wages. The economics of pursuing a legal claim and the impact of medical malpractice reforms have served to impose a modicum of self-regulation and limitation on medical malpractice claims, reducing claims for minor injury and claims that might be frivolous.

Weak physician-patient relationship. A third trait of the potential plaintiff is the absence of a strong relationship with his or her physician. The single greatest deterrent to litigation remains a strong physician-patient relationship rich with positive interactions and communication. A recent study analyzing the demographics and risk of malpractice concludes that a physician's gender, specialty, and age affect the risk of a suit. Of note, male physicians were three times as likely to be in a high claims group as female physicians. The investigators surmised that female physicians may interact more effectively with patients than their male colleagues.[15]

Uncertain financial future. Many plaintiffs are individuals who face an uncertain financial future. They are often unable to withstand the financial burden of medical expenses attendant with a poor or unexpected result. Therefore potential plaintiffs are frequently unemployed, underemployed, recently retired, single or recently divorced, or students.

Strong support group. The last trait frequently found among potential plaintiffs is the presence of a strong support group, especially if there are family members who are directly or indirectly associated with medicine or law. As socially acceptable as litigation may be in the United States, persevering through the process of selecting an attorney and initiating legal action still requires a certain degree of motivation and strength, which can be buttressed by supportive family and friends.

In preparing themselves to initiate a lawsuit, potential plaintiffs commonly use similar phrases, with which most risk managers quickly become familiar. Many potential plaintiffs, instead of making a direct threat to sue, often use expressions such as "I want to make sure that this never happens to another patient," "I want to teach you a lesson," and "I am not interested in the money, it's the principle."

Conducting investigations

In conducting investigations, risk administrators need to be aware of legally imposed limits and restrictions. For example, some courts have ruled that risk administrators may not interview subsequent caregivers of an injured patient. Some courts have extended this theory to prohibit discussions even with members of a hospital's house staff and nursing staff. The rationale is that such ex parte discussions violate the sanctity of the physician-patient relationship and are prohibited under physician-patient privilege statutes.[16] A second rationale offered is that a physician has a fiduciary duty to refrain from assisting his or her patient's adversary.

Although the aforementioned rationales may be persuasive regarding subsequent providers who care for the patient and are not used by the health care organization, application of a rule that bars an organization from interviewing employees creates a number of practical problems. Such a restriction would prevent the organization from being able to respond to a complaint, develop litigation strategy, provide accurate or complete responses to discovery requests, prepare employees adequately for depositions or trial, depose experts adequately, and prepare the best presentation at trial.

Of equal concern to an attorney is the protection of investigative reports and interviews from disclosure. There are two avenues by which such protection may be ensured. A recognized principle is that such information constitutes "work product." The work product principle protects an attorney's representation of his or her client's interest and requires that good cause be shown before a court will allow discovery of an attorney's preparation of the client's case. Generally, work product includes information prepared by an attorney or his or her representative (e.g., a risk manager) in anticipation of litigation. Such information includes personal knowledge and legal theories, as well as statements of witnesses. This principle, though, does not necessarily protect information about the location of such information and the names and addresses of witnesses. In applying this principle to the protection of reports and interviews made by attorneys and risk managers, care should be taken to follow the general rules of the work product principle. Disclosure of such information to a third party may result in loss of ability to assert the principle to defeat discovery requests by the other party. If information is gathered by nonattorney risk administrators, the information should be forwarded to the attorney, sometimes with the inclusion of a statement that it is being sent to assist the attorney in contemplated litigation.

A second means of protecting such information from discovery by the other party may be available under state statutes that prohibit disclosure of information used internally to improve patient care or to reduce morbidity and mortality. Precise adherence to the rules set forth in a statute usually is critical to protect the information from disclosure. Some statutes may address only hospitals and have not been updated to incorporate HMOs. Generally, information is protected when used and discussed within recognized health care organization committees for quality improvement purposes.

Notifying insurance carriers

Risk administrators have the responsibility to properly notify an insurance carrier of a claim or possible claim that exposes its coverage. Reference to the exact wording of the insurance policy, of course, is critical as to the necessary timing and scope of notification. Generally, the notice requirement is phrased in one of two ways: A policy may require that the insured give the carrier "immediate notice of a lawsuit" or may require notice "when it appears that an occurrence is likely to involve indemnity" under the policy. The second type of notice language can be particularly problematic for a health care organization because it is vulnerable to a subjective interpretation as to when an occurrence is "likely to involve indemnity." The phrase may be interpreted from both an objective and a subjective standard. The controlling rule in insurance law is that if the language of an insurance policy is ambiguous or otherwise susceptible to more than one reasonable interpretation, it is to be construed in favor of the insured. Notwithstanding this rule, insureds may wish to be cautious and provide notification at the earliest possible moment that it appears a carrier's insurance policy may be exposed.

Selecting defense counsel

The skills expected of a litigator are likely to be different from those of a corporate attorney. Of course, competency, truthfulness, honesty, and responsiveness are important traits in both, as well as the ability to communicate effectively with the client. On the other hand, a certain aggressiveness that might be expected of a litigator might be inappropriate in a corporate attorney. Undoubtedly, one of the greatest assets of a litigator is that he or she possesses the capabilities to take a case to trial, advocate the position of the defendant(s), and, of course, obtain a favorable verdict.

As with the selection of any other consultants, in selecting defense counsel a health care organization would do well to keep in mind the following:

1. Selection should not be made solely on the basis of price.
2. Expectations should be made clear to the defense counsel from the outset.
3. A new defense counsel, regardless of his or her reputation, should always be started on a small project or a single case to ensure that a positive working relationship will result.

4. The defense counsel should be allowed reasonable professional latitude to do his or her best job, although giving defense counsel freedom of action does not eliminate the organization's responsibility to monitor defense counsel's progress.
5. The results achieved by defense counsel should be fairly evaluated because both the organization and defense counsel deserve honest feedback from each other.

Assisting defense counsel

A medical malpractice action may be costly to an organization, but it can be extraordinarily disturbing to a health care provider named as a defendant. Generally speaking, physicians and nurses are unaccustomed to the confrontation and adversity that characterize the litigation process. They may be frightened and intimidated by the procedures that may appear to them to be geared more toward proving them culpable than determining what actually happened.

In the discovery or fact-finding stage of the litigation proceeding, risk administrators have a dual role. Both roles reduce the cost of use of outside litigation counsel and the possibility of loss to an adverse verdict or disadvantageous settlement. Risk administrators should assist outside defense counsel in discovery. This task may be easy or difficult, depending on the thoroughness with which the initial investigation was conducted. Equally important, risk administrators should help guide the defendant through the litigation process.

Clarification of expectations. The first step in assisting legal counsel is to express the expectations of the organization's risk administrators about how defense counsel will handle the claim. Expectations are best clarified in advance and with a single attorney charged with managing the case. It is important that direction be given to defense counsel in the following five areas: assignment of file, initial review, conduct of discovery, conduct of trial, and arrangement for billing.

If the relationship involves multiple claims, the defense firm and risk administrator should mutually designate an attorney who will have overall responsibility for supervising the various cases referred to that firm. If because of a conflict or another reason the defense firm to which a case has been sent is unable to represent the organization, this fact should be communicated immediately to the organization by telephone and the file should be returned promptly. As to the assignment of a case to a particular attorney, some organizations defer to the supervising attorney at the defense firm. Conversely, some risk administrators prefer matching particular cases to the skills, styles, or personalities of particular attorneys and will retain the right to make the selection. An assignment letter should include the name of the risk administrator working on the file. If a defense attorney other than the one selected to handle the case works on the case, this fact should be communicated to the organization.

As soon as possible after a claim is assigned to a defense firm, the primary defense attorney should send an acknowledgment, as well as his or her assessment of the case, to the risk administrator. This review should include a summary of the pertinent facts revealed to date, a review of medical records, a recitation of the issues presented in the complaint, a mention of areas that will require additional research and investigation, and, if there is sufficient information available, a statement of opinion as to liability, verdict potential, and settlement value.

Any motions filed on behalf of the organization should be limited to meaningful issues and receive prior approval from the risk administrator. Any requests by the defense attorney to interview employees of the organization or to retain outside experts should also receive prior approval from the risk administrator. The risk administrator should obtain a status report from the defense attorney at least twice a year.

Defense attorney requests for approval of travel expenditures should be made in writing and should include the purpose of the trip; the travel destination; the time period required to complete the work; the exact means and the cost of travel; the specific identification, location, and cost of lodgings; and the cost of car rental, if required. In any event reimbursement should always be supported by receipts. The billing cycle also should be clearly understood, and the hourly fees of all defense attorneys working on the case should be provided in writing. Changes in those fees should not be made without the approval of the risk administrator. To enable evaluation of the charge, the bill should provide details of the legal services rendered, including (1) the date of service, (2) a clear description of the service rendered, (3) the actual time expended, and (4) the identity of the attorney who rendered the service. Charges for review of files should be kept at a minimum, and interoffice conferences between attorneys of the defense firm should be discouraged or prohibited. Finally, the defense firm should be informed of which legal expenses will not be reimbursed. Such items might include interoffice conferences, time spent filing papers with the court, secretarial time, copying charges, and unsupported charges for travel.

Distribution of responsibilities. The manner in which the risk administrator and the primary defense attorney share responsibilities during discovery should be clear to both. The risk administrator should help compile answers to interrogatories, if he or she is not entirely responsible for their completion. It is cost-effective for risk administrators to undertake as much of this task as possible. Similarly, risk administrators should be responsible for the production of documents, such as medical records, billing statements, policy and procedure manuals, incident reports, photographs, laboratory reports, logs, scheduling reports, and other physical evidence.

In most risk management programs, risk administrators automatically assume primary responsibility for drafting answers and producing documents. However, they are probably not as involved as they should be in preparing witnesses for depositions. This task is too often left to defense counsel. As with drafting answers to interrogatories and producing documents, witness preparation should be a shared responsibility between defense counsel and the risk administrator.

A common complaint of deponents is that they have not been adequately prepared. Unfortunately, at times defense counsel may not have or may not take the time to prepare each witness adequately. To avoid this situation, risk administrators should be trained and ready to prepare witnesses. The two important aspects of this preparation are to provide the general rules of demeanor and conduct of a witness in a deposition and to review in detail the care and treatment rendered by the deponent, relying in particular on office or hospital records.

Some organizations have shown prospective deponents videotapes of staged depositions. Such tapes are commercially available. In addition, various articles and monographs have been written on the subject. In their excellent book, *Preventing Malpractice. The Co-Active Solution,* Dr. Thomas Leaman and attorney James Saxton provide 10 rules for deposition preparation (Box 19-2).[17] Although the rules are directed to physicians, they are equally applicable to other health care providers or for that matter to any person who is required to give a deposition.

RECENT DEVELOPMENT: USE OF ALTERNATIVE DISPUTE RESOLUTION

Alternative dispute resolution has been used successfully in a variety of settings to bring people to agreement. Now, physicians and hospitals are adapting these same methods of reconciling differences to medical malpractice cases to avoid the hassle and expense associated with trial preparation. The two forms of alternative dispute resolution with which most people are familiar are mediation and arbitration. Mediation is the process whereby a neutral third party assists parties in a dispute to reach a voluntary settlement of their differences. In arbitration a neutral third party hears the evidence and arguments of each party and then renders a final and generally binding decision.

Rush-Presbyterian-St. Luke's Medical Center in Chicago has developed an interesting model for the use of mediation in medical malpractice litigation. In 1995 it began the first hospital-based mediation program in Illinois and one of the first in the country in response to the excessive costs, adversarial nature, and unpredictable outcomes associated with jury trials in Cook County. The program was created in an effort to resolve disputes in a rational and reasoned manner and as an alternative to trials by juries, which are susceptible to emotional appeals.

One of the unique features of the Rush model is the use of co-mediators. These individuals are drawn from the ranks of the most prominent and active trial attorneys from both the

---

BOX 19-2. **TEN RULES FOR THE PHYSICIAN'S DEPOSITION**

1. The physician must know the records intimately—office records, hospital charts, any statements by other health care professionals, medical literature, and alternative treatments.
2. The physician must listen to the question carefully and respond only when he or she understands it completely. If the physician does not understand it, then the attorney must be asked to rephrase it. Never help to rephrase it or suggest a more appropriate question.
3. The physician should respond thoroughly, but directly and to the point, and not tell stories, ramble, digress, or volunteer information. On certain topics one may need to be more comprehensive if appropriate to the theme of the defense.
4. The physician should use the medical record. If the record is in order, it can be the best defense tool. For example, the plaintiff's attorney may describe the client's level of pain and suffering. If the physician's records do not confirm this, the chart can be used to demonstrate it.
5. The theatrics of the plaintiff's attorney should be disregarded. Sometimes the attorney will act surprised and shocked by a response, use body language, or repeat certain phrases in an attempt to irritate the defendant. Such theatrics are intended to make the physician uncomfortable and unsure of the response.

    At times the plaintiff and defense attorneys may resort to arguing with each other. It is important for the physician not to misinterpret the defense attorney's anger to mean that something has gone wrong or that there is a problem with the responses. Such battles may be a technique for the defense attorney to maintain control of the deposition. If such tactics are to be used, they should be discussed with the physician before the deposition. Their use should also be minimal; professional courtesy is an important part of legal ethics.
6. The physician should be consistent. If the physician does not give the desired response to a question from the plaintiff's attorney, the attorney may ask the question over and over, each time phrasing it a bit differently, looking for an inconsistent response. The physician should remember that the plaintiff's attorney has been working on these questions for weeks before the deposition. The physician's failure to give the anticipated response can be devastating; the attorney will work hard to get the needed response or at least neutralize the damage from an unfavorable, unanticipated response.
7. The physician should wait for the next question after finishing a response. Often the plaintiff's attorney will pause, using body language to urge the physician to say more. The physician should not try to fill the void, but should simply wait patiently for the next question.
8. The physician should be extremely cautious in responding to leading questions, such as "Is it a fair statement . . .," "Let me summarize your testimony as follows . . .," and "Doctor, just so I understand what you are saying. . . ." Statements like these mean the plaintiff's attorney is about to reinterpret the physician's testimony. Usually there is a slight twist to that interpretation, which the attorney is hoping to have affirmed. The physician should remember that fairness has nothing to do with this process; the interpretation may not correctly reflect what was said. The physician should agree only with those statements with which he or she is comfortable. If the physician disagrees, then he or she must simply say so, and repeat the previous response.
9. The physician should be careful of conversation during breaks. Although inappropriate, the plaintiff's attorney may try to engage the physician in conversation. This could have an impact on the case. A deposition is not the time for social niceties. Breaks should be used to relax and regain composure. One must be on guard from arrival at the deposition until departure.
10. The physician should be courteous, professional, firm, and credible. Demeanor should be professional and serious, for a physician's professional ability has been challenged. As such, a deposition is neither the time nor the place for chitchat and humor. However, under no circumstances should a physician be offensive, insulting, or argumentative.

From T. Leaman & J. Saxton, *Preventing Malpractice: The Co-Active Solution* 68-70 (Plenum, New York 1993).

---

plaintiff and defense bar. They undergo mediation training offered by the medical center in association with local law schools. As an indication of the fairness and neutrality of that training, the Rush program allows the plaintiff to pick both of the mediators. Plaintiffs agree to mediation when it is offered largely because they can see the benefits of a fast, less expensive resolution.

The mediation process begins with both parties voluntarily agreeing to participate in the program. Premediation submissions, including a statement of the facts, description of the injury, claim of special damages, and past and future expenses, are exchanged. A neutral location is selected in which the mediation will take place. To once again enhance the neutrality of the process, the mediation proceedings generally are held in a location away from the hospital.

The experiment in the use of alternative dispute resolution by Rush-Presbyterian-St. Luke's Medical Center these last 4 years has been positive. An average of 12 cases have been submitted to the Rush program each year, with close to 90% of the cases being resolved, many on the same day of the mediation. The operational costs of the mediations have been nominal and, in the event a lawsuit has been resolved, there have been substantial savings through the elimination of additional defense costs.[18]

RISK PREVENTION

Effective risk prevention depends on the reliable recognition of risk exposure, determination of its causes, implementation of corrective action, and continual monitoring of risk indicators to determine if risk exposure resolves. This process requires close and active cooperation of risk administrators and clinical managers.

Assessing risk exposure

Risk exposure is identified either by examination of the facts of an individual case, which could reveal a continuing source of liability risk, or from examination of data, which can be trend data of a particular risk indicator or clinical performance data. Once risk exposure is identified, quantitative measures, or indicators, reflective of that exposure should be developed to enable risk administrators to determine the presence of similar risk in other areas of the organization and to be used as a measuring stick to gauge the success of interventional efforts. Literally hundreds of indicators can be measured, so risk administrators must identify a manageable number that will yield the required information.

Indicators are usually rates of selected events, such as hospital falls, medication errors, and adverse clinical outcomes. They may be measured in targeted areas or throughout the entire organization. Data for indicators can be obtained from a wide variety of sources in an organization. Unique data bases are often found in claims and billing (whose data bases typically contain patient encounter data consisting of at least ICD-9-CM codes, visit status, care delivered, and patient disposition), utilization management (often a rich source of data), the pharmacy, medical staff offices (including the credentialing data base), the patient relations department (which might have a detailed data base of patient complaints and corrective actions), and quality management (which should have all available clinical performance data). The risk administrator should have in his or her own department data on lawsuits, risk cases, incident reports, and specified occurrence reports and screening.

As an example, if a hospital risk administrator identifies falls by patients, staff, and visitors as a source of risk exposure, he or she might determine that much of the problem relates to travel on floors that are wet from cleaning. Further analysis may lead to the identification of a number of interventions that would serve to minimize or eliminate travel on wet floors. Interventions might include using large yellow plastic warning signs placed six feet apart around the wet area, confining routine floor cleaning to evenings (after visiting hours), and cleaning no more than 50% of the width of a walkway at one time. Appropriate indicators for monitoring risk exposure could include the monthly rates of a series of measurements based on routine, random walk-around inspections, such as the percentage of just-mopped floors without proper warning signs, the percentage of floors actually cleaned during visiting hours, and the percentage of floor

cleanings in which more than half the hallway was mopped. These three represent "process" indicators that reflect the success in executing the interventions. Of course, if the hypothesis that these three interventions will be effective in reducing the rate of falls is wrong, then successful implementation of the interventions will have no effect on the rate of falls. Therefore it is crucial to include measurement of an "outcome" indicator that will provide information about whether the problem was ameliorated by the interventions. A useful outcome indicator would be the monthly number of falls by patients, staff, and visitors. Outcome indicators, as opposed to process indicators, should be reflective of the level of risk exposure and thus should be the measure of success of any risk prevention effort.

Clinical quality indicators are often but not always risk indicators. Clinical risk indicators are limited to those aspects of medical care that present risk. Quality management, however, encompasses the improvement of medical care that is not considered to present any legal risk. For example, a hospital with the lowest rate of surgical complications in town may seek to lower it even further through an aggressive quality improvement project. If no risk exposure in that area had been identified, the indicators developed to monitor surgical complications would be clinical quality indicators but not clinical risk indicators. Similarly, not all risk indicators are clinical quality indicators. An institution may identify risk exposure because of the failure of its medical staff to consistently obtain proper written informed consent before certain procedures, as required by the staff bylaws. The indicator of percentage of procedures with written informed consent forms completed beforehand would be useful to assess risk in this situation. However, failure of the physician to obtain written informed consent to a procedure is a legal rather than a medical issue, so an indicator of this failure would be an indicator of legal risk but not of clinical quality.

Risk indicators should be valid reflections of the clinical or operational activity they are intended to measure. They should be free from measurement bias, and each measured event should be reliably observed. Poorly crafted risk indicators prevent the accurate recognition of risk exposure and the understanding of its causes and doom to failure many risk avoidance efforts.

Defining performance expectations

The next step in risk reduction is to establish for each indicator a target level that will be used as the measure of success in risk reduction. For example, a project to reduce medication errors could establish a target of a 50% reduction in errors over 3 months, and a rate in subsequent months of no higher than 10 incidents per month throughout the organization. These targets are the standards against which the success of the project should be measured, and if the indicator target rate is not met, further corrective action is warranted. Many risk reduction and quality improvement projects ultimately fail despite initial promise because of inadequate long-term monitoring of the risk exposure and the lack of a predetermined commitment to further action if expected results are not achieved.

Monitoring the results of action is so important that the necessary indicators and their expected values over time should be established before any action is taken. The measuring sticks (the indicators) and the criteria for success (the expected values) should be established before taking action so that the determination of whether an intervention is successful will not be biased by the personal stakes acquired by staff in the development and implementation of the corrective action plan.

In particularly troublesome areas, performance expectations can be formalized and reinforced through operational protocols and clinical practice guidelines. These guides are written formal expressions of courses of action expected in defined circumstances. Classic examples are nursing protocols for initiating blood transfusions and physician practice guidelines for pacemaker insertion. Care must be taken, however, to avoid the interpreting of clinical practice guidelines as strictly defined standards of care. Nevertheless, protocols and guidelines, when properly and carefully designed, can be an effective way of standardizing selected features of operations and clinical care and reducing risk exposure. Adherence to them can be measured through indicators.

Taking specific action to reduce risk

Risk prevention depends on the accurate identification of those clinical and operational processes in need of corrective efforts. In their efforts to diagnose the causes of risk exposure, risk administrators should adopt a structured problem-solving technique predicated on an organized approach to identifying all of the clinical and operational processes that affect the clinical area with risk exposure. This approach may include the construction of process flow diagrams and cause-and-effect diagrams. Input should be obtained from staff with daily working knowledge of each relevant clinical and operational process.

Once an operational or clinical process has been identified as a problem, corrective interventions should be crafted, and each step necessary for their successful implementation should be detailed in a written "corrective action" plan. The plan's formulation should be made with multidisciplinary input, and specific responsibilities and times for completion of each task should be specified. Successful implementation of a corrective action plan will often depend on widespread, continual staff education and committed involvement of managers in all relevant clinical and operational departments.

Adopting general risk avoidance strategies

Risk administrators should develop a general risk avoidance plan that includes organization-specific strategies. Two universally important components deserve specific mention. The first is to provide regular general risk management education to all staff. This program need not go into detail about legal principles but should keep all staff—clinical and nonclinical—aware of the constant need to avoid risk and report it whenever discovered. This education is particularly important for physicians, given the greater risk exposure encountered in their work. Periodic (e.g., annual) seminars should review the essentials of risk prevention in clinical practice, stressing the crucial elements of good communication and proper medical record keeping. The presentation of recent organizational and comparative trend data on risk indicators can be an effective tool to stimulate physician interest and maintain attention.

A second important component of a risk avoidance plan is to strengthen the medical staff credentialing criteria and procedures. Criteria for good standing should be far beyond mere possession of current licensure and malpractice insurance. Data on quality of care, risk cases, patient complaints, and particularly the clinical outcomes of the physician's care (e.g., surgical mortality and complication rates) should play a role. It is becoming increasingly perilous for health care organizations to ignore such data in their credentialing process. In their review of the impact of performance data on medical practice, physicians Topol and Califf comment that:

The problem of too many physicians [doing procedures, many of whom perform too few each year to achieve competency,] is compounded by the lack of adequate training for many, who too frequently derive their "training" by attendance at a demonstration course. Careful consideration should be given to the criteria for privileges of individual physicians. Low-volume physicians whose patients have poor outcomes should be prohibited from doing procedures. The minimum number of cases per year should be strictly enforced. [For example,] the Joint American College of Cardiology and American Heart Association Task Force recommends that cardiac surgeons do at least 100 bypass operations per year, but in a review of the data now available in New York and Pennsylvania, more than one third of cardiac surgeons did not meet this criterion. Volume is not the only issue; guidelines are necessary for the actions that should be triggered when indicators of poor-quality medicine are evident. Indeed, availability of outcome data would likely alter the behavior of low-volume or poor-outcome practitioners. However, if these measures are unsuccessful, strategies ranging from admonitory communication to frank termination of procedural privileges could be used.[19]

Continually reassessing risk exposure: the cycle of continuous risk reduction

Risk reduction is a continuous cyclical process (Fig. 19-1). The first step of the cycle is the assessment of risk, which includes the identification of risk exposure and its measurement through risk indicators. In doing this step, an organization is determining its degree of exposure to a certain risk, which is referred to as *point A* in the diagram. The second step is the creation of expectations of where the level of risk exposure should fall to over time; in this step the organization determines its risk reduction goal (referred to as *point B*). The

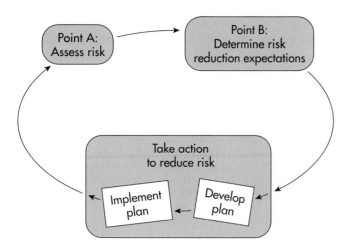

Fig. 19-1. Cycle of continuous risk reduction.

third and final step is taking action to reduce the risk exposure, that is, to reduce risk exposure from point A to point B. This step requires the development of a corrective action plan and its successful implementation. Once action is taken, the steps of the cycle are repeated as necessary. Risk exposure is reassessed to gauge the success of the intervention and the need for further action. If risk reduction expectations are not met, they are revised as appropriate and further action is taken. Failure to monitor known risk exposure, especially once improvement begins, can allow attention and resources to be diverted to other projects and lead to the ultimate failure of an initially successful intervention.

RISK FINANCING

A health care organization finances the risk of loss from liability in one of two ways. It may retain the risk, or it may seek to shift or transfer the risk.[20]

Retaining risk

The use of internal funds to pay losses is referred to as *loss retention* or *retaining risk*. Under this arrangement, a health care organization may either fund or not fund the cumulative value of the risks retained. Of course, the more fiscally responsible approach is to fund the losses in a self-insurance program by which a trust fund is established and the organization makes annual contributions according to actuarial studies as to the estimated value of losses retained. A self-insurance program is most appropriate when a hospital (1) wishes to achieve an advantageous cash flow, (2) has the capacity to satisfy actuarial funding requirements, (3) possesses the sophistication to set appropriate reserves, (4) is able to maintain a reasonably low level of self-retention or deductible, and (5) finds it otherwise impossible or impractical to transfer the risk.

On occasion an organization that has a fully funded self-insurance program, nevertheless, may elect to assume a risk

for a type of loss not covered under the self-insurance program if insurance for such a risk is either unavailable or the price is prohibitive. The organization, despite accepting responsibility for it, may neglect to fund it. In the event a loss does materialize, the organization would have to fund it from general operating funds. An alternative is to fund a loss reserve or consider alternative approaches to self-insurance.

Self-insurance programs pose some inherent problems for the institution. Pressures to achieve short-term financial objectives can jeopardize long-term financial viability of the self-insurance program. For example, some institutions limit the funding of a self-insurance fund to actual lawsuits as opposed to probable claims. This approach eventually could result in an inadequate surplus in the trust fund. A similar tendency is for organizations to accept coverage of losses in cases in which the losses are less clear or more unpredictable. Such losses would more prudently be either transferred or covered under a commercial insurance policy. Yet another disadvantage of a self-insurance program is the inability to counteract pressures by excess carriers to increase the self-insured retention limits.[21]

Other insurance arrangements might serve as alternatives to developing a self-insured retention program. These arrangements include insurance purchasing groups, risk retention groups, and offshore captive insurance companies.[22] However, these alternative structures may be more expensive and time-consuming to implement and operate than a self-insured trust and may be more applicable to a multihospital system or a physician hospital organization as opposed to a single hospital entity.

Transferring risk

For most organizations the transfer of risk in whole or in part takes place in one of three ways. Most commonly, risk is transferred to a commercial insurance company under a primary or excess policy. A second approach is to share risk by requiring physicians who are members of the medical staff or network to maintain minimum levels of insurance. These two approaches are commonplace and do not require further elaboration.

The third approach is also fairly common but has been the subject of misunderstanding and misuse. It attempts to shift liability by use of an indemnification or "hold harmless" agreement in a contract. Such a provision allows one party to transfer the legal liability to another contracting party and is frequently insisted on by vendors, insurers, and managed care programs. Health care organizations should not unwittingly accept such provisions. First of all, many malpractice insurance policies expressly exclude such transfers of liability so that the acceptance of the liability of another may be an uninsured loss. In addition, such provisions are typically worded in an overly broad fashion. An even worse alternative is a mutual indemnification clause. Neither should be accepted by an organization. A one-way agreement unfairly shifts liability to the hospital, whereas mutual indemnification ensures that both parties will become entangled in the question of liability.

When faced with an indemnification provision, an organization's legal counsel should endeavor to have it deleted, should not accept a mutual indemnification, and may suggest the following alternative wording:

It is understood and agreed that neither of the parties to this agreement shall be liable for any negligent or wrongful act chargeable to the other and that this agreement shall not be construed as seeking to either enlarge or diminish any obligation or duty owed by one party against the other or against third parties. In the event of a claim for any wrongful or negligent act, each party shall bear the cost of its own defense.

EXTERNAL REQUIREMENTS

The environment within which a health care organization's risk management program operates is a fabric of loosely connected laws, regulations, and accreditation requirements. Voluntary accreditation is available from a number of organizations, including the JCAHO and the National Committee for Quality Assurance (NCQA). This environment continues to be one of constant change, with, for example, revisions to some accreditation requirements released annually. Risk administrators must vigilantly monitor the ever-changing external regulatory environment and ensure organizational compliance with all risk management–related requirements.

CONCLUSION

Health care organizations are dynamic entities in which programs, personnel, priorities, and external requirements are in a constant state of flux. As a result, legal risks often can assume a fluid state. A successful approach to the prevention of injuries caused by a certain set of circumstances may ultimately fail when those circumstances change. The benefits of a fall prevention program successfully instituted in a geriatric unit might be undermined by a reduction in nursing staff, expansion of the unit, change in patient mix, or physical reconfiguration of the unit. When that happens, new solutions and alternative approaches will be required. Risk management programs must be modifiable, adapting to changing patterns and trends. Risk administrators must realize that problems once solved may reappear and require new

solutions, sometimes repeatedly. Constant vigilance through monitoring is essential. Effective risk management requires continual attention to the ever-changing organizational realities and legal milieu.

ENDNOTES

1. Joint Commission on Accreditation of Healthcare Organizations, *Accreditation Manual for Hospitals* 262 (JCAHO 1992).
2. G. Troyer & S. Salman, *Handbook of Healthcare Risk Management* 81 (Aspen Systems, Germantown, Md. 1986).
3. B.L. Brown, *Risk Management for Hospitals: A Practical Approach* 2 (Aspen Systems, Germantown, Md. 1979).
4. M. Holoweiko, *What Are Your Greatest Malpractice Risks?* Medical Economics 144 (1992).
5. E. Hirshfeld, *Should Practice Parameters Be the Standard of Care in Malpractice Litigation?* 266 J.A.M.A. 2886-2891 (1991).
6. E. Topol & R. Califf, *Scorecard Cardiovascular Medicine: Its Impact and Future Directions,* 120 Ann. Intern. Med. 68 (1994).
7. *See* A. Southwick, *The Law of Hospital and Health Care Administration* 554-578 (2d ed, Health Administration Press, Ann Arbor, Mich. 1988) for a more detailed discussion of corporate negligence.
8. *Fox v. Health Net of California,* Calif. Super. Ct. (Riverside), No. 219692 (1993).
9. L. Harpster & M. Veach eds., *Risk Management Handbook for Health Care Facilities* 255 (American Hospital Publishing, Chicago 1990).
10. H. Rubin et al., *Watching the Doctor-Watchers: How Well Do Peer Review Organization Methods Detect Hospital Care Quality Problems?* 267 J.A.M.A. 2349-2354 (1992).
11. A. Localio et al, *Identifying Adverse Events Caused by Medical Care: Degree of Physician Agreement in a Retrospective Chart Review,* 125 Ann. Intern. Med. 457-464 (1996).
12. R. Balsamo & M. Pine, *Twelve Questions to Ask about Your Outcomes Monitoring System,* 20 Physician Executive 13-16, 22-25 (1994).
13. R. Balsamo & M. Pine, *Important Considerations in Using Indicators to Profile Providers,* 21 Physician Executive 38-45 (1995).
14. J. Orlikoff, *Preventing Malpractice: The Board's Role in Risk Management,* Trustee 9 (1991).
15. M. Tragin et al, *Physician Demographics and Risk of Medical Malpractice,* 93 Am. J. Med. 541 (1992).
16. *Petrillo v. Syntex Laboratories, Inc.,* 148 Ill. App. 3d 581, 499 N.E. 2d 952 (1st Dist. 1986).
17. T. Leaman & J. Saxton, *Preventing Malpractice: The Co-Active Solution* 68-70 (Plenum, New York 1993).
18. M. Brown, *Rush Hospital's Medical Malpractice Mediation Program: An ADR Success Story,* 86 Illinois Bar Journal 432 (1998).
19. Topol & Califf, *supra* note 6.
20. A. Sielicki, *Current Philosophy of Risk Management,* Top. in Health Care Financing 6 (Spring 1983).
21. J. Hamman, J. Ziegenfuss, & J. Williamson eds., *Risk Management Trends and Applications* 73 (American Board of Quality Assurance and Utilization Review Physicians, Sarasota, Fla. 1988).
22. B. Youngberg, *Essentials of Hospital Risk Management* 145-147 (Aspen Publishers, Rockville, Md. 1990).

APPENDIX 19-1   Top 10 allegations by average cost*

1998 Rank	1999 Rank	Allegation	Claims (no.)	Average cost
1	1	Improper treatment—Birth-related	309	$260,300
6	2	Failure to diagnose—Hemorrhage	91	$221,900
9	3	Failure to diagnose—Abdominal problems/other	91	$167,600
2	4	Failure to diagnose—Myocardial infarction	150	$166,100
3	5	Surgery—Postoperative death	109	$160,800
5	6	Failure to diagnose—Cancer	379	$149,500
8	7	Failure to diagnose—Pregnancy problems	75	$147,100
+	8	Surgery—Unnecessary	64	$141,400
4	9	Failure to diagnose—Circulatory problem	170	$128,600
7	10	Failure to diagnose—Infection	232	$125,900

From St. Paul Fire and Marine Insurance Co. (1999).
*Table did not appear in 1998 Allegations Review.

APPENDIX 19-2   Top 10 allegations by frequency

1998 Rank	1999 Rank	Allegation	Claims (no.)	Average cost
1	1	Surgery—Postoperative complications	901	$ 85,800
2	2	Failure to diagnose—Cancer	379	$149,500
5	3	Improper treatment—Insufficient therapy	364	$ 64,000
3	4	Improper treatment—Birth-related	309	$260,300
4	5	Surgery—Inadvertent act	265	$107,000
6	6	Improper treatment—During examination	240	$ 51,000
8	7	Failure to diagnose—Infection	232	$125,900
9	8	Improper treatment—Drug side effect	221	$ 89,200
7	9	Failure to diagnose—Fracture/dislocation	189	$ 54,100
10	10	Improper treatment—Infection	178	$101,200

From St. Paul Fire and Marine Insurance Co. (1999).

APPENDIX 19-3   All allegations by location

Location	Claims (no.)
Hospital	
Emergency department	846
Labor/delivery/nursery	363
Other	298
Outpatient surgery	200
Patient care area	643
Surgery	1517
SUBTOTAL	3867
Office	
Physician office/clinic	2446
Other	217
Surgicenter	20
SUBTOTAL	2683
TOTAL	6550

From St. Paul Fire and Marine Insurance Co. (1999).

APPENDIX 19-4 Unusual Incident Report

THIS IS AN INTERNAL QUALITY CONTROL DOCUMENT
DO NOT PLACE IN PATIENT RECORD

I. NAMEPLATE

I. _____ PATIENT _____ VISITOR _____ OTHER (check one)

Date of incident: _____ Time of incident: _____ A.M. _____

P.M. _____

Location of incident: _____

(Unit/Area)

If NO addressograph, print   Attending physician:_____

name, DOB, unit, patient number;   Witness: _____ Phone no.: _____

if visitor, give address.   Witness: _____ Phone no.: _____

II. TYPE OF INCIDENT: (check at least one)

_____ Reaction to contrast/dye

Type:_____

_____ Wrong blood given

_____ Unexpected return to the operating room

_____ Brain damage that could be the result of treatment or medical intervention

_____ Neurological deficit, nerve injury or paralysis that could be the result of treatment or medical intervention

_____ Unexpected patient death

_____ Inaccurate needle or sponge count

_____ Unplanned hospital admission subsequent to outpatient surgery procedure

_____ Informed consent form not signed or inaccurate

_____ Total or partial loss of limb or the use of limb

_____ Needle stick to patient or visitor

_____ Burns from food, liquid, or mechanical equipment

_____ Central line complication/problem resulting in patient injury

_____ Intubation/extubation injury

_____ Damage to or disappearance of personal property

_____ I.V. infiltration (provide detail in Section III)

_____ Fall (provide detail in Section III)

_____ Medication error (provide detail in Section III)

_____ OTHER (provide detail in Section III)

_____ Serious illness or injury (including death) to patient that might have been caused by medical device* (see Section IV)

III. INCIDENT FACTS/DATA: (should be consistent with what is written in the medical record)

_____

_____

_____

_____

IV. PRODUCT IDENTIFICATION: (this information is required by the FDA through The Safe Medical Device Act of 1990 if the Medical Device has caused serious illness or injury [including death] to patient)

List all products/devices connected to the patient at the time of the incident:

Product/Device name	Lot #/Expiration date	Serial #	Manufacturer
1. _____	_____	_____	_____
2. _____	_____	_____	_____
3. _____	_____	_____	_____
4. _____	_____	_____	_____
5. _____	_____	_____	_____
6. _____	_____	_____	_____

Disposable items *should not be discarded* until cleared by Risk Management.

Location of medical device/product: _____

V. Preparer's signature: _____ Date: _____ Time: _____ A.M. _____

P.M. _____

Title: _____

Unit Leader's Signature: _____ Date: _____ Unit: _____

Routing instructions: 1. Submit original to Office of Risk Management (ORM)

2. Original must be received by the ORM within 24 hours of incident.

3. For Patient Care Units, carbon to be maintained by Quality Improvement Coordinating Committee Chairperson.

4. For Ancillary Units, carbon to be maintained by Ancillary Care Evaluation Committee Chairperson.

SERIOUS INCIDENTS—CALL OFFICE OF RISK MANAGEMENT DIRECTLY

THIS FORM MAY NOT BE DUPLICATED

FORM/n0325 Rev. 2/92   FOR OFFICE USE ONLY

From Rush-Presbyterian-St. Luke's Medical Center, Chicago, 1997.

Medicolegal and Ethical Encounters

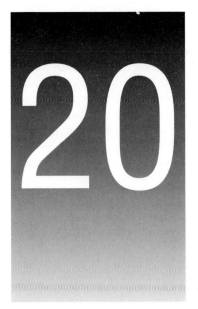

Physician-patient relationship

MATTHEW L. HOWARD, M.D., J.D., F.C.L.M

Physician-patient relationships (PPRs) presumably have been a source of concern since some forgotten ancestor first claimed special talent as a healer. The Hippocratic oath can be thought of as a codification of rules governing the PPR, the existence of which suggests that some physicians at least needed to be bound by oath to enforce adherence to the social norm.[1] The sanctions[2] of the Code of Hammurabi may be the earliest expression of the idea that physicians should be liable for harm to patients.[3]

Modern professional negligence law has arisen by application of elements of English common law of contracts and torts to the same concerns expressed by Hippocrates and Hammurabi.[4] Changes in the structure of the medical profession, which began in 1964 with the passage of Medicare legislation and are proceeding at an increasingly accelerated pace through legislative mandates, corporate initiatives, and technological change, continue to modify the traditional approaches. This chapter is intended to provide an overview of the issues, generally stating the majority view. Case law varies between jurisdictions; both case law and statutes should be examined for variance before taking any action with potential legal consequences.

The PPR traditionally has been considered contractual. Written contracts are the exception; the contract is implied by the actions of the parties in seeking and providing advice and care. The physician is deemed to have promised that professionally acceptable care will be provided, with no guarantee. Unless a specific warranty has been made, courts will not infer that a physician has guaranteed treatment success.[5] The fact that a patient does not pay for services does not affect the existence of the contract or lessen the physician's duties, obligations, responsibilities, or liabilities.[6]

For a person to be professionally liable to another, four conditions must be met. A person claiming compensation for malpractice must show that the professional owed a duty of care to that person (duty owed), the duty was not met (an accepted professional standard of care was breached), and the breach of duty resulted (causation) in otherwise avoidable damages (injury) to the person making the claim. Each one of these elements (duty, breach of the duty, causation, and injury) must be proven for the plaintiff to prevail, which is true whatever the profession. The law applied to physicians or other health care professionals is fundamentally the same as that applied to architects, engineers, and attorneys.

Before a professional duty can be established, the traditional and general rule has been that a professional relationship must exist. Demonstrating the existence of a relationship between the physician and the person claiming to have been harmed is the keystone of every medical malpractice action.[7]

Under certain statutes, duties may arise from hospital-patient relationships, which, once established in accordance with the terms of the law, impose duties on the physician. When a physician becomes involved in a legal problem that stems from a hospital-patient relationship, it is usually because of a special relationship between the hospital and physician. Managed care and telemedicine are further altering the traditional analysis.

NATURE AND CREATION

In the absence of a PPR or some other special relationship, physicians are not legally compelled to treat strangers, even during an emergency, in almost all states.[8] When a person seeks the services of a physician for the purposes of medical or surgical treatment, that person becomes a patient and the traditional PPR is established.[9] A contract is implied by the mutuality of the relationship.[10] The physician is not an employee of the patient.[11] This traditional relationship is consensual, meaning the patient has consciously sought out a physician who has affirmatively agreed to provide care. The mutuality of the relationship is independent of who solicits the relationship or who pays for the services provided.[12] As we shall see, many problems arise in situations in which the physician is held to a duty to a person for whom he or she has not consciously agreed to provide care.

Creation of the PPR usually requires some form of physical contact with the patient. It may be created by a single telephone conversation. Pathologists[13] and radiologists,[14] however, have a duty to the patient to exercise reasonable and ordinary skill and care while rendering their services even though they generally have no personal contact with the patient.

Whether a PPR legally exists is a factual determination. For public policy reasons, courts give persons alleging injury from medical malpractice considerable latitude as to the evidence required to establish the existence of the relationship.[15] Courts will determine whether the patient entrusted care to the physician and whether the physician indicated acceptance of the duty to render care. If the circumstances of the contact caused the patient to have a reasonable expectation of treatment or if the physician undertook to render treatment, then the courts will infer the existence of a relationship.[16]

One legal definition of treatment is "the broad term covering all steps taken to effect a cure of an injury or disease. The word includes examination and diagnosis as well as application of remedies."[17] This broad interpretation and the willingness of most courts to interpret almost any action as an undertaking-to-treat may result in a PPR that the physician did not intend to create.

LIMITING THE DUTIES IMPOSED

Once established, unless limited or conditioned by agreement, the relationship continues until the services are no longer needed or are properly terminated. Once the relationship has been terminated, the physician is generally not obligated to follow the patient's progress.[18]

Courts are quick to find a PPR yet generally recognize the physician's ability to qualify or limit the relationship.[19] Agreements to treat may be limited to one particular treatment or procedure.[20] Physician availability may be restricted, if clearly understood and accepted by the patient, to certain times and places.[21]

Physicians generally are free to choose their patients[22] and are not obligated to treat anyone with whom they have no special relationship.[23] Absent statutorily imposed requirements, physicians are not compelled to practice, to practice under terms other than those the physician may choose to accept, or to provide care to any or all prospective patients. This principle is recognized by the Principles of Medical Ethics of the American Medical Association and supported by case law.[24]

An established relationship renders the physician liable for damages legally caused by any breach of the resulting duty. The fundamental duty is to exercise the same degree of knowledge, skill, diligence, and care that an ordinary competent physician would exercise under the same or similar circumstances. There is a concomitant duty to suggest a referral if the physician knows or should know that he or she does not possess the requisite knowledge or skill to properly treat the patient.[25] Failure to make a referral is negligence.[26]

The patient is obligated to cooperate by following reasonable instructions for further evaluation and treatment.[27] A patient's failure to do so may preclude holding the physician solely liable for any resulting injuries.[28] The physician, however, must provide the patient with information necessary to explain why physician recommendations ought to be followed.[29] The physician's relative liability will be determined from the facts and circumstances by the trier of fact. A patient's failure to follow instructions does not, of itself, terminate the relationship or relieve the physician of obligations, nor does failure to pay the physician's fees relieve the physician from further responsibility.[30]

BREACH OF CONTRACT

Because the relationship is contractual in nature, an injured party may allege a breach of contract.[31,32] As a general rule, when the presumptive patient declines the contract, no physician duty exists.[33] Some courts have come to opposing conclusions.[34] In the medical setting, this claim arises where the physician is alleged to have guaranteed a particular result or has promised to perform in a certain manner.[35] If the physician does not reasonably live up to the guarantee, then a valid action for breach of contract may exist, even if the physician's performance was not negligent or deficient under the measure of meeting usual professional standards.[36]

Claims arising in breach of contract are rare because the law allows only compensation for actual damages caused by the breach of contract, because tort damages are far more lucrative for the patient, and because most physicians understand the risks of offering guarantees and do not make statements that could be interpreted as a guarantee. Guarantees of physician availability, especially in the obstetrical context, have been a source of litigation, and are discussed next.

SPECIAL SITUATIONS

Once outside the traditional confines of a patient voluntarily approaching a physician at the physician's office or clinic, innumerable variations on the theme occur, some of which lead to unexpected results.

"Curbstone" and "sidewalk" consultation

Physicians are not obligated to give gratuitous advice.[37] Having given advice, however, physicians owe a duty of due care to anyone who might reasonably rely on such advice. If the gratuitous advice causes injury, the physician may be liable for the injury.[38] The degree of contact may be determinative.[39] Where a consultant offered advice to the treating physician but charged no fee and never examined the patient, no duty to the patient was created.[40]

"Second opinion" programs

When a physician receives a referral from a third party for the purposes of a "second opinion," a claim against that physician grounded in medical malpractice can succeed if the patient can demonstrate that the physician either affirmatively treated or affirmatively advised how treatment should proceed and harm resulted.[41]

Substitute and covering physicians

As a general rule, physicians may use substitute physicians if they are unavailable. The substitute physician must be competent[42] and qualified,[43] and the patient must be aware, especially where services are particularly personal, that a substitution may take place.[44] Without this understanding, a cause of action for breach of contract and for abandonment may exist. Because the fact that physicians share after-hours call duty is so widely known, in most instances the courts will impose constructive knowledge and consent on the patient, even in the absence of express consent. To be certain that the patient understands and agrees, written consent to on-call coverage arrangements and substitution should be obtained.

When called on to treat another physician's patient, the substitute physician establishes a separate and independent PPR, which includes a duty to diagnose, treat, and manage any identifiable and detrimental condition that may have been negligently caused by the primary physician. Failure to do so may lead to an independent malpractice action against the substitute.[45] Merely signing a prescription form for another physician has been held insufficient to establish such an independent relationship.[46] The attending physician will not be liable for the acts of the covering physician[47] unless there is some control of the treatment by the attending physician, agency or concert of action between the two physicians, or negligence in the referral.[48]

House staff

Generally, interns, residents, and employed staff physicians are treated as employees of their hospital, and as such their liability is vicariously imputed to the hospital. Employees are essentially indemnified by the hospital for acts performed within the usual course of their duties.[49] Physicians working as fellows may not enjoy the hospital's indemnification; their status depends on their contractual agreement with the hospital. Nevertheless they have duties to all hospital patients with whom they establish a relationship.

Part-time, volunteer, and clinical faculty

Clinical faculty not employed by the hospital, functioning in an educational capacity for students and house staff, may be liable to patients who serve as teaching examples. In determining whether a PPR was created during contact with a patient seen during a teaching session or on rounds, courts look at the nature of the physician's contact with the patient and whether the patient had a reasonable expectation that the teaching physician's role included treatment.[50]

As a general rule, the court will determine whether the physician had actual contact with the patient and whether any examination or treatment of the patient was done for the patient's benefit.[51] If an examination causes the patient to reasonably believe that the examination was made for treatment purposes, the court may infer a relationship.[52] In contrast, if a physician conducting a lecture merely discusses a patient's case and recommends a course of treatment that, when followed, results in injury, courts have found no PPR and insufficient contact.[53] A teaching physician supervising physicians-in-training may be held responsible for any negligent care that the instructor ordered and also may be held liable for negligent supervision of the trainee.

Emergency department physicians and emergency situations

Generally, physicians are not under a duty to treat anyone with whom no relationship exists, even in emergencies where death or disability will result.[54] The public policy implications of this rule have led to institution of "Good Samaritan" laws in many states, providing for immunity from professional liability for intervening physicians. Physicians often view these protections as deficient because immunity is predicated on physician abstention from seeking payment for care rendered and because protection exists against liability for "ordinary" negligence but not against "gross" negligence. Physicians understandably may be reluctant to risk a court determination as to whether an error committed in the heat of an emergency was ordinary or gross negligence.

Freedom to refuse treatment does not extend to hospitals, which have a duty to render reasonable emergency medical aid to the extent that hospital facilities will allow.[55] The law in this area has been substantially modified by the Emergency Medical Treatment and Active Labor Act (EMTALA). The law was enacted out of congressional concern that hospitals were refusing to provide care for uninsured patients, sending them instead to public or charity facilities that might be miles away, and thus it was characterized as an "antidumping" law.

As enacted, EMTALA provides for fines and suits against hospitals, but only for fines against physicians. Because the law characterizes the fines as civil penalties, trial by jury is not required. Proof of negligence is not required. Each violation may cost a physician $50,000, and this fine may not be covered by medical malpractice insurance policies.

As case law is developing, EMTALA's scope is being broadened beyond the inappropriate transfer out of emergency departments of indigent patients or women in labor. It is reasonable to assume that increased physician liability will follow. EMTALA has been superimposed on the preexisting rule that the private physician who has agreed to be on-call for the emergency department is presumed to have a relationship with the patient based on the public's reasonable expectation of emergency care.[56]

Telephone contacts

Although physical contact is usually required, a relationship may be established even from a telephone call if the court interprets the physician's comments as treatment. Where a covering physician's contact with the patient was limited to informing the patient that his or her admission could be arranged only by the family physician and commenting that the family physician's earlier diagnosis seemed reasonable, the court ruled that no relationship had been established.[57] Where a physician questioned a caller and advised hospital admission, a relationship was considered established.[58] Similarly, where a patient made an appointment after talking to a physician but was then refused care when she arrived for her appointment, the appointment made for the specific purpose of treating the condition that had been discussed over the telephone was deemed sufficient to establish a PPR.[59]

Where a physician had not seen a patient for more than two years and seven months, a telephone call to discuss treatment options was deemed sufficient to reestablish a PPR, precluding a statute of limitations defense against a subsequent negligence suit.[60]

Sexual contacts

A sexual component to the PPR is universally condemned.[61] Numerous states have passed laws providing for disciplinary action against physicians who engage in such relationships.[62] Although the American Medical Association's standard states flatly that all sexual contact between physicians and patients is misconduct, some courts have declined to adopt this view, holding that the sexual relationship must arise out of the PPR to fall within the purview of the statute.[63] In other instances, suits grounded in medical malpractice because of sexual conduct have been brought by patients, with conflicting results.[64] The increasing social pressure to end such contacts should suggest to the prudent physician that social relationships should be strictly confined to nonpractice situations.

Managed care relationships

Additional complications have been introduced by the increased role of third-party payors in determining the care provided. Where a third-party payor did not approve a physician's plan of treatment and declined to pay for continued hospitalization, the court held that the third-party payor could be held liable when medically incorrect decisions resulted from institutional obstacles present because of attempts to reduce costs. However, the third-party payor escaped liability in the particular case because the physician failed to press

the patient's case with the payor.[65] In a similar situation, a patient committed suicide after being discharged when the insurer declined to pay for further hospitalization.[66] The appellate court reversed a summary judgment for the hospital and remanded for trial on the issue of whether the actions of the insurer led to the death.

Telemedicine

Has a relationship been established by an exchange of information on an Internet site? A court may conclude that an Internet site that appears to have been established for the purposes of bringing in new patients may establish a relationship.

It is a fundamental rule of due process that a court may not exert jurisdiction over a person unless that person has some "minimal contacts" with the state seeking jurisdiction.[67] A person living and working in Illinois who is involved in an automobile accident in Illinois with a California resident cannot be called to a California court to respond to a personal injury suit brought by the Californian. Neither can he or she be called to any court in the United States other than an Illinois court. Where a physician has provided personal services to an out-of-state patient, as happens frequently in our mobile society as patients seek out major medical centers or well-known physicians, the courts treat the resulting malpractice claim as they would the automobile accident. Jurisdiction resides in the state where the incident took place. However, where the physician has attracted out-of-state patients through marketing schemes, personal jurisdiction in the patient's home state has been established.[68] Where the PPR was based on the mail-order nature of the business, the court found jurisdiction. The applicability of this decision to advice provided over a "chat" site or Internet site should be clear. Several states have enacted statutes that forbid prescribing for patients where the only contact has been by telecommunications, so-called "reaching into another state." Penalties ranging from reprimand to loss of license to practice may apply.[70]

Relationships imposed by statute

An increased duty to treat is being imposed by some states as a condition of licensure. For example, physicians have been forbidden to refuse care to patients who have tested positive for human immunodeficiency virus.[71]

LIABILITY FOR INJURY TO THIRD PARTIES
Nonpatient relationships with physicians

Not every patient contact results in the creation of a PPR. When a physician performs an examination at the request of a third party for sole use by the third party (e.g., to determine eligibility for employment or for the issuance of life insurance), courts differ in their interpretation of the physician's duty to the patient. If a physician is employed to perform pre-employment examinations, then the physician's duty is owed to his or her employer; no PPR is implied. Absence of therapeutic intent is often the key issue.[72] Courts have said that the employed physician owes no duty to the examinee other than to avoid causing an injury[73] and is under a duty to use reasonable care to avoid same.[74] Failure to do so may lead to a claim based on ordinary negligence rather than medical malpractice. Another court assumes no duty unless advice is offered.[75] No liability exists for a negligently performed examination, but the employer may be liable to the examinee for the negligent acts of a physician-employee under the doctrine of respondeat superior.[76] The physician may in turn be liable to the company under a contract theory for any resulting damages.

As a general rule, a third-party employed physician is not bound to disclose abnormal findings to an examinee. Possible exceptions to this rule occur if the physician conducts an examination on a person with whom he or she has a prior existing PPR or if the physician completes an attending physician's statement for an insurance company and is paid a fee for doing so (contrast with physician as salaried employee).[77] Under such circumstances, the physician might have a duty to disclose significant findings to the examinee. This traditional rule was explicitly abandoned and physician liability expanded in a case in which a preemployment physical included a chest x-ray examination. The physician, failing to detect what later proved to be a lung carcinoma, reported to the employer that the person was employable. This court ignored traditional intent to treat and patient expectation rules in finding the physician liable.[78]

If a physician gratuitously elects to discuss findings with the examinee, he or she must not misrepresent the examinee's medical condition. If the physician recommends treatment, liability may result if substandard advice causes injury to the examinee.[79] Third parties other than employers may employ physicians to examine or treat a patient. The courts distinguish between liability to the third party (for the examination itself) and liability to the patient (for the treatment once it has begun).[80]

Indirect relationships with physicians

Recognizing the fundamental principle that all must use ordinary care not to injure others, violations of that duty occur when an injury results that is reasonably avoidable and is a foreseeable consequence of a person's actions. All physicians have a duty to warn patients about aspects of their medical condition or treatment that could injure others.[81] The physician treating a seizure patient, for example, may be liable for injury to a nonpatient if the injury is indirectly caused by negligent treatment, failure to diagnose the condition, or failure to advise the patient of the risks of engaging in dangerous activities.[82]

Although the courts reject creating a PPR with the third-party victim, they freely apply ordinary negligence principles and hold that the injury to the nonpatient was a foresee-able consequence of the patient's condition, which imposed on the physician a duty to avoid injury to foreseeable victims.[83] Lack of foreseeability was at issue where a physician treated a police officer for a pituitary gland tumor. A citizen later shot by the officer was not permitted to maintain an action either under malpractice or negligence theories against the treating physician.[84]

Liability has resulted when physicians have failed to advise patients of the danger of performing certain acts while taking medications, such as driving while using sedatives or decongestants,[85] or have failed to properly caution patients with communicable diseases to avoid transmitting the disease to third parties.[86] The Michigan Court of Appeals considered a suit against a physician brought by the family of a motorist killed in an automobile accident with the physician's patient. The patient had received a sedating medication by injection and was given no warning against driving. The Michigan court permitted the suit to proceed not in negligence as described previously but as a medical malpractice action, ruling that dismissing the suit because of the absence of a PPR between the physician and the deceased would "exalt form over substance."[87] To date, no other court has followed this example.

Where a patient's relative who was permitted to remain in an emergency department treatment area fainted at the sight of blood and sustained significant permanent sequelae from the resulting head injury, the physician was held to have no liability to the injured relative.[88]

Courts have imposed liability on physicians who bear a special relationship to a dangerous person and a subsequent victim.[89] Such a relationship may support affirmative physician duties for the benefit of a nonpatient third party.[90] The duty to the nonpatient stems from the physician's special relationship with the patient, and the potential for harm to the third party is a result of the patient's behavior. The leading case is *Tarasoff v. Regents of the University of California,*[91] which imposed liability on a psychotherapist whose patient had repeatedly expressed hostile intent toward a specific person who was subsequently murdered. Most subsequent cases have limited that liability to the facts of the Tarasoff case, although the victim need not be a patient. Where hostile intent has not been limited to a specific, readily identifiable person, no liability has been found when harm subsequently resulted.[92] The duty to protect endangered third persons has been extended to the protection of endangered property.[93]

RELATIONSHIPS FORMED BY CONTRACT WITH OTHERS

If a physician contracts with a third party to treat a patient, then the PPR is not established with the patient until there is some overt undertaking. If the physician does not treat the proposed patient, then no duty to the expectant patient is created. However, physician liability to the third party who relies on the physician's assurance to treat may exist.[94] When a third party contracts with a physician to treat a particular patient and the treatment is undertaken, the PPR is established and the physician's duty is now to the patient rather than the third party.[95] If the physician's agreement to provide care to a patient leads the third party to believe that the patient is being competently cared for, and because they are reasonably restrained by this belief the third party does not seek care elsewhere, then the physician could be liable to both patient and third party. Liability to the patient would be based on medical malpractice, and liability to the third party would be based on breach of contract. Such a situation could arise in the case of a minor student at college being treated at the request of a parent living elsewhere.

A physician employed by a third party for the sole purpose of obtaining evidence to support the third party's challenge to a claim of injury is under no duty to the examinee.[96] The physician is generally under no duty to inform the examinee of the results of the examination and is not liable to the examinee if a negligent examination or negligently prepared report of the examination later causes injury to the examinee, provided the report was not, as postulated, prepared for the use or benefit of the examinee.[97]

TERMINATION

The duties imposed on the physician by the creation of a PPR continue until the relationship is terminated. This termination may occur through completion of the treatment by virtue of patient recovery,[98] dismissal of the physician by the patient, mutual consent, or formal physician withdrawal.[99] Like any other contract, the parties may terminate the agreement by mutual consent. The patient may unilaterally terminate the relationship for any reason and at any time. This termination may be express or implied by the patient's actions.[100] Even though dismissed, the physician is under a duty to warn the patient of any risk of discontinuing treatment. A prudent physician will carefully document the basis and circumstances of dismissal as protection against a later claim by the patient of abandonment. The relationship may be considered terminated once a patient's care has been properly and completely transferred to another physician so that the services of the transferring physician are no longer needed and the duty of continuing care ends.[101] Once services are terminated, the traditional rule has been that the physician is under no duty either to provide future care or to reestablish the relationship.[102] However, some courts have mandated such liability on the grounds that the physician is in a better position than the patient to keep abreast of changing knowledge.[103]

If during the course of treatment a physician concludes that he or she lacks the requisite skill or knowledge to treat the patient competently or for other acceptable reasons determines that the patient would be more properly treated by another

physician or at another facility, then the patient should be so informed. As a practical matter, patients readily accede to their physician's judgment in these circumstances and termination of the relationship by a mutually agreed on transfer usually results. If transfer is declined, then the treating physician is required to inform the patient of the consequences of the refusal, to carefully document the refusal and appropriate counseling, and to continue care until a proper unilateral termination of the relationship has been accomplished.

Unilateral termination by the physician is permitted. The patient must be provided sufficient time to arrange for care to be provided by another physician. Written notice[104] should be provided, preferably by certified mail.[105] The notice should provide an explanation of the patient's condition and the further services needed, as well as a description of the likely consequences of failure to obtain continuing care. The physician should continue to provide care for such time as it will reasonably take for the patient to secure further care, and this length of time should be specified in the notice letter.[106] Improper withdrawal[107] by physicians has resulted in suits for breach of contract,[108] professional negligence, and abandonment.[109]

Abandonment

Abandonment is the unilateral severance of the PPR by the physician without reasonable notice to the patient at a time when continued medical care is still necessary.[110] If physician illness or disability is the cause of the withdrawal, then abandonment has not occurred. Liability for abandonment may be found where the physician intends to terminate the relationship without the patient's consent, as well as where the court finds physician failure to attend the patient as frequently as due care in treatment would demand. Such failure denies the patient the benefit of the PPR and is referred to as *constructive abandonment.*

Abandonment may give rise to an action for either negligence or breach of contract.[111] If a patient is injured because the physician failed to see the patient often enough or if the physician improperly concluded that the patient's condition required no further treatment, the patient has a cause of action in negligence alone.[112] In an action for negligence the patient must present expert testimony; such testimony is not required in an action for breach of contract. The remedies vary, however, and negligence is the action generally preferred. Because abandonment can occur only if there is a valid PPR, it does not result if a physician permissively refuses to enter into such a relationship with a particular person.[113]

EXPECTATIONS OF THE FUTURE: TRENDS

Society's perception of the PPR is generally reflected in the law. During the past several years, both legislation and case law have tended to perceive the physician as being so able to bear the costs of compensation to injured patients that expansion of physician liability to provide for compensation to more patients has been a justifiable public policy. Recent court decisions support a conclusion that such expansion of physician liability is continuing and equally support a conclusion that the pendulum is beginning to swing in the opposite direction.

Supporting the idea that liability expansion is continuing is the series of cases discussed earlier with regard to EMTALA and its extension beyond the situations that presumably led to its adoption, as well as recent cases in which physicians have been prosecuted under criminal statutes in circumstances that once would have been treated solely as civil professional negligence issues.[114] A case that initially appears to reduce a physician's right to exercise judgment in accepting patients for care, by permitting criminal prosecution for negligently exercising the option to refuse to accept a patient for care, led to conviction of a resident physician. The trial court refused to dismiss the indictment.[115] New York State created a new area of physician liability when its court of appeals found that a physician may be liable in malpractice for providing false testimony during a patient's suit against his or her health insurer.[116] A summary judgment for a physician has been reversed where suit was brought by the children of the patient on grounds that their parent was never informed that his hereditary disease could affect his children.[117]

Supporting the opposite point of view is a case in which a deceased patient's family brought suit against treating physicians on the theory that the physicians' failure to inform the patient of his prognosis led him to engage optimistically in financial dealings that because of his subsequent early death harmed his heirs.[118] The court declined to hold the physicians liable.

Telemedicine is likely to be a continuing source of controversy. When will contacts through the Internet or other electronic means suffice to establish a PPR? The offering of specific treatment is likely to be the key factor. More important, where will the case be tried? The trial locale will depend on whether the patient can claim sufficient contact between the physician and the patient's home state.

CONCLUSION

Physician liability depends on the existence of a PPR. Such a relationship may be explicit, implicit, or statutorily imposed. Numerous situations arise in our complex society in which physician, patient, government, and third-party payor interact in ill-defined ways, such that PPRs can arise by implication and without conscious physician intent. Physicians should be cautious in their statements and in their behavior to avoid creating a relationship that contrary to their intentions imposes legal obligations.

The legal obligation imposed is the requirement to exercise ordinary professional care in the discharge of professional duties. The plaintiff patient alleging malpractice must establish the existence of the PPR, a breach of the duty created by that relationship, and the existence of an injury caused by the breach. Reasonable differences of opinion as to these elements may subject the physician to all the financial and emotional stress of a lawsuit and its aftermath. Proof of the elements stated, which requires a mere preponderance of the evidence, will subject the physician to liability, will trigger National Practitioner Data Bank reports, and may precipitate disciplinary action.

ENDNOTES

1. Attributed to Hippocrates, Greek physician, fourth century, B.C.
2. A physician whose patient loses an eye under treatment has his own eye put out.
3. Hammurabi, Babylonian king, lived in the twenty-seventh century, B.C.E., roughly 4700 years before the publication of this work.
4. *Thomas v. Corso,* 265 Md. 84, 288 A. 2d 379 (1972) (abandonment is a contract issue, no expert required).
5. *Pike v. Honsinger,* 155 N.Y. 201, 49 N.E. 760 (1898); *Greenstein v. Fornell,* 275 N.Y.S. 673 (1932).
6. *Vitta v. Dolan,* 155 N.W. 1077 (Minn. 1916) (patient need not pay; physician duty remains).
7. *Kennedy v. Parrot,* 243 N.C. 355, 90 S.E. 2d 754 (1956) (preference for tort law over contract law in "due care" situations).
8. *Childs v. Weis,* 440 S.W. 2d 104 (Tex. 1969) (physician may arbitrarily refuse to render care to a nonpatient).
9. *Traveler's Ins. Co. v. Bergeron,* 25 F. 2d 680, 49 S.Ct. 33 (1928) (relationship established when professional services are accepted by another person for purposes of medical or surgical treatment).
10. *Findly v. Board of Supervisors,* 230 P. 2d 526 (Ariz. 1951) (consensual relationship); *Brumbalow v. Fritz,* 183 Ga.App. 231, 358 S.E. 2d 872 (1987) (patient refused advised admission, then was injured while leaving emergency department; suit against physician dismissed).
11. *In re Estate of Bridges,* 41 Wash. 2d 916, 253 P. 2d 394 (1953) (physician not employee).
12. *Hoover v. Williamson,* 236 Md. 258, 203 A. 2d 861 (1964) (services paid for by employer but duty to employee).
13. *Walters v. Rinker,* 520 N.E. 2d 468 (Ind.Ct.App. 1988) (examination of tumor removed from patient establishes PPR).
14. *Rule v. Cheeseman,* 181 Kan. 957, 317 P. 2d 472 (1957) (radiologist's duty of care).
15. *Viita, supra* note 6 (not necessary for patient to know physician, engage his or her services, or pay for them in ordinary way).
16. *Betesh V. United States,* 400 F.Supp. 238 (D.C. 1974) (in the context of a preinduction physical, physician's recall of rejected examinee to check on progression of disease was sufficient act to indicate treatment).
17. *Kirschner v. Equitable Life Assurance Soc.,* 284 N.Y.S. 506 (1935) (defines "treatment").
18. *Fleischman v. Richardson-Merrell, Inc.,* 266 A. 2d 639, 558 N.Y.S. 2d 688 (1990) (no duty to follow patient's progress once relationship is terminated).
19. *Osborne v. Frazor,* 425 S.W. 2d 768 (Tenn. 1968) (relationship by its terms may be limited); *Mozingo v. Pitt County Memorial Hosp, Inc.,* 415 S.E. 2d 134 (N.C. 1992).
20. *Markley v. Albany Medical Center,* 163 A. 2d 539, 558 N.Y.S. 2d 688 (1990) (duty may be limited to those medical functions undertaken by physician and relied on by patient).
21. *Sendjar v. Gonzales,* 520 S.W. 2d 478 (Texas 1975) (physician had right to refuse hospital calls).
22. *Hoover, supra* note 12 (no duty to nonpatient unless physician affirmatively acts).

23. *Hiser v. Randolph,* 617 P. 2d 774 (Ariz. 1980), *overruled on other grounds,* 688 P. 2d 605 (1988) (may refuse to treat patient). The author must distinguish between duty for professional liability purposes, discussed here, and duties imposed as a condition of licensure. In various states, duties as a condition of continued licensure have been imposed that restrict a physician's right to freely choose those for whom he or she will provide care. Included are abstention from balance billing of Medicare patients, acceptance of Medicaid patients, and acceptance of HIV-positive patients. Additional restrictions are created by federal civil rights laws and the Americans with Disabilities Act.

24. *Childs, supra* note 8 (right of physician to refuse intoxicated patient); *Childers v. Frye,* 158 S.E. 744 (N.C. 1931) (may refuse to treat nonpatient); *Coss v. Spaulding,* 126 P. 468 (Utah 1912) (physician employed by third party to examine also gratuitously advised, thereby establishing a relationship).

25. Malpractice: Physician's Failure to Advise Patient to Consult Specialist or One Qualified in a Method of Treatment which Consultant Is Not Qualified to Give, 35 A.L.R. 3d 349 (failure to get consultation).

26. *Shoemaker v. Crawford,* 78 Ohio App. 3d 53, 603 N.E. 2d 1114 (1991), *appeal denied,* 64 Ohio 3d 1434, 595 N.E. 2d 943 (1992) (physician's admitted lack of experience in managing postoperative patient establishes negligence where that lack of experience was proximate cause of patient's injury).

27. Malpractice: What Constitutes Physician-Patient Relationship for Malpractice Purposes, 17 A.L.R. 4th 132 (PPR for malpractice purposes).

28. Medical Malpractice: Patient's Failure to Return, as Directed, for Examination or Treatment as Contributory Negligence, 100 A.L.R. 3d 723 (patient contributorily negligent for failure to return).

29. *Truman v. Thomas,* 27 Cal. 3d 285, 611 P. 2d 902, 165 Cal.Rptr. 208 (1980) (physician liable for failure to warn of consequences of refusing Pap smear).

30. *Rule, supra* note 14.

31. *Osborne, supra* note 19 (contractual relationship between patient and physician).

32. *Alexandridis v. Jewett,* 388 F. 2d 829 (1968) (obstetrician breached contract when he did not deliver infant).

33. *Thor v. Superior Court,* 5 Cal. 4th 725, 855 P. 2d 375, 21 Cal.Rptr. 357 (1993) (physician has no duty toward quadriplegic who refuses medically necessary feeding tube).

34. *Laurie v. Senecal,* 666 A. 2d 806, 808 (1995) (physician's duty persists despite refusal).

35. *Guilmet v. Campbell,* 385 Mich. 57, 188 N.W. 2d 601 (1971) (physician's representations interpreted as guarantees); *Stewart v. Rudner,* 349 Mich. 459, 84 N.W. 2d 815 (1957) (family practitioner breached contract by promising cesarean section that was not performed). N.B. Michigan law was later amended to require such contracts to be in writing.

36. *Greenwald v. Grayson,* 189 S. 2d 204 (Fla. 1976) (ability to recover in contract even though no negligence shown).

37. *Oliver v. Brock,* 342 S. 2d 1 (Ala. 1976) (no obligation to practice or to accept professional employment).

38. *Osborne, supra* note 19.

39. *Ingber v. Kandler,* 128 A.D. 2d 591, 513 N.Y.S. 2d 11 (1987) (informal opinion offered without review of records or even knowledge of patient's name does not establish relationship); *Grassis v. Retik,* 25 Mass.App.Ct. 595, 521 N.E. 2d 411 (1988) (admitting resident not responsible for later negligence of treating physicians where resident had no further contact with patient).

40. *Reynolds v. Decatur Memorial Hosp.,* 277 Ill.App. 3d 80, 660 N.E. 2d 235, 214 Ill. Dec. 44 (1996) ("[t]he rules . . . cannot, as a matter of law, require a physician to enter into a PPR with every person treated in the hospital whose treating physician might make an informal inquiry about that case.").

41. *Hickey v. Travelers Ins. Co.,* 158 A.D. 2d 112, 558 N.Y.S. 2d 554 (1990) (cause remanded for trial to determine whether physician was guilty of "negligent omission" for which apparently no liability would be imposed, or "negligent commission" for which liability would be imposed).

42. *Reed v. Gershweir,* 160 Ariz. 203, 772 P. 2d 26 (Ct. App. 1989) (physician not liable for malpractice of covering physician where reasonable care in selecting coverage was exercised).

43. *Blackshear v. Calis,* L-01240-93 (N.J. Super. Ct. Middlesex Cnty., July 16, 1996) (obstetricians left inexperienced resident to do difficult forceps delivery).

44. *Alexandridis, supra* note 32 (obstetrician breached contract when resident delivered infant).

45. *Perna v. Pirozzi,* 457 A. 2d 431 (N.J. 1983) (patient should be informed of substitution in advance).

46. *Baird v. National Health Foundation,* 144 S.W. 2d 850 (Mo. 1940) (substitute physician cannot use other physician's negligence as excuse for own actions).

47. *Bass v. Barksdale,* 671 S.W. 2d 476 (Tenn.Ct.App. 1984) (covering physician signed prescription at request of primary physician).

48. *Steinberg v. Dunseth,* 631 N.E. 2d 809 (Ill.App., 4th Dist. 1994).

49. *McKenna v. Cedars of Lebanon Hosp.,* 93 Cal.App. 282, 155 Cal.Rptr. 631 (1979) (malpractice action against resident physician for emergency care rendered to in-patient with whom resident had no prior contract allowed protection of Good Samaritan statute); *Leathers v. Serrell,* 376 F.Supp. 983 (1979) (intern loses hospital's immunity because he did not function within strict interpretation of statute when he treated nonpatient).

50. *Smart v. Kansas City,* 105 S.W. 709 (1907), *overruled on other grounds,* State ex. rel. McNutt v. Keet, 432 S.W. 2d 597 (Mo. 1968) (where clinical professor examined patient on ward with patient's knowledge, consent, and belief the purpose was for treatment, a relationship was implied).

51. *Rogers v. Horvath,* 65 Mich. App. 644, 237 N.W. 2d 595 (1975) (no relationship because examination not conducted for patient's benefit and no advice offered).

52. *Perna, supra* note 45.

53. *Rainer v. Grossmen,* 31 Cal.App. 3d 539 (1973) (lecturing physician gave advice in response to question; no attempt to treat; no relationship).

54. *Pearson v. Norman,* 106 P. 2d 361 (Colo. 1940) (license to practice does not require physician to accept all comers).

55. *Clough v. Lively,* 186 Ga.App. 415, 367 S.E. 2d 295 (1988) (emergency department nurse checked patient's vital signs and drew blood at police request; patient dies after transfer to jail; PPR established by consent to draw blood).

56. *Hiser v. Randolph,* 617 P. 2d 774 (Ariz. 1980), *overruled on other grounds, Thompson v. Sun City Comm. Hosp.,* 141 Ariz. 597, 688 P. 2d 605 (1984) (assenting to hospital bylaws, which required participation in emergency room call, altered physicians' right to refuse to treat a patient).

57. *Wilmington General Hosp. v. Manlove,* 54 Del. 15, 174 A. 2d 135 (1961) (more than public reliance on hospitals to provide care is required to establish PPR); *Weaver v. University of Michigan Board of Regents,* 506 N.W. 2d 264 (Mich. App. 1993) (telephone call to make appointment does not create PPR).

58. *Fabran v. Matzko,* 236 Pa. Super. 267, 344 A. 2d 569 (1975) (telephone contact insufficient to establish relationship); *St. John v. Pope,* 901 S.W. 2d 420 (Tex. Sup. Ct. 1995) (telephone discussion about postoperative fever, followed by physician advice to seek care from surgeon who performed surgery, insufficient to establish relationship).

59. *Hamil v. Bashline,* 224 Pa. Super. 407, 305 A. 2d 57 (1973) (telephone contact constituted advice and treatment); *Lyons v. Grether,* 218 Va. 630, 239 S.E. 2d 103 (1977) (appointment arranged by telephone to treat created duty where patient was not permitted to enter with guide dog).

60. *Swift v. Coleman,* No. 68488 (N.Y. App. Div., 3d Dept., Mar 10, 1994) (anticipation of future treatment created by single telephone call sufficient to establish a "continuous relationship of trust and confidence"); *Cogswell v. Chapmen,* 672 N.Y.S. 2d 460 (App. Div. 1998) (giving medical advice in response to query from patient is sufficient to establish PPR).
61. Council on Ethical and Judicial Affairs, American Medical Association, *Sexual Misconduct in the Practice of Medicine,* 266 J.A.M.A. 2741 (1991).
62. *See, e.g.,* Colo. Rev. Stat. Ann. 12-36-117(1)(r); Fla. Stat. Ann. 458.331(1)(j); Ariz. Rev. Stat. Ann. 32-1401(21)(z); Doering's Calif. Bus. and Prof. Code §756.
63. *Gromus v. Medical Board of California,* 8 Cal.App. 4th 589, 10 Cal.Rptr. 452 (1992) (sexual interaction must breach professional duty in a way "substantially related to the qualifications, functions, or duties of the occupation for which a license was issued."); *Larsen v. Comm. on Medical Competency,* 585 N.W. 2d 801 (N. D. 1998) (consensual relationship for 3 months grounds for revocation of license).
64. *New Mexico Physicians Mutual Liability Co. v. LaMure,* 116 N.M. 92, 860 P. 2d 734 (1993) (insurance company not required to indemnify physician found liable in medical malpractice by jury for sexual misconduct with patient); *Patricia C. v. Mark D.,* 12 Cal.App. 4th 1211, 16 Cal.Rptr. 2d 71 (1993) (psychotherapist not liable in malpractice for sexual misconduct with patient). *But, see Benavidez v. United States,* 177 F. 3d 927 (10th Cir. 1997) (homosexual relations between therapist and patient under the influence of drugs and alcohol is malpractice).
65. *Wickline v. State,* 192 Cal.App. 3d 1630, 239 Cal.Rptr. 810 (1986) (physician has duty to advocate for his or her patient and to challenge inappropriate payor decisions).
66. *Wilson v. Blue Cross,* 222 Cal.App. 3d 660, 271 Cal.Rptr. 876 (1990) (insurer may be liable if refusal to pay for continued hospitalization was clearly contrary to informed medical opinion).
67. *International Shoe v. State of Washington,* 325 U.S. 310, 66 S.Ct. 154 (1945).
68. *Bullion v. Gillespie,* 895 F. 2d 213 (5th Cir. 1990) (mailing drugs to patient in another state attracted to the physician's practice through nationally distributed literature establishes jurisdiction in patient's state); *Kenndy v. Freeman,* 919 F. 2d 126 (10th Cir. 1990) (processing and reading biopsy specimens from out-of-state physicians).
69. *See, e.g.,* Calif. Business and Professions Code § 2234 (g).
70. *In re B.T. Taylor, M.D.,* Action Report, Medical Board of California (Oct 1999) (reprimand from Medical Board of California after Colorado disciplined physician for prescribing over Internet and by telephone for patients never personally examined by him).
71. *Cahil v. Rosa,* 89 N.Y. 214, 674 N.E. 2d 274 (1997) and *Lasser v. Rosa,* 237 A.D. 361 (N.Y. 1997) (New York State human rights law forbids a dentist from turning away patients because of positive HIV tests).
72. *Lotspeich v. Chance Vought Aircraft,* 369 S.W. 2d 705 (Tex.App. 1963) (employer has liability under respondeat superior to employee for physician's negligence; no PPR); *Mracheck v. Sunshine Biscuit,* 308 N.Y. 116, 123 N.E. 2d 801 (1954) (employer liability for acts of negligent physician; no PPR).
73. *Lotspeich, supra* note 71 (no duty to employee except not to injure); *Mero v. Sadoff,* 31 Cal.App. 4th 1466, 37 Cal.Rptr. 2d 769 (1995) (physician who injuries patient during worker's compensation examination is liable in malpractice even in absence of PPR).
74. *Beadling v. Sirotta,* 41 N.J. 555, 197 A. 2d 857 (1964) (preemployment examination, duty of reasonable care; not entitled to results of examination, but entitled to not be injured during examination).
75. *Fleishman, supra* note 18.
76. *Wilmington General Hosp., supra* note 57.
77. *Dowling v. Mutual Life Ins. Co. of N.Y.,* 168 So. 2d 107 (La. 1964) (prior relationship may impose duty).
78. *Green v. Walker,* 910 F. 2d 291 (1990) (physician has responsibility "to the extent of the tests conducted").
79. *Keene v. Wiggins,* 69 Cal.App. 3d 308, 138 Cal.Rptr. 3 (1977) (no duty where examination is for report to employer but voluntary care or attempt to treat or benefit worker creates a duty).
80. *Maltempo v. Cuthbert,* 504 F. 2d 325 (5th Cir. 1974) (promise to parents to treat imprisoned son).
81. *Myers v. Quisenberry,* 144 Cal.App. 3d 888, 193 Cal.Rptr. 733 (1983) (failure to warn diabetic patient of driving risk).
82. *Lemmon v. Freese,* 210 N.W. 2d 576 (Ia. 1973) (liable for foreseeable injury to third party resulting from failure to warn patient of dangers of seizures).
83. *New Mexico Physicians, supra* note 64.
84. *Joseph v. Shafey,* 580 So. 2d 160 (Fla. 1991) (no duty or privity of contract between citizen shot by officer and officer's physician).
85. *Wilschinsky v. Medina,* 108 N.M. 511, 775 P. 2d 713 (1989) (physician's duty extends to members of the public who may be injured by sedated driver; the duty is met by warning the patient not to drive); *Zavalas v. State of Oregon,* 861 P. 2d 1026 124 Or. App. 166 (1993) (physician liable in negligence to people injured by patient driving under the influence of drug prescribed by physician); *Kaiser v. Suburban Transporation System,* 398 P. 2d 14 (Wash. 1965) (failure to warn bus driver of sedating effect of decongestant).
86. *DiMarco v. Lynch Homes Chester County, Inc.,* 559 A. 2d 330 (Pa. 1989) (injured third party relied on incorrect advice provided by physician to patient regarding communicability of hepatitis).
87. *Welke v. Kuzilla,* 144 Mich.App. 245, 375 N.W. 2d 403 (1985) (malpractice action allowed despite absence of PPR).
88. *McElwain v. Van Beek,* 447 N.W. 2d 442 (Minn.Ct.App. 1989) (duty to warn third parties applies only to dangers arising from the patient).
89. *Duvall v. Goldin,* 363 N.W. 2d 275 (Mich. 1984) (special relationship imposes duty on physician that benefits third party).
90. *Id.* (special relationship with dangerous person imposes a duty to warn public).
91. *Tarasoff v. Regents of the University of Calif.,* 17 Cal. 3d 425, 551 P. 2d 344, 131 Cal.Rptr. 14 (1976) (failure to warn third party of known threat presented by patient).
92. *Thompson v. County of Alameda,* 27 Cal. 3d 741, 614 P. 2d 728, 167 Cal.Rptr. 70 (1980) (endangered third party not readily identifiable; no duty to warn); *Sellers v. United States,* 870 F. 2d 1098 (6th Cir. 1989) (no duty to injured third party where in-patient psychiatric service had no knowledge of patient's harmful intent to a particular person).
93. *Peck v. Counseling Service of Addison County, Inc.,* 499 A. 2d 422 (Vt. 1985) (duty to warn nonpatient third party of possible property damage).
94. *Supra* note 59.
95. *Hoover, supra* note 12, at 250 (relationship between physician and patient no matter who pays).
96. *Davis v. Tirrell,* 443 N.Y.S. 2d 136 (1981) (psychiatrist employed by school district to examine student and advise district about handicap; no PPR).
97. Council on Ethical and Judicial Affairs, *supra* note 61.
98. *Thiele v. Ortiz,* 165 Ill.App. 3d 983, 520 N.E. 2d 881 (1988) (duty to evaluate possible complication of surgery 2 weeks postoperatively exists despite presence of other treating physicians).
99. *Peterson v. Phelps,* 123 Minn. 319, 143 N.W. 793 (1913) (termination of duties).
100. *Millbaugh v. Gilmore,* 30 Ohio St. 2d 319, 285 N.E. 2d 19 (1972) (patient's conduct terminated relationship).
101. *Brandt v. Grubin,* 131 N.J.Super. 182, 329 A. 2d 82 (1972) (referral of psychiatric patient terminates care).
102. *Hoemke v. New York Blood Center,* 720 F.Supp. 45 (S.D.N.Y. 1989) (physician had no duty to contact past recipients of blood tranfusions to warn them that they could be HIV infected and that they could spread the virus to others); *Boyer v. Smith,* 345 Pa.Super. 66, 497 A. 2d 646 (1985) (no duty to contact past recipient of medications when new risks discovered).

103. *Tresemar v. Burke,* 86 Cal.App. 3d 656, 150 Cal.Rptr. 384 (1978) (physician required to notify patients of risks of Dalkon shield once such risks became known).

104. *Burnett v. Laymon,* 181 S.W. 157 (Tenn. 1915) (definition of reasonable notice dictated by circumstances of case).

105. *Groce v. Myers,* 224 N.C. 165, 29 S.E. 2d 553 (1944) (reasonableness of notice).

106. *Miller v. Dore,* 154 Me. 363, 148 A. 2d 692 (1959) (must notify with sufficient time for patient to find substitute).

107. *Collins v. Meeker,* 198 Kan. 390, 424 P. 2d 488 (1967) (improper withdrawal from case).

108. *See* Measure and Elements of Damages in Action Against Physician to Achieve Particular Result or Cure. 99 A.L.R. 3d 303 (breach of contract).

109. *See* Liability of Physician Who Abandons Case, 57 A.L.R. 2d 432.

110. *Stohlman v. Davis,* 220 N.W. 247 (Neb. 1928); *Mucci v. Houghton,* 57 N.W. 305 (Iowa 1894); *Groce v. Myers,* 224 N.C. 165, 29 S.E. 2d 553 (1944) (abandonment defined).

111. *Chase v. Clinton County,* 217 N.W. 565 (Mich. 1928); *Alexandridis, Supra* note 32 (causes of action in abandonment).

112. *Thomas v. Corso,* 265 Md. 84, 288 A. 2d 379 (1972) (negligent care distinguished from abandonment).

113. *Easter v. Lexington Memorial Hosp.,* 303 N.C. 303, 278 S.E. 2d 253 (1984) (PPR required).

114. *State v. Warden,* 813 P. 2d 1146 (Utah 1991) (conviction for negligent homicide of infant upheld); *People v. Holvey,* 205 Cal.App. 3d 51, 252 Cal.Rptr. 335 (1988) (statute providing for criminal prosecution for "contributing to death of elderly dependent" is constitutional and applies to physicians; case remanded for trial; subsequently modified with respect to nonphysicians by *People v. Heitzman,* 9 Cal. 4th 189, 886 P. 2d 1229 (1994).

115. *People v. Anyakora,* 162 Misc 2d 47, 616 N.Y.S. 2d 149 (1993), *summary affirmation,* 238 A.D. 2d 216, 656 N.Y.S. 2d 253 (1997) (chief obstetrical resident convicted for failure to admit and for falsifying records used to justify refusal; action brought by Committee of Interns and Residents to obtain malpractice defense dismissed), 86 N.Y. 2d 478, 657 N.E. 2d 1315, 634 N.Y.S. 2d 32 (1995).

116. *Aufrichtig v. Lowell,* 85 N.Y. 2d 540, 650 N.E. 2d 401, 626 N.Y.S. 2d 743 (1995) (PPR creates a fiduciary duty that implies requirement to offer truthful testimony); *see also Hammond v. Aetna Casualty & Surety Co.,* 243 F.Supp. 793 N.D. Supp 793 (1965).

117. *Safer v. Estate of Pack,* 291 N.J.Super. 619, 677 A. 2d 1188 (1996), appeal denied, 146 N.J. 568, 683 A. 2d 1163 (1996) (physician has duty to warn those at known risk of avoidable harm from genetically transmissible condition, and duty extends to patient, as well as to members of immediate family of patient who may be adversely affected by breach of duty).

118. *Arato v. Avedon,* 5 Cal. 4th 1172, 858 P. 2d 598, 23 Cal.Rptr. 2d 131 (1993) (physician's duty does not extend to liability for inaccurate prognosis as to life expectancy).

Consent to and refusal of medical treatment

It is a fundamental principle of our legal system that all persons have the right to make major decisions regarding their bodies. The doctrine that a patient who is subject to medical treatment without consent has a cause of action against the physician or surgeon comes from two principles basic to our belief in the inalienable rights of all people. The relationship between patient and physician is one known to the law as a "fiduciary relationship" (good faith and trusting). The other principle involved in the doctrine of the right to consent to medical treatment is that a person of sound mind has the right to make the decision about what becomes of his or her body. Neither the state nor another individual has the right to compel someone to accept treatment that he or she does not want.

The Editorial Committee updated this chapter. The committee gratefully acknowledges the past contributions of Emidio A. Bianco, M.D., J.D., and Harold L. Hirsh, M.D., J.D.

CONSENT

One who consents to being touched cannot later complain that he or she has been battered, even though the touching may have caused actual harm. Valid consent of the person touched therefore is a complete defense to an action of battery.[1] However, an authorization of consent induced by misrepresentation, fraud, or duress is void and of no legal effect. Similarly a consent may be invalid if the act consented to is unlawful or if the consent was given by one who had no legal authority to give it.[2,3]

Opportunities for a battery in a medical care setting are considerable. A battery can occur in the absence of hands-on contact (e.g., the administration of medication, the application of x-rays and sound waves, or any procedure under the physician's control that does not involve actual body contact). Where the aforementioned conduct occurs in the absence of consent, the courts will probably find a constructive touching that is sufficient for a battery.

To be liable for battery, a person must commit some positive and affirmative act that results in an unpermitted contact.[4] Courts provided the action for battery as a means to keep the public peace by providing a legal substitute for private (physical) retribution.[5] Expert medical testimony is not required in a battery action. Because recovery may be based on the invasion of one's dignitary interest, one may recover from battery even in the absence of physical harm.[6] Physician-attorneys, physicians, and attorneys who are familiar with medicolegal issues know that an action against a physician based solely on the issue of battery is extraordinarily rare.

Expressed consent

Expressed consent occurs when a patient specifically grants the physician permission to undertake the diagnosis and treatment of a specific problem. Expressed consent may be given either in writing or by voice. Written permission creates less of a proof problem in court; vocal permission is legal but may create a credibility problem in the legal arena.

Implied consent

Consent may be implied by the conduct of the patient in a particular case or by the application of existing law in certain situations. A patient who voluntarily submits to treatment under circumstances that would indicate awareness of the planned treatment authorizes the treatment by implication, even without express consent. A patient who presents himself or herself at the physician's office for a routine procedure implies his or her consent to treatment.

Implied consent, particularly in the light of informed consent, is risky for physicians and should be relied on only for simple, routine procedures. To avoid the legal risks of implied consent, the physician should carefully document the circumstances of treatment in the patient's record or document the explanation given to the patient concerning the proposed treatment. However, there are many medical circumstances in which courts will readily find that consent was implied.

Under certain circumstances, the law, either by court opinion or by statute, creates an implication of consent.[7] For example, the courts generally find implied consent in a medical emergency. It is presumed as a matter of law that a conscious reasonable person suffering from a condition requiring emergency medical treatment would consent to treatment. When expressed consent may not be apparent by voice or writing, implied consent will be found in most cases, which is probably the reason that traditional consent cases remain extraordinarily rare despite an aggressively litigious society. Implied consent is frequently apparent (e.g., by some manifestation, by an overt sign, or by the patient's failure to object to being touched).

Some medical situations in which implied consent is readily apparent include an emergency, an emergency involving a minor child, a comatose patient requiring immediate treatment, a mentally incompetent patient requiring treatment when a legal guardian is unavailable, an intoxicated patient who temporarily lacks the capacity to reason (consent) yet requires care, and a patient who did not sign the consent form but nevertheless allowed treatment to proceed without objection.

SCOPE OF CONSENT

When a patient consents to medical therapy, the performance of a procedure, or a surgical operation, the scope of the consent is limited to whatever parameters were expressed before the medical intervention; nevertheless, in the appropriate clinical circumstances an extension of the scope of the consent would be permissible.

As a general rule, a physician commits a battery if he or she exceeds the scope of consent given by a patient. The problem usually occurs when a surgeon extends a surgical procedure beyond the limits previously discussed with the patient. If the surgeon performs the wrong procedure, clearly he or she is outside the scope of the patient's consent. If he or she performs the wrong procedure in addition to the one authorized by the patient, the surgeon may be liable for battery. Thus a physician who performed a nonemergent hysterectomy when he found infected fallopian tubes during surgery on a patient who had consented only to a repair of a lacerated uterus was held liable.[8]

Most jurisdictions have ruled that a physician may extend a procedure beyond the scope of consent to treat an emergency.[9] In many states a surgeon may extend the surgery if he or she discovers an unexpected abnormal condition during the operation, and if prompt treatment is reasonably advisable for the welfare of the patient.[10] If the patient authorizes a physician to remedy a condition rather than to perform a specific procedure, the courts will generally allow the physician to render treatments reasonably necessary to correct the condition.[11] The patient's consent to one procedure does not imply consent to a prohibited extension of such procedure.[12] An operative permit (the consent form) cannot use vague language, such as "anything the physician thinks is necessary." The carte blanche assumed by some physicians of a previous generation is a thing of the past.

CONSENT BY MINORS

The general rule of law is that a minor (age defined by the particular jurisdiction in which one resides) must obtain the consent of a parent or guardian before a physician may proceed with nonemergency treatment. Most jurisdictions have enacted exceptions, however, that allow a minor to consent to selected or limited medical care without the advice or consent of parents. Some examples of minor consent exceptions include the following:
- A minor who is married
- A minor who is a parent but unmarried

- Statutory therapeutic exceptions (e.g., treatment for chemical abuse, treatment of sexually transmitted diseases, provision of contraceptives, physical examination for rape, abortion, and psychotherapy)
- A minor who requires emergency care

Most of the statutory exceptions are self-evident; however, the emergency medical situation deserves further consideration. Most physicians understand that where there is imminent danger of death without emergency treatment, consent will be implied. On the other hand, what reasonable action can a physician undertake when the medical circumstances require that he or she anticipate the need to intervene to prevent an impending medical disaster? For example, a 14-year-old boy is brought to the emergency department for the evaluation and treatment of a displaced, compound comminuted fracture of the femur. The orthopedist quickly straightens the lower extremity to reduce the potential for permanent neurovascular damage. The patient requires treatment as soon as possible, but the clinical circumstances are not a matter of life and death. The first step is for the physician to comfort the patient. The second step is for him or her to use all reasonable means, with administrative assistance, to contact the patient's parents. The third step is for the physician to make a reasonable medical judgment, in the best interest of the patient, as to how long treatment can be postponed before encountering a high risk of bone infection or neurovascular damage. Let us assume that in this case the orthopedist reasonably concluded that 30 minutes was a safe interim. After the 30 minutes have passed, the parents are still nowhere to be found. The physician talks to the boy, explaining the necessity for the procedure, then proceeds. Two hours later the parents appear in the emergency department and confront the orthopedist about operating without their consent. The orthopedist has two defenses: (1) A reasonable effort was made to contact the parents, who were unavailable (from a legal point of view, they had constructively abandoned their child), and (2) the physician was put in the position of acting in locus parentis (became the parent on-the-spot) and acted in the best interest of the child based on his orthopedic expertise, which led him to anticipate immediate danger of permanent injury.

Another case involves a 12-year-old Jehovah's Witness who sustained a ruptured spleen during a Little League football game. On arrival at the emergency department the patient is momentarily stable; the ruptured spleen is recognized immediately, and potential disaster is anticipated. Blood transfusions are medically necessary. The parents will not consent to treatment because of their religious convictions. Suddenly the child takes a turn for the worse. The immediate diagnosis is recurrence of bleeding. The physician instructs hospital administration to obtain a court order, but treatment cannot be postponed until the order becomes available. The physician wheels the child into the operating room, starts a blood transfusion, performs a splenectomy, and saves the child's life. Because the state has a compelling interest in saving innocent third parties, courts will invariably override the parental right to consent even in the face of a First Amendment right. Most courts assert that a minor does not possess the maturity and experience required to exercise an unfettered religious right to refuse lifesaving treatment.

CONSENT BY SPOUSE

Consent to treatment by one spouse for the other spouse is not generally recognized by American law, even when the other spouse is incompetent, unless the spouse has been appointed legal guardian by a court of proper jurisdiction. Physicians tend to be intimidated by a patient's aggressive spouse. Both physicians and spouses frequently and mistakenly believe that marriage compromises a person's right to consent, believing that marriage somehow endows one spouse with the right to co-consent for the other spouse or to veto the other spouse's given consent.

In 1974 the Oklahoma Supreme Court reviewed a case in which J.C. Murray, the husband of Artie V. Murray, sued Dr. D.C. Vandevander, alleging that Vandevander performed a panhysterectomy on his wife without his consent.[13] The question on appeal was whether a husband could recover from a physician and hospital for damage to a marital relationship resulting from an operation on his wife. The court stated that a married woman, even though living with her husband, has a statutory right to separate earnings and a natural right to her health, strength, skill, and capacity to earn and that the natural right of a married woman to her health is not qualified by requiring that she have the consent of her husband to receive surgical care from a physician.

The husband has no inherent power to consent for his wife, nor does he have a right of refusal that can override his wife's consent to treatment.

In 1976, in *Danforth v. Planned Parenthood of Central Missouri,* the U.S. Supreme Court reviewed the constitutionality of a Missouri statute on abortion, which among other things stated:

1. Before submitting to an abortion during the first 12 weeks of pregnancy, a woman must consent in writing to the procedure and certify that her consent is informed and freely given and is not the result of coercion.
2. A woman seeking an abortion must have the co-consent in writing of the spouse unless a licensed physician certifies that the abortion is necessary to preserve the mother's life.
3. An unmarried woman younger than 18 years must have the written consent of a parent or person in loco parentis.[14]

The court had no problem with the requirement that a woman give informed consent before undergoing an abortion. Justice Blackmun delivered the opinion of the court.[14] In *Roe v. Wade* the Supreme Court held that, before approximately the end of the first trimester, the abortion decision and its effectuation must be left to the medical judgment of the pregnant woman's attending physician; subsequent to approximately the end of the first trimester, the state may regulate abortion procedure in ways reasonably related to maternal health; and at the stage subsequent to viability, the state may regulate and even proscribe abortion except where an abortion is deemed medically necessary for the preservation of the life or health of the mother.[15]

Applying this reasoning to *Danforth,* Justice Blackmun, speaking for the court, stated:

The spousal consent provision . . . which does not comport with this standard enunciated in *Roe v. Wade* is unconstitutional, since the State cannot delegate to a spouse a veto power which the state itself is absolutely and totally prohibited from exercising during the first trimester of pregnancy. The state may not constitutionally impose a blanket parental consent requirement . . . as a condition for an unmarried minor's abortion during the first 12 weeks of her pregnancy for substantially the same reasons as in the case of the spousal consent provision.

In the absence of constitutionally acceptable legislation regulating spousal consent, the common law recognizes a person's natural right to consent for treatment and that this natural right is not conditioned by marriage. In *Danforth* the Supreme Court ruled that, during the first 12 weeks of gestation, the requirement for co-consent by a spouse or parental consent for a minor was unconstitutional on the basis that a state cannot grant to a person veto power that the state itself does not possess.

Although a physician acting in the best interest of a patient may rely on the consent of the spouse of an unadjudicated incompetent patient, the consent of a competent patient's spouse is not a valid substitute for the consent of the patient. Nor is spousal consent a prerequisite for treatment of a competent patient, even if the treatment involves procedures that may affect the patient's marital relationship.[16] However, it is advisable to discuss thoroughly with the patient and his or her spouse any procedure that may compromise the patient's ability to reproduce or perform sexually. Although the husband's consent is not required for artificial insemination of his wife, a husband who is not consulted and does not consent may not be liable for support of the resulting child and a subsequent divorce may be based on adultery.[17] Because the welfare of the child resulting from artificial insemination may be at stake, the physician should not perform such a procedure without the consent of both husband and wife.

CONSENT BY FAMILY MEMBERS

For reasons similar to those cited in the three preceding cases, a family member's right to consent for another family member is not recognized by American law unless the family member is a legal guardian appointed by a court of proper jurisdiction or is the natural guardian of a minor child.[18] Karen Quinlan, approximately 21 years of age, overdosed with phenobarbital and chlordiazepoxide (Librium). After it

became apparent that she would not regain consciousness, Joseph Quinlan (Karen's father) was appointed her legal guardian, and he ordered the withdrawal of treatment; however, Karen's physicians refused to comply. Eventually the New Jersey Supreme Court ruled that Joe Quinlan, acting as Karen's legal guardian, could order the withdrawal of treatment and that such withdrawal of treatment would not be considered homicide but rather the exercise of a legitimate consent right to refuse treatment in Karen's best interest.

LEGAL DIMENSIONS

At least three legal dimensions surround a person's right to self-determination. The first dimension involves the law of battery, which implies that any unpermitted contact or offensive touching is a personal indignity. The second dimension of modern consent law—informed consent—is concerned with whether a physician imparts that amount of information that a patient has a right to expect before making an intelligent, informed choice about whether to accept or reject medical recommendations. The third dimension of modern consent law is based on the right to privacy (right against the invasion of one's privacy). From a medical perspective the right against the invasion of one's privacy is a doctrine that usually deals with the right of a patient to refuse lifesaving treatment. The Supreme Court found that the right to privacy was evident from the penumbras (shadowed regions) formed by emanations from the Bill of Rights, specifically the First, Third, Fourth, Fifth, and Ninth Amendments.[19]

INFORMED CONSENT

The purpose of the doctrine of informed consent, implicit in its name, is to give the patient sufficient information so that he or she has the opportunity to make a knowledgeable and informed decision about the use of a drug or device in the course of treatment. It is part of the duty to warn the patient. The development of the doctrine of informed consent during the past two decades is evidence of the recent enforcement of this duty to warn.

Informed consent implies joint decision-making. The patient's right of self-decision can be effectively exercised only when the patient possesses enough information to enable him or her to make an intelligent choice. Informed consent is a basic social policy for which exceptions are permitted where risk disclosure poses such a serious psychological threat or detriment to the patient as to be medically contraindicated.[20]

Physicians should be mindful of the fact that the legal doctrine of informed consent has very strong moral and ethical overtones. The American Medical Association's (AMA's) first, second, and fifth Principles of Medical Ethics imply the ethics of informed consent as follows: "A physician shall be dedicated to provide competent medical service with compassion and respect for human dignity, and shall deal honestly with patients and colleagues, . . . [and] make relevant information available to patients, colleagues, and the public."[21]

According to the American College of Physicians' Ethics Manual, the patient should be informed and educated about his or her condition, should understand and approve of his or her treatment, and should participate responsibly in his or her own care.[22] One can reasonably conclude that physicians have a moral, ethical, and legal duty to impart to a patient whatever relevant information is necessary to make an informed decision either to reject or to accept treatment.

This background information should make it clear that the physician must obtain the patient's consent to touch or treat, and the patient should have enough information to provide consent that is based on an informed, intelligent choice to either accept or reject a physician's recommendations. Whereas traditional consent emanates from the law of battery, the prevailing view is that treatment administered in the absence of informed consent is actionable under a negligence rather than a battery theory.[23] In other words, a physician's failure to provide a patient with information necessary to make an informed, intelligent choice is a breach of the standard of disclosure, which if found to be the cause of the alleged injury, makes a prima facie case for negligence (breach of a duty causing an injury). Thus an action against a physician for the lack of informed consent may prevail even though traditional consent was obtained and even though the physician's performance otherwise remained within acceptable standards of medical practice. Because the doctrine of informed consent is grounded in the law of negligence, a physician's duty to disclose is more than a call merely to speak at the patient's request or merely to answer the patient's question; it is a duty to volunteer, if necessary, that information needed by the patient to make intelligent decisions.[24]

Whether to disclose

Once the physician-patient relationship is established, the physician has a duty to inform the patient of his or her condition, the presumptive diagnosis, the differential diagnoses, the purposes of tests, the treatment options, the associated risks, the alternatives, the prognosis, and the expectations.[25]

Patients have a right to know everything that they need to know to decide for themselves whether to undergo therapy, surgery, or even a diagnostic procedure. The doctrine of informed consent recognizes that patients have the right to know and to understand their diagnoses and the right to choose or refuse therapy.

The physician should rarely, if ever, withhold material information or pressure the patient into making a decision, regardless of the patient's personality makeup or any scientific or medical facts. The test for the sufficiency of disclosure is not the length of a catalog of all information; it is the relevance of the information to the decision being made. When properly informed, the patient cannot say, "If I had only known this, that, or the other, I would have decided differently"—the so-called but for assertion. Of course, the law recognizes that a responsible relative or other person may receive information that, if told to the patient, might harm the patient's physical or emotional condition. Physicians' invoking the so-called therapeutic professional discretion is now accepted. In an emergency situation nothing should be allowed to interfere with prompt treatment.

Materiality is the touchstone for determining the adequacy of the disclosure. There are numerous definitions and tests as to what constitutes materiality. In any such test the crux of the issue is the effect of the nondisclosure on the patient's ability to make an intelligent choice, and as such each case presents the issue as a question of fact.

To give an informed consent to medical treatment, a patient should be told his or her diagnosis, the differential diagnosis, the nature of the diagnosis, the nature of the therapeutic procedure to be performed, the material risk associated with his or her care and management, the prospect of success of the treatment (i.e., the prognosis or expectations), and the detail of alternative courses of treatment that are available. The physician has the duty to inform the patient of the adverse consequences of any proposed treatment or procedure so as to enable the patient to make an intelligent decision about whether or not to consent to the treatment. This duty is particularly compelling when the recommended treatment includes a type of elective surgery and the probability of the risk might dissuade a person from submitting to the treatment.

Elements of informed consent

Based on a number of appellate decisions, the following elements of informed consent should be understood by practicing physicians[26,27]:

1. A physician should explain to the patient the nature of the procedure, treatment, or disease.
2. The patient should be informed about the expectations of the recommended treatment and the likelihood of success.
3. The patient should know what reasonable alternatives are available and what the probable outcome would be in the absence of any treatment.
4. The patient should be informed about the particular known inherent risks that are material to the informed decision about whether to accept or reject medical recommendations.

The first and second elements are commonly followed by physicians and are rarely, if ever, pivotal issues in an informed consent action. The third element generally is not a pivotal issue unless one of the reasonable alternatives might have been safer or the outcome of no treatment would not have been significantly different from that of treatment. The fourth element requires basic understanding because most physicians probably do not read cases written by appellate judges; thus most physicians probably are not familiar with the legal distinction between an inherent risk and a material risk. This distinction is rarely taught in medical schools or at medical conferences unless an attorney or physician familiar with informed consent has the opportunity to point out the distinction. For purposes of understanding, an inherent risk can be considered a medical concept; that is, an inherent risk is one of a number of known adverse effects (or injuries) that may result from the mere use of an indicated drug or the mere proper performance of a diagnostic procedure or surgical operation. A material risk is a particular inherent risk a physician knows or ought to know would be a significant factor in a reasonable person's decision whether to reject or accept treatment.[28] The scope of the disclosure (inherent risks that are material) must be measured by the patient's need to know whether a potential peril is material in making an intelligent informed choice.

SCOPE OF DISCLOSURE

The scope and propriety of the disclosure depend on the state of medical knowledge at the time of the disclosure. When appropriate, the patient also should be informed of the identities and responsibilities of other persons who will participate in the patient's care and management. A physician who specializes in psychiatry has the same legal duty as any other physician to exercise reasonable care in selecting, administering, and obtaining informed consent for treatment. A valid consent may be exercised only if the patient giving it is competent enough to engage in the informed consent process. Competency can be a particularly critical element for psychiatrists because they commonly treat patients whose cognitive capacity may be at issue.

Under the common law and in some states by statute, a competent adult has the fundamental right to control decisions relating to his or her own medical care, including decisions regarding the provision, withholding, or withdrawal of medical or surgical means or procedures calculated to prolong life.[29] Thus a physician's diagnosis, even if terminal, must be disclosed to a competent adult patient because the patient has a statutory right to make all necessary decisions concerning health care. Moreover, there is a recognized fiduciary, confidential physician-patient relationship in Florida that imposes on the physician the duty to disclose known facts.[30]

Courts have imposed on physicians a duty to inform a patient of an unfavorable diagnosis.[31] Some courts recognize the existence of a therapeutic privilege to withhold the diagnosis in certain situations.[32] In determining whether disclosure of an unfavorable diagnosis is required, the courts have considered factors such as the emotional status of the patient and in particular whether disclosure would seriously jeopardize the chances of recovery—even if slim.[33,34] However, in an ordinary case there would appear to be no justification for suppressing facts, and the physician should make a substantial disclosure to the patient or risk tort liability.[35] Although the Current Opinions of the Judicial Council of the American Medical Association does not specifically mention the issue of unfavorable diagnosis, Opinion 8.11 provides, "The physician must properly inform the patient of the diagnosis and of the nature and purpose of the treatment undertaken or prescribed. The physician may not refuse to inform the patient."[36]

Moreover, a patient's right to know is not necessarily confined to a situation in which "disease is present and has been conclusively diagnosed."[37] In one recent case a 37-year-old man had seen his physician about symptoms of exertional chest pain of several weeks' duration, and his physician prescribed nitroglycerin therapy. The court found that the physician had a duty to inform the patient that he suspected coronary artery disease, despite inconclusive tests.[38] Thus the duty of disclosure arises any time a treating physician is aware of abnormalities that indicate risk or danger, and it is premised on the belief that a patient needs to know such information to make an intelligent, informed decision about the future course of medical care.

Test results

The right to know also extends to test results. If an abnormal test has clinical significance, such as a Pap smear that suggests malignancy, the physician is obligated to notify the patient. Mere failure to notify in itself is not actionable. If a physician has made reasonable notification attempts and the patient has related incomplete or misleading identifying information, the patient's negligence might relieve the physician from liability for the failure to disclose significant test results.[39]

Risks

The disclosure must be viewed in the context of anticipated risks that fall within the expertise of the physician. Discretion consistent with this expertise is greater when the risk of adverse result is relatively slight. Similarly a full disclosure is not required where the disclosure of all risks would be impractical for therapeutic reasons (i.e., where the risk is very rare and not material to a patient's decision or would unduly frighten the patient into refusing to undergo necessary treatment that would definitely reduce morbidity or mortality).

A certain minute incidence of idiosyncratic allergic reactions and unexpected deaths has occurred in nearly all treatments and surgeries, and full disclosure of these unexpected risks has not been required. A minority view holds that all risks potentially affecting the patient's decision should be disclosed.

Complicated medical problems and treatments usually carry more risks and require a more complete explanation. The patient's questions, intelligent or not, need to be answered by the physician to the patient's satisfaction. Medically unknown risks clearly cannot be disclosed to the patient. All material risks of treatment that are not remote or merely theoretical must be explained to ensure that the patient understands.

When a physician wishes to treat a patient's complaint by a method that entails certain definite risks and knows that a safer alternative treatment exists, the physician is obliged to advise the patient to that effect. The patient has the right to decide which course of action he or she prefers. He or she may choose not to have any treatment at all. Failure to explain an alternative, if one exists, might be construed as negligence. In particular, when therapy is new, experimental, or unusual, there is a particular duty to warn the patient that all the effects of the treatment may not be completely known. As the probability or severity of risk to the patient increases, the physician's duty to inform increases. When a physician does not want to perform a procedure that interests the patient because he or she is not entirely convinced that it is the best or safest approach, as long as respectable medical opinion would consider it acceptable, the physician should at least tell the patient that the treatment is available elsewhere and help the patient contact those who perform it.

Alternatives

The physician's duty of disclosure has been held to encompass alternative modes of diagnosis and treatment. In other words, there is a duty to apprise the patient of those procedures that represent feasible alternatives to the method initially selected. He or she has a duty to explain available alternatives and to brief the patient as to the significant pros, cons, disadvantages, and dangers. Physicians should attempt to "walk in the patient's shoes" and consider the patient's hobbies, occupation, and the actual incidence of risks. Chloramphenicol's potential to cause a fatal aplastic anemia (1 in 25,000 to 40,000) has limited its use to the treatment of serious infections in which the location of the infection or the susceptibility of the organism limits or prevents the use of less toxic agents. This is particularly true in the treatment of typhoid fever caused by *Salmonella typhi* and meningitis caused by ampicillin-resistant *Haemophilus influenzae*. In a clinical situation where chloramphenicol is the best and most effective drug and is probably lifesaving, the indication for using chloramphenicol outweighs the risk of developing aplastic anemia, which in this case arguably is not a material risk. On the other hand, when prescribing chloramphenicol in a clinical situation in which another agent would be just as effective and safer, the incidence of aplastic anemia would be material.

An archetypal case involving informed consent is the treatment of hyperthyroidism. Three modes of treatment are still in vogue—drug therapy, radioactive iodine, and subtotal thyroidectomy. The material risks of drug therapy are a recurrence of hyperthyroidism (up to 72% of patients) and agranulocytosis (less than 1% of patients). The once-feared adverse effect of developing thyroid tumors in later years has not proved to be more likely in patients treated with radioactive iodine than in patients from a randomly selected population; however, the incidence of postradioactive hypothyroidism at 10 years ranges from 40% to 70%.[40] Laryngeal nerve injuries are a well-known risk of thyroidectomy that cause hoarseness. Consequences of superior laryngeal nerve injury are more subtle than recurrent laryngeal injury because vocal cord failure usually does not occur until after protracted use of the voice, such as opera singing, for approximately 60 minutes.[41] The most famous case illustrating this point is that of Amelita Galli-Curci, one of the world's great lyric sopranos of the 1920s whose voice would inevitably fail during the last act of an opera.[42] Vocal cord failure is an inherent material risk of subtotal thyroidectomy that should be disclosed, not only to persons such as Placido Domingo and Luciano Pavarotti, but to everyone because the "loss of voice" is a devastating injury.

Referrals or consultations

The duty to refer a patient to a specialist is most often imposed on general medicine practitioners. Under some circumstances, however, courts may impose a duty on a specialist to refer the patient to a subspecialist if a higher degree of skill and training is necessary in the management of the patient.[43] An illustrative case is *Logan v. Greenwich Hospital Association*.[44] In this case an internist suggested that a patient suffering from systemic lupus erythematosus undergo a kidney biopsy to determine the extent of her kidney disease. After referral to a urologist, the biopsy was performed, but the procedure was complicated by a punctured gall bladder requiring cholecystectomy.

The court agreed with the plaintiff's contention that the urologist, as the specialist who would perform the procedure, had a duty to disclose all viable alternatives to the method selected, regardless of whether such alternatives might prove more hazardous.[45] In this way the patient would possess all material information necessary for making an informed decision. On the other hand, one should seriously doubt that a reasonable patient would choose a more hazardous procedure or treatment. The referring internist was found to have reasonably relied on his colleague, a specialist in such matters, to present all viable alternatives.

Similarly, if a physician is not qualified to render necessary treatment, he or she bears a duty to advise the patient to consult an appropriate specialist who can provide the therapy.[46] The physician's duty to consult arises when he or she knows or reasonably should know that he or she does not possess the required knowledge and skill to treat the condition.[47] Some courts have held that this duty arises when a physician realizes that a method of therapy is ineffective and alternative modes of treatment are available.[48]

Uncertainty about the nature of the patient's condition is a material fact that must be communicated to a patient when obtaining informed consent. If consultation with a specialist would help clarify the diagnosis, this must be disclosed to the patient. Furthermore, failure to communicate uncertainty about the nature of the patient's condition in a timely manner is not defensible on grounds that the uncertainty was not disclosed until it was deemed appropriate to do so. This duty of disclosure extends to consulting physicians when their services are sought by an attending physician and paid for by the patient. In this situation consulting physicians, even though they may be indirect providers of medical care to the patient, owe a duty to exercise due care and diligence in communicating favorable or unfavorable findings or diagnoses to the attending physician and to the patient, if necessary. Generally, communication of findings by telephone or by written report to the attending physician will be sufficient. However, in some situations it may be necessary for the consulting physician to both call and write the treating physician and to communicate to the patient directly. The type and urgency of the communication depend on considerations such as the severity of the condition, the potential for harm caused by the delay in proper diagnosis and treatment, and the extent of the patient's knowledge of his or her injury or illness so as to avoid any unnecessary delay in diagnosis and treatment.

PROGNOSIS

Patients are entitled to know the full prognosis, complications, sequelae, discomforts, cost, inconveniences, and risks of each option, including no treatment or no action. Patients have a right to know what to expect and what might happen to them. All of this is predicated on the reasonable foreseeability of events by the physician. Rare or exotic events are not part of informed consent.

Disclosure standards developed by courts

Two approaches—the professional disclosure standard and the general disclosure standard, or reasonable patient standard—have been adopted by the courts in delineating the scope of the physician's disclosure obligation. The objective or reasonable patient disclosure standard, which is set forth by statute or common law in a significant minority of jurisdictions, imposes a duty on the part of the physician to disclose any information that would reasonably bear on the patient's decision-making process. It should be tailored to the ability of the patient to comprehend. Even in the face of supportive expert medical testimony, a physician may be found to have breached the proper disclosure standard in these jurisdictions if a jury were to conclude that specific information that was not disclosed would have influenced significantly the reasonable patient's decision whether to undergo a particular form of therapy or treatment. The general standard permits the jury to decide whether the physician disclosed enough information for a reasonable patient to make an informed choice about treatment, whereas the professional standard permits physicians to testify whether the physician defendant disclosed sufficient information, according to community standards of medical practice. The modern trend is for courts to adopt the general standard.

Who discloses?

Who is responsible for obtaining the patient's informed consent?[49] The courts generally have placed the duty on the pa-

tient's attending physician at the time in question.[50,51] The courts generally recognize that the physician rather than a nurse or other health care provider is best qualified to discuss care and management. The nurse or other provider may only supplement or complement the physician's specific information with general information regarding the patient's situation. A substitute physician covering for the patient's original physician has an independent obligation to inform the patient of the risks, benefits, and alternatives to the part of the treatment that he or she is to administer.

Courts are eminently clear in their written opinions that the responsibility to obtain informed consent from a patient clearly remains with the physician, and this responsibility cannot be delegated. The physician may delegate authority to obtain informed consent to another physician but cannot delegate his or her responsibility for obtaining a proper informed consent. Apparently, appellate courts believe that a physician is in the best position to decide what information should be disclosed for the patient to make an informed choice, notwithstanding the fact that courts do not provide practical standards of disclosure. The scope of disclosure in any given case is a physician's responsibility. It is hoped that thoughtful discussion will be sufficient at trial to overcome an action for a lack of informed consent. On the other hand, appellate courts have furnished physicians with formidable defenses against an action for a lack of informed consent (discussed later).

Hospital role

A question that frequently arises, particularly for those practicing in a hospital setting, is, "Does the hospital have a responsibility to ensure that the patient received adequate disclosure even though the courts have placed the primary duty in the physician's hands?"[52]

Under the theory of respondeat superior, an employer-hospital could be held jointly liable with an employee-physician whose failure to obtain informed consent can be shown to have caused injury and damage to a patient. Yet, hospitals are not uninvolved in the consent process. Physicians must be supplied with the medical records, forms, or other documents needed to record the patient's informed consent. A hospital policy must govern the procedure by which consents are obtained, and deviation from such a procedure is admissible evidence.[53] Hospital liability can arise when the hospital knew or should have known that the physician did not obtain the patient's informed consent or when the hospital failed to prevent surgery or another treatment from proceeding without the informed consent of the patient. If consent previously given is withdrawn by the patient, nurses or other hospital personnel must delay planned physician treatment so that the physician can clarify the patient's decision. A nurse's or other hospital employee's dialogue with a patient concerning informed consent or procurement of a written authorization from the patient does not relieve the attending physician of the duty to disclose and is likely to be viewed as a mere ministerial act of the hospital employee.

Another development that renews the focus on the hospital's role in informed consent is the courts' tendency to impose stricter obligations on hospitals to ensure that physicians obtain consent before performing a procedure. With a nurse acting as its agent, a hospital should monitor whether consent has been obtained.

CONSENT FORMS

The mere fact that the hospital supplies consent forms does not suffice to impose a duty on the hospital to make a disclosure. The nurse may supplement or complement the physician's specific information with general information regarding the patient's situation. Hospitals have the duty to ensure that informed consent is properly obtained.[54] One court called a hospital's failure to ensure that informed consent was properly obtained a "fraudulent concealment."[55]

A patient who consents to surgery performed by a specific surgeon and is operated on by another surgeon can successfully sue the surgeon who did not operate for malpractice based on lack of informed consent and can sue the operating surgeon for battery.[56] One court has allowed recovery on a claim of unnecessary surgery based on lack of informed consent.[57]

A consent form is not essential but may be helpful in establishing at trial that consent was obtained; however, it is not determinative of the issue. The mere signing of a written consent form constitutes only some evidence of a valid consent; the consent must be based on all the elements of true informed consent—knowledge, voluntariness, and competency.

General-purpose consent forms that allow for insertion of specific information also can be used for numerous procedures and treatments. Most states prohibit by statute or by common law any provisions under which the patient releases in writing the physician or hospital from prospective liability that arises from actions or inactions involving the patient's medical care.

Some hospitals and many physicians have developed consent forms that summarize such information and also constitute a permanent record, usually in the patient's medical chart, of the communication between physician and patient. Formats vary considerably according to the treatment setting and particular procedures involved. The AMA and other organizations have published consent form manuals that provide sample forms.[58] Witnesses and signed permits are not required; however, a witnessed form is an attestation that an informed consent session took place (although it is not an attestation that the patient necessarily received adequate disclosure). Even well-drawn consent forms may not prevent allegations of failure to obtain consent in cases involving complex or high-risk treatments.[59] Adequate informed consent is best established by an accurate narrative documentation by the attending physician.[60]

When a patient alleges that a physician failed to obtain valid consent to treatment, the primary question is likely to be, "What did the physician tell the patient?" Because most professional negligence actions do not reach litigation until several years after the treatment was rendered, it is important to document the information communicated to the patient concerning the proposed treatment.

Authority to give consent

Adults are presumed competent and therefore must consent to proposed treatment. An incompetent adult patient who is incapacitated by physical or mental illness and is unable to understand the nature and consequences of his or her actions cannot give a valid informed consent to proposed treatment. As a result, consent must be obtained from someone who is authorized to consent on behalf of the patient. The same is true for minors, who in most instances lack the legal capacity to consent. Where a court has adjudicated the patient to be incompetent, the patient's court-appointed guardian or conservator must authorize the treatment proposed for the patient. If the physician has determined that the patient is incapable of comprehending the nature and consequences of his or her conduct, but the patient has not been judged incompetent, most courts may decide to accept the consent of the patient's next of kin (the closest known relative). In such cases the courts view the guardian or relative as standing in the shoes of the patient.

Substituted consent gives rise to a number of problems. The authority of one to consent to treatment for an incompetent patient necessarily implies the right to refuse such treatment. However, the courts have restricted this right of refusal in cases in which consent was unreasonably withheld.[61] In such cases the physician or hospital may treat the case as an emergency and seek a court order authorizing the necessary treatment. Two issues must be considered: (1) Is there a demonstrable need to proceed before the patient will be able to consider the matter, assuming he or she will become lucid, and (2) is the proposed treatment appropriate for the patient' condition? If there is not enough time to seek a court order, it is wise for the physician to consult with one or more colleagues and document their concurrence with the proposed therapeutic measures and the need to proceed with the treatment.[62]

If the patient's next of kin disagrees with the proposed treatment or if the patient, although incompetent, takes a position contrary to the family's wishes, the physician must be extremely cautious. There is some indication that the courts will consider the wishes of the patient, even though he or she may be unable to give valid consent.[63] In most cases it is best to proceed quickly with treatment (1) if a near relative has consented, (2) if it is medically necessary to proceed quickly with treatment, and (3) if there is no applicable prohibitive statute.[64]

The best way to avoid the legal risks of substituted consent for an incompetent adult patient is to place the matter before a court. In most states any adult citizen of the state, including a near relative of the patient, may petition the court to establish a conservator or guardian of the patient.[65] The process is usually simple and inexpensive. If there are conflicts of interest involving the relative who would consent for the patient or if the patient has strong views on the matter, they will be considered in the conservatorship or guardianship hearing and will be weighed by the court in appointing a person authorized to consent for the patient.

Ability to consent

Consent must be given by a patient who is mentally and physically capable of comprehending the information provided by the physician during the dialogue and making a decision concerning the course of treatment. The physical effects of pain or medication must not be so great as to diminish the patient's mental abilities to comprehend the consent process. The fact that the patient is suffering from mental illness or transitory episodes of nonlucidity does not necessarily vitiate the mental capacity to consent to treatment. The mere fact that the patient refuses diagnosis or treatment does not reflect lack of mental capacity to consent to treatment. Coercion must not be used to induce consent. Those patients lacking mental capacity to give informed consent require a surrogate, usually a close family member or guardian, to give substitute consent.

In the absence of a court-appointed guardian, a third party may be empowered to act on behalf of a principal under the terms of a written power of attorney. Such a document confers authority on a third party to handle specific personal or financial matters on behalf of the principal. In recent years these documents have been used to permit a third party to make health care decisions on behalf of a principal who has become functionally incompetent. Under numerous state statutes, these powers of attorney are legally effective until there has been a judicial declaration of incompetence or disability. Case law and statutory law do not generally mandate appointment of a guardian to provide consent if interested family members of the patient are available to provide consent for routine day-to-day procedures. No decisions have been reported wherein physicians or hospitals have been found liable for not resorting to court processes to obtain consent. However, certain types of patients and procedures, such as sterilization of a mentally incompetent patient, will usually require the appointment and consent of a guardian under the statutes of certain jurisdictions. These statutes must be consulted before unusual procedures, such as sterilization, electroconvulsive therapy, psychosurgery, or investigational treatments, are undertaken.

The physician whose patient has already received the appointment of a guardian must obtain the informed consent of the guardian through the same process of dialogue that the physician would have had with the patient if he or she were competent. Where the court has not previously appointed a guardian for the incompetent patient, the physician's decision to obtain informed consent for nonemergency diagnosis or treatment from family or from a court-appointed guardian will depend on the policy of the hospital.

Issues of informed consent and competency may be among the first to arise when plans are being made for patients with mental disabilities. The determination of competency is a legal issue decided by the courts, and the courts apply different standards of competency in different situations (the degree of competency needed to make a valid will is different from the degree of competency needed to execute a valid power of attorney or to give effective consent for medical treatment). Thus, for example, a psychiatrist may perform a mental status examination and render an opinion regarding the ability of a patient to make a reasoned judgment about a particular matter, but the actual decision about competency is a legal determination made by the courts. Where the patient is considered incompetent to make medical decisions and treatment is indicated on a medical basis, courts can authorize or reject treatment based on the doctrine of substituted judgment.

In most states, if the patient is incompetent, the spouse may give consent for the patient in emergency and certain nonemergency situations (custodial medical care). Children, grandchildren, parents, grandparents, siblings, nieces, nephews, or cousins, however, may or may not legally give consent for incompetent patients in medical matters, and court proceedings to designate a guardian may be necessary. In some situations in which there is a difference of opinion among family members regarding a patient's care or if family members are distant emotionally or geographically, formal legal proceedings may be advisable to determine who can give consent for the incompetent patient.

An exception to the requirement of informed consent is recognized when the patient is incompetent and the procedure contemplated is more of a routine, remedial measure. For example, daily custodial care of incompetent institutionalized psychiatric patients is excepted. However, if informed consent would be required for a specific treatment (e.g., the administration of electroconvulsive therapy) the consent of a guardian or appointed substitute decision-maker is required. If the physician has determined that a patient is incapable of comprehending the nature and consequences of his or her conduct but the patient has not been judged legally incompetent, most courts will accept the consent of the patient's next of kin as defined by local law.

If the patient is not competent to understand his or her illness, in all probability any consent that he or she gives will be held to be legally invalid. Because mental disability may alter the patient's ability to understand and cope with the implications of the diagnosis, the physician must tailor his or her explanation according to the individual patient's condition. Most patients can be told that they have a memory problem, that they will need to trust and rely on others to assist them, that they will receive continuing care from the physician, and that research is underway for long-term solutions. If the patient is incompetent to consent, family members should be told the full details of what to expect.

Exceptions to material disclosure

There are four generally recognized exceptions to the physician's duty to make prior disclosure of material risks, although all four might not necessarily be available in a particular state. First, in his or her professional judgment a physician may conclude that disclosure of a risk poses such a threat of detriment to the patient that it is contraindicated from a medical point of view. This is known as *therapeutic privilege* or *professional discretion*.[66] The physician may choose to use therapeutic professional discretion to keep medical facts from the patient or surrogate when the physician believes disclosure would be harmful, dangerous, or injurious to the patient. Depending on the circumstances, the physician may make the revelations to the next of kin, although he or she is not required to do so.[67,68] However, the privilege will not be upheld simply because the physician believes that a patient would probably refuse treatment if informed of the material risks. Withholding information must be based on the physician's established knowledge that his or her patient will be unduly alarmed by a full disclosure. Second, a competent patient may specifically ask not to be informed.[69] A patient may waive his or her right to make an informed consent. In other words, a physician need not disclose the nature and risks of a treatment to a patient who specifically requests that he or she not be told. The patient may reject disclosure out of a desire to remain ignorant, or the patient may have already had a similar medical experience. Third, a physician is privileged not to advise the patient of matters that are common knowledge or of which the patient has actual knowledge, particularly on the basis of past experience.[70] Fourth, no duty to inform arises in an emergency in which the patient is unconscious or otherwise incapable of giving valid consent and harm from failure to treat is imminent and outweighs any harm threatened by the proposed treatment.[71]

Opinion 8.07 of the AMA's *Current Opinions of the Judicial Counsel,* regarding informed consent, could justify by analogy exercising therapeutic privilege by withholding grave prognostic information on the same basis as withholding information regarding risks of treatment.[72]

"The patient's right of self-decision can be effectively exercised only if the patient possesses enough information to enable an intelligent choice. The patient should make his own determination of treatment. Informed consent is a basic social policy for which exceptions are permitted . . . [as] when risk disclosure poses such a serious psychological threat or detriment to the patient as to be medically contraindicated. Social policy does not accept the paternalistic view that the physician may remain silent because divulgence might prompt the patient to forego needed therapy."

EMERGENCY CARE AND INFORMED CONSENT

Generally the law implies patient consent during emergency situations.[73] The courts generally hold that conditions requiring immediate treatment for the protection of the patient's life or health justify the implication of consent if it is impossible to obtain express consent from the patient or from one who is authorized to consent on his or her behalf.[74] The courts simply assume that a competent, lucid adult would consent to lifesaving treatment. It is essential to document the circumstances that created the emergency.[75] In such cases the physician must document the following facts: (1) the treatment was for the patient's benefit, (2) an actual emergency existed, and (3) there was an inability to obtain the express consent of the patient or someone authorized to consent on his or her behalf.[76-78] An emergency is defined as a condition in which there is an immediate threat to the life, person, or health of the patient, and the hazard to the patient will increase without immediate treatment.[79]

The fact that the proposed treatment may be medically advisable or may become essential at some future time is not sufficient to allow nonconsensual treatment.[80] If the physician is uncertain whether the patient's condition warrants immediate action without consent, he or she should seek confirmation of the emergency from a colleague. In one case the court, deciding in favor of the treating physician, relied heavily on the fact that the treating physician had obtained concurring consultations from four surgeons before amputating the patient's crushed foot after a train accident.[81] Generally the courts have decided in favor of the physician in cases in which immediate treatment was necessary to eliminate an imminent threat of death or harm to the patient.

The general rule concerning consent for emergency treatment applies to the treatment of minors, as well as adults.[82] The courts have consistently held in favor of physicians who have treated "mature" minors (usually older than 15 years) who have consented to their own emergency treatment.[83] The courts tend to favor any medical or surgical treatment that is necessary to prevent serious injury to or impairment of the health of a child. However, in any case involving emergency treatment of a minor, it is prudent to make and document an effort to contact the minor patient's parents or another legally responsible person.

CAUSES OF ACTION

Conceptually, informed consent merges into and derives from the following:
   Assault and battery
   Negligence involving the duty to disclose
   Simply the tort of lack of informed consent
   The ethical and legal respect for dignity, autonomy, and life
Within the context of informed consent, the theories of battery and medical malpractice concepts are not inconsistent, and it is not necessary to require that the patient make an election of the theory of the case. In jurisdictions allowing alternative pleading, both battery and negligence allegations may be asserted for a claimed lack of informed consent. However, as a matter of proof these two torts are essentially mutually exclusive. It is difficult to prove by a preponderance of the evidence that the physician intentionally and carelessly failed to obtain the patient's informed consent.

The failure to achieve an informed consent can raise a negligence claim based on the physician's failure to disclose material information to the patient, which is a duty imposed by virtue of the physician-patient relationship. To establish such a claim, however, there must be evidence that the physician knew or should have known that the undisclosed information was material to an informed decision. Recovery is appropriate under an informed consent claim only if the undisclosed information is proved to have caused the patient's alleged injury. The fact that the procedure was the most appropriate or best treatment possible or that it was not administered negligently is immaterial.

The early and even some later cases involving patient consent spoke almost exclusively of battery and were concerned with a physician's intentional, unauthorized touching of the patient.[84] A few of the early cases, however, raised the question of whether the action for failure to obtain patient consent ought properly to lie in negligence rather than battery.[85] In 1957 the California Supreme Court held that an action arising from a physician's failure to give a patient sufficient information to make an informed decision should sound in negligence not battery.[86] The court held that a physician violates his or her duty to the patient and subjects himself or herself to liability if he or she withholds any facts necessary to form the basis of an intelligent consent. Courts now appear to agree that negligence is the proper cause of action for failure to inform a patient properly about a procedure for which consent is sought.[87] Actions grounded in battery are still found but usually involve cases in which (1) the patient consented to one procedure and another was actually performed, (2) the physician failed to disclose a disability that was certain to result from a proposed nonemergency procedure, or (3) the physician performed an experimental procedure without advising the patient of its experimental nature.[88-90]

An increasing number of courts allow the jury to determine whether the physician withheld information necessary to form a reasonable and intelligent decision about proposed treatment. Some courts require no expert testimony, but others allow expert testimony on the question of the materiality of the information withheld and whether the alleged injury is related to the therapeutic or diagnostic process.[91,92] Depending on the jurisdiction, one of two tests is used by the jury when determining whether the plaintiff patient would have refused treatment: (1) The subjective test, which requires the jury to ascertain whether the actual patient would have refused, or (2) the objective test, which requires the jury to ascertain whether a reasonable person standing in the patient's shoes would have refused treatment. The fact that the injury has occurred often will color the jury's finding. Courts have recognized this problem.[93] At the time of trial the uncommunicated risk has been revealed; therefore it would be surprising if the patient plaintiff did not claim that had he or she been informed of the dangers he or she would have declined treatment. Subjectively the plaintiff must believe so

with the 20/20 vision of hindsight (otherwise the case is lost); therefore it is doubtful that justice will be served by placing the physicians in jeopardy of the patient's bitterness and disillusionment. Thus an objective test is preferable (i.e., What would a prudent person standing in the patient's position have decided if adequately informed of all material perils?)

The ever-present and difficult question for physicians is how much information is legally sufficient. The courts have attempted to give the medical profession some guidance. In *Cobbs v. Grant* the California Supreme Court stated further that a "lengthy polysyllabic discourse on all possible complications" or a "mini-course of medical science" is not required.[94] The court required, as a minimum, disclosure of risks (meaning probability or likelihood) of death and serious bodily harm resulting from more perilous procedures. The concept of disclosure of the serious risks presumably would not be confined or determined by professional standards. However, the *Cobbs* court also required disclosure of "such information as a skilled professional would provide," thereby interjecting a form of medical community standard into the test. Disclosure of the nature and purpose of the proposed treatment, the risks and benefits reasonably expected, any alternative methods, and the risks of no treatment at all is required.

Another view is found in *Canterbury v. Spence,* in which the court stated[95]:

The scope of the physician's communication to the patient must be measured by the patient's need, and that need is the information material to the decision. Thus the test for determining whether a particular peril must be divulged is its materiality to the patient's decision: All risks potentially affecting the decision must be unmasked. And to safeguard the patient's interest in achieving his own determination on treatment, the law must itself set the standard for adequate disclosure.

In *Canterbury* the physician was held liable for failure to divulge a 1% risk of paralysis associated with a laminectomy. The court stressed the serious nature of the undisclosed risk rather than the mathematical possibility of its occurrence. In a more recent case the court stated:

The rule that the issue is to be decided by the jury, not on a medical standard, but on a reasonable man standard reflects concern for two problems: on the one hand, the rule preserves the patient's dignity in choosing his own course; on the other hand, by requiring only that information that would be relevant to a reasonable man, a doctor is not required to give every patient a complete course in anatomy and to explain every risk, no matter how remote before a consent would be valid.

Ultimately, the test for determining whether a particular peril must be divulged is its materiality to the patient's decision: Thus all risks potentially affecting the decision should be unmasked. In a broad outline, we agree that a risk is material when a reasonable person in the patient's position would likely attach significance to the risk or cluster of risks in deciding whether or not to forego the proposed therapy.

In light of the *Canterbury* court's discussion on "materiality" a practitioner is likely to have provided adequate information if the following are disclosed: diagnosis (description of the patient's condition or problem), nature and purpose of proposed diagnosis and treatment, risks and consequences of the proposed treatment, viable alternatives to the proposed treatment (if any), risks of not being treated, and prognosis. After *Canterbury,* numerous courts have followed the reasonable patient standard, but in general the states are pretty much split between the two standards, with a few jurisdictions adopting hybrids of one test or the other.[96,97]

EVIDENTIARY PROOF OF ADEQUATE DISCLOSURE

Written documentation of the informed consent is of key importance for both parties should litigation later arise. The weight to be accorded to such documentary evidence versus a mere oral consent is a question for the trier of fact. However, a written consent form signed by the patient often provides strong documentary evidence, which in at least one state forms a rebuttable presumption that valid consent was obtained. It may be necessary to establish the time, location, and persons present; the content of the dialogue; and the treatment authorized. Much of this information may be contained within the actual consent form if the patient signs it. The evidentiary value of a written consent form that is signed by the patient depends on the specificity of the information in the form viewed in conjunction with the discussions between the physician and the patient. Therefore, standing alone, the form may be insufficient to prove consent. However, any such question of the effect of the form is a factual issue to be determined by the fact finder.[98] Where the form speaks only in general terms and fails to comply with the relevant statutory provisions requiring specificity, additional evidence is necessary to establish the validity of the consent.

Consent forms and the physician's progress notes should include a statement by the physician, explaining that the patient was capable of understanding the nature of his or her physical condition, the proposed diagnostic or therapeutic procedures, and the risks of proceeding with the proposal, not proceeding with the proposal, or proceeding with alternative diagnostic or therapeutic procedures. Such statements often contain the acknowledgment that the physician answered all of the patient's questions. The signing of a blank consent form will not support a finding of informed consent. Informed consent also will not be found if the signer is functionally illiterate and if there is no indicia that a proper disclosure has been made. An informed consent statute codifies that there is a presumption of validity where there is a written and signed consent form.

In handling issues relating to instructions or informed consent in the medical record, any language limitations should be noted, as should attempts to work with translators. Notations should be made concerning literature provided to the patient or his or her representative. Notations are necessary to confirm that copies of instructions were relayed to the patient, and any failure to comply with the instructions, as well as confirmation that the patient was informed of risks of noncompliance, should be noted.

Burden of proof

In a medical malpractice case injury is alleged to have occurred as the result of a treatment error or omission.[99] In the informed consent context, however, litigation may be initiated even where there has been no treatment error or omission (e.g., where treatment that entails foreseeable material risks causes injury). The patient thus complains not that the treatment was negligently provided but that had there been full disclosure of the material risks or available alternatives, he or she would not have undergone the treatment and thus would not have been injured (the but for rule). As in other medical malpractice cases, it is essential for the plaintiff in an informed consent action to establish that the harm or injury suffered is the proximate result of a breach of duty or violation of the standard of care. If a patient does not receive enough material information to make an informed decision and is subsequently injured, the patient could successfully sue the physician, even if traditional consent was obtained and the physician's performance was flawless. The patient must show that the lack of informed consent (failure to receive sufficient information) was the cause of the injury.

But for rule

As to proximate cause using a lack of consent tort analysis, the patient must show that an undisclosed risk caused the injury, in the sense that the injury would not have occurred but for the consent, which would have been withheld had the patient known of the risk. If he or she had known of the risk, no consent would have been given.[100]

Because virtually any patient confronted with a severe disability resulting from treatment will testify in good faith that, if he or she had known of the risk, he or she would have refused the procedure, the courts have invoked the so-called but for rule. Realistically the patient cannot testify otherwise, or the case will be lost. The patient must establish this fact. Some states have adopted what is known as the *prudent patient rule;* that is, they determine what a prudent person in the patient's position would have decided if adequately informed of all reasonably foreseeable significant and serious though insignificant perils. Thus evidence of what the particular patient plaintiff would have done is immaterial if it is not what the ordinary reasonable patient would have done. This rule, of course, protects the physician from having to anticipate or know the idiosyncrasies of each patient. But given the theoretical basis for informed consent (protection of the patient's autonomy and self-determination), the prudent patient rule substitutes the standard of the "community of patients" for the old rule of the medical community's standard of disclosure. It therefore protects individual autonomy to a noticeable degree.

Depending on the jurisdiction involved, courts have taken at least two different approaches in determining whether a lack of informed consent caused an injury—the subjective standard (i.e., would the actual patient have refused to consent had the alleged lack of information been disclosed) and the objective standard (i.e., would a reasonably prudent person in the same or similar community and circumstances have refused to consent). From a practical point of view, irrespective of which standard is applied, the jury decides whether the patient would have refused treatment if the physician had imparted the alleged missing information.

Understanding of the varied medical risks that are inherent to the practice of medicine is ordinarily outside the knowledge of the layman and therefore requires the introduction of expert testimony. The expert witness must set forth in testimony that the claimed injury was a result of the diagnosis and treatment and that the injury is a known inherent risk of the treatment that had been rendered. Obviously, if the risk was not a known inherent risk or if there was no medically scientific relationship of the risk to the alleged injury, a lack of informed consent could not have caused the claimed injury.[101] Applying either standard, the patient has to proffer testimony that would convince a jury that the treatment would have been refused if the withheld information had been disclosed. In those jurisdictions in which a subjective standard is applicable, the law requires that the materiality of the nondisclosure to an informed decision be viewed solely from the point of view of the particular patient; in other words, the materiality of a risk to a reasonably prudent person in the patient's shoes cannot be considered.[102]

STATUTORY REQUIREMENTS AND DISCLOSURE

The analysis of any disclosure issue necessarily includes an examination of any statutes of the jurisdiction in which the patient was treated; any statutory requirements (or exceptions) of adequate disclosure should be reviewed thoroughly.[103] In some states the duty of obtaining informed consent is codified, giving rise to an additional negligence action for violation of statute.[104] These statutes frequently provide that the health care provider is obligated to inform the patient of the common risks and reasonable alternatives to the proposed treatment or procedure and that but for the physician's failure to do so the claimant would not have consented to the proposed treatment or procedure.

Particular attention must be paid to any statute wherein the risks required to be disclosed are defined by an administrative agency of the executive branch. Disclosure by the physician of such defined risks provides a rebuttable presumption that an adequate disclosure was made by the physician. In at least one state (Hawaii) a physician is not required to explain the realm of potential risks and complications associated with the proposed treatment because by statute the physician is required to explain only the intended result of the treatment.

DEFENSES TO AN ACTION FOR A LACK OF INFORMED CONSENT

One of the best and most cogent defenses against a lack of informed consent is a documented counseling session. The collective experience of those in the medical profession indicates that many patients forget or misinterpret what physicians say during an informed consent session. There is no question that documentation enhances physician credibility. The note need not be in great detail but should be a convincing statement that the patient received informed consent, reading, for example, "The adverse affects of subtotal thyroidectomy were discussed with John Doe, including such things as the 'loss of voice' and the loss of his parathyroid glands requiring lifelong therapy to maintain appropriate serum calcium levels." Having a third person, such as the nurse or technician who will be involved in performing a procedure, should be helpful in ensuring informed consent. Patients are reluctant to ask physicians questions about a procedure because they do not want to appear "stupid" or "offensive," especially the night before surgery is to be performed. Conversely, such patients will readily discuss their lack of understanding with a third party who in turn can inform the physician that his or her patient lacks understanding about the procedure.

A second defense may involve the lack of immediate capacity for the person to consent, for example, coma, transitory intoxication, psychosis, or being a minor (who may be competent but lacks the legal capacity to consent). Informed consent is not an issue during a medical emergency. A third defense involves the "so what" defense. When asserting the so what defense, the court will give the physician an opportunity to contend that even if his or her patient had been informed of the risk at issue, the patient would have consented to treatment.

The unduly alarming defense provides the defendant physician with an opportunity to contend that material information was withheld because he or she was acting in the patient's best interest. For example, a middle-aged man passed a kidney stone, which testing revealed was composed of uric acid. A complete clinical evaluation revealed that the man had primary gout with associated hypertension and a uric acid level of 10 mg/dl. Several examinations of the urine revealed no evidence of proteinuria. The blood urea nitrogen and creatinine levels were normal. A respectable group of physicians would view this conglomeration of signs as evidence of urate nephropathy without renal failure. This same group of physicians would probably alkalinize the urine, urge the patient to maintain hydration, and prescribe allopurinol as a general treatment plan to prevent further stone formation and prevent or reduce the chance of renal failure developing from chronic urate nephropathy. Six weeks later, the patient developed acute toxic epidermal necrolysis, which caused multiple body scars and scarring of both corneas. Toxic epidermal necrolysis is a known and rare adverse reaction to allopurinol. In this case the physician can assert two defenses based on his or her long-term familiarity with the patient. The first defense would be the so what defense. The second defense would be the unduly alarming defense; that is, the physician did not tell the patient because he would have accepted the treatment in any event and because the patient might have developed severe anxiety associated with extreme worry, insomnia, diarrhea, and anorexia. Acceptance of the unduly alarming defense by a jury would depend on a physician's ability to establish a credible knowledge of the patient's emotional character. The unduly alarming defense has become somewhat sophisticated in terminology by placing it under the rubric of therapeutic privilege. The physician must prove that he or she exercised the therapeutic privilege in the best interest of the patient, otherwise the patient would have refused necessary and effective treatment, or there would have been deleterious effects on the patient's well-being.

Assumption of risk

The doctrine of assumption of risk means that the patient understands the possibility of all risks of untoward unpreventable results of treatment or no treatment and knowingly consents to the course selected.[104] Where it applies, this doctrine is usually a good defense to an action for negligence. It is related to the doctrine of informed consent and refusal. If all risks that occur have not been revealed to the patient, as a matter of law the doctrine of assumption of risk is not applicable. Where statutes codify the requirement for informed consent, there are available defenses to this action (e.g., not disclosing very remote or commonly known risks, not disclosing information to a patient who did not want to be informed, or being unable to make disclosure under the circumstances, such as surgery).

A signed consent form or a note in the chart made contemporaneously with the event is presumptive evidence that a valid consent has been obtained. The patient may rebut that presumption if he or she can demonstrate that the quality of the consent was faulted as follows:

The language was too technical.
The physician's manner was hostile, antagonistic, pontifical, or condescending.
The patient was emotionally distressed.
The patient was sedated.
There was no time for contemplation and consultation.
There are several statutory defenses to informed consent as follows:

The patient does not want to be informed or would have undergone the procedure anyway (in at least 12 states).
The known risks are so commonly appreciated or the risk is too remote a possibility to be substantiated (in 8 states).
Therapeutic privilege prevails when the physician wishes to avoid a substantial adverse impact on or detriment to the patient's health (in at least 10 states).
The situation is an emergency, or there are other compelling circumstances (in at least 15 states).

COUNSELING TIPS ON OBTAINING INFORMED CONSENT

The following list provides some tips for obtaining informed consent:

1. Document the counseling session: The physician should have documented evidence that informed consent was given to the patient.
2. Accept the doctrine: Many physicians resist acceptance of the doctrine of informed consent on practical grounds. On the other hand, there is little or no chance that the doctrine will ever be abolished because informed consent emanates from the right of self-determination and the right to guard against the invasion of one's privacy. Furthermore, informed consent has strong moral and ethical overtones.
3. Have a third person (health care provider) present at the counseling session: Patients may be reluctant to question their physicians but will likely question the witness who in turn can inform the physician about the patient's lack of understanding.

A COMPETENT PATIENT'S RIGHT TO REFUSE TREATMENT

The sources of the right to refuse treatment, even when lifesaving, are the following:

1. The law of battery that prevents touching unpermitted by the patient.
2. Informed consent that is grounded in negligence and emanates from the right of self-determination.
3. The spirit of American democracy: Americans have an almost unfettered right to act, provided the act does not interfere with another person's right and does not violate a specific statute or some applicable common law.
4. The U.S. Constitution: According to the U.S. Supreme Court, the right to privacy (right against invasion of privacy) is evident from the Bill of Rights, specifically the First, Third, Fourth, Fifth, and Ninth Amendments.[106] The Supreme Court has found the right against the invasion of one's privacy to include the right to marry irrespective of race, color, or creed and the right to possess pornographic literature in the privacy of one's home, even though virtually every process that leads to such possession could be declared illegal.[107,108]

RIGHT TO REFUSE LIFESAVING TREATMENT IS NOT ABSOLUTE

The right to refuse treatment is not absolute. Occasional exceptions to this principle occur where certain refusals conflict with compelling state interests, such as the preservation of life, the prevention of suicide, the protection of third parties, and the protection of the ethical integrity of the medical profession. Increasingly, however, there is a recognized right to die.

A person's right to refuse lifesaving treatment is balanced by the state's interest in human life. When a court is petitioned to override a patient's right to refuse treatment, the process of reviewing the case is not arbitrary. Most courts use at least four compelling state interests to determine whether a state should override a patient's right to refuse treatment. The existence of just one interest is enough to override a patient's right to refuse:

1. Preservation of human life is a paramount state interest.
2. The state has a compelling interest to override a person's right to refuse lifesaving treatment to protect innocent third parties (minor children, adult incompetents, and spouses) from not having the opportunity to benefit from having a live healthy parent, guardian, or spouse.
3. The state has a duty to prevent suicide. From a legal perspective, suicide is a direct act or violent measure against one's self, which is specifically designed to end life.
4. The state has an interest in maintaining the ethical integrity of the medical profession. The courts will protect physicians from being forced to treat or not treat without a hearing or the opportunity to withdraw from the case.

Abe Perlmutter, a 73-year-old man with quadriplegia from progressive amyotrophic lateral sclerosis, was unable to breathe without a mechanical respirator.[109] Perlmutter requested withdrawal of the respirator. His physicians refused to do so because of potential liability for homicide (unlawful killing of another human being). Perlmutter pleaded with his physicians to withdraw treatment because he was suffering needlessly. His physicians were sympathetic but pointed out that withdrawal of artificial life support might be viewed as homicide in Florida. Perlmutter decided to exercise his right in court. The trial judge held that Perlmutter's request had not triggered a compelling state interest; that is, (1) there was no duty to preserve human life in the presence of progressive incurable illness; (2) there were no innocent third parties involved (no minor children and Mrs. Perlmutter had died recently); (3) the court rejected suicide as a countermanding state interest because withdrawal of the respirator was not a direct act to end Mr. Perlmutter's life (the respirator was merely suspending the act of dying); and (4) there was no compromise of professional integrity because the physicians had nothing to offer. The court stated that a mentally and legally competent patient, having full knowledge of the consequences, may request removal of artificial life support where there is no compelling state interest. When a Perlmutter situation arises, however, there is no need to act precipitously, and wisdom would recommend consulting the hospital attorney.

Ernestine Jackson was admitted to Mercy Hospital in Baltimore on an emergency basis in February 1984.[110] She was 25- to 26-weeks' pregnant and was in preterm labor; the fetus was lying in an oblique to transverse position. Cesarean section was recommended. Jackson was counseled that there was a 40% to 50% chance she would need a blood transfusion; nevertheless, she steadfastly refused to compromise her religious beliefs and was wholeheartedly supported by her husband. Backed by the medical staff from the University of Maryland Hospital, Mercy Hospital petitioned the Circuit Court of Baltimore City to appoint a guardian with authority to consent to a blood transfusion for Jackson. All the physicians agreed that there was a high risk of mortality if Jackson did not permit transfusion. After hearing medical testimony, the Circuit Court found that, despite the risks to the mother, delivery by cesarean section without blood transfusion posed virtually no threat to the fetus. The Maryland Court of Appeals concluded that a competent, pregnant adult has a right to refuse a blood transfusion in accordance with her religious beliefs, if such decision is made knowingly and voluntarily and will not endanger the delivery, survival, or support of the fetus. The court pointed out that its conclusion was consistent with a patient's right of informed consent to medical treatment and that whether an individual has a right to refuse a blood transfusion necessarily turns on facts existing at the moment.

Hubert Hamilton, a 35-year-old Jehovah's Witness, was shot through the chest in 1973. Surgery without transfusion involved a serious risk of death. The judge authorized transfusion after ascertaining that Hamilton fully understood the ramifications of his decision not to consent to a blood transfusion, was separated from his wife, and had a 2-year-old child for whom he provided the sole support. This case is an example of the state overriding a person's right to refuse treatment based on religious grounds to protect an innocent third party (loss of sole support).[111]

The state steadfastly guards a person's right to refuse treatment, even when lifesaving. A state will not override the person's right to refuse unless it can find at least one applicable compelling state interest. The Jackson and Hamilton cases are examples of how the same right (right to refuse transfusion on religious grounds) was upheld in one case because there was no compelling state interest and was overridden in the other case because there was an innocent third party. The right of an incompetent patient to refuse treatment is discussed elsewhere in this text.

REFUSAL OF CONSENT

The corollaries of the patient's right to consent to treatment are the right to refuse recommended treatment, after due disclosure by the physician, and the right to withdraw consent previously granted before the inception of treatment. The courts generally agree that in the absence of an emergency a competent adult patient may refuse medical or surgical treatment.[112]

In the majority of states the law upholds a competent adult's right to refuse even lifesaving treatment. The courts generally apply the traditional battery law principle of freedom from unauthorized touching or hold that the First Amendment right to free practice of religion precedes a physician's duty to render care.[113,114] Members of the Jehovah's Witness religious sect, for example, refuse blood transfusions on the basis of their literal interpretation of the Bible's prohibition against drinking blood. However, some courts try to find grounds on which to order the necessary treatment. These courts will usually authorize treatment to protect the life or health of a child or fetus on the grounds that the child will be "neglected" under applicable state statutes if treatment is refused or that the state owes a paramount duty to protect its children.[115] A number of courts have ordered necessary treatment over the objections of competent adult patients.[116] Several courts have held that terminally ill elderly patients could refuse treatment that would prolong their lives, particularly if the treatment is extremely painful, and that the hospital and physician involved would incur no criminal or civil liability for acknowledging refusal.[117]

The courts generally leave refusals of treatment undisturbed. The patient's fundamental right of inviolability of the person is controlling in the absence of a compelling state interest. Just as consent to treatment should be properly documented in the patient's medical record, the refusal to consent should be documented. The content of the dialogue in which the patient refused to consent to treatment should be explained. The physician is under no legal duty to persuade a competent patient to undergo recommended treatment, even though the refusal to consent will likely result in serious health impairment or death.

INFORMED REFUSAL

The corollary of the doctrine of informed consent is often referred to as the requirement of *informed refusal*. Courts are expanding the concept of informed consent to include informed refusal. The courts generally agree that in the absence of an emergency a competent adult patient may refuse medical or surgical treatment. When a patient or his or her surrogate rejects diagnosis or treatment, he or she should be advised in a discreet, professional manner of the consequences of the refusal.[118]

Both the medical and the legal professions have accepted that the physician has a duty as they say to "lead the patient to the water but not to make him or her drink." This may no longer be completely accurate. Recent rulings render the physician liable for any injury legally resulting from the patient's refusal to take treatment. The courts based their findings on the fact that the physician had a duty to inform the patient of the perils and pitfalls of refusing care in a discreet, human, ethical, moral, and professional manner, and he or she failed to do so.

If a patient indicates that he or she is going to decline the risk-free test or treatment, the physician has the additional duty to disclose all material risks of which a reasonable person would want to be informed before deciding not to undergo the care or procedure. Failure of the physician to disclose to the patient all relevant information, including the

risks to the patient if the care or test is refused, renders the physician liable for any injury legally resulting from the patient's uninformed refusal to take the treatment or test if a reasonably prudent person in the patient's position would not have refused had he or she been adequately informed. This rationale has been applied in at least 11 states and is typified by the ruling of a California court that held that a patient has the right to be informed of reasonably foreseeable risks that may arise if he or she refuses treatment. In that California case a woman who refused to have a Pap smear subsequently developed metastases and died of cervical cancer. Her survivors sued based on the argument that her physician had failed to inform her of the attendant risks in refusing to have the test. The physician was found liable for failure to disclose the amount of information that was needed for an adequate informed refusal.

No code order for competent patient

A no code order merely cancels the need to perform routine cardiopulmonary resuscitation in the event of cardiopulmonary arrest. If a patient is capable of authorizing or rejecting a do-not-resuscitate order, a no code designation should not be issued without the patient's consent. A physician may be liable in damages for failing to determine that a patient is competent and terminally ill before he or she authorizes the entry of a no code on the patient's chart.[119]

PHANTOM PHYSICIAN

A patient who consents to medical care by a specific physician and is treated by another physician may successfully sue the physician who did not provide treatment based on lack of informed consent and can sue the treating physician for battery or negligence predicated on risk of informed consent.[120] Courts have allowed recovery on a claim of unnecessary surgery or medical care based on lack of informed consent. The physician responsible for negotiating informed consent with a patient should perform the procedure for which consent is being obtained (i.e., not a phantom surgeon or physician). In some jurisdictions the physician may, if he or she sees fit, delegate this duty, but it is still his or her legal responsibility to ensure that the patient has been properly informed and understands.

ROLE OF PHYSICIAN

Two issues of concern to medical personnel arise in connection with tests and physical examinations that police request for criminal suspects: (1) Do such tests constitute a battery for which an examining physician may be held liable, and (2) do such tests constitute a violation of the suspect's constitutional rights?

The extent to which a physician may be liable in battery for performing an examination or test at the request of police but without the patient's consent is unclear. In such cases a technical battery has surely occurred.[121] But the statutes of some states provide that one who operates a motor vehicle on the state's public ways has consented by implication to tests to determine alcohol content in blood.[122] Some of these statutes declare specifically that a person may refuse to take such tests. At least one state, however, provides that an unconscious person is presumed to have consented to such tests.[123] Some states grant immunity to practitioners from any liability arising from obtaining blood samples at the request of a police officer pursuant to applicable state statutes.[124] In the absence of statutes that create such immunity or give rise to implied consent, a physician may be liable for technical battery if he or she performs a test without the patient's consent. However, liability would probably be limited to nominal (extremely small) damages, unless unreasonable force was used or the patient was negligently injured.

The U.S. Constitution places certain restraints on the power of government to interfere with the liberty and property of its citizens. In cases involving the examination of criminal suspects, several of these restrictions arise, including the prohibition against unreasonable search and seizure established by the Fourth Amendment, the privilege against self-incrimination contained in the Fifth Amendment, the right to due process set forth in the Fifth and Fourteenth Amendments, and the right to counsel guaranteed by the Sixth Amendment.

The federal courts have held that a simple physical examination of a suspect does not violate constitutionally based protections against self-incrimination.[125] The admission into evidence of test results from a blood sample taken at the request of a police officer from an unconscious criminal suspect does not violate the Fourth Amendment prohibition against unreasonable search and seizure or the due process clause of the Fourteenth Amendment.[126] Nor does evidence based on a blood test violate the constitutional prohibition against self-incrimination if a person suspected of violating a motor vehicle code expressly refuses to consent to such a test on advice of counsel.[127] However, the blood sample must be obtained in a simple, medically acceptable manner under the supervision of a physician in a hospital setting. The suspect's request for blood alcohol testing by another acceptable method must be allowed, and the physician and police must refrain from using unreasonable force in administering the test.

Scientific analysis of the accused's blood, hair, or other similar body material samples does not require the presence of the accused's counsel.[128] A search of body cavities for illegally possessed substances is constitutionally permissible as long as there is a clear probable cause and the physician performs the examination under hygienic conditions and in a reasonable manner.[129] Generally, physicians and police officers are given latitude in conducting body examinations during customs searches at U.S. borders.[130]

If a blood sample is obtained by misrepresentation, the results are inadmissible in evidence, and the treating physician may be subject to liability in battery. In a case in which the police told a suspect that a blood sample was needed to determine intoxication, the suspect's consent was held to be invalid because the police actually wanted the sample to determine the suspect's blood type in connection with a rape investigation.[131]

A physician who performs medical examinations or tests at the request of police should remember that the tort liability and constitutional issues involved are usually independent. A test that does not violate the suspect's constitutional rights may nonetheless constitute a technical battery and may subject the physician to tort liability. Although the courts have provided exquisite guidance concerning the constitutional rights of suspects who undergo medical examination, the question of tort liability for those conducting the examination still remains unclear.

Mohr v. Williams, cited earlier, established that a physician who exceeds the scope of consent commits a battery.[132] It is common practice for physicians to obtain a group of tests when confronted with a patient in the emergency department. If a physician obtains a blood alcohol test that is not medically necessary to evaluate the patient, such an act would constitute a technical battery. A technical battery is apparent anytime a physician exceeds the scope of consent by obtaining blood tests that are not medically necessary for diagnosis and treatment. Physicians have an overriding concern about whether they should honor police requests or can be ordered by the police to obtain body fluids that might be used as incriminating evidence when the extraction of such body fluids is not medically necessary. In other words, under what circumstances can the police direct the suspect to allow the extraction of body fluids (pumping the stomach, examining the rectum for glassine bags containing drugs, or obtaining blood specimens) that is medically unnecessary but may uncover incriminating evidence?

As mentioned earlier, the U.S. Constitution places certain restraints on the power of government to interfere with the liberty and property of its citizens. In cases involving the examination of criminal suspects, several of these restrictions arise, including the prohibition against unreasonable search and seizure established by the Fourth Amendment, a privilege against self-incrimination contained in the Fifth Amendment, the right to due process set forth in the Fifth and Fourteenth Amendments, and the right to counsel guaranteed by the Sixth Amendment.[133] Three U.S. Supreme Court cases help to illustrate the boundaries that surround state authority when obtaining body fluids for the purpose of garnering incriminating evidence.

SPECIAL SITUATIONS
Research involving human subjects

The National Research Act (P.L. 93-348), enacted July 12, 1974, gave the U.S. Department of Health, Education, and Welfare (now the Department of Health and Human Services and the Department of Education) the responsibility for regulating the use of human subjects in biomedical and behavioral research. On March 13, 1975, the Department issued its final regulations, entitled *Protection of Human Subjects,*[134,135] containing regulations that establish in detail the manner in which federally funded research involving human subjects shall be approved and the methods by which subjects are protected. The regulations require that the subject's informed consent be obtained before the research commences. Informed consent is defined as follows:

(c) "Informed consent" means the knowing consent of an individual or his legally authorized representative, so situated as to be able to exercise free power of choice without undue inducement or any element of force, fraud, deceit, duress, or other form of constraint or coercion. The basic elements of information necessary to such consent include:
1. A fair explanation of the procedure to be followed and the purposes, including identification of any procedures which are experimental;
2. A description of any attendant discomforts and risks reasonably to be expected;
3. A description of any benefits reasonably to be expected;
4. A disclosure of any appropriate alternative procedures that might be advantageous for the subject;
5. An offer to answer any inquiries concerning the procedures; and
6. An instruction that the person is free to withdraw his consent and to discontinue participation in the project or activity at any time without prejudice to the subject.[136]

The regulations require documentation of the subject's consent in either a "long" or "short" form.[137] The documentation of consent will take one of the following two forms:

1. Provision of a written consent document embodying all of the basic elements of informed consent. This may be read to the subject or to his legally authorized representatives, but in any event he or his legally authorized representatives must be given adequate opportunity to read it. This document is to be signed by the subject or his legally authorized representatives. Sample copies of the consent form as approved by the Board are to be retained in its records.
2. Provision of a "short form" written consent document indicating that the basic elements of informed consent have been presented orally to the subject or his legally authorized representatives. Written summaries of what is to be said to the patient are to be approved by the Board. The short form is to be signed by the subject or his legally authorized representatives and by an auditor witness to the oral presentation and to the subject's signature. A copy of the approved summary, annotated to show any additions, is to be signed by the persons officially obtaining the consent and by the auditor witness. Sample copies of the consent form and of the summaries as approved by the Board are to be retained in its records.

Either of these forms may be modified, provided that (1) the risk to the subject is minimal, (2) the use of the forms described would invalidate objectives of considerable immediate importance, and (3) any reasonable alternative means for attaining such objectives would be less advantageous to the subject than modifying the consent procedure.[138] If a physi-

cian wishes to treat a patient using medical procedures that depart from established and accepted methods, he or she must be familiar with the federal regulations discussed earlier and with any applicable laws or regulations of the state.

Consent to experimental procedures

All experimental research involving diagnosis, treatment, and the use of investigational drugs or devices must be carefully conducted in conformance with research protocols approved by a hospital's investigations review board or research committee. Experimental treatments and procedures are those that have not yet been established to be reliable and acceptable in medical practice. Investigational drugs or devices are those that the Food and Drug Administration (FDA) has not yet approved for commercial distribution. The conduct of such investigational diagnosis and treatment, as well as the procurement of informed consent to such treatment, is closely regulated by federal authority. Treatment should not exceed the scope of the patient's consent, unless emergency treatment or a closely related extension of the treatment becomes therapeutically necessary during the performance of the authorized experimental treatment.

Drug research

The Food, Drug, and Cosmetic Act authorizes the Department of Health and Human Services to regulate the use of investigational drugs.[139] The regulations issued by the department require the investigator to certify that:

[H]e will inform any patients or their representatives that drugs are being used for investigational purposes, and will obtain the consent of the subject or their representatives, except where this is not feasible or, in the investigator's professional judgment, is contrary to the best interest of the subjects.[140]

The regulations define the term *consent* to mean:

[t]hat the person involved has legal capacity to give consent, is so situated as to be able to exercise free power of choice, and is provided with a fair explanation of pertinent information concerning the investigational drug, and/or possible use of a control, as to enable him to make a decision on his willingness to receive said investigational drug. This latter element means that before the acceptance of an affirmative decision by such person the investigator should carefully consider and make known to him (taking into consideration such person's well-being and his ability to understand) the nature, expected duration, and purpose of the administration of said investigational drug; the method and means by which it is to be administered; the hazards involved; the existence of alternative forms of therapy, if any; and the beneficial effects upon his health or person that may possibly come from the administration of the investigational drug.[141]

Consent is required in all cases in which an investigational drug is administered "primarily for the accumulation of scientific knowledge" or is administered to patients who are otherwise receiving medical treatment.

Any time a patient is enrolled as part of a clinical trial, the duty of the research physician to disclose all possible risks, benefits, and potential consequences must be taken seriously. Where a court finds that the decision to continue a patient in a control group was negligent, serious questions may arise about the validity of exposing control groups to a potentially noxious agent or environment, which in turn may cast doubt on the validity of the concept controlled or the double-blind study.[142]

Elective sterilization using federal funds

To perform a nonemergency sterilization on a patient in a program supported by federal funds administered by the U.S. Public Health Service, a physician must obtain the patient's informed consent. The applicable regulations define the *informed consent* as:

[t]he voluntary, knowing assent from the individual on whom any sterilization is to be performed after he has been given (as evidenced by a document executed by such individual):
1. A fair explanation of the procedures to be followed;
2. A description of the attendant discomforts and risks;
3. A description of the benefits to be expected;
4. An explanation concerning appropriate alternative methods of family planning and the effect and impact of the proposed sterilization including the fact that it must be considered to be an irreversible procedure;
5. An offer to answer any inquiries concerning the procedures; and
6. An instruction that the individual is free to withhold or withdraw his or her consent to the procedure at any time prior to the sterilization without prejudicing his or her future care and without loss of other project or programs benefits to which the patient might otherwise be entitled.[143]

Such consent must be documented in one of two ways: (1) a written consent form describing in detail the information listed in subsections 1 through 6 of the regulations or (2) a short form written consent form that indicates that the six basic elements of consent have been presented orally to the patient, supplemented by a written summary of the oral presentation. The written summary must be signed by the person obtaining the consent and by a witness. Each consent document must prominently display the following language: "NOTICE: Your decision at any time not to be sterilized will not result in the withdrawal or withholding of any benefits provided by programs or projects."[144]

Physicians who perform sterilization procedures should be thoroughly familiar with current federal regulations applicable to sterilization. Regulations change so frequently that the previous discussion and extracts are provided only as examples.

Uniform Anatomical Gift Act

The Uniform Anatomical Gift Act, adopted in all states, generally provides that persons 18 years of age or older may donate all or part of their bodies after death for research, transplantation, or placement in a tissue bank. Survivors may give authorization for donation, if the decedent had not done so. Consents for donations may be superseded by decisions of state officials to conduct autopsies in accordance with local statutes or ordinances.

EPILOGUE

The scope and propriety of disclosure to patients are dependent on the state of medical knowledge at the time of the disclosure. When appropriate, the patient also should be informed of the identity and responsibility of other persons who will participate in the patient's care and management. A physician who specializes in psychiatry has the same legal duty as any other physician to exercise reasonable care in selecting, administering, and obtaining informed consent for treatment. A valid consent may be exercised only if the patient giving it is competent enough to engage in the consent process. This can be a particularly critical element for psychiatrists, because they commonly treat patients whose cognitive capacity may be at issue. Once the physician-patient relationship is established, a physician has a duty to inform the patient of his or her condition and of the presumptive and differential diagnoses.[145]

The law in all states requires a physician to obtain the consent of a patient or his or her surrogate before treating that patient. In the absence of that consent the physician may be held liable in a civil lawsuit for battery, assault, and professional negligence or medical malpractice.

At least 13 states have professionally articulated disclosure standards (i.e., by physician custom or standard).

At least 4 states have a reasonable patient standard. This standard requires no expert witness testimony.

At least 10 states have no specified standards.

At least 10 states have a patient comprehension standard (i.e., the reasonable person or all questions answered).

Two states, Georgia and Arizona, have abolished or modified the informed consent requirement, the latter possibly by implication.

The process of obtaining a patient's informed consent to a medical procedure requires balancing the need to disclose complete, reliable, up-to-date medical information with the practical concern of avoiding undue alarm to patients. The physician may exercise his or her professional judgment with respect to the scope of the disclosure where such is in the best interest of the patient. This exception should be closely limited because it can be contrary to the very basis of the informed consent requirement, that is, the right of self-determination.

CONCLUSION

Physicians have a moral, ethical, and legal duty to disclose sufficient information to patients in obtaining a valid informed consent to perform a recommended procedure or treatment. The moral duty arises from the individual's natural desire to be free to make personal choices about what shall become of his or her body—the right to refuse or accept treatment. Thus the assumption of a definite risk is a highly private and personal matter rather than a scientific matter. The ethical duty arises from the collective wisdom of the medical profession, mainly the beliefs that patients are necessary partners in the diagnostic and therapeutic processes, that physicians have an inherent professional duty to respect a patient's wishes to know about his or her disease, and that patients have a right to know all necessary facts before making a choice about whether to follow medical recommendations. The legal duty arises from the common law, statutes, and the U.S. Constitution, which recognize that patients have a dignitary interest that does not allow them to be touched in the absence of consent and that Americans have a right to privacy, a right to refuse treatment, and a right to be informed about the benefits and adverse effects inherent in proposed medical care. The transcending American principle that controls the nature of consent to treatment is the right of self-determination.

ENDNOTES

1. W. Prosser, *Handbook of the Law of Torts* 102 (3d ed. 1964).
2. *Hancock v. Hullett,* 203 Ala. 272. 82 So. 522 (1919).
3. *Moss v. Rishworth,* 222 S.W. 225 (1920).
4. W.P. Keeton et al., *Prosser and Keeton on Law of Torts* 41 (5th ed. 1984).
5. *Id.*
6. J.H. King Jr., *The Law of Medical Malpractice in a Nutshell* 130 (2d ed. 1986).
7. *See, e.g.,* Ill. Ann. Stat. ch. 95, para. 11-501.1 (Smith-Hurd Supp. 1976).
8. *King v. Carney,* 204 P. 270 (1922).
9. *Wheeler v. Barker,* 92 Cal. App. 2d 776, 208 P. 2d 68 (1949); *Jackovach v. Yocom,* 212 Iowa 914, 237 N.W. 444 (1931).
10. *Barnett v. Bachrach,* 34 A. 2d 626 (N.J. 1943).
11. *McGuire v. Rix,* 118 Neb. 434, 22 N.W. 120 (1929).
12. *Chambers v. Nottebaum,* 96 So. 2d 716 (1957).
13. *Murray v. Vandevander,* 522 P. 2d 302 (1974).
14. *Danforth v. Planned Parenthood of Central Missouri,* 428 U.S. 52 (1976).
15. *Roe v. Wade,* 410 U.S. 113 (1973).
16. *Id.*
17. *Gursky v. Gursky,* 39 Misc. 2d 1083, 242 N.Y.S. 2d 406 (1963).
18. *In re Quinlan,* 335 A. 2d 647 (1976).
19. *Griswold v. Connecticut,* 381 U.S. 479 (1965); also *see Loving v. Virginia,* 388, U.S. 1 (1967) (the right to marry irrespective of race, color, or creed) and *Stanley v. Georgia,* 394 U.S. 557 (1969) (right to possess pornographic literature in the privacy of one's home).
20. 49 A.L.R. 3rd 501, 505 (1970).
21. American Medical Association's Judicial Council, *Principles of Medical Ethics* ix (1984).
22. Ad Hoc Committee on Medical Ethics, *American College of Physicians' Ethics Manual,* 101 Ann. Intern. Med. 121-137 (1984).
23. *Supra* note 8, at 154-155.
24. *Canterbury v. Spence,* 464 F. 2d 772 (D.C. Cir. 1972).
25. *Supra* note 8, at 131.
26. *Cobbs v. Grant,* 502 P. 2d 1 (Calif. 1972).
27. *Sard v. Hardy,* 379 A. 2d 1014 (M.D. 1977).
28. *Id.*
29. Civil Rights § 765.02.
30. *Tetstone v. Adams,* 373 So. 2d 362; *Brooks v. Cerrato,* 355 So. 2d 119 (1978).
31. *Dowlings v. Mutual Life Insurance Co.,* 373 So. 2d 362; Brooks, *supra* note 30.
32. *Nathanson v. Kline,* 350 P. 2d 1093 (1960).
33. *Nathanson v. Kline,* 354 P. 2d 670 (1969).
34. *Sinkev v. Surgical Assoc.,* 186 N.W. 2d 658 (1971).
35. *Supra* note 32.
36. AMA Current Opinions of the Judicial Counsel 8.11 (1984).
37. *Gates v. Jensen,* 92 Wash. 2d 246, 250, 595 P. 2d 919, 922 (1979).
38. *Keogan v. Holy Family Hosp.,* 95 Wash. 2d 306, 622 P. 2d 1246 (1980).
39. *Ray v. Wagner,* 286 Minn. 354, 176 N.W. 2d 101 (1970) (physician not liable when patient's contributory negligence resulted in her failure to learn of suspicious Pap smear result).
40. T.S. Harrison, *Hyperthyroidism,* in *Textbook of Surgery* 585-593 (D.C. Sabiston ed., W.B. Saunders, Philadelphia 1986).
41. *Id.*
42. *Id.*
43. *Phillips v. United States,* 566 F.Supp. 1 (D.S.C. 1981) (an infant's manifestation of signs of congestive heart failure obligated referral to a pediatric cardiologist under the applicable standard of family practice or pediatric care); *Larsen v. Yelle,* 246 N.W. 2d 841 (Minn. 1976); *Id.* at 845 (if a physician has every reasonable indication that he or she is fully capable of treating the patient, however, there is no duty to consult another physician); *see Collins v. Itoh,* 503 P. 2d 36 (Mont. 1972).
44. *Logan v. Greenwich Hosp. Ass'n.,* 191 Conn. 282, 465 A. 2d 294 (1983).
45. *Id.* The case was remanded for a new trial on the issue of whether an open kidney biopsy represented a viable alternative.
46. *Osborne v. Frazor,* 58 Tenn.App. 15, 425 S.W. 2d 768 (1968). See Annotation, *Malpractice: Physician's Failure to Advise Patient to Consult Specialist or One Qualified in a Method of Treatment which Physician is Not Qualified to Give,* 35 A.L.R. 3d 349 (1971).
47. *Kelly v. Carrol,* 36 Wash. 2d 482, 219 P. 2d 79 (1950) (a duty to refer exists when a practitioner knows that a therapy will be of no benefit to the patient and that an alternative mode of treatment is available elsewhere that is more likely to be successful).
48. *Rahn v. United States,* 222 F.Supp. 775 (S.D. Ga. 1963) (if current therapy is unsuccessful, and if specialty assistance is available, a duty to consult exists).
49. President's Commission for the Study of Ethical Problems in Medicine and Biomedical and Behavioral Research, Making Health Care Decisions: The Ethical and Legal Implications of Informed Consent in the Patient-Practitioner Relationship, 1-3 (Government Printing Office, Washington, D.C. 1982).
50. *Price v. Neyland,* 320 F. 2d 674 (D.C. Cir. 1963).
51. *Harris v. Robert C. Groth, M.D., Inc., P.S.,* 99 Wash. 2d 438, 663 P. 2d 113 (1983).
52. *See Cobbs v. Grant,* 104 Cal.Rptr. 505, 502 P. 2d 1 (1972); *Green v. Hussey,* 127 Ill.App. 2d 174, 262 N.E. 2d 156 (1970).
53. *Cowman v. Hornaday,* 329 N.W. 2d 422 (Iowa 1983).
54. *Roberson v. Menorah Medical Center,* 588 S.W. 2d 134 (Mo. Appl. 1979).
55. *Garcia v. Presbyterian Hosp. Center,* 593 P. 2d 487 (N.M. Ct.App. 1979).
56. *Estrada v. Jacques,* S.E. 2d (N.C. Ct.App. 1984).
57. *Lipsus v. White,* 458 N.Y.S. 2d 928 (N.Y. App.Div. 1983).
58. AMA, *Medicolegal Forms* (1976); Hospital Ass'n of N.Y. State, *Manual of Consent Forms* (1974).
59. *Cross v. Trapp,* 294 S.E. 2d 446 (W. Va. 1982).
60. *Archer v. Galbraith,* 567 P. 21 115 S (Wash. Ct. App. 1980).
61. *Collins v. Davis,* 44 Misc. 2d 622. 254 N.Y.S. 2d 666 (1964).
62. *Consent to Medical or Surgical Procedures,* I Health Law Manual 14-11 (1975).
63. Petition of Nemser, 51 Misc. 2d 616, 273 N.Y.S. 2d (1966).
64. *E.g.,* the Illinois statute concerning autopsy provides that if one close relative prohibits autopsy, the autopsy may not be performed, even though another close relative had given consent. See Ill. Ann. Stat. ch. 91, para. 18-12 (Smith-Hurd 1976).

65. *See, e.g.,* Ill. Ann. Stat. ch. 3. para 112 et seq. (Smith-Hurd 1961).

66. *E.g., Schultz v. Rice,* 809 F. 2d 643 (10th Cir. 1986); *Pardy v. United States,* 783 F. 2d 710 (7th Cir. 1986).

67. *See Lester v. Aetna Casualty & Surety Co.,* 240 F. 2d 676 (5th Cir. 1957).

68. *Nishi v. Hartwell,* 52 Haw. 188 and 296, 473 P. 2d 116 (1970).

69. *Putenson v. Clay Adams, Inc.,* 12 Cal.App. 3d 1062, 91 Cal.Rptr. 319 (1st Dist. 1970).

70. *E.g., Wachter v. United States,* 877 F. 2d 257 (4th Cir. 1989).

71. *Crouch v. Most,* 78 N.M. 406, 432 P. 2d 250 (1967).

72. AMA Current Opinions of the Judicial Counsel 8.07 (1984).

73. *Dunham v. Wright,* 423 F. 2d 940 (1970); *Berlinger v. Lackner,* 331 Ill.App. 591. 73 N.E. 2d 620 (1947); *Pratt v. Davis,* 224 Ill. 300, 79 N.E. 562 (1906).

74. 61 Am. Jur. 2D Physicians and Surgeons § 159 (1972); 56 A.L.R. 2d 695 § 3.

75. Restatement of Torts § 62 (1934).

76. *Luka v. Lowrie,* 171 Mich. 122, 136 N.W. 1106 (1912).

77. *Tabor v. Scobee,* 254 S.W. 2d 474 (Ky. Ct.App. 1952).

78. Jackovach, *supra* note 9.

79. *Supra* note 75.

80. *Supra* note 76; *Mohr v. Williams,* 95 Minn. 261, 104 N.W. 12 (1905).

81. *Supra* note 75.

82. *Wells v. McGehee,* 39 So. 2d 196 (1949); *Sullivan v. Montgomery,* 279 N.Y.S. 575, 17 N.E. 2d 446 (1935).

83. *Lacey v. Laird,* 166 Ohio St. 12, 139 N.E. 2d 25 (1956); *Gulf and Ship Island R.R. v. Sullivan,* 155 Miss. 1, 119 So. 501 (1928); *Bishop v. Shurly,* 237 Mich. 76. 211 N.W. 75 (2926). *But see contra. Bonner v. Moran,* 126 F. 2d 121 (D.C. Cir. 1941), which held that a 15-year-old could not alone consent to donation of blood for benefit of another.

84. *Pizzlotto v. Wilson,* 444 So. 2d 143 (La. 1983); *Mercer v. Chi,* 282 N.W. 2d 697 (Iowa 1979).

85. *See, e.g., Mohr v. Williams,* 95 Minn. 261, 104 N.W. 12 (1905).

86. *Salgo v. Leland Stanford, Jr.,* Univ. Board of Trustees, 154 Cal.App. 2d 560, 317 P. 2d 170 (1957).

87. Waltz & Scheuneman *Informed Consent to Therapy,* 64 NW.U.L. Rev. 628 (1970).

88. *Bang v Charles T. Miller Hosp.,* 251 Minn. 427, 88 N.W. 2d 188 (1958); Plante, *An Analysis of Informed Consent,* 36 Fordham L. Rev. 639 (1968); McCoid, *A Reappraisal of Liability for Unauthorized Medical Treatment,* 41 Minn. L. Rev. 381 (1957); Leg. Med. Ann. 203.

89. Bang, *supra* note 87.

90. *Fiorentino v. Wenger,* 19 N.Y. 2d 407, 227 N.E. 2d 296 (1967).

91. *Green v. Hussey,* 127 Ill.App. 2d 173, 262 N.W. 2d 156 (1970); *Aiken v. Clarey,* 396 S.W. 2d 668 (Mo. 1965); Bucklin, *Informed Consent: Past, Present, and Future,* Leg. Med. Ann. 203 (1975).

92. Green, *supra* note 90, at 174.

93. *Cobbs v. Grant,* 104 Cal.Rptr. 505, 502 P. 2d 1 (1972).

94. *Id.*

95. *Supra* note 24.

96. *Flannery v. Georgetown Univ. Hosp.,* 79 F. 2d 960 (D.C. App. 1980).

97. *Jeffries v. McCague,* 363 A. 2d 1167 (Pa. 1970).

98. *Haynes v. Hoffman,* 164 Ga.App. 236, 296 S.E. 2d 216 (1982).

99. *See, e.g.,* Alfidi, *Informed Consent, A Study of Patient Reaction,* 216 J.A.M.A. 8 (1971); Johnrude, *Informed Consent: An Objective Evaluation of or a Possible Solution,* Radiology (1971).

100. *Small v. Gifford Memorial Hosp.,* 133 Vt. 552. 349 A. 2d 703 (1975); *Hunter v. Brown,* 4 Wash. App. 899, 484 P. 2d 1162 (1971); *Getchell v. Mansfield* 260 Or. 174. 489 P. 2d 953 (1971).

101. R.D. Miller, *Treatment Authorization and Refusal, Problems in Hospital Law* 224-225 (Aspen Publications, Rockville, Md. 1990).

102. C.L. Spring & B.J. Winick, *Informed Consent, in Legal Aspects of Medicine,* 61-63 (J.R. Vevaina, R.C. Bone & E. Kossoff eds., Springer-Verlag, New York 1989).

103. Alaska Statute § 09.55.556; § 09.55.556 (b).(5); Cal. Health & Safety Code § 1704.5 (1980); Connecticut General Statute § 52-582; Delaware Annotated Code Title 18 § 6852; 18 § 6852(b); Florida Statutes Annotated § 768.46(3)(a); Georgia Annotated Code § 88-2906; Georgia Code Ann. § 31-9-6(d)(1985); Georgia Code Ann. § 31-9-6.1 (1988 Supp.); Hawaii Revised Statutes § 671-3(b); Idaho Revised Statutes § 939-4304; § 939-4304; § 939-4305; Iowa Code Annotated 9 147.137. Iowa Code Ann. § 147.137; Kentucky Revised Statutes § 304 40-320; Louisiana Revised Statutes § 1299 40. A(a); Maine Revised Statutes Annotated Title 24 § 2905; Title 24 § 2905.2; Missouri Statutes 516.280; Revised Statutes Missouri (1978); Nebraska Revised Statutes § 44-2816; Nevada Revised Statutes. § 41 A. 110; New Hampshire Revised Statutes Annotated § 507-c.211. § 507-c:2(b) (4); New York Public Health Law § 2805-d.1 Civ. Procedure Law § 4401-a; North Carolina General Statutes § 90-21.13; § 90-21.13(b); North Dakota Central Code § 26-401-025; Ohio Revised Code § 2317 54A, § 231754; Oregon Revised Statutes § 671.097; Pennsylvania Statutes Annotated Title 40, § 1301.103; Tennessee Annotated Code rd § 23-3417; Texas Revised Civil Statutes Article 4590; § 6.02 § 98-14-5(2)(d); Utah Code Annotated § 78-14-5(d)(e); Vermont Statutes Annotated Title 12, § 1909(a)(1); 12, § 1909(e) 12 § 1909(d); Washington Code Annotated § 7.70.050.

104. Florida Statutes, § 381.3712(4) (M), (485,324,459.0125) (1984); Georgia Code Section 43-34-21 (G) (1984); Hawaii Revised Statutes, § 671-3 (C) (1983); Kansas Statutes Annotated, § 65-2836(O) (1984); Kentucky House Bill 609 (1984); Louisiana H. Con. Resolution 125 (1983); Massachusetts General Laws Annotated ch. III, § 70E (1979); Minnesota Statutes, § 144.651, Subdivision 9 (1984); New Jersey Revised Statutes, Title 45, ch. 9 (1984); Pennsylvania H.B. 1972 (1984); Virginia Code, Section 54-325.2:2 (1985).

105. *Rochester v. Katalan,* 320 A. 2d 704 (Del. 1974). *See* Annotation, *Patient's Failure to Reveal Medical History to Physician as Contributory Negligence or Assumption of Risk in Defense of Malpractice Action,* 33 A.L.R. 4th 790 (1984).

106. *Griswold v. Connecticut,* 381 U.S. 439 (1965).

107. *Loving v. Virginia,* 388 U.S. 1 (1967).

108. *Stanley v. Georgia,* 394 U.S. 557 (1969).

109. *Satz v. Perlmutter,* 362 SO. 2d 160 (Fla. 1978).

110. *Mercy Hosp. v. Jackson,* 489 A. 2d 1130 (M.D. 1985).

111. *Hamilton v. McAuliffe,* 353 A. 2d 634 (M.D. 1976).

112. *Schloendorff v. New York Hosp.* 211 N.Y. 125, 105 N.E. 92 (1914).

113. *Id.*

114. *In re Estate of Brooks,* 32 Ill. 2d 361, 205 N.E. 2d 435 (1965).

115. *Raleigh Fitkin-Paul Morgan Memorial Hosp. v. Anderson,* 42 N.J. 421, 201 A. 2d 537 (1964); *State v. Perricone,* 37 N.J. 462, 181 A. 2d 751 (1962); *People ex rel Wallace v. Labrenz,* 411 Ill. 618, 104 N.E. 2d 769 (1952); *In re Vasco,* 263 N.Y.S. 552 (1933).

116. *Kennedy Hosp. v. Heston,* 58 N.J. 569, 279 A. 2d 670 (1971); *Application of President of Georgetown College, Inc.,* 331 F. 2d 1000 (D.C. Cir.), *cert. denied,* 377 U.S. 978 (1964); *Collins v. Davis,* 254 N.Y.S. 2d 666 (1964).

117. *Palm Springs General Hosp. v. Martinez,* No. 71-12687 (Dade County Ct. Fla. 1971).

118. *Truman v. Thomas,* 165 Cal.Rptr. 308, 611 P. 2d 902 (1980).

119. *Payne v. Marion General Hosp.,* 549 N.E. 2d 2043.

120. *Perna v. Pirozzi,* 92 N.J. 446, 457, A. 2d 431 (1983).

121. *See, e.g., Bednarik v. Bednarik,* 18 Misc. 633, 16 A. 2d 80 (1940).

122. *See, e.g.,* Ill. Ann. Stat. ch. 95, para. 11-501.1 (Smith-Hurd Supp. 1976).

123. Fla. Stat. Ann. § 322.261 (c) (West 1975).

124. *See, e.g.,* N.Y. Veh. & Traf. Law § 1194.7.b (McKinney Supp. 1976).

125. *McFarland v. United States,* 150 F. 2d 593, *cert. denied,* 325 U.S. 788, *reh'g denied,* 327 U.S. 814 (1945); *Leeper v. Texas,* 139 U.S. 462 (1891); *Battle v. Cameron,* 260 F.Supp. 804 (1966).

126. *Breithaupt v. Abram,* 352 U.S. 432 (1957).

127. *Schmerber v. California,* 384 U.S. 757 (1966).
128. *United States v. Wade,* 388 U.S. 218 (1967).
129. *Rochin v. California,* 342 U.S. 165 (1952); *Rivas v. United States* 368 F. 2d 703, *cert. denied,* 386 U.S. 945 (1966); *Hugues v. United States,* 406 F. 2d 366 (9th Cir. 1968).
130. *See* 22 L. Ed 2d 909 (1970); 16 L. Ed. 2d 1332 (1967).
131. *Graves v. Beto,* 424 F. 2d 524 (5th Cir. 1970).
132. *Supra* note 85.
133. *Supra* note 8, at 131.
134. *Supra* note 7.
135. 45 C.F.R. § 46.1 et seq. (1976).
136. 45 C.F.R. § 46.3 (1976).
137. 45 C.F.R. § 46.10 (1976).
138. 45 C.F.R. § 46.10(c) (1976).
139. 21. U.S.C.A. § 321 et seq. (West 1972).
140. 21 C.F.R § 312.1 (A) (13) (1976).
141. 21 C.F.R. § 310.102(b)-(c) (1976).
142. *Burton v. Brooklyn Doctors Hosp. et al.,* 452 N.Y.S. 2d 875 (1982).
143. 42 C.F.R. § 50.202(d) (1976).
144. 42 C.F.R. § 50.202(d) (7) (iii) (1976).
145. *Dowling v. Mutual Life Insurance Co. of New York,* 168 So. 2d 107 (La. App. 1964) (physician's failure to inform patient that chest radiograph revealed tuberculous infiltration was actionable in tort).

SELECTED CASES

In an effort to provide the reader with recent significant case law from various jurisdictions regarding application of legal principles in connection with the doctrine of informed consent, the editors have compiled the following list of cases. These cases offer interesting and useful insights. Accordingly, practitioners in the various jurisdictions listed below likely will benefit from review of these cases.

Gorab v. Zook, 943 P. 2d 423 (Colo. 1997).
Albany Urology Clinic v. Cleveland, 2000 Ga. LEXIS 214 (Ga. 2000).
Carr v. Strode, 904 P. 2d 489 (Hawaii 1995).
Hernandez v. Schittek, 713 N.E. 2d 203 (Ill. App. 1999).
Bowman v. Beghin, 713 N.E. 2d 913 (Ind. App. 1999).
Cacdac v. West, 705 N.E. 2d 506 (Ind. App. 1999).
Capel v. Langford, 734 So. 2d 835 (La. App. 1999).
Leger v. Louisiana Medical Mutual Ins. Co., 732 So. 2d 654 (La. App. 1999).
Herrington v. Spell, 692 So. 2d 93 (Miss. 1997).
Duttry v. Patterson, 741 A. 2d 199 (Pa. Super. 1999).
Boutte v. Seitchik, 719 A. 2d 319 (Pa. Super. 1998).
Flanagan v. Wesselhoeft, 712 A. 2d 365 (R.I. 1998).
Ashe v. Radiation Oncology Associates, 9 S.W. 3d 119 (Tenn. 1999).
Shadrick v. Coker, 963 S.W. 2d 726 (Tenn. 1998).
Moates v. Hyslop, 480 S.E. 2d 109 (Va. 1997).
Mello v. Cohen, 724 A. 2d 471 (Vt. 1998).
Backlund v. Univ. of Washington, 975 P. 2d 950 (Wash. 1999).
Brown v. Dibbell, 595 N.W. 2d 358 (Wis. 1999).
Schreiber v. Physicians Insurance Co., 588 N.W. 2d 26 (Wis. 1999).

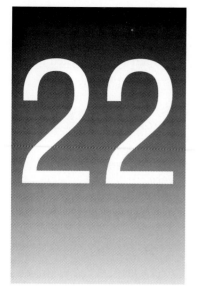

Medical records and disclosure about patients

FILLMORE BUCKNER, M.D., J.D., F.C.L.M.

PURPOSE AND FUNCTION OF MEDICAL RECORDS
STANDARDS OF RECORD-KEEPING
OWNERSHIP AND PATIENT ACCESS
CONFIDENTIALITY AND PRIVACY
PRIVILEGE AND ADMISSIBILITY
COMPUTERIZED MEDICAL RECORDS

Medical records are an integral part of patient medicolegal and ethical encounters care—medically, legally, and administratively. They must be up to standard in every way. The medical record of a hospital, clinic, or private physician's patient is often essential to the resolution of issues in nearly every branch of the law. Medical evidence is estimated to play a part in about three fourths of all civil cases and in about one fourth of criminal cases brought to trial.[1]

A properly kept medical record can serve as the physician's best friend and witness. The medical record has frequently been called the "the malpractice witness that never dies." If improperly maintained, the record may prove to be his or her worst enemy.[2] Despite continued emphasis by medical schools, insurers, and hospital risk managers, physicians simply do not do an adequate job of maintaining medical records. One Australian pediatric teaching hospital's study revealed that in only 3% of medical records were more than 50% of entries properly authenticated and that legibility and abbreviations made understanding the patient's course and actions taken time consuming and less than optimal.[3]

PURPOSE AND FUNCTION OF MEDICAL RECORDS

The *Accreditation Manual for Hospitals* of the Joint Commission on Accreditation of Healthcare Organizations (JCAHO) has outlined the purposes of medical records as follows[4]:

- To serve as the basis for the patient's care and for continuity in the evaluation of the patient's treatment
- To furnish documentary evidence of the course of the patient's medical evaluation, treatment, and change in condition during the hospital stay, during an ambulatory care or emergency visit to the hospital, or while being followed in a hospital-administered home care program

- To document communication between the practitioner responsible for the patient and any other health care professional who contributes to the patient's care
- To assist in protecting the legal interests of the patient, the hospital, and the practitioner responsible for the patient
- To provide data for use in continuing education and research

However, this definition gives a rather abbreviated and one-sided view of the modern functions of medical records. Today, medical records serve a multitude of functions. There is no doubt that the primary function of medical records remains the same, but medical records are an increasingly important tool in the care and treatment of the patient. In the present medical environment, a patient rarely sees a single health care provider. A good medical record is the premier tool for providing different members of the health care team and successive health care providers a working knowledge of the patient's care and treatment.

Second, the medical record is an important economic tool. It serves as documentation for reimbursement. Third, as the JCAHO recognizes, the medical record functions as an essential tool in medical education and clinical research. Fourth, in a closely related area, the record functions as a peer review tool for the utilization and quality review organizations and the risk management reviewers employed by the hospital and insurance companies. Fifth, the medical record functions as an essential tool in the process whereby the hospital or private organization credentials and recredentials physicians. It serves an identical function in state physician licensing reviews. Sixth, the medical record serves several legal functions. As mentioned previously, it is "the witness that never dies" in professional liability suits against health care providers. A patient with a record that demonstrates a well-documented course of care and treatment may not be less likely to sue, but defense attorneys know that a well-documented, complete, and unambiguous medical record makes a case infinitely easier to defend. The medical record also functions to document the injuries of crime victims, victims of domestic violence, victims of elder or child abuse, victims of workplace accidents, and personal injury litigants. In addition, the medical record may play a vital role in courtroom competency issues in a variety of estate, criminal, and civil commitment cases. Finally, the medical record functions as a source of public health data and vital statistics.

STANDARDS OF RECORD-KEEPING

The standards for medical record-keeping are determined by three overlapping bodies of regulations. Individual state statutes or administrative regulations furnish the first layer of requirements. These state statutes and administrative regulations usually are extensive and detailed. Medical records may be covered under specific health regulations, regulations for business records, or both. For example, the Washington state administrative code has four pages of health regulations detailing what should be entered and contained, the mechanics of entry, and the authentication of the records.[5] Local regulations may place some differing burdens on hospital records in contrast to physician or clinic records, but the trend is for all three of the regulatory bodies to treat medical records seamlessly from the out-patient setting to the extended care facility. The next layer of control is exerted by the JCAHO. The JCAHO also has extremely extensive and detailed standards for medical records located in two sections of their accreditation manual, *Assessment of Patients and Information Management Planning*.[6] However, the JCAHO standards are more concerned with the content and handling of the medical records entry than with the mechanics of entry. The JCAHO standards also attempt to incorporate the third layer of control, federal regulations, including those of Medicare.[7] Hospital staffs, managed care organizations, and clinics may assert institutional requirements applicable to their records that exceed or are in addition to the three layers of control described previously.

Because the state and JCAHO standards are so extensive,* it behooves the practitioner to review these requirements and draw up a checklist to use in creating, maintaining, and signing out records. Although most of the requirements are what would be expected, it is the rare practitioner who does not find requirements that he or she never contemplated. There-

fore, without such a checklist, all but a rare handful of practitioners will have records that are in compliance with medical record requirements and will be vulnerable to disciplinary action if the hospital or clinic staff so chooses. The following generalities concerning the mechanics of medical record entry and the contents of medical records may be considered national standards from a practical standpoint.

Mechanics of medical record entry

The mechanics of entering data into a medical record are simple and well known but frequently overlooked by the busy practitioner. First, medical record entries are to be made contemporaneously with the event. Writing entries is not to be postponed until a more convenient time or until the end of the day. When entries are written or dictated contemporaneously with the care or treatment provided, the record is in chronological order naturally. There is no justifiable reason not to keep records in chronological order. Medical record entries should aim at conveying all relevant, objective, accurate information concerning the patient. Subjective conjecture or opinions should not be entered or entered only as necessary. Abbreviations and acronyms routinely should be avoided to eliminate the possibility of confusion. However, if abbreviations are a necessity, only approved abbreviations should be used. Entries must be legible if entered by hand and in most jurisdictions may be entered by typewriter or computer to ensure legibility. Most jurisdictions require that the records be written in ink and in English. The entries should be direct, concise, clear, complete, and unambiguous. No entry should be altered or backdated. All entries should be signed or otherwise authenticated in a legal manner and timed and dated.*

Contents of the record

Simply reviewing the requirements outlined by the JCAHO and Medicare/Medicaid provides a fair picture of the minimal requirements for the contents of medical records. Combining the requirements of the two leads to a chart that contains the following items:

- Identification and demographic information
- Evidence of informed consent
- Evidence of known advance directives
- Admitting complaint or diagnosis
- History of the present illness
- Past history (including social history)
- Family history
- Orders
- Laboratory reports
- Imaging reports
- Consultations
- Reports of procedures or tests

---

*In Washington state there are 92 requirements and subrequirements applicable to the nonpsychiatric hospital record. (See Louis Vontver & Fillmore Buckner, *Medical Record Requirement Checklist,* 1995.)

*Some states allow notes to be authenticated with a rubber stamp or some combination of computer keyboard strokes.

- Progress notes that include the following:
  Clinical observations
  Results of treatment
  Complications
- Final diagnosis
- Discharge summary

The contents listed do not include items that may be required by local statutes or regulations or a hospital, institution, or specialty organization's specific requirements. In addition, a thoughtful risk manager might add the following requirements:

- Notations concerning lack of patient cooperation, failure to follow advice, or failure to keep appointments, as well as records of follow-up telephone calls and letters
- For any laboratory, radiographic, diagnostic test or consult ordered, the dates ordered, received, and reviewed
- Copies of records, instructions, diets, or directions given to the patient or to the patient's representative

Additions, corrections, and statements of disagreement

A great deal of misinformation has been published and passed from physician to physician as to how medical record corrections and additions should be made. No medical record should ever be altered or backdated. Corrections or additions should be made as outlined in the Uniform Health Care Information Act.[8] The procedure described in the act is simple. The health care provider should never expunge or obliterate any material. Instead, the provider should add the correction or addition to the medical record as a new chronological entry. The provider also should make a note in the margin, indicating that the record has been corrected or amended, and indicate where the correction or amendment may be found.[9]

Both the Uniform Health Care Information Act and the Kennedy-Kassebaum–generated Department of Health and Human Services proposed regulations allow patients to view their medical records and offer corrections or amendments for any errors they encounter.[10] If the provider agrees with the proposed correction or amendment, the provider corrects or amends the record as described previously. If the provider disagrees with the proposed correction or amendment, the provider must notify the patient of his or her refusal to correct or amend the record and offer the patient the opportunity to add a concise statement of disagreement. On receipt of the statement of disagreement, the provider enters it in the medical record, marks the disputed entry as disputed, and identifies where the statement of disagreement is located.

Alteration, destruction, or loss of medical records

In the law of evidence the loss, destruction, or significant alteration of evidence is termed *spoliation of evidence.* Thus, when medical records that have been altered or have had portions removed or when cases in which the record cannot be found come before the court, the evidentiary concept of spoliation of evidence is invoked. Wigmore explains the common law evidentiary inference concept or remedy for spiloation as follows:

It has always been understood—the inference, indeed, is one of the simplest in human experience—that a party's . . . suppression of evidence by . . . spiloation . . ., is receivable against him as an indication of his consciousness *that his case is a weak or unfounded one;* and from that consciousness may be inferred the fact itself of the cause's lack of truth and merit. The inference does not apply itself necessarily to any specific fact in the cause, but operates, indefinitely though strongly, against *the whole mass of alleged facts constituting his cause.*[11]

Therefore alterations to records can prove to be disastrous. Records with alterations are absolutely deadly in court. Document examination is now a sophisticated science. With skill and uncanny accuracy, experts may be able to determine the time that entries were made in medical records and who made them.[12]

Courts reason that destroying or altering records in anticipation of or in response to a discovery request falls under the umbrella of misuse of discovery. Discovery rules provide a broad range of sanctions for the misuse of discovery. Sanctions can include monetary fines, contempt charges, establishing or precluding the facts at issue, striking pleadings, dismissing all or parts of the action, and even granting a default judgment against the offending party. In addition to these evidence and discovery sanctions, many penal codes include criminal penalties for perjury and spoliation. In several jurisdictions, spoliation of evidence itself is a cause of action in tort.[13]

Therefore tampering with medical records may make a malpractice case impossible to defend. Further, providers who falsify a patient's record may be found civilly and criminally liable. Proof of such charges will result in loss of hospital privileges and even loss of license to practice.[14]

Retention of medical records

The increased complexity of health care delivery has heightened the importance of medical record retention. If at all possible, medical records should be maintained indefinitely. If the health care provider continues to see the patient, the records should be retained indefinitely. A general guideline is to maintain medical records for at least 10 years after the *last* time the patient was seen by the health care provider. In the case of minors, medical records should be kept for a minimum of 10 years or until the patient reaches the age of majority plus the applicable statute of limitations, whichever is longer. The presence of a latent injury may extend the statute of limitations until the injury is discovered. Discovery rules in some states extend malpractice liability beyond the statute of limitations. These rules usually allow a period of time, most often 1 year, after discovery of the malpractice to bring a suit. In states with such discovery rules, minors' records should be retained for sufficient time for the minor to reach majority and for the statute of repose, if there is one, to expire. If there is no statute of repose, minors' and adults' records must be kept indefinitely because there is no time limit to bringing a suit under the discovery rule.

It is imperative, apart from any statutory mandates, that physicians maintain comprehensive patient records as long as the threat of a medical malpractice suit exists. During this period of vulnerability, a physician requires complete and accurate medical records to successfully defend himself or herself in a malpractice action.

In some instances it is impossible for a health care provider to retain medical records indefinitely. Records may be stored at a commercial facility or microfilmed.[15] However, both of these alternatives are expensive, especially for the physician leaving practice. Many times, local clinics or hospitals agree to maintain the records of a physician who is retiring or leaving the community to establish at least a marginal contact with the physician's former patients. Either as partial consideration in a sale of medical records or as total consideration for the unremunerated transfer of records, a binding written agreement should be made. The agreement should specify the following, at a minimum[16]:

- That the transferee will act as trustee of the records for the transferor
- That the records must be retained for a specific term of years or indefinitely
- That the trustee will honor the confidentiality of the patient
- That the patient's requests for copies of all information will be honored
- That the original provider, his or her attorney-in-fact, and his or her personal representative will have access to and may copy any record
- That the records may be microfilmed, scanned, or otherwise reduced or compacted at no expense to the original provider
- That the agreement is binding on the transferee's successors and assigns

The original chart must be maintained securely in the event that there is a claim or lawsuit. The patient relies on the records to provide information about his or her care and treatment. Also, medical research relies heavily on access to medical records from decades before.

State regulations. State law may dictate specific medical record retention requirements. For example, Maryland law provides that, unless the patient is notified, a health care professional cannot destroy an adult's medical record, laboratory report, or x-ray film for 5 years after the record or report is made.[17] In the case of a minor patient, a medical record, laboratory report, or x-ray film cannot be destroyed until the patient attains the age of majority plus 3 years or for 5 years after the record or report is made,

whichever is the longer period of time, unless the parent or guardian of the child is notified or the minor patient is notified, if the care provided is care for which the minor is permitted to consent.[18] Employee health records should be retained according to specific state retention requirements. Some state laws guarantee patients or their representatives the right to review and copy their medical records.[19]

Federal regulations. Federal regulations governing the Medicare program require participating hospitals to keep patient records for at least 5 years or that period determined by the appropriate state regulation governing the retention of records, whichever is longer.[20] All of the following categories of Medicare records are required to be maintained for at least 5 years after a Medicare cost report is filed with the fiscal intermediary: building materials; cost report materials; and reviews, reports, and other records.[21] All records pertaining to any reimbursement issue that is on appeal with the Medicare program should be retained until the conclusion of the appeal.[22]

The federal regulations protecting confidentiality of alcohol and drug abuse treatment records do not have specific general retention periods. However, the regulations require that the records be maintained in a secure room, locked file cabinet, safe, or other similar container when not in use.[23] Methadone treatment programs must maintain records traceable to specific patients, showing dates, quantities, and batch or code marks of the drug dispensed for 3 years after the date of dispensing.[24] Likewise, when narcotic drugs are administered for treatment of narcotic-dependent, hospitalized patients, the hospital must maintain accurate records, showing dates, quantities, and batch or code marks for the drug administered for at least 3 years.[25] The Occupational Safety and Health Administration (OSHA) requires that a provider maintain, for years after the end of the year to which it relates, documentation consisting of a log and descriptive summary, a supplementary record detailing the injuries and illnesses, and an annual summary, which is to be posted, of an employee's occupational injuries and illnesses.[26]

Other regulations, recommendations, and requirements. JCAHO provides that the length of time for which medical records are to be retained is dependent on the need for their use in continuing patient care, legal research, or educational purposes and on law and regulation.[27] A provider may wish to consider the recommendations of professional associations regarding record retention times. For example, three such associations—the American Hospital Association, the American Medical Association, and the American Medical Record Association—have recommended that the complete patient medical record (in original or reproduced form) be retained for 10 years. This period would commence upon the last encounter with a patient. These associations further suggest that after 10 years such records may be destroyed, unless statute, ordinance, regulation, or law specifically prohibits destruction and provided that the institution retains certain information for specified purposes.[28]

Destruction of medical records

Some states have specific regulations governing the destruction of medical records.[29] Usually these regulations call for incineration or shredding as a means of protecting patient confidentiality. If a health care entity destroys its own records, it should establish written policies covering the destruction and require a written declaration from the person responsible for record destruction that the prescribed policies were followed. However, unless a provider, clinic, or hospital has its own commercial incinerator or shredding facility, the destruction of records will require the use of a commercial document disposal company. It is important that the record destruction by such a commercial entity be covered by a written agreement. That agreement should include provisions that cover the following points:

- The method of destruction
- Warranties that the confidentiality of the records will be honored
- Indemnification for any unauthorized record disclosures
- A certificate of destruction from the commercial entity, certifying the date, method, and the complete destruction of the record, which should be retained as a permanent record

Record security and protection

Although reason would dictate that a certain degree of record security and protection is necessary to prevent unauthorized access to medical records and ensure the integrity of the information contained therein, there are few specific guidelines regulating record security and protection.[30] The general provisions of the Uniform Health Care Information Act call for providers to effect "reasonable" safeguards for the security of medical records but do not specify what those reasonable safeguards should be.[31] However, the comments to the chapter indicate that the safeguards should be reasonable for the sensitivity of the information contained, the type of provider maintaining the information, and other factors particular to the information's environment. It would behoove the health care provider to understand the following recommendations for record security and protection and make note of those that can be incorporated into their program:

- Maintain a written health care management policy, with security and protection provisions.
- Require background checks and bonding of all record personnel.
- Keep the door locked, allowing only those authorized with access to records.
- Ensure locked, fireproof record storage.
- Change locks on a regular basis or with a change of personnel.

- Use passwords, access codes, or advanced recognition technology and firewalls for automated systems*
- Do not keep confidential material on a publicly accessible system, and do not run a publicly accessible system on the institution's internal system.
- Change passwords and access codes on a regular basis.
- Maintain written or electronic access and print logs.
- Archive and backup records stored off-site.
- Allow zero tolerance for security violations regardless of the form of the records. No record security violation should go unrecorded or unpunished.

Record retrieval

No record system is complete without an organized method for retrieval. In the United States, medical record systems are based on retrieval by identification number and/or alphabetical names. Strange as it may seem, there seem to be few if any regulations governing the retrieval system used, but there are cases reflecting damages for retrieval failures.[32]

OWNERSHIP AND PATIENT ACCESS
Ownership

There is little controversy about who owns the tangible medical record, that is, the paper, film, or recording that contains the medical information; the health care provider who is responsible for creating, compiling, and maintaining the medical record owns it.[33] In facilities where records are compiled by several individual health care providers, the facility is the owner rather than the assorted individual health care providers.[34] Ownership is established by statute in several states and by contract in others.[35]

However, the ownership interest in the medical record differs from the ownership interest in most other personal property and is governed by a large body of ethical, administrative, statutory, and common law controls, some of which are detailed in the section on record retention and others that are detailed next. The concept of ownership is further complicated by two federal court cases that hold that the patient has a limited "property right" in the record.[36] However, most court cases reflect the patient's right to access the medical record and the medical information therein rather than their ownership rights to the physical record.

Patient access to medical records

The distinct trend since the 1970s is to assure patients the right to access their own medical records. The principal arguments in favor of this position are (1) that access to the records will allow the patient to become better informed about his or her medical condition and improve the patient's participation in medical decision-making and compliance, (2) that patient access to medical records is the only way to allow errors in the record to be

---

*See the section on computerized medical records for a more complete discussion of security for electronic records.

corrected and error perpetuation stopped, and (3) that patients have the right to be informed about their medical care and that provider reluctance to allow them access to their records is a reflection of a paternalistic and outdated profession.

The Uniform Health Care Information Act certainly is in agreement with these arguments. It provides for patient access to medical records under all but a few circumstances[37] and allows patients to copy those records or to seek correction of errors in their record.[38] If the physician will not correct the error, the patient has the right to insert a statement of disagreement in the medical record.[39] The act provides civil and criminal sanctions for physician failure to allow access or correction to the record.[40] These same provisions are mirrored in the proposed Confidentiality of Individually Identifiable Health Recommendations of the Secretary of Health and Human Services.[41] This trend is also reflected in legislative action. More than 30 states now have statutes allowing some degree of patient access to personal medical records.[42] These statutes vary widely, and space limitations preclude a complete discussion of all jurisdictions. The reader is urged to research the applicable statutory law carefully in his or her jurisdiction.

This trend to allow patients access to their medical records is also reflected in case law. Even in the absence of statute, courts have tended to grant patients the right to review and copy their medical records.[43] Courts reflect some of the same concerns reflected in the Uniform Health Care Information Act and have tended to deny patients access to their medical records if there was danger that the information would harm the patient. This denial usually has been in connection with psychiatric records.[44] At least one court has levied sanctions against a provider who failed to allow a patient legitimate access to his or her medical records.[45]

CONFIDENTIALITY AND PRIVACY

The medical record is apt to contain more personal information than any other single document. It contains sensitive health care information and demographic, sexual, behavioral, dietary, and recreational information. Because of the vast amount of highly sensitive information in the medical record, patients expect that the information therein will be held in privacy. The mirror image of that expectation—loss of personal privacy—is the greatest concern of more than one fourth of our population.[46]

The privacy v. confidentiality conflict

Patient privacy advocates look for a model based on access only by informed patient consent and question the need to circulate health care information beyond the health care provider. Professor Alan Westin[47] calls this concept *privacy.*

On the other hand, Westin defines *confidentiality* as the question of how medical data shall be held and used by the provider who collected it, what other further uses will be made of it, and if or when the patient's consent will be re-

quired. Confidentiality advocates, hospitals, insurers, managed care organizations, educators, researchers, public health agencies, government agencies, utilization review organizations, and risk managers hold to the premise that access to and sharing of health care data are critical to a well-functioning, cost-efficient health care system and are essential to the discovery and monitoring of disease trends.

The conflict between the concepts of "privacy" and "confidentiality" then, reduced to its basics, is whether we support privacy, recognizing that the greater social good will be negatively affected, or whether we believe that the greater social good is important enough to negatively affect the privacy of the medical records and the information therein. There appears to be little doubt that current legal theory supports the concept of confidentiality, and in this day of third-party payors, fourth-party auditors, and the multiple legitimate needs for health care information, classic patient privacy is a myth.

Constitutional privacy protections

Privacy advocates relying on constitutional privacy protection get little support. First, the right to privacy under the Constitution offers protection only from intrusions by the government.[48] Therefore constitutional remedies do not reach breaches by private health care information holders. Furthermore, a whole series of federal court cases have demonstrated that even when there is government intrusion into individually identifiable health care information, individuals cannot rely on constitutional protections to preserve their privacy. The strong public interest represented by the need for the information outweighs the individual's need for privacy.

The seminal case in this series is *Whalen v. Roe.*[49] In an attempt to stem the illegal distribution of prescription drugs, the New York legislature passed a law requiring that all prescriptions for Schedule II drugs be logged and information concerning the prescription, including the identity of the patient, be transmitted to the State Department of Health. Public disclosure of the information was forbidden, and access to the information was confined to department and investigative personnel. Patients receiving Schedule II drugs and their physicians brought suit, questioning the constitutionality of the law. They argued that the physician-patient relationship was one of the zones of privacy accorded constitutional protection. A unanimous United States Supreme Court held that the patient identification process was reasonable exercise of the state's broad police powers.[50] In *United States v. Westinghouse Electric Corp.*[51] the United States Court of Appeals for the Third Circuit elucidated the following seven factors to be considered in determining "whether an intrusion into an individual's privacy is justified . . .:"[52]

- The type of record requested
- The type of information it does or might contain
- The potential for harm in any subsequent nonconsensual disclosure

- The injury from disclosure to the relationship in which the record was generated
- The adequacy of safeguards to prevent unauthorized disclosure
- The degree of need for access
- Whether there is an express statutory mandate, articulated public policy, or other recognizable public interest militating toward access

The test appears to have survived the test of time[53] and offers pragmatic evidence that even under constitutional protections, privacy is dead and confidentiality reigns.

Confidentiality

Section 5.05 of the AMA Code of Ethics adopts a standard for confidentiality.[54] It directs the physician not to reveal information about the patient without the patient's consent or as required by law. It then goes on to say some "overriding social considerations" will make revelations "ethically and legally justified." Although the text and the 65 annotations may give a member physician some idea of the scope of the problem, the broadness, vagueness, and double speak of Section 5.05 reflect the current confused state of medical record confidentiality in the United States.

State regulation. State statutes have developed piecemeal across the country. All states require health care providers to report some types of patients to state agencies.[55] However, universality ends with that statement. State confidentiality rules are dramatically inconsistent in their regulations and even their presence.[56] In pre–World War II America this inconsistency was not a problem. The population was not tremendously mobile, and health care information was essentially local. However, since World War II the American population has become increasingly mobile, and coincident with both that mobility and the development of regional and national payers, health care information has crossed state lines as never before. In addition, the expanded use of electronic health care information has no regard for state boundaries. The patchwork effect of strikingly different state confidentiality regulations or the complete lack thereof became a major problem. The National Commissioners for Uniform State Laws attempted to remedy this problem in the early 1970s with the Uniform Health Care Information Act (UHCIA).[57]

The UHCIA was a comprehensive set of nine articles of health care information management regulations designed to be passed by state legislatures. Article I defines the scope of the problem and principles involved. Article II deals with disclosures of health care information with and without the patient's consent.[58] Article III permits patients access to their medical records and permits copying of the records. Article IV deals with the correction and amendment of the medical record. Article V requires that notice of information practices be given patients. Article VI details persons authorized to act for patients. Article VII requires security for records, and Article VIII de-

fines the civil and criminal penalties for failure to adhere to the regulations. Article IX is essentially legislative boilerplate. Unfortunately, in the 24 years since the commissioners first drafted the UHCIA, only two states have adopted it.[59]

In most states the state common law becomes the principal protector of medical record confidentiality. Not surprisingly, there is no great number of suits dealing with breach of confidentiality. Most health care providers attempt to honor the patient's confidentiality and frequently have justifications that are persuasive to juries when violations of confidentiality do occur. In addition, a suit will frequently make the very facts the patient does not want revealed part of the public record. Finally, many violations of confidentiality do not generate sufficient economic damages to justify the cost of litigation. However, suits for breach of confidential relationship,[60] breach of fiduciary duty,[61] breach of implied contract,[62] defamation,[63] negligence,[64] intentional infliction of emotional distress,[65] and invasion of privacy[66] have all been used as common law causes of action to enforce medical record confidentiality.

The lack of consistent state regulations and the limitations of state common law remedies have resulted in repeated calls for a comprehensive federal law governing medical record confidentiality. Despite widespread support for such an enactment and general agreement on the nature of the principles to be supported, no truly comprehensive federal statute or regulation has been put in force.

Proposed federal regulations. Much like the state confidentiality regulations, existing federal regulations have been enacted piecemeal, affecting one industry or special situation at a time but failing to address an overall plan for the health care industry. The only existing federal regulations specific to the health field are those concerning alcohol and drugs. Some of the regulations enforcing these acts were outlined earlier in the section on retention of records.

In the 1950s and 1960s in a series of incidents medical records of drug and alcohol abuse were disclosed without authorization to law enforcement officers and employers. As a result of the furor over these incidents, Congress enacted the Comprehensive Alcohol Abuse and Alcohol Prevention and Treatment Act of 1970.[67] This act was followed in 1972 by the Drug Abuse Office and Treatment Act.[68] The regulations apply to all categories of providers and are not limited to drug or alcohol treatment facilities. All information, even the information that the patient has been a patient, is considered nondisclosable. The prohibition is broad and applies even if the inquirer has secured a subpoena.[69] A patient's consent must be obtained for each specific release of information, including disclosures to third-party payors and the patient's family.[70] To be valid, the consent must be made voluntarily, be in writing, clearly identify the patient, specify the material to be released, clearly identify the provider supplying the information, clearly identify who is to receive the information, state the purpose and extent of the disclosure, inform the patient that the consent may be revoked at any time, and contain an expiration date. It goes without saying that the consent must be signed and dated.[71]

Beginning with the 96th Congress, numerous health care privacy and confidentiality bills have been introduced. Most of those bills have included many or all of the features of the UHCIA. Senator Bennett (R-Utah) introduced one of the most important of these bills in 1994. The Bennett bill was a well-conceived confidentiality statute with only one significant shortcoming—it failed to take into account current electronic health information practices. It was doomed to failure under the dual attacks of the privacy advocates who thought it allowed too easy access to personal information and the health care's electronic services industry that thought it squashed needed electronic financial services.

In 1996, Congress passed the Kennedy-Kassebaum Bill,[72] which called for the enactment of a privacy statute within 3 years. The legislation also called for the Secretary of Health and Human Services to send recommendations for protecting the confidentiality of health care information to Congress. The secretary sent those recommendations in September 1997. The secretary listed the following framework for federal privacy legislation:

Such legislation should:
- Allow for the smooth flow of identifiable health information for treatment, payment and related operations, and *for specified additional purposes related to health care that is in the public interest.*
- Prohibit the flow of identifiable information for any additional purposes, unless specifically and voluntarily authorized by the subject of the information.
- Put in place a set of fair information practices that allow individuals to know who is using their health care information and how it is being used.
- Establish fair information practices that *allow individuals to obtain access to their records and request amendment of inaccurate information.*
- Require persons who hold identifiable health information to safeguard that information from inappropriate use or disclosure.
- Hold those who use individually identifiable health information accountable for their handling of this information, and to provide legal recourse to persons harmed by misuse.

Again, Congress failed to enact a comprehensive health care privacy law but instead instructed the Secretary of Health and Human Services to develop a set of regulations. The secretary published the proposed regulations in November 1999.[73]

The proposed regulations and their accompanying notes cover just under 300 typewritten pages of extreme complexity but again fail to produce a comprehensive set of federal confidentiality regulations for the entire health care industry. Section 160.102 of the proposed rules indicates that the rule applies only to health plans, health care clearinghouses, and health care providers who transmit health information elec-

tronically. Thus paper and film records are not covered and nonprovider, nonplan, nonclearinghouse holders of health care information are not included, and the regulations do not fulfill the framework the secretary recommended to Congress. Section 164.522, Compliance and Enforcement, does not allow for a private action against violators or spell out specific penalties the secretary may impose.

The principal regulations are as follows:

Section 164.506 permits any authorized disclosure and unauthorized disclosures to carry out treatment, payment, or health care operations when required by the secretary, required by law, or required by audits. It also specifies how information may be de-identified.

Section 164.508 requires an authorization to release information at the patient's request or for the health care entity to secure information. It also specifies that authorization is necessary to release information to a non-health-care–related division of the same entity or the patient's employer. To be valid an authorization must contain the following:
  (i) A specific and meaningful description of the information to be disclosed.
  (ii) The name of the entity to make the disclosure.
  (iii) The name of the entity to receive the information.
  (iv) An expiration date.
  (v) Signature and date.
  (vi) If made by a representative, a description of authority.
  (vii) A statement that acknowledges that the patient knows he/she has the right to revoke the authorization.
  (viii) A statement that a patient knows that information disclosed to any entity other than a health plan or health care provider will no longer be protected by the federal privacy law.

Section 164.510 permits unauthorized disclosure for public health activities, health oversight activities, judicial and administrative proceedings, coroners and medical examiners, law enforcement purposes, research purposes, and government health data systems. It also details disclosures for directory purposes, emergency situations, and specialized classes.

Section 164.512 requires notice to patients of the entity's information practices.

Section 164.514 allows patients to access and copy their medical records with much the same exception provisions as the UHCIA.[74]

Section 164.515 provides patients with an accounting of disclosures except those for treatment, payment, and health care operations and those to health oversight or law enforcement agencies.

Section 164.516 allows patients to make amendments and corrections to medical records.

Section 164.518 requires the covered entities to designate an individual responsible for privacy issues, have a contact person or office, train personnel in health information policies, and have in place administrative, technical, and physical safeguards for health care information.

Section 164.520 requires documentation of all policies and procedures and retention of that documentation for at least 6 years.

Section 164.524 requires all covered entities to be in compliance within 2 years of the effective date of the regulations.

The preceding summary does little to illustrate the complexity of the multiple qualifying clauses in each of the sections. This compounding complexity is probably the most discouraging feature of the proposed regulations. It will be the rare health care provider who can take the time to read the regulations and their comments let alone understand and absorb them. It is unfortunate that the secretary could not learn from the clear concise wording used by the National Commissioners for Uniform State Laws in the UHCIA. It appears, at the time of this writing, that the limited applicability of the proposed regulations together with the complexity of their presentation makes it unlikely that they can satisfy the need for national confidentiality guidelines. Congress must fill the vacuum as soon as possible.

PRIVILEGE AND ADMISSIBILITY
Provider-patient privilege

An issue closely related to privacy and confidentiality is how confidential health care information is treated by the courts. As might be surmised from the preceding discussions, it would seem apparent that nowhere is the release of confidential health care information more in the public interest than in the court of law. In addition, there is no physician-patient testimonial privilege in the common law. It seems incongruous therefore that since 1828 all but three states have passed some sort of provider-patient testimonial privilege statute.[75] The statutes vary widely from state to state, but all offer some degree of protection to the patient by not allowing the provider to testify in court about the patient's medical information. Many states do not recognize the privilege in criminal cases, others limit the privilege to psychotherapists, and still others include a variety of health care providers in addition to physicians. Under Section 501 of the Federal Rules of Evidence, if a claim in federal court arises under state law, that state's privilege rule will apply. However, if a claim arises under federal law, no privilege will be recognized.[76] There has been a definite trend in both federal and state courts to look at the health care testimonial privilege skeptically. Even in that bastion of privilege, the psychiatric record, courts have questioned the merits of confidentiality. Critics see the privilege as nothing more than a litigation tactic and doubt that testimony deters people from seeking psychiatric care or for that matter any health care. The current uses of group therapy and the fact that people in states without the privilege seek care at the same rate as in privilege states are frequently asserted arguments.

Nonetheless, a general body of law has developed in regard to the provider-patient privilege. The privilege extends to the entire medical record, including x-ray films, laboratory reports, billing records, and all other documents compiled and maintained by the provider.[77] The communication must be made in confidence for the privilege to apply. The communication also must be made within the context of the provider-patient relationship and be made in regard to diagnosis or treatment. Therefore situations in which the communicator is a nontraditional patient, such as when he or she is undergoing an independent medical examination, or relating facts unrelated to diagnosis or treatment are not covered by the privilege.[78]

The privilege and the benefit thereof belong to the patient, although anyone with an interest may assert it. Only the patient may waive the privilege. The waiver may be express or implied. An express waiver is made when the patient signs an authorization directing the provider to disclose the information. Implied waivers may be made in several different ways. The patient may voluntarily introduce the medical evidence to the court; the patient may voluntarily place his or her medical condition at issue in litigation, or the patient may fail to assert his or her privilege when the medical information is placed into evidence. A good rule of thumb for health care providers is to always assert the privilege when faced with a subpoena that is not accompanied by a patient's authorization to disclose the information. As already mentioned, this is required by the federal alcohol and drug regulations and even in cases not involving alcohol or drugs, failure to assert the privilege has resulted in liability in at least one state court.[79]

Admissibility

As is the case with all evidence, medical records must be relevant and material to the issues before the court to be admitted into evidence. However, depending on the document, a variety of objections may be raised to the admission of even relevant and material health care information. In addition to the privilege objection discussed previously, some medical information, such as incident reports, may be protected because they were made in anticipation of litigation or fall within the attorney-client privilege or are part of the attorney's work product. However, the most common objection to admission is that the medical record is hearsay. It is an out of court statement being introduced to prove the truth of the matter asserted in the statement. However, medical records tend to fall into any one of a number of exceptions to the hearsay rule. First, medical records are business records[80] or records of regularly conducted activity and fall under that exception to the hearsay rule.[81] Second, statements made for the purposes of medical diagnosis or treatment[82] are exceptions to the hearsay rule. Finally, dying declarations[83] and declarations against interest[84] are also exceptions that may apply to medical records. For practical purposes, records made in accordance with the record-keeping mechanics outlined previously are admitted as evidence over the hearsay objection.

COMPUTERIZED MEDICAL RECORDS

The computerized medical record is an electronically stored data base containing a patient's health care information from one or multiple sources. The health care industry has become the last industry in the United States to become computerized. In every other industry the electronic record has become the norm. Whether this rejection of the computer is a result of some inbred reactionary trait on the part of the medical profession or truly an objective look at a new technology is open to debate because computerized records have some well-known problems. Critics cite hardware crashes and breakdowns, power failures, software glitches, sabotage of the system by both disgruntled employees and hackers, unauthorized access, viruses, Trojan horses, and a host of other real and imagined problems. On the other hand, the health care industry is hard pressed to deny that computerized medical records facilitate and many times are essential to effective quality assurance, analysis of practice patterns, and research activities; speed the retrieval of data and expedite billing; reduce the number of lost records; expedite the transfer of data between facilities; and are a proven cost reducer.

Computerized medical records as a legal aid

From a legal standpoint, however, some other factors weigh more heavily in favor of the computerized medical record. First and foremost, a computerized record system produces a legible record. Many of the problems of wrong medication, wrong dose, wrong directions, and wrong procedure caused by illegible and misinterpreted records will be eliminated. Second, a properly planned medical record system can incorporate practice guidelines that are automatically triggered by a diagnosis or symptom syndrome.[85] Adherence to practice guidelines has been an effective defense in many malpractice actions. Guidelines also have been championed as the most effective method of eliminating unnecessary and costly defensive medicine practices.[86] In a like manner, the effective computerized medical record system will have connections to the pharmacy and pharmacy data banks. Computerized prescriptions and orders will not permit prescriptions or orders for drugs for which the patient has a known allergy, and the system will alert both provider and pharmacist of potentially harmful drug-drug interactions or incompatibilities with the patient's physical or laboratory findings.[87] Adverse drug events are now the No. 1 adverse hospital event[88] and are second only to birth injuries in the amount of damages paid in malpractice claims. Reducing these adverse events would be an significant risk management accomplishment. Fourth, computerized medical record systems can track ordered laboratory, diagnostic, or imaging

tests; alert the provider of abnormal tests; and even notify the patient of the need or lack thereof for future tests, diagnosis, or treatment.[89] Fifth, computerized medical records automatically confirm the date and times of all entries and keep a dated and timed log of all individuals who have accessed the record. Many individuals think these features make medical records more secure than paper records. In any case, such entries offer great protection against accusations of Medicare or Medicaid fraud and abuse. Finally, most computerized record systems automatically generate patient educational materials tailored to the patient's diagnosis and treatment. These defensive features are hard to beat in a paper system.

Computerized record criteria

As mentioned previously, properly compiled and maintained medical records are business records. Electronic medical records also are business records.[90] As such they must meet certain criteria to ensure their admissibility as evidence in court. The most critical element in the admissibility of electronic records is reliability. When a paper record is prepared, it is fixed in form and content. In most cases changes may be detected. The electronic media may be changed, and the changed product may be indistinguishable from the original. Therefore the first criterion to be met is that the electronic medical record must place each entry as made in a "read only" mode. That is, once the entry is made, it cannot be altered. Any changes must be made by a new note entered in order, dated, and timed.

Although no formal criteria have been published to date, the following criteria must be adhered to for electronic data to be considered "records" in the evidentiary sense:

- Compliant: Information-keeping must adhere to local jurisdictional requirements for admissibility as "business records."
- Responsible: Written policies and procedures for record storage and maintenance are established and maintained.
- Implemented: The written policies and procedures are employed at all times.
- Consistent: Record-maintenance systems ensure that records stored and maintained are managed in a uniform fashion to enhance credibility.
- Comprehensive: All business records are stored and maintained.
- Identifiable: All business records for a discrete transaction are readily identifiable and accessible.
- Complete: Stored records preserve the content and structure of the business transaction creating them to ensure accuracy and understanding.
- Authorized: All maintained records must have been stored under the auspices of an authorized creator.
- Preserved: Records must be inviolate to preserve their original content. No records may be audited without a concise audit trail that preserves relevant information of the original content.

- Removable: Records may be removed from storage only with the consent of an authorized entity. All removals must be evidenced by an audit trail that preserves the content of the record being removed.
- Usable: The information in the stored records must be accessible for general business purposes, for exportation to reporting functions, and for redaction when necessary. Any and all accesses (even simple reading) must create an audit trail.[91]

A careful analysis of these requirements will stress that, in addition to reliability, both a functioning archival system and a secondary, preferably off-site, backup system are essential to a well-functioning medical records system. Unfortunately, the backup system is the most commonly overlooked element of computerized medical records.

The Federal Rules of Evidence have long recognized the admissibility of electronic business records.[92] In addition, the Rules recognize a computer printout as an "original" for the purposes of admission.[93] Most state courts have followed the federal leads on both issues.[94]

Security issues

The privacy issue is the most common concern voiced about computerized medical records. As already discussed, privacy can no longer be a consideration in medical records of any type. What the health care industry must consider are reasonable rules of confidentiality. Computerized records have all the confidentiality concerns of their paper counterparts and the added concerns of preserving the integrity of the record and preventing unauthorized remote access to the information. Although medical record security in general has already been discussed, some issues specific to the security of electronic records are discussed next.

Access. With paper records one of the principal security measures used is limiting access to records to a limited number of individuals and in some situations limiting access to only the attending physician. However, one of the great advantages of the electronic medical record is that it can offer seamless recording from any number of sources. It also can offer access to a nonfragmented medical record to the same number of sites. Therefore traditional criteria of limiting access to a single physician or group of physicians or limiting access by job criteria will limit the benefits of the electronic record. All providers involved in the care of the patient should have access to and be able to make notes in the record. It is as important for the dentist caring for the patient to know about the patient's rheumatic fever as it is for the pharmacist or clinical pharmacologist to know about the patient's renal function. When the patient comes to the emergency department in the middle of the night, the triage person needs immediate access to the complete record. Thus access must be spread across a wider range of provider and job categories and cannot be limited by current "attending" criteria.

Authorizations. The access issues described previously mandate that a system of blanket category authorizations to enter the system must be made. For instance, "all licensed providers" (which would include licensed practical nurses in many states), "all licensed providers except . . . ," or "all licensed providers and . . . ."

Authentication. In the field of computerized medical records, authentication is defined as the system for determining the identity of an individual seeking access to the system to enter or retrieve data. The simplest authentication system is the combination of user identification name and password. If the individual enters the combination of symbols making up the user name followed by the proper password, entry is allowed. User identification names are usually permanent and are frequently numerical. Passwords generally are changed periodically, monthly, or quarterly. Another relatively simple system combines the user identification name with a smart card not unlike a credit card or mechanized gate card. As computers have become more sophisticated, so have authentication systems. Commercial authentication systems are now available based on "digital signature," fingerprints, retinal patterns, facial biometrics, and voice recognition. Authentication systems need constant upkeep to remove people who leave the system and add new people to the system.

Firewalls. Another advantage of electronic records is that they allow remote access to medical records. Therefore providers may access and enter data from remote sites, such as physician offices and outlying clinics. The access ports for these remote sites are vulnerable to unauthorized individuals entering the system. They must be guarded by firewalls. A firewall is a point of entry for remote users that can be configured and controlled. A firewall normally restricts access by denying entry to incoming messages arising from an unapproved source and limiting access to approved sources, such as a list of approved phone numbers or identified computers. A firewall also may limit the functions it allows an incoming source to perform.

Transmission control protocol wrappers. Wrappers serve somewhat the same function as firewalls. Wrappers may be thought of as functioning within the server rather than at the port of entry, as does the firewall. It too will intercept incoming data and check it against a programmed security protocol. In addition to denying entry to the system or preventing a proposed function, wrappers can audit the source, date, and time of the entry.

Audit trails. As already discussed, an audit trail (formerly known as _audit log_) logs all access to electronically stored medical information. An effective audit trail records the identification of the individual accessing the record, the time and date of record access, the record or records accessed, the portion of the record accessed, and the action made. The audit trail must be secured against modification and provide for periodic analysis for unauthorized access.

Audit trails that meet or exceed these criteria appear to be an effective tool in preventing unauthorized access to records. It would appear from the proposed federal regulations that audit trails for individual patient records are going to be available for review by patients and that there are few presently proposed exceptions to allowing that review.

Encryption. If health care information is to be sent over public networks, such as the Internet, it must be encrypted to ensure confidentiality.

Virus control. Viruses must be controlled by strict rules against downloading unauthorized software programs from the Internet or bringing in software from home. In addition, antivirus software must be installed and updated on a regular basis. Regular checks of the software configurations and unauthorized service ports will help control the problem as well.

ENDNOTES

1. Matte J., *Legal Implications of the Patient's Medical Record*, in *Legal Medicine Annual* 345-375 (C.H. Wecht ed., 1971).
2. *See Schwartz v. Board of Regents of the State of New York et al.*, 453 N.Y.S. 836 (1982); *Peterson v. Tucson General Hospital, Inc.*, 559 P. 2d 186 (1976).
3. Dawson et al., *The Pediatric Hospital Medical Record: A Quality Assessment*, 12 Aust. Cain. Rev. 89-93 (1993).
4. Joint Commission on Accreditation of Healthcare Organizations, *Accreditation Manual for Hospitals* 79-92 (JCAHO 1990).
5. Washington Administrative Code, Title 246: Department of Health §246-318-440, Records and Reports—Medical Record System.
6. Joint Commission on Accreditation of Health Care Organizations, *Accreditation Manual for Hospitals: Standards* 5-10, 54-63 (JCAHO 1995).
7. 42 C.F.R. Ch. IV §482.24.
8. National Conference of Commissioners on Uniform State Laws, *Uniform Health Care Information Act,* 9 U.La. Ann. 478 (1988).
9. *Id.* §4-102.
10. *Id.* §4-101; D.H.H.S. Proposed Standards for Privacy of Individually Identifiable Health Information, Federal Register, Nov 3, 1999, pp 59917-60065 to be codified at 45 C.F.R. Parts 160-164.
11. *Thor v. Boska,* 113 Cal.Rptr. 296, 302 (1974); 2 Wigmore (3d ed. 1940) §278 at 120 (emphasis added).
12. *See* Anderson, *Counterfeit, Forged and Altered Documents,* 32 Law Society J. 48 (1994); Fortunato & Stewart, *Sentence Insertion Detected Through Ink, ESDA, & Line Width,* 17 J. Forensic Sciences 1702 (1992); Schwid, *Examining Forensic Documents,* 64 The Wisconsin Lawyer 23 (1991).
13. Buckner F., *Cedars-Sinai Medical Center v. Superior Court and the Tort of Spoliation of Evidence,* 6 Legal Medicine Perspectives 1-3 (1999).
14. *Ritter v. Board of Commissioners of Adams County Public Hospital,* 637 P. 2d 940 (1981). *See also,* Buckner F., *Medical Records and Physician Disciplinary Actions,* 11 J. Medical Practice Management 284-290 (1996); Hirsh H., *Tampering with Medical Records,* 24 Med. Trial Tech. Q. 450-455 (Spring 1978); Preiser, *The High Cost of Tampering with Medical Records,* Medical Economics 84-87 (Oct 4, 1986); Gage, *Alteration, Falsification, and Fabrication of Records in Medical Malpractice Actions,* Med. Trial Tech. Q. 476-488. (Spring 1981); Mich. Stat. Ann. § 14.624(21) (Callaghan 1976); Tenn. Code Ann. § 63-752(f) 14(Supp. 1976); Tenn. Code Ann. § 39-1971 (1975) (making it a crime to falsify a hospital medical record for purposes of cheating or defrauding).
15. Several states specifically authorize the microfilming of records. *See* Cal. Evid. Code §1550 (West 1986).
16. Buckner F., *Closing Your Medical Office,* 4 J. Med. Pract. Mgmt. 274-280 (1989).
17. §403(b) of Health General Article Ann. Code of Maryland (LEXIS 199).
18. *Id.* §403(c).
19. Rev. Code Wn. §70.02.080.
20. 42 C.F.R. §482.24(b)(1) (1990).
21. Medicare & Medicaid Guide (CCH) §6420.85 (1990).
22. *Id.*
23. 42 C.F.R. §2.16.
24. 21 C.F.R, §291.505(d)(13)(ii).
25. 21 C.F.R. §291.505(f)(2)(v).
26. 29 C.F.R. §§1904.1-1904.6.
27. Standard MR 4.2 JCAHO, *supra,* note 4.
28. American Hospital Association and American Medical Record Association, *Statement on Preservation of Medical Records in Health Care Institutions* (1975).
29. *See* Tenn. Code Ann. §68-11-3058 (1987).
30. *See supra,* note 23.
31. §7-101, Uniform Health Care Information Act, *supra,* note 8.
32. *See Fox v. Cohen,* 406 N.E. 2d 178 (1980); *Bondu v. Gurvich,* 473 So.2d 1307 (1985).
33. Dewitt et al., *Patient Information and Confidentiality: Treatise on Health Care Law,* Matthew Bender, 1991.
34. *Parsley v. Associates in Internal Medicine,* 484 N.Y.S. 2d 485 (1985).
35. *See* Tenn. Code Ann. §68-11-304 (1990).
36. *See Bishop Clarkson Memorial Hospital v. Reserve Life Insurance Co.,* 350 F. 2d 1006 (8th Cir. 1965); *Pyramid Life Ins. Co. v. Masonic Hosp. Assn.,* 191 F.Supp. 51 (W.D. Okla.1961).
37. §3-102 Uniform Health Care Information Act, *supra,* note 8. Denial of Examination and Copying
    (a) A health care provider may deny access to health care information by a patient if the provider reasonably concludes that:
    (1) the disclosure of information may be injurious to the health of the patient;
    (2) knowledge of the health care information could reasonably be expected to lead to the patient's identification of an individual who provided the information in confidence and under circumstances in which confidentiality was appropriate;
    (3) knowledge of the health care information could reasonably be expected to endanger the life of any individual;
    (4) the information was compiled and is used solely for litigation, quality assurance, peer review or administrative purposes; or
    (5) the health care information is otherwise prohibited by law.
38. §4-101 Uniform Health Care Information Act, *supra,* note 8.
39. §4-102 Uniform Health Care Information Act, *supra,* note 8.
40. §§ 8-101,8-102, 8-103, Uniform Health Care Information Act, *supra,* note 8.
41. *Supra,* note 10; *See also* Health Privacy and Confidentiality Recommendations (National Committee on Vital and Health Statistics, Washington, D.C. June 25, 1997).
42. *For examples see* Wn. Rev. Code 70.02.080 (1993); Fla. Stat. Ann. §455.241 (1985); Or. Rev. Stat. Ch.192 §525 (1993); Nev. Rev. Stat. Ch. 629, §061 (1983); N.Y.M.H.L §33.16 (1988).
43. *See State v. Bickman,* 414 N.E. 2d 37 (1980); *Stregel v. Tofane,* 399 N.Y.S. 2d 584 (1977); *Pierce v. Penman,* 515 A. 2d 948 (1986).
44. *See Gotkin v. Miller,* 379 F.Supp. 859 (E.D.N.Y. 1974); *Cynthia B.v. New Rochelle Hosp. Medical Center,* 458 N.E. 2d 363 (1983).
45. *Penman, supra,* note 43.
46. Wall Street Journal/ABC poll Sept 16, 1999, quoted in *Standards for Privacy of Individually Identifiable Health Information: Proposed Rule,* 64 Federal Register 59917 at 59919 (Nov 3, 1999).
47. Alan Westin, *Computers, Health Records and Patient's Rights* (1976).
48. Barefoot, *Enacting a Health Information Confidentiality Law: Can Congress Beat the Deadline?* 77 N. C. Law Rev. 283 (1998).
49. 429 U.S. 589 (1977); *See also U.S. v. Miller,* 425 U.S. 435 (1976).

50. Held:
 1. The patient-identification requirement is a reasonable exercise of the State's broad police powers, and the District Court's finding that the necessity for the requirement had not been proved is not a sufficient reason for holding the statute unconstitutional. Pp. 596-598.
 2. Neither the immediate nor the threatened impact of the patient-identification requirement on either the reputation or the independence of patients for whom Schedule II drugs are medically indicated suffices to constitute an invasion of any right or liberty protected by the Fourteenth Amendment. Pp. 598-604.
    (a) The possibility that a physician or pharmacist may voluntarily reveal information on a prescription form, which existed under prior law, is unrelated to the computerized data bank. Pp. 600-601.
    (b) There is no support in the record or in the experience of the two States that the New York program emulates for assuming that the statute's security provisions will be improperly administered. P. 601.
    (c) The remote possibility that judicial supervision of the evidentiary use of particular items of stored information will not provide adequate protection against unwarranted disclosure is not a sufficient reason for invalidating the entire patient-identification program. Pp.601-602.
    (d) Though it is argued that concern about disclosure may induce patients to refuse needed medication, the 1972 statute does not deprive the public of access to Schedule II drugs, as is clear from the fact that about 100,000 prescriptions for such drugs were filed each month before the District Court's injunction was entered l. Pp. 602-603.
 3. Appellee physicians' contention that the 1972 statute impairs their right to practice medicine free from unwarranted state interference is without merit, whether it refers to the statute's impact on their own procedures, which is no different from the impact of the prior statute, or refers to the patients' concern about disclosure that the Court has rejected (see 2 *(d)*,URA). P. 604. 403 F. Supp. 931, reversed. STEVENS, J., delivered the opinion for a unanimous court. BRENDAN, J., *post,* p. 606, and STEWART, J., *post,* p. 607, filed concurring.
51. *United States v. Westinghouse Electric Corp.,* 638 F. 2d 570 (1980).
52. *Id.* at 578.
53. *See Doe v. Southern PA Transportation Authority,* 72 F. 3d 1133 (1995).
54. AMA Council on Ethical and Judicial Affairs, *Code of Medical Ethics: Current Opinions and Annotations,* §5.05 (1997).
55. Buckner F., *The Uniform Health-Care Information Act: A Physician's Guide to Record and Health Care Information Management,* 5 J. Med. Pract. Mgmt. 207 (1990).
56. *See* §1-101 Uniform Health Care Information Act, *supra* note 8; *see also* Barefoot, *supra* note 48.
57. *Supra* note 8.
58. U.H.C.I.A. §2-101 Disclosure by Health-Care Providers; §2-101 Patient Authorization to Health-Care Provider for Disclosure; §2-103 Patient's Revocation of Authorization for Disclosure; §2-104 Disclosure Without Patient's Authorization; §2-105 Compulsory Service.
59. Montana and Washington.

60. *See Vassilades v. Garfindel's,* 492 A. 2d 580 (1985).
61. *See,* Barefoot, *supra* note 48.
62. *See, Geisberger v. Willuhn,* 390 N.E. 2d 945 (1979).
63. *See, Cobb v. Tinsley,* 243 S.W. 1009 (1922).
64. *See, Massengil v. Yuma County,* 456 P. 2d 376 (1969).
65. *See Whitmire v. Woodbury,* 267 S.E. 2d 783, *rev'd on other grounds,* 271 S.E. 2d 419 (1980).
66. *See, Mikel v. Abrams,* 716 F. 2d 907 (1982).
67. *See* 42 U.S.C.A. §290.
68. *Id.*
69. 42 C.F.R. 2.13(b).
70. *Id.* at §§2.36, 2.37.
71. *Id.* at §2.31.
72. Health Insurance Portability and Accountability Act of 1996, 42 U.S.C.§1320 (emphasis added).
73. Standards for Privacy of Individually Identifiable Health Information, *supra* note 46.
74. *Supra* note 41.
75. South Carolina, Texas, and Vermont.
76. Rule 501, General Rule, Federal Rules of Evidence for United States Courts and Magistrates Effective July 1, 1975 as Amended to September 1, 1991 (West).
77. *See, Tucson Medical Center v. Rowles,* 520 P. 2d 518 (1974).
78. *See, Polsky v. Union Mutual Stock Life Ins. Co.,* 436 N.Y.S. 2d 744, (1981); *See also, Chiasera v. Mutual Ins. Co.,* 422 N Y.S. 2d 341 (1979); *Griffiths v. Metropolitan St. Ry. Co.,* 63 N.E. 808 (1902)
79. *Smith v. Driscoll,* 162 P. 572 (1917).
80. *See,* Fla. Stat. Ann. §90.803(6).
81. Rule 803(6) Federal Rules of Evidence, *supra* note 76.
82. *Id.,* Rule 803(4).
83. *Id,* Rule 804(b)(2).
84. *Id.* Rule 804(b)(3).
85. *See,* van Wingerde et al, *Linking Multiple Heterogenous Data Sources to Practice Guidelines,* 391 A.M.I.A. Annual (1998).
86. *See,* Kapp, *Our Hands are Tied: Legal Tensions and Medical Ethics* (Auburn House, Westport, Conn. 1998).
87. *See,* Evans et al., *Preventing Adverse Drug Events in Hospitalized Patients,* 28 Ann. Pharmacother. 523 (1994).
88. *Id.,* at 523.
89. *See* Buckner F., *The Duty to Inform, Liability to Third Parties and the Duty to Warn,* 100 J. Med. Pract. Mgmt. (1998).
90. Rule 803(6) Federal Rules of Evidence, *supra* note 76.
   (6) **Records of Regularly Conducted Activity.** A memorandum, report, record, or data compilation, *in any form* of acts, events, conditions, opinions or diagnoses, made at or near the time by, or from information transmitted by, a person with knowledge, if kept in the course of a regularly conducted business activity . . .
91. *From* Apgood, *Electronic Evidence,* 53 Washington State Bar News 46, 47 (1999).
92. *See* Rule 34 Federal Rules of Civil Procedure; *See also* Rule 803(6) Federal Rules of Evidence, *supra* note 76.
93. Rule 1001(3) Federal Rules of Evidence, *supra* note 76.
94. *See Bray v. Bi-State Development,* 949 S.W. 2d 93 (1997).

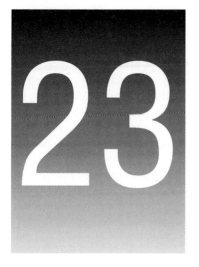

Telephone contact and counseling

THE IMPACT OF THE TELEPHONE ON MEDICAL PRACTICE
DEVELOPMENT OF STRUCTURED TELEPHONE MANAGEMENT
PRINCIPLES OF TELEPHONE MANAGEMENT
ANATOMY OF A TELEPHONE CALL
MEDICAL AND LEGAL IMPLICATIONS OF TELEPHONE MEDICINE
CONCLUSION

THE IMPACT OF THE TELEPHONE ON MEDICAL PRACTICE

The telephone is an integral part of medical practice. Patients naturally turn to the telephone to obtain prompt medical advice. Reliance on the telephone in all phases of medical care is increasing dramatically. Telephone contacts regarding medical concerns are so frequent that procedures used for telephone advice must be closely scrutinized to avoid causing patient dissatisfaction and giving improper advice.

The impact of the telephone on medical practice cannot be denied. The telephone is relied on for prompt access to medical care. Physicians schedule both professional and nonprofessional activities around telephone accessibility. A patient's most immediate access to his or her physician is the telephone. Telephone contacts account for between 11% and 50% of all medical encounters.[1] Another study reported that 12% to 28% of all primary medical care is delivered over the phone, and up to one half of physician-patient telephone contacts result in further evaluation.[2] In 1971, 13% of all patient-care contacts in the United States were reported to be by telephone. A decade later, "among primary care specialties, telephone calls account for 19.4% of all patient encounters in family/general practice, 24.6% in general internal medicine, 28.5% in pediatrics, and 19.6% in obstetrics/gynecology."[3] Although the telephone is used extensively in all primary care specialties, most studies regarding physician-patient telephone contacts are related to pediatric care. During the average pediatrician's day, he or she spends 1 to 2 hours receiving incoming calls seeking medical advice.[4] In a busy primary practice of six physicians, an average of one new phone call is received every 90 seconds.[5] In a 1987 study of Denver and Baltimore pediatricians, approximately 51% of the respondents considered the telephone the most frustrating part of their practice.[6] After-hours phone calls generally are inconvenient, and the sheer volume of calls can be overwhelming.

DEVELOPMENT OF STRUCTURED TELEPHONE MANAGEMENT

Telephone contacts in primary practice run the gamut from requesting care for medical emergencies to handling routine administrative details. Because the volume of calls is large, telephone management is an essential part of every medical practice. Phone calls must be managed so as not to be obtrusive during office hours. Patient telephone contacts must be handled promptly and efficiently, and coverage must be provided at all times when physicians are away from the office.

It is impractical, if not impossible, for a physician to speak to every patient who calls. Delegation of telephone responsibility to nonphysicians occurs whether or not it is planned. Although there is some controversy about whether nurses or other trained personnel should do telephone triage or give advice, it is clear that nonphysician personnel already perform both functions.[7] In many settings the delegation of telephone responsibility to nonphysicians is unstructured. Telephone advice given without procedural parameters encourages assumption of more responsibility by nonphysicians than the physician assumes. Lack of documentation and inappropriate follow-up may occur even when a physician gives advice. In this context it is clear that a structured approach to telephone advice and counseling is required.

Concerns about telephone management began to appear in the literature in the late 1960s and early 1970s. The early literature involved time motion studies and frequency of physician-patient phone contacts. These topics progressed to recognition of the need for training, specialization of

The Editorial Committee updated this chapter. The committee gratefully acknowledges the past contribution of William Wick, M.D., J.D.

personnel, and development of protocols and procedures to handle telephone contacts.

Beginning in the early 1970s and with more emphasis recently, attempts were made to formalize telephone counseling procedures. Systems were developed to allow nonphysician personnel to handle telephone contacts. These systems recognized that a registered nurse or other personnel specifically trained for telephone counseling could provide prompt, accurate advice to meet the patient's needs, allowing more efficient use of the physician's time for direct patient care.[8]

In 1972 the American Academy of Pediatrics in its work, *Standards of Child Health Care,* included a chapter on telephone techniques.[9] The academy said "the handling of telephone calls concerning minor illness is the most urgently felt pressure of pediatric practice and the patient care-taking task most frequently delegated by pediatricians to allied health personnel."[10] Guidelines were developed for handling patient telephone contacts. Physicians were advised to ensure that every pediatric setting formulated its own decision-making rules and standing orders and that a set of written guidelines was available.

A registered nurse, Sally Tripp, was one of the early authors and advocates of guidelines for telephone counseling systems.[11] She found nurses were making health care decisions over the telephone and the time had come to establish guidelines to determine when patient care could be managed via the phone. A system to evaluate the effectiveness of that management was also needed. Tripp focused on the use of the telephone in pediatric practice. The guidelines she developed were to assist the nurse in decision-making concerning whether a child should be seen immediately by a physician or should be seen by the physician but not immediately, whether the physician should talk to the mother, or whether the situation was appropriate for home management.

During the 1970s Dr. Harvey Katz recognized the role of the nurse practitioner in pediatric health care and the need for assessing the quality of telephone care given by nonphysician personnel.[12-14] Comprehensive works in the field of pediatric telephone management by Dr. Jeffrey L. Brown and Dr. Barton Smith appeared in 1980.[15,16] In 1982 Katz published the *Telephone Manual of Pediatric Care.*[17] Katz recommended that pediatricians develop procedures for dealing with patient problems over the telephone. In this context, guidelines were developed for commonly encountered questions and symptoms. The materials were developed in response to a lack of published material on telephone use. This need was particularly evident in pediatrics, where a high volume of patient contact was by telephone. According to Brown, programs for training physicians and nurses either ignored or gave only cursory attention to the principles of screening and treating patients over the phone.[18]

In a 1986 publication, *Management of Pediatric Practice,* the American Academy of Pediatrics observed that the office telephone system was "an integral part of pediatric practice, yet too often it is neglected or left to chance."[19] Organization

of a telephone system that included specialized training, protocols, and supervision was advocated.

In 1990 Scott and Packard authored *Telephone Assessment with Protocols for Nursing Practice* in response to perceived needs in nursing practice.[20] They viewed their work as a tool for nursing management rather than a medical tool for use by nurses. The procedures were designed to be used by experienced nurses in a formalized telephone consultation setting.

Once protocols and systems were developed to handle telephone management, attention shifted to evaluation of the effectiveness of the system and the performance of personnel. Simulations were used to evaluate telephone decision-making by primary care physicians. The hypothesis was that experienced physicians would make correct management decisions more frequently when performing telephone triage. The study concluded that most physicians obtained information sufficient to determine the severity of the illness but that factors other than the type or amount of information obtained could account for deficiencies in telephone management.[21] A recent study of an after-hours pediatric telephone triage system in Denver was analyzed retrospectively. In four years, 107,938 phone calls were managed without adverse clinical outcome.[22] Given the volume of medical care delivered over the telephone, the volume of literature evaluating the success of this form of medical management is surprisingly small.

PRINCIPLES OF TELEPHONE MANAGEMENT

After the medical community acknowledged that patients were managed over the telephone, organized and efficient methods for appropriately handling this aspect of medical practice were needed. Although the physician is the most qualified person to give medical advice, the focus of telephone management has been on procedures for nonphysician personnel. Delegating telephone management allows for more efficient use of the physician's time and provides better access to medical services.

An organized procedure for telephone management separates patient calls related to routine administrative matters from those needing medical assessment. The procedure developed is in essence one of timing, prioritizing, or triage. The person performing the telephone function, whether a physician or nonphysician, determines if the call presents a true emergency; if the patient must be seen immediately, later in the day, or in the near future; if home management is appropriate; or if the caller should be referred elsewhere.

The telephone system is an extension of the physician and the practice. The effectiveness of a practice is often judged by its telephone encounters. Procedures for telephone management must reflect the overall patient care philosophy of the practice. These procedures should provide efficient access to appropriate care, continuity of that care, and the necessary follow-up.

In reality, telephone management is triage. The purpose of a telephone encounter is to assess the need for medical care in terms of immediacy rather than to diagnose and treat. Standard procedures should help decide the immediacy of the need for health care and assist the patient in making health care decisions.

The elements of a telephone management system include the following:

1. Delegation of responsibility to a person specifically designated for the function
2. Standard protocols and guidelines for telephone assessment
3. Specialized training for telephone assessment
4. A system for documentation specifically designed for telephone encounters
5. Proper coverage, supervision, review, and evaluation

Delegation of responsibility

Most procedural systems for telephone management involve delegating the majority of telephone calls to an individual other than a physician. In many settings this person is a nurse or a nurse practitioner. However, some physicians use specially trained, nonnurse personnel in this capacity. Qualifications for the position generally include intelligence, warmth and compassion, a calm personality, and sound judgment. If a person is to be trained for this function, some experience or interest in the area of practice is helpful.

Telephone management requires that the individual involved be a skilled communicator. This skill is often a product of personality and requires a "people orientation." Any telephone encounter has the usual requirements of any interpersonal contact. The person with telephone responsibility must be polite, interested, and businesslike and must speak clearly and distinctly.

Standard protocols and guidelines for telephone assessment

Protocols have been developed for use in telephone encounters to provide guidelines for assessing callers and assisting in their management. A number of manuals have been developed for telephone counseling and triage.[23-26] Each practice should formulate its own decision-making guidelines and rules, and the persons responsible for telephone assessment should be familiar with these guidelines. Protocols should provide suggestions for patient teaching and self-evaluation when home management is elected. These protocols will aid in providing consistent patient care and appropriate prioritizing. However, protocols cannot teach assessment skills and do not diagnose. They simply provide a means to assess problems and direct appropriate care.

Although the telephone encounter has been described as a triage or "sorting out," it is more than that. Telephone assessment involves an exercise in independent and informed judgment. Not all patients who are ill need to see a physician. In many cases all the patient needs is assurance and directions for personal assessment.

The primary purpose of a telephone encounter is to identify the immediacy of the patient's need. Telephone decision-making either by a physician, nurse, or other trained telephone counselor attempts to determine the appropriate disposition of the problem. Calls requesting health care advice are separated by degree of urgency. Telephone management personnel must be able to differentiate among severe life-threatening emergencies, in which the patient should be seen immediately; dangerous conditions, in which the person can be transported to an office or emergency room within 20 to 30 minutes; and those situations that can be handled either by immediate appointment, appointment on the same day, or a future appointment. Guidelines and protocols are designed to assist the telephone manager in identifying the urgency of each situation.

Specialized training for telephone assessment

Effective telephone systems incorporate training programs to familiarize personnel with the telephone system, techniques for telephone management, and the protocols and guidelines. Such training is required before the person is placed in the position and should be an ongoing part of any telephone management system. Training methods include a review of protocols and manuals, formal lectures, role-playing, monitoring actual patient contacts, and enactment of troublesome situations.

In addition to the professional education generally required of all health care personnel, ongoing training and evaluation specifically directed toward telephone management must be part of any telephone system.

A system of documentation specifically for telephone encounters

Documentation of the telephone encounter is essential. The method of documenting telephone contacts is no different from the documentation required for any other medical assessment. Entries should be made in ink, errors noted as such, late entries designated, and significant information noted. An adequate medical record requires that a history be obtained and recorded and the disposition specified. Entries should be made immediately after the encounter.

The form of document used for the telephone encounter must be adapted to the needs of the practice. In some cases entries are made in a telephone logbook. Other practices use a form with self-adhesive backing. A specialized telephone encounter notepad that can be carried in a lab coat pocket allows for easier reporting.

The reasons for documenting the telephone encounter are obvious. Information conveyed during a phone conversation may be essential to future medical care. If additional information needs to be conveyed or if instructions need to be modified, this information is available. Without a record of the encounter, the appropriateness of the care cannot be evaluated and the effectiveness of the system cannot be assessed.

Procedures for coverage, supervision, review, and evaluation

Every telephone management system that delegates calls to nonphysician personnel requires physician availability. Telephone management systems must ensure that someone is available to take calls at all times. A physician also must be available or on call continuously. In addition, physician supervision in terms of review and follow-up is essential.

Although protocols provide assistance in proper management, certain calls invariably must be referred to a physician. These situations include an emergency call, a nonemergency call that the patient feels is an emergency, and any time the patient asks to speak to a physician.

Every telephone system should be monitored on a regular basis. It has been recommended that a physician should review the charts related to telephone dispositions at least twice a day, and calls should be reviewed with the nurse or nurses handling them before they go off duty.[27] The frequency of review is best determined by the requirements of the individual practice, the personnel involved, and the degree of responsibility that has been delegated, but every telephone system staffed by nonphysician personnel must have a system for physician review.

ANATOMY OF A TELEPHONE CALL

The basic anatomy of a telephone call is as follows:
1. Identification
2. History and assessment
3. Disposition

The conversation usually begins with a greeting and identification of the caller and the person receiving the call. The next step is an inquiry about the reason for the call and an offer of help.

Taking a history and obtaining relevant information are obviously more difficult over the telephone than in face-to-face encounters. Visual clues and physical findings are absent. During the telephone encounter, the person providing telephone support must rely on tone and expression, how messages are phrased, and the choice of words. Information must be obtained to make an appropriate assessment and recommendation. Protocols are used after sufficient information is obtained about the problem to direct the focus of the inquiry. Major concerns and symptoms should be recorded. The telephone counselor must be alert to situations in which the first reason given for the call may not be suggestive of the ultimate problem.

Telephone responsibility for nonnurse medical assistants is to provide access to care rather than treatment. Therefore diagnosis is not the goal. The patient must join in and assist the decision-making process. The major goal of the nonphysician is to assist the caller in the decision-making. The initial approach is open ended in an attempt to determine the general reason for the call. When the general reason for the call has been ascertained, questions can be asked to focus the inquiry. These questions should lead the caller to elaborate on significant points. Silence may also encourage the caller to elaborate.

Based on the information received, a mutual decision should be reached on how to proceed. A record must be made of the instructions given. If information was given from a reference source, it should be noted. When home care is suggested, instructions should be given and reviewed with the caller to ensure that the instructions are understood. The caller must be advised of what to look for, why it is significant, and that any change in circumstances should be reported immediately. It has also been recommended that every phone call have an alternate solution, for example, a directive that there be a call back if the symptoms do not improve within a specified period.[28]

MEDICAL AND LEGAL IMPLICATIONS OF TELEPHONE MEDICINE
Special concerns with telephone encounters

As soon as a medical practice gives advice and counseling over the telephone, a legal duty to the patient arises. Medicolegal aspects of patient care extend to advice given over the telephone and provide yet another avenue of potential liability. Procedures for telephone practice have been developed in an effort to ensure that patients are handled appropriately and in a way that will be scrutinized favorably when challenged in court.

Like any other aspect of medical practice, the telephone encounter may provide the basis for a malpractice claim. To be liable for action taken in a telephone encounter, the health care provider must violate the standard of care. The standard of care is generally considered to be the degree of care, skill, and judgment usually exercised by the average practitioner in the circumstances presented. The same standard, that of average care, applies to advice given in person or over the telephone.

The difficulty of telephone assessment cannot be denied. The telephone encounter has been described as assessing a patient with your eyes closed and hands tied. There are health care providers who advise against telephone assessment. If no advice is given, no duty arises.[29]

The board of directors of the Emergency Nurses Association (ENA) approved the following position statement on telephone advice on April 27, 1991:

ENA believes that, in the best interest of the patient, the nurse should not render opinions regarding diagnosis or treatment by the telephone. The emergency nurse should inform the person calling that conditions cannot be diagnosed by telephone and that the caller should either come to the emergency department for examination and treatment or see a private physician or health care provider. In some cases, it may be necessary for the nurse to assess the urgency of the situation and determine if it is life threatening. In life-threatening situations, it may be appropriate for the nurse to teach cardiopulmonary resuscitation (CPR) or other life-saving measures by phone. In these situations, emergency medical services should be assessed. The nurse should carefully document each conversation.

ENA recognizes that some institutions have developed sophisticated telephone triage programs. These programs should be predicated on clearly defined protocols, with medical direction by experienced, professional emergency staff members. Staff members should have specialized education in triage, telephone assessment, legal aspects and limits, and capabilities of the service. A quality assurance program is essential to ensure quality control of the telephone triage program.[30]

Although controversy exists as to whether telephone advice should be given, studies evaluating telephone care have generally demonstrated that the systems function well. As mentioned earlier, the Denver study showed that in four years 107,938 cases were successfully managed without an adverse clinical outcome.[31] Evaluation of primary care physicians indicated that inadequate telephone triage may be related to factors other than type or amount of information obtained.[32] The inability to obtain adequate information by telephone may correlate with an inability to elicit information with the patient present.

Three basic rules should be followed in telephone contacts:
1. If there is any doubt about the seriousness of the condition, a physician should see the patient.
2. If more than one phone call is received about one individual on the same day, a physician should see the patient.
3. If the patient requests an examination, a physician should examine the patient.

As long as patients contact physicians by telephone, advice will be given, and whenever assessments are made that require judgment, the potential exists for a claim that the judgment is in error. In telephone encounters, like all other aspects of medical care, judgments will be required. Organized procedures, protocols, training, and an evaluation system can reduce the potential for claims but cannot eliminate them. Exposure to liability for telephone encounters is no different from other aspects of medical practice, and the potential for liability does not justify abandoning this form of access to health care.

Recording phone calls

In some multispecialty clinics, all telephone encounters are tape recorded to document patient contacts. Although this recording may be helpful to the practice, it may not be legally useful or practical. In some jurisdictions, recorded telephone calls are inadmissible unless the caller is specifically aware that the telephone conversation is being recorded. For example, Wisconsin has a statute that provides that evidence obtained from recording a telephone conversation is "totally inadmissible in civil actions unless the person is informed that the conversation is being recorded and that it may be used in court."[33] As a practical matter, most medical practitioners do not wish to provide this type of information to their patients. In some jurisdictions a recorded telephone encounter may not be admissible in the defense of a medical negligence claim.

Inquiry about medication

Questions about medications present a potential for liability. Health care providers may provide advice about medications commensurate with their training. A physician can give directions concerning the use of prescription medications. Registered nurses cannot prescribe but can engage in teaching about the appropriate use of medications.[34] A consistent policy for handling questions related to medications should be part of any telephone management system.

Cases involving telephone encounters

Few appellate court decisions deal specifically with the issue of whether telephone management has met the standard of care. Reported cases have considered legal issues raised in the context of telephone management. There are decisions that consider whether a telephone contact is sufficient to create the physician-patient relationship necessary for liability and whether telephone calls extend the statute of limitations. A telephone encounter may determine the place of trial. Improper telephone advice may provide the factual basis on which liability is predicated.

A telephone call for the purpose of initiating treatment may be sufficient to create a physician-patient relationship. Most courts dealing with the issue have decided that telephone advice, depending on the content of the conversation, may create such a relationship. A telephone call made merely to schedule an appointment with a health care provider does not itself establish a physician-patient relationship where there is no ongoing relationship and no medical advice is sought.[35]

A physician's refusal to see a patient in response to a late-night phone call may not create a physician-patient relationship sufficient to provide the basis for liability. In *Clanton v. VonHamm* the patient went to a hospital emergency room complaining of back pain, was examined by a physician, and was released.[36] Later, the patient called the physician at home. After listening to the symptoms, the physician, according to the plaintiff's allegations, refused to see her, told her it was too late, and that she should see him in the morning. The plaintiff's back condition resulted in paraplegia. The issue was whether the telephone conversation created a physician-patient relationship. The plaintiff interpreted her conversation with the physician as a "total refusal" of her efforts to secure (the physician's) medical services. The plaintiff did not believe the physician took her case, did not rely on any medical advice, and was not dissuaded from seeking medical attention as a result of anything the physician said. In denying liability, the court concluded that a physician-patient relationship did not arise from the phone call.

Consultation on a treatment plan over the phone may be sufficient to allow the jury to consider whether a physician-patient relationship exists. A medical malpractice action was initiated to recover damages for severe birth injuries suffered by the infant plaintiff.[37] The defendant, an obstetrician/gynecologist, rendered prenatal care to the plaintiff but did not attend the delivery. The mother was admitted to the hospital after her membranes ruptured. She remained in the hospital for two days. Labor did not progress, and she was discharged. The plaintiff later contacted the defendant physician, who advised her to return to the hospital. He then called the attending physician and made recommendations for treatment, including induction of labor. The plaintiffs based their allegations of medical negligence on the telephone recommendations. The court concluded there was at least a question of fact on the negligence issue in light of the defendant's participation in the treatment through the telephone recommendations.

Factual disputes may relate to medical advice given over the telephone. In *Howat v. Passaretti* an action was commenced by the deceased's estate seeking damages for improper treatment of a fractured left leg.[38] The defendant orthopedic surgeon made the diagnosis. Unfortunately, the patient died from massive pulmonary emboli. The facts concerning phone calls to the defendant physician's office were disputed. There was evidence that the deceased made two calls and was told each time by the physician's receptionist to keep his leg elevated, take aspirin, and keep his next appointment. The defendant denied receiving the calls and denied that any of his employees gave such advice.

The plaintiff's expert witness testified that, if the calls were made, the patient should have been told to come in for examination. The receptionist had no recollection of any contact with the decedent, and there were no telephone message slips regarding the decedent's calls. The jury found for the health care provider, and the verdict was sustained on appeal.

A claim of medical malpractice for loss of a testicle was allegedly the result of improper telephone advice.[39] The patient contacted the physician and complained of testicular and abdominal pain. The patient's pain persisted, and he had a number of telephone contacts with the defendant physician. The physician assumed the patient had recurring subacute prostatitis. It was subsequently discovered that the patient had an infarcted testicle caused by torsion. The plaintiff's claim presented an issue of fact for the jury on whether it was negligent to provide treatment over the telephone without insisting on a physical examination.

Another factual dispute concerning information given over the phone arose in an emergency room setting.[40] The patient was brought to the emergency room after an automobile accident. The hospital had no residents or interns. Physicians voluntarily made themselves available on a rotating basis to treat patients in the emergency room.

After the emergency room nurse telephoned the physician on call, it was his duty to diagnose the patient's condition, prescribe treatment, and determine whether to admit the patient to the hospital. As frequently happens, the nurse and the physician disputed the frequency of the telephone contacts and the information conveyed. The patient died, and the death was attributed to traumatic shock. The physician on call did not come to the emergency room to examine the patient, stating that he relied on information given by the nurse over the phone. There was no dispute that the physician was told that the patient had been in an accident and had sustained more than a slight or insignificant injury. The conflicting testimony about the phone call may have led to the jury verdict in favor of the patient.

In determining whether actions are barred by the statute of limitations, courts have considered telephone calls. Although the plaintiff in one case did not have a firm appointment for future treatment when she left the hospital, the patient's telephone call to arrange a further appointment indicated a continuous relationship necessary to extend the statute of limitations.[41]

In another case a telephone call to a physician requesting a release letter that involved no advice or consultation did not create an issue as to whether or not the statute of limitations was extended.

Factors considered in determining whether treatment ceases include the following[42]:

1. Whether there is a relationship between the patient and physician with regard to the condition
2. Whether the physician is attending and examining the patient
3. Whether there is something more to be done

Telephone consultations may constitute proof of a continuing physician-patient relationship.[43]

Whether the statute of limitations is extended depends on the statutory language, which can vary from jurisdiction to jurisdiction. In some states the statute of limitations does not begin to run until the end of a continuing course of treatment. A telephone call may be considered part of the continuing treatment or may provide evidence of a continuing physician-patient relationship, which extends the statute.

A telephone call also may create an issue regarding the place of trial. Advice given in a telephone call made from the patient's home in one county to the health care provider in another county provided the basis for a malpractice claim. The plaintiffs initiated the action in the county where they placed the call and where they received the advice. The court concluded that the proper venue was in the county where the caller received the advice.[44]

At least one unreported case focused directly on the procedural system for telephone advice given by a registered nurse working in a pediatric group practice. A trained pediatric nurse counselor gave the advice. The counseling system had been in existence for two years before the incident that gave rise to the medical negligence action. The suit was brought 10 years after the incident. The nurse counseling system included specialized training, a training manual, and protocols and guidelines. The nurses worked closely with the pediatricians, who were available for consultation if questions arose and for appointments if examinations were necessary.

The case involved a claim of misdiagnosis of *Haemophilus influenzae* type B meningitis. A 27-month-old girl came to her pediatrician with a temperature of 104° F. She was diagnosed as having the flu, and aspirin was prescribed. The child did not improve, and her parents called the pediatric office 48 hours after her initial evaluation. The testimony differed as to the telephone encounter. The nurse felt it was acceptable for the parents to observe the child and call the next morning if there was no improvement. The log entry did not document the offer of an appointment or the parents' refusal. The clinic was not contacted the next morning, but a day later (four days after the original visit and two days after the telephone call) the child's condition worsened. The parents contacted the on-call physician, who suspected meningitis and directed the parents to take their daughter to the local hospital where a lumbar puncture confirmed the diagnosis.

The child responded to antibiotic therapy but sustained significant neurological sequelae, including profound deafness, mental retardation, right-sided hemiparesis, poor speech, and retarded language development. The jury found the clinic negligent and awarded $2.5 million in damages.

From a survey of the jurors, it was learned that the liability finding was based not on the fact that advice was given over the telephone but on the nurse's failure to follow the practice's established guidelines and protocols. The jury felt it was reasonable and appropriate to give medical advice over the telephone. They were not critical of the organization and structure of the nurse counseling system. The jurors responding to the inquiry felt that people seeking advice from a medical clinic did not always need to speak to a physician and that it is appropriate for a person with a nursing background to perform telephone counseling. The criticisms offered by the jurors are those frequently heard in medical negligence litigation: The assessment was inadequate, and the documentation needed improvement.[45]

CONCLUSION

From the standpoint of potential liability, telephone counseling systems do not differ significantly from other aspects of medical practice. An organized procedure must be adopted and implemented by well-trained and skilled personnel. Identification of potential high-risk problems can serve as "red flags" for the phone counselor. Certain circumstances are more likely to lead to serious adverse outcomes. These tend to be life-threatening diseases that are difficult to diagnose at early stages because of nonspecific symptoms. These potential cases must be identified so that phone counselors can be trained to be aware of them and respond appropriately.

A number of measures can be taken to improve the quality of telephone encounters and reduce liability. All medically relevant telephone encounters must be documented. Specific personnel must be designated and trained for the function. Guidelines and procedures must be adopted. High-risk situations must be identified and discussed. The system needs a low threshold for examination and appointment. When nonphysician personnel are performing the telephone counseling function, physicians must be available for supervision, consultation, and examination. The system must provide a procedure for evaluation of quality and service, as well as follow-up.

Finally, it has been recognized for more than two decades that medical advice is given over the telephone. In that time it also has been recognized that nonphysician personnel can be specifically trained to deal successfully with telephone evaluation and management. In the same period, litigation involving medical assessment and evaluation has skyrocketed. As long as health care providers are required to make judgments over the telephone, lawsuits are likely to follow. However, no data are available to suggest that telephone management emerged as an area of greater medicolegal concern than any other area of practice.

ENDNOTES

1. P.D. Sloane et al., *Physician Decision-Making Over the Telephone*, 20 J. Family Pract. 279 (1985).
2. S.Z. Yanovski et al., *Telephone Triage by Primary Care Physicians*, 89 Pediatrics 701 (Apr 1992).
3. S.E. Radecki et al., *Telephone Management by Primary Care Physicians*, 27 Med. Care 817 (Aug 1989).
4. A.B. Bergman et al., *Time Motion Study of Practicing Pediatrics*, 38 Pediatrics 254 (1966).
5. H.P. Katz, *Telephone Manual of Pediatric Care* (Slack, New York 1982).
6. P. Fosarelli & B. Schmitt, *Telephone Dissatisfaction in Pediatric Practice: Baltimore and Denver*, 80 Pediatrics 28-31 (1987).
7. J.M. Dunn, *Warning: Giving Telephone Advice Is Hazardous to Your Professional Health*, Nursing 40-41 (Aug 1985).
8. J. Strain & J. Miller, *The Preparation, Utilization, and Evaluation of a Registered Nurse Trained to Give Telephone Advice in Private Pediatric Office*, 47 Pediatrics 1051-1056 (1971).
9. Committee on Standards of Child Health Care, *Telephone Techniques in Pediatric Practice*, in *Standards of Child Health Care* (2d ed., American Academy of Pediatrics, Evanston, Ill. 1972).
10. *Id.*
11. S. Tripp, *Telephone Techniques in Pediatric Practice*, 71 Am. J. Nursing 1722-1724 (1971).
12. H.P. Katz et al., *Quality of Telephone Care: Assessment of a System Utilizing Non-Physician Personnel*, 68 Am. J. Public Health 31-37 (1978).
13. H.P. Katz, *Telephone Utilization in a Prepaid Multispecialty Group Practice*. Abstract presented at Eleventh Annual Meeting, Ambulatory Pediatric Association, 42 (1971).
14. H.P. Katz et al., *Night Call—An Extended Role for the Nurse Practitioner*. Abstract presented at Fourteenth Annual Meeting, Ambulatory Pediatric Association 70 (1974).
15. J.L. Brown, *Telephone Medicine: A Practical Guide to Pediatric Telephone Advice* (Mosby, St Louis 1980).
16. B.D. Schmitt, *Pediatric Telephone Advice: Guidelines for the Health Care Provider on Telephone Triage and Office Management of Common Childhood Symptoms* (Little, Brown and Company, Boston 1980).
17. *Supra* note 5.
18. J.L. Brown, *Pediatric Telephone Medicine: Principles, Triage and Advice* vii (J.B. Lippincott, Philadelphia 1989).
19. E.J. Saltzman & D.W. Shea, *Management of Pediatric Practice* 28 (American Academy of Pediatrics, Evanston, Ill. 1986).
20. M.P. Scott & K.P. Packard, *Telephone Assessment with Protocols for Nursing Practice* (W.B. Saunders, Philadelphia 1990).
21. *Supra* note 2, at 705.
22. S.R. Poole et al *After Hours Telephone Coverage: The Application of an Area-Wide Telephone Triage and Advice System for Pediatric Practices*, 92 Pediatrics 670 (Nov 1993).

23. J.L. Brown, *Pediatric Telephone Medicine: Principles, Triage, and Advice* (J.B. Lippincott, Philadelphia 1989).
24. *Supra* note 16.
25. H.P. Katz, *Telephone Medicine Triage and Training: A Handbook for Primary Health Care Professionals* 4 (Slack, New York, 1990).
26. *Supra* note 20.
27. *Supra* note 16, at 11.
28. *Supra* note 20, at 11.
29. *Supra* note 7, at 40.
30. Emergency Nurses Association, *Position Statement: Telephone Advice,* 17 J. Emergency Nursing 52A (Oct 1991).
31. *Supra* note 22.
32. *Supra* note 2.
33. Wis. Stat. § 885.365.
34. *Supra* note 20, at 9.

35. *Weaver v. Univ. of Michigan Board of Regents,* 506 N.W. 2d 264 (Mich. App. 1993).
36. *Clanton v. VonHaam,* 177 Ga. App. 694, 340 S.E. 2d 627 (1986).
37. *DeJesus By Negron v. Parkchester General,* 161 A.D. 2d 465, 555 N.Y.S. 2d 374 (1990).
38. *Howat v. Passaretti,* 11 Conn. App. 518, 528 A. 2d 834 (1987).
39. *Craft v. Wilcox,* 180 Ga. App. 372, 348 S.E. 2d 894 (1986).
40. *Thomas v. Corso,* 265 Md. 84, 288 A. 2d 379 (1972).
41. *Ward v. Kaufman,* 120 A.D. 2d 929, 502 N.Y.S. 2d 883 (1986).
42. *Giles v. Sanford Memorial Hosp. & Nursing Home,* 371 N.W. 2d 635 (Minn. App. 1985).
43. *Grondahl v. Bulluck,* 318 N.W. 2d 240 (Minn. App. 1982).
44. *Anthony v. Forgrave,* 337 N.W. 2d 546 (Mich. App. 1983).
45. K.P. Katz & W. Wick, *Malpractice, Meningitis, and the Telephone,* 20 Pediatric Annals 85-89 (1991).

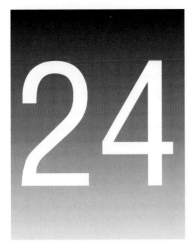

Ethics and bioethics

JOHN R. CARLISLE, M.D., LL.B., F.C.L.M.

TRUTH TELLING
THE PRINCIPLES OF BIOMEDICAL ETHICS
AUTONOMY
BENEFICENCE (AND ITS COUNTERPART, NONMALFEASANCE)
JUSTICE

It may seem strange to some that there is a chapter touching on bioethics in a textbook of legal medicine. Many physician readers might think that the practice of law has little to do with ethics, and the legal readers might be forgiven for failing to perceive much effect of ethical discourse in contemporary medical practice. Both these viewpoints are unfair, and it is consistent with the role and mission of the American College of Legal Medicine (ACLM) to show how ethical discourse has a significant influence on the interface between law and medicine.

At their simplest, both law and medicine, when practiced at their best, seek to do what is right and good, and ethics helps both disciplines better define and ultimately achieve that objective. The contemporary construction of bioethics was first well formulated in the United States in the mid 1970s by the statement of the four principles of bioethics elucidated by Beauchamp and Childress.[1] These principles, which are intended to guide the resolution of all ethical dilemmas in biomedicine, have become at once the mantra of ethicists and the generally accepted guiding principles for all bioethical discourse. They are as follows:

1. Autonomy of the person
2. Beneficence
3. Nonmalfeasance (which some see as an element of beneficence)
4. Justice

With these goals to guide personal morality, directing as it does all aspects of professional behavior, the performance of physicians, attorneys, and medicolegal specialists will generally tend toward the good and urge others to do so as well.

There is considerable need for ethical thought in the twenty-first century as the practice of both medicine and law tends more and more to regard commercial concerns as an appropriate if not a principal concern. As a result, professionals training for practice in these fields should certainly be given a basis for understanding ethical issues and generating ethical discourse in their medical and law schools so that an effective balance between commercial concerns and moral principles may suffuse medicolegal problem solving. It has been widely argued that the resurgent feeling of need for ethical evaluation has resulted from the rapid progression of medical technologies in various fields, making it technically possible to do so many things that previously were not considered because they could not be done. The thesis is that because we can do so many more things, we are ever more impelled to ask ourselves whether we ought to do those things. Although clearly those issues have been involved in the needed resurgence of ethical discourse, in the twenty-first century different and perhaps even more profound changes appeared in our society and in the way we delivered health and legal services. These changes have worked even more strongly to bring ethical issues into relevance. Certainly many of the issues posed by the exponential growth of "managed care" involve intense ethical concerns and have prompted a resurgence of interest in the subject.

In addition the rise in general levels of education and the broad sweeping prominence of concepts of autonomy have driven the idea of benevolent paternalism, which in the past had been a large part of the ethos of both law and medicine, into the background. The desire, in fact the demand, of patients, families, and clients to understand all of the alternatives and to make meaningful choices whether or not they are considered wise by professional advisors has forced physicians and attorneys to think in ever more ethically oriented terms about what they tell people, what they counsel them about, the alternatives they put to them, and the way in which they interact with patients' choices. As with any change, there is some resistance within the professions, but many believe that overall these changes in attitude will be a great advantage to the professions, their patients and clients, and society in general.

Evermore physicians and attorneys will need to concern themselves as much with what ought to be as with what could be, and it is hoped that, together with colleagues in other interested disciplines, they will be equipped to engage in an ethical discourse that will effectively inform and guide those deliberations.

In recognition of the increasing importance of ethical guidance in medical and medicolegal practice, many organizations interested in those fields publish codes of ethics and ethical opinions designed to assist professionals in considering bioethical issues. Guidance is offered by the American Medical Association's Ethical Code and supplanted by the published opinions of the Council on Judicial and Ethical Affairs. The Canadian Medical Association has promulgated a new Code of Ethics following up on a several-year study by its Committee on Ethics. These general guidelines are supplanted by ethical codes provided by a number of medical, medicolegal, and legal societies. The ACLM recently adopted its own Code of Ethics for medicolegal practice, which it is hoped will be of assistance at the interface of law and medicine. In addition there are international codes, such as the Declaration of Geneva, the International Code of Medical Ethics, the Declaration of Tokyo, the Declaration of Oslo, and the Declaration of Helsinki. In their latest revised editions, many of the codes provide additional guidance to supplement traditional medical texts, such as the Oath of Hippocrates. A number of governmental agencies and research funding bodies also have devised and made available ethical guidelines that will be helpful.

TRUTH TELLING

As previously indicated, there is much in the obligation between a physician and patient that is like the fiduciary relationship with which attorneys are familiar. The imbalance of power between the physician and the patient dictates that society must hold the physician to owe the highest duty of fidelity, honesty, and lack of self-interest to his or her patient. The physician must tell the patient the truth, the whole truth, and nothing but the truth and must act at all times in the best interests of the patient, forsaking any personal interest that conflicts with that of the patient. He or she must not deal secretly with others who are contrary in interest to the patient and must at any time reasonably account to the patient for his or her activity on their behalf. Physicians' duties related to confidentiality and conflict of interest arise from this fiduciary relationship.

What then should be the obligation of the physician when he or she knows that a serious mistake has been made in the patient's treatment? One might think that it would be the clear obligation of the physician to disclose any error made, to assist the patient as much as possible to recover from that error, and to seek any recompense to which he or she might be entitled. Indeed most learned professions, including the law, recognize such obligations in their ethical codes and guidelines. It is interesting and somewhat regrettable, however, that the medical profession by and large does not recognize this obligation and certainly does not in the large part practice as if it were recognized. The culture

of blaming, which is part of medical training; the litigious nature of the medicolegal field; and physicians' abhorrence of the idea that they could be responsible through simple human error for adverse outcomes suffered by patients make physicians reluctant to discuss errors and certainly reluctant to disclose them. The recently published study from the Institute of Medicine, edited by Linda Kohn, Janet Corrigan, and Molla Donaldson,[2] discusses this phenomenon at length and points out how far the medical profession has to go in recognizing and dealing with error and in prescribing and fostering open communications with patients and their families when error occurs.

Generally it is the burden of learned professions to spend time and considerable effort assisting patients in understanding complex and unfamiliar concepts (e.g., during the process of obtaining informed consent and directions for action). As physicians continually improve their skills and attitudes in this aspect of their practices, it would serve them well to consider how those same skills might be applicable to honest communication with patients and families when adverse outcomes occur. If physicians truly believe themselves to be obligated to act as advocates for their patients in the health care system and if the profession wishes to retain the good reputation for honesty and skill and the public trust that it thereby enjoys, this issue should certainly be on the front burner of professional discussion in the next few years. Without pointing any fingers from a professional corner that is far from entirely blameless, attorneys and ethicists may be able to help in this consideration and should make every effort to do so.

Telling the truth surely must be one of the principal hallmarks of all professional callings, particularly in the field of legal medicine. All trainees in that field should recognize this fact and should work through the complicated discussions that surround this seemingly simple concept. Competence to deal with such issues should be seen as a prerequisite for entering independent professional practice.

The fiduciary nature of the relationship between physician and patient represents that fundamental trust that is the essence of the interaction between physicians and the community. It is the basic reason that people trust physicians. Much in the rest of this book describes the legal result of the outrage people exhibit when they feel that their trust has been betrayed, and this backlash serves as evidence of a basic public expectation that physicians will honor that ethical trust. In an era when so many influences and so much money seek to draw the physician's loyalty to agendas other than those of the patient, there is a growing need for frank discussion among physicians, attorneys, and social policymakers as to what these expectations are and should be.

For physicians, the trust between them and their patients is fundamental to patients seeking care and to their compliance during the provision of care. For the medical profession, the settling of public expectations when moves are afoot to divide physicians' loyalties in the health care system is essential, and to that end, considerable public discussion and ethical discourse must happen.

THE PRINCIPLES OF BIOMEDICAL ETHICS

The basic principles set out and elucidated in ethical codes serve to guide decision-making. They are often individually imprecise or indecisive and may even be in conflict, and thus ethical discourse serves to analyze and determine the best approach to the good in individual cases and factual situations. The study of ethics thus involves the development of facility in ethical discourse, mostly through the study of worked case examples rather than as a general philosophical discussion. It is perhaps for this reason that bioethical analysis has become so helpful and popular in the medicolegal context, mirroring in its methods as it does the way in which the substantive elements of the medical and legal disciplines are generally analyzed.

The classic sources of medical ethics were in the continental line of humanist philosophy, which had as its goal to seek rules capable of universality. Modern examples of this line of thought are the Declarations of the World Medical Association and the World Health Organization, arising from the Universal Declaration of Human Rights of 1948. This set of fundamental principles is rooted in an analysis of the evils of World War II and is declared to be of fundamental and universal applicability. The principles are equality among human beings, protection of individual liberties, respect for the dignity of all persons, and privacy. The more modern formulation of fundamental principles has been largely adopted for bioethical discourse and considers autonomy, beneficence, nonmalfeasance, and justice, although many would consider nonmalfeasance a part of beneficence and some would add compassion.

AUTONOMY

The word *autonomy* is derived from the Greek *auto nomos,* or self-rule, and involves in essence the idea of individual free choice or what citizens of Western democracies often call *freedom* or *liberty.* In the bioethical sense the concept is that physicians and attorneys have an obligation to respect the free choice of the patient or client and more than that to facilitate in every reasonably possible way the making of such a free choice by each client or patient. In medical terms the concept is that the patient should control what happens to him or her in a medical sense by the exercise of free will and free choice. As early as 1914, Justice Cordozo pronounced the most famous and lasting statement of this principle when he wrote, "Every human being of adult years and sound mind has a right to determine what shall be done with his own body."[3]

Western societies have put a high value on free choice and liberty, and thus respect for even foolish or eccentric decisions is ultimately required because of the perception that the sort of society that does not require respect for autonomy is profoundly unacceptable. In practical terms, relating to medical encounters, a patient is often not in a position without the assistance of the physician to marshal enough information about the choice to be made that his or her unassisted preference could be considered genuinely autonomous. Thus for physicians and patients the concept of autonomy resolves itself into the patient's right to receive information sufficient to allow a reasonable person to make an intelligent decision and the patient's right to make a decision as to whether to accept or refuse the recommended medical treatment. From this practical interpretation of the importance of autonomy arise our legal rules relating to informed consent and what has come to be called *informed refusal.* This is but one example of how law takes ethical discourse and makes it into a practical requirement for everyone involved. An understanding of the ethical analysis of autonomy makes it easier to understand why informed consent is required and easier to enter into a legal debate about what the elements of that consent should be and how the law should characterize and implement the requirement.

Law is mostly about limits on autonomy, for clearly autonomy is limited. Whereas each individual should be free to make autonomous decisions about issues that affect only his or her own rights and interests, there must be limits on purely autonomous decision-making when the rights and interests of others are affected. To use a popular phrase, "Your rights end where my nose begins." Many of the issues that arise from "hard times" in medicine and the need to consider prioritizing and rationing available medical services are about the proper limits on autonomous decision-making, and this is discussed in the following section.

Wishes

In medicine, encounters between physicians and patients in which treatment recommendations would ordinarily be made often occur in circumstances in which the patient is not, at the time of treatment, able to express his or her wishes or exercise the right of autonomy. Increasingly in today's society, patients are able to foresee that there may be a time later in life when they are in a situation in which they wish to influence the decisions about their care but are unable to articulate their wishes at the time. Contemporary thought dictates that if wishes were previously expressed and are known to those recommending treatment, the previously expressed wishes ought to be respected as the best available indicator of the patient's autonomous choice. Previous wishes also must be interpreted carefully, and an attempt should be made to understand how those wishes might apply to current circumstances that significantly differ from what the patient might have been contemplating when the previous wishes were expressed.

Various types of formal advance directives have become popular and are now part of most health care settings. Many forms of living wills or advance directives are available, and many jurisdictions have dealt in statute with the way in which such documents should be used and interpreted. There does not seem to be any ethical reason that a person should not be able to contemplate at one point in his or her life circumstances he or she believes may occur later and exercise autonomous choice regarding responses to those circumstances at an earlier time. Equally there does not seem to be any obvious reason why physicians should not respect choices made at an earlier time provided there is no reasonable ground to believe that they have changed in the interval.

Many early living wills were quite simple and did not give much detail about the patient's wishes. Physicians often had difficulty interpreting these simple directives, and this limited their utility in facilitating the autonomy expressed. A patient's statement that he or she "did not wish to be kept alive artificially" did not provide much practical guidance to physicians treating the patient in a later critical illness. Did the patient mean that he or she did not want cardiopulmonary resuscitation but did want other supportive treatments? Did the patient mean that he or she did not want only any supportive treatments or any treatment at all? Did the patient mean that he or she did not wish to be kept alive by artificial means only when suffering from a predictably terminal illness for which no reasonable treatment is available, or did the patient mean that he or she did not wish to be given a brief, although admittedly artificial, form of treatment that would quickly bring an acute episode under control? In the last few years, all of these questions have resulted in much more well-thought-out forms of advance directives that ask patients more detailed questions about their preferences and give much more helpful guidance to physicians. A number of bioethical institutes have issued such documents, which seem to be both helpful and in high demand.

In the event of the apparent need for acute intervention to save life or limb, the default condition, at least in the bioethics of the Western world, has been generally accepted as being in favor of lifesaving treatment. The majority of ethical discourse suggests that it is reasonable to presume that most people wish to be saved at least from acute danger. This presumption must be interpreted carefully, however, against the zeal of the physician to provide care that he or she knows may be curative but may have been prohibited. The physician, whose personal feelings may strongly dictate in favor of treatment, must not be allowed to cavalierly ignore the principle of patient autonomy. A recent Canadian case illustrates this principle.[4]

A 57-year-old woman was brought unconscious to the emergency room. She had suffered significant injuries, including a head injury and multiple lacerations of her upper body, face, and scalp, in a severe motor vehicle accident. The attending physician conscientiously believed that the patient would die from exsanguination quite shortly and that he must administer a blood transfusion to save her life. In searching the patient's belongings, nurses found a card in her wallet stating that she was a Jehovah's Witness and would never wish to receive blood products or transfusions. Although this card was signed, places provided for a date and for a witness' signature were blank. The attending physician knew about the card and administered the transfusion anyway. The patient recovered and sued, alleging battery. The court found that the transfusion had been necessary from a medical standpoint and that it had saved the patient's life. The court also found that the physician was fully aware that this treatment was against the patient's wishes and contravened her direction. The physician was found to have committed battery, and damages were awarded in the amount of $20,000. The court held that, where the patient's refusal was based on religious grounds, it would not apply a test of reasonableness to them. The court held that it could not and would not absolve the physician from his responsibility to respect the patient's autonomous choice by finding the patient's religious convictions to be unreasonable.

Substitute decision-makers

The principle of autonomy should not be considered to be restricted to the patient's own choice whether personally expressed or expressed by advance directive. The patient may appoint a substitute decision-maker to serve in the event of his or her incapability, and in many jurisdictions statute law provides for decisions to be made on behalf of the patient by others. The decisions made by substitutes are to be treated in all respects as if the patient made them personally. Most of the laws recognize that the substitute decision-maker is in as much need of information from the physician as the patient would be if making the decision and require disclosure of such information. Most such statutes provide that if the physician is persuaded that the substitute decision-maker is not acting in the best interest of the patient or is not acting in accordance with the best knowledge available of the patient's actual wishes, he or she may seek the guidance of a court when practical.

Although it is clear that the principle of autonomy should be respected as a fundamental principle of medical ethics, it is equally clear that the respect for that principle does not mean that the patient's wishes must be accepted and complied with in every case. Medical ethics does not require physicians to accede to patient choices that are illegal, illicit, or self-destructive. For example, patient demands to illegally prescribe drugs or to assist the patient in self-destruction or self-destructive activity may properly be resisted. It is more difficult to analyze the physician's proper response to a patient's choice that is unhealthy or foolish but falls short of impropriety. It is nevertheless clear that freedom of choice includes freedom to make foolish choices, even choices that may be quite harmful or destructive, and these freedoms are not limited to choices in medical care but extend to lifestyle choices, such as the use of drugs, alcohol, tobacco, and other unhealthy lifestyles.

Of particular concern is the patient's request that the physician end his or her life or assist him or her in ending his or her own life. In most jurisdictions it is not a criminal offense to commit suicide, but in some jurisdictions it is an offense to assist or counsel another person to commit suicide. The principle of autonomy, as we have discussed, should not be interpreted as a requirement to always do what the patient wants, but at the same time the physician is dedicated to making the patient better if possible or making the patient feel as much better as possible, and classic texts dictate against the taking of life or the doing of harm.

Good palliative care often requires extreme measures to relieve pain and suffering, using powerful drugs that also may shorten the patient's life. This double effect has come to be accepted as a proper approach both ethically and legally in most jurisdictions, and treatment designed to reduce the suffering of a patient of a reasonable character is not interpreted by most as the doing of harm even though it may be reasonably foreseen to shorten the patient's life.

Positive actions taken by the physician to end or shorten the patient's life are criminal in most jurisdictions and are seen as sufficiently significant breaches of the principle of nonmalfeasance that many feel they cannot be justified by claims of respect for a patient's autonomous decision to die. In several European countries tentative steps have been taken to relax the legal rules surrounding euthanasia, and there is a fierce discussion in the ethical community and an equally fierce political and legal dispute in North America regarding the proper response to this situation. The proper ethical principle to apply and the societal determination of the conflict of principles between respect for autonomy and nonmalfeasance are yet to be resolved in most jurisdictions and will continue to be the subjects of intense ethical discourse and litigation for some years to come.

This debate will indeed be exacerbated by the fact that patients with serious life-ending illnesses survive longer because of the efficacy of their treatments and their states of reduced function; thus reduced ability to exercise their autonomous choice creates problems. As patients' ability to express their choice is reduced by their illness, it often becomes more and more difficult to determine whether their expressed wishes are their genuine choice or whether their apparent capability to make choices is illusory.

Refused autonomy

Sometimes patients, particularly those with long-term, chronic illnesses that have made them dependent in many ways, do not wish to make choices and do not wish to have information about their illness. The state of dependency extends to the patient's stated desire to simply depend on the physician to provide treatment in his or her best interest (in a maternalistic way) rather than be told all of the facts on which choices might be based. The principle of autonomy requires respect for patient wishes and decisions but should not be interpreted as requiring patients to make those decisions if they do not want to make them.

Ethical issues that arise from the principle of autonomy

A number of ethical issues in law and medicine are not directly part of the principle of autonomy but arise from it. Prominent among these are privacy, confidentiality, and its limits; the duty to warn; and the physician-patient relationship as a fiduciary obligation.

Privacy and confidentiality. Most authors include consideration of privacy and confidentiality in the discussion of the principle of autonomy because privacy is viewed as a principle closely related to autonomy. The right of self-determination or self-rule, particularly in today's society, in many ways revolves around the right to keep to oneself intimate information and thought. Dissemination of a person's most closely held secrets and thoughts robs the individual in many cases of the ability to exert self-determination and violates the self of the individual in a way that destroys autonomy. In both medicine and law the ancient texts require the maintenance of patients' or clients' secrets to the exclusion of all others, and almost every licensing and self-governing authority in both professions enforces strict rules to ensure the maintenance of patient or client confidences.

This principle is generally thought to be more than just an ethical precept; it is indeed a practical necessity for the practice of the profession. The attorney cannot effectively represent a client who out of fear of disclosure fails to tell the attorney every relevant detail about the matter, and similarly the physician must obtain from the patient a history, including every relevant detail no matter how embarrassing it may be or how much it might subject the patient to public odium if disclosed. For these reasons, patients and clients clearly must know that the ethics of the profession prohibit the practitioner from disclosing any information obtained through the physician-patient or attorney-client relationship. Only in this way will the patient or client be encouraged to be forthcoming, and only in this way will optimal services be delivered.

In contemporary society there is so much health information electronically shuttled around the world in computer banks for the purpose of billing, quality management, statistical analysis, and research it perhaps is not surprising that there have been a number of notable incidents in which privacy has not been accorded the value that it once was, and the confidentiality interests of the patient or client have been violated or ignored. A large Royal Commission Inquiry in Ontario, Canada, several years ago revealed widespread abuses of patient confidentiality by attorneys, insurance companies, and government agencies; similar improprieties have been disclosed from time to time all over the Western world. Given the devastating effects that inappropriate disclosures may have on patients and given the ever-increasing spread of this information by electronic means, it perhaps is not surprising that there has been a resurgence of interest in the confidentiality of health information, and a number of jurisdictions have attempted various legislative means of ensuring privacy through regulations. From the point of view of the physician and attorney, the privacy rights of the patient as part of the ethical principle of autonomy should be viewed as extremely important and, wherever possible, should be highly respected. Rules requiring the maintenance of patient and client confidentiality should be carefully respected and should be broken only for a good reason or when required by law.

Of course, some overriding public interests will require breaches of confidentiality on the established principle that autonomy always has its limits and that in appropriate circumstances the autonomy of the individual must yield to the higher interests of the public and the state.

Most professional rules provide that confidentiality may be breached when such breach is required by law; mandatory reporting laws related to infectious disease, unfit drivers, unfit commercial pilots, and gunshot and grievous wounds are proper legal and ethical justifications for breach of confidentiality.

The duty to warn. Of particular interest are situations in which the autonomy and confidentiality interests of a patient or client conflict with the personal safety interests of another person. When a patient indicates to a attorney, therapist, or physician that he or she intends to kill or seriously harm another person, it is often difficult to balance these interests. On the one hand, attorneys and physicians know that normal people often casually make statements of that kind without any real intent of carrying them out. They also are aware of a number of widely reported and tragic circumstances in which patients or clients who made such threats, which were not reported, went on to carry them out at the cost of the life of the threatened person. Because the prediction of general dangerousness is so difficult and may be impossible, it will often be extremely problematic for the practitioner to determine any reasonable basis on which to make a prediction as to when such threats might be carried out and when they might safely be treated as merely part of a normal, if strained, professional interview.

In many jurisdictions the law now requires that practitioners err on the side of safety by imposing a duty to warn individuals who are the subject of such threats in breach of confidentiality even if it does not seem likely that the threats will be carried out. This erring on the side of prevention of harm is favored by most ethicists as a sound decision, erring toward the achievement of the good. The literature now discloses reasonably good consensus as to warning signs suggesting that such threats are more likely to be carried out. Such warning signs are a definite and an immediate plan to take action, the apparent means to take action, a recent acquisition of the named weapon, availability of the victim to the perpetrator, and the description of a detailed plan of attack. If such signs are present, the knowledge that an actual attack is more lkely will further ethically justify warning the putative victim.

The physician-patient or attorney-client relationship as a fiduciary relationship. The ethical requirement to respect autonomy of the patient as the principal pillar of bioethics causes consideration of the nature of that relationship. This is one of the areas where the professions of law and medicine have somewhat divergent views as to the implications of the ethical principle for the relationship of the professional with the patient or client.

In the legal profession, most codes of ethics of the bar and most legal licensing statutes establish clearly that the attorney-client relationship is a fiduciary relationship of utmost trust and fidelity and requires complete disclosure, utmost honesty, and utmost fidelity. For example, most bar codes strictly require the attorney to inform the client if any mistake, error, or misconduct occurs and to advise the client to obtain independent counsel. In most bar rules the records and papers pertaining to a transaction, when properly paid for, belong to the client and must be delivered forthwith, and in the attorney-client relationship everything that passes between the attorney and his or her client must be strictly accounted for and a full accounting must be delivered at any time it is demanded.

In contrast, the relationship between the physician and patient is not viewed by most medical societies and licensing authorities as so clearly of a fiduciary nature. Although the physician is expected to do his or her best for the patient and to see himself or herself at all times as principally obligated to the patient, many ordinary features of a fiduciary relationship are not accorded as much importance. The ownership and delivery of medical records are not nearly so clear, and there is no recognized obligation on the part of the physician in most jurisdictions to inform the patient of any error or misconduct or to suggest the obtaining of an independent and alternate caregiver. The concept of therapeutic privilege, which allows the physician the privilege in some circumstances to withhold the truth from the patient on the basis of his or her opinion that the truth might hurt the patient psychologically or make him or her resort to rash action such as refusing treatment, still seems to have some currency in sectors of the medical profession. There also continues to be some legitimacy accorded the idea that the use of placebos and other therapeutic fibs is necessary for cure in some situations. All of this speaks interestingly of the somewhat different approach to the incidents of autonomy in the two professions.

BENEFICENCE (AND ITS COUNTERPART, NONMALFEASANCE)

Beneficence is the duty to do good, be caring, and to help and support on all occasions. Nonmalfeasance is the duty to endeavor to do no harm, and both concepts certainly date at least from the time of the Hippocratic oath in which the physicians swore, "I will follow that system of regimen which according to my ability and judgment I consider for the benefit of my patients and abstain from whatever is deleterious and mischievous."[5]

Every medical student is taught that the first precept of medicine is to do no harm and that secondarily everything should be done to benefit the patient and to be supportive, caring, and helpful whenever possible. The physician is meant to relieve suffering, produce beneficial outcomes wherever possible, avoid bad outcomes, and enhance the patient's quality of life if possible. This concept is connected with the concept of autonomy, which directs that the physician do what the patient wishes whenever possible and most often that will be to relieve the patient's suffering and provide a cure. Doing no harm is a value inculcated in all physicians, but some have considerable difficulty recognizing when unreasonable persistence in treatment that is designed to do good in the face of a clinical situation in which further treatment is useless because it cannot alter the ultimate and inevitable outcome is not beneficent and may be malfeasant.

Although it is true that there are often great difficulties in determining in medical terms when a treatment passes from the therapeutic to the futile, it will often be a function of patient autonomy to make that decision with the best information the practitioner can provide. In any event the principle of nonmalfeasance requires that the physician be alert to circumstances in which futility may supervene beneficent attempts at a cure, and unreasonable persistence in treatment stops being beneficent and starts constituting malfeasance.

JUSTICE

The fourth principle of bioethics is justice, and in simple terms justice can be thought of as fair play or at the very least freedom from unfair discrimination. As resources to provide health care become more constrained, problems related to the principle of justice will become more important in the ethical discourse of biomedicine. It is likely in the future that the discussion of this fourth principle will assume an ever-greater predominance in the discourse and may approach the prominence heretofore accorded to autonomy.

In many ways the issues that flow from the principle of justice may be seen as the antithesis of those that flow from autonomy. Justice deals with the fair distribution of the system, with whether patients get what they reasonably may consider their due from the health care system, and with the definition of what is a fair distribution of the resources that are available. If autonomy dictates that the patient's interest is always foremost and what is best for the patient should be first in the physician's mind, the principle of justice dictates that the physician must have concern for the fair distribution of the system's resources and for ensuring that they are not distributed in a way that depends on inappropriate discrimination.

A common formulation designed to distribute services fairly is that patients should exercise their autonomy to receive such services as they desire provided that the system can and will provide only those services that are judged to be medically necessary. Of course, many years of experience in health administration and health insurance administration

demonstrate that determining what is medically necessary is the most difficult and problematic determination that must be made within those systems. What is really needed? Are treatments that are designed to make the patient better necessary, and are those that are designed to make the patient feel better unnecessary? How would it be reasonably determined whether a treatment designed to make a patient get better has a sufficient and reasonable likelihood of doing so that the resources of the system should be directed to it in preference to meeting some other patient's needs or demands? To what extent may treatment be denied to patients because there is no scientific evidence that it will make them better in the face of their persistent and apparently honest assertion that the receipt of the treatment makes them feel better?

Are some patients entitled to a greater share of the system's resources because of their station in life or contributions to society? Are highly intelligent contributors to science worth more than poorly educated workers? Are wealthy persons who have made huge contributions to the public welfare to be given preference over the poor? Is it legitimate to consider a patient less entitled to system resources if he or she suffers from a disease to which his or her own behavior, such as alcoholism or smoking, has avoidably contributed? Is a patient's entitlement to health care cumulative over a lifetime? Does there come a point where the patient has used so much of the resources of the system that he or she is not entitled to any more until the needs of others have been satisfied?

In determining whether to allocate resources to the patient it may be legitimate to consider the likely benefit to the patient and to increase the allocation of resources to those who are more likely to benefit or whose quality of life is likely to be improved. Is it legitimate to increase the allocation of resources where the duration of the benefit is likely to be greater rather than lesser or where the patient's condition is more urgent than that of a competing patient? Are some treatments, although likely to be successful and very beneficial, simply so resource intensive that they should not be given because they just consume too much of the available pie for the benefit of one individual? Box 24-1 lists the opinion of the Council on Ethical and Judicial Affairs of the American Medical Association with respect to some of these issues.[6]

BOX 24-1. ACCEPTABLE CRITERIA FOR RESOURCE ALLOCATION AMONG PATIENTS

Likelihood of benefit to the patient
Improvement in the patient's quality of life
Duration of benefit
Urgency of the patient's condition
Amount of resources required for successful treatment

How should the independent practitioner allocate his or her time as a resource between the many patients who will assert demands for care? Is it inevitable that physicians will give more time and effort to patients they like or whose disease is treatable than to those who are obnoxious or whose condition is intractable?

Can a physician properly participate in organizations for the delivery of care that insert into the physicians' attempts to do justice to his or her patient's questionable incentives? Is it appropriate for a physician to participate in a managed care plan that provides a large percentage of his or her yearly remuneration as a bonus, which the physician receives only if he or she meets a goal to restrain service delivery, meaning he or she will have to work hard not to give care and not to refer patients? Is it appropriate for a physician to practice within a scheme that forbids him or her to discuss with the patient alternatives for care that are not offered by the patient's benefit plan? Should society permit or prohibit those sorts of schemes? If it is not possible to achieve optimal justice in every patient encounter, ethical discourse suggests that at the very least inappropriate discrimination must not be tolerated.

All professional practitioners understand that their practice must be as free as possible from inappropriate discrimination and bias, and certainly all are aware of the inappropriateness of discrimination based on race, religion, national origin, gender, sexual orientation, or political opinion. However, there is considerable literature to suggest that the practice of medicine, perhaps without intention, has contained a good deal of bias on some, if not all those grounds, in particular on the basis of age, race, and gender.

Numerous variance studies done in a number of jurisdictions demonstrate that there appear to be variations in relation to access to care between patients of different ages, genders, and racial origins for no reason that appears to be grounded in science or medicine. It must be presumed that many subtle factors that are hard to identify often combine to produce such discrimination. Clearly, in the name of the justice principle, bioethics requires each practitioner to search his or her practice and all practice protocols in which he or she is involved for the subtle influence of prejudice and discrimination and

to eliminate it whenever and wherever possible. Of course it is sometimes extremely difficult for practitioners to perceive these differences or to even be aware of the possibility of their existence. Thus it will be the role of the bioethicist and bioethics committees to assist practitioners in identifying elements of their practices or programs in which infractions of the justice principle may exist. This use of the ethical discourse ought not to be seen as a search for "bad apples" or rule infractions but as a necessary assistance to practitioners, groups, and health institutions in eliminating these most subtle but important infractions of the justice principle.

At the same time there are a few circumstances where scientific principles properly discriminate between age groups, gender groups, and races on the basis of demonstrable real differences between them. Considerable study will often be required to distinguish between situations of subtle discrimination and situations in which scientific and medical considerations dictate an appropriate discrimination between persons and groups with regard to access to, or the nature of, treatment offered.

Limitations of space have permitted only a brief outline of the basic principles of bioethics in a medicolegal context. It is hoped that this chapter and the way in which ethical discourse presents an opportunity to reflect in a different way on the medicolegal dilemmas evident elsewhere in this book may stimulate the interest of the reader in further exploring ethics as a medicolegal tool.

ENDNOTES

1. T.L. Beauchamp & J.F. Childress, *Principles of Bio-Medical Ethics* (Oxford University Press, London 1979).
2. Community on Quality of Health Care in America, Institute of Medicine, *To Err Is Human: Building a Safer Health System* (Linda Kohn, Janet Corrigan, & Molla Donaldson eds., National Academy Press, Washington, D.C. 2000).
3. *Schoendorf v. Society of New York Hospital,* 1914, 105 N.E. 92 (N.Y.C.A.).
4. *Malette v. Shulman* 63O. R. 2d, 243, 72O. R. 2d, 417 (O.C.A.).
5. Mason & McCall-Smith, *Oath of Hippocrates,* in *Law and Medical Ethics* 251 (Butterworths, London 1983).
6. AMA Council on Ethical and Judicial Affairs, *Ethical Considerations in the Allocation of Organs and Other Scarce Medical Resources Among Patients,* 155 Arch. Intern. Med. 401 (1995).

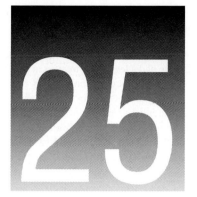

Fetal interests

ETHICAL CONSIDERATIONS
THE LAW

Although in legal contexts the term *fetus* has been used to refer to the conceptus throughout all stages of development, fetus more properly refers to "the product of conception from the end of the eighth week to the moment of birth."[1] Before this (i.e., from the moment of conception until approximately the end of the eighth week) the developing human is more properly referred to as an *embryo*. Herein, the terms *fetus* and *conceptus* are used interchangeably.

ETHICAL CONSIDERATIONS
The moral standing of the unborn

Underlying the legal controversy over fetal interests is an essentially ethical question: Does the human fetus have moral standing? "To attribute moral standing to a creature . . . is to say that it deserves or merits or qualifies for the protections of morality."[2]

Under one approach, moral standing is equated with "personhood."[3] Under this approach a fetus has moral standing and thus a right to life and freedom from infliction of bodily harm, if he or she is a person. Thus it is morally relevant to ask, "When does the embryo/fetus become a person?" Three answers to this question have been suggested. One answer is that the embryo is a person from the moment of conception. A second answer is that personhood is not achieved until the moment of birth, when "independent life and human relationships are possible. [A] third . . . adopts the middle ground . . . recogniz[ing] the status of the embryo as linked to certain stages of biological development."[4] Under this third view the fetus becomes a person somewhere between conception and birth—perhaps when he or she becomes recognizably human, heart or brain activity appears, or he or she becomes viable (capable of surviving outside the womb).

Alternatively it might be argued that, even assuming the fetus is not yet a person, he or she is a potential person and that this potential to become a person endows the fetus with the same basic moral rights enjoyed by persons.

A second approach recognizes that deciding on when the developing human achieves personhood does not answer the ethical question because nonpersons may still have moral standing. Stated otherwise, personhood is a sufficient but not necessarily a necessary condition for having moral rights.

Personhood is important as an inclusion criterion for moral equality: Any theory that denies equal moral status to certain persons must be rejected. But personhood seems somewhat less plausible as an exclusion criterion, as it appears to exclude infants and mentally handicapped individuals who may lack the mental and social capacities typical of persons.[5]

Under this second approach the moral standing of the fetus might be grounded in respect for the intrinsic value or inherent dignity of life in general or human life in particular (because, "while there may be an ongoing discussion as to [the] personhood [of the embryo/fetus], no one denies that the human embryo constitutes human life").[6] Alternatively the moral standing of the fetus, beginning in the second trimester, might be grounded in respect for sentient beings.[7]

Metaethics

What is being determined when a judgment is made that the fetus has moral standing? Is it determined that, for example, abortion is immoral?

Moral skeptics espouse those ethical theories asserting "that there are no right answers to moral questions, such as abortion, only accepted answers" and include moral nihilists, as well as irrealists. Nihilists believe that there are no such things as moral facts and "that without moral facts moral practice is all a sham."[8] Irrealists agree that there are no such things as moral facts but maintain that such facts are not necessary for moral practice. There are several different versions of irrealism, including subjectivism, which asserts that in making a moral judgment about abortion people are doing nothing more than expressing their personal feelings on the subject (i.e., "I don't like abortion"), and relativism, which

The Editorial Committee updated this chapter. The committee gratefully acknowledges the past contribution of Frederick A. Paola, M.D., J.D., F.A.C.P., F.A.C.L.M.

asserts that moral truth exists only in relation to one's particular society or culture.

In contrast to moral skepticism is the view epitomized by the idea of natural law, "the view that there is an unchanging normative order that is a part of the natural world, . . . that there is a natural foundation to moral beliefs."[9]

Clearly an individual's understanding of what it means to make a moral judgment will affect the way he or she answers the question, "How ought I act toward those whose judgment on the moral standing of the fetus is different from my own?" Corresponding to the metaethical theories discussed previously are normative theories addressing this question.

Consider the position of those who believe that abortion is morally wrong because it is the taking of life that has moral status. Within this group some seem undisturbed by the fact that there is deep disagreement over the moral status of the fetus. They wish to prohibit abortion. But others in this group, while holding that abortion is wrong, [maintain] that reasonable persons could disagree with them and that human reason seems unable to resolve the question. For this reason, they oppose legal prohibitions of abortion. The former believe that the latter do not take the value of human life seriously, while the latter believe that the former fail to recognize the depth and seriousness of the disagreement among reasonable persons.[10]

Thus normative relativists are likely to believe that it is wrong to judge those who hold different values or to try to make them conform to another's values because their values are as valid as another's. At the other end of the spectrum, universalists or absolutists, taking the position that both sides of the abortion debate cannot be right and that there is only one moral truth with regard to the moral standing of the unborn, are likely to believe that whatever intrinsic value an ethic of nonjudgmental tolerance may have is outweighed by the gravity of the fetal interests at stake.

THE LAW
Constitutional rights of the unborn

In *Roe v. Wade* the U.S. Supreme Court determined that the unborn were not "persons" as far as the U.S. Constitution was concerned.[11] Consequently the unborn were denied constitutional protection from deprivation of life, liberty, and property.

The *Roe* court also found a constitutionally fundamental "right of privacy . . . broad enough to encompass a woman's decision whether or not to terminate her pregnancy." Such a right could be abridged only where such abridgment was necessary to achieve a compelling state interest. Although Roe recognized the state's interest in the "potential" human life represented by the fetus, *Roe* did not recognize any rights of the unborn themselves; *Roe* asserted that the state's interest in protecting potential human life becomes compelling only at the point of fetal viability. The effect of *Roe* was to strike down state laws criminalizing abortion.

In the 1992 decision dealing with the abortion issue, *Planned Parenthood v. Casey,* the U.S. Supreme Court reaffirmed a woman's constitutional right to abort a fetus before viability without "undue" state interference, as well as the state's right to prohibit abortion after viability except to preserve the life or health of the woman.[12,13]

[T]he Casey Court held that the state had a legitimate interest in protecting fetal life from the onset of pregnancy. Accordingly, it was legitimate for government to act throughout pregnancy to undermine abortion, so long as it did not . . . "unduly burden" the woman's ability to choose it. This position contrasted sharply with *Roe v. Wade's* holding that only during the third trimester could government enact regulations designed to preserve the life of the fetus.[14]

Fetal rights under tort law

Although the early common law recognized fetal rights under criminal law and property law, it did not recognize fetal rights under tort law. The first American case to address an individual's right to bring an action for harm sustained while in utero was *Dietrich v. Inhabitants of Northampton.*[15] In this case a woman who was 5 months pregnant slipped and fell on the defendant's negligently maintained road. She prematurely delivered an infant that lived only about 15 minutes. The legal issue was whether the child could maintain a cause of action in negligence. The Massachusetts Supreme Judicial Court, in an opinion by Justice Holmes, answered in the negative, reasoning that the "unborn child did not have standing to sue because it was part of its mother, and not a separate being, at the time of the injury."

In *Allaire v. St. Luke's Hospital* a pregnant patient was severely injured by a negligently operated hospital elevator.[16] The infant was born severely and permanently disabled several days later. The Illinois Supreme Court, citing *Dietrich,* denied a cause of action.

In a vigorous dissent, however, Justice Boggs distinguished *Dietrich* by narrowly interpreting its holding as applicable to only the nonviable fetus. Boggs argued that the fetus in *Allaire,* being viable, had an existence separate from that of the mother, and he concluded that the hospital therefore owed the fetus a duty of due care.

Finally, in *Bonbrest v. Kotz* the Federal District Court for the District of Columbia held that a child sustaining an injury while a viable fetus could maintain a cause of action against a third party.[17] The court, as had Justice Boggs, distinguished *Dietrich* on the ground that in *Bonbrest* the infant plaintiff was viable at the time of the injury.

The *Bonbrest* decision opened the floodgates to what is now the majority rule favoring recovery for prenatal injuries. Every jurisdiction now permits recovery for prenatal injuries if the child is born alive. Furthermore, even the conditions considered key for recovery in *Bonbrest*—that the fetus be viable at the time of injury and that the plaintiff survive delivery—have been removed in some jurisdictions. Thus the majority of state courts has now rejected the viability requirement of *Bonbrest* and now allows recovery for prenatal injuries inflicted at any point during gestation.[18]

Preconception tort liability. The rejection of the viability requirement has made it possible for courts to recognize tort liability before viability and even before conception. Preconception tort liability refers to "those situations in which the defendant's tortious actions before the plaintiff's conception result in harm to the infant plaintiff."[19]

In *Jorgensen v. Meade Johnson Laboratories* the U.S. Court of Appeals for the Tenth Circuit held that plaintiff children, who were alleging that their mothers' preconception use of defendant Johnson's oral contraceptives had caused their Down syndrome, could maintain a cause of action for preconception tort liability.[20] Likewise, the Supreme Court of Illinois, which in *Allaire* had denied recovery to an infant plaintiff on the basis of no separate legal existence at the time of injury (a decision overruled in 1953 by *Amann v. Faidy*), has now broadened its range of potential plaintiffs to include those not yet conceived at the time of the injury. In *Renslow v. Mennonite Hospital* the court found "a right to be born free from prenatal injuries foreseeably caused by a breach of duty to the child's mother."[21] Emma Renslow was 13 years old and Rh negative when she negligently received transfusions of Rh-positive blood. Her daughter was born nearly 8½ years later and required exchange transfusions because of her mother's sensitization. Permanent damages were alleged to have occurred because of blood incompatibility and resulting hemolysis. In extending a tortfeasor's duty to those who have not yet been conceived, the court termed it "illogical to bar relief for an act done prior to conception where the defendant would be liable for this same conduct had the child, unbeknownst to him, been conceived prior to his act."

In contrast, the New York Court of Appeals, *Albala v. City of New York*, concluded that New York law did not recognize a cause of action for preconception negligence.[22] Likewise, the Appellate Division of the Supreme Court of New York has held that New York does not recognize a preconception strict liability cause of action.[23]

A relatively new subset of preconception tort claims is illustrated by the so-called third-generation diethylstilbestrol (DES) lawsuits. In *Enright v. Eli Lilly & Co.* a plaintiff injured as a result of preterm birth alleged that her grandmother's ingestion of DES while pregnant with her (plaintiff's) mother damaged her mother's reproductive system and in turn caused the plaintiff's preterm birth.[24] The New York Court of Appeals, citing *Albala,* held that the plaintiff had no cause of action. Likewise, in *Sorrels v. Eli Lilly & Co.* a woman and her infant daughter alleged that use of DES by the infant's grandmother had caused the infant's preterm birth and consequent severe hearing loss.[25] The U.S. District Court for the District of Columbia, saying that Maryland law did not recognize a preconception duty, dismissed the plaintiff's preconception claims.

Wrongful death of fetuses. Historically under the common law, although liability was imposed on tortfeasors whose victims survived, tortfeasors who killed their victims escaped liability because the cause of action "died" with the victim. Wrongful death statutes were enacted as a legislative response to this perceived loophole in the common law and allowed survivors to seek compensation for the death of the victim.

If an injured fetus is born alive and dies subsequently, every state now permits a wrongful death action to be brought on his or her behalf.[26] If the victim is stillborn, courts have disagreed over whether a fetus is a "person" within the meaning of states' wrongful death statutes. *Verkennes v. Corniea* was the first opinion to allow a wrongful death action on behalf of a stillborn child.[27] Recovery was still conditional on fetal viability at the time of the injury. As of 1996 the majority of states allow recovery for the wrongful death of a fetus. The majority of these jurisdictions, like *Verkennes,* have held that only a viable fetus is protected under wrongful death statutes; only six states (Georgia, Louisiana, Illinois, Missouri, West Virginia, and South Dakota) have indicated that recovery is not conditional on fetal viability. Nine other jurisdictions still deny recovery to the stillborn infant, concluding that even the viable fetus is not a "person" within the meaning of the applicable wrongful death statute.[28]

Parental tort liability. Although courts have been willing to compensate the unborn for injuries caused by negligent acts of tortfeasors, especially professionals responsible for the care of the mother and fetus, few have imposed liability on those individuals whose actions are most commonly hazardous to the unborn. Pregnant women who, for example, smoke, use cocaine, or abuse alcohol impair the development of their infants. Most who do so are aware of the potential for harm to the infant.

The reluctance to compensate children injured prenatally by their mother's conduct stems largely from a desire to avoid intruding on the privacy interest of the pregnant woman but also reflects the parental immunity doctrine. Intrafamily tort immunity was intended to promote the societal goal of family harmony and unity.

In 1980 in *Grodin v. Grodin* the Michigan Court of Appeals overruled the doctrine of parental immunity and expanded fetal rights to allow a cause of action for damages against a mother for her negligence during pregnancy.[29] In holding that "the litigating child's mother would bear the same liability for injurious, negligent [prenatal] conduct as would a third person," the court in essence "pitted the legal rights of the pregnant woman and the fetus against each other, rather than conceptualizing them as one legal entity."[30]

Fetal rights and criminal law

Crimes against a fetus. Early Anglo-American law recognized fetal rights under criminal law. As early as 1628,

Lord Coke proposed that an individual should be criminally liable for injuring a child in utero if that child were later born alive. "Thus, if a pregnant woman took a harmful potion or if a man beat a pregnant woman, the wrongdoer would be charged with murder if the woman later delivered an infant who subsequently died of the resulting injury."[31]

The criminal law continues to recognize the fetus as a person with regard to the criminal acts of third parties. Eighteen states now have "feticide" statutes, and another two states recognize a common law crime of "feticide," thus treating the killing of a pregnant woman as two counts of homicide.[32] In the 1984 case *Gloria C. v. William C.* a New York family court recognized a fetus as a person for the purpose of issuing a protective order.[33] In that case a pregnant woman had sought a protective order to protect her fetus from her allegedly abusive husband.

Criminal prosecution of pregnant women. Regarding recognition of the fetus as a person with regard to the criminal acts of mothers, the Center for Reproductive Law and Policy has reported that as of 1996, approximately 200 women in more than 30 different states had been charged with crimes against their fetuses. Because no state has a statute specifically criminalizing drug abuse by the pregnant woman, prosecutors have unsuccessfully attempted to prosecute maternal substance abuse under the guise of other laws, such as those dealing with child abuse, child support, manslaughter, or the delivery of a controlled substance.

Pamela Rae Stewart-Monson, for example, had placenta previa. She was advised by her physician to stay off of her feet, to abstain from sexual intercourse, and to seek medical attention if she bled vaginally. She delivered a brain-damaged infant that died within 6 weeks.

Stewart-Monson was arrested and charged under Section 270 of the California Penal Code, an 1872 child support statute that prohibited the intentional omission of "necessary . . . medical attendance [to children]." Since its enactment, the statute had been extended in 1925 to cover fathers who failed to support "a child conceived but not yet born" and in 1974 to cover mothers.

California alleged that Stewart-Monson failed to maintain bed rest, engaged in sexual intercourse, used amphetamines on the day of delivery, and failed to seek medical attention promptly once vaginal bleeding began. The indictment was dismissed on a pretrial motion that the child support statute did not encompass the conduct alleged.[34]

Likewise, Elizabeth Levey was 8½ months pregnant when she crashed her car, allegedly driving while intoxicated. On the day after the accident, she delivered a stillborn infant. The district attorney charged Levey with vehicular homicide, relying on the Massachusetts rule that a fetus is a person under the homicide law.[35] The charges were later dropped.[36]

Diane Pfannenstiel was charged under a Wyoming statute that prohibits intentionally or recklessly injuring a child. Pfannenstiel was 4 months pregnant when arrested. The case therefore differed from the aforementioned cases in that the mother was charged with child abuse before the child was even born. The court dismissed the charges against Pfannenstiel because the district attorney could not prove that the fetus, still in utero and thus unavailable for examination, had been injured.

In 1989 Floridian Jennifer Johnson was charged with and convicted of delivering (postnatally through the umbilical cord) a controlled substance (cocaine) to a minor (her infant), notwithstanding the defense counsel's argument that the drafters of the applicable Florida delivery law did not intend for that law to apply to the unborn.[37] The conviction was upheld by Florida's Fifth District Court of Appeals but was reversed unanimously by the Florida Supreme Court.[38] The court found that there was insufficient evidence to support the trial court's finding that cocaine had been delivered postnatally to the neonate through the umbilical cord and that the state legislature had not intended to treat drug-dependent mothers as criminals.

Indeed, most such cases have been dismissed. In July 1996, however, the South Carolina Supreme Court, in *Whitner v. South Carolina,* became the first state appeals court to uphold a guilty verdict in such a case, ruling that a pregnant woman who had taken drugs could be prosecuted for child abuse.[39]

In 1996 Florida's Second District Court of Appeals became the first appellate court to rule that a pregnant woman can be prosecuted for homicide in the death of that child. In *State of Florida v. Kawana M. Ashley* the accused was about 26 weeks pregnant when, allegedly unable to afford a legal abortion, she shot herself in the abdomen with a .22-caliber pistol.[40] The bullet struck the fetus in the wrist; she was delivered but died 15 days later of organ failure, a consequence of her preterm birth. The court said that the mother's act of shooting herself while pregnant could support a finding of criminal negligence and therefore a charge of manslaughter.

Also in 1996, Wisconsin prosecutors became the first to use a murder statute in a case in which the fetus did not die. In *Wisconsin v. Zimmerman,* Deborah Zimmerman was charged with attempted murder after giving birth, via emergency cesarean section, to a girl with fetal alcohol syndrome and a blood alcohol level of 0.199 (nearly two times the legal limit in Wisconsin). Refusing the attachment of a fetal monitor preoperatively, she had announced, "I'm just going to go home and keep drinking, and drink myself to death, and I'm going to kill this thing because I don't want it anyways."[41]

Forced medical intervention on behalf of the unborn

Judicial intervention and the viable fetus. It has been reported that, since 1981, health care providers have on more than 21 occasions asked courts to order unwilling women to submit to cesarean sections and that 86% of these requests have been granted.[42] The following cases are illustrative.

In *Raleigh Fitkin-Paul Morgan Memorial Hospital v. Anderson* a court ordered a Jehovah's Witness woman, who was 8 months pregnant and hemorrhaging, to submit to a blood transfusion to save her life and the life of her fetus.[43] Likewise, in *Jefferson v. Griffin Spaulding County Hospital* a court ordered a full-term woman with placenta previa to submit to a cesarean section after her physicians informed her of a 99% chance that her infant would not survive a vaginal delivery.[44]

In contrast, in *In re A.C.* the mother (A.C.) was in her twenty-sixth week of gestation and dying of cancer.[45] The District of Columbia District Court ordered a cesarean section against the wishes of A.C. and her husband, and the surgery was performed. The infant girl lived less than 3 hours, and A.C. died within 2 days.

The District of Columbia Court of Appeals vacated the district court's order and held that "in virtually all cases [where maternal and fetal health interests conflict] the question of what is to be done is to be decided by . . . the pregnant woman . . . on behalf of herself and the fetus," regardless of the age (i.e., viability) of the fetus.[46]

More recently, a maternal-fetal medicine specialist told a 22-year-old Illinois woman that her 32-week-old fetus was not receiving enough oxygen. The physician advised the woman to undergo either induction of labor or a cesarean section. The woman, a Pentecostal Christian, refused for religious reasons, insisting that the child be born naturally and asserting that God would protect her unborn child. The hospital informed Cook County officials, who sought to have a court order the pregnant woman to undergo the cesarean.[47] An Illinois Appellate Court confirmed a lower court ruling that the state could not force the woman to undergo a cesarean section. The case was appealed to the Illinois Supreme Court; however, on December 16, 1993, the court refused to enter the dispute. On December 18, 1993, the U.S. Supreme Court declined the request of the fetus' representative (the Cook County public guardian) that they hear the case.[48] On December 29, 1993, a boy was delivered to the couple, identified as Mircea and Tabita Bricci. Although the infant appeared to be well physically, obstetricians warned that "it will be more than 6 months before any signs of any mental abnormalities or retardation would be detectable."[49]

Judicial intervention and the previable fetus. In *Taft v. Taft* the husband of a woman 16 weeks' pregnant sought a court order requiring his wife to submit to "purse string sutures" to maintain cervical competency and save the fetus' life.[50] Although the appellate court refused to override the mother's (religious) objections, it did so on the narrow grounds that no evidence was offered to support the medical necessity of the treatment in question.

In a second case, *In re Jamaica Hospital,* the court ordered a woman 18 weeks' pregnant to submit to a blood transfusion to save both her own life and the life of her fetus.[51] The woman had refused for religious reasons. The court determined that, although the fetus was not yet viable and the state's interest in protecting his or her potential life therefore was not yet compelling, the state's interest was "highly significant" and outweighed the mother's right to refuse treatment for religious reasons.

Fetal protection by third parties

An interesting area of the law of fetal interests concerns its treatment of fetal protection by third parties. As a general rule, "[t]he duty to do no wrong is a legal duty, . . . [whereas t]he duty to protect against wrong is, generally speaking and excepting certain intimate relations in the nature of a trust, a moral obligation only, not . . . enforced by law."[52] American law, although traditionally imposing no affirmative duty on individuals to rescue strangers, is "in a steady movement toward requiring acts of Good Samaritanism . . . by whittling away at the concept of 'stranger.'"[53]

As such, although not penalizing the failure to rescue complete strangers, the law recognizes rescue as a normal human reaction. As Judge Cardozo wrote in *Wagner v. International Railway Co.,* "Danger invites rescue. The cry of distress is the summons to relief. The law does not ignore these reactions of the mind in tracing conduct to its consequences. It recognizes them as normal."[54] The law's tendency is to compel men to act like good neighbors and to leave heroism to individual option."[55] Against this background, the law's treatment of the fetus' right to be abetted by third parties is somewhat uneven, a phenomenon no doubt attributable to the unique nature of the "maternal-fetal dyad."[56]

Johnson Controls. In *Johnson Controls,* a company excluded from employment in its battery factory all women younger than 70 unwilling or unable to produce medical documentation of sterility.[57] The company, concerned that lead used in the battery-making process would result in fetal abnormalities, professed an interest in the health of its employees' fetuses, as well as concern about legal liability. The U.S. Court of Appeals for the Seventh Circuit upheld the policy.

Determining that protecting the safety of fetuses (or other noncustomer third parties) is not reasonably related to either the "essence of the [battery-making] business" or the "essence of the job," the U.S. Supreme Court held that Johnson Controls' fetal protection policy was illegal under Title VII of the Civil Rights Act of 1964 as amended by the Pregnancy Discrimination Act of 1978.[58,59] In essence the effect of the court's restrictive interpretation of Title VII was the following: Whereas before *Johnson Controls* employers were free to act so as to protect fetal safety (though they had no duty to do so), after *Johnson Controls* employers were legally prohibited from doing so.

Rights of Conscience

Congress and 44 state legislatures have enacted so-called conscience clauses, "statutes intended to protect health care providers' rights to refuse to provide or participate in certain procedures including abortion] to which they have moral or religious objections."[60] Although these clauses exist to protect the rights of health care providers with moral objections to abortion, fetuses clearly have an interest in seeing such rights protected. Unfortunately, the existing statutory protection of rights of conscience is inadequate from the point of view of fetal protection.

For example, not all conscience clauses protect all classes of persons. Some state conscience clauses protect "individuals" but not institutions.[61] Many of the conscience clauses that do extend their protection to institutions protect only private institutions.[62] Only 10 states' conscience clauses prohibit discrimination in admission to residency training programs because of an applicant's refusal to participate in "the controversial service."[63] Furthermore, there is a substantial body of evidence that the existing rights of conscience of health care providers are being ignored, and to make matters worse, most courts view conscience clauses with disfavor and interpret the involved statutory language narrowly.[64,65]

Frozen embryos

Ethical and legal issues. The development of technology for creating embryos through in vitro fertilization (IVF) and freezing those embryos for later disposition has created new ethical and legal issues. Once they are created, what may ethically be done with these so-called preembryos? What does existing law have to say on the subject? What should the law have to say on the subject?

It should be pointed out that American constitutional law, as interpreted by *Roe* and later abortion cases, has nothing to say about what may or may not be done with preembryos.

First, the viability standard cannot be applied to a technology that allows an embryo to be sustained indefinitely outside the mother's body; second, when an embryo is outside the mother's body and frozen, its existence is no longer in conflict with [the woman's] constitutionally protected privacy interests.[66]

Specifically, *Roe* and progeny do not preclude the state from protecting these preembryos. "*Roe* merely holds that the state cannot force a woman to physically bear a child . . . until the point of viability has been reached."[67]

In assessing the constitutionality of laws regulating the disposition of frozen embryos, the standard to be applied by the courts will depend on whether they view the right to avoid genetic parentage as a fundamental right. If that right is determined not to be fundamental, state action will be upheld if reasonably related to a legitimate state interest. In contrast, if that right is deemed to be fundamental, state action "unduly burdening" that right will be struck down as unconstitutional unless such action is necessary to achieve a compelling state interest.

In perhaps the most famous IVF case to date, the Tennessee Supreme Court, in *Davis v. Davis,* was forced to decide on the custody of seven cryopreserved embryos in a divorce case.[68] The trial court had held that the embryos were "children in vitro" and, invoking the doctrine of *parens patriae,* granted temporary custody to the mother. The Court of Appeals of Tennessee reversed and, in granting joint legal custody to Mr. and Mrs. Davis, implied that the cryopreserved embryos were property to be distributed equitably rather than persons.[69] The Tennessee Supreme Court, in affirming the decision of the appeals court, held that the embryos were not persons under the law but that neither were they property. Rather, they were something in between, deserving of special respect. In addition, the court wrote[70]:

[T]he gamete providers should execute prior agreements [dealing with the disposition of the embryos] that may be modified later by agreement. Absent such modification, the agreement is enforceable. If no prior agreement is made, . . . where the gamete providers disagree on disposition . . . the case should be decided in favor of the party objecting to becoming a parent if the opposing party has any other reasonable way to become a parent.

In effect the court found that the right to avoid genetic parenthood is a fundamental right and seemed to echo the American Fertility Society's characterization of preembryos as something in between person and property.

The preembryo deserves respect greater than that accorded to human tissue but not the respect accorded to actual persons. The preembryo is due greater respect than other human tissue because of its potential to become a person and because of its symbolic meaning for many people. Yet, it should not be treated as a person, because it has not yet developed the features of personhood, is not yet established as developmentally individual, and may never realize its biological potential.[71]

Louisiana has a statute that treats cryopreserved embryos as legal persons before implantation.[72] Under this statute, transfers of frozen embryos are treated as adoptions.

Protection for preembryos under criminal law. It has been suggested that preembryos might possibly enjoy protection under the criminal law of certain jurisdictions. Thus Missouri implicitly affords preembryos the protection of its homicide statute by defining them as legal "persons."

[T]he laws of this state shall be interpreted . . . to acknowledge on behalf of the unborn child at every stage of development, all the rights, privileges, and immunities available to other persons, citizens and residents of this state, subject only to the Constitution of the United States, and decisional interpretations thereof by the United States Supreme Court.[73]

In contrast, under New York State law a "person" is one "who has been born and is alive."[74] A fetus therefore could not claim to be a "person" for the purposes of New York's homicide law. Nevertheless the destruction of a fetus beyond

24 weeks of gestation is considered a homicide under New York law. Theoretically the reach of the homicide law could be extended to include other nonpersons, such as preembryos.

Wisconsin illustrates another approach. Under Wisconsin law, the destruction of an unborn child (a human being from the time of conception until live birth), though not characterized as a homicide, is punishable by a $5000 fine and up to three years in prison where the offender is not the mother and $200 and six months in prison where the offender is the mother.[75]

ENDNOTES

1. *Stedman's Medical Dictionary* (23d ed, Williams and Wilkins, Baltimore 1976).
2. T. Beauchamp, *The Moral Standing of Animals in Medical Research,* 20 Law Med. Health Care 7-16, at 9 (1992).
3. "Persons" generally are capable of reason, self-awareness, social involvement, and moral reciprocity. *See supra* note 2.
4. B.M. Knoppers & S. LeBris, *Recent Advances in Medically Assisted Conception,* 17 Am. J. L. Med. 329-361, at 333 (1991). The embryonic heart begins to beat by about day 21 of gestation. Brain waves are detectable by day 40. There is evidence of fetal respiratory movement ("breathing" amniotic fluid) by the end of the third month of gestation, which is thought to prepare the lungs for extrauterine life.
5. M.A. Warren, *Abortion,* in *A Companion to Ethics,* 311 (P. Singer ed., Blackwell, Cambridge, Mass. 1993).
6. *Supra* note 4, at 337.
7. "Many neurophysiologists believe that normal human fetuses begin to have some rudimentary capacity for sentience at some stage in the second trimester of pregnancy." *See supra* note 5, at 309.
8. M. Smith, *Realism,* in *A Companion to Ethics,* 403 (P. Singer ed., Blackwell, Cambridge, Mass. 1993).
9. S. Buckle, *Natural Law,* in *A Companion to Ethics,* 162, 170 (P. Singer ed., Blackwell, Cambridge, Mass. 1993).
10. D. Wong, *Relativism,* in *A Companion to Ethics,* 448 (P. Singer ed., Blackwell, Cambridge, Mass. 1993).
11. *Roe v. Wade,* 410 U.S. 113 (1973).
12. *Planned Parenthood v. Casey,* No. 91-744 and 91-902, U.S. Sup. Ct., (1992).
13. Under the "undue burden" test, state laws are invalid if they have the purpose or effect of placing a substantial obstacle in the path of a woman seeking to abort a nonviable fetus.
14. M.A. Field, *Abortion Law Today,* 14 J. Legal Med. 13 (1993).
15. *Dietrich v. Inhabitants of Northampton,* 138 Mass. 14 (1884).
16. *Allaire v. St. Luke's Hospital,* 184 Ill. 359, 56 N.E. 638 (1900).
17. *Bonbrest v. Kotz,* 65 F.Supp. 138 (D.D.C. 1946).
18. *See, e.g., Kelly v. Gregory,* 125 N.Y.S. 2d 696 (App. Div. 1953).
19. M.L. Mascaro, *Preconception Tort Liability: Recognizing a Strict Liability Cause of Action for DES Grandchildren,* 17 Am. J. L. Med. 435-455, at 437 (1991).
20. *Jorgensen v. Meade Johnson Laboratories,* 483 F. 2d 237 (10th Cir. 1973).
21. *Renslow v. Mennonite Hosp.,* 67 Ill. 2d 348, 367 N.E. 2d 1250 (1977).
22. *Albala v. City of New York,* 54 N.Y. 2d 269, 429 N.E. 2d 786, 445 N.Y.S. 2d 108 (1981).
23. *Catherwood v. American Sterilizer Company,* 126 A.D. 2d 978, 511 N.Y.S. 2d 805 (N.Y. App. Div. 1987).
24. *Enright v. Eli Lilly & Co.,* 77 N.Y. 2d 377, 570 N.E. 2d 198, 568 N.Y.S. 2d 550 (1991).
25. *Sorrels v. Eli Lilly & Co.,* 737 F.Supp. 678 (1990).
26. W. Prosser & W. Keeton, *The Law of Torts,* § 55 at 368 (5th ed. 1984).
27. *Verkennes v. Corniea,* 38 N.W. 2d 838 (Minn. 1949).
28. *See Farley v. Sartin,* 195 W.Va. 671, 466 S.E. 2d 522, 528 n.13 (W.Va. 1995); *see also* G.A. Meadows, *Wrongful Death and the Lost Society of the Unborn,* 13 J. Legal Med. 99-114, at 103 (1992).
29. *Grodin v. Grodin,* 102 Mich. App. 396, 301 N.W. 2d 869 (1980).
30. R.I. Solomon, *Future Fear: Prenatal Duties Imposed by Private Parties,* 17 Am. J. L. Med. 411-434, at 412 (1991).
31. E. Coke, *The Third Part of the Institutes of the Laws of England* 50 (Printed by W. Rawlins, for Thomas Basset at the George near St. Dunstans church in Fleetstreet, London 1628), photo reprint (1979).
32. *Supra* note 30, at 413.
33. *Gloria C. v. William C.,* 124 Misc. 2d 313, 476 N.Y.S. 2d 991 (N.Y. Fam. Ct. 1984).
34. G.J. Annas et al., *American Health Law,* 978 (Little, Brown & Co., Boston 1990).
35. *Commonwealth v. Cass,* 392 Mass. 799, 467 N.E. 2d 1324 (1984), construing Mass. Gen. Laws Ann. ch. 90, § 246(a) (1984 & Supp. 1991) to include a fetus as a person.
36. Washington Post, Nov 25, 1989, at A4.
37. *Florida v. Johnson,* No. E89-890-CFA slip op. (Seminole Cnty., Cir. Ct. July 13, 1989)
38. *Johnson v. Florida,* No. 89-1765 (Dist. Ct. App., 5th Dist., Apr. 18, 1991).
39. *Whitner v. South Carolina,* op# 24468, 1996 SC LEXIS 120.
40. *Florida v. Kawana M. Ashley,* 670 So. 2d 1087.
41. St. Petersburg Times, Aug 18, 1996, p. 9A, col. 1.
42. M.A. Field, *Controlling the Woman to Protect the Fetus,* 17 Law, Med. & Health Care 114 (1989).
43. *Raleigh Fitkin-Paul Morgan Memorial Hospital v. Anderson,* 201 A. 2d 537; *cert. denied,* 377 U.S. 985 (1964).
44. *Jefferson v. Griffin Spaulding County Hosp.,* 274 Ga. 86, 247 S.E. 2d 457 (1981).
45. *In re A.C.,* 573 A. 2d 1235 (D.C. 1990).
46. *Id.* at 1237.
47. Patrick T. Murphy, the public guardian in Cook County, Ill., and the representative of the fetus, maintained that the woman should not be physically compelled to undergo a cesarean; rather, it was his position that if she disobeyed a court order to have the operation, she should be fined.
48. New York Times, Dec 15, 1993, at A22, col. 5; *see also* New York Times, Dec 19, 1993, at 35, col. 1.
49. Newsday, Dec 31, 1993, at 7, col. 1.
50. *Taft v. Taft,* 446 N.E. 2d 395 (Mass. 1983).
51. *In re Jamaica Hosp.,* 491 N.Y.S. 2d 898 (S.Ct. Queens Co. 1985).
52. *Buch v. Armory Mfg. Co.,* 69 N.H. 257, 44 A. 809, 1897.
53. F. Cahn, *The Moral Decision,* 190 (Indiana University Press, Bloomington, Ind. 1955). These "intimate relations" or exceptions to the no-duty rule, which have been deemed to create or impose an affirmative duty to rescue, include the following situations: (1) cases where a special relationship exists between the plaintiff and defendant; (2) cases where the defendant is bound contractually to rescue the plaintiff; (3) cases where the danger or injury to the plaintiff is due to the defendant's own conduct; (4) cases where the defendant has already undertaken to rescue the plaintiff; and (5) cases where the defendant is required statutorily to rescue the plaintiff.
54. *Wagner v. International Railway Co.,* 232 N.Y. 176 (1921).
55. *Supra* note 53, at 191.
56. S.S. Mattingly, *The Maternal-Fetal Dyad,* 22 Hastings Center Report 13-18 (Jan/Feb 1992).
57. International Union, *UAW v. Johnson Controls,* 886 F. 2d 871 (7th Cir. 1989) (en banc), *cert. granted,* 110 S.Ct. 1522 (1990), *rev'd* 111 S.Ct. 1196 (1991).
58. 42 U.S.C.A. § 2000e (West 1981 & Supp. 1991).
59. Pub. L. No. 95-555, § 1, 92 Stat. 2076 (codified as amended at 42 U.S.C.A. § 2000e(k)).
60. L.D. Wardle, *Protecting the Rights of Conscience of Health Care Providers,* 14 J. Legal Med. 177-230 (1993).

61. *See, e.g.,* Iowa Code Ann. § 146.1; 42 U.S.C. § 300a-7(a).

62. *Supra* note 60, at 184-185.

63. *Id.* at 193.

64. *Id.* at 219-221.

65. *Id.* at 199.

66. Saltarelli, *Genesis Retold: Legal Issues Raised by the Cryopreservation of Preimplantation Human Embryos,* 36 Syr. L. Rev. 1021 (1985-1986).

67. C. Perry & L.K. Schneider, *Cryopreserved Embryos: Who Shall Decide Their Fate?* 13 J. Legal Med. 463-500, at 471 (1992).

68. *Davis v. Davis,* No. 34, slip op. (Tenn. Sup. Ct., June 1, 1992).

69. *Davis v. Davis,* 1990 Tenn. App. LEXIS 642 (13 Sept. 1990).

70. *Supra* note 68.

71. Ethics Committee of the American Fertility Society, *Ethical Considerations of the New Reproductive Technologies,* 53 Fertil. Steril. 37S, 58S (Supp. 2, June 1990).

72. La. Rev. Stat. Ann. § 9:123 (West 1991).

73. Mo. Rev. Stat. § 1.205(2) (Supp. 1992).

74. N.Y. Penal Law § 125.05 (McKinney 1987).

75. Wis. Stat. Ann.§ 940.04 (West 1982).

GENERAL REFERENCES

R.H. Blank, *Maternal-Fetal Relationship: The Courts and Social Policy,* 14 J. Legal Med. 73-92 (1993).

A.M. Capron, *Fetal Alcohol and Felony,* 22 Hastings Center Report 28-29 (May/June 1992).

A.M. Capron, *Parenthood and Frozen Embryos: More Than Property and Privacy,* 22 Hastings Center Report 32-33 (Sept/Oct 1992).

S.A. Garcia, *Drug Addiction and Mother/Child Welfare: Rights, Laws, and Discretionary Decisionmaking,* 13 J. Legal Med. 129-203 (1992).

J.C. Merrick, *Maternal Substance Abuse During Pregnancy,* 14 J. Legal Med. 57-71 (1993).

J.A. Robertson, *Casey and the Resuscitation of Roe v. Wade,* 22 Hastings Center Report 24-28 (1992).

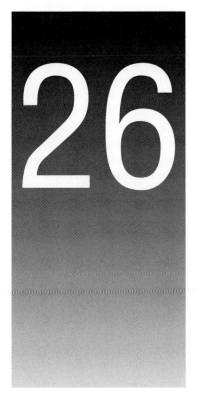

Organ donation and transplantation

Transplantation has been a viable treatment for end-stage renal disease (ESRD) since the late 1960s, and within the last decade it has become viable treatment for other organ failure, particularly since the advent of the immunosuppressant cyclosporine in the mid-1980s. Newer immunosuppressants, such as FK506 and mycophenolate (CellCept), have expanded therapeutic options and helped improve graft and patient survivals. Transplantation for most solid organs has moved beyond the experimental stage.

In 1995 there were 11,818 kidney transplants, 2361 heart transplants, 3923 liver transplants, 871 lung transplants, and 1027 pancreas transplants (majority were combined kidney-pancreas transplants) in the United States.[1] Transplants for all organs except heart-lung have increased each of the past several years, but growth has been limited by a shortage of donors. Pancreas transplantation has seen the most dramatic growth, doubling since 1990. In addition, 45,000 corneas and countless other tissues, such as heart valves, blood, skin, bone, and dural tissue, were transplanted.[2]

The 1-year patient survival rate for kidney transplants in which the organ is donated by a living relative is now 93%, and for cadaveric kidney transplants it is 85%, up from 50% one decade before. The 1-year survival rate is 84% for heart transplants, 76% for liver transplants, and 79% for pancreas transplants.[3]

Transplantation centers have multiplied and no longer are limited to academic institutions. As of early 1997, 281 medical institutions were operating organ transplant programs, including more than 255 kidney centers, 164 heart centers, 121 liver centers, 94 lung centers, and 124 pancreas centers. Approximately 63 organ procurement organizations operate in 11 designated regions.[4]

In general the demand for tissue and organs far outstrips the supply. In the United States as of June 1997, more than 36,000 patients were on kidney waiting lists, 3800 on heart lists, 2000 on pancreas or kidney-pancreas lists, and 8500 on liver waiting lists.[5]

Potential demand for vital organs is likely to increase as the indications for transplantation expand. Age limitations, for example, have become a relative contraindication. As procedures and immunosuppressives are refined and reimbursement mechanisms become better established, more potential recipients will seek transplantation. The U.S. Senate report on the National Organ Transplant Act (NOTA) stated, "It is estimated that with

The Editorial Committee updated this chapter. The committee acknowledges the past contribution of Mary Jo Wiley, M.S.N., J.D.; S. John Swanson III, M.D., F.A.C.S.; and Victor Walter Weedn, M.D., J.D., F.C.L.M.

recent improvements in transplantation surgery and medical management as many as 10% of our population at some time may be candidates for transplantation surgery in the future."[6]

The traditional procurement policy of "voluntarism" has been inadequate. The potential supply of organs is limited to the estimated 20,000 patients declared brain dead in the United States each year, but organs are actually harvested from only about 15% of these.[7] The increasing need for organs and the inadequacy of initial voluntary efforts have been the driving forces behind much of the legislation concerning transplantation. In 1968 the Uniform Anatomical Gift Act (UAGA) was promulgated to facilitate cadaver donations. Later statutes were amended to allow for donation by a signature on the back of drivers' licenses. Brain death statutes were passed to allow removal of vital organs from artificially maintained bodies. Medicare funding and the Joint Commission on Accreditation of Healthcare Organizations (JCAHO) standards now mandate that hospitals have protocols for routinely approaching families for organ donations. States have passed required request and routine injury laws. Implied consent for corneas from medical examiner cases has been adopted in many states. As the pressure for organs mounts, policymakers will increasingly move away from voluntary to compulsory systems of procurement.

The major legal problems pertinent to transplantation are consent or authorization to donate, the determination of death in the case of procurement from a cadaver, and the rationing of organs and medical resources.

STATE ANATOMICAL GIFT ACTS

The foundation for the law on organ procurement in the United States is the UAGA, which provides the legal authorization for the system of voluntary donations and specifically defines the legal mechanisms for organ and tissue donations. In an effort to promote organ and tissue procurement, the National Conference of Commissioners on Uniform State Laws (NCCUSL) and the American Bar Association, after 3 years of deliberation, drafted the model act in 1968.[8] By 1972 all 50 states, the District of Columbia, and Puerto Rico had adopted the UAGA, spurred on by the excitement over heart transplantation. Many of the states modified the UAGA during enactment or by later amendments. A substantially altered 1987 version of the UAGA, embodying new legal developments and other legislation, has been promulgated by the NCCUSL (Appendix 26-2).[9] As of August 1996 it had been adopted by 19 states (Arizona, Arkansas, California, Connecticut, Hawaii, Idaho, Iowa, Minnesota, Montana, Nevada, New Mexico, North Dakota, Oregon, Rhode Island, Utah, Vermont, Virginia, Washington, and Wisconsin), and the remaining states have all retained some version of the 1968 UAGA. However, many states that have not formally adopted the 1987 UAGA and that effectively repealed the 1968 UAGA have amended their UAGA several times over the years, blurring the distinctions. Therefore every state has adopted some version of the 1987 UAGA.[10]

The UAGA authorizes persons or their families to make an "anatomical gift" of all or part of his or her body to take effect upon death. The legally binding right to direct the disposition of one's own remains after death is a new right created by the UAGA. Previously, as a carry-over from the original common law of England, one had no property rights in his or her body after death. Individuals could not clearly bequeath their bodies, and heirs could nullify or overrule bequests. Even families did not have full property rights in bodies but rather a limited right to possess the body for burial purposes. Bodies were considered "quasiproperty."[11,12]

According to the 1968 UAGA, any person 18 years of age or older and "of sound mind" can execute an anatomical gift. Many states have substituted different age requirements. The requirement for a sound mind has been deleted from the 1987 UAGA. An anatomical part includes organs, tissues, eyes, bones, arteries, blood, other fluids, and other portions of the human body. Any condition can be imposed on the gift, but if the condition is inappropriate or unacceptable, it should be declined.

Gifts by a decedent

The decedent's wishes, if known, are to be carried out despite the wishes of the next of kin. Knowledge of religious beliefs may constitute knowledge of the decedent's intentions. In *In re Moyer's Estate* the Utah Supreme Court found that this posthumous control over one's body was "in the public interest" as long as it was not "absurd" or "preposterous."[13] In *Holland v. Metalious,* the deceased willed her eyes to an eye bank and her body to one of two medical schools.[14] The New Hampshire Supreme Court stated that the wishes of the decedent should usually be carried out, but because the medical schools had declined to accept the donation (because of objections of the spouse and children), the court ruled that the surviving spouse could determine the disposition of the body. No survivor has the legal right to veto a valid gift by the decedent; however, as a practical matter, if the family objects to the donation over the expressed desire of the decedent, it may be prudent to decline the decedent's donation.

Gifts by next of kin

When the deceased has not indicated his or her intentions, the UAGA spells out specifically who among those available at the time of death may make an anatomical gift of the body or body parts. The UAGA first designates the spouse, and if the spouse is not available at the time of death, then an adult son or daughter, followed by either parent, then an adult sibling. If none of the aforementioned is available, a guardian of the decedent at the time of the death or any other person authorized or under an obligation to dispose of the body (e.g., the medical examiner or anatomical board) may donate the body or body parts.

Consent by one next of kin (e.g., one brother) is legally negated by the objection of another of the same class of next of kin (e.g., another brother), although inquiry of all in a class is not required to exclude the possibility that someone might object, as confirmed in *Leno v. St Joseph Hospital*.[15] New York allows any family member to veto a gift by any other family member; in Florida a spouse cannot make a donation over the objection of an adult son or daughter.

The statute does not address the status of divorced or separated spouses, stepparents, stepchildren, other dependents, designated caregivers, those appointed power of attorney, and others. The list of next of kin to be approached for organ donation in the UAGA is not necessarily the same as that for inheritance, autopsy consent, or even required request statutes. Consent by next of kin must be timely; the specified individuals must make the gift "after or immediately upon death." This provides little guidance as to the time and diligence necessary in attempting to contact these persons before considering them "unavailable." Time limits for the harvest of particular organs and tissues are clearly relevant.

Execution of the gift

The gift may be executed by a will or other document. Such provisions in typical estate wills are discouraged because they are usually not immediately available at the time of death. The use of "living wills" is preferred because they are immediately available as part of the medical record. Two witnesses are necessary to validate a gift during the donor's lifetime, but none is required in the case of a gift by next of kin. Some states have relaxed or eliminated (as in the 1987 UAGA) this witness requirement, whereas other states have statutorily specified witness requirements. The next of kin can make gifts by a signed document or by telegraphic or recorded message. The 1987 UAGA would also allow other forms of communication reduced to writing and signed by the recipient. Neither delivery nor public filing is necessary to make the gift effective. The gift can be revoked or amended by a signed statement, an oral statement in the presence of two witnesses, or a statement to an attending physician.

Any card, form, or even sticker may be carried by the donor to evidence the intention of the gift. During the mid-1970s, 44 states incorporated legislation to enable organ and tissue donation by the mere signing of the back of a driver's license. Most organ procurement agencies and transplant surgeons do not accept such a signature by itself (so-called pocket wills) but rather require the contemporaneous consent of the next of kin. They speculate that the decedent may have changed his or her mind since the signing and that they could not afford the negative publicity that might occur in the face of objections by the family. Use of donor cards is mandated in the 1987 UAGA, which requires law enforcement officers and emergency rescue personnel to make a reasonable search for a document of gift and then requires the hospital to cooperate in the implementation of the anatomical gift. Routine inquiry further emphasizes acceptance of documents of a decedent's wishes and provides a mechanism to check the currency of the card.

Persons accepting a gift

Any specified person, physician, hospital, accredited medical school or university, tissue bank, or procurement agency can accept an anatomical gift for education, research, therapy, or transplantation. Several states additionally allow donation to anatomical boards, which generally receive unclaimed bodies for educational purposes. In Connecticut the state commissioner of health must approve recipients. The attending physician is the presumed donee, if a donee is not specified. The attending physician who makes a determination of death is excluded from participating in any part of the transplant procedures, although it does not prevent him or her from communicating with the transplant team. The term *hospital* is substituted for the term *attending physician* in the 1987 version of the act.

The intentions of the donor must be respected, including any condition imposed on the gift. A donee can accept or reject a gift. The donee of the entire body can authorize embalming and funeral services. One provision authorizes any postmortem examination necessary to ensure medical acceptability of the donated organ, including an autopsy. The donee of a part must remove the part without unnecessary mutilation and then relinquish custody to the next of kin or other person under obligation to dispose of the body. The drafters chose not to deal with the issue of compensation for processing the gift.

The UAGA does not qualify in any way the legal right of a physician, organ procurement organization, or transplant team who receives a donated organ to do with it what they perceive as properly carrying out the intentions of the family. It has been argued that the donee holder of an organ is the owner of the organ and thus has the absolute right, limited only by any express covenant of purpose, to choose the ultimate organ recipient. It also has been argued that the intermediary party is an agent of the donor or the donor's family and is liable for failure to comply with their wishes. It has even been espoused that the donee is a public trustee who is liable for negligence (or perhaps conversion) to a prospective recipient for an inappropriate selection.

Medical examiners

Most vital organs are retrieved from patients who are declared brain dead because most natural deaths render organs unsuitable for transplants. Approximately 50% of brain deaths result from motor vehicle accidents or other violence and therefore fall under the jurisdiction of the coroner or medical examiner. The UAGA states that it is subject to other state laws governing autopsies; thus medical examiner and coroner laws take precedence. Comments to the original 1968 NCCUSL act state that it

is necessary to preclude the frustration of the important medical examiner's duties in cases of death by suspected crime or violence. . . . It may prove desirable in many if not most states to reexamine and amend the medical examiner statutes to authorize and direct medical examiners to expedite their autopsy procedures in cases in which the public interest will not suffer.

The 1986 National Task Force on Transplantation also recommended enactment of laws that would encourage coroners and medical examiners to give permission for organ and tissue procurement from cadavers under their jurisdiction.

Many states have "implied consent" statutes that allow harvest of corneas from medical examiner cases when no known objection to the harvest exists. The 1987 version of the UAGA provides that the medical examiner may authorize removal of an organ or tissue for transplant purposes if it will not interfere with the postmortem investigation and if the medical examiner does not know of an objection to the donation after making a reasonable effort, and taking into account the useful life of the part, to find documentation of the decedent's intention and to contact the next of kin.

Immunity

The physician who removes an organ in good faith is protected from civil and criminal liability by the UAGA. Mississippi and Montana grant civil immunity only; South Carolina makes an exception for malpractice. In *Nicoletta v. Rochester Eye and Human Parts Bank,* parties recovering organs were protected when they relied on the good faith belief that a person consenting to donation was a surviving spouse when in fact she was not.[16] This provision of immunity withstood constitutional attack in *Williams v. Hofmann.*[17]

The provision applies only to valid gifts. The UAGA takes effect only after death has been declared; it does not afford protection to the pronouncement of death itself. Failure to comply with the provisions of the act (e.g., no unnecessary mutilation of the body) may demonstrate bad faith. However, the act's provisions are to be construed liberally to achieve its stated goal of promoting organ and tissue donations. In *Ravenis v. Detroit General Hospital* the Michigan Court of Appeals ruled that the protection did not preclude liability for the negligent failure of a hospital to screen a donor adequately for disease that was subsequently transmitted to a recipient.[18] Thus courts may interpret this provision of immunity to be inapplicable to malpractice.

Most states also have protective clauses in their blood banking statutes that specifically maintain that blood transfusions, organ procurement procedures, and transplants are to be regarded as services rather than sales of products; accordingly, members of the transplant team are exempt from strict product liability.

The 1987 UAGA revision

The 1987 NCCUSL model act, among other things, added provisions for routine inquiry, required requests, presumed consent for medical examiner cases, and prohibition of the sale of organs (Appendix 26-2).[19] These substantial new provisions codify in the UAGA legislation what has to some extent been adopted elsewhere. These issues are discussed in the following sections.

ROUTINE INQUIRY OR REQUIRED REQUEST

Possible policy solutions to increase voluntary organ and tissue donations include routine inquiry, required request, and presumed or implied consent legislation. Only 1 of 25 hospital deaths provides material suitable for organ donation, although 24 of 25 deaths provide material suitable for tissue donations.[20] An estimated 17,000 to 26,000 potential organ donors die each year in the United States.[21] Only 15% to 20% of potential donors become actual donors (about 2600 in 1984).[22,23] However, approximately 70% to 75% of families were approached for permission to grant donation.[24] The limiting factor appears to be the inadequate request and referral by the health care team.[25-28]

Recognizing the problem, Arthur Caplan called for "required request" legislation, which would force providers to approach families for donation in appropriate cases.[29] This legislation focuses on the consent of surviving family members. "Routine inquiry," on the other hand, refers to asking a patient on hospital admission if he or she is an organ donor. This method focuses on the advance decision of the individual and his or her right to self-determinism, which is the proper priority according to the UAGA. Furthermore, it saves valuable time by preempting the need to contact the family before procurement. However, some have argued that queries during admission to the hospital are poorly timed because potential patients may feel apprehensive either that the care they receive might be substandard if they fail to comply with a request for donations or that medical providers might be less vigorous in resuscitative attempts if they do comply.[30]

Required request is now found in the laws of most states, in federal Medicare and Medicaid conditions of participation, and in JCAHO standards of accreditation.[31,32] Both the JCAHO and Medicare merely require that a hospital have written protocol. Most current state legislation has been enacted in the form of amendments to state anatomical gift acts and rather closely tracks the federal law. State laws are typically more detailed and sweeping and apply to unaccredited, nonparticipating hospitals. However, state laws are generally weak and vary greatly; few states even require documentation of the request, which would allow for enforcement, and several create institutional exemptions and wide discretionary exceptions for requests. Approximately half the states have weak versions of required request in which the sole requirement is a mere written hospital policy of routine requests of family members. In some states the request must be made by the physician, whereas in others the request must be made by a designated member of the hospital staff or of the regional organ procurement agency. Appropriate training of the requester is sometimes required. Half the states require documentation of the inquiry and its disposition; in many states this documentation is in a log book, a central registry, or a place other than the medical record.

There are numerous exceptions to the requirement of request based on considerations such as medical criteria, known objection, or religion. In Alabama the attending physician can decide that inquiry should not be made. In Massachusetts, exception is allowed when discussion would cause the family undue emotional distress. Lobbying efforts have exempted hospitals in several states.[33]

Early measures requiring request have doubled and tripled overall tissue procurement, but vital organ procurement, which was the target of the legislation, has increased only modestly. Legal sanctions may be imposed if these provisions are not followed or are insufficient. The Health Care Financing Administration (HCFA) is seeking ways to assess compliance with Medicare and Medicaid required request regulations.[34]

The 1987 UAGA has provisions for both routine inquiry and required request (Section 5). Documentation is to be placed in the medical record. The hospital administrator is responsible for implementation, and the Commissioner of Health is responsible for oversight. Furthermore, the legislation mandates that donor cards be sought and respected. Law enforcement agents, emergency personnel, and hospital personnel are to make a reasonable search for a donor card or other documentation of gift at the time of death or "near" the time of death. When evidence of a desire to donate is found, the hospital is to cooperate in the implementation of the gift. Administrative (but not criminal or civil) sanctions are to be imposed.

In an effort to increase public awareness of and improve hospital participation in the donor program, Pennsylvania Act 102 amended the state's UAGA in 1994. The new law changed the way hospitals handle the identification and referral of potential donors and the request for anatomical donations, requiring hospitals to work with the organ procurement organization after every hospital death. In addition to formalizing the process of required request, the new law allows Pennsylvania drivers to indicate donor consent on the front of their driver's license; state Department of Transportation computer records are accessible 24 hours a day. The new law also created an Organ Donation Awareness Trust Fund for educational purposes and set up a contribution system tied to driver's license renewal and state income tax filings. To ensure compliance, Act 102 stipulates that a hospital can be fined up to $500 for every death not reported. The legislation also mandates that the state Department of Health conduct medical reviews to compare organ procurement organizations' referral records to hospitals' death records, which can be used to measure compliance rates.[35]

Pennsylvania's routine referral law has increased referrals and donations dramatically throughout the state. Since the law was enacted, the state has experienced a 26% increase in the number of donors and a 36% increase in the number of transplants.[36] The legislation's success has marked an important milestone in addressing the organ shortage in Pennsylvania and has sent a message to other states that enacting similar legislation may be a key to increasing their donation rates. As of June 1997 at least eight states had enacted routine referral laws, and several more are expected to follow suit.[37]

PRESUMED OR IMPLIED CONSENT

Presumed consent laws, in which consent is presumed in the absence of actual knowledge of objection, are common in Europe. It is a policy of "opting out" instead of "opting in." It has not been a popular notion in the United States, but as demand continues to outstrip the supply for organs and tissues, presumed consent will be increasingly favored by policymakers. Even in countries with implied consent laws, families are regularly asked permission for donations.[38]

A number of states have enacted legislation authorizing medical examiners to have corneas removed based on presumed consent. These laws allow removal of the corneas when the death falls under the jurisdiction of the medical examiner, when removal of the corneas will not interfere with the investigation or disturb the appearance of the body, and when there is no known objection from the next of kin. Maryland passed the first such law in 1975. These presumed consent laws have been highly effective in increasing the supply of corneas.

Statutes vary remarkably in the degree of diligence required in attempting to locate family members. Some states require no effort, others require reasonable effort, some require a good faith effort, some specify attempts for a 4-hour period, and some specify attempts for a 24-hour period unless the organ or tissue would become unfit earlier. Numerous instances of families becoming outraged after corneas have been retrieved from loved ones have resulted in litigation and in Texas in a change in the law.[39]

In *Powell v. Florida* the implied consent statute for removal of corneas by medical examiners was upheld by the Florida Supreme Court.[40] Two sets of parents sued when the corneas of their sons were removed by medical examiners without their consent or without any attempt to give them notice. The court found that the legislation was reasonable, did not violate due process or equal protection requirements, and served a public purpose. It noted that the state of Florida was spending $138 million per year to support its blind citizenry, that corneal transplantation is in great demand, and that it is frequently successful in restoring sight. The court determined that recovery from medical examiner autopsy cases was the most important source of quality tissue and that removal of the corneal tissue, which did not affect the decedent's appearance, was an insignificant bodily intrusion compared with the autopsy itself. The court cited California statistics that approximately 80% of the families of decedents could not be located in time for medical examiners to remove usable corneal tissue. The court further held that the next of kin has no property right in the remains of the decedent but merely a limited right to possess the body for burial purposes. Similarly, medical examiner implied consent statutes have withstood constitutional challenge in Georgia and Michigan.[41,42]

In *Kirker v. Orange County* a mother was awarded damages for the intentional infliction of emotional distress caused by the "mutilation of her daughter's body" when the medical examiner granted permission to remove the child's eyeballs despite an expressed refusal for corneal donation in the medical record.[43] The medical examiner should have known of the objection. An attempted coverup was also shown.

As previously mentioned, the 1987 model act includes a provision authorizing any organ or tissue donation by a medical examiner for transplantation based on a presumed consent provided that a reasonable effort is made to discover any appropriate objection. Maryland and California have expanded presumed consent beyond medical examiner situations to include patients dying in hospitals.

CADAVER ORGANS: DETERMINATION OF DEATH

Most kidneys (80%), most livers (except those from living parental donors), and all hearts for transplantation are harvested from patients who have been declared brain dead and maintained on life support. In such cases a determination of death is necessary. Patients experiencing traumatic deaths often are not brain dead but die of cardiac arrest. An estimated five to six times more donors have no heartbeat than are brain dead.[44] Protocols for such donors have been established in several centers; rapid, timely management of the cadaver may allow organ recovery after the heart has stopped and the patient has been declared dead. The premature removal of organs may subject the physicians to civil and criminal liability.

The law has always held that a person is dead when a licensed physician pronounces him or her dead, if the determination is based on accepted medical standards. Brain death has become an accepted standard, and every court that has examined the question has held it a legally proper determination, regardless of the presence or absence of a state brain death statute. However, medical standards for determination of brain death have become rigorous in many jurisdictions, and failure to adhere to methods for determination specified by such standards may result in liability.

The physician who removes an organ in good faith may be protected from civil and criminal liability by the UAGA. This act appears to take effect only after death has been declared. However, it is to be construed liberally so that its stated goal of promoting organ and tissue donations may be achieved and conflicts of interest avoided (Section 7). The act specifically states that the physician who makes the determination of death "shall not participate in the procedures for removing or transplanting a part."

In *Tucker v. Lower* the brother of an organ donor alleged that the organs had been removed before the donor was legally dead.[45] At the time, Virginia had not yet adopted a brain death standard. The jury found for the surgeon based on the instruction that death could be determined if there was complete and irreversible loss of brain function.

However, in *Strachan v. John F. Kennedy Memorial Hospital* the court ruled that the hospital was liable for delaying the release of a body while attempting to change the parent's decision not to donate. An emergency department physician had diagnosed brain death 3 days before the official pronouncement of death and disconnection of the respirator.[46]

ORGANS AND TISSUES FROM FETUSES AND ANENCEPHALIC INFANTS

The national organ shortage is much more critical for pediatric organs (especially livers) than for adult organs. Less than 6% of organ donations are from donors 5 years of age and under.[47] It has been estimated that the potential demand each year for infant organs is approximately 1000 livers and 500 hearts and kidneys.[48] This is a conservative estimate because approximately 7500 infants with life-threatening congenital heart defects are born each year.[49] As of June 1997 the United Network for Organ Sharing listed 89 patients under 5 years of age who were waiting for a kidney, 355 patients waiting for a liver, 90 patients waiting for a heart, and 14 patients waiting for a heart-lung block.[50] Half the transplant candidates die before an organ becomes available. In comparison with adults, a very small number of infants and children die with transplant-suitable organs.

Anencephalic infants represent an important potential source of fetal organs. Organs from such infants could meet the bulk of the current demand for infant organs. Organs from stillborns and infants dying from other diseases generally are not suitable for procurement and transplantation.

Anencephaly is an abnormality of primary neurulation commencing within the first month of gestation and resulting in the congenital absence of a major portion of the brain, skull, and scalp. Cranial neural tissue is exposed and often protrudes from the skull defect. Both cerebral hemispheres are absent or unrecognizable. Although some rudimentary cerebral development can occur, there is no functioning cerebral cortex. Anencephalic children cannot reason and presumably cannot suffer. The term *monster* has been applied to this anomaly, which represents the most severe form of neural tube defect (spina bifida). Anencephaly is a universally fatal condition. Two thirds of anencephalic infants die in utero. Very few survive beyond 1 week after birth. Infants provided maximal support may survive somewhat longer, but when strict diagnostic criteria are applied, survival still does not exceed 2 months. Longer survival periods have been reported; however, the diagnostic criteria were not well documented. Cases of amniotic band syndrome, ruptured encephalocele, and iniencephaly are sometimes confused with the diagnosis of anencephaly and probably account for the rare cases of prolonged survival reported in the literature.

Between 13% and 33% of infants born with anencephaly have defects of the nonneural organs. These defects may complicate care and render their organs unsuitable for donation.

Estimates of the incidence of anencephaly have varied from 0.3 to 7 per 1000 births.[51] Differences result from, among other things, different diagnostic criteria, true geographical differences, and prenatal screening programs. Prenatal detection of anencephaly usually results in early termination of pregnancy; thus screening programs can dramatically reduce the incidence of anencephaly at birth. The Centers for Disease Control and Prevention (CDC) cites an incidence of 0.3 per 1000 births (live births and stillbirths).[52] Extrapolation of this figure would indicate that more than 1000 infants are born with anencephaly annually in the United States, but this figure would drop to less than 100 if screening and induced abortion were uniformly applied.

The first transplant of the heart of an anencephalic infant occurred in October 1987 at the Loma Linda University Medical Center in California without legal incident. Subsequently, other parents requested that their anencephalic children be used as donors to help other children. This meant that the pregnancies were carried to term rather than terminated. With parental permission, the live-born anencephalic children were then placed on respiratory support and their organs donated if brain death criteria were fulfilled within 1 week. Only 1 of 12 anencephalic newborns met brain death criteria, and no recipient could be found for his organs; consequently the program was suspended. One of the infants survived for 2 months after the respirator was removed.[53]

The Medical Task Force on Anencephaly reported in March 1990 that it was able to identify 80 anencephalic infants who were involved in transplantation protocols.[54] Only 41 of the infants were used as sources of organs, providing 37 kidneys, two livers, and three hearts.

A major problem with organ donation from anencephalic infants is that legal criteria for brain death are not easily applied. Brain death criteria are derived from the Uniform Determination of Death Act, in which a declaration of brain death is based on irreversible cessation of all brain functions, including those of the brainstem (so-called whole brain death). Although anencephalic infants have no higher cortical function, they may have good brainstem function. Therefore they have intact circulatory and respiratory function; have good reflexes; may cry, swallow, and regurgitate; and may respond to pain, vestibular stimuli, and sometimes sound. Frequent malformations of special sense organs and facial muscles may complicate neurological evaluations or render them impossible.[55]

Although technically incorrect, some have argued that anencephalic infants are "brain absent" and that the brain death concept is not applicable. Others have argued that anencephalic infants have no capacity to reason and thus are not "persons" within the meaning of governing statutes. They may be considered nonviable fetuses. Several states have introduced bills to allow a determination of death in anencephalic infants. One approach is for states to amend their brain death acts to declare anencephalic babies brain dead. Another approach is to change the UAGA so that the term *donor* includes those diagnosed as either brain dead or anencephalic. If an anencephalic child is a person born alive, the Baby Doe handicapped-infant regulations, requiring appropriate nutrition, hydration, and medication, may apply and arguably may prevent organ procurement until natural death.

Many commentators have alluded to a "slippery slope"; that is, creating a special category of brain death for anencephalic infants may open Pandora's box. If anencephalic babies are considered to have a marginal existence that can be sacrificed for the good of society, who else can be sacrificed? Why not extend brain death equivalence to other handicapped infants, particularly to those who are suffering from their handicap? Why limit such rationalization to neonates? What of other "brain-dead" patients, such as those in chronic persistent vegetative states? These commentators believe that the law should be consistent and that less fortunate persons should not be treated with lesser justice. If an anencephalic infant is a person and is alive, he or she is ethically worthy of respect and has legal rights.

The Medical Task Force on Anencephaly noted that anencephaly differs from a persistent vegetative state (PVS) in that (1) anencephaly is an embryological malformation, whereas PVS is an acquired condition with various etiologies; (2) in anencephaly the extent of neurological malformation is readily demonstrable by clinical examination, whereas in PVS the extent of permanent neurological damage is not always observable; (3) anencephaly can be diagnosed with certainty, whereas the diagnosis of PVS may be problematic; and (4) the prognosis for anencephaly is measured in days to weeks, whereas patients with PVS may live for months to years.[56]

The Medical Task Force on Anencephaly recognized four general approaches to organ procurement from infants with anencephaly, as follows:

1. The infant is immediately placed on maximal life-support systems at birth, and the organs are removed as soon as possible without regard to presence or absence of brainstem function.
2. The infant is immediately placed on maximal life-support systems at birth, and the organs are removed after brainstem functions are observed to stop.
3. The infant is given standard (minimal) care until he or she develops hypotension, hypoxia, bradycardia, or cardiac arrest; the infant is then placed on maximal life-support systems, and the organs are removed after brainstem functions are observed to stop.
4. The infant is given standard (minimal) care until he or she dies, and then the organs are harvested.

Of 34 anencephalic infants who were on transplantation protocols and could be thus categorized, the success rate for transplantation was 100% for the first approach but 0% to 11% for the other three approaches.[57] There is a conflict of interest between the clinician's duty to maintain the health of the donor and the duty to preserve organs for a potential recipient.

Fetal tissue has uses other than pediatric organ transplants. Fetal tissue is plastic, immunoprivileged, and available. It has been used to treat diabetes and bone marrow disorders and is a possible consideration for the treatment of Parkinson's disease, Alzheimer's disease, and almost any genetic metabolic disease.

The 1973 *Roe v. Wade* decision did not deprive the fetus of all legal protections, and subsequent regulations and judicial case law have furthered fetal rights. In particular, federal regulations regarding the protection of human subjects may apply. The 1975 Department of Health and Human Services (DHHS) Section 46.201 states that DHHS regulations apply to "research, development, and related activities involving . . . the fetus." The 1985 Health Research Extension Act prohibits federally supported research on nonviable, living fetuses ex utero unless (1) that research is for the benefit or health of the fetus; (2) the research will pose no added risk of suffering, injury, or death to the fetus; and (3) the research cannot be accomplished by other means. Some states limit experimentation on aborted fetal remains, although transplantation research is arguably not research on the remains themselves, within the meaning of the statutes. The Fifth Circuit Court of Appeals has declared Louisiana's statute prohibiting experimentation on an unborn child or a child born as a result of abortion unconstitutional.[58]

Potential sources of human fetal tissue include tissue from stillbirths, ectopic pregnancies, spontaneous abortions, and elective abortions. The tissue must be viable; sufficiently differentiated for use; of sufficient quantity for extraction and implantation; free from major genetic abnormalities or diseases; and free from bacterial, fungal, and viral contamination. These requirements generally render all fetal tissue useless, except that derived from elective abortions. In other words, as a practical matter, only tissue from elective abortions is of sufficient availability and quality to serve as a significant source of fetal tissue for transplantation.

On March 22, 1988, then DHHS Secretary Robert Windom, sparked by an National Institutes of Health (NIH) proposal to implant fetal tissue into patients with Parkinson's disease, imposed a moratorium on further NIH funding of experiments using fetal tissue pending a report from a special NIH advisory panel to examine the medical, ethical, and legal implications of using aborted fetuses for research. After several meetings, 18 of 21 panel members concluded that the use of fetal tissue from induced abortions for transplantation research would be acceptable. The panel recommended that appropriate guidelines be established and that the decision to terminate a pregnancy be kept independent from the decision to use the tissue for research. Nonetheless, on November 2, 1989, DHHS Secretary Louis Sullivan disregarded the panel's recommendations and extended the moratorium indefinitely. He indicated that such research might provide justification for women to decide to have an abortion and would likely result in an increased incidence of abortions across the country.[59-61]

The moratorium did not affect use of fetal tissue not involving transplantation into human subjects with NIH funds. The NIH could fund research using fetal tissue from spontaneous abortions or fund transplants of human fetal tissue (even from induced abortions) into animals. Moreover, the policy letter had no legal bearing on transplantation of any fetal tissue that was not federally funded.

Concern has also been raised over a market in fetal tissue for transplantation, which might result in conceptions and abortions for profit or in manipulation of abortion decisions at the risk of pregnant women. Hana Biologicals of Alameda, California, applied to the Food and Drug Administration (FDA) for permission to market fetal pancreatic tissue. Jeremy Rifkin petitioned the DHHS to declare such a sale prohibited by the NOTA.[62]

The National Institutes of Health Revitalization Act of 1993, enacted to amend the Public Health Service Act and revise and extend programs of the NIH, addresses the issue of research on transplantation of fetal tissue. According to the act, the secretary may conduct or support research on the transplantation of human fetal tissue for therapeutic purposes, regardless of whether the tissue is obtained pursuant to a spontaneous or induced abortion or pursuant to a stillbirth.[63] Under the statute, federally funded projects require a statement in writing from the woman providing the tissue, stating that she is donating the tissue for use in research, that the donation is made without any restriction regarding the identity of any recipients, and that the woman has not been informed of the identity of any recipient. In addition, the attending physician is required to make a statement in writing that the abortion was not planned to coincide with the need for the tissue. The statute also prohibits the purchase of human fetal tissue or the use of donated tissue from a specified donor (e.g., a relative).

In a report issued by the General Accounting Office, extramural projects using fetal tissue that are funded by the NIH follow federal guidelines, including informed consent requirements, and there have been no reports of violations in the methods used to obtain fetal tissue at sites conducting transplantation research.[64]

The NIH awarded more than $6 million to five extramural research projects involving therapeutic uses of human fetal tissue between fiscal 1993 and 1996; of this, $5.9 million supported human fetal tissue transplantation activities. Researchers have found that human fetal tissue can be used to treat a number of illnesses, including juvenile diabetes, leukemia, and Parkinson's disease.[65]

The British Medical Association has promulgated guidelines on the use of fetal tissue, including the condition that tissue may be obtained only from dead fetuses resulting from therapeutic or spontaneous abortion. Death of a fetus was defined as an irreversible loss of function of the organism as a whole.[66]

LIVING DONORS: DONOR CONSENT

Legal requirements for transplantation by a living donor primarily revolve around issues of consent of the donor for organ procurement. The rights of privacy and self-determination demand that adults of legal age and sound mind must give informed consent for donation of their organs or tissues. Competent adults should give consent voluntarily, knowingly, and intelligently after being fully informed of potential risks.

In the typical case the HLA-matched sibling is asked to donate a kidney. The sibling may have considerable trepidation concerning the risk, pain, and disfigurement of the surgery, as well as the potential future compromise of his or her remaining kidney. Although consent is usually granted, the potential donor may decide to refuse. There is no legal duty to be a Good Samaritan. Family and community pressure may significantly cloud the voluntariness of this consent. The issue of living, unrelated kidney donors, which was once viewed with suspicion, has now become common practice. Spousal donation is the most common, but it has been extended to friends. Again the donor shortage has prompted attempts to increase the donor pool. Living-donor protocols include extensive education and psychological evaluation to ensure informed consent.

In the case of *McFall v. Shrimp,* Robert McFall, a victim of aplastic anemia in need of a bone marrow transplant, sued to compel his cousin, David Shrimp, the only person found on initial testing to be a compatible donor, to complete his compatibility testing and if compatible to donate a portion of his marrow.[67] The marrow harvest was described to Shrimp as consisting of inserting a curved needle into his hip at least 200 times. McFall's counsel argued that there is a duty to aid another in peril of his life; the court disagreed. McFall never received a transplant and died shortly thereafter.

In the case of a vital organ transplant, a psychiatric or psychological assessment of the donor and donee may be advisable to negate possible future allegations of duress and also because of the high rates of psychiatric morbidity and suicide in recipients.

Organ donors have failed in their suits against transplant surgeons because of the absence of a physician-patient relationship. In *Sirianni v. Anna* a mother, who donated a kidney to her son after his kidneys were negligently removed by a surgeon, was not allowed to recover against the surgeon for her impairment of health, which she sustained as a result of the loss of her kidney.[68] She undertook the operation with full knowledge of the consequences.

MINORS AND INCOMPETENT DONORS

In the case of minors and incompetent (e.g., mentally impaired) persons a court order is usually necessary for the organ transplantation. Although parents and guardians gener-

ally may consent to medical treatment of their children and wards, it is not clear that they have the same authority when surgery is not medically indicated. As a practical matter, most surgeons refuse to perform such surgery without a court order. The consent of guardians or parents is often additionally sought, but the court may overcome their refusal.

In most cases involving intrafamilial transplants, judicial approval has been granted. Judges conducting these hearings in chambers have almost always allowed the harvest procedure and foregone the need for a written explanation of the court's findings. Even where a record is present, courts have not always articulated well the basis for their decision. This may be categorized best as simple judicial approval of parental consent.

In a 1972 Connecticut case, *Hart v. Brown,* the court approved a transplant between two identical 7-year-old twins, considered the medical ramifications, and stated that the parents' motivation and reasoning had met with approval of the guardians ad litem, physicians, clergy, and the court.[69]

Courts also invoke the equitable doctrine of parens patriae to give consent on behalf of minors and incompetent persons. The court often appoints a guardian ad litem in such cases to argue on behalf of the incompetent person.

If the court focuses on the interests of the potential donor with a protective eye, it may find that no objective reason exists for the donor to submit to the risk and bodily intrusion of an organ harvest. It has been argued that the court has no power to authorize the surgery in the absence of specific enabling legislation.

In the 1973 Louisiana case *In re Richardson* a husband brought suit against his wife to compel her consent to the removal of a kidney from their mentally retarded son for donation to his older sister.[70] The Fourth Circuit Court held that neither the parents nor the courts could authorize surgical intrusion on a mentally retarded minor for the purpose of donating organs, that such an authorization would invade the minor's right to freedom from bodily intrusion, and that it was not shown to be in the minor's best interest.

In 1975 the Supreme Court of Wisconsin in *In re Guardianship of Pescinski* held that the court had no power to compel a 39-year-old catatonic schizophrenic patient to donate a kidney to a 38-year-old sister in the absence of any showing of benefit to the incompetent: "[The] incompetent particularly should have his own interests protected. Certainly no advantage should be taken of him."[71] Medical testimony indicated that the risk to the donor at that time was one death in 4000 kidney transplants. The dissent stated that requirement of consent was inappropriate as applied to an incompetent person without lucid intervals.

Other courts have authorized donation by applying a "best interest" test and finding psychological benefit (or absence of detriment) and asserting consent.

In a 1979 Texas case, *Little v. Little,* a mother sought judicial consent for the removal of a kidney from her 14-year-old daughter with Down syndrome for her son.[72] The guardian was opposed. The mother argued that the daughter was the only suitable donor for her brother, that there was no threat to her life, and that the daughter would have wanted this for her ill brother. Medical testimony alleged that the daughter was a perfect match (despite brother and sister not being identical twins) and that the chance of finding a suitable cadaver kidney was extremely remote. The judge authorized the transplant on the basis of "substantial psychological benefit" to the donor.

Courts have increasingly used the doctrine of "substituted judgment" to decide medical cases involving difficult ethical issues with incompetent persons. Specifically, the court must substitute itself, as nearly as possible, for the incompetent person to act with the same motives and considerations as would have moved the individual.

In the 1969 case *Strunk v. Strunk,* the mother of a 27-year-old mentally retarded man with an IQ of 35 petitioned the court for a kidney removal to be used for his 28-year-old brother.[73] The court, based on psychiatric testimony that the death of the donor's brother would have an extremely traumatic effect on the donor, allowed the transplantation to avoid the detriment. The court reached this result despite testimony from the director of the renal division at the local institution; the director stated that, if something happened to the retarded donor's remaining kidney, he would not meet the selection criteria necessary for hemodialysis or transplantation. The dissent stated that "it is common knowledge that the loss of a close relative or a friend to a 6-year-old is not of major importance." Opinions concerning psychological trauma at best are nebulous.

CONFIDENTIALITY OF POTENTIAL DONORS

Potential donors are often HLA matched to find an immunocompatible host and thereby achieve a greater chance of graft survival. Modern immunosuppressive therapies generally obviate this need except in the case of bone marrow transplantation. The need for matched organs has given rise to expensive HLA registries. There is great pressure to give names of those individuals with matching phenotypes to potential recipients.

In the case of *Head v. Colloton* the plaintiff, William Head, had leukemia and sued to demand disclosure of the identity of the only potential donor in the institution's bone marrow transplant registry who had a matching HLA type.[74] The potential donor had been HLA typed as a possible platelet donor for an ill family member. She was telephoned by the registry and asked in general terms if she would be interested in being a bone marrow donor; she responded that she would be interested only if it was for a family member. The court maintained the anonymity of the potential donor and refused further inquiry but did so on narrow legal grounds relating to the interpretation of the Iowa Freedom of Information Act. The plaintiff died during the court proceedings without having had a marrow transplant.

Names of potential donors should be placed on registries only after they have given informed consent, and donors should be able to withdraw their names at any time. Disclosures should be restricted to necessarily involved medical personnel only.

ARTIFICIAL AND ANIMAL TRANSPLANTS

In the immediate future, organs from animals (xenografts), except porcine heart valves, will continue to play only a minor role in transplantation and will remain largely experimental. Important strides have been made in the understanding of xenograft rejection, but a major barrier to this technique remains. Genetically engineered animals, probably pigs, will incorporate human immunological factors. Baboon hearts and livers have always been rejected and thus have fallen from favor. Simians will not meet the need because of low numbers. An additional concern is the transmission of animal diseases (zoonoses).

Artificial hearts also have a poor overall record but are increasingly used for temporary replacement until a human transplant can be performed. Left ventricular assist devices, on the other hand, have become popular.

Failure to obtain adequate informed consent has been a major criticism of most pioneering efforts. Today, this issue is better recognized, and more appropriate consent procedures are being followed. All human experimentation must be reviewed by a medical institution's internal review board. The first artificial heart transplant precipitated a lawsuit, *Karp v. Cooley,* which remains the leading authority on the issue of informed consent for an experimental therapy.[75]

Special considerations exist regarding artificial organs. The Medical Device Amendment enacted in 1976 ensures the safety of medical devices and imposes strict regulations on manufacturers of artificial organs regarding interstate commerce.[76] The DHHS and FDA have responsibility to promulgate regulations under this act. These regulations were not enforced in cases of early artificial heart transplants but have since been and will continue to be enforced. Also, strict product liability may be applied to these implants.

DONOR SCREENING

Donors must be screened to determine suitability of donation. Transmission of disease from an organ or tissue donation is an important concern. Transplantation personnel must maintain constant vigilance against bacterial and fungal infections resulting from organs and tissue derived from septic patients and from contamination during handling. The implant may act as a nidus for infection. Cytomegalovirus (CMV) is the most common problem and can be clinically significant. Other serious diseases that can be transmitted via transplantation include cancer and infections with the human immunodeficiency virus (HIV), hepatitis B, tuberculosis, toxoplasmosis, and Jakob-Creutzfeldt disease. Cancer, except low-grade brain malignancies, obviates a patient as a donor. The organ may be impaired by nontransmissible disease, such as atherosclerosis; however, the donor shortage has led to expanded donor criteria, including older donors (over age 60); treated, controlled hypertensive patients; and even diabetic persons without evidence of renal disease.

Screening for transmissible disease involves chart review, specific laboratory tests, and examination of the donor. The United Network for Organ Sharing, discussed later in this chapter, requires documentation of certain tests and evaluations as minimal acceptable standards for an independent organ procurement agency.

Inadequate screening can give rise to litigation. Ordinary negligence liability results if the disease or defect is discoverable by standard medical practices. Failure to test for HIV antibody would be a breach of standard medical practice in cases of heart transplantation, but it would result in liability only if the donee subsequently developed an HIV infection. If no results were available by the time a transplantation would need to proceed, liability might not attach because a court might find that a surgeon acted reasonably. However, a court may find that the brain-dead cadaver should have been maintained until a result could have been obtained or that, if a risk factor were present in the donor's record, the donation ought to have been declined. Liability should not attach if, as can happen, HIV is transmitted despite a negative HIV antibody test; donor screening is imperfect. Faulty testing or specimen mix-ups may result in incompatible organs being transplanted, in which case liability is likely. The immunity statutes previously mentioned may protect an organ procurement agency or a transplantation team.

In *Ravenis v. Detroit General Hospital* the hospital was found negligent in two cases in which patients lost the sight remaining in an eye after transplantation of an infected cornea.[77] No hospital official was responsible for selection; slit-lamp examinations were not performed despite availability of equipment, and the appropriate information for the surgeon to determine the unsuitability of the tissue for transplantation was missing from the patient's chart.

In *Good v. Presbyterian Hospital* a medical malpractice action was brought under the informed consent theory against a transplant surgeon who performed a heart and lung transplant on a 5-year-old patient.[78] The plaintiff, the patient's mother, alleged that the surgeon failed to advise her that the organs to be transplanted had tested positive for CMV and that the virus caused the 5-year-old child's death. The court found that the transplant surgeon did not violate the New York informed consent standards, since the universal practice of reasonable medical practitioners in 1990 under similar circumstances was not to discuss specifically the CMV status of organs with the patient or the patient's representatives.[79]

FEDERAL LEGISLATION

Health matters are generally the province of state law. Because of ongoing developments in the field, the need for cen-

tralized national allocation of organs, and funding issues, however, the federal government has become increasingly involved in transplantation and has attempted to enhance and coordinate private and local government initiatives. For example, the federal government sponsored the establishment in 1983 of the American Council on Transplantation, a group of private sector organizations and individuals to promote organ donation (dissolved in the early 1990s).

The National Organ Transplant Act (NOTA) was enacted in 1984.[80] It called for the creation of a national Organ Procurement and Transplantation Network (OPTN) to match prospective donors to prospective recipients, the creation of a special advisory task force, and the prohibition of the sale of organs. The OPTN was to create a fair and equitable system of organ allocation that could optimize matches between organs and patients throughout the United States by facilitating regional independent organ procurement agencies (IOPAs). Grants for the establishment of new agencies and the improvement of existing IOPAs were authorized to form an adequate base of a truly national network. This network was then to "assist organ procurement organizations in the distribution of organs which cannot be placed locally, to develop organ procurement standards, and to help coordinate transport."

The United Network for Organ Sharing (UNOS), a private, nonprofit entity solely devoted to organ procurement and transplantation, was awarded the federal contract to run the OPTN in September 1986. Federal oversight of UNOS is provided by the Division of Organ Transplantation under the Health Resources and Services Administration, within the Public Health Service and the DHHS.

The Task Force on Organ Transplantation was created by DHHS Secretary Heckler in January 1985. It rendered its final report in April 1986 and was dissolved. The 78 recommendations largely define federal policy.

The Omnibus Budget and Reconciliation Act (OBRA) of 1986 built on the 1984 legislation and the task force's recommendations by amending the Social Security Act.[81] First, it mandated as Medicare and Medicaid conditions of participation that hospitals institutionalize a required request policy (as previously explained) to increase the voluntary supply of organs. Second, also as Medicare and Medicaid funding requirements, it stated that hospitals performing transplantations must be members and must abide by the rules and policies of the OPTN (i.e., UNOS).

The statutory requirement that transplantation centers must be members and abide by the OPTN gives UNOS great regulatory power. Many consider UNOS as a unique experiment in self-regulation within the health care field. UNOS requirements are more stringent than DHHS regulations. The policies of UNOS, equivalent to conditions of participation, are subject to review and approval by the DHHS and are subjected to public "notice and comment" in the *Federal Register.* Despite lip service to the contrary, the system appears to operate in a very centralized manner, rather than the flexible, pluralistic decentralized system originally envisioned in the 1984 NOTA.[82]

Membership in UNOS as a qualified IOPA was a great organizational challenge. The task force recommended that competition between organ procurement organizations be discouraged. IOPAs were required to have defined and exclusive service areas. The response was for all IOPAs in given areas to merge into single entities. A regional system of IOPAs is now in place. Anticipated litigation never materialized.

Membership in UNOS as a transplantation center qualified by procedure will continue to be problematic. To become members, new programs must already have performed a particular procedure many times, which is almost impossible without federal funding. Thus the UNOS membership guidelines tend to entrench existing members who helped establish the guidelines. The governmental umbrella over UNOS might shield its members from antitrust considerations.

Sale of organs

The NOTA of 1984 prohibited the transfer of "any human organ for valuable consideration if the transfer affects interstate commerce."[83] The term *human organ* is defined as the human kidney, liver, heart, lung, pancreas, bone marrow, cornea, eye, bone, skin, and any other organ included by the secretary of the DHHS for regulation. It is not intended to include replenishable tissues, such as blood or semen. The term *valuable consideration* does not include the "reasonable payment associated with removal, transportation, implantation, processing, preservation, quality control, and storage, or the expenses of travel, housing, or lost wages in connection with donation of the organ."

The commerce clause reflects an attempt to fit the regulation into the federal constitutional commerce powers. In other situations this language has been interpreted so broadly as to include almost any interstate or intrastate transaction. Nonetheless, several states have also passed such prohibitions.

A 38-year-old leukemia patient needed a bone marrow transplant but could not find a suitable donor. His older brother was homeless and earned money by serving as a subject in medical experiments. He initially refused to be tested for compatibility. An anonymous donor offered him $1000 to undergo testing and $2000 to donate. He was tested and was found not to be an HLA match. If he had matched, the prohibition against "the transfer of any human organ for valuable consideration" arguably would have been applicable and would have barred his marrow donation to his brother.[84]

Food and Drug Administration

The FDA has jurisdiction over tissue banking and has maintained a task force on transplantation since 1983. The regulation of the safety and efficacy of human tissue is analogous to regulation of manufactured materials for use in therapy. The agency is developing proposals for regulating cryopreserved semen, dura mater, and heart valves. The FDA is not concerned with solid organs except possibly for disease transmission by improper screening of donors. The FDA is also concerned with organ perfusion solutions.[85]

In October 1993 the U.S. House of Representatives passed H.R. 2659, the Organ and Bone Marrow Transplantation Amendments of 1993, to revise and extend programs relating to the transplantation of organs and bone marrow. The proposals amended 42 U.S.C., Sections 273 and 274. The amendments extended for 3 fiscal years the authorization of appropriations for the NOTA. In November 1995 the Senate favorably reported the proposed Solid Organ and Bone Marrow Transplant Reauthorization Act of 1995 to revise and reauthorize funding for transplantation programs.[86] This legislation, which is administered by the Health Resources and Services Administration of the DHHS, would provide for continued operation of the transplant network and scientific registries and provide rules for transplant network governance and administration. In addition, appropriations would establish a patient advocacy and case management office for the bone marrow transplantation program.

The secretary of the DHHS is required to issue regulations establishing enforceable procedures for the procurement, allocation, and transplantation of solid organs and bone marrow. Such regulations also would establish the criteria that must be satisfied for membership in OPTN. In issuing such regulations, the secretary is directed to consider existing policies and guidelines issued by UNOS and the National Bone Marrow Registry.

The secretary is required to review and approve any changes in the amount of patient registration fees imposed by the private contractor administering the system of solid organ procurement.

Organ allocation policies of the OPTN and the member organ procurement organizations (OPOs) require maintenance of a single list of patients referred for transplants for each solid organ and give preference to patients who are U.S. citizens or permanent resident aliens.

Expansion of the system of patient advocacy for bone marrow transplant patients is provided with an inclusion for case management services. The General Accounting Office is required to perform studies of the National Marrow Donor Program.

Last, the secretary of the DHHS is required to study the feasibility, fairness, and enforceability of allocating solid organs to patients based solely on the clinical need of the patient involved and the viability of organs involved.

Legislation and administrative rule-making in the areas of organ donation and transplantation are undergoing continual revisions. The reader should consult the appropriate federal and state reference source materials, in addition to current medicolegal periodicals, to keep apprised of these revisions and updates.

SELECTION OF ORGAN RECIPIENTS

The scarce supply of organs and tissues relative to demand and the economic considerations of transplantation force the medical community to confront ethical issues on rationing. The public must perceive the allocation of organs as fair and equitable, or the national organ and tissue supply (which depends on voluntary contributions) will be jeopardized.

Regulation of recipient selection for organs is now imposed nationally through funding requirements. The NOTA of 1984 created the OPTN for the equitable distribution of all available organs in the United States.[87] The OBRA of 1986 requires all hospitals to abide by the policies of the OPTN as conditions of Medicare and Medicaid payment.[88] The federal OPTN contract was awarded to UNOS.

The basis of the UNOS system is a computerized point system for allocation. The point system is an objective method of patient selection determined primarily by probability of success, time on the waiting list, logistic factors, and medical need, modified from the proposal by Starzl.[89] Variances can be granted for fair patient selection criteria to accommodate local concerns.

Kidneys require more stringent testing than other solid organs because potential donees can be maintained on dialysis while awaiting an optimal kidney. Difficult choices must be made for nonpaired vital organs. Kidneys will be offered first to the recipient located anywhere in the country who has a perfect antigenic match. Only 15% to 25% of kidneys will have such a match. Otherwise, cadaveric kidneys will be allocated on a point system based on time of waiting, quality of antigen match, and panel-reactive antibody screen (a measure of sensitization). Medical urgency is not considered for kidney allocation.

Extrarenal organs will be allocated based on organ size, ABO typing, time of waiting, degree of medical urgency, and logistic factors. Pancreata will be offered solely on the basis of distance to a potential recipient and time on a waiting list.

Pediatric organs and patients are given special consideration. Dual transplants (e.g., simultaneous kidney-pancreas) are also handled outside the usual schema.

Patients on local waiting lists are offered organs in descending sequence, with the highest number of points receiving the highest priority. Only if an organ is not accepted locally will it be offered regionally, and then nationally. Organ sharing arrangements between interregional and intraregional OPOs may be entered into on approval of UNOS. The OPTN (UNOS) patient waiting list is open only to direct UNOS-member OPOs, and such members cannot offer organs to non-UNOS member transplantation centers. A potential recipient may be placed on multiple listings, even though this confers some advantage.

The final decision to accept an offered organ remains the prerogative of the transplantation surgeon, physician responsible for the care of the patient, or both. A transplantation center has 1 hour to accept an offered organ, or the offering procurement agency will be free to offer the organ to another recipient.

The issue of whether the patient with the greatest chance of survival or the one with the greatest urgency should receive an organ has been a source of continuing debate. A potential heart recipient deteriorates and becomes suddenly much more ill, so he or she is at once more critically in need of a new heart and less likely to survive the transplantation. This question is largely moot with respect to kidneys because patients can be placed on dialysis (except in the rare case of exhaustion of vascular access sites). However, the issue of deterioration is paramount with respect to hearts and livers. Medical urgency determines the status for liver and heart recipients in the UNOS system. The potential for manipulating the system as a result of its subjectivity has led to extensive efforts to develop listing criteria for liver transplantation. Criteria for all organs are being considered by UNOS and its membership.

Highly sensitized patients, or "responders," have antibodies against most histocompatibility antigens. A negative crossmatch may give a responder his or her only chance to receive a surviving transplantation. However, the chance of organ acceptance is lower than that for similarly matched nonresponders. The transplantation community generally feels an obligation to offer to this patient his or her last small chance at a tolerable organ.

Matching is a significant criterion based on sound immunological principles. HLA compatibility is unavoidably discriminatory against African-Americans and Hispanics (who have a several times higher rate of ESRD) because most available kidneys have been donated by whites. On the basis of histocompatibility alone, most kidneys from large urban centers would go to white suburban areas. HLA compatibility is of debatable significance to other organs.

Other criteria, such as age and lifestyle, although not a part of the UNOS point system, may be locally operative. Valid medical justifications for these gray areas exist; for instance, is a young patient a better surgical risk than an older alcoholic patient who continues to drink and is likely to damage the new liver and unlikely to take medications regularly? However, discrimination based on age or social position raises issues of fairness. Such subjective criteria are also prone to capriciousness. These do not seem to be primary selection criteria.

After a patient receives a transplant, he or she is usually given greater consideration for a subsequent organ, but the chances for long-term success fall as a patient receives more transplants.

Persons from other countries may not come to the United States and pay for a transplant and deplete national organ resources. Payment for organs is now prohibited. Currently, aliens are held to about 5% of current waiting lists, but those on the lists are to be treated as American citizens and not to be discriminated against based on political influence, national origin, race, gender, religion, or financial status. UNOS members are not to enter into contractual arrangements with foreign agencies or governments or perform transplants on nonresident aliens for financial advantage. Exportation and importation of organs are to be strictly arranged and coordinated through UNOS. Although thousands are maintained on the United States waiting lists, several hundred kidneys are shipped abroad because they are unacceptably old by rigorous U.S. standards.

Lawsuits can be filed against hospitals, transplant surgeons, and committees on behalf of patients who fail to obtain vital organs because others have received the organs first. This is increasingly likely because criteria might be attacked as arbitrary, capricious, or otherwise unreasonable. The implication that one recipient is chosen over another for financial reasons might be argued as an illegal sale of an organ and thus a basis of liability. Another problem area involves cases in which a sudden decline in health precipitates a recipient's "jumping the queue" (being ranked higher priority) and receiving an organ that would have gone to another. Although the sudden deterioration may suggest a poorer prognosis, others in the queue are at increasing risk for sudden death. The potential liability for choosing between who lives and dies is enormous, and the absence of suits to date is surprising.

COST AND PAYMENT CONSIDERATIONS

Vital organ transplantation is extremely expensive. The approximate range for a typical kidney transplant is $25,000 to $30,000; for a heart transplant procedure, $57,000 to $110,000; for a heart-lung transplant, $130,000 to $200,000; for a liver transplant, $135,000 to $238,000; and for a pancreas transplant, $30,000 to $100,000.[90]

Transplantation failures and ancillary costs (e.g., transportation and lodging for the patient and family when the patient does not live near the transplantation center) greatly elevate these figures. Almost all vital organ transplant patients require lifelong maintenance on immunosuppressant therapy, although this may be changing. The cost of conventional immunosuppression maintenance (steroids and azathioprine) averages $1000 to $2000 per year and $5000 to $7000 per year for cyclosporine. However, because cyclosporine decreases overall complications, it does not raise overall costs. The OBRA of 1986 enabled Medicare and Medicaid to cover out-patient immunosuppressive therapy, particularly cyclosporine, for 3 years after transplant.[91]

The cost of transplantation is generally prohibitive, and individuals must rely on third-party reimbursement. Furthermore, many if not most of those in need of a solid organ transplant are incapable of employment. Thus transplants can be viewed as treatment for a catastrophic life-threatening illness.

Established in 1972, the Medicare End-Stage Renal Disease Program (ESRDP) provides treatment to patients with kidney failure regardless of their ability to pay.[92] ESRD was the first disease targeted for funding through a special program by the federal government. This program established the standard acquisition charge for transplantable kidneys, allowing each transplant center to predict its organ charges regardless of the location of origin of the organ or complicating expenses attributable to an individual donor. Over the

years the method of payment for transplantable kidneys has been extrapolated to all solid organ transplants.

The cost of the ESRDP, primarily for long-term dialysis, continues to escalate as the number of beneficiaries, now 275,000, increases.[93] Transplantation costs in the United States in 1994 were approximately $4 billion, or 0.04% of total health care expenditures.[94] This amount is much greater than anticipated, and the ESRDP is often cited as an expensive program run amok.[95,96]

Kidney transplants are cost effective (with the initial large investment generally being paid back in 3 years) compared with the alternative, hemodialysis. The long-term costs of maintaining patients with functioning grafts are only one third of those for dialysis patients.[97,98] Furthermore, the quality of life is improved, allowing more people to become productive citizens again. No alternative exists for heart or liver transplants.

In this era of cost containment, many find it difficult to justify the expense of transplantation for the few while sacrificing more widespread financing of health care. The juggernaut is not easily stopped because U.S. society typically responds to individual pleas for a specific and lifesaving treatment. Increasingly the federal government is asked to subsidize transplants, but federal fiscal restraints make this difficult.

At present the costs of transplantation are high but not higher than the costs of taking care of the typical AIDS patient or cancer patient, and the results are much better. As a result of the organ shortage, the total costs to the government are now relatively low and predictable. However, the government's ability to pay for organ transplants may not continue, particularly because of a growth in the supply of organs, increase in demand, and technological innovations, such as usable artificial organs. Over time, pressures will grow to relax the standards for patient reimbursement. The history of the ESRDP demonstrates this process of ever more lenient selection standards tending toward universal access.

Medicare coverage of services furnished to individuals with ESRD who require dialysis or kidney transplantation is authorized under Section 1881 of the Social Security Act. Medicare also covers other organ transplants that the HCFA has determined are "reasonable and necessary" (Section 1862) and pays for those transplant and related organ procurement services.[99] Based on a report by the Office of Health Technology Assessment that liver transplants are no longer experimental, the HCFA reported that it will cover the cost of some adult liver transplants, including those needed because of alcoholic cirrhosis.[100] As of February 2, 1995, lung transplants and heart-lung transplants were added to the list of medically reasonable and necessary services covered under Medicare, when specific established criteria were met.[101] Medicare considers pancreas transplantation experimental but will fund the kidney portion of a combined kidney-pancreas transplantation, whereas private insurers cover the entire procedure.

States pay for transplantation procedures for low-income persons through Medicaid (subsidized by the federal government). The states vary greatly in their coverage and payment policies. In 1990, of the 50 states and the District of Columbia, only 12 states reimbursed pancreas transplants, 15 provided for lung transplants, and 23 paid for heart-lung transplants but 40 provided reimbursement for heart transplants, 48 for liver transplants, and 50 for kidney transplants. Only Wyoming offered no transplantation reimbursement.[102]

For Medicare and Medicaid (and most private health insurance plans) the funding eligibility trigger is "medical necessity" for the treatment. Thus the government will pay for a transplantation if, like other medical therapy, it can be shown that the procedure is reasonable and necessary for the illness and that such treatment is not experimental.

Patients have successfully sued for reimbursement from state agencies when policies or administrative regulations have unfairly denied coverage. In *Brillo v. Arizona,* Mrs. Brillo successfully sued the state to provide coverage for her liver transplantation.[103] The service director's policy determination was that the state would not pay for adult liver transplants because they were experimental, although they would pay for pediatric liver transplants. The court found the policy to be arbitrary, capricious, and a denial of equal protection of the law.

In *Allen v. Mansour* the Michigan court ordered Medicaid funding for an alcoholic with cirrhosis, holding that the recipient selection criterion of a 2-year abstinence from alcohol in cases of cirrhosis caused by alcoholism was arbitrary and unreasonable as formulated and applied.[104] The court noted that this criterion was developed on meager experience and that "medical necessity" of the procedure is the touchstone for evaluating the reasonableness of standards in state Medicaid plans.

In *Lee v. Page* the Florida Medicaid program refused to fund a liver transplant to be performed at the University of Nebraska for a medically qualified 26-year-old woman with a fatal liver disease. The state's position was that the high cost of the liver transplant procedure, which would divert substantial funds from other needy persons, and the minimal benefit to the population of all eligible recipients made the refusal to pay reasonable. The court indicated that states have considerable leeway to implement federally backed Medicaid programs. States must adopt "reasonable standards," but they cannot exclude coverage for "medically necessary treatments." A state can legitimately argue in support of its refusal to fund a treatment as unnecessary either because the treatment is experimental or because it is inappropriate. The court held that liver transplantation is no longer experimental. The court also held that an unfavorable cost-benefit determination is not a medical appropriateness criterion and thus is not a reasonable standard from which to refuse funding.

This is not a question of the limits on the amount Medicaid will pay for a procedure, but rather a case where Medicaid refuses to pay the entire amount based on the cost of the procedure. . . . [Medicaid] cannot eliminate one health-related service while leaving others intact. . . . It does not appear that federal law permits Florida to refuse to fund all liver transplants. . . . Florida voluntarily entered the federal Medicaid cooperative program and must comply with the standards.[105]

In *Todd v. Sorrell.* a Virginia child was determined to be a suitable candidate for a liver transplantation by the Children's Hospital of Pittsburgh.[106] Because of cancer, 85% of the child's liver had been removed, and secondary biliary cirrhosis had developed. The hospital required an advance payment ($162,000). The Virginia Medicaid program refused to pay because its policy was to pay for pediatric liver transplants only in cases caused by biliary atresia. The U.S. Court of Appeals for the Fourth Circuit overturned a district court's holding and granted an injunction ordering the state to pay for the transplantation pending a final three-judge panel review. Nonetheless, citing the high costs of liver transplants ($250,000), other priorities, and the poor outcomes of liver transplants, Virginia decided to stop Medicaid funding of all liver transplants (May 1988).

Oregon decided not to spend Medicaid monies on transplantations except for kidneys and corneas. It reversed its controversial stand after public protest.[107,108]

MALPRACTICE SUITS

For a number of reasons, malpractice suits involving transplantation of vital organs have been almost nonexistent. First, in the past, transplantations were considered largely experimental, and thus customary standards were not well established. Second, failure was a well-recognized risk. Third, the careful attention by physicians in these cases resulted in generally good relationships and good communication with patients and their families. Fourth, the surgeons and institutions involved were of high stature and esteem. Fifth, transplant physicians were few and closely knit, making opposition testimony difficult to find. Sixth, damages were difficult to prove, given the ill health of the patients. However, a marked increase in suits may be anticipated in the future because these conditions will no longer hold true as vital organ transplants become commonplace.

In *McDermott v. Manhattan Eye, Ear & Throat Hospital* the appellate court reversed a lower court's finding of negligent corneal transplant, holding that evidence was insufficient to support a malpractice claim that the surgeon lacked the skill or experience to perform the operation, that the operation was of extreme delicacy with a high incidence of failure, and that the situation was one of desperation.[109]

The degree to which courts are reluctant to find liability in favor of transplant efforts can be found in *State of Missouri ex rel. Wichita Falls General Hospital v. Adolph.*[110,111] A Missouri transplant team flew to Wichita Falls, Texas, to harvest a heart from a donor and then returned to Missouri to transplant the heart into a recipient. During the transplant they discovered that the Texas hospital had incorrectly typed the donor as type A rather than type B. The patient died shortly thereafter, despite a second transplant. A Missouri appeals court refused to allow a Missouri trial court assert jurisdiction over a Texas hospital because of the potential adverse effect on future transplants.

Several problem areas are likely to be litigated in the future, especially the issues of informed consent and suitability of the organ for transplant.

Theoretically, *strict liability* (in which the court may award damages without a finding of fault by the defendant) might apply to injuries sustained from implants of diseased or defective organs as an unreasonably dangerous defective product or from an implied warranty. Plaintiffs in early cases of hepatitis and adverse reactions to transfusions of blood and blood products successfully argued theories of strict liability. Later decisions rejected the notion, holding that provision of blood is a service and not the sale of a product.

Most states now have statutes that specifically protect hospitals and blood banks from strict liability. Such laws hold that transfusions of blood and blood products are not sales, so no warranties attach, and that liability may be imposed only for negligence or willful misconduct. Many statutes further include transplantations of other tissues and organs in these provisions. The states that specifically mention blood but fail to mention other tissues and organs might risk the interpretation that their legislatures intended to exclude organ transplantations from such protection. Otherwise, strict liability is unlikely to be applied to organ transplantation because transplantation will be construed to be a hospital and physician service instead of the sale of a product, in light of the blood banking court decisions and the federal and state proscriptions against sales of organs. Statutory immunity conferred by the UAGA also might apply to negligent procedures, as discussed earlier.

RECENT DEVELOPMENTS

On December 7, 1993, The House of Delegates of the American Medical Association (AMA) adopted a report from the Council on Ethical and Judicial Affairs that was subsequently revised in response to comments received from peer reviewers.[112] This report recommended that mandated choice, in which individuals would be required to state their preferences regarding organ donation when they renew their driver's licenses, file their income tax return, or perform some other task mandated by the state, should be pursued by the AMA in working with state medical societies to draft model legislation for adoption by state legislatures. The report raised ethical objections to the alternative of presumed consent, in which it is assumed that an individual would consent to be an organ donor at death unless an objection from the individual before death or from his or her next of kin after death is known to the health care provider. A federal circuit court has adopted this approach.[113] In this case the circuit court of appeals, in reversing the district court's ruling, determined that a widow could maintain a civil rights action filed against the coroner based on his removal of the decedent husband's

corneas for use in transplantation without the widow's consent. The court held that consent was presumed when the coroner claimed a lack of knowledge as to any objection to such removal of organs for transplantation before performing the procedure.

Medical examiners and transplant coordinators are cooperating to maximize the lawful retrieval of organs and tissues for transplantation.[114,115] Representatives from the Association of Organ Procurement Organizations, the North American Transplant Coordinators Organization, the American Society of Transplant Surgeons, and the National Association of Medical Examiners have met to agree on guidelines for their respective members. This need for cooperative efforts is underscored by the estimate that currently approximately one suitable transplant candidate in the United States is dying every 4 hours because of lack of a suitable organ for recommended transplantation. These guidelines are needed to protect concerns that forensic evidence will not be lost or affected by the subsequent transplantation surgery. The results of a retrospective study (from 1990 to 1992) of information received from responding organ procurement organizations indicated that as many as 2979 individuals may have been denied transplants because of medical examiner denials.[116] Such denials were generally the result of a perceived need by the medical examiner to preserve forensic evidence that could be necessary later in documenting the cause of an individual's death.

Multiple efforts to increase organ donation are underway. Virginia has become the latest in a growing number of states to offer an organ donation license plate. In the spring of 1997, Ohio residents were encouraged to discuss their decision to donate over breakfast. As part of a National Organ and Tissue Donor Awareness Week milk cartons carried the donation message. Organ donor networks across the country sponsor a variety of activities from relay races to formalized studies designed to identify and standardize effective strategies that improve donation.[117] The 104th Congress passed the Organ Donation Insert Card Act as part of the health insurance portability law enacted in 1996. The new law required the Treasury Department to include information on organ and tissue donation with each refund check. In addition, the campaign included print ads and radio public service announcements recorded by members of Congress. The new law was enacted with the goal of increasing the number of potential organ donors and encouraging potential donors to discuss their decisions with family members.[118]

In the current managed care environment, with intensified scrutiny of health care costs, questions surround the possible surplus of transplantation centers, as discussed at the first joint annual meeting of UNOS and the DHHS Division of Organ Transplantation.[119] Statistics indicated that 40% of kidney transplant centers were performing fewer than 25 transplants a year and that 40% of liver transplant centers were performing fewer than 15 transplants per year, accounting for only 8% of livers transplanted in the United States. In contrast, the 20 largest liver transplant centers were performing 76% of the liver transplants. Since centers with a higher volume of cases seemed to have better outcomes, performance criteria were suggested as a basis for determining whether a new transplant program should be approved and whether an existing program should be allowed to continue with government support. Evidence also indicated that the cost of a transplant generally decreases as the volume of cases increases at a center. For many U.S. citizens, availability of transplant centers will be determined by these considerations.

The HCFA published a final rule in May 1996 setting performance standards for organizations that procure organs for transplantation under the Medicare and Medicaid programs. The final rule modified some of the requirements contained in the interim final rule, allowing greater flexibility regarding performance criteria. Flexibility is important to transplantation, a field of medicine that continues to develop and adapt

ENDNOTES

1. United Network of Organ Sharing (UNOS) Update (Richmond, Va., Summer 1997).
2. Tissue Banking Data (Washington Regional Transplant Consortium, Washington, D.C. Summer 1997).
3. *UNOS 1996 Annual Report on The Scientific Registry of Transplant Recipients and The Organ Procurement and Transplantation Network,* (Richmond, Va. 1996).
4. UNOS Membership Data, http://www.ew3.att.net/UNOS.
5. 2 The UNOS Bulletin (July 1997).
6. National Task Force on Organ Transplantation, *Organ Transplantation: Issues and Recommendations* (DHHS, Washington, D.C., GPO # 1986-O-160-709, 1986).
7. *Id.*
8. Uniform Anatomical Gift Act (1968), National Conference of Commissioners.
9. Uniform Anatomical Gift Act (1987), National Conference of Commissioners on Uniform State Laws (Chicago 1987); § 8A U.L.A. 16 (Supp. 1989).
10. § 8A U.L.A. 2 (Supp. 1996); § 8A U.L.A. 9 (Supp. 1996).
11. *New Developments in Biotechnology: Ownership of Human Tissues and Cells—Special Report* (Office of Technology Assessment, U.S. Government Printing Office, Washington, D.C. 1987).
12. P. Matthews, *Whose Property?: People as Property,* Current Legal Problems 193-239 (1983).
13. *In re Moyer's Estate,* 577 P. 2d 108 (1978).
14. *Holland v. Metalious,* 198 A. 2d 654 (1964).
15. *Leno v. St Joseph Hospital,* 302 N.E. 2d 58 (1973).
16. *Nicoletta v. Rochester Eye and Human Parts Bank,* 519 N.Y.S. 2d 928 (1987).
17. *Williams v. Hofmann,* 223 N.W. 2d 844 (1974).
18. *Ravenis v. Detroit General Hospital,* 234 N.W. 2d 411 (1976).
19. *Supra* note 9.
20. Maximus, Inc., *Assessment of the Potential Organ Donor Pool: Report to Health Resources and Services Agency* (DHHS, Washington, D.C. 1985).
21. *Organ Transplantation Q & A* (DHHS, Division of Organ Transplantation, Washington D.C., DHHS Pub. No. [HRS-M-SP] 89-1, 1988).
22. K.J. Bart et al., *Increasing the Supply of Cadaveric Kidneys for Transplantation,* 31 Transplantation 383-387 (1981).
23. S.W. Tolle et al., *Responsibilities of Primary Physicians in Organ Donation,* 106 Ann. Int. Med. 740-744 (1987).
24. J. Prottas, *The Structure and Effectiveness of the U.S. Organ Procurement System,* 22 Inquiry 365-376 (1985).
25. J.M. Prottas, *The Organization of Organ Procurement,* 14 J. Health Politics, Pol. & L. 41-55 (1989).
26. A.L. Caplan, *Professional Arrogance and Public Misunderstanding,* 18 Hastings Center Report 34-37 (1988).
27. S.J. Youngner et al., *Brain Death and Organ Retrieval,* 261 J.A.M.A. 2205-2210 (1989).
28. J. Prottas & H.L. Batten, *Health Professionals and Hospital Administrators in Organ Procurement: Attitudes, Reservations, and Their Resolution,* 78 Am. J. Pub. Health 642-645 (1988).
29. A. Caplan, *Ethical and Policy Issues in the Procurement of Cadaver Organs for Transplantation,* 314 N. Engl. J. Med. 981-983 (1984).
30. J.F. Childress, *Ethical Criteria for Procuring and Distributing Organs for Transplantation,* 14 J. Health Politics, Pol. & L. 87-113 (1989).
31. Omnibus Budget and Reconciliation Act (OBRA) of 1986, Pub. L. 99-509, § 9318 *amending* Title XI of the Social Security Act *adding* § 1138, *Hospital protocols for organ procurement and standards for organ procurement agencies; further clarification* in 53(40) Federal Register 6526-6551 (Mar 1, 1988).
32. *Joint Commission on Accreditation of Healthcare Organizations Standards,* R.I.2 (1995).
33. V.W. Weedn & B. Leveque, *Routine Inquiry for Organ and Tissue Donations,* 84 Tex. Med. 30-37 (1988).
34. *Transplant Action* (American Council on Transplantation, Alexandria, Va., July/August 1989).
35. *Pennsylvania Governor Signs Legislation to Increase Voluntary Organ Donation,* Health Care Daily (BNA, Dec 5, 1994); *available in* WESTLAW, BNA-HCD.
36. *Supra* note 1.
37. *Id.*
38. A. Caplan, *Organ Procurement: It's Not in the Cards,* 14 Hastings Center Report 9-12 (1984).
39. *Supra* note 33.
40. *Powell v. Florida,* 497 So. 2d 1188, 1986, *cert. denied,* 107 S.C. 2202 (1986).
41. *Georgia Lions Eye Bank v. Lavant,* 335 S.E. 2d 127, 1985, *cert. denied,* 475 U.S. 1084 (1986).
42. *Tillman v. Detroit Receiving Hospital,* 360 N.W. 2d 275 (1984).
43. *Kirker v. Orange County,* 519 So. 2d 682 (1988).
44. J.A. Light et al., *A Rapid Organ Recovery Program for Non-Heartbeating Donors* (Washington Hospital Center and Medlantic Research Institute [abstract *presented at* Congress] Summer 1997).
45. *Tucker v. Lower,* No. 2831, Law & Eq. Ct. (Richmond, Va., May 23, 1972).
46. *Strachan v. John F. Kennedy Memorial Hospital,* 538 A. 2d 346 (1988).
47. *Supra* note 3.
48. J.R. Botkin, *Anencephalic Infants as Organ Donors,* 82 Pediatrics 250-256 (1988).
49. J.W. Walters, *Anencephalic Organ Procurement: Should the Law Be Changed?* 2 BioLaw S83-S89 (1987).
50. *Supra* note 5.
51. D.A. Stumpf et al. (The Medical Task Force on Anencephaly), *The Infant with Anencephaly,* 322 N. Engl. J. Med. 669-674 (1990).
52. Centers for Disease Control, *Congenital Malformations Surveillance, January 1982-December 1985* (DHHS, Washington, D.C. 1988).
53. *Loma Linda Stops Program to Retrieve Transplantable Organs from Anencephalic Newborns,* BioLaw § 13-1, U:1127 (1988).
54. *Supra* note 51.
55. H.H. Kaufman, *Pediatric Brain Death and Organ/Tissue Retrieval* (Plenum Medical Book, New York 1989).
56. *Supra* note 51.
57. *Supra* note 51.
58. P. King & J. Areen, *Legal Regulation of Fetal Tissue Transplantation,* 36 Clin. Res. 187-222 (1988).

59. J. Palca, *Fetal Tissue Transplants Remain Off Limits,* 246 Science 752 (1989).

60. M.W. Danis, *Fetal Tissue Transplants: Restricting Recipient Designation,* 39 Hastings L. J. 1079-1152 (1988).

61. C. Marwick, *Committee to Be Named to Advise Government about Fetal Tissue Transplantation Experiments,* 259 J.A.M.A. 3099 (1988).

62. *Committee on Fetal Tissue Transplantation Established,* BioLaw § 13-1, U:965 (1988).

63. National Institutes of Health Revitalization Act of 1993, Pub. L. No. 103-43, 107 Stat. 122 (1993).

64. United States General Accounting Office, *NIH-Funded Research: Therapeutic Human Fetal Tissue Transplantation Projects Meet Federal Requirement* (GAO HEHS-97-61, March 1997).

65. *Id.*

66. *BMA Guidelines on the Use of Fetal Tissue,* The Lancet 1119 (May 14, 1988).

67. *McFall v. Shrimp,* Allegheny Cnty Ct. Common Pleas, 10 Pa.D.&C. 3d 90 (1980).

68. *Sirianni v. Anna,* 285 N.Y.S. 2d 709 (1967).

69. *Hart v. Brown,* 289 A. 2d 386 (1972).

70. *In re Richardson,* 284 So. 2d 185 (1975).

71. *In re Guardianship of Pescinski,* 226 N.W. 2d 180 (1975).

72. *Little v. Little,* 576 S.W. 2d 493 (1979).

73. *Strunk v. Strunk,* 445 S.W. 2d 145 (1969).

74. *Head v. Colloton,* 331 N.W. 2d 870 (1983).

75. *Karp v. Cooley,* 349 F.Supp. 827 (1972), *aff'd,* 493 F. 2d 408 (1974).

76. Medical Device Amendment, Pub. L. 94-295 (1980).

77. *Supra* note 18.

78. *Good v. Presbyterian Hospital,* 934 F.Supp. 107 (1996).

79. *Id.*

80. National Organ Transplant Act, Pub. L. 98-507, 98 Stat 2339, 42 U.S.C. 201 (Oct 1984).

81. *Supra* note 31.

82. J.F. Blumstein, *Government's Role in Organ Transplantation Policy,* 14 J. Health Politics, Pol. & L. 5-39 (1989).

83. *Supra* note 80.

84. *Payment to Homeless Man to Donate Bone Marrow to Brother,* Bio-Law § 13-3, U:881 (1988).

85. *Transplant Action 2* (American Council on Transplantation, Alexandria, Va., Sept/Oct/Nov 1989).

86. *Senate Labor Panel Reports Out Bill Reauthorizing Funding for Programs,* Health Care Daily (BNA, Nov 15, 1995); *available in* WEST-LAW, BNA-HCD.

87. *Supra* note 80.

88. *Supra* note 31.

89. T.E. Starzl et al., *A Multifactorial System for Equitable Selection of Cadaver Kidney Recipients,* 257 J.A.M.A. 3073-3075 (1987).

90. *From Here to Transplant . . . Introductory Information for Patients and Families* 19 (American Council on Transplantation, Alexandria, Va., *rev'd* Oct 1989).

91. *Supra* note 31.

92. End-Stage Renal Disease Program (ESRDP), Pub. L. No. 603, § 86 Stat. 1329 (1972).

93. United States Renal Data Systems (DHHS/PHS, Washington, D.C. 1995).

94. J.S. Wolf, *Financial Support of Organ Procurement in the United States,* 29 Transplantation Proceedings 1631-1632 (1997).

95. M. Angell, *Cost Containment and the Physician,* 254 J.A.M.A. 1203-1207 (1985).

96. J. Aroesty & R. Rettis, *The Cost Effects of Improved Kidney Transplantation,* Rand Rep. No. R-3099-NIH/RC (1984).

97. *Id.*

98. P.E. Eggers, *Effect of Transplantation on the Medicare End-Stage Renal Disease Program,* 318 N. Engl. J. Med. 223-229 (1988).

99. 42 C.F.R. § 405 (1996).

100. *HCFA Notice,* 55 Fed. Reg. 8547 (Mar 8, 1990).

101. 60 F.R. § 6537 (1995).

102. Congressional Research Services, 103rd Cong., 1st Sess *Medicaid Source Book: Background Data and Analysis (A 1993 Update)* 605 at 292-295.

103. *Brillo v. Arizona,* cited in ACT Transplant Action (July/Aug, 1986).

104. *Allen v. Mansour,* 681 F.Supp. 1232 (D. Ct. E. D. Mich., 1986).

105. *Lee v. Page,* No. 86-1081-Civ-J-14, U.S. Dist. Ct. (Middle Dist. of Florida, Jacksonville Division, Dec 19, 1986).

106. *Todd v. Sorrell,* No. 87-3806, U.S. Ct. of App. (4th Cir., Mar 4, 1988).

107. H.G. Welch & E. B. Larson, *Dealing with Limited Resources: The Oregon Decision to Curtail Funding for Organ Transplantation,* 319 N. Engl. J. Med. 171-173 (1988).

108. R. Crawshaw et al., *Organ Transplants: A Search for Health Policy at the State Level,* 150 West. J. Med. 361-363 (1989).

109. *McDermott v. Manhattan Eye, Ear & Throat Hospital,* 270 N.Y.S. 2d 955, *aff'd without opinion* 224 N.E. 2d 717 (1966).

110. *State of Missouri ex rel. Wichita Falls General Hospital v. Adolph,* 728 S.W. 2d 604 (1987).

111. R.M. Baron, *Asserting Jurisdiction Over the Providers of Human Donor Organs:* State of Missouri ex rel. Wichita Falls General Hospital v. Adolph, 92 Dick. L. Rev. 393 (Winter 1988).

112. Council on Ethical and Judicial Affairs (AMA), *Strategies for Cadaveric Organ Procurement Mandated Choice and Presumed Consent,* 272 J.A.M.A. 809-812 (1994).

113. *Brotherton v. Cleveland,* 923 F. 2d. 477 (6th Cir., 1991).

114. D. Jason, *The Role of the Medical Examiner/Coroner in Organ and Tissue Procurement for Transplantation,* 15 Am. J. Forensic Med. & Path. 192-202 (1994).

115. R. Voelker, *Can Forensic Medical and Organ Donation Co-exist for Public Good?* 271 J.A.M.A. 891-892 (1994).

116. T. Shafer et al., *Impact of Medical Examiner/Coroner Practices on Organ Recovery in the United States,* 272 J.A.M.A. 1607-1613 (1994).

117. *Supra* note 1.

118. UNOS Update (Richmond, Va., Spring 1997).

119. A. Skolnick, *Are There Too Many US Transplantation Centers?: Some Experts Suggest Fewer, Cheaper, Better,* 271 J.A.M.A. 1062-1064 (1994).

APPENDIX 26-1   Organs used in transplantation

CORNEAS

The cornea is the clear "window" in front of eye allowing light to enter.

The first cornea transplant was performed in 1905.

At any given time, 3000 to 5000 people await corneas.

The body does not reject a transplanted cornea.

Cornea donors range in age from newborn to age 70 or older.

KIDNEYS

The kidney is the most frequently transplanted organ.

More than 73,000 kidney transplants were performed in the United States between 1988 and 1995.

Approximately two thirds of kidneys are from unrelated, deceased donors; approximately one third come from living-related donors.

More than 31,000 people in the United States are on waiting lists for kidney transplants.

Kidneys have functioned normally after transplantation for more than 30 years with living-related donors.

Kidneys have functioned normally after transplantation for more than 20 years with nonrelated cadaver donors.

HEART

More than 16,700 heart transplants were performed in the United States between 1988 and 1995.

In 1996, about 4000 people were awaiting heart transplants in the United States.

The 1-year survival for heart transplants currently averages 84%.

Survival rates of up to 17 years have been documented for heart recipients.

Currently, several thousand heart transplants are being performed annually in the United States.

LIVER

An estimated 5000 people die each year in the United States from end-stage liver disease who would have been acceptable candidates for liver transplantation.

Patient survival for more than 15 years is documented.

Modified from Pub. L. 98-507, 98th Congress.

More than 10,000 liver transplants have been performed since 1986.

The 1-year success rate for liver transplants is about 75%.

Living-related partial liver transplants usually involve a parent donating a portion of his or her liver to a child.

LUNGS

The lung is the most complicated type of transplant performed and may be transplanted along with the heart, depending on the nature of the illness.

About 900 lung transplants are performed annually in the United States.

The success rates of single-lung and double-lung transplants are improving dramatically.

PANCREAS

A pancreas transplant can cure diabetes.

If a patient undergoing a kidney transplant has diabetes, the pancreas may be transplanted along with the kidney.

More than 4900 pancreas transplants were performed in the United States between 1988 and 1995.

BONES

Most bone transplants last the life of the individual.

Bone can be preserved and stored indefinitely by a "bone bank."

SKIN

Skin can be used as a temporary covering for severe burns.

Donor skin is generally from the back or thigh.

Skin can be cryopreserved for up to 4 weeks for use with burn victims. It can be preserved via a freeze-drying process for up to 5 years for use in periodontal work.

BONE MARROW

Transplanted bone marrow is used to treat patients with leukemia or other forms of cancer, certain types of anemia, and certain genetic diseases.

Close relatives are the best potential donors.

When a match cannot be found from a relative, the odds of an unrelated person being a close match are 20,000 to 1.

APPENDIX 26-2   Amended Uniform Anatomical Gift Act of 1987

SECTION 1. DEFINITIONS

As used in this [Act]*:

(1) "Anatomical gift" means a donation of all or part of a human body to take effect upon or after death.

(2) "Decedent" means a deceased individual and includes a stillborn infant or fetus.

(3) "Document of gift" means a card, a statement attached to or imprinted on a motor vehicle operator's or chauffeur's license, a will, or other writing used to make an anatomical gift.

(4) "Donor" means an individual who makes an anatomical gift of all or part of the individual's body.

(5) "Enucleator" means an individual who is [licensed] [certified] by the [State Board of Medical Examiners] to remove or process eyes or parts of eyes.

(6) "Hospital" means a facility licensed, accredited, or approved as a hospital under the law of any state or a facility operated as a hospital by the United States government, a state, or a subdivision of a state.

(7) "Part" means an organ, tissue, eye, bone, artery, blood, fluid, or other portion of a human body.

(8) "Person" means an individual, corporation, business trust, estate, trust, partnership, joint venture, association, government, governmental subdivision or agency, or any other legal or commercial entity.

(9) "Physician" or "surgeon" means an individual licensed or otherwise authorized to practice medicine and surgery or osteopathy and surgery under the laws of any state.

(10) "Procurement organization" means a person licensed, accredited, or approved under the laws of any state for procurement, distribution, or storage of human bodies or parts.

(11) "State" means a state, territory, or possession of the United States, the District of Columbia, or the Commonwealth of Puerto Rico.

(12) "Technician" means an individual who is [licensed] [certified] by the [State Board of Medical Examiners] to remove or process a part.

SECTION 2. MAKING, AMENDING, REVOKING, AND REFUSING TO MAKE ANATOMICAL GIFTS BY INDIVIDUAL

(a) An individual who is at least [18] years of age may (i) make an anatomical gift for any of the purposes stated in Section 6(a), (ii) limit an anatomical gift to one or more of those purposes, or (iii) refuse to make an anatomical gift.

From National Conference of Commissioners on Uniform State Laws (July 1986).

*Words or phrases enclosed in brackets indicate instances in which each state is to supply its own appropriate terms.

(b) An anatomical gift may be made only by a document of gift signed by the donor. If the donor cannot sign, the document of gift must be signed by another individual and by two witnesses, all of whom have signed at the direction and in the presence of the donor and of each other, and state that it has been so signed.

(c) If a document of gift is attached to or imprinted on a donor's motor vehicle operator's or chauffeur's license, the document of gift must comply with subsection (b). Revocation, suspension, expiration, or cancellation of the license does not invalidate the anatomical gift.

(d) A document of gift may designate a particular physician or surgeon to carry out the appropriate procedures. In the absence of a designation or if the designee is not available, the donee or other person authorized to accept the anatomical gift may employ or authorize any physician, surgeon, technician, or enucleator to carry out the appropriate procedures.

(e) An anatomical gift by will takes effect upon death of the testator, whether or not the will is probated. If, after death, the will is declared invalid for testamentary purposes, the validity of the anatomical gift is unaffected.

(f) A donor may amend or revoke an anatomical gift, not made by will, only by:

(1) a signed statement;

(2) an oral statement made in the presence of two individuals;

(3) any form of communication during a terminal illness or injury addressed to a physician or surgeon; or

(4) the delivery of a signed statement to a specified donee to whom a document of gift had been delivered.

(g) The donor of an anatomical gift made by will may amend or revoke the gift in the manner provided for amendment or revocation of wills, or as provided in subsection (f).

(h) An anatomical gift that is not revoked by the donor before death is irrevocable and does not require the consent or concurrence of any person after the donor's death.

(i) An individual may refuse to make an anatomical gift of the individual's body or part by (i) a writing signed in the same manner as a document of gift, (ii) a statement attached to or imprinted on a donor's motor vehicle operator's or chauffeur's license, or (iii) any other writing used to identify the individual as refusing to make an anatomical gift. During a terminal illness or injury, the refusal may be an oral statement or other form of communication.

(j) In the absence of contrary indications by the donor, an anatomical gift of a part is neither a refusal to give other parts nor a limitation on an anatomical gift under Section 3 or on a removal or release of other parts under Section 4.

(k) In the absence of contrary indications by the donor, a revocation or amendment of an anatomical gift is not a refusal to make another anatomical gift. If the donor intends a revocation to be a refusal to make an anatomical gift, the donor shall make the refusal pursuant to subsection (i).

SECTION 3. MAKING, REVOKING, AND OBJECTING TO ANATOMICAL GIFTS BY OTHERS

(a) Any member of the following classes of persons, in the order of priority listed, may make an anatomical gift of all or a part of the decedent's body for an authorized purpose, unless the decedent, at the time of death, has made an unrevoked refusal to make that anatomical gift:
(1) the spouse of the decedent;
(2) an adult son or daughter of the decedent;
(3) either parent of the decedent;
(4) an adult brother or sister of the decedent;
(5) a grandparent of the decedent; and
(6) a guardian of the person of the decedent at the time of death.

(b) An anatomical gift may not be made by a person listed in subsection (a) if:
(1) a person in a prior class is available at the time of death to make an anatomical gift;
(2) the person proposing to make an anatomical gift knows of a refusal or contrary indications by the decedent; or
(3) the person proposing to make an anatomical gift knows of an objection to making an anatomical gift by a member of the person's class or a prior class.

(c) An anatomical gift by a person authorized under subsection (a) must be made by (i) a document of gift signed by the person or (ii) the person's telegraphic, recorded telephonic, or other recorded message, or other form of communication from the person that is contemporaneously reduced to writing and signed by the recipient.

(d) An anatomical gift by a person authorized under subsection (a) may be revoked by any member of the same or a prior class if, before procedures have begun for the removal of a part from the body of the decedent, the physician, surgeon, technician, or enucleator removing the part knows of the revocation.

(e) A failure to make an anatomical gift under subsection (a) is not an objection to the making of an anatomical gift.

SECTION 4. AUTHORIZATION BY [CORONER], [MEDICAL EXAMINER], OR [LOCAL PUBLIC HEALTH OFFICIAL]

(a) The [coroner] may release and permit the removal of a part from a body within that official's custody, for transplantation or therapy, if:
(1) the official has received a request for the part from a hospital, physician, surgeon, or procurement organization;

(2) the official has made a reasonable effort, taking into account the useful life of the part, to locate and examine the decedent's medical records and inform persons listed in Section 3(a) of their option to make, or object to making, an anatomical gift;
(3) the official does not know of a refusal or contrary indication by the decedent or objection by a person having priority to act as listed in Section 3(a);
(4) the removal will be by a physician, surgeon, or technician; but in the case of eyes, by one of them or by an enucleator;
(5) the removal will not interfere with any autopsy or investigation;
(6) the removal will be in accordance with accepted medical standards; and
(7) cosmetic restoration will be done, if appropriate.

(b) If the body is not within the custody of the [coroner] or [medical examiner], the [local public health officer] may release and permit the removal of any part from a body in the [local health officer's] custody for transplantation or therapy if the requirements of subsection (a) are met.

(c) An official releasing and permitting the removal of a part shall maintain a permanent record of the name of the decedent, the person making the request, the date and purpose of the request, the part requested, and the person to whom it was released.

SECTION 5. ROUTINE INQUIRY AND REQUIRED REQUEST; SEARCH AND NOTIFICATION

(a) On or before admission to a hospital, or as soon as possible thereafter, a person designated by the hospital shall ask each patient who is at least [18] years of age: "Are you an organ or tissue donor?" If the answer is affirmative the person shall request a copy of the document of gift. If the answer is negative or there is no answer and the attending physician consents, the person designated shall discuss with the patient the option to make or refuse to make an anatomical gift. The answer to the question, an available copy of any document of gift or refusal to make an anatomical gift, and any other relevant information must be placed in the patient's medical record.

(b) If, at or near the time of death of a patient, there is no medical record that the patient has made or refused to make an anatomical gift, the hospital [administrator] or a representative designated by the [administrator] shall discuss the option to make or refuse to make an anatomical gift and request the making of an anatomical gift pursuant to Section 3(a). The request must be made with reasonable discretion and sensitivity to the circumstances of the family. A request is not required if the gift is not suitable, based upon accepted medical standards, for a purpose specified in Section 6. An entry must be made in the medical record of the patient, stating the name and affiliation of the individual making the request, and of the name, response, and relationship to the patient of the person to whom the request was made. The [Commissioner of Health] shall establish guidelines] and [adopt regulations] to implement this subsection.

(c) The following persons shall make a reasonable search for a document of gift or other information identifying the bearer as a donor or as an individual who has refused to make an anatomical gift:

   (1) a law enforcement officer, fireman, paramedic, or other emergency rescuer finding an individual who the searcher believes is dead or near death; and

   (2) a hospital, upon the admission of an individual at or near the time of death, if there is not immediately available any other source of that information.

(d) If a document of gift or evidence of refusal to make an anatomical gift is located by the search required by subsection (c)(1), and the individual or body to whom it relates is taken to a hospital, the hospital must be notified of the contents and the document or other evidence must be sent to the hospital.

(e) If, at or near the time of death of a patient, a hospital knows that an anatomical gift has been made pursuant to Section 3(a) or a release and removal of a part has been permitted pursuant to Section 4, or that a patient or an individual identified as in transit to the hospital is a donor, the hospital shall notify the donee if one is named and known to the hospital; if not, it shall notify an appropriate procurement organization. The hospital shall cooperate in the implementation of the anatomical gift or release and removal of a part.

(f) A person who fails to discharge the duties imposed by this section is not subject to criminal or civil liability but is subject to appropriate administrative sanctions.

SECTION 6. PERSONS WHO MAY BECOME DONEES; PURPOSES FOR WHICH ANATOMICAL GIFTS MAY BE MADE

(a) The following persons may become donees of anatomical gifts for the purposes stated:

   (1) a hospital, physician, surgeon, or procurement organization, for transplantation, therapy, medical or dental education, research, or advancement of medical or dental science;

   (2) an accredited medical or dental school, college, or university for education, research, advancement of medical or dental science; or

   (3) a designated individual for transplantation or therapy needed by that individual.

(b) An anatomical gift may be made to a designated donee or without designating a donee. If a donee is not designated or if the donee is not available or rejects the anatomical gift, the anatomical gift may be accepted by any hospital.

(c) If the donee knows of the decedent's refusal or contrary indications to make an anatomical gift or that an anatomical gift by a member of a class having priority to act is opposed by a member of the same class or a prior class under Section 3(a), the donee may not accept the anatomical gift.

SECTION 7. DELIVERY OF DOCUMENT OF GIFT

(a) Delivery of a document of gift during the donor's lifetime is not required for the validity of an anatomical gift.

(b) If an anatomical gift is made to a designated donee, the document of gift, or a copy, may be delivered to the donee to expedite the appropriate procedures after death. The document of gift, or a copy, may be deposited in any hospital, procurement organization, or registry office that accepts it for safekeeping or for facilitation of procedures after death. On request of an interested person, upon or after the donor's death, the person in possession shall allow the interested party to examine or copy the document of gift.

SECTION 8. RIGHTS AND DUTIES AT DEATH

(a) Rights of a donee created by an anatomical gift are superior to rights of others except with respect to autopsies under Section 11(b). A donee may accept or reject an anatomical gift. If a donee accepts an anatomical gift of an entire body, the donee, subject to the terms of the gift, may allow embalming and use of the body in funeral services. If the gift is of a part of a body, the donee, upon the death of the donor and before embalming, shall cause the part to be removed without unnecessary mutilation. After removal of the part, custody of the remainder of the body vests in the person under obligation to dispose of the body.

(b) The time of death must be determined by a physician or surgeon who attends the donor at death or, if none, the physician or surgeon who certifies the death. Neither the physician or surgeon who attends the donor at death nor the physician or surgeon who determines the time of death may participate in the procedures for removing or transplanting a part unless the document of gift designates a particular physician or surgeon pursuant to Section 2(d).

(c) If there has been an anatomical gift, a technician may remove any donated parts and an enucleator may remove any donated eyes or parts of eyes, after determination of death by a physician or surgeon.

SECTION 9. COORDINATION OF PROCUREMENT AND USE

Each hospital in this State, after consultation with other hospitals and procurement organizations, shall establish agreements or affiliations for coordination of procurement and use of human bodies and parts.

SECTION 10. SALE OR PURCHASE OF PARTS PROHIBITED

(a) A person may not knowingly, for valuable consideration, purchase or sell a part for transplantation or therapy, if removal of the part is intended to occur after the death of the decedent.

(b) Valuable consideration does not include reasonable payment for the removal, processing, disposal, preservation, quality control, storage, transportation, or implementation of a part.

(c) A person who violates this section is guilty of a [felony] and upon conviction is subject to a fine not exceeding [$50,000] or imprisonment not exceeding [five] years, or both.

SECTION 11. EXAMINATION, AUTOPSY, LIABILITY

(a) An anatomical gift authorizes any reasonable examination necessary to assure medical acceptability of the gift for the purposes intended.

(b) The provisions of this [Act] are subject to the laws of this State governing autopsies.

(c) A hospital, physician, surgeon, [coroner], [medical examiner], [local public health officer], enucleator, technician, or other person, who acts in accordance with this [Act] or with the applicable anatomical gift law of another state [or a foreign country] or attempts in good faith to do so is not liable for that act in a civil action or criminal proceeding.

(d) An individual who makes an anatomical gift pursuant to Section 2 or 3 and the individual's estate are not liable for any injury or damage that may result from the making or the use of the anatomical gift.

SECTION 12. TRANSITIONAL PROVISIONS

This [Act] applies to a document of gift, revocation, or refusal to make an anatomical gift signed by the donor or a person authorized to make or object to making an anatomical gift before, on, or after the effective date of this [Act].

SECTION 13. UNIFORMITY OF APPLICATION AND CONSTRUCTION

This [Act] shall be applied and construed to effectuate its general purpose to make uniform the law with respect to the subject of this [Act] among states enacting it.

SECTION 14. SEVERABILITY

If any provision of this [Act] or its application thereof to any person or circumstance is held invalid, the invalidity does not affect other provisions or applications of this which can be given effect without the invalid provision or application, and to this end the provisions of this are severable.

SECTION 15. SHORT TITLE

This [Act] may be cited as the "Uniform Anatomical Gift Act (1987)."

SECTION 16. REPEALS

The following acts and parts of acts are repealed:
    (1)
    (2)
    (3)

SECTION 17. EFFECTIVE DATE

This [act] takes effect _____.

APPENDIX 26-3   National Organ Transplant Act*

AN ACT

To provide for the establishment of the Task Force on Organ Transplantation and the Organ Procurement and Transplantation Network, to authorize financial assistance for organ procurement organizations, and for other purposes.

Be it enacted by the Senate and House of Representatives of the United States of America in Congress assembled, That this Act may be cited as the "National Organ Transplant Act."

From *UNOS 1996 Annual Report on the U.S Scientific Registry of Transplant Recipients and The Organ Procurement and Transplantation Network* (Richmond, Va., 1996).

*The opinions or assertions contained herein are those of the authors and are not to be construed as official or as representing those of the U.S. Army or the Department of Defense.

TITLE I—TASK FORCE ON ORGAN PROCUREMENT AND TRANSPLANTATION
Establishment and duties of task force

Sec. 101. (a) Not later than ninety days after the date of the enactment of this Act, the Secretary of Health and Human Services (hereinafter in this title referred to as the "Secretary") shall establish a Task Force on Organ Transplantation (hereinafter in this title referred to as the "Task Force").

(b)(1)   The Task Force shall—
    (A) conduct comprehensive examinations of the medical, legal, ethical, economic, and social issues presented by human organ procurement and transplantation.
    (B) prepare the assessment described in paragraph (2) and the report described in paragraph (3), and

(C) advise the Secretary with respect to the development of regulations for grants under section 371 of the Public Health Service Act.

(2) The Task Force shall make an assessment of immunosuppressive medications used to prevent organ rejection in transplant patients, including—

(A) an analysis of the safety, effectiveness, and costs (including cost-savings from improved success rates of transplantation) of different modalities of treatment;

(B) an analysis of the extent of insurance reimbursement for long-term immunosuppressive drug therapy for organ transplant patients by private insurers and the public sector;

(C) an identification of problems that patients encounter in obtaining immunosuppressive medications; and

(D) an analysis of the comparative advantages of grants, coverage under existing Federal programs, or other means to assure that individuals who need such medications can obtain them.

(3) The Task Force shall prepare a report which shall include—

(A) an assessment of public and private efforts to procure human organs for transplantation and an identification of factors that diminish the number of organs available for transplantation;

(B) an assessment of problems in coordinating the procurement of viable human organs including skin and bones;

(C) recommendations for the education and training of health professionals, including physicians, nurses, and hospital and emergency care personnel, with respect to organ procurement;

(D) recommendations for the education of the general public, the clergy, law enforcement officers, members of local fire departments, and other agencies and individuals that may be instrumental in affecting organ procurement;

(E) recommendations for assuring equitable access by patients to organ transplantation and for assuring the equitable allocation of donated organs among transplant centers and among patients medically qualified for an organ transplant;

(F) an identification of barriers to the donation of organs to patients with special emphasis upon pediatric patients, including an assessment of—

(i) barriers to the improved identification of organ donors and their families and organ recipients;

(ii) the number of potential organ donors and their geographical distribution;

(iii) current health care services provided for patients who need organ transplantation and organ procurement procedures, systems, and programs which affect such patients;

(iv) cultural factors affecting the facility with respect to the donation of the organs; and

(v) ethical and economic issues relating to organ transplantation needed by chronically ill patients;

(G) recommendations for the conduct and coordination of continuing research concerning all aspects of the transplantation of organs;

(H) an analysis of the factors involved in insurance reimbursement for transplant procedures by private insurers and the public sector;

(I) an analysis of the manner in which organ transplantation technology is diffused among and adopted by qualified medical centers, including a specification of the number and geographical distribution of qualified medical centers using such technology and an assessment of whether the number of centers using such technology is sufficient or excessive and of whether the public has sufficient access to medical procedures using such technology; and

(J) an assessment of the feasibility of establishing, and of the likely effectiveness of, a national registry of human organ donors.

Membership

Sec. 102. (a) The Task Force shall be composed of twenty-five members as follows:

(1) Twenty-one members shall be appointed by the Secretary which:

(A) nine members shall be physicians or scientists who are eminent in the various medical and scientific specialties related to human organ transplantations;

(B) three members shall be individuals who are not physicians and who represent the field of human organ procurement;

(C) four members shall be individuals who are not physicians and who as a group have expertise in the fields of law, theology, ethics, health care financing, and the social and behavioral sciences;

(D) three members shall be individuals who are not physicians or scientists and who are members of the general public; and

(E) two members shall be individuals who represent private health insurers or self-insurers.

(2) The Surgeon General of the United States, the Director of the National Institutes of Health, the Commissioner of the Food and Drug Administration, and the Administrator of the Health Care Financing Administration shall be ex officio members.

(b) No individual who is a full-time officer or employee of the United States may be appointed under subsection (a)(1) to the Task Force. A vacancy in the Task Force shall be filled in the manner in which the original appointment was made. A vacancy in the Task Force shall not affect its powers.

(c) Members shall be appointed for the life of the Task Force.

(d) The Task Force shall select a Chairman from among its members who are appointed under subsection (a)(1).

(e) Thirteen members of the Task Force shall constitute a quorum, but a lesser number may hold hearings.

(f) The Task Force shall hold its first meeting on a date specified by the Secretary which is not later than thirty days after the date on which the Secretary establishes the Task Force under section 101. Thereafter, the Task Force shall meet at the call of the Chairman or a majority of its members, but shall meet at least three times during the life of the Task Force.

(g)(1) Each member of the Task Force who is not an officer or employee of the United States shall be compensated at a rate equal to the daily equivalent of the annual rate of basic pay in effect for grade GS-18 of the General Schedule under section 5332 of title 5, United States Code, for each day (including travel time) during which such member is engaged in the actual performance of duties as a member of the Task Force. Each member of the Task Force who is an officer or employee of the United States shall receive no additional compensation.

(2) While away from their homes or regular places of business in the performance of duties for the Task Force, all members of the Task Force shall be allowed travel expenses, including per diem in lieu of subsistence, at rates authorized for employees of agencies under sections 5702 and 5703 of title 5, United States Code.

Support for the task force

Sec.103. (a) Upon request of the Task Force, the head of any Federal agency is authorized to detail, on a reimbursable basis, any of the personnel of such agency to the Task Force to assist the Task Force in carrying out its duties under this Act.

(b) The Secretary shall provide the Task Force with such administrative and support services as the Task Force may require to carry out its duties.

Report center

Sec.104. (a) The Task Force may transmit to the Secretary, the Committee on Labor and Human Resources of the Senate, and the Committee on Energy and Commerce of the House of Representatives such interim reports as the Task Force considers appropriate.

(b) Not later than seven months after the date on which the Task Force is established by the Secretary under section

101, the Task Force shall transmit a report to the Secretary, the Committee on Labor and Human Resources of the Senate, and the Committee on Energy and Commerce of the House of Representatives on its assessment under section 101(b)(2) of immunosuppressive medications used to prevent organ rejection.

(c) Not later than twelve months after the date on which the Task Force is established by the Secretary under section 101, the Task Force shall transmit a final report to the secretary, the Committee on Labor and Human Resources of the Senate, and the Committee on Energy and Commerce of the House of Representatives. The final report of the Task Force shall include—

(1) a description of any findings and conclusions of the Task Force made pursuant to any examination conducted under section 101(b)(1)(A),

(2) the matters specified in section 101(b)(3), and

(3) such recommendations as the Task Force considers appropriate.

Termination

Sec. 105. The Task Force shall terminate three months after the date on which the Task Force transmits the report required by section 104(c).

TITLE II—ORGAN PROCUREMENT ACTIVITIES

Sec. 201. Part H of title III of the Public Health Service Act is amended to read as follows:

PART H—ORGAN TRANSPLANTS
Assistance for organ procurement organizations

Sec.273. (a)(1) The Secretary may make grants for the planning of qualified organ procurement organizations described in subsection (b).

(2) The Secretary may make grants for the establishment, initial operation, and expansion of qualified organ procurement organizations described in subsection (b).

(3) In making grants under paragraphs (1) and (2), the Secretary shall—

(A) take into consideration any recommendations made by the Task Force on Organ Transplantation established under section 101 of the National Organ Transplant Act, and

(B) give special consideration to applications which cover geographical areas which are not adequately served by organ procurement organizations.

(b)(1) A qualified organ procurement organization for which grants may be made under subsection (a) is an organization which, as determined by the Secretary, will carry out the functions described in paragraph (2) and—

(A) is a nonprofit entity,

(B) has accounting and other fiscal procedures (as specified by the Secretary) necessary to assure the fiscal stability of the organization,

(C) has an agreement with the Secretary to be reimbursed under title XVIII of the Social Security Act for the procurement of kidneys,

(D) has procedures to obtain payment for non-renal organs provided to transplant centers,

(E) has a defined services area which is a geographical area of sufficient size which (unless the service area comprises an entire State) will include at least fifty potential organ donors each year and which either includes an entire standard metropolitan statistical area (as specified by the Office of Management and Budget) or does not include any part of such an area,

(F) has a director and such other staff, including the organ donation coordinators and organ procurement specialists necessary to effectively obtain organs from donors in its service area, and

(G) has a board of directors or an advisory board which—

  (i) is composed of—

    (I) members who represent hospital administrators, intensive care or emergency room personnel, tissue banks, and voluntary health associations in its service area,

    (II) members who represent the public residing in such area,

    (III) a physician with knowledge, experience, or skill in the field of histocompatibility,

    (IV) a physician with knowledge or skill in the field of neurology, and

    (V) from each transplant center in its service area which has arrangements described in paragraph (2)(G) with the organization, a member who is a surgeon who has practicing privileges in such center and who performs organ transplant surgery,

  (ii) has the authority to recommend policies for the procurement of organs and the other functions described in paragraph (2), and

  (iii) has no authority over any other activity of the organization.

(2) An organ procurement organization shall—

  (A) have effective agreements, to identify potential organ donors, with a substantial majority of the hospitals and other health area entities in its service area which have facilities for organ donations,

  (B) conduct and participate in systematic efforts, including professional education, to acquire all usable organs from potential donors,

  (C) arrange for the acquisition and preservation of donated organs and provide quality standards for the acquisition of organs which are consistent with the standards adopted by the Organ Procurement and Transplantation Network under section 274(b)(2)(E),

  (D) arrange for the appropriate tissue typing of donated organs,

  (E) have a system to allocate donated organs among transplant centers and patients according to established medical criteria,

  (F) provide or arrange for the transportation of donated organs to transplant centers,

  (G) have arrangements to coordinate its activities with transplant centers in its service area,

  (H) participate in the Organ Procurement Transplantation Network established under section 274,

  (I) have arrangements to cooperate with tissue banks for the retrieval, processing, preservation, storage, and distribution of tissues as may be appropriate to assure that all usable tissues are obtained from potential donors, and

  (J) evaluate annually the effectiveness of the organization in acquiring potentially available organs.

(c) for grants under subsection (a) there are authorized to be appropriated $5,000,000 for fiscal year 1985, $8,000,000 for fiscal year 1986, and $12,000,000 for fiscal year 1987.

Organ procurement and transplantation network

Sec.274. (a) The Secretary shall by contract provide for the establishment and operation of an Organ Procurement and Transplantation Network which meets the requirements of subsection. (b) The amount provided under such contract in any fiscal year may not exceed $2,000,000. Funds for such contracts shall be made available from funds available to the Public Health Service from appropriations for fiscal years beginning after fiscal year 1984.

(b)(1) The Organ Procurement and Transplantation Network shall carry out the functions described in paragraph (2) and shall—

  (A) be a private nonprofit entity which is not engaged in any activity unrelated to organ procurement, and

  (B) have a board of directors which includes representatives of organ procurement organizations (including organizations which have received grants under section 273), transplant centers, voluntary health associations, and the general public.

(2) The Organ Procurement and Transplantation Network shall—

(A) establish in one location or through regional centers—

  (i) a national list of individuals who need organs, and

  (ii) a national system, through the use of computers and in accordance with established medical criteria, to match organs and individuals included in the list, especially individuals whose immune system makes it difficult for them to receive organs,

(B) maintain a twenty-four-hour telephone service to facilitate matching organs with individuals included in the list,

(C) assist organ procurement organizations in the distribution of organs which cannot be placed within the service areas of the organizations,

(D) adopt and use standards of quality for the acquisition and transportation of donated organs,

(E) prepare and distribute, on a regionalized basis, samples of blood sera from individuals who are included on the list and whose immune system makes it difficult for them to receive organs, in order to facilitate matching the compatibility of such individuals with organ donors,

(F) coordinate, as appropriate, the transportation of organs from organ procurement organizations to transplant centers,

(G) provide information to physicians and other health professionals regarding organ donation, and

(H) collect, analyze, and publish data concerning organ donation and transplants.

Scientific registry

Sec. 274a. The Secretary shall, by grant or contract, develop and maintain a scientific registry of the recipients of organ transplants. The registry shall include such information respecting patients and transplant procedures as the Secretary deems necessary to an ongoing evaluation of the scientific and clinical status of organ transplantation. The Secretary shall prepare for inclusion in the report under section 274b an analysis of information derived from the registry.

General provisions respecting grants and contracts

Sec. 274b. (a) No grant may be made under section 273 or 274a or contract entered into under section 274 or 274a unless an application therefore has been submitted to, and approved by, the Secretary. Such an application shall be in such form and shall be submitted in such manner as the Secretary shall by regulation prescribe.

(b)(1) In considering applications for grants under section 273—

(A) the Secretary shall give priority to any applicant which has a formal agreement of cooperation with all transplant centers in its proposed service area,

(B) the Secretary shall give special consideration to organizations which met the requirements of section 273(b) before the date of the enactment of this section, and

(C) the Secretary shall not discriminate against an applicant solely because it provides health care services other than those related to organ procurement.

(D) The Secretary may not make a grant for more than one organ procurement organization which serves the same service area.

(2) A grant for planning under section 273 may be made for one year with respect to any organ procurement organization and may not exceed $100,000.

(3) Grants under section 371 for the establishment, initial operation, or expansion of organ procurement organizations may be made for two years. No such grant may exceed $500,000 for any year and no organ procurement organization may receive more than $800,000 for initial operation or expansion.

(c)(1) The Secretary shall determine the amount of a grant made under section 273 or 274a. Payments under such grants may be made in advance on the basis of estimates or by the way of reimbursement, with necessary adjustments on account of underpayments or overpayments, and in such installments and on such terms and conditions as the Secretary finds necessary to carry out the purposes of such grants.

(2)(A) Each recipient of a grant under section 273 or 274a shall keep such records as the Secretary shall prescribe, including records which fully disclose the amount and disposition by such recipient of the proceeds of such grant, the total cost of the undertaking in connection with which such grant was made, and the amount of that portion of the cost of the undertaking supplied by other sources, and such other records as will facilitate an effective audit.

(B) The Secretary and the Comptroller General of the United States, or any of their duly authorized representatives, shall have access for the purpose of audit and examination to any books, documents, papers, and records of the recipient of a grant under section 273 or 274a that are pertinent to such grant.

(d) For purposes of this part:

(1) The term "transplant center" means a health care facility in which transplants of organs are performed.

(2) The term "organ" means the human kidney, liver, heart, lung, pancreas, and any other human organ

(other than corneas and eyes) specified by the Secretary by regulation and for purposes of section 274a; such term includes bone marrow.

Administration

Sec. 274c. The Secretary shall, during fiscal years 1985, 1986, 1987, and 1988, designate and maintain an identifiable administrative unit in the Public Health Service to—

(1) administer this part and coordinate with the organ procurement activities under title XVIII of the Social Security Act,

(2) conduct a program of public information to inform the public of the need for organ donations,

(3) provide technical assistance to organ procurement organizations receiving funds under section 273, the Organ Procurement and Transplantation Network established under section 274, and other entities in the health care system involved in organ donations, procurement, and transplants, and

(4) one year after the date on which the Task Force on Organ Transplantation transmits its final report under section 104(c) of the National Organ Transplant Act, and annually thereafter through fiscal year 1988, submit to Congress an annual report on the status of organ donation and coordination services and include in the report an analysis of the efficiency and effectiveness of the procurement and allocation of organs and a description of problems encountered in the procurement and allocation of organs.

Report

Sec. 274d. The Secretary shall annually publish a report on the scientific and clinical status of organ transplantation. The Secretary shall consult with the Director of the National Institutes of Health and the Commissioner of the Food and Drug Administration in the preparation of the report.

TITLE III—PROHIBITION OF ORGAN PURCHASES

Sec. 274e. (a) It shall be unlawful for any person to knowingly acquire, receive, or otherwise transfer any human organ for valuable consideration for use in human transplantation if the transfer affects interstate commerce.

(b) Any person who violates subsection (a) shall be fined not more than $50,000 or imprisoned not more than five years, or both.

(c) For purposes of subsection (a):

(1) The term "human organ" means the human kidney, liver, heart, lung, pancreas, bone marrow, cornea, eye, bone, and skin, and any other human organ specified by the Secretary of Health and Human Services by regulation.

(2) The term "valuable consideration" does not include the reasonable payments associated with the removal, transportation, implantation, processing, preservation, quality control, and storage of a human organ or the expense of travel, housing, and lost wages incurred by the donor of a human organ in connection with the donation of the organ.

(3) The term "interstate commerce" has the meaning prescribed for it by section 201(b) of the Federal Food, Drug and Cosmetic Act.

TITLE IV—MISCELLANEOUS
Bone marrow registry demonstration and study

Secs. 274f and 274g. (a) Not later than nine months after the date of enactment of this Act, the Secretary of Health and Human Services shall hold a conference on the feasibility of establishing and the effectiveness of a national registry of voluntary bone marrow donors.

(b) If the conference held under subsection (a) finds that it is feasible to establish a national registry of voluntary donors of bone marrow and that such a registry is likely to be effective in matching donors with recipients, the Secretary of Health and Human Services, acting through the Assistant Secretary for Health, shall, for purposes of the study under subsection (c), establish a registry of voluntary donors of bone marrow. The Secretary shall assure that—

(1) donors of bone marrow listed in the registry have given an informed consent to the donation of bone marrow; and

(2) the names of the donors in the registry are kept confidential and access to the names and any other information in the registry is restricted to personnel who need the information to maintain and implement the registry, except that access to such other information shall be provided for purposes of the study under subsection (c).

If the conference held under subsection (a) makes the finding described in this subsection, the Secretary shall establish the registry not later than six months after the completion of the conference.

(c) The Secretary of Health and Human Services, acting through the Assistant Secretary for Health, shall study the establishment and implementation of the registry under subsection (b) to identify the issues presented by the establishment of such a registry, to evaluate participation of bone marrow donors, to assess the implementation of the informed consent and confidentiality requirements, and to determine if the establishment of a permanent bone marrow registry is needed and appropriate. The Secretary shall report the results of the study to the Committee on Energy and Commerce of the House of Representatives and the Committee on Labor and Human Resources of the Senate not later than two years after the date the registry is established under subsection (b).

Approved October 19, 1984.

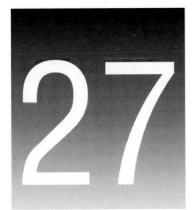

The process of dying

WHEN DEATH OCCURS
THE DYING PATIENT
CONCLUSION

One of the most difficult situations in the practice of medicine is the management of the dying patient. In caring for the dying patient, physicians confront not only the limits of their medical capabilities and the mortality of the patient, but also their own mortality:

And death means being no more. It cuts me off from all relation to the world and other human beings. It hurls me into non-being. Death teaches me that just as other things have ceased to be, so must I. Death tells me that all life is a flight to non-being. Human existence is a brief moment of light . . . Death . . . is my supreme possibility (for it leads me to authentic concern about the things which really matter) but it is also the limit of all my possibilities. A man who realizes he is to die cannot give supreme concern to any other event. Man must face death every moment and every day.[1]

Traditionally, physicians have been taught that their prime duties were the alleviation of pain and the prolongation of life. Success in achieving these goals has been variable at best, and physicians often are forced to choose between them.

Death has generally been defined as the cessation of life. Historically, the law has always accepted medicine's definition of death. Technological developments in medicine have precipitated the need for a legal reevaluation of the medical definition, since death has both a medical and a legal status. The interests of the deceased and family, health care providers, and society all require a reliable process of determining when death occurs.

WHEN DEATH OCCURS

As a first consideration, there is no specific moment of dying. Humans die in stages. During the ebbing of life there is a progression from clinical death to brain death, biological death, and then cellular death. *Clinical death* occurs when the body's vital functions (respiration and circulation) cease.

When the brain is deprived of oxygen because of cessation of circulation, brain death is inevitable. *Brain death* follows clinical death almost immediately unless resuscitative procedures are started promptly, because under normal conditions the human brain cannot survive loss of oxygen for more than 6 to 10 minutes. If resuscitative measures are instituted at the moment of clinical death, brain death may be averted and the patient may recover fully. On the other hand, brain death may follow despite reanimation efforts.

The brain also dies in steps. First the cerebral cortex, the site of the highest centers, ceases to function. Then successively, the cerebellum (older part of brain developmentally, associated with equilibrium) and the so-called lower brain centers die. Ultimately the brainstem and the vital centers (controlling respiration, heart rate, and blood pressure) die. If irreversible destruction of the highest centers of the brain occurs without damage to the vital centers, there is permanent loss of consciousness but cardiorespiratory functions can continue, sometimes unaided but most often only with artificial assistance. This is the so-called persistent vegetative state (PVS). When the lower areas of the brain are damaged in addition to the cerebrum, it still may be possible to maintain cardiovascular function for some time.

Ultimately, when all the components of the brain are dead, biological death, or permanent extinction of bodily life, occurs. Thereafter the process of cellular death begins, and because of differences in cellular composition, the death of different parts of the body occurs at different times and stages. That is why viable organs such as the heart or kidneys can be removed immediately after biological death and transplanted successfully. Also, even after biological death, organs within the lifeless body can be maintained for a time by means of mechanical and chemical support.

The transfer from one state of viability to another may be slow or very rapid. This decline depends on age; physical, constitutional, and environmental factors; and the life-extinguishing cause. In the sequence of dying there comes a point of irreversibility, which physicians diagnose as death.

The Editorial Committee updated this chapter. The committee gratefully acknowledges the past contribution of Frederick Adolf Paola, M.D., J.D., F.A.C.P., F.C.L.M., and John A. Anderson, M.D., J.D., F.C.L.M.

When this point has been reached, nothing further can be done to restore life. In many instances, physicians can slow the process but cannot prevent its ultimate conclusion—death.

Pronouncement of death

A formulation of death consists of (1) a definition of death, (2) criteria for determining that death has occurred, and (3) specific medical tests that show whether those criteria have been met.

Traditional formulation of death. A definition of death must "accurately show the quality so essentially significant to a living organism that its loss is termed death."[2] Traditionally, death was defined as the irreversible cessation of vital fluid (air and blood) flow. The corresponding ("heart-lung") criteria are the cessation of heart and lung function. Specific medical tests available to the physician to determine whether this criterion had been met included palpation for a pulse, auscultation for heart and breath sounds, use of a mirror held under the nares for evidence of condensation from exhaled breath, visualization of the optic fundus for vessel pulsation, and an electrocardiographic examination. If those examinations confirmed that vital functions had ceased, the physician would state that death had occurred. If the patient were young and the asystole or apnea promptly discovered, the physician might have delivered a precordial "thump" or injected intracardiac epinephrine in an attempt to stimulate the heart. If such methods were not employed or were unsuccessful, the physician pronounced the patient dead.

Impingement of technology. In the late 1950s and early 1960s the medical community became aware that in some cases of apparent cardiac arrest, the patient was actually in a ventricular tachyarrhythmia and that prompt establishment of an airway, conversion of the cardiac rhythm, and reestablishment of an adequate cardiac output might sustain life. Efforts to perform cardiopulmonary resuscitation (CPR) began to be undertaken widely and became medically fashionable. About this same time, cardiac care units came into nationwide vogue, with the medical community realizing that, with proper monitoring, many patients who had experienced asystole or arrhythmia after myocardial infarction, respiratory arrest, or other sudden catastrophe, and who would otherwise have expired, might survive to leave the hospital.

With the great mushrooming of medical technology that was occurring, including the development of defibrillators, ventilators, newer antibiotics and chemotherapeutic agents, hemodialysis and peritoneal dialysis, and transplantation, medicine had expanded capabilities to support and sustain the lives of those who previously would have died. Driven by the twin duties of pain alleviation and prevention of death, the physician enthusiastically embraced these new advances with little attention given to ethical, sociological, or economic consequences.

Brain death. With the development of modern resuscitation technology, it became possible to maintain heart and lung function for hours or days after all brain function had ceased. This created a dilemma for physicians. Discontinuing ventilatory support in such patients would cause the "death" of the patient, under the traditional formulation of death, and might be deemed the equivalent of a homicide.

The senselessness of maintaining patients in this hopeless condition and the increasing success of organ transplant programs led to a reexamination of the formulation of death.

This issue was first addressed by an ad hoc committee at the Harvard Medical School, convened to examine the definition of brain death. Its report appeared in an article entitled "A Definition of Irreversible Coma."[3] Using this term as synonymous with brain death, that article listed a series of criteria (the "Harvard Criteria") to be employed in pronouncing brain death. These criteria included the following:

1. Unreceptivity *and unresponsivity:* a total unawareness of externally applied stimuli and inner need and complete unresponsiveness, despite application of intensely painful stimuli.
2. *No spontaneous movements or breathing:* absence of all spontaneous muscular movement or breathing, as well as absence of response to stimuli such as pain, touch, sound, or light.
3. *No reflexes:* fixed, dilated pupils; lack of eye movement despite turning the head or ice-water stimulus; lack of response to noxious stimuli; and generally, lack of elicitable deep tendon reflexes.

Additionally, the committee recommended that the preceding observations be confirmed by two electroencephalograms (EEGs), taken at least 24 hours apart, documenting the absence of cortical electrical activity above baseline. It was also deemed necessary to exclude the presence of any metabolic state, hypothermia, or drug intoxication that might cause or contribute to a reversible loss of brain activity or function.[4]

These criteria proved to be extremely reliable and provided a strong impetus for physicians, attorneys, and policymakers to examine the propriety of bringing the then-accepted legal definition of death into conformity with then-current medical knowledge.

President's Commission recommendation

In 1978, Congress authorized the formation of a blue-ribbon panel of medical researchers and practitioners, other health care specialists, ethicists, attorneys, and public representatives to investigate troublesome areas in medicine.[5] In 1979, President Carter appointed the President's Commission for the Study of Ethical Problems in Medicine and Biomedical and Behavioral Research. The commission's investigation included the "definitions of death."

In their report "Defining Death" the commissioners urged all U.S. jurisdictions to accept a Uniform Determination of

Death Act, which would establish the "irreversible cessation of all functions of the entire brain, including the brain stem,"[6] as the criterion of death. This would provide guidelines for physicians to determine that death had occurred and to assist in its pronouncement. Members of the commission, the American Bar Association (ABA), the American Medical Association (AMA), and the National Conference of Commissioners on Uniform State Laws met to propose such a model act.

1. Determination of Death. An individual who has sustained either [a] irreversible cessation of circulatory and respiratory functions or [b] irreversible cessation of all functions of the entire brain, including the brainstem, is dead. A determination of death must be made in accordance with accepted medical standards.
2. Uniformity of Construction and Application. This act shall be applied and construed to effectuate its general purpose to make uniform the law with respect to the subject of this Act among states enacting it.

This model statute has since been approved by the AMA, the ABA, and the Uniform Law Commissioners and endorsed by the American Academy of Neurology and the American Electroencephalographic Society. The President's Commission urged all states to adopt the use of brain death criteria in the determination of death.

Newer technology has allowed additional refinements in the physician's ability to demonstrate "irreversible cessation of all functions of the entire brain." In cases where the Harvard criteria or similar guidelines have established brain death, absence of cerebral circulation has been demonstrated using angiographic techniques. Similarly, absence of brain metabolism (lack of glucose uptake by the brain) has been verified by applying nuclear medicine techniques and positron emission tomography (PET). When the brain is receiving no circulation and is not metabolizing the only substrate it is capable of utilizing, the conclusion must be that there has been "irreversible cessation" of brain function and therefore brain death. These techniques have validated the concept of brain death, the determination of which is made "in accordance with accepted medical standards," as described in the Uniform Determination of Death Act.

The President's Commission used a *whole-brain formulation,* under which death is defined as the irreversible loss of an organism's ability to "'function as a whole' (to integrate, regulate, and organize important organ systems)."[7] Whole-brain theorists posit that "the entire brain (cerebral hemispheres, brain stem, cerebellum, and diencephalon [thalamus and hypothalamus]) must be rendered permanently functionless to determine death."[8] Nevertheless, referring to this formulation as "whole brain" is somewhat of a misnomer because under the definition the essential quality (i.e., the loss of which constitutes death) is the brainstem's ability for "noncognitive integration of vegetative functions."[9] Loss of the so-called higher brain functions of consciousness and cognition is irrelevant.

In 1991, New Jersey enacted a law with a conscience clause permitting competent adults with religious beliefs to designate in advance that the traditional, heart-oriented definition of death should be applied to them.[10]

Consequences for the criminal law. The brain death criterion has been applied in unusual circumstances in criminal homicide cases. In an Arizona case the defendant argued that it was not his criminal actions that caused the death of the victim, but rather those of the physician who terminated the life-support systems.[11] He alleged that evidence was insufficient to warrant his conviction for murder. However, the court ruled that the murder conviction was justified because (1) brain death was also a valid test of death in Arizona, and (2) the victim's brain function had ceased as a result of the defendant's action and before life support was discontinued.

In a comparable California case the victim had been shot in the head during a robbery attempt.[12] There was evidence of brain death by EEG, although the victim's heart and lungs continued to function on a ventilator. The victim's family agreed to have him serve as a donor for cardiac transplantation surgery at Stanford University Hospital. The victim was pronounced dead using the Harvard criteria and then flown to Stanford, where the heart was removed for transplantation. The defendant's attorney objected when the charge against his client was changed from assault with intent to murder to murder in the first degree. The defense attorney claimed that the surgeon who removed the heart actually "murdered" the victim by his surgical act. In this case, again the court disagreed. The patient (victim) had died and was considered brain dead as a result of the criminal act itself and nothing else. On the basis of this case, California judicially adopted the concept of brain death as had Arizona.[13] The brain death formulation was subsequently adopted by statute in California and is now contained in Chapter 3.7, Section 7180 of that state's Health and Safety Code.

In most cases, within 3 to 10 days after brain death per se occurs, total cardiovascular collapse usually ensues. In only a few reported cases has survival been prolonged beyond that point in adults. In children, however, cardiac and circulatory functions may continue for a considerably longer period after electrocerebral silence occurs and the Harvard criteria for brain death have been met.[14] Few civil cases have turned on the diagnosis of death by brain death criteria.

The higher brain formulation of death. Why is the definition of death important?

The definition of death debate is actually a debate over the moral status of human beings. . . . [While] humans are [still alive], full moral and legal human rights accrue. Saying people are alive is simply shorthand for saying that they are bearers of such rights. That is why the definition of death debate is so important.[15]

The traditional (heart-lung) definition of death measured the point at which clinical death occurred. The biological life of the human organism was taken as a sine qua non for personhood, and therefore the traditional definition allowed one to identify specifically those cases in which humans ceased to be persons.

Some suggest that the "whole-brain" formulation's definition of death is inadequate and should be replaced by one defining death as "the irreversible loss of consciousness and cognition."[16] "Defining death to include irreversible PVS would merely require extending the definition to include situations in which the brainstem is functioning but the neocortex is dead."[17] Under this formulation, permanent "failure of [those] brain areas responsible for consciousness and cognition" would be the criterion of death.[18] Although practical obstacles remain to the implementation of this "higher-brain"[19] formulation of death (including the subjective nature of consciousness[20] and the nonspecificity of confirmatory laboratory tests[21]), the consciousness formulation retains its theoretical appeal because consciousness and cognition, unlike the ability to integrate vegetative functions, are "irreplaceably spontaneous and innate" and thus "essential to the definition of human life."[22]

Although one criticism of higher brain formulation of death has been the inability of clinicians to determine precisely the irreversible loss of higher brain functions, the AMA's Council on Scientific Affairs and Council on Ethical and Judicial Affairs have concluded that a diagnosis of PVS can be made with an error rate of less than one in a thousand.[23]

Veatch has suggested the following:

An individual who has sustained irreversible loss of consciousness is dead. A determination of death must be made in accordance with accepted medical standards. However, no individual shall be considered dead based on irreversible loss of consciousness if he or she, while competent, has explicitly asked to be pronounced dead based on irreversible cessation of all functions of the entire brain or based on irreversible cessation of circulatory and respiratory functions.

Unless an individual has, while competent, selected one of these definitions of death, the legal guardian or next of kin (in that order) may do so. The definition selected by the individual, legal guardian or next of kin shall serve as the definition of death for all legal purposes.[24]

Death certificate

After the patient has been pronounced dead, the attending physician should prepare the working copy of the death certificate, which includes most of the following data: name and address of the decedent, age, place and date of birth, names of parents (including mother's maiden name), birthplace of parents, race, and decedent's occupation. These data are included primarily for statistical and epidemiological purposes. The death certificate also provides space for the attending physician to indicate how long he or she has treated the patient, when he or she last saw the patient alive, and the immediate and contributing causes of death, together with their duration.

Other conditions affecting the patient are also listed, even though they may not have contributed to the cause of death. Most states also provide for inclusion of data regarding surgery and/or biopsy and autopsy as indicative of the cause of death. The immediate cause of death is not always necessarily the mechanism of death, such as cardiac arrest or ventricular fibrillation, but rather the condition that eventually resulted in death, such as myocardial infarction with arrhythmia.

Using this working document, the mortician types the final death certificate, which is then presented to the physician for signature and dating. Burial or other disposition of the remains is not permitted in most states until the attending physician has signed the completed death certificate.

Cause of death

As noted previously, the cause of death listed on the death certificate should be the immediate cause, the condition that resulted in death rather than the mechanism of death.

When the cause of death may be obscure or the physician has not seen the patient in a specified time (which varies from state to state), state law usually requires that the medical examiner or coroner be contacted. The case then becomes a medical examiner's or coroner's case. State laws differ considerably with respect to circumstances under which the coroner or medical examiner must be notified regarding the death and will determine whether an autopsy is appropriate. Most states specify that such notification is essential in following situations: dead-on-arrival (DOA) cases; cases in which the cause of death cannot be determined because of an inadequate hospital stay; cases in which death occurred following hospitalization for less than 24 hours; all cases of sudden, violent, suspicious, unexpected, unexplained, and medically unattended death; all intraoperative or perioperative deaths (including preoperative and immediate postoperative); death related to industrial employment; death resulting from therapeutic misadventure; death resulting from alleged, suspected, or known criminal activity; and death resulting from vehicular traffic accidents as well as train or airplane accidents.

The physician must understand the critical importance of contacting the medical examiner or coroner in his or her jurisdiction when there is any doubt about the circumstances surrounding the death. The physician should be willing to speak with the medical examiner or the staff to discuss the case with them at length. Requests for results or data on the medical examiner's autopsy or a copy of the autopsy protocol for the physician's records are usually honored.

Custody of body, authorization for autopsy, and disposal of remains

Although the individual may indicate before death that he or she wishes to have an autopsy performed, such a statement is advisory or directive only, not mandatory. As soon as death occurs, the next of kin are recognized by law to have a property interest in the decedent's body. According to a schedule prescribed by state law, they are the ones who may consent to autopsy. The ranking order of individuals who may grant such permission for autopsy or have custody of the remains is usually as follows: surviving spouse, eldest living child of the decedent (if of age), parent(s) of the decedent, legally appointed guardian, eldest living sibling of the deceased (if of age), aunt(s) and uncle(s) of the decedent, and other kin in order of consanguinity.

Before autopsy can be requested, the physician must pronounce the patient dead and appropriate family members or next of kin must be contacted. When death occurs in a hospital, the death pronouncement note must be written in the hospital record and the autopsy request form completed and signed before the performance of that procedure. It is also appropriate to indicate on the permission form any restrictions on the extent of the examination, such as head excluded, chest only, or abdomen only. The more extensive the autopsy and the more tissues examined, the more accurate, valuable, and complete will be the information gathered for the benefit of the physicians, surviving family members, and society.

When controversy arises over consenting to autopsy among members of a group of equal consanguinity, it is probably inadvisable or imprudent to accept the consent of only one member of the group who is willing to give it. Often the original permit may have been obtained from a low-priority relative only because that individual was the one first located after the death of the patient, and one of closer consanguinity subsequently objects. When there are no known relatives, custody of the body and responsibility for its disposition may be accepted by a friend, a lodge, or similar organization. However, such a casual custodian of a dead body may have no legal authority to grant permission for an autopsy.

Although it has occurred occasionally, it is considered unprofessional for a physician to use the threat of medical examiner contact as a tool to pry autopsy consent from a family when the death is from natural causes, which would not otherwise require medical examiner involvement or investigation. Cooperation with the medical examiner, provision of appropriate information, access to physicians' and hospital records, and so on allow as much knowledge as possible to be gained to help elicit the cause of death in confusing cases.

The medical examiner is not empowered to function as a watchdog over the clinical performance of physicians in the community. However, by the nature of the work, the medical examiner or coroner may become involved in cases of alleged professional negligence or incompetence. The investigations and examinations in such situations should be conducted in the same careful, thorough manner as in any other case. The final report should be prepared in a highly professional manner and should be available to all appropriate parties. A competent, careful, thorough, scientific, unbiased investigation and report serve the cause of justice in any medicolegal situation, whether civil or criminal.

Additional cases of death appropriate for medical examiner investigation are violent, accidental, and mysterious deaths, including suspected homicide or suicide. Those that may be caused entirely or partly by any factor other than natural causes are also reportable. These include but are not limited to death associated with burns, chemicals, or electrical or radiation injury; death under suspicious circumstances; death of patients of public institutions not hospitalized primarily for organic disease; death of persons in the custody of law enforcement officers; all deaths that occur during, in association with, or as a result of diagnostic, therapeutic, or anesthetic procedures; any death resulting from neglect; and death of persons not disabled by recognizable disease.

Once the autopsy has been completed, or once death is pronounced when no autopsy is to be performed, the remains may be turned over to next of kin or surviving family members, a mortician, an embalmer, or a funeral director for burial, cremation, or other disposition. As noted previously, such final disposition cannot take place until the attending physician, or the coroner or medical examiner, has completed and signed the death certificate. It is critical that the physician's signature be added to the death certificate only after that certificate has been completed by a mortician or funeral director. Signing a blank death certificate or one that is incomplete may create serious problems for the attending physician.

THE DYING PATIENT
Traditional physician role: "Hippocratic Oath"

From the historical beginnings of medicine, the physician's goal was twofold: to preserve life and to relieve suffering. From the days of the Greek and Roman physicians through the early 1960s, these goals did not conflict. Physicians might have been tempted to hasten the patient's demise by giving an excessively large dose of morphine for "pain relief" or to provide some other method of inducing the patient's death. However, the constraints of the Judeo-Christian religions with their proscriptions against killing, the various ethical codes for physicians (Hippocrates, Maimonides), and the possibility of criminal prosecution for euthanasia usually prevented physicians from undertaking such activities. Often, physicians could provide only psychological and emotional support for dying patients, because complete pain relief was not possible without jeopardizing vital functions.

The double effect. A patient with metastatic cancer requires narcotic analgesics for control of pain. In this example showing the double effect, as the patient's narcotic requirements escalate, it becomes increasingly difficult to control the pain without depressing the patient's respiratory drive. Because relieving pain and maintaining compromised function are both legitimate goals of medicine, what should the physician do when these goals conflict? Such situations are often analyzed in terms of the "double effect":

Some actions have several effects that are inextricably linked. One of those effects is intended by the agent and is ethically permissible (e.g., relief of pain); the other is not intended by the agent and is ethically questionable (e.g., respiratory depression). Proponents of this argument state that ethically permissible effect can be allowed, even if the ethically questionable one will inevitably follow, when the following conditions are present:

(a) The action itself is ethically good or at least indifferent, that is, neither good nor evil in itself (in this case, the action is the administration of a drug, a morally indifferent act).

(b) The agent must intend the good effects, not the evil effects, even though these are foreseen (in this case, the intention is to relieve pain, not to compromise respiration).

(c) The morally objectionable effect cannot be a means to the morally permissible one (in this case, respiratory compromise is not the means to relief of pain).[25]

The 1993 Michigan ban against assisted suicide contains an exemption contemplating the double effect; it exempts the prescription, dispensing, or the administration of medication designed "to relieve pain or discomfort and not to cause death, even if the medication or procedure may hasten or increase the risk of death."[26]

Effects of technology and a changing patient population

As already described in discussing the evolution of the concept of brain death, resuscitation techniques and technology began to be applied in the late 1960s, and their use was not limited to that group for whom resuscitation was originally recommended. As early as 1973 the American Heart Association (AHA) and the National Academy of Sciences (NAS) reinforced the original recommendations regarding CPR, urging that CPR be employed in the case of young individuals with sudden, unexpected arrest, or victims of drowning or electrocution. The 1973 AHA and NAS statements noted that "[CPR] is not indicated in certain clinical situations, i.e., terminal irreversible illness where death is not unexpected." CPR was also considered an inappropriate modality for the chronically ill individual with no hope of recovery.

Unfortunately, with the passage of time, resuscitation techniques and life-support measures were applied to a progressively sicker, older, more infirm population. CPR became a commonplace activity on the hospital scene whenever an arrest occurred. Its performance was straightforward and almost rote, frequently with no consideration given to patient selection or therapeutic aim.

In many cases, patients were resuscitated with no subsequent return of cognitive (higher brain) functions. Families and society were left with a burgeoning population of patients, maintained on ventilators, with no hope of return to a normal, sapient state. In those cases in which brain death criteria were applicable, death might be pronounced using those criteria and the patient then withdrawn from the ventilator to "let nature take its course." In those cases where brain death criteria were not met and ventilator support could not be removed, the burden continued, and the patient was maintained in his or her noncognitive state.

Not surprisingly, concerns arose that resuscitation was being inappropriately used, in many cases on patients who were

harmed rather than benefited. The physician's goals of prolonging life and easing suffering had come into conflict with each other.

Withholding and withdrawing treatment: the patient with capacity

A legal consensus exists that the adult with capacity has a legally protected right to refuse life-sustaining[27] treatment. Historically, courts have grounded this right either in the common-law right to self-determination, or the privacy and liberty guarantees of the federal or state constitutions, or in statutes, rather than in exceptions to homicide laws.[28]

Courts have characterized the termination of life support as permissible "letting die,"[29] distinguishing it from impermissible "killing" (murder, suicide, or assisted suicide). Courts have generally given two reasons for this distinction: (1) the intention of the patient in refusing treatment is not self-destruction but rather control of his or her care, and (2) the cause of death in the patient who refuses life-sustaining treatment is the patient's illness, not the patient's refusal. A better explanation for this distinction is

[t]hat if liability is not to be imposed on physicians who withhold or withdraw life support, it is because they have no duty to provide it. The absence of a duty arises from the fact that the treatment has been declined by a competent patient or for an incompetent patient by a surrogate legally authorized to do so.[30]

The right of the patient with capacity to refuse unwanted medical treatment gained constitutional recognition in *Cruzan v. Director, Missouri Dept. of Health,* with the majority's assertion that "[t]he principle that a competent patient has a constitutionally protected liberty interest in refusing unwanted medical treatment may be inferred from our prior decisions."[31] The practical effect of the court's characterization of the patient's claim to refuse unwanted medical treatment as a "liberty interest" (rather than a fundamental right) is that the state need not have a compelling countervailing interest to overcome that claim.

The right of patients with capacity to refuse life-sustaining treatment applies even to those who are not terminally ill. In *Elizabeth Bouvia v. Riverside General Hospital,* Elizabeth Bouvia was a young woman with cerebral palsy and virtually no use of her voluntary muscles. As a result, she was unable to take her own life. She had hospitalized herself and "disclosed her intent to discontinue sufficient caloric intake so that she would eventually succumb to starvation." Bouvia asked the court to enjoin the defendant hospital from administering artificial nutrition and hydration against her will and from transferring or discharging her.

The court, while stating that Bouvia "[did] have a fundamental right to terminate her own life and to terminate medical intervention," framed the issue differently. The issue was, according to the court, "whether or not a severely handicapped, mentally competent person who is otherwise physically healthy and not terminally ill has the right to end her life *with the assistance of society*" (emphasis added).[32] They held she did not.

In a later case involving Ms. Bouvia, where the issue was framed as whether she had the right to refuse life-sustaining medical treatment, the California Court of Appeals held that she indeed had a right to refuse nutrition and hydration to end her life.[33]

Withholding and withdrawing treatment: the patient who has lost capacity

There seems to be a legal consensus that, in theory, the right of a patient without capacity to refuse medical treatment should be coextensive with the corresponding right of a patient with capacity. The effective exercise of that right, however, is problematic. Thus some patients without capacity may be unable to express any preference with regard to treatment; other patients without capacity, although able to express treatment preferences, may be expressing preferences that are not authentic expressions of their will. Consequently, a decision concerning the treatment of the patient without capacity must be made by a surrogate decision-maker.

As indicated earlier, the patient with capacity has the right to refuse life-sustaining treatment irrespective of that patient's medical condition or prognosis. Although the same is theoretically true regarding patients who have lost decision-making capacity,

[c]ourts . . . understandably look carefully at the patient's medical condition or prognosis before sanctioning surrogate decisions for nonautonomous patients who have not expressed a clear position of abating treatment. The clearest cases [have] involved patients who are terminally ill. . . . Courts have [also] upheld numerous decisions to abate treatment for patients in a persistent vegetative state. . . . Few courts have yet to grapple with the charged issue of abating treatment for nonvegetative, nonterminally ill patients [without capacity].[34]

Decision-making for the patient without capacity and with an advance directive. Advance directives include "living wills, durable powers of attorney, appointment of health care proxies, . . . and other devices that allow a competent person to give directions concerning [his/]her medical treatment if [he/]she becomes incompetent."[35]

To better inform patients about their legal rights to execute advance directives and refuse treatment, Congress in 1990 enacted the Patient Self-Determination Act (PSDA).[36] This act, which took effect on December 1, 1991, mandated that health care institutions (including nursing homes, hospitals, home health agencies, hospices, clinics, and HMOs) in receipt of federal funds under Medicare and/or Medicaid provide each patient with written information regarding his or her rights under the laws of his or her state to participate in the medical decision-making process and to formulate an advance directive. The PSDA encourages the use of advance

directives by requiring hospitals to inform patients of their right to execute such directives.

LIVING WILL STATUTES. California was the first state to enact living will legislation, with its own Natural Death Act[37] in 1977. By 1992, all but three states had enacted living will laws providing a statutory mechanism for persons to exercise their legal right to refuse life-sustaining treatment in the event they lose decision-making capacity.[38] Living will statutes are problematic:

Most of these statutes include fairly rigorous standards for preparing a binding directive. Many statutes provide, for example, that a directive becomes binding only if and when the patient is determined to be terminally ill (and typically that determination must be made by more than one physician. In some states, a directive is legally binding only if, after the onset of terminal illness but before the onset of incompetence (a fleeting moment for some patients), the patient reaffirms the directive. Increasingly, physicians and lawyers alike have criticized these statutory models both for their procedural obstacles and for failing to make clear which forms of care are to be foregone and [under] what circumstances.[39]

For these reasons, an increasingly attractive option for patients is to delegate the legal authority to make health care decisions to another person in the event that the patient becomes unable to make such decisions.

DURABLE POWER OF ATTORNEY AND HEALTH CARE PROXIES. Normally a power of attorney executed by an individual allows another, acting as his or her agent, to make decisions for him or her. In the event of the incompetence of the original declarant, the power of attorney lapses and becomes void; in other words, the agent can no longer act for the principal should the principal become incompetent after the original delegation of authority.

The *durable* power of attorney, on the other hand, permits decision-making by the agent in the event that the principal becomes incompetent. When extended to health care situations, it delegates to the agent the authority to make health care decisions for the principal, in the event of the latter's incapacity or incompetence.

As of 1987, all 50 states had general durable power of attorney statutes that were "probably adequate authority to empower a health care proxy decision-maker."[40] Further, as of 1992, all states except Alabama had enacted statutes that either explicitly authorized the delegation to a proxy of the legal authority to make health care decisions or that had been specifically interpreted as authorizing such a delegation (so-called "health care proxy" acts).[41] In *Cruzan* the U.S. Supreme Court suggested that the Constitution might require that states give legal effect to the health care decisions of a duly appointed surrogate decision-maker.

Decision-making for the patient without capacity and without a formal advance directive. The problem remains of how to make medical decisions for patients who have lost capacity without ever having executed a formal advance directive. Under these circumstances, different states use different procedures and different substantive criteria for surrogate decision-making. In general, "[t]he consensus view is that there is a hierarchy of three standards to be applied in making decisions under these circumstances] . . . : the subjective standard, the substituted judgment standard, and the best interests standard."[42]

Thus the decision-making process in such a case begins with an inquiry into whether the patient has executed an informal advance directive by expressing a desire either to accede to or decline treatment under the present circumstances.

THE SUBJECTIVE STANDARD. The strictest standard is the subjective standard, under which the surrogate's decision is based on the patient's own preferences as expressed before his or her loss of capacity. The surrogate asks, "What did the patient in fact decide before losing decision-making capacity?"[43] Expressions of those preferences are to be found, for example, in "oral directions to family members, friends, or health-care providers, reactions of the patient to medical treatment administered to others, the individual's religious beliefs, and the patient's previous pattern of behavior concerning his or her own medical care"[44] before the patient's loss of decision-making capacity.

New York,[45] Missouri,[46] and Michigan[47] adhere to the subjective standard, and Michigan's *In re Martin* illustrates this approach.

In *In re Martin* the Supreme Court of Michigan took up the question of whether life-sustaining treatment in the form of a gastrostomy tube could be withdrawn from a patient who was neither terminally ill nor unconscious, but who was (irreversibly) cognitively and communicatively impaired and without decision-making capacity. Although Michigan common law recognizes a right to refuse life-sustaining medical treatment, the court held that that right only survives the patient's loss of capacity to the extent it is actually exercised before the loss of capacity. The court concluded that, because the evidence showing that Martin had actually decided, before losing capacity, to decline life-sustaining treatment in his present condition was not clear and convincing, the gastrostomy tube could not be withdrawn.

In *Cruzan v. Director, Missouri Dept. of Health,*[48] the U.S. Supreme Court held that the "liberty interest" protected by the Fourteenth Amendment's due process clause does not preclude states from requiring, as a prerequisite for forgoing life-sustaining treatment of patients without capacity, "that there be clear and convincing evidence that the patient herself decided prior to losing decision-making capacity that life-sustaining treatment should be stopped."[49] The state's adoption of this decision-making standard was justified by the state's interests in "preserving life and personal choice, preventing abuse by the surrogate, and ensuring accurate fact finding and reducing the risk of error."[50] It is important to understand that *Cruzan* permits, but does not require, states to insist upon "clear and convincing" proof that the subjective

standard has been satisfied. *Cruzan* states that the "challenging task of creating appropriate procedures for safeguarding incompetents' liberty interests is entrusted to the 'laboratory' of the states. . . ."[51]

SUBSTITUTED JUDGMENT STANDARD. Under this standard the surrogate asks, "What would the patient decide if the patient were able to decide?"[52] New Jersey's famous *Quinlan*[53] case illustrates this approach.

Karen Quinlan was originally brought to a New Jersey hospital in a comatose state, where her consent to treatment was implied by the emergency doctrine. She was intubated and maintained on a respirator. Despite such treatment, she remained in a persistent vegetative state[54] from which it became clear that she would not emerge. Because Karen would thus never have the capacity to assert her right to be free of unwanted physical intrusions, her father sought to assert this right for her and asked that mechanical ventilation be stopped. Invoking the doctrine of "substituted judgment," the court held that "the only practical way to prevent destruction of Karen Quinlan's right [of privacy] is to permit the guardian and family of Karen to render their best judgment . . . as to whether she would exercise it in these circumstances."[55]

BEST INTERESTS STANDARD. When it is unclear what the patient would decide if he or she were able to decide, most courts allow the surrogate to forgo life-sustaining treatment if doing so is in the patient's best interests. Meisel has pointed out that "no court that permits the use of the substituted judgment standard has rejected the application of a best interests standard if the evidence is insufficient to meet the former," although not all courts that permit the use of the substituted judgment standard have had to decide whether to permit the use of the best interests standard when the substituted judgment standard cannot be met.[56]

It is well accepted that "continued life-sustaining treatment per se is not always in a patient's best interests, and forgoing [such] treatment is not always contrary to a patient's interests."[57]

Although the preceding three "standards" establish the facts that must be proved to enable a surrogate to forgo life-sustaining treatment, a separate consideration is, "How convincingly must these facts be established?" In other words, what standard of proof must be met?

Most states, irrespective of which of the preceding three standards for surrogate decision-making they use, require that those standards be met with "clear and convincing evidence."[58] As noted earlier, New York, Missouri, and Michigan, for example,

[r]equire clear and convincing evidence that the patient himself or herself authorized the forgoing of life-sustaining treatment before losing decision-making capacity. . . . Other states require clear and convincing evidence that the patient would have decided to forgo treatment—in effect, clear and convincing evidence of the substi-

tuted judgment standard. In other states what is required is clear and convincing evidence that it is not in the patient's best interests . . . that treatment be continued.[59]

DECISION-MAKING BY FAMILIES. Some 20 states have enacted "family decision" acts, which codify the "age-old custom of turning to the next of kin for guidance about treatment when a patient is unable to make decisions personally."[60] Such acts are based on the twin assumptions that first, when a patient's preferences are knowable, family members are the persons most likely to know them; and second, that when those preferences are not knowable, family members are the persons most likely to act in the patient's best interests. In 1992, in response to recommendations made by the New York State Task Force on Life and the Law,[61] New York State enacted legislation controlling do-not-resuscitate (DNR) decision-making by surrogates for incapacitated patients who have executed neither an advance directive nor a health care proxy.[62] Under this legislation, such a patient is represented by a surrogate chosen from a prioritized list (court-appointed guardian, spouse, adult child, parent, adult sibling, or close friend). The surrogate decides about CPR on the basis of the patient's wishes, to the extent that these wishes can be determined, and failing that, in accordance with the patient's best interests.

Deciding for the patient who never had capacity. The *Cruzan* case articulates no standards governing surrogate refusal of treatment on behalf of persons who have never been competent, and the U.S. Supreme Court has not yet been faced with this issue.

Massachusetts grappled with this issue in *Superintendent of Belchertown State School v. Saikewicz.*[63] Joseph Saikewicz was a 67-year-old mentally retarded man in urgent need of treatment for acute leukemia. However, because of the severity of his mental retardation (he had an IQ of 10 and a mental age of about 2 years and 8 months), he was unable to give informed consent to treatment. A court-appointed guardian ad litem recommended "that not treating Mr. Saikewicz would be in his best interests." The probate judge agreed with the guardian ad litem.

The appeals court affirmed. The court used as the starting point of its analysis the principle that "a general right . . . to refuse medical treatment . . . must extend to the case of an incompetent, as well as a competent, patient because the value of human dignity extends to both." The court reasoned therefore that in refusal-of-treatment cases involving never-competent persons, courts should attempt

[t]o ascertain the incompetent person's actual interests and preferences. In short, the decision in cases such as this should be that which would be made by the incompetent person, if that person were competent, but taking into account the present and future incompetency of the individual as one of the factors which would necessarily enter into the decision-making process of the competent person.

New York dealt differently with a similar case in the *Matter of Storar.*[64] John Storar was a 52-year-old mentally retarded man with a mental age of about 5 years. He had bladder cancer and a secondary anemia necessitating periodic blood transfusions, but he was unable to give informed consent to the transfusions. His mother refused to give consent because the transfusion process distressed her son and his illness was terminal.

The New York Court of Appeals reasoned that since John Storar had never had capacity, he was in essence a child. Since, under New York law, "no parent can withhold a blood transfusion from a child when without it the child will die,"[65] the court ruled that the blood transfusions could not be withheld. The court reasoned that "it was unrealistic to try to determine what [John Storar] would want done under the circumstances." The court also rejected the substituted judgment test adopted by other courts because it believed that no third party should be permitted to make a quality-of-life judgment for another.

Do-not-resuscitate orders

In recent years an individual's right to self-determination is foremost in the resuscitation decision. Both the legal and the medical communities have recognized that this is a corollary to the patient's right of informed consent. This right comes before the interests of the physician and hospital and includes the right of informed refusal of resuscitation in any care setting.

When patients did not wish to be but were still resuscitated, physicians were considered to have violated the dictum enunciated by Justice Cardozo in the *Schloendorff* case[66] in 1914: "Every human being of adult years and sound mind has a right to determine what shall be done with his own body."

As with the right to refuse other unwanted medical treatment, constitutional support for the individual's right to refuse unwanted resuscitation is derived from the "right to privacy" and from the liberty interest protected by the Fourteenth Amendment. Decisions not to resuscitate may be thought of as a subdivision of decisions to withhold medical treatment.

Although they have been perceived as a new development, DNR[67] orders form part of the long-range picture in the evolution of our current awareness of mutual rights and responsibilities in the area of death and dying. In this context, it is relevant to consider the memorandum that appeared more than 30 years ago on the bulletin board of a large, respected teaching hospital: "The following patients are not to be resuscitated: those who are very elderly (over 65 years of age); those who are suffering from malignant disease; those with chronic chest disease; and those with chronic renal disease."

This memo was posted at the Neasden Hospital in Britain in 1965. When it came to public notice, the news spread like wildfire through the British press. A great public hue and cry ensued. The hospital administration said that it did not intend the message the memo appeared to convey, or perhaps it was mistyped, or incorrectly interpreted; regardless, hospital administration did not mean what was stated in the memo. This was apparently the first attempt to apply any type of protocol in nonresuscitation cases.

Currently, most hospitals have policies under which all patients will be resuscitated unless a written DNR order has been entered on their chart. In addition, the Joint Commission on Accreditation of Healthcare Organizations (JCAHO) required, effective January 1, 1988, that all facilities seeking accreditation must have a DNR policy, without defining the limits or criteria to be included within that policy.[68] The consensus now seems to be that patients have the right and should be afforded the opportunity to exercise their autonomous decision not to be resuscitated. The "reflex resuscitation" of anyone experiencing an arrest is now disappearing in favor of antecedent decisions to forgo it or to have positive orders for resuscitation, if needed.

New York was the first state to comprehensively regulate DNR orders. New York's DNR law presumes consent to resuscitation in the absence of an *order not to resuscitate* (ONTR). A physician may not write such an order without first obtaining the patient's consent, if the patient has decision-making capacity, or the consent of a duly appointed surrogate if the patient lacks decision-making capacity. The New York DNR law also provides a statutory list of acceptable surrogates when the patient is incompetent and has not, before losing capacity, appointed a surrogate. The surrogate must base his or her decision regarding CPR on the patient's wishes or, if the patient's wishes are unknown and unknowable, on the patient's best interests. Furthermore, a surrogate may consent to an ONTR only if an attending physician has determined to a reasonable degree of medical certainty that (1) the patient has a terminal condition, (2) the patient is permanently unconscious, (3) resuscitation would be medically futile, or (4) resuscitation would impose an extraordinary burden on the patient in light of the patient's medical condition.

DNR laws such as New York's do not create a duty to resuscitate where none previously existed. Rather, they create a presumption that all patients who have not expressly consented to an ONTR would consent to resuscitative measures.

Futility

Medical futility is not easily defined, but "generally, the term means care that serves no useful purpose and provides no immediate or long-term benefit."[69] More specifically, futile care

[m]ay be that which does not address . . . the underlying illness . . . that in time will cause death, [or] . . . it may be care that does not achieve its immediate purpose. Whether . . . performing an appendectomy on a patient with incurable cancer would be futile depends on which of these two meanings one adopts.[70]

In discussing futility, one must be careful to distinguish between physiologically futile treatment (defined as treatment that is "clearly futile in achieving its physiologic objective and so [of] no physiologic benefit to the patient"[71]) and treatment with "important physiologic effects which medical judgment concludes [nonetheless] are nonbeneficial to the patient as person."[72] Futility is an increasingly important issue in end-of-life medicine.

In re Wanglie. The case of Helga Wanglie was hailed in a *New England Journal of Medicine* editorial as "a new kind of right to die case."[73] In earlier "right to die" cases it had been families and patients seeking to have life-sustaining treatment withheld or withdrawn over the objections of the health care providers, whereas in the *Wanglie* case it was the patient's physicians who sought to withdraw life-sustaining treatment over the objections of the patient's family. Helga Wanglie was an 86-year-old, ventilator-dependent Minneapolis woman in PVS. In November 1990, her physicians informed the Wanglie family that continued mechanical ventilation was "nonbeneficial" to Mrs. Wanglie as a person and that it should be discontinued.

Mrs. Wanglie's husband (an attorney), daughter, and son rejected the idea of withdrawing ventilatory support, saying "that physicians should not play God, that the patient would not be better off dead, that removing life support showed moral decay in our civilization, and that a miracle could occur."[74] Although the husband initially "told a physician that his wife had never stated her preferences concerning life-sustaining treatment" in the setting of PVS, he later "asserted that the patient had consistently said she wanted respirator support for such a condition."

The hospital asked that the court appoint an independent conservator to decide whether continued use of the respirator was beneficial to the patient; and in the event the conservator found its use was not beneficial, the hospital asked that a second hearing be held on the question of whether it was legally obliged to provide the respirator. On July 1, 1991, the court appointed the husband as conservator and, noting that no request had yet been made for permission to stop treatment, declined to address the matter.[75] The hospital, unclear about its legal duty to continue to provide ventilatory support, announced that it would not discontinue such support. Three days later, Mrs. Wanglie died of sepsis-induced multisystem organ failure.

In the matter of Baby K. In 1993 the U.S District Court for the Eastern District of Virginia took up the question of whether a hospital was required to provide ventilator treatment for an anencephalic infant (Baby K) suffering repeated episodes of respiratory distress. The hospital and physicians insisted that such treatment was futile; the infant's mother rejected this position and refused to consent to a DNR order. The district court held that under the federal antidumping law (the Emergency Medical Treatment and Active Labor Act [EMTALA]) "the hospital would be liable . . . if Baby K arrived [in the ER] in respiratory distress . . . and the Hospital failed to provide [the] mechanical ventilation . . . necessary to stabilize her acute medical condition."[76] EMTALA, the court wrote, "does not admit of any 'futility' . . . exceptions"; further, the court seemed to equate medical futility with physiological futility when it wrote in dictum that "[e]ven if EMTALA contained [a futility exception] . . . , [it] would not apply here. The use of a mechanical ventilator to assist breathing is not 'futile' . . . in relieving the acute symptoms of respiratory difficulty which is the emergency medical condition that must be treated under EMTALA."

In 1994 a panel of the U.S. Court of Appeals for the Fourth Circuit affirmed two to one.[77]

Gilgunn v. Massachusetts General Hospital. Catherine Gilgunn was a 71-year-old patient with Parkinson's disease, diabetes, and heart disease; she had experienced a cerebrovascular accident (CVA) 1 year earlier. She had had a mastectomy for breast cancer in June 1989, when she was admitted to the Massachusetts General Hospital for surgery for a hip fracture. There she developed irreversible brain damage.[78]

Despite the daughter insisting that her mother had always said she wanted "everything possible done medically," the attending physician asked for and received from the ethics committee permission for a DNR order, which was then entered on the chart. Three days later, Mrs. Gilgunn was weaned from the respirator and died.

In a jury trial the Suffolk County Superior Court ruled that the hospital and its physicians were not guilty of negligently imposing emotional distress on the daughter. The judge had asked the jury to consider whether the patient, had she been able, would have requested CPR and mechanical ventilation. The jury answered in the affirmative but agreed with the defendants that such treatment would have been futile.

DNR orders and futility. When resuscitation is considered futile therapy (some suggest that CPR for patients who will not survive to be discharged from the hospital is futile[79]), advance decisions about CPR should be considered and DNR orders written. If no reasonable expectation exists that the patient will benefit from resuscitation, it may then be considered an inappropriate (if not unethical) modality to use, especially without having first consulted the patient and obtaining his or her consent.

Some even argue that when the physician has determined that attempts at CPR would be futile in a particular patient, the physician has the authority to enter a DNR order without the consent of the patient or the patient's family.[80] This follows from the principle that physicians have no duty to provide useless therapy to patients or to discuss useless therapy with them. Patients for whom CPR might arguably be deemed futile include the following:

1. Patients who are brain dead.
2. Anencephalic newborns.
3. Patients with . . . metastatic cancer in [its] agonal stage.
4. Elderly patients with acute stroke, sepsis, or pneumonia.
5. Patients with severe cardiomyopathy.
6. Elderly patients with renal failure who are found pulseless and apneic.
7. Elderly patients with asystole, electro-mechanical dissociation, or agonal rhythms.
8. Very low birth weight newborns who suffer a cardiac arrest in the first 72 hours following birth.
9. Patients with severe chronic lung disease.[81]

Analysis of the relevant case law lends credence to the argument that physicians' liability for not providing futile CPR is remote and that physicians expose themselves to greater liability by providing such treatment. Nevertheless, when unilateral DNR orders are to be written, it would be prudent to do so under the auspices of hospital or medical staff guidelines for their issuance.

CONCLUSION

Currently accepted guidelines involving the process of dying are as follows:

1. Early communication between physician and patient (or patient's family or surrogate where appropriate) regarding diagnosis, prognosis, and therapeutic options together with reasonable expected goals is critical.
2. Patients should be encouraged to execute advance directives regarding their choices about treatment options or goals.[82] This would ensure that the proper locus of decision-making would be in its traditional place: at the bedside, between patient (family) and physician.
3. The patient's decision-making capacity should be carefully assessed.
4. An attempt should be made to seek unanimity among the members of the health care team.
5. It is a legal myth that "it is permissible to terminate extraordinary treatments, but not ordinary ones." Decisions about forgoing or discontinuing life-support measures on terminally ill patients must balance the benefit of the proposed therapy against the burden imposed on the patient. Such decisions must take into proper consideration the patient's constitutional liberty interests and common-law right of informed consent. These rights must be juxtaposed against the state's interests as articulated in the U.S. Supreme Court decision in *Cruzan.*
6. When families or surrogates must be involved, decisions should not be rushed. Time to deliberate must be provided, together with appropriate pastoral or social work support or psychological counseling as appropriate.

ENDNOTES

1. A.T. Padovano, *The Estranged God* 26 (Sheed and Ward, New York 1966).
2. S.J. Youngner & E.T. Bartlett, *Human Death and High Technology: The Failure of the Whole-Brain Formulations,* 99 Ann. Int. Med. 252 (1983).

3. A. Beecher, *A Definition of Irreversible Coma: Report of the Ad Hoc Committee of the Harvard Medical School to Examine the Definition of Death,* 205 J.A.M.A. 337 (1968).
4. *Id.*
5. Public Law 95-622 (1978).
6. Report of the President's Commission for the Study of Ethical Problems in Medicine and Biomedical and Behavioral Research, *Defining Death: Medical, Legal and Ethical Issues in the Determination of Death* (1981).
7. *Supra* note 2, at 252.
8. J.L. Bernat, *How Much of the Brain Must Die in Brain Death?* 3 J. Clinical Ethics 21-26 (1992).
9. *Supra* note 2, at 253.
10. 26 N.J. Stat. 6A-4 (Declaration of Death Act). *See also* R.M. Veatch, *The Impending Collapse of the Whole-Brain Definition of Death,* 23 Hastings Center Report 18-24, at 22 (1993).
11. *State v. Fierro,* 124 Ariz. 182, 603 P. 2d 74 (1979).
12. *People v. Saldana,* 47 Cal. App. 3d 954, 121 Cal. Rptr. 243 (1975).
13. *People v. Lyons,* Cal. Super. Ct., Oakland (May 21, 1974), *cited in* Friloux, *Death: When Does It Occur?* 27 Baylor L. Rev. 10 (1975).
14. J. Korein, *Brain Death, in Anesthesia and Neurosurgery,* 282, 284, 292-293 (J. Cottrell & H. Turndorf eds., Mosby, St Louis 1980).
15. Veatch, *supra* note 10, at 22.
16. *Supra* note 2; *see also* R.M. Veatch, *The Whole-Brain Oriented Concept of Death: An Outmoded Philosophical Formulation,* 3 J. Thanatol. 13-30 (1975).
17. C.H. Baron, *Why Withdrawal of Life-Support for PVS Patients Is Not a Family Decision,* 19 Hastings Center Report 73-75 (1991).
18. *Supra* note 2, at 253.
19. R.M. Veatch, *Brain Death and Slippery Slopes,* 3 J. Clinical Ethics 187 (1992).
20. J. Miller, *Trouble in Mind,* Sci. Am. 180 (Sept 1992).
21. J.L. Bernat, *The Boundaries of the Persistent Vegetative State,* 3 J. Clinical Ethics 176-180 (1992).
22. *Supra* note 2, at 257.
23. Council on Scientific Affairs and Council on Ethical and Judicial Affairs, *Persistent Vegetative State and the Decision to Withdraw or Withhold Life Support,* 263 J.A.M.A. 428 (1990).
24. Veatch, *supra* note 10, at 23.
25. A.R. Jonsen et al., *Clinical Ethics* 112-113 (3d ed., McGraw-Hill, New York 1992).
26. Y. Kamisar, *Are Laws Against Assisted Suicide Unconstitutional?* 23 Hastings Center Report 32, at 33 (1993).
27. Life-sustaining treatment means "any medical intervention, technology, procedure, or medication that is administered . . . in order to forestall the moment of death, whether or not the treatment is intended to affect the underlying life-threatening disease(s) or biologic processes." *See* Hastings Center, *Guidelines on the Termination of Life-Sustaining Treatment and the Care of the Dying* 4 (1987).
28. D.W. Brock, *Voluntary Active Euthanasia,* 22 Hastings Center Report 19 (1992).
29. Forgoing life-sustaining treatment at the patient's behest is sometimes called "voluntary passive euthanasia" (VPE).
30. A. Meisel, *Legal Myths About Terminating Life Support,* 151 Archives Int. Med. 1498 (1991).
31. *Cruzan v. Director, Missouri Dept. of Health,* 110 S.Ct. 2851 (1990).
32. *Elizabeth Bouvia v. Riverside General Hospital,* No. 159780 Riverside Co., Cal. (Sup. Ct., Dec 19, 1983).
33. *Bouvia v. Superior Court,* 225 Cal. Rptr. 287 (Cal. App. 1986).
34. L. Gostin & R.F. Weir, *Life and Death Choices after* Cruzan: *Case Law and Standards of Professional Conduct,* 69 The Milbank Q. 143, at 159-160 (1991).
35. J.A. Robertson, *Second Thoughts on Living Wills,* 21 Hastings Center Report 9 (1991).

36. Omnibus Reconciliation Act of 1990, Pub. L. 101-508, 4206, 4751, 104 Stat. 1388, *codified at* 42 U.S.C. 1395 cc(a)(1)(Q), 1395mm(c)(8), 1395cc(f), 1396a(a)(57), (58), 1396a(w). *See also* regulations at 57 Fed. Reg. 8194-8204 (March 6, 1992).
37. *The California Natural Death Act: an Empirical Study of Physicians' Practice,* 31 Stan. L. Rev. 913 (1979).
38. A. Meisel, *A Retrospective on* Cruzan, 20 L. Med. & Health Care 342, 344 (1992); *see also* J. Areen, *Advance Directives Under State Law and Judicial Decisions,* 19 L. Med. & Health Care 91-100 (1991).
39. Areen, *supra* note 38, at 92; *see also* J.A. Robertson, *Second Thoughts on Living Wills,* 21 Hastings Center Report 6-9 (1991).
40. J. Areen, *The Legal Status of Consent Obtained from Families of Adult Patients to Withhold or Withdraw Treatment,* 258 J.A.M.A. 229 (1987).
41. Meisel, *supra* note 38, at 344.
42. Meisel, *supra* note 38, at 342.
43. *Id.*
44. *Supra* note 34, at 158.
45. 72 N.Y. 2d 517, 531 N.E. 2d 607, 534 N.Y.S. 2d 886 (N.Y. 1988).
46. *Cruzan by Cruzan v. Harmon* 760 S.W. 2d 408 (Mo. 1988).
47. *In re Martin,* 450 Mich. 204 (Mich. 1995).
48. *Supra* note 31, at 2841.
49. Meisel, *supra* note 38, at 343.
50. *Supra* note 34, at 146.
51. *Supra* note 31, at 2857.
52. Meisel, *supra* note 38, at 342.
53. *In The Matter of Karen Quinlan,* 70 N.J. 10, 335 A. 2d 647, *cert. denied,* 429 U.S. 922 (1976).
54. Persistent vegetative state (PVS) is defined as "the irreversible loss of all neocortical functions [with] brainstem functions intact." It is an eyes-open unconsciousness." *See* R.E. Cranford, *Neurologic Syndromes and Prolonged Survival: When Can Artificial Nutrition and Hydration Be Forgone?* 19 L. Med. & Health Care 13, at 14 (1991).
55. *Supra* note 53; *see also Matter of Farrell,* 108 N.J. 335, 529 A. 2d 404 (1987).
56. Meisel, *supra* note 38, at 343.
57. *Id.*
58. *See,* however, *In re Fiori,* No. J-67-95, 4/2/96, in which the Pennsylvania Supreme Court rejected the "clear and convincing" evidence test as one that would thwart the right of the unsophisticated or uneducated PVS patient to be free of unwanted medical care.
59. Meisel, *supra* note 38, at 343.
60. A.M. Capron, *Where Is the Sure Interpreter?* 22 Hastings Center Report 26-27 (Jul/Aug 1992).
61. The New York State Task Force on Life and the Law, *When Others Must Choose: Deciding for Patients Without Capacity* (New York State Task Force on Life and the Law, New York 1992).
62. *N.Y. Consolidated Laws Service,* Public Health 2965.2.(a).
63. *Superintendent of Belchertown State School v. Saikewicz,* 373 Mass. 728, 370 N.E. 2d 417 (1977).
64. *Matter of Storar,* 52 N.Y. 2d 363, 438 N.Y.S. 2d 266, 420 N.E. 2d 64, *cert. denied,* 454 U.S. 858, 102 S.Ct. 309, 70 L.Ed. 2d 153.
65. S. Wachtler, *A Judge's Perspective: the New York Rulings,* 19 L. Med. & Health Care 60, at 61 (1991).
66. *Schloendorff v. Society of New York Hospital,* 211 N.Y. 125, 105 N.E. 92 (1914).
67. DNR orders are sometimes referred to as *orders not to resuscitate* (ONTR).
68. *JCAHO 1989 Accreditation Manual,* M.A. 1.4.11, at 82 (1988).
69. F.H. Marsh & A. Staver, *Physician Authority for Unilateral DNR Orders,* 12 J. Legal Med. 115-165, at 117 (1991); *see also* S.J. Youngner, *Who Defines Futility?* 260 J.A.M.A. 2094 (1988).
70. L.A. Albert, Cruzan v. Director, Missouri Dept. of Health: *Too Much Ado,* 12 J. Legal Med. 331-358, at 335 (1991).

71. Hastings Center, *Guidelines on the Termination of Life-Sustaining Treatment and the Care of the Dying,* 32 (Indiana University Press, Bloomington, Ind. 1987).

72. J.H. Miles, *Medical Futility,* 20 L. Med. & Health Care 310 (1992).

73. M. Angell, *The Case of Helga Wanglie: A New Kind of Right to Die Case,* 325 N. Engl. J. Med. 511-512 (1991).

74. S.H. Miles, *Informed Demand for "Non-Beneficial" Medical Treatment,* 325 N. Engl. J. Med. 513 (1991).

75. *In re Helga Wanglie,* Fourth Judicial District (Dist. Ct., Probate Ct. Div.) PX-91-283, Minn., Hennepin County.

76. *Matter of Baby K,* 832 F.Supp. 1022 (E.D.Va. 1993).

77. *In the Matter of Baby K,* 16 F. 3d 590 (4th Cir. 1994).

78. N. Hentoff, *A Doctor Alone Could Decide When You Should Die,* St. Petersburg Times A:12 (Sept 5, 1995).

79. *Supra* note 69, at 118.

80. *Supra* note 69.

81. *Supra* note 69, at 119.

82. *See,* however, J. Lynn, *Why I Don't Have a Living Will,* 19 L. Med. & Health Care 101-104 (1991).

GENERAL REFERENCES

L.A. Albert, Cruzan v. Director, Missouri Dept. of Health: *Too Much Ado,* 12 J. Legal Med. 331 (1991).

M. Battin, *Voluntary Euthanasia and the Risks of Abuse: Can We Learn Anything from The Netherlands?* 20 L. Med. & Health Care 133-143 (1992).

D.W. Brock, *Voluntary Active Euthanasia,* 22 Hastings Center Report 10-22 (1992).

B. Brody, *Special Ethical Issues in the Management of PVS Patients,* 20 L. Med. & Health Care 104 (1992).

C.B. Cohen & P.J. Cohen, *Required Reconsideration of DNR Orders in the Operating Room and Certain Other Treatment Settings,* 20 L. Med. & Health Care 354-363 (1992).

D.K. McKnight & M. Bellis, *Foregoing Life-Sustaining Treatment for Adult, Developmentally Disabled Public Wards: A Proposed Standard,* 18 Am. J. L. & Med. 203-232 (1992).

A. Meisel, *A Retrospective on* Cruzan, 20 L. Med. & Health Care 340-353 (1992).

R.J. Miller, *Hospice Care as an Alternative to Euthanasia,* 20 L. Med. & Health Care 127-132 (1992).

T.E. Miller, *Public Policy in the Wake of* Cruzan: *A Case Study of New York's Health Care Proxy Law,* 18 L. Med. & Health Care 360-367 (1990).

S.G. Pollack, *Identifying Appropriate Decision-Makers and Standards for Decision,* 19 Hastings Center Report 63-65 (1989).

F. Rouse, *Advance Directives: Where Are We Heading After* Cruzan? 18 L. Med. & Health Care 353-359 (1990).

S. Wachtler, *A Judge's Perspective: the New York Rulings,* 19 L. Med. & Health Care 60-62 (1991).

R.F. Weir, *The Morality of Physician-Assisted Suicide,* 20 L. Med. & Health Care 116-126 (1992).

R.F. Weir & L. Gostin, *Decisions to Abate Life-Sustaining Treatment for Nonautonomous Patients,* 264 J.A.M.A. 1849-1852 (1990).

S.M. Wolf, *Final Exit: the End of Argument,* 22 Hastings Center Report 30-33 (1992).

S.J. Youngner & E.T. Bartlett, *Human Death and High Technology: the Failure of the Whole-Brain Formulations,* 99 Annals Int. Med. 252-258 (1983).

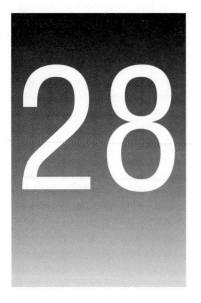

Physician-assisted suicide

S. SANDY SANBAR, M.D., Ph.D., J.D., F.C.L.M.

AID-IN-DYING, PHYSICIAN-ASSISTED SUICIDE, AND EUTHANASIA
SUICIDE AND ATTEMPTED SUICIDE
ASSISTED SUICIDE
QUILL V. VACCO
COMPASSION IN DYING V. STATE OF WASHINGTON
BRIEF AMICUS CURIAE OF THE AMERICAN COLLEGE OF LEGAL MEDICINE
U.S. SUPREME COURT DECISIONS
RECENT DEVELOPMENTS

On June 26, 1997, the Supreme Court of the United States decided two cases dealing with physician-assisted suicide. In *Vacco v. Quill* the Supreme Court held that New York's prohibition on assisted suicide does not violate the equal protection clause of the Constitution.[1] And in *State of Washington v. Glucksberg* the Supreme Court held that Washington's prohibition against causing or aiding a suicide does not violate the due process clause of the Constitution.[2] These two cases are discussed subsequently. First, however, this chapter includes brief introductory discussions of aid-in-dying, suicide, attempted suicide, and assisted suicide. The two physician-assisted suicide decisions of the U.S. Courts of Appeals for the Second and Ninth Circuit Courts are also discussed.[3,4] These two cases were granted certiorari in 1996 and subsequently were decided in 1997 by the U.S. Supreme Court. The chapter includes recent developments in and the future of physician-assisted suicide.[5]

AID-IN-DYING, PHYSICIAN-ASSISTED SUICIDE, AND EUTHANASIA

Physicians generally have consistently and compassionately aided and comforted dying patients, particularly those who suffer excruciating, agonizing, slow, and very painful deaths, by allowing them to die "comfortably," principally through use of pain medications. Physicians' orders not to resuscitate, turning off the respirator in a respirator-dependent patient, withholding needed medications (e.g., antibiotics and anticancer drugs), and not administering hydration and nutrition are methods by which the patient and often the immediate family agree to a course of treatment or "nontreatment" aimed at hastening the death of the terminally ill patient. In the case of hospitalized patients, however, the attending physician bears the responsibility of ordering that course of "medical therapy," thereby "letting the patient die." The

physician is clearly playing an active, compassionate role in hastening the terminally ill patient's death. The methods used, however, are perfectly legal and are based on laws that involve legal advance medical directives and living wills (see Chapter 27).

Another example of aid-in-dying with physician involvement is *terminal sedation*. This method of "physician-aided dying" includes the administration of large doses of morphine and similar medications, which has a dual effect of relieving the pain and hastening the death of the terminally ill patient. This form of aid-in-dying is both legal and deemed ethically acceptable by the medical community at large, the American Medical Association (AMA), and most recently (June 1997) the U.S. Supreme Court, simply because the intent of the treatment is not to kill or hasten death but rather to relieve the intractable pain and suffering of the terminally ill patient.[6] This practice has been used for the conscious, mentally competent, terminally ill patient, as well as for the comatose or not fully conscious terminally ill patient.

Consent for aid-in-dying is provided by the patient or surrogate decision-maker. The attending physician, who is directly involved, often concurs with the patient's decision and provides medical treatment at the end of life, which is designed to ease the suffering and agony of a painful death. If the physician does not agree with the patient and family for whatever reason (e.g., religious beliefs), he or she must transfer the care to another physician whose personal beliefs would not interfere with the terminal care of the patient. Medical treatment in this context may include administration of drugs that have a *dual effect,* one of which may hasten the death of the patient, thereby terminating the pain and suffering. If the physician orders or administers the dual-effect treatment, it is considered aid-in-dying. On the other hand, if the patient requests the same medical treatment with its known dual effect, and if the physician knowingly provides that medication by prescription so that the patient can end his or her life, it is considered physician-assisted suicide. In this scenario the intent of the patient, which is communicated to the prescribing physician, is to end his or her life prematurely by unnatural means. The dual effect of sedation and relief of pain and suffering is no longer the primary consideration.

In contrast to aid-in-dying, *physician-assisted suicide* refers to the practice whereby the physician provides the patient with the medical information (e.g., discussing painless and effective pharmacological means of committing suicide) or the means (e.g., writing a prescription) enabling that patient to end his or her own life.

On the other hand, if the physician's intent is merely to provide pain medication to ease the suffering of the terminally ill patient, and if the physician is unaware that the patient intends to end his or her own life, the physician is not assisting the patient's death because the physician lacks knowledge of the patient's intent to commit suicide.

Finally, a physician or other health care provider who provides a medical treatment intended to cause the death of a terminally ill patient without that patient's or a family member's consent may be charged with murder, manslaughter, or criminal homicide. The physician would be committing *voluntary active euthanasia,* in which the physician actively and directly (e.g., by administering a lethal injection of morphine or potassium) causes the death of a competent patient. Such active euthanasia is illegal in all 50 states. Neither the patient's consent nor the physician's motivation by mercy are relevant in a criminal proceeding; criminal law exists to protect the public interest, as opposed to the private interests, and the perpetrator's motive for killing is not an element of homicide.

SUICIDE AND ATTEMPTED SUICIDE

Presently in America, no state has a statute prohibiting suicide or attempted suicide, but the majority of the states have enacted laws imposing criminal sanctions on individuals who assist in a suicide.[7] Historically, suicide, attempted suicide, and assisted suicide have been considered crimes. In seventeenth-century England, suicide had been declared murder.[8] In America, in 1798, seven of the thirteen colonies had penalties for suicide. In 1816, *Commonwealth v. Bowen* was the leading case on suicide, which was described by the Massachusetts judge as self-destruction and a crime of "awful turpitude" and was considered in the eyes of the law to be equally as heinous as the murder of one by another.[9] In New York, for example, in the 1843 case of *Breasted v. Farmers' Loan & Trust Co.* the crime of suicide was described by the Superior Court as a "criminal act of self-destruction."[10]

By 1868, however, the crime of suicide was no longer punishable in America, although attempted suicide remained punishable. In 1877 the court held in *Commonwealth v. Mink,* another case from Massachusetts, that any attempt to commit suicide was unlawful and criminal.[11] In 1881 the new Penal Code of New York provided that an intentional attempt to commit suicide was a felony with a maximum penalty of 2 years' imprisonment.[12]

In 1901, New Jersey declared that suicide was not a crime. In 1919 the New York Legislature removed the prohibition against attempted suicide, which was no longer a crime but was declared a "grave public wrong."[13] In 1965 the New York Legislature deleted this declaration.[14]

ASSISTED SUICIDE

Most states now have laws against assisting suicide, even though suicide and attempted suicide are no longer considered crimes. "States that specifically prohibit assisted suicide either classify it as a unique offense or define it as a type of murder or manslaughter."[15]

In 1828, New York enacted its first prohibition of assisted suicide. The statute punished any individual who assisted another in committing "self-murder" for first-degree manslaughter.[16] Since 1919, however, not a single physician has been convicted of assisting a patient to commit suicide in the state of New York.

In 1996 the state of Iowa enacted a law forbidding assisted suicide, but the law does not prohibit "the responsible actions of a licensed health professional to administer pain medication to a patient with a terminal illness."[17]

QUILL V. VACCO

In New York a person who intentionally aids another person to commit suicide or who intentionally aids another person to attempt suicide may be convicted of a felony. This law led three physicians and their three patients to pursue a claim in which they asserted that prohibiting physicians from acceding to requests from their terminally ill, mentally competent patients for help in hastening their deaths violated their civil rights. All three patients died from their terminal illnesses during the course of the litigation. In April 1996 the three-judge panel of the Second Circuit Court of Appeals, based in New York, unanimously held as follows[18]:

- The controversy was justiciable.
- No fundamental right to assisted suicide existed.
- The law prohibiting assisted suicide, which was challenged by the physicians and their patients, violated the equal protection clause of the U.S. Constitution to the extent that the laws prohibited a physician from prescribing medication to be self-administered by a mentally competent, terminally ill person.

Controversy

In *Quill* the physicians had not been charged with commission of any crimes, but the court noted that Dr. Quill had a criminal proceeding instituted against him in the past, and the other two physicians faced the threat of criminal prosecution. In the usual course of events a court will not consider mere hypothetical, academic, or moot questions. The court found in *Quill* that a sufficiently concrete, justiciable controversy was presented that permitted the court to address the issue without first requiring the physicians to expose themselves to actual criminal prosecution.

Right to assisted suicide

The due process clause of the Fourteenth Amendment of the U.S. Constitution prohibits deprivation of life, liberty, or property without due process of law. Consistently the courts have been reluctant to recognize new rights. Instead, courts have chosen to analyze a controversy by determining whether the claim or right falls within those rights mentioned in the text of the U.S. Constitution, including freedom of association; the right to participate in the electoral process and to vote; the right to travel interstate; the right to procedural fairness with regard to claims for governmental deprivations of life, liberty, or property; and the right to privacy. In *Quill* the court reviewed cases from other jurisdictions and found that no state has recognized a right to assisted suicide, and it refused to recognize such a right as a result of this case.

Violation of equal protection clause

Because the court found no fundamental right to assisted suicide, it concluded that the New York law did not impinge on any fundamental right or involve suspect classifications of individuals. However, the court concluded that the New York laws prohibiting assisted suicide were not rationally related to a legitimate state interest.

The court noted that New York has recognized, both by statutes and legal cases dealing with this issue, that a person has the right to decide what will be done with his or her own body. This right extends to the right of the competent, terminally ill patient to hasten death with proper proof of a desire to do so.

The discussion by the court of equal protection in *Quill* contrasted the 1990 holding by the U.S. Supreme Court in *Cruzan v. Director, Missouri Dept. of Health,* holding that it could be inferred from earlier Supreme Court opinions that a competent person has a constitutionally protected interest in refusing unwanted medical treatment.[19]

The Second Circuit Court saw no distinction between disconnecting life support, which is permissible in New York, and writing a prescription to hasten death, which is not legally permitted. The court said that by either procedure death does not result from natural causes. The court noted that the disconnection of life support is "nothing more or less than assisted suicide." The *Quill* court rejected the state's argument that the laws are rationally related to the state's interest in preserving the lives of all its citizens at all times and under all conditions. The court said:

But what interest can the state possibly have in requiring the prolongation of a life that is all but ended? Surely, the state's interest lessens as the potential for life diminishes. And what business is it of the state to require the continuation of agony when the result is imminent and inevitable?

To the questions raised, the *Quill* court gave no answer.

COMPASSION IN DYING V. STATE OF WASHINGTON

In the state of Washington the statute (similar to that of New York) that made it a felony to "aid" another to attempt suicide was challenged by three patients, four physicians, and the nonprofit organization Compassion in Dying. The latter provides free information, counseling, and assistance to mentally competent, terminally ill adults. This organization has strict eligibility criteria: the patient must be terminally ill, a competent adult, and capable of understanding his or her own decision. As in the previous case, all three patients were suffering painful, debilitating, and terminal illnesses and died before this decision was announced in 1996.

The Ninth Circuit Court held that the "provision of statute that prohibited aiding another person to commit suicide violated due process clause as applied to terminally ill patients who wished to hasten their own death with medication prescribed by their physicians."[20] The court answered affirmatively the question of whether it is permissible to aid in killing oneself and recognized a liberty interest that must be constitutionally protected. The court made it clear, however, that the only conduct it was holding constitutional was physician-assisted suicide (i.e., the prescribing of medication by a physician for the purpose of enabling the patient to end his or her life). The court discussed the relevant factors and interests, including interests of the state, the means by which the state furthers its interests, the importance of the liberty interest, the burden on the liberty interest, and the consequences of upholding or overturning the statutory provision. The court considered the following state interests:

- Preservation of life
- Prevention of suicide
- Avoiding the involvement of third parties and precluding the use of arbitrary, unfair, or undue influence
- Protection of family members and loved ones
- Protection of the integrity of the medical profession
- Avoiding adverse consequences that might ensue if the statutory provision at issue is declared unconstitutional

Each of the legitimate interests asserted by the state was resolved in favor of the plaintiffs. The Ninth Circuit Court noted that the state of Washington already permits a competent, terminally ill patient to direct the withdrawal or withholding of life-sustaining treatment. The state interest in preventing suicide is diminished in situations involving terminally ill, competent adults. The court said that the decision of a "terminally ill adult who ends his life in the final stages of an incurable and painful degenerative disease in order to avoid debilitating pain and humiliating death" is not senseless and does not come too early. The involvement of third parties (i.e., the physicians) to provide the terminally ill patient with supervised and directed treatment aimed at terminating life was not arbitrary, unfair, or constituting undue influence.

The Ninth Circuit Court held that there was a liberty interest in the choice of how and when one dies and that the Washington law banning assisted suicide, as applied to competent, terminally ill adults who wish to hasten death by obtaining medication prescribed by their physicians, violated the due process clause. The court was convinced that it was not opening "Pandora's box" and that sufficient safeguards could be put in place to prevent a slide down the "slippery slope" to a society that embraces death for those who pose a burden.

BRIEF AMICUS CURIAE OF THE AMERICAN COLLEGE OF LEGAL MEDICINE

Friend-of-the-court briefs to the U.S. Supreme Court were submitted by several organizations, including the AMA, with whom 45 other organizations signed on to the brief in opposition to physician-assisted suicide. The American College of Legal Medicine (ACLM) was also granted consent to file a brief amicus curiae in the two cases submitted to the U.S. Supreme Court.

U.S. SUPREME COURT DECISIONS

Chief Justice Rehnquist delivered the opinion of the Supreme Court that upheld the laws prohibiting assisted suicide in the states of New York and Washington. The Chief Justice stated in *Washington v. Glucksberg,* "To hold for respondents, the Court would have to reverse centuries of legal doctrine and practice, and strike down the considered policy choice of almost every state."[21] The Supreme Court noted that "the overwhelming majority of state legislatures have drawn a clear line between assisting suicide and withdrawing or permitting the refusal of unwanted lifesaving medical treatment by prohibiting the former and permitting the latter." The Supreme Court also noted that "nearly all states expressly disapprove of suicide and assisted suicide either in statutes dealing with durable powers of attorney in health-care situations, or in 'living will' statutes. Thus even as the states move to protect and promote patients' dignity at the end of life, they remain opposed to physician-assisted suicide."

Letting versus making the patient die

The Supreme Court pointed out that it also has recognized, at least implicitly, the distinction between "letting" a patient die and "making" that patient die. In *Cruzan v. Director, Missouri Dept. of Health,* the Supreme Court concluded that "[t]he principle that a competent person has a constitutionally protected liberty interest in refusing unwanted medical treatment may be inferred from our prior decisions."[22] The Supreme Court stated that Cruzan provided no support for the notion that refusing life-sustaining medical treatment is "nothing more or less than suicide."

Opinion by Justice Stevens

In a separate opinion, Justice Stevens was not persuaded that in all cases there will be a significant difference between the intent of the physicians and that of the patients or the families in the two situations. He stated:

There may be little distinction between the intent of a terminally ill patient who decides to remove her life-support and one who seeks the assistance of a doctor in ending her life; in both situations, the patient is seeking to hasten a certain, impending death. The doctor's intent might also be the same in prescribing lethal medication as it is in terminating life support. A doctor who fails to administer medical treatment to one who is dying from a disease could be doing so with an intent to harm or kill that patient. Conversely, a doctor who prescribes lethal medication does not necessarily intend the patient's death, rather that doctor may seek simply to ease the patient's suffering and to comply with her wishes. The illusory character of any differences in intent or causation is confirmed by the fact that the American Medical Association unequivocally endorses the practice of terminal sedation, the administration of sufficient dosages of pain-killing medication to terminally ill patients to protect them from excruciating pain even when it is clear that the time of death will be advanced. The purpose of terminal sedation is to ease the suffering of the patient and comply with her wishes, and the actual cause of death is the administration of heavy doses of lethal sedatives. This same intent and causation may exist when a doctor complies with a patient's request for lethal medication to hasten her death.

Opposition by President Clinton

In 1997 the U.S. Supreme Court decision pertaining to physician-assisted suicide is correct both politically and from the standpoint of public policy in the majority of the states that have laws prohibiting assisted suicide. The Supreme Court noted that on April 30, 1997, President Clinton signed the Federal Assisted Suicide Funding Restriction Act of 1997, which prohibits the use of federal funds in support of physician-assisted suicide.

The Supreme Court also noted that "the states are currently engaged in serious, thoughtful examinations of physician-assisted suicide and other similar issues." California voters rejected an assisted-suicide initiative similar to Washington's in 1993. On the other hand, in 1994, voters in Oregon enacted (through ballot initiative) that state's Death with Dignity Act, which legalized physician-assisted suicide for competent, terminally ill adults. Is the Oregon state law unconstitutional? That question may require another decision by the U.S. Supreme Court.

Justice Stevens, who agreed with the holding but wrote a separate opinion in the cases of assisted suicide, would not "foreclose the possibility that an individual plaintiff seeking to hasten her death, or a doctor whose assistance was sought, could prevail in a more particularized challenge." The Supreme Court appears to be leaving the door open for a "particularized" challenge in the future. One can foresee the creation of an exception to the laws prohibiting assisted suicide for the terminally ill, competent adult who is in excruciating agony and extreme pain and suffering with no hope of survival beyond a few days or weeks or even up to 6 months.

Justice O'Connor, who also concurred with the holding and wrote a separate opinion in the cases of assisted suicide, encouraged the states to resolve this matter by stating that, "There is no reason to think the democratic process will not strike the proper balance between the interests of terminally ill, mentally competent individuals who would seek to end their suffering and the state's interests in protecting those who might seek to end life mistakenly or under pressure." Justice O'Connor, quoting from Cruzan, stated that in such circumstances "the challenging task of crafting appropriate procedures for safeguarding liberty interests is entrusted to the 'laboratory' of the states in the first instance."[23]

Right of the terminally ill to terminal sedation

The U.S. Supreme Court made it clear that the administration of terminal sedation to a competent, terminally ill patient by the physician, which by its dual effect may hasten that patient's death, is both ethical and legal as long as the terminal treatment is intended to relieve the pain and suffering of an agonizing terminal illness. Arguably, terminal sedation in some cases may represent active euthanasia or physician-assisted suicide. Nevertheless, terminal sedation is ethical and legal as long as the physician claims that the intent of the medical treatment is to relieve the pain and suffering and not to hasten death or kill.

This construction of terminal sedation by the U.S. Supreme Court may be interpreted as representing a significant step toward physician-assisted suicide. The opinion of Justice Stevens in the matter of terminal sedation is particularly meaningful. It remains for the states to do their homework, as suggested by Justice O'Connor, and craft appropriate procedural safeguards in dealing with the right of terminally ill patients to hasten death.

RECENT DEVELOPMENTS
Oregon Death with Dignity Act

In the general election of November 1994, voters in the State of Oregon passed by 52% to 48% the Oregon Death with Dignity Act,[24] a citizens' initiative petition placed on the state's ballot. The act was also referred to as the "physician-aid-in-dying law."[25] The act was promptly challenged in court by its opponents as violating the due process and the equal protection clauses of the Fourteenth Amendment,[26] and the U.S. District Court for the District of Oregon enjoined enforcement of the act. In 1997, however, the U.S. Court of Appeals for the Ninth Circuit Court[27] reversed the injunction for failure of the plaintiffs to establish actual injury. On October 27, 1997, the Oregon voters rejected a ballot initiative[28] that would repeal the Oregon Death with Dignity Act, thereby legalizing physician-assisted suicide.

The Oregon Death with Dignity Act allows qualified, terminally ill state residents who have a life expectancy of less than 6 months to request medications to end their lives. Two oral requests and one written request are required. There is a mandatory 15-day waiting period between the first oral request and the date when the patient may receive the prescription from the physician. Before prescribing the lethal drugs, the physician who is counseling the patient should be convinced that the terminally ill patient has made an informed decision and is not suffering from a psychiatric or psychotic disorder or depression. The diagnosis by the attending physician must be confirmed by a consulting physician. Both the attending and the consulting physicians must determine that the patient is mentally competent and capable of making a voluntary decision. Physicians are under no obligation to participate in the patient's act. Neither the physician nor other individuals may directly administer the lethal drugs to the terminally ill patient; euthanasia is not permitted under the act. However, the concept of physician-assisted suicide does sanction physician participation, but not administration of the lethal drugs.[29,30]

On March 24, 1998, Oregon recorded the case of Mrs. A as the first legal physician-assisted death/suicide under the Oregon Death with Dignity Act. Under the Act, a "good faith standard" rather than the more usual negligence standard immunizes physicians from civil and criminal liability.[31]

In 1998 a total of 23 patients received prescriptions for lethal drugs and were reported to the Oregon Health Division.[32] Of the 23 patients, 15 died after taking the lethal drugs, six died from underlying diseases, and two were alive as of January 1, 1999. Of the 15 patients who took the lethal drugs, 13 had cancer. None of the 15 patients expressed concern about the financial impact of their illness, and only one expressed concern about pain control. The decision to request and use a prescription for lethal drugs by the 15 patients was associated with concern about loss of autonomy or control of bodily functions, not with fear of intractable pain or concern about financial loss. The choice of physician-assisted suicide by the terminally ill patients was not associated with level of education or health insurance coverage.

In 1999 a total of 33 patients received prescriptions for lethal drugs and were reported to the Oregon Health Division.[33] Of the 33 patients, 26 died after taking the lethal drugs, five died of their underlying illnesses, and two were alive as of January 1, 2000. Another patient who received the prescription of lethal drugs in 1998 died after ingesting the lethal drugs in 1999. Of the 27 patients who died in 1999 (nine per 10,000 deaths in Oregon), 17 had cancer, four had amyotrophic lateral sclerosis (Lou Gehrig's disease), and four had chronic obstructive pulmonary disease. The reasons for requesting assistance with suicide included loss of autonomy, loss of control of bodily functions, an inability to participate in activities that make life enjoyable, and a determination to control the manner of death.

Physician-assisted suicide in Michigan

Dr. Jack Kevorkian, a retired pathologist in Michigan, crusaded in the 1990s for assisted suicide, stimulating much public attention. He admitted to assisting about 130 persons commit suicide. In *People v. Kevorkian* the Supreme Court of Michigan addressed the murder charges against Dr. Kevorkian as to whether the imposition of criminal charges by those who assist others in committing suicide was constitutional.[34] The court held that the due process clause of the U.S. Constitution did not encompass a fundamental right to commit suicide, with or without assistance, and regardless of whether the would-be assistant was a physician. The state of Michigan tried Dr. Kevorkian by juries on three occasions but was unable to convict him for assisting people in committing suicide.

In November 1998, Dr. Kevorkian videotaped himself administering a lethal dose of barbiturates to a terminally ill man with Lou Gehrig's disease. The videotape was given to the CBS-TV news program *60 Minutes* for broadcast. On March 26, 1999, Dr. Kevorkian was convicted of second-degree murder and sentenced to 10-25 years in prison.[35] He had gone far beyond assistance in suicide to actual performance of active euthanasia; he had slid down the slippery slope.

In 1994, right-to-die organizers in Michigan fell short of the required 256,457 signatures by approximately 50,000 names; their assisted-suicide initiative remained off the ballot.

Physician-assisted death in The Netherlands

Oregon is the only place in the world where physician-assisted suicide is legal. The Netherlands, however, is the only country in which physicians openly assist suicides; the government has turned a blind eye to physician participation in patient suicide. The Netherlands has experienced no great increase in the numbers of assisted deaths, thereby allaying fears of the slippery slope. In 1990 and 1995, nationwide surveys in The Netherlands revealed that physician-assisted suicide and euthanasia on explicit patient request rose from 2.1% to 2.7% of all deaths.[36] The rates of euthanasia in patients unable to make explicit requests fell, from 0.8% to 0.7% of all deaths.

Physician-assisted suicide in psychiatry

In 1994 the Dutch Supreme Court ruled that in exceptional instances, physician-assisted suicide might be justifiable for patients with no physical illness but with intolerable and unbearable mental suffering.[37] In 1997 in The Netherlands an estimated 320 psychiatric patients a year requested physician-assisted suicide; only two to five psychiatric patients per year were granted such a request. In The Netherlands, psychiatric consultation for medical patients who request physician-assisted death is relatively rare.

Physician-assisted suicide among AIDS patients

Among patients with acquired immunodeficiency syndrome (AIDS) in North Holland between 1984 and 1993, 23% of all deaths were reported as cases of euthanasia or physician-assisted suicide, a much greater percentage than found among other patients.[38]

Between November 1994 and January 1995, 228 physicians in the Community Consortium, an association providing health care to patients infected with human immunodeficiency virus (HIV) in the San Francisco Bay area, were interviewed regarding their attitudes and practices toward assisting with suicide of AIDS patients. Results were compared with a 1990 survey of consortium physicians. Within the group of physicians caring for HIV patients, the acceptance of assisted suicide increased from 28% in 1990 to 48% in 1995. A majority of the physician respondents in 1995 said that they had granted a request for assisted suicide from a patient with AIDS at least once.

Patients with amyotrophic lateral sclerosis

A survey of patients with amyotrophic lateral sclerosis (ALS) was conducted between 1995 and 1997 in Oregon and Washington to determine their attitudes toward assisted suicide.[39] ALS is a debilitating neuromuscular disorder that results in gradual paralysis, respiratory failure requiring a respirator, and death, usually within 3 to 5 years from disease onset or diagnosis. Most patients with ALS in that study would consider assisted suicide, and many would request a prescription for a lethal dose of medication well before they intended to use it.

Attitudes of countries worldwide and medical professionals

Euthanasia and related practices were examined worldwide based on questionnaires completed by 49 national representatives of the International Association for Suicide Prevention.[40] Active euthanasia was said to occur in 12 of the 49 countries, with widespread acceptance of passive euthanasia.

Only a minority of Italian primary care physicians endorsed euthanasia or assisted suicide, based on the euthanasia questionnaire completed by 336 general practitioners.[41] Agreement with the practice of euthanasia or assisted suicide was correlated with non-Catholic religious affiliation, inexperience in treating terminally ill patients, and the burnout dimension of depersonalization. Similarly, among German physicians of all specialties and medical activities, 81.7% were against physician-assisted suicide, and all rejected it for nonmoribund patients.[42] German neurologists, intensivists, anesthetists, and oncologists were among the specialists most likely be confronted with terminally ill patients, and they tended to agree more readily to physician-assisted suicide.

Another investigation compared the attitudes of 62 Japanese and 72 American psychiatrists toward hospital patients who wished to die.[43] The majority of both Japanese and American psychiatrists agreed that suicidal ideation or completed suicide in hospitalized patients could be a reasonable choice in certain cases.

In a 1998 U.S. survey of physician-assisted suicide and euthanasia, 1902 of 3102 physicians in 10 specialties completed mailed questionnaires.[44] A substantial proportion of physicians reported that they received requests for physician-assisted suicide and euthanasia, and approximately 7% complied with the patient's requests at least once.

Most general internists, especially minority physicians, in six urban areas of the United States indicated that they were personally reluctant to participate in physician-assisted suicide.[45]

White physicians in the United States were more likely than black physicians to accept physician-assisted suicide as a treatment alternative.[46]

For American physicians to perform euthanasia or physician-assisted suicide, the patient almost always must have intractable pain or poor physical functioning. Although most physicians seemed comfortable with their actions, some experienced adverse consequences.[47]

Overall, residents in internal medicine, psychiatry, and emergency medicine expressed opposition or uncertainty regarding assisted suicide and euthanasia, but emergency medicine residents were more likely to support assisted suicide.[48] The majority of Oregon emergency medical technicians who responded to a survey expressed support for physician-assisted suicide, and almost three fourths of them had confronted at least one terminally ill patient who had attempted suicide.[49]

In a study by the Department of Social and Preventive Medicine at the University of Queensland, Australia, critical care nurses, more than any other professional group, indicated that they supported the right of terminally ill patients to euthanasia or physician-assisted suicide, and their responses were similar to those of community members.[50] In a pilot study of gerontological nurses in New York regarding legalization of assisted suicide, 58% favored its legalization for elderly patients and 46% for all ages.[51]

It is important to remember that "the patient's request to die is a situation that requires the physician to engage in a dialogue to understand what the request means, including whether the request arises from a clinically significant depression or inadequately treated pain."[52]

The Pain Relief Promotion Act of 1999, a bill introduced in the U.S. Congress, would criminally punish those who used controlled substances to cause or assist in causing a patient's death. This would discourage physicians from engaging in experimentation and innovation in palliative care.[53] If this act were to become the law in the United States, American physicians would no longer be able to consider the patient's request to die.

ENDNOTES

1. *Vacco v. Quill,* 117 U.S. 2293 (1997).
2. *Washington v. Glucksberg,* 117 U.S. 2258 (1997).
3. *Quill v. Vacco,* 80 F. 3d 716 (2nd Cir., 1996).
4. *Compassion in Dying v. State of Washington,* 79 F. 3d 790 (9th Cir., 1996).
5. *Brief Amicus Curiae of the American College of Legal Medicine,* submitted to the U.S. Supreme Court, October Term, in *Vacco v. Quill,* and *Washington v. Glucksberg* (1996).
6. *Supra* note 2.
7. M.T. CeloCruz, *Aid-in-Dying: Should We Decriminalize Physician-Assisted Suicide and Physician-Committed Euthanasia?* 18 Am J. L. Med. 377 (1992).
8. *See* References in *Quill v. Vacco,* 80 F. 3d 716 at 732 (2nd Cir., 1996).
9. *Commonwealth v. Bowen,* 13 Mass. 365 (1816).
10. *Breasted v. Farmers' Loan & Trust Co.,* 4 Hill 73, at 75 (Sup. Ct., 1843).
11. *Commonwealth v. Mink,* 123 Mass. 422, 428 (1877).
12. Act of July 26, 1881, ch. 676 §§ 174, 178, 3 1881 N.Y. Laws 42-43.
13. Act of May 5, 1919, ch. 414, § 1, 2 1919 N.Y. Laws 1193.
14. Act of July 20, 1965, ch. 1030, 1965 N.Y. Laws 2355 (*codified at* N.Y. Penal Law § 35, 10(4).
15. L.O. Gostin, *Drawing a Line Between Killing and Letting Die: the Law, and Law Reform, on Medically Assisted Dying,* 21 J. L. Med. & Ethics 94-101, at 96 (1993).
16. Act of Dec. 10, 1828, ch. 20, 4 1828 N.Y. Laws 19 (*codified at* N.Y.Rev.Stat. pt. 4, ch. 1, tit. 2 art. 1, sec. 7 [1829]).
17. Iowa Code Ann. §§ 707A.2, 707A.3 (Supp. 1997).
18. *Supra* note 3.
19. *Cruzan v. Director, Missouri Dept. of Health,* 497 U.S. 261 (1990).
19a. *See In re Quinlan,* 70 N.J. 10, 41, 355 A. 2d 647, *cert. denied,* 429 U.S. 922, 97 S.Ct. 319, 50 L.Ed. 289 (1976).
20. *Supra* note 4.
21. *Supra* note 2.
22. *Supra* note 19.
23. *Id.*
24. Or. Rev. Stat. s 127.800-807 (1995).
25. Simon M. Canick, *Constitutional Aspects of Physician-Assisted Suicide after Lee v. Oregon,* 23 Am. J. L. & Med. 69 (1997).
26. *Lee v. Oregon,* 869 F. Supp. 1491 D.Or. 1994).
27. *Lee v. Oregon,* 107 F. 3d 1382 (9th Cir. 1997).
28. Ballot Measure 510 Or. H.B. 2954-1997.
29. K. Haley & M. Lee eds., *The Oregon Death with Dignity Act: a Guidebook for Health Care Providers* (Oregon Health Sciences University, Portland 1998).
30. A.E. Chin, K. Hedberg, G.K. Higginson, & D.W. Fleming, *Oregon's Death with Dignity Act: the First Year's Experience* (Oregon Health Division, Portland 1999).
31. H. Hendin, K. Foley, & M. White, *Physician-Assisted Suicide: Reflections on Oregon's First Case,* 14 Issues L. Med. 243-270 (1998).
32. A.E. Chin, K. Hedberg, G.K. Higginson, & D.W. Fleming, *Legalized Physician-Assisted Suicide in Oregon (the First Year's Experience),* 340 N. Engl. J. Med. 577-583 (1999).
33. A.D. Sullivan, K. Hedberg, & D.W. Fleming, *Legalized Physician-Assisted Suicide in Oregon (the Second Year),* 342 N. Engl. J. Med. 598-604 (2000).
34. *People v. Kevorkian,* 447 Mich. 436, 527 N.W. 2d 714 (1994).
35. L.L. Emanuel ed., *Regulating How We Die: the Ethical, Medical, and Legal Issues Surrounding Physician-Assisted Suicide* (Harvard University Press, Cambridge, Mass. 1998).
36. J.H. Groenewoud, A. van der Heide, J.G.C. Kester et al., *A Nationwide Study of Decisions to Forego Life-Prolonging Treatment in Dutch Medical Practice,* 160 Archives Int. Med. 357-363 (2000).
37. J.H. Groenewoud, P.J. van der Maas, G. van der Wal, et al., *Physician-Assisted Death in Psychiatric Practice in The Netherlands,* 336 N. Engl. J. Med. 1795-1801 (1997).
38. L.R. Slome, T.F. Mitchell, E. Charlebois, et al., *Physician-Assisted Suicide and Patients with Immunodeficiency Virus Disease,* 336 N. Engl. J. Med. 417-421 (1997).
39. L. Ganzini, W.S. Johnston, B.H. McFarland, et al., *Attitudes of Patients with Amyotrophic Lateral Sclerosis and Their Care Givers Toward Assisted Suicide,* 339 N. Engl. J. Med. 967-973 (1998).
40. M.J. Kelleher, D. Chambers, P. Corcoran, et al., *Euthanasia and Related Practices Worldwide,* 19 Crisis 109-115 (1998).
41. L. Grassi, K. Magnani, & M. Ercolani, *Attitudes Toward Euthanasia and Physician-Assisted Suicide Among Italian Primary Care Physicians,* 17 J. Pain Symptom Mgmt. 188-196 (1999).

42. H. Csef & B. Heindl, *[Attitude Toward Physician-Assisted Suicide Among German Doctors: a Representative Survey of the Medical District Association of Wurzburg],* 123(50) Dtsch. Med. Wochenschr. 1501-1506 (1998).

43. D. Berger, I. Fukunishi, M.A. O'Dowd et al., *A Comparison of Japanese and American Psychiatrists' Attitudes Toward Patients Wishing To Die In The General Hospital,* 66(6) Psychother. Psychosom. 319-328 (1997).

44. D.E. Meier, C.E. Emmons, S. Wallenstein et al., *A National Survey of Physician-Assisted Suicide and Euthanasia in the United States,* 338(17) N. Engl. J. Med. 1193-1201 (1998).

45. D.P. Sulmasy, B.P. Linas, K.F. Gold, & K.A. Schulman, *Physician Resource Use and Willingness in Assisted Suicide,* 158(9) Archives Int. Med. 974-978 (1998).

46. E.W. Mebane, R.F. Oman, L.T. Kroonen, & M.K. Goldstein, *The Influence of Physician Race, Age, and Gender on Physicians' Attitudes Toward Advance Care Directives and Preferences for End-of-Life Decision-Making,* 47(5) J. Am. Geriatr. Soc. 579-591 (1999).

47. E.J. Emanuel, E.R. Daniels, D.L. Fairclough, & B.R. Clarridge, *The Practice of Euthanasia and Physician-Assisted Suicide in the United States: Adherence to Proposed Safeguards and Effects on Physicians,* 280(6) J.A.M.A. 507-513 (1998).

48. L.W. Roberts, B.B. Roberts, T.D. Warner, et al., *Internal Medicine, Psychiatry, and Emergency Medicine Residents' Views of Assisted Death Practices,* 157(14) Archives Int. Med. 1603-1609 (1997).

49. T.A. Schmidt, A.D. Zechnich, & M. Doherty, *Oregon Emergency Medical Technicians' Attitudes Toward Physician-Assisted Suicide,* 5(9) Acad. Emerg. Med. 912-918 (1998).

50. C. Cartwright, M. Steinberg, G. Williams, & J. Najman, *Issues of Death And Dying: the Perspective of Critical Care Nurses,* 10(3) Aust. Crit. Care 81-87 (1997).

51. J. Beder, *Legalization of Assisted Suicide: a Pilot Study of Gerontological Nurses,* 24(4) J. Gerontol. Nurs. 14-20 (1998).

52. P.R. Muskin, *The Request to Die: Role for a Psychodynamic Perspective on Physician-Assisted Suicide,* 279(4) J.A.M.A. 323-328 (1998).

53. D. Orentlicher, A. Caplan, *The Pain Relief Promotion Act of 1999: a Serious Threat to Palliative Care,* 283(2) J.A.M.A. 255-258 (2000).

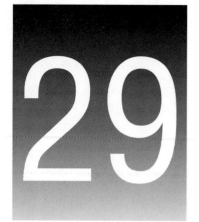

Reproduction patients

PRECONCEPTION ISSUES
CONCEPTION ISSUES
POSTCONCEPTION ISSUES
BIRTH-RELATED ISSUES

This chapter reviews some of the most frequently encountered issues involving reproduction patients.

PRECONCEPTION ISSUES
Genetic counseling

Approximately 3% to 5% of all infants are born with a congenital or hereditary disorder. More than one fourth of all pediatric hospitalizations and deaths beyond the perinatal period are caused by such disorders. More than 3500 genetic diseases have been described. Only in the past two decades has significant prenatal detection of congenital birth defects and genetic disease been possible.

Routine genetic screening has become the standard of care in many situations. Most states have enacted legislation requiring phenylketonuria (PKU) testing immediately after birth to allow effective treatment. The federal government has established voluntary screening centers for sickle cell trait.[1] Several states have also established blood screening as a prerequisite to marriage or attendance at school. Screening may also occur at birth, or the states allow departments of health or school authorities to designate segments of the population for screening.[2] Prenatal screening for neural tube defects has been the subject of policy consideration. In the private sector, some companies use genetic screening to detect hypersusceptibility to certain occupational exposures, although this is controversial because of the potential for discriminatory practice or abuse.[3] Donors of semen for artificial insemination are usually screened for genetic diseases (see Conception Issues).

Family practitioners and obstetricians may be liable if they fail to administer the prenatal care that is the standard practice within their medical community. This prenatal care might include testing for rubella titers or serum alpha-fetoprotein (AFP) to show a risk of congenital defect. In *Monusco v. Pos-*

tle a physician was held liable to an infant for failure to test and immunize her mother for rubella before the child was conceived.[4] Liability may also be found for failure to obtain a genetic history or to recognize a genetic disease in the parents or siblings that would suggest a risk of genetic disease in the fetus. Once a risk is identified, there is a duty to inform the prospective parent or pregnant patient that further workup or referral might be indicated or that termination of the pregnancy may be an option. Further, recognition of a genetic disease requires counseling about future offspring.

Wrongful birth and wrongful life cases have involved genetic counseling for known teratogens[5,6]; autosomal dominant conditions that would be apparent in the parents[7-9]; autosomal recessive conditions,[10-14] many of which could be discovered by carrier or prenatal testing; and X-linked conditions that could be discovered by prenatal testing.[15-18] There might be a duty to refer a patient to a specialist in the field of genetic counseling if a case falls beyond the expertise of the attending physician. The American Medical Association (AMA) Council on Scientific Affairs' indications for such a referral are (1) genetic or congenital anomaly in a family member; (2) family history of an inherited disorder; (3) abnormal somatic or behavioral development in a child; (4) mental retardation of unknown etiology in a child; (5) pregnancy in a woman over the age of 35; (6) specific ethnic background suggestive of a high rate of genetic abnormality; (7) drug use or long-term exposure to possible teratogens or mutagens; (8) three or more spontaneous abortions, early infant deaths, or both; and (9) infertility.[19]

An important aspect of current genetic counseling is prenatal blood testing, most often employed on maternal serum in the fifteenth week of gestation, although it can be performed from the fifteenth week up to the twenty-first week. If the serum screen is positive, an amniocentesis may be indicated. The indications for genetic amniocentesis include advanced maternal age, abnormal AFP levels, and previously recognized genetic disorders.

The Editorial Committee updated this chapter. The committee gratefully acknowledges the past contribution of Michael S. Cardwell, M.D., J.D., M.P.H., M.B.A., and Thomas G. Kirkhope, M.D., J.D.

Genetic amniocentesis is considered a low-risk procedure with a complication rate of about 0.5%, or lower if performed under ultrasound guidance and after at least the sixteenth week of gestation. The mother risks uterine infection, intestinal perforation, and possible Rh sensitization. The fetus risks infection, hemorrhage, and trauma to the vital organs. *Chorionic villus sampling* (CVS) is a prenatal diagnostic alternative to amniocentesis. CVS can be performed in the first trimester, 7 to 10 weeks earlier than amniocentesis; the results are often known within a few days. This could allow decisions to abort to be made within the first trimester. The first large collaborative study to compare the two procedures showed CVS to be associated with a slightly elevated but statistically insignificant risk of fetal loss compared with amniocentesis.[20]

Contraception

When the first birth control clinic in the United States opened in New York City in 1916, local authorities acted to shut it down within 10 days as a violation of obscenity laws.[21] Today, in contrast, the Social Security/Medicaid Act,[22] the federal Population Research and Voluntary Family Planning Programs Act,[23] and related federal regulations, along with state laws and regulations, provide for federal and state funding for family planning services and programs. In 1987 the federal and state governments spent $386 million to provide family planning services.[24]

Contraception issues affect a significant proportion of American society; 78% of married couples and 69% of unmarried women aged 18 to 44 are exposed to the risk of unintended pregnancy.[25] One of every 10 women aged 15 to 19 becomes pregnant each year.[26] A contraceptive method with an annual failure rate of 1% will leave one woman in seven with an unintended pregnancy.

The U.S. Supreme Court has created a constitutional right of privacy that protects individual procreative choices from governmental intrusion. The right to use contraception was, in 1965, the earliest of these rights to be defined.[27] Specifically, neither laws nor regulations can abridge access to and use of contraceptives by adults, married or single.[28] The court struck down the federal Comstock Law and similar state laws that prohibited obscenity, contraception, and abortion. As early as 1970, congressional action, such as the Family Planning Services and Population Research Act, indicated the shift toward governmental support of contraception and family planning.[29]

Contraception-related litigation has involved physician liability under theories of negligence in prescribing, negligence during a procedure, and inadequate or defective informed consent. A physician who fails to impress on the patient that the chosen contraceptive method is not foolproof may be liable for costs associated with an unwanted pregnancy. In one case, personnel at a clinic misrepresented that an intrauterine device (IUD) had been recovered, and the patient was allowed to bring an action alleging fraud.[30] Manufacturers have also been found liable for inadequate warnings and defective products.

Minors and contraception. Family planning involving minors remains a controversial issue. Availability and provision of contraceptives present slightly different issues when minors are involved because the state has a more reasonable interest in controlling the behavior of minors. In 1981, Congress enacted the Adolescent Family Life Act and regulations to fund innovative demonstration programs addressing the problems of teenage pregnancy and childbearing.[31,32] The act was designed to provide funding to various organizations, including and involving religious organizations, for services and research involving premarital adolescent sexuality and pregnancy. Grantees under the act were not allowed to use the funds for certain services, such as family planning services and abortion counseling. In several opinions the Supreme Court cautioned that minors might not have rights equal to those of adults.[33] In *Doe v. Blum* a court held that minors to whom family planning and abortion information was not sent because they were not "heads of household," although they were eligible for AFDC benefits and Medicaid, did not state a cause of action.[34] In *Bowen v. Kendrick* the U.S. Supreme Court found that the Adolescent Family Life Act of 1981 did not create excessive entanglement of church and state and thus was found to be constitutional on its face, but not necessarily constitutional as applied.[35]

Oral contraceptives. Most lawsuits involving oral contraceptive agents are product liability cases brought against manufacturers for inadequate warning of potential adverse reactions. The reactions that have most often given rise to suits are stroke, pulmonary thromboembolism, myocardial infarction, and ruptured hepatic adenoma. In a 1985 Massachusetts Supreme Court case the court, in contrast to some other jurisdictions, held that the duty to warn a consumer of adverse reactions goes beyond mere compliance with a U.S. Food and Drug Administration (FDA) labeling requirement or reliance on a physician's warning. The court ruled in favor of the plaintiff, declaring that the manufacturer must provide the patient directly with a written warning.[36]

Physicians also have been found liable for their negligence in prescription of oral contraceptives (birth control pills). The physician must fully inform the patient of the possible side effects and alternatives. The presence of a contraceptive package insert does not absolve the physician of otherwise discussing the potential hazards with the patient in plain language. Documentation of these discussions is desirable. To conform with standard medical practice, a prescription must be based on accepted indications and contraindications. Before writing a prescription, the physician must perform an adequate physical examination and order relevant laboratory testing, including cervical cytology.

In *Klink v. G.D. Searle & Co.* a 19-year-old woman who had never had normal menstrual periods sought birth control.[37] The physician explained the alternative methods but did not discuss possible side effects. Nearly a year and a half later the woman had a stroke. The court ruled in the plaintiff's favor, stating that birth control pills were not a proper method of treatment for her primary amenorrhea. If used as a diagnostic method to establish uterine hormonal responsiveness, they should not have been continued longer than 6 months.

In *Hamilton v. Hardy* a woman had moved to a different city. Her new physician saw no reason to discourage her from taking her birth control pills but did change her prescription.[38] She returned with migraine headaches and was told to continue the pills and not to worry. She then suffered a stroke. At no time did the physician discuss adverse side effects. The court held that this was a breach of the physician's duty to warn of possible hazards. In *Hamilton* the plaintiff sought to recover for a stroke allegedly caused by the use of oral contraceptives. An expert witness for the plaintiff had indicated that the "average" gynecologist would have stopped use of the pills when the patient complained of headaches. The defendant established that "some" physicians in the community would have continued their use.

The plaintiff stated that she had not given informed consent because she was not told about the risk of stroke. The physician argued that no expert testimony had established a duty to disclose. The trial court judge dismissed the action.

On appeal the higher court reversed and remanded. It held that the case could be taken from the jury only when a "respectable minority" of physicians approved the treatment selected by the defendant. It also stated that the duty to disclose was a "duty imposed by law" and did not have to be established by expert testimony.[39]

Intrauterine devices. Most lawsuits involving IUDs are product liability cases against the manufacturer for a product unreasonably dangerous because of defective design. The complications that have most often given rise to lawsuits are uterine and pelvic infections, infertility, uterine perforation, and ectopic pregnancy.

Litigation over the Dalkon Shield forced a recall of the product in 1984.[40] By mid-1985 the Dalkon Shield manufacturer, A.H. Robins Company, had paid out $520 million to 9500 women for claims of pelvic inflammatory disease (PID), sterility, septic spontaneous abortion, and other injuries, with many other claims still outstanding and unfiled. Robins filed for bankruptcy and in July 1988 the U.S. District Court for the Eastern District of Virginia confirmed a bankruptcy reorganization plan, which provided for the establishment of a trust fund of at least $2.475 billion to pay the qualified outstanding claims and allowed for consideration of some claims that did not originally meet the April 1986 filing deadline. Various attempts were made, through individual and class action lawsuits against third parties such as Robins' insurer, to circumvent the effects that the bankruptcy action might have on claimants. In November 1989 the U.S. Supreme Court denied review of a Fourth Circuit opinion upholding an injunction in connection with Robins' bankruptcy reorganization plan that barred suits against such third parties.[41]

In 1986, Searle and Ortho withdrew from the IUD market in the United States because of the costs of litigation, even though their products did not have the high complication rate of the Dalkon Shield.[42] At the time of the decision to withdraw, 775 cases had been filed against Searle in connection with its Copper-7 IUD.[43] It has been generally noted that the resulting unavailability of the IUD to American women was unfortunate, because the Dalkon Shield was the only unreasonably unsafe product.[44]

For a few years the Progestasert, a hormone-producing IUD by Alza Corporation with an effective lifetime of 1 year, was the only IUD marketed in the United States. In 1988, GynoPharma, in cooperation with The Population Council, introduced the ParaGard T380, a copper IUD that is effective for up to 10 years, according to the American College of Obstetricians and Gynecologists (ACOG). Marketing involves a seven-page patient informed consent form. Use of the device is limited: specifically, it is not to be used in women who have never been pregnant, who have a history of PID, or who engage in sex with multiple partners.

Physicians have also been found liable for negligent use and care of IUDs. As with oral contraceptives, the physician must fully inform the patient of risks and alternatives. The physician must prescribe in conformity with accepted medical indications and contraindications. A physical examination and pertinent laboratory tests must be performed before insertion. The patient must be monitored, initially within 3 months after insertion and then at least once a year.

In *Killebrew v. Johnson* a patient became pregnant with an IUD in place.[45] Her gynecologist was to perform an abortion, ligate the fallopian tubes, and remove the IUD. The IUD could not be found at surgery and was not seen on postoperative x-ray films. The physician told the patient that the device was gone. Subsequently she developed abdominal pain, dysuria, and other complaints that progressed during the next 2 years. It was eventually determined that the IUD was in the peritoneal cavity, and that it was visible on the original postoperative films. The IUD was removed and her symptoms disappeared. The court held that the physician should have personally examined the x-ray films to determine the presence or absence of the IUD instead of relying on the radiologist's report.

Other methods

SPERMICIDAL CHEMICALS. The U.S. Supreme Court refused to hear and thereby has let stand the case of *Wells v. Ortho Pharmaceutical Corp.*, in which the manufacturer was found liable for the birth defects allegedly caused by its spermicidal jelly.[46]

SUBDERMAL IMPLANTS. Norplant is a long-acting contraceptive that uses flexible capsules of levonorgestrel. Product liability cases are pending at the appellate level.

INJECTABLES. Depot medroxyprogesterone acetate (Depo-Provera) is a long-acting synthetic progestational agent that, when injected intramuscularly, prevents ovulation for approximately 12 weeks.[47] Although used for contraception in other countries for many years,[48] this drug did not receive FDA approval for use as a contraceptive agent until 1992 in the United States,[49] although it had been used for other purposes.[50]

The timing of administration of both Norplant and Depo-Provera is important because it is possible to give either drug when the patient is already pregnant or has already ovulated. There is some evidence of teratogenesis of these drugs on a developing fetus. Their use without checking for possible pregnancy could lead to physician liability. To avoid this problem, the drug is given during menses.

Sterilization

Surgical sterilization (e.g., tubal ligation, vasectomy) is usually regarded as a voluntary procedure to confer permanent contraception; however, it can also be therapeutic, incidental, or involuntary. When a woman's physical or mental health would be threatened by a pregnancy, sterilization is medically indicated, and the procedure is considered *therapeutic*. Sterilization is incidental when it results from therapy performed for another purpose. Examples include chemotherapy for cancer, hysterectomy for endometriosis, and bilateral orchiectomy for prostatic carcinoma. Involuntary sterilization most often involves mentally retarded wards.

Voluntary sterilization. Contraceptive sterilization has become the most popular method of birth control in the United States, possibly because fewer birth control options are available in the United States than in other developed countries. Contraceptive sterilization among young U.S. women (aged 20 to 29) is about 50% higher than comparable rates in Great Britain and The Netherlands.[51] Tubal ligation accounts for 40% of the contraception practiced by married U.S. women aged 25 to 34.[52] An additional 16% are protected by sterilization of the male partner.[53] In 1987, federal and state governments spent $65 million to subsidize contraceptive sterilization services. Of this amount, 97% was from federal sources (88% through Medicaid).[54]

The right of privacy, which protects an individual's procreative decisions from an unjustified intrusion of law and which has been applied to contraception and abortion, logically extends to sterilization. In general, public hospitals cannot abridge choices of pregnancy, abortion, or sterilization. Public hospitals may not prohibit elective sterilization unless there is a state statute to the contrary.[55]

In contrast, private hospitals can limit the procedures they perform. Private hospitals may refuse to engage in abortion or sterilization procedures. Even public funding in a private hospital does not necessarily force it to perform abortions or sterilizations.

Individual health care workers can also limit the procedures in which they participate. Some state laws contain "conscience clauses" that permit individual physicians and nurses to refuse to take part because of religious or moral beliefs.

The general rules of informed consent apply to sterilization procedures. It is advisable to have a separate consent form for sterilization. This form should, among other things, emphasize (1) that the procedure intends a permanent condition and (2) that a small but real chance of failure may result in an unintended pregnancy.

Failure of sterilization procedures is the most common basis for the birth-related actions called "wrongful conception" or "wrongful pregnancy" cases, as discussed later.

Tubal ligation can be performed by a number of surgical techniques with different failure and complication rates. Patients should normally be informed of failure rates and of alternative treatments. Faulty physician-patient communication is a frequent source of liability in this area. In cases such as *Sard v. Hardy*,[56] *Gowan v. Carpenter*,[57] and *Wilsman v. Sloniewicz*,[58] in which physicians performed tubal ligations using techniques associated with high failure rates, patients were allowed to sue, alleging that they were not informed of alternative sterilization procedures. In *Dohn v. Lovell* the Court of Appeals of Georgia elaborated on the Georgia Voluntary Sterility Act's description of a "full and reasonable medical explanation" in favor of a patient who told her physician that she wanted her tubes "cut, tied and burnt."[59] The physician used clips without informing her, and she became pregnant.

In addition to informed consent requirements, some states have other statutory requirements. In Virginia the procedure can be performed only in a hospital or licensed facility.[60] In Georgia the physician must consult with at least one other physician before the operation.[61] Some courts have held that spousal consent cannot be required.[62]

If the elective sterilization procedure is to be paid by Medicaid, detailed regulations apply. To obtain federal funds, a written consent using a special Department of Health and Human Service (DHHS) form signed 30 days (but not more than 180 days) before surgery must be obtained except in a certified emergency.[63] At least one state, California, has regulations similar to those of the federal government, including a mandatory waiting period between the time of consent and the performance of the sterilization.[64]

Where the sterilization is performed under the auspices of government authority, the physician is viewed as an agent of the state and may be subject to constraints. In *Downs v. Sawtelle* a single, deaf-mute mother of two instituted a civil rights action alleging that physicians and several social service workers conspired to sterilize her against her will.[65] State action was found in the functioning of the private community hospital because the town and the hospital were so intertwined.[66]

Involuntary sterilization. In the early 1900s, involuntary sterilization was authorized and mandated by state legislations for "imbeciles, idiots, sexual perverts, epileptics, the insane, and recidivist criminals."[67] The term *eugenic sterilization* was used to denote control of procreation to prevent what were considered undesirable genetic traits. The constitutionality of compulsory sterilization for mentally retarded persons was first upheld in the landmark 1927 U.S. Supreme Court case *Buck v. Bell.* Writing for the court, Justice Oliver Wendell Holmes stated:

It is better for all the world, if, instead of waiting to execute degenerate offspring for crime, or let them starve for their imbecility, society can prevent those who are manifestly unfit from continuing their kind. The principle that sustains compulsory vaccination is broad enough to cover cutting the Fallopian tubes . . . [T]hree generations of imbeciles are enough.[68]

Most of these statutes have now been found constitutionally invalid because they were considered cruel and unusual punishment, violative of the equal protection clause, or lacking due process. Exceptions have been made for limited situations involving mentally retarded persons who would be unable to appreciate the consequences of their acts or care for their children and who might pass on a hereditary form of retardation.

Many states, however, legislatively authorize involuntary sterilization of wards who are genetically retarded.[69] These current statutes generally require the following findings: permanence of the condition; capacity of the ward to function sexually; high probability of transmission of the genetic disease (recent research has shown that most forms of mental retardation are not hereditary); inability of the ward to care for offspring; inability of the ward to use less drastic forms of birth control; and minimal risk of personal injury to the ward.[70] Often the court must find that the sterilization is in the best interests of the ward.[71] In many jurisdictions, these findings must be based on clear and convincing proof rather than a mere preponderance of the evidence.[72] Most statutes include provisions that exculpate physicians and administrative officials from civil and criminal liability when acting in accordance with the law, although some allow civil liability in the case of a negligently performed procedure.[73]

Many of the statutes fail to cover noninstitutionalized mentally retarded persons. In these jurisdictions some courts have failed to grant sterilization because of the absence of legislative authority to do so; other courts have been willing to grant the sterilization so as not to discriminate against those who are cared for at home.[74]

Courts have recently begun to authorize involuntary sterilization on incompetent wards in the absence of any legislation on the subject.[75] This change has been promoted in part by the *Sparkman* decisions by lower federal courts and the Supreme Court. From these it has become clear that, contrary to prior case law, judges are protected by judicial immunity, and the private individuals instituting suit are not subject to liability for violation of federal civil rights law.[76]

CONCEPTION ISSUES
Assisted conception and nontraditional parentage

Infertility is a common problem, occurring in about 15% of all U.S. couples. Assisted reproductive technologies can now offer alternatives to adoption that can provide otherwise infertile couples with emotional, biological, and genetic involvement in pregnancy.

These technologies are giving rise to a host of nontraditional parentage situations and an entirely new conceptual legal notion of "family." It is now possible for a child to have five "parents": the biological or genetic father (a sperm or testicle donor), the rearing or social father (the traditional father), the genetic mother (the ovum donor), the gestational or birthing mother (the surrogate mother), and the rearing or social mother (the traditional mother).[77]

Legal issues surrounding these various nontraditional parenting arrangements include questions of lineage, inheritance, legitimacy, adultery, confidentiality, status of residual legitimacy, status of residual embryos, responsibility for diseases and defects, and the correlative rights of the different parties. Now that cytological analysis is technically feasible, legal and ethical issues also are involved in preimplantation genetic screening.[78] In general the laws governing these family and health issues are state laws, rather than federal laws, with the exception of federal constitutional provisions and federal fetal research regulations. Specific state legislation regarding the new reproductive possibilities is beginning to be promulgated. Other state laws that may affect this area include laws on adoption, paternity, legitimacy, inheritance, "baby selling," child custody and support, homicide, feticide, abortion, fetal experimentation, and child abuse and neglect.

Artificial insemination. Artificial insemination (AI) is now relatively common. It consists of inoculation of the semen of the husband (AIH) or another donor (AID) into the reproductive tract of the woman. An estimated 40,000 cases of AID are performed each year in the United States. The process is so simple that women have performed the procedure on themselves.

Approximately half the states have enacted legislation dealing with AI. Although AI has been used for decades, Georgia enacted the first statute in 1964.[79] In general, these statutes deal with the legal status of the resulting child, donor selection, practitioner licensing, and the confidentiality of records. In addition, most state legislation requires that AI be performed by a licensed physician. Even without specific legislation prohibiting insemination by nonphysicians, such an act might be considered unauthorized practice of medicine.

In addition to statutes, many states have dealt judicially with questions of parental rights and obligations resulting from AIH and AID. Some early court cases held that AID was adulterous and the child illegitimate. The clear majority view today is to consider AID not to be adulterous (unless sexual intercourse has occurred) and the children to be legitimate, based on public policy considerations and the desire not to stigmatize innocent children.[80]

Most legislation codifies this judicial trend but creates a presumption of legitimacy *only* when the husband has given written permission for AID. In the absence of a written agreement, the AI donor will be considered the legal father and responsible for child support. In *In re Baby Doe,* however, the Supreme Court of South Carolina concluded that a husband who encouraged and assisted his wife in AI could be held liable for support of the resulting child even if he had not consented to the procedure in writing.[81] In other jurisdictions, consent of the husband is presumed. A number of states expressly relieve the sperm donor of all obligations and rights to the child unless he is also the husband of the woman inseminated. As discussed later, these statutes can prove problematic when applied to cases in which the donor actually intends to raise and be responsible for the child, as in surrogacy arrangements.

Some courts have imputed parentage rights and obligations on the husband in times of conflict in an effort to preserve traditional family mores. In a 1968 California Supreme Court case, *People v. Sorenson,* the court upheld a criminal prosecution of a man for failure to pay child support for the child born to his former wife after he had given his consent for AID.[82] In *C.M. v. C.C.* the unmarried biological father sued for visitation rights after the mother refused visitation or any other parental role to him.[83]

Infertility programs in governmental settings may not abridge the constitutional rights of privacy and procreative choice. A single woman sued the Wayne State University AI clinic for restricting insemination to married couples.[84] The suit was settled on the condition that the restriction be dropped.

The confidentiality of donor records is a potential problem area in AID. The child may claim the right to know his or her biological father. The sperm donor usually does not want responsibility for parentage and relies on the confidentiality of the physician's records. The mother and her spouse usually do not want the identity of the donor known in order to protect the family unit. At least eight states (California, Colorado, Hawaii, Minnesota, Montana, North Dakota, Washington, and Wyoming) have adopted the portion of the Model Uniform Parentage Act that allows the identity of a sperm donor to be obtained only on court order for "good cause."[85]

In vitro fertilization. In vitro fertilization (IVF) is now an accepted alternative method of conception. The sperm and ovum are allowed to incubate outside the human body, and the resulting embryo is then implanted back into the uterus. Indications for IVF include absent or nonpatent fallopian tubes, inadequate motile sperm count, hostile cervical mucus, refractory endometriosis, and unexplained infertility. IVF has been called "the final common pathway of infertility therapy."[86] Approximately 40% of the attempts result in a pregnancy; the live birth rate is in the range of 25%.

The first "test-tube baby" was Louise Brown, born in England in 1978. The first successful IVF program in the United States was established at the Eastern Virginia Medical School in Norfolk, which led to the first American IVF pregnancy in 1993. By 1993, there were more than 200 such programs in the United States.

If the intended parents supply the sperm and the ova, and if the natural mother is the woman who receives the embryos, traditional family legal principles would apply. If the sperm are not from the intended father, new and existing family law principles concerning paternity and AID and perhaps adoption should apply. When, however, an ovum is donated, or when a surrogate mother is utilized, whether or not she is also the source of the ovum, legal relationships are less clear.

State legislation on AI may also directly or implicitly apply to IVF. Physicians in many states have resorted to approaching their state or local district attorneys for their legal opinions (to ensure that they would not be prosecuted under state statutes) before proceeding with IVF programs.

Pennsylvania requires certain information to be filed with the state department of health by persons conducting or experimenting in IVF but imposes no direct regulations or limitations on the practice of IVF.

The Illinois Abortion Act of 1975, as amended in 1984, includes the provision, "Any person who intentionally causes the fertilization of a human ovum by a sperm outside the body of a living human female shall with regard to the human being thereby produced be deemed to have the care and custody of a child for the purposes of Section 4 of the Act to Prevent and Punish Wrongs to Children."[87] Section 4 states, "It shall be unlawful for any person having the care or custody of any child, willfully to cause or permit the life of such child to be endangered, or the health of such child to be injured, or willfully cause or permit such child to be placed in such a situation that its life or health may be endangered."[88] The statute would seem to prohibit the destruction of unused embryos. In fact, the very process of placing an embryo in a petri dish and supplying adequate nutrients might be construed as a situation that may be so life endangering as to create liability.

The constitutionality of this law was unsuccessfully challenged in *Smith v. Hartigan.*[89] The statutes were interpreted such that the attorney general's office would not prosecute, allowing IVF programs to proceed. The position of the court was that the laws applied to the physicians only during the preimplantation stage when they had custody, and that if a conceptus was found to be defective, destruction of the fetus would be considered a lawful pregnancy termination and not a willful injury. Then, in April 1990, the U.S. District Court of the Northern District of Illinois ruled that Section 6(7) of the law, prohibiting any experimentation using a human embryo that is not "therapeutic to the fetus," is unconstitutionally vague because it fails to define "experimentation" and "therapeutic."

The risk of congenital malformations associated with IVF is apparently no higher than in a conventional birth.[90] If a child is born with a genetic defect, a program will not likely be found liable as long as the program followed accepted standards and did not have an above-normal rate of defective products. Nonetheless, it would seem prudent to perform some genetic screening, if only a history, on the husband and wife. The American Fertility Society published new Minimal *Standards for Programs of In vitro Fertilization* in 1990.[91] These standards list the skills required of personnel, the services offered, and the necessary facilities and may be used as evidence of the standard of care in a malpractice suit. Preimplantation screening is now feasible and may allow the detection of cytogenetic disorders and certain metabolic disorders. A single cell is removed from the blastomere and analyzed via the usual cytogenetic methods. Polymerase chain reaction (PCR) assaying can be used for detection of single-gene disorders.

Surrogate motherhood. When a woman is physically incapable of bearing a child, a surrogate mother or "gestational mother" may be an alternative to adoption. The infertile client, usually a married couple but possibly a single man or woman, contracts for the services of a woman to bear a child and then to relinquish her parental rights in favor of the contracting parents. Most often the baby's biological father and his wife, the prospective adopting or "rearing" mother, are the contracting parents. Conception by AI of the surrogate mother is the usual procedure contemplated. Recently however, implantation has been performed after IVF. This may or may not make use of the oocytes of the proposed rearing mother. Attorneys, physicians, or surrogate agencies often act as brokers in these arrangements. Although surrogacy has been practiced for centuries,[92] open consideration of surrogate motherhood with the advent of medically sanctioned artificial procreative methods has become an option only in the last decade. Increasing public attention has prompted competing legislative proposals that would either sanction or outlaw these arrangements.

Public policy arguments against surrogate mothering may provide a basis for finding a surrogacy contract unenforceable. Such arguments may include that it (1) undermines the traditional notions of family and threatens the sanctity of marriage; (2) disregards and undervalues the strong attachment of the maternal bond; and (3) is morally repugnant because children are treated like chattels. It is also argued that poor women would be economically exploited. In one US. study, 40% of volunteer surrogate mothers were found to be unemployed or on welfare.[93] Some of the public policy arguments against this form of collaborative reproduction are reminiscent of public policy arguments originally made against AI.

Even if surrogacy contracts are not considered contrary to public policy, courts would not specifically enforce performance; that is, they would not force a woman to bear a child. In general, contracts are not enforceable when law prohibits them. State laws against baby bartering, paid adoption, or surrogate arrangements might apply. The Thirteenth Amendment's prohibition against slavery and the sale of one person by another might also be applied to find a contract unlawful and therefore unenforceable. Even if the contract is deemed unenforceable, however, suit may still be brought against the surrogate for emotional suffering by the contracting couple.

The majority of surrogacy arrangements proceed without judicial involvement, with few reported instances of parties reneging on their agreements.[94,95] Courts have uniformly refused to enforce surrogacy contracts, although custody is often awarded to the biological father and his wife under a "best interests of the child" analysis.

Problems result, however, when combinations of public policy arguments, contract law principles, state laws and constitutions, and federal constitutional doctrines are put to the test, as follows:

1. The surrogate develops a maternal attachment and decides to keep the baby.
2. The surrogate decides not to go through with the contract and terminates her pregnancy by an abortion.
3. The surrogate inadvertently or wantonly exposes the child to noxious or teratogenic agents.
4. The baby has defects, and none of the potential parents wants the baby.

If the contract is upheld, then contractual provisions are controlling; on the other hand, if the contract is unenforceable or void, then the courts would offer little or no help in disentangling the multiple difficulties.

BABY M. The most significant and publicized surrogate motherhood case to date is *In re Baby M,* decided by the New Jersey Supreme Court in 1988. The high court reversed the lower appellate decision and declared the contract unenforceable because such contractual surrogate arrangements are otherwise against the public policy and interests.[96] Nonetheless, custody was taken from Mary Beth Whitehead, the surrogate mother, and given to the Sterns, the contracting couple, on the basis of the best interests of the child.

The New Jersey Supreme Court largely reversed the holding of the trial court judge, ruling that the contract was invalid and unenforceable on two bases: direct conflict with existing state statutes and conflict with public policy.

The New Jersey Supreme Court reestablished parental rights in Mrs. Whitehead, who was by that time Mrs. Whitehead-Gould, but under a "best-interests" analysis, the court granted continuing custody of the child to the Sterns. Further proceedings at the trial court level granted extended visitation rights to Whitehead-Gould. The Sterns did not appeal.

OTHER SURROGACY CASES. Other reported cases of surrogacy indicate how surrogacy can distort traditional concepts of the family.[97] In California, Alejandro Munoz bore a child as a "favor" for her second cousin, Nattie Haro. Munoz had inseminated herself with a plastic syringe using sperm from Haro's husband. Later she sued for shared custody of the child, and her claim was upheld by the Supreme Court. In another California case a lesbian woman bore a child after inseminating herself with sperm donated by the homosexual brother of her lover. After the lesbian couple separated, the judge granted visitation rights to both women and the semen donor. In a midwestern state, two homosexual men made arrangements through a surrogate agency to have someone else bear a child whom they would raise. The first reported case of surrogacy in South Africa involved a 48-year-old grandmother who delivered triplets for her daughter. She had been implanted with four embryos produced from her daughter's ova and her son-in-law's sperm, because the daughter had previously had a hysterectomy for uncontrolled hemorrhage during a delivery. In a 1989 case an Alaska court upheld the surrogacy arrangements that had been made between sisters when the biological mother changed her mind about giving the baby up for adoption after the maximum time period allowed by the Alaska adoption statute.[98]

As complications develop, the artificial nature of these arrangements will be tested. In Texas a surrogate mother reportedly died in the eighth month of pregnancy because of pregnancy-related heart failure.[99] In Washington, D.C., an HIV-positive child was born, and both the contracting couple and the surrogate refused to claim the child. Future issues may include such topics as a female employee's decision to "moonlight" as a surrogate by making use of the health insurance benefits and pregnancy-leave policy provided by her primary employer; violation of constitutional rights of the surrogate with respect to enforcement of contract provisions concerning her behavior during pregnancy; the prospective rearing parents' rights to have those provisions enforced; and the possibility of physician liability for both the surrogate and the contracting couple when surrogacy arrangements do not proceed as planned.

Courts in the future may respond to the apparent and significant need filled by surrogate arrangements, as judged by their general and growing popularity, success, and public acceptance. As illustrated in the Baby M case, however, three guiding sets of principles must always be addressed: (1) contract law statutes and principles, (2) state statutes and principles related to family law, including criminal statutes, and (3) constitutional considerations. Clearly, however, regardless of how the validity of the contract or agreement is decided, the custody of the child will always be based on a "best-interests" test.

Cryopreservation of embryos and gametes. The preservation of embryos and gametes by freezing is an integral part of IVF. The first successful births after freezing, thawing, and implantation of a human embryo were in 1984 by groups in Australia and The Netherlands. Cryopreservation has now become routine for preserving multiple embryos for use in subsequent cycles.

Some special issues involved in cryopreservation have been exemplified in court cases. A wealthy couple died in an airplane crash, leaving millions of dollars and two frozen embryos in Australia.[100] In a scenario that is likely to be repeated, a Tennessee couple who had cryopreserved seven embryos separated, and the husband filed a court action seeking to enjoin the wife from having the embryos implanted against his will. The Tennessee Supreme Court ruled that the biological father of the cryopreserved embryos had an absolute right not to become a birth father against his will.[101]

Only the beginnings of these complex problems have been seen. Cryopreservation of unfertilized oocytes would minimize the legal and ethical concerns; unfortunately, this procedure has proved to be more technically difficult.

POSTCONCEPTION ISSUES
Prenatal injury issues

It is surprising how seldom traumatic injury to a pregnant woman causes injury to a fetus. The most common situation resulting in a liability for prenatal injury follows blunt abdominal trauma that is secondary to a motor vehicle collision.

In the past, there was no criminal liability for the prenatal injury of a stillborn infant; recently, however, several states have enacted statutes allowing criminal prosecution for fetal death. Most state penal codes, while statutorily prescribing criminal punishment for wrongful death of a person, define a "person" as a human being who has been born and is alive. This rule follows from Lord Coke's restatement of English law: "If a woman is quick with child and takes a potion, or if a man beats her, and the child is born alive and dies of the potion or battery, this is murder." However, approximately half of the states have specifically legislated a crime of feticide/homicide or involuntary manslaughter for the death of a fetus. The Supreme Judicial Court of Massachusetts decided in 1984 in *Commonwealth v. Cass* that a viable fetus is a "person" within the meaning of the Massachusetts vehicular homicide statute.[102] For the first time a state levied a criminal punishment, absent specific legislation, for the death of a fetus not born alive. In *State v. Wickstrom* the defendant, who beat his pregnant girlfriend, was convicted of first-degree criminal abortion, a violation of the criminal statute prohibiting the performance of abortions by nonphysicians.[103]

There is a clear trend toward liberalizing civil liability for prenatal injury. The right to sue for damages for the death of another is based on wrongful death statutes that have been enacted in some form by all 50 states.

Most states have extended civil liability to persons causing intrauterine injury resulting in stillbirth. A few courts have limited liability for prenatal injury to those cases in which the fetus was viable (defined in the sense of *Roe v. Wade* as a fetus so developed as to be capable of a separate existence[104]) at the time of injury. In 1989, in *Cowe by Cowe v. Forum Group, Inc.,* the Court of Appeals of Indiana established a cause of action for prenatal injury because the defendants' negligent failure to diagnose the pregnancy of their retarded ward and their subsequent failure to render prenatal care resulted in injury to the child.[105] Although these cases have dealt with direct trauma to the infant, the rationale would appear to extend to toxic chemicals and even to teratogenic agents.

There is increasing interest in holding mothers responsible for the health of their offspring. At the same time, injunctive relief has usually been granted in emergency situations (see later section on court-ordered obstetrical interventions). In San Diego a woman was charged for failing to summon medical help when she began to hemorrhage during her pregnancy. She delivered a son with severe brain damage later that day, who died approximately a month later. The municipal court judge dismissed criminal charges because the 1926 law with which she was charged was intended to force fathers to pay for the support of their children and did not apply to this situation. A woman in Toledo, Ohio, was charged with felony endangerment of her child for regularly using cocaine during her pregnancy. The grand jury returned an indictment when her daughter developed withdrawal symptoms a few days after birth. The mother tested positive for cocaine. The child was placed in a foster home, and the mother was placed in a drug rehabilitation program. The case was eventually dropped.

On the other hand, a child was allowed to maintain a civil action against his mother and her physician for prenatal negligence in *Grodin v. Grodin* for the unreasonable exercise of parental discretion in the use of tetracycline, resulting in damage to her son's teeth.[106] Much discussion has surrounded mandatory treatment of drug-addicted obstetrical patients; however, most commentators agree that such treatment is ineffective.[107]

Abortion

The history of legalized abortion is one of controversy. The first step toward legalization came in 1965, through the Supreme Court case of *Griswold v. Connecticut.*[108] In that case, the U.S. Supreme Court created a "zone of privacy" for married persons that prevented states from regulating their choice to use contraception. Then in *Roe v. Wade* the Supreme Court declared that the right of privacy was broad enough to encompass a woman's decision to terminate her pregnancy.[109] In *Roe* a Texas abortion statute, similar to those of 31 other states, was struck down in its entirety as unconstitutional. The court reasoned that the state could invade the privacy of the mother to a limited extent when the state's interest in protecting the health of the mother or the life of the fetus became sufficiently strong. The court imposed the following limitations:

1. Before the end of the first trimester, the decision to abort is strictly between the woman and her physician.

2. Beginning in the second trimester but before the fetus becomes viable, the state may impose regulations reasonably related to the mother's health.

3. During the period of fetal viability (generally the third trimester), the state may regulate or prohibit all abortions except when necessary to preserve the health of the mother.

A wave of restrictive state and municipal abortion legislation was promulgated in reaction to *Roe.* Most were quickly struck down as unconstitutional. Gradually, in the wake of this activity, the Supreme Court seemed to retreat from its "strict scrutiny" standard toward the more lenient "rational basis" analysis to determine the constitutionality of legislation and regulations. This retreat led to a most significant trio of decisions that helped to define the outer limits of the right to abortion. In the *Maher v. Roe, Poelker v. Doe,* and *Harris v. McRae* decisions, the Supreme Court upheld government spending statutes that reimburse an indigent woman for the cost of childbirth but not for the cost of an abortion.[110]

Then, in *City of Akron v. Akron Center for Reproductive Health, Inc.,* the Supreme Court, despite the urgings of the U.S. solicitor general to relax standards of review, reaffirmed its *Roe v. Wade* analysis of strictly scrutinizing abortion regulations to protect the fundamental right of privacy.[111] In *Akron,* regulations requiring that all second-trimester abortions be performed in a hospital were found to be invalid without evidence that such routine hospitalization was medically necessary. Without a compelling state interest, the regulations were held to unconstitutionally decrease the availability of abortions by substantially increasing the cost.

Under the Reagan and Bush administrations a partially new U.S. Supreme Court became increasingly dissatisfied with the rationale of the *Roe v. Wade* opinion on abortion. In *Thornburgh v. American College of Obstetricians and Gynecologists,* after the appointment of two Reagan-appointed justices and shortly before the appointment of a third, the Supreme Court granted review in a case that did not present substantially novel issues but rather was viewed as a chance to review the subject.[112] In a close 5-to-4 decision the court struck down the Pennsylvania Abortion Control Act of 1982 and thereby affirmed its previous stance, with the dissent questioning the validity of *Roe v. Wade.*

In 1988 the prolife administration was successful in pushing through regulations under Section 1008 of Title X of the Public Health Service Act that prohibit the counseling of clients concerning abortion or the referral of any patient to a physician for an abortion, even if requested, by any program receiving federal Title X funds. Further, the regulations require that if such a clinic provides for abortions or abortion counseling or referral from private funding sources, those services must be financially and physically separate.

In 1991 the U.S. Supreme Court upheld the validity of the regulations in *Rust v. Sullivan.*[113] In January 1993, however, President Clinton used an executive order to abrogate the so-called Gag Rule. The restrictions on federal funding of abortions remain.

Webster. In 1989 the Supreme Court ruled on *Webster v. Reproductive Health Services.*[114] In *Webster* the Court opened the door for greatly increased government regulation and restriction of abortions without actually overturning *Roe, Akron, Thornburgh,* or *Commonwealth.* Following the rationale of *Maher, Poelker,* and *Harris,* the court upheld the constitutionality of a Missouri statute that, inter alia, forbids the use of state employees and of state facilities to perform or assist in any nontherapeutic abortions. Citing *Harris* and relying on *Roe's* philosophy that the states are free to make value judgments favoring childbirth over abortion, the court reasoned that "the State's decision here to use public facilities and staff to encourage childbirth over abortion places no governmental obstacle in the path of a woman who chooses to terminate her pregnancy"; rather, "Missouri's refusal to allow public employees to perform abortions in public hospitals leaves a pregnant woman with the same choices as if the State had chosen not to operate any public hospitals at all. The court declined to reassess the validity of *Roe* on the additional grounds that the Missouri statute was not a criminal statute forbidding all abortions. Unlike *Akron,* the Missouri statute was found to cause an insignificant increase in the cost of an abortion; furthermore, the statute did not contain any of the same flaws as the statute in *Thornburgh.*

Before *Webster* the U.S. Supreme Court and lower federal courts disallowed a number of state and local statutory requirements that impermissibly restricted access to abortion: requirements for establishing a waiting period between the time of counseling and the performance of the abortion; the requirement that a physician must provide lengthy and detailed information specified by an ordinance; restrictive zoning ordinances[115] and building permits[116]; and requirements that fetal remains be disposed of in a humane and sanitary manner.[117] They have allowed requirements of the presence of a second physician during postviability abortions; requirements that physicians performing abortions maintain surgical privileges at an appropriate hospital[118]; and licensing criteria of medical facilities in which abortions are performed that include licensure of outpatient facilities and that are consistent with accepted medical practice.[119] More recently, however, the Supreme Court has upheld state statutes involving "pre-abortion" issues. In 1992 the court decided *Planned Parenthood v. Casey.*[120] In Casey the court allowed the following issues to stand: state-required pre-abortion counseling, a wait of 24 hours before obtaining the abortion, parental or judicial consent for a minor, and state-required statistical reporting to public authorities.

Abortion and minors. Women under 21 years old account for a significant portion of all abortions in the United States.[121] In several opinions the Supreme Court cautioned that minors might not have rights equal to those of adults.[122] The rationale for a more restrictive view of minors' rights is based on the states' more compelling interest in protecting the minors from their own uninformed or less-than-mature choices. Although no federal court has allowed parental consent or notice as a prerequisite to access to contraceptives by an unemancipated minor, the U.S. Supreme Court has, with increasingly well-defined restrictions, approved state parental notification and consent requirements for abortion.

The Supreme Court has not said that the failure to provide bypass alternatives in every instance is an undue burden.[123] These statutes can pose a significant hindrance to unemancipated minors who seek abortions, especially in rural areas, and so must be carefully and narrowly crafted to withstand strict judicial scrutiny. The Supreme Court has held that, for such a statute to be upheld, it "also must provide an alternative procedure whereby authorization for the abortion can be obtained."[124] Such a bypass mechanism provides that the minor's parent does not necessarily have a "right" to veto the abortion, and it is most likely to be applied when, for example, (1) the minor is shown to be mature enough to give valid consent for the procedure; (2) when notification of the minor's parent or parents is shown to be in conflict with the minor's best interests, as in the case of the parents' abuse of the minor; or (3) despite the incapacity of the minor to give valid consent, the abortion is shown to be in the minor's best interests. Bypass procedures must also afford expedited appeals processes and ensure confidentiality throughout the process. A parental involvement statute must also have acceptable provisions concerning the burden of proof, waiting periods, and determination of court-appointed counsel.[125]

The practical differences between a statute requiring "consent" of a parent and a statute requiring "notice" to a parent are often insignificant. By requiring only that a minor notify a parent before receiving an abortion, a statute clearly does not give the parent veto power; however, parents may possess veto power independent of the existence of the statute because of their parental control over the minor. The same requirements generally apply to each type of parental involvement statute. The AMA's Council on Ethical and Judicial Affairs concluded that minors seeking abortions should not be required to involve their parents before the procedure.[126]

Paternity suits

Paternity suits are civil actions requiring proof by a preponderance of the evidence. The evidentiary laws on the admissibility of blood testing to determine paternity are of two types: inclusionary or exclusionary. Traditionally, state laws have been exclusionary, in which they allow the admission of blood test results only when they conclusively exclude an accused man as the father. When paternity testing evidence is inadmissible, the courtroom proceeding focuses on the unsubstantiated allegation of the mother that a man is the father against his assertion that he is not.

Approximately half the states have statutorily departed from admitting only exclusionary testing and have created an *inclusionary* rule that allows the admission of any serological tests, even when they indicate only a statistical likelihood of paternity. In many states this has been accomplished by the adoption of model legislation proposed by the Commission on Uniform State Laws: the Uniform Act on Blood Tests to Determine Paternity (1975), the Uniform Act on Paternity (1960), and the Uniform Parentage Act (1973). Additionally, case law in some states has created a judicial adoption of the inclusionary rule, often overcoming exclusionary status. In *Cramer v. Morrison* the court found that the histocompatibility leukocyte antigen (HLA) test results were admissible as possible proof of paternity despite a statute that seemed to allow only exclusionary blood tests.[127] The court reasoned that HLA testing is not the "blood test" contemplated by the statute; rather, the drafters had in mind the testing of red blood cell antigens (Landsteiner blood grouping tests) available at the time the law was enacted.

Evidence of biological paternity is not necessarily controlling.[128] The constitutionality of a state statute that refuses men the opportunity, in some situations, to prove their paternity has been upheld by the U.S. Supreme Court.[129]

Although the awarding of primary custody to fathers has become much more common in recent decades, "paternity rights" have far to go before reaching the level of constitutional protection that is afforded maternity-related rights, such as the right to abortion. To date, the right to choose to end a pregnancy within statutory limits has been deemed to be exclusively that of the mother, whose body is directly affected by the decision, despite a number of attempts by fathers to prevent the abortion.[130] The U.S. Supreme Court denied review of states' appellate court opinions, which state that a putative father may not prevent a pregnant woman from aborting his child.[131]

Pregnancy discrimination

The U.S. Civil Rights Act of 1964 was amended by the Pregnancy Discrimination Act (PDA) to prohibit discrimination on the basis of pregnancy. This act was passed in response to the U.S. Supreme Court decision in *Gilbert v. General Electric Co.,* which held that employment disability insurance programs that excluded coverage of pregnancy and disability did not discriminate on the basis of sex and thus did not violate Title VII.[132] Congress heard testimony on extensive discrimination against pregnant women and intended the PDA to provide relief for working women. In *California Savings and Loan Association v. Guerra* the court considered the case of Lillian Garland, who had taken pregnancy disability leave in 1982 but was not reinstated afterward because her position as a receptionist had been filled during her absence.[133] The trial court held that the California employers were subject to reverse discrimination by the application of the state law requiring an employer to provide leave and reinstatement to a pregnant employee. The U.S. Supreme Court then held that the California statute was consistent with the PDA.

The final word as to whether employers could discriminate against pregnant women on the basis of fetal concerns was given by the U.S. Supreme Court in *International Union v. Johnson Controls.*[134] The "fetal protection policy" of Johnson Controls was found to be in direct violation of the PDA. Pregnant women may be discriminated against only if the pregnancy affected their ability to do their job. If pregnancy would affect the essence of the business then the employer could use "nonpregnancy" as a qualification.

Wrongful conception or wrongful pregnancy

Actions by parents against physicians for negligent contribution to unplanned pregnancies are termed "wrongful conception" or "wrongful pregnancy" cases. The injury in these specialized malpractice cases is the unplanned pregnancy, usually followed by the birth of a normal, healthy baby. The plaintiffs generally attempt to prove that the unplanned pregnancy is caused by the negligence of the physician. Primarily, four situations result in wrongful pregnancy cases: (1) a failed sterilization or failure to ascertain the success of a sterilization operation, (2) the ineffective prescription of contraceptives or counseling on contraception, (3) the failure to diagnose pregnancy in time for an elective abortion, and (4) an unsuccessful abortion.

Failure of sterilization procedures is the most common basis for a wrongful pregnancy action. A small number of tubal ligations and vasectomy procedures become recanalized and result in regained fertility. In the case of tubal ligation, fallopian tissue on histological sections and the length of the specimen are important factors. Patients should normally be informed of alternative treatments. In the case of vasectomy, standard practice generally requires the use of contraception until the establishment of two aspermic postvasectomy specimens. The patient's noncompliance is often the reason for failure to obtain the specimens, but a physician may have the duty to warn the patient of the consequences of his noncompliance.

Initially, these cases met with little success.[135] The birth of a healthy baby was not considered to be a legal injury. As a matter of public policy, life was preferred over nonlife. Furthermore, the courts alluded to the inability to assess damages for the birth of a child. The first successful wrongful pregnancy case was the California case, *Custodio v. Bauer.*[136] This suit was brought by a woman who became pregnant soon after she underwent a tubal ligation. The award was considered the logical extension of a malpractice action; to deny the claim would be to allow the injury from a physician's negligent act to go uncompensated.

Wrongful pregnancy cases have also been brought under contract and warranty theories, based on declarations by the physician that the sterilization was irreversible, that the patient would have no more children, or that the sterilization was successful. In most cases these nonnegligence claims have been rejected, because the courts are reluctant to find such warranties without separate contracts for consideration other than the usual physician fees.[137]

Other wrongful pregnancy cases have been brought with some success under theories of informed consent based on the physician's failure to inform the patient that the sterilization procedure might not be successful. In *Sard v. Hardy* a physician performed a cesarean section for the delivery of the plaintiff's third child and also a bilateral tubal ligation.[138] The patient and her husband were assured by the physician that she could not become pregnant again, although the Madlener technique used was associated with an unusually high failure rate. Two years later, after the patient again became pregnant, she successfully sued despite the signing of a consent form, alleging that the physician negligently failed to inform her that the procedure might not result in permanent sterility as intended and alleging that she was not informed of alternative sterilization procedures.

In the unusual case in which a child is both conceived as a result of a physician's negligence and also born with a congenital deformity, disease, or mental impairment, then virtually all courts allow for the special costs pertinent to raising a handicapped child. Some courts in the past have allowed financial support to extend, not just until majority, but for the lifetime of the child. In these cases, both "wrongful pregnancy" and "wrongful birth/life" causes of action and related measurement of damages might be appropriate.

BIRTH-RELATED ISSUES
Wrongful birth

Claims of liability have been made for negligence that results in a defective child being born when that child is unwanted solely because of the defect. In such a claim, referred to as a "wrongful birth" claim, the negligence of the physician does not cause the defect itself. Rather, a physician may be liable when the defect is foreseeable or discoverable, and when the physician fails to foresee or test for the defect. The plaintiff parents argue that they would have prevented the birth of the child, through the use of contraception or abortion, had they been properly informed and counseled.

When a child is born with a congenital defect, such as a hereditary disease or a physical or mental handicap, the physician might be found liable for wrongful birth for these reasons: failure to take a genetic history or otherwise screen for genetic disease, failure to correctly inform the parents of their chances of producing defective offspring, failure to recognize a genetic disease or teratogenic risk and so inform the parents of the possible consequences, failure to perform prenatal testing when indicated, failure to perform the testing or interpret the results properly, failure to inform the parents of possible prenatal testing or recommended amniocentesis, or failure to perform an abortion or refer to a willing physician.

The history of wrongful birth actions is parallel to but less well developed than that of wrongful pregnancy. The earliest cases were brought alleging illegitimacy as a compensable defect, but courts always rejected this as the basis for a claim.[139] The first cases involving an impaired infant were rejected based on the public policy preferring life over non-life and the inability to assess damages.[140] Courts were also reluctant to find in the physician a duty to advise the parents of all possible genetic defects. Furthermore, they felt that the judicial proceedings themselves would engender a perception of the child as being unwanted and create a negative stigma in the child's mind.

The first successful recovery for wrongful birth was in the Texas case *Jacobs v. Theimer*.[141] This case was brought by a woman who had contracted rubella during pregnancy and gave birth to a deformed child. The court found negligence in the physician's failure to warn of the potential harm of rubella to a fetus. Since the *Theimer* decision, wrongful birth claims have ultimately been recognized by every court that has considered the issue.

Most suits in the 1960s and 1970s resulted from inadequate counseling based on maternal risk factors, such as advanced maternal age, ethnic factors, or rubella exposure. Subsequent cases have focused on failure to recognize a genetic defect in the parent or older sibling.[142] Many cases involve naive or false reassurances offered by physicians to mothers that minimized the possible effects of a drug, illness, or disease on the pregnancy. The defense has largely centered on the facts of the case and, in particular, that (1) the parents failed to disclose all relevant facts that might have indicated the genetic predisposition or fetal risk and (2) the mother still would have given birth to the child, especially if the defect is first discoverable after abortion is no longer an option.[143] Wrongful birth has been limited to legal actions against health care providers as opposed to employers.[144]

The doctrinal turning point allowing general acceptance of wrongful birth suits came in the *Roe v. Wade* decision, clarifying that there was no public policy prohibiting abortions.[145] States were free to adopt policies preferring childbirth to abortion. Many states have passed or considered legislation prohibiting wrongful birth suits because of the fear that the wrongful birth cause of action will force physicians to identify defective fetuses and promote abortions. Dictum in the Webster case indicated that such policies and legislation would be upheld as long as the state did not thereby create any affirmative barriers for a woman who is seeking an abortion.[146] In *Hickman v. Group Health Plan, Inc.*, the Minnesota Supreme Court in a 4-to-3 decision held that the state statute that prohibited the maintenance of an action for damages based on a wrongful birth theory does not contravene the right of a pregnant woman to choose an abortion.[147] The court found no state action and no interference with the right to an abortion.

Wrongful life

The main difference between a "wrongful birth" and a "wrongful life" claim is the identity of the plaintiff. Unlike a wrongful birth suit, in which the plaintiffs are the parents of the disabled child, a suit claiming wrongful life is brought by or on behalf of the disabled child, based on theories of physician negligence similar to the negligent actions alleged in wrongful birth cases. Essentially, the child argues that he or she should never have been born—that nonexistence is preferable to the life of an individual so handicapped by a congenital disability. These cases are in many ways quite similar to the "right-to-die" cases.

Only a small number of states recognize wrongful life as a valid cause of action. In most states an inability to assess damages is perceived to exist as the result of an inability to place a value on nonlife, so that the various values of life and nonlife cannot be compared and contrasted. Furthermore, public policy generally favoring life over death is a barrier to wrongful life actions in many states. Overall, wrongful life has been an unpopular jurisprudential notion explicitly rejected in the majority of states that have considered it. Several states have passed legislation prohibiting wrongful life suits.

Court-ordered obstetrical interventions

With medical advances in obstetricians' ability to monitor fetal conditions and with increased knowledge about the effects of maternal behavior on infant health, intervention becomes more acceptable to physicians and judges who perceive some preventable risk to an unborn child. One of the first cases involving court-ordered obstetrical intervention was *In re A.C.*[148] Although the court initially ordered a cesarean section on a dying mother to save the fetus, it eventually reversed itself.

More recently in *Baby Boy Doe v. Mother Doe* the U.S. Supreme Court refused to order a lower Illinois court to convene an emergency hearing on whether to order an emergency cesarean section.[149] The mother refused on religious grounds to undergo the procedure. The ACOG, American Civil Liberties Union (ACLU), and others have issued statements opposing court-ordered treatment for pregnant women on grounds of maternal rights, medical uncertainty, and the irregularity of the judicial proceedings involved.[150]

A national survey investigated obstetrical procedures ordered by the court in the interest of fetuses over the objections of pregnant women in 21 cases during a 5-year period.[151] Cesarean sections constituted the bulk (15) of the judicially mandated procedures, but hospital detentions and transfusions were also ordered. Court orders for cesarean sections had been obtained in 11 states, and among the 21 cases in which court orders were sought, orders were obtained in 86%. Some conclude that court-ordered intervention is ethical provided if (1) it poses insignificant or no health risks to the woman or would promote her interests in life or health and (2) compelling reasons exist to override her autonomy.[152]

ENDNOTES

1. National Sickle Cell Anemia Control Act, 86 Stat. 136 (1972).
2. P. Reilly, *Genetics, Law, and Social Policy* 50-52 (Harvard University Press, Cambridge, Mass. 1977); and *State Laws and Regulations Governing Newborn Screening* (American Bar Foundation, Chicago 1985).
3. Jecker, *Genetic Testimony and the Social Responsibility of Private Health Insurance Companies,* 21 J. L. Med. & Ethics 109-116 (1993).
4. *Monusco v. Postle,* 437 N.W. 2d 367 (1989).
5. *Jacobs v. Theimer,* 519 S.W. 2d 846 (Tex. 1975).
6. *Harbeson v. Parke-Davis,* 656 P. 2d 483 (1983), 746 F. 2d 517 (1984).
7. *Speck v. Finegold,* 439 A. 2d 110 (1981).
8. *Brubaker v. Cavenaugh,* 542 F.Supp. 944 (1982).
9. *Moores v. Lucas,* 405 S. 2d 1022 (1981).
10. *Schroeder v. Perkel,* 432 A. 2d 834 (1981).
11. *Park v. Chessin,* 400 N.Y.S. 2d 204 (1976), 440 N.Y.S. 2d 110 (1977).
12. *Turpin v. Sortini,* 174 Cal. Rptr. 128 (1981), 643 P. 2d 954 (1982).
13. *Curlender v. Bioscience Laboratories,* 165 Cal. Rptr. 477 (1980).
14. *Mellis v. Chicago Memorial Hosp.,* No. 70L-15177 (Ill Cir. Ct. Cook County, June 18, 1974).
15. *Nelson v. Krusen,* 635 S.W. 2d 582 (1982).
16. *Lininger v. Eisenbaum,* 764 P. 2d 1202 (Colo. 1988).
17. *Call v. Kezirian,* 185 Cal. Rptr. 103, 1982.
18. *Siemieniec v. Lutheran Gen. Hosp.,* 512 N.E. 2d 691.
19. American Medical Association, Council on Scientific Affairs, *Genetic Counseling and Prevention of Birth Defects,* 248 J.A.M.A. 221-224 (1982).
20. 21 Fam. Plan. Perspect. 188 (1989).
21. 21 Fam. Plan. Perspect. 282 (1989).
22. Title XIX of the Public Health Service Act, 42 U.S.C. 1396a.
23. Title X of the Public Health Service Act, 42 U.S.C. 300 et seq.
24. 20 Fam. Plan. Perspect. 288 (1988).
25. 20 Fam. Plan. Perspect. 112 (1988).
26. 20 Fam. Plan. Perspect. 262 (1988).
27. *Griswold v. Connecticut,* 381 U.S. 479, 85 S.Ct. 1678 (1965).
28. *Eisenstadt v. Baird,* 405 U.S. 438, 92 S.Ct. 1029(1972).
29. An act for the suppression of trade in and circulation of obscene literature and articles of immoral use: 17 Stat. Ch. 258 § 148 (1873); The Family Planning Services and Population Research Act, Pub. Law No. 91-572 (Title X of the Public Health Services Act).
30. *Gaines v. Preterm-Cleveland, Inc.,* 514 N.E. 2d 709 (Ohio 1988).
31. Title XX of the Public Health Service Act, 42 U.S.C. 42 C.F.R. 59.5 et seq.
32. 21 Fam. Plan. Perspect. 123 (1989).
33. *E.G. Carey v. Population Services Internat'l,* 431 U.S. 678 (1977).
34. *Doe v. Blum,* 729 F. 2d 186 (1984).
35. *Bowen v. Kendrick,* 108 S.Ct. 2562 (1988).
36. *MacDonald v. Ortho Pharmaceutical Corp.,* 475 N.E. 2d 65 (Mass. 1985).
37. *Klink v. G. D. Searle & Co.,* 614 P. 2d 701 (Wash. 1980).
38. *Hamilton v. Hardy,* 549 P. 2d 1099 (Colo. 1976); 9 A.L.R. 4, 586 (1986).
39. This "respectable minority" test has been used many times since then in medical malpractice cases. See, e.g., *State Board of Medical Examiners v. McCroskey,* 880 P. 2d 1188 (1989).
40. Peterson, *Women Face Birth Control Confusion,* USA Today, Feb 5, 1986 at A1-2; Katz, *Dalkon Case Floods the Court,* USA Today, April 21, 1981 at A1; Middleton, *I.U.D. Discontinuation Seen as Unlikely to Affect Litigation,* 8 Nat. L.J. 13 (Feb 17, 1986).
41. 58 U.S.L.W. 3307; 21 Fam. Plan. Perspect. 246 (Nov 7, 1989).
42. 20 Fam Plan. Perspect. 288, 292 (1988).
43. *Searle Takes Two IUD's off U.S. Market,* Galveston Daily News, Feb 1, 1986, at B7.
44. Klitsch, 20 Fam. Plan. Perspect. 19 (1988).

45. *Killebrew v. Johnson,* 404 N.E. 2d 1194 (Ind. 1980).

46. *Wells v. Ortho Pharmaceutical Corp.,* 788 F. 2d 741 (1986) *writ denied,* 107 S.Ct. 437 (1986).

47. Kaunitz, *Long-acting Injectable Contraception with Depot Medroxyprogesterone Acetate,* 170 Am. J. Obstet. Gynecol. 1543-1549 (1994).

48. *Id.*

49. Federal Drug Administration, *F-D-C Reports ("The Pink Sheet"),* Oct 29, 1992.

50. Cullins, *Non-contraceptive Benefits and Therapeutic Uses of Depot Medroxyprogesterone Acetate.*

51. 20 Fam. Plan. Perspect. 288, 293 (1988).

52. *Id.*

53. 20 Fam. Plan. Perspect. 112, 116 (1988).

54. 20 Fam. Plan. Perspect. 288 (1988).

55. *Hathaway v. Worcester City Hosp.,* 475 F. 2d 701 (CCA1 1973); *Padin v. Fordham Hospital,* 392, F.Supp. 447 (D.C. N.Y. 1975).

56. *Sard v. Hardy,* A. 2d 1014 (Md. 1977).

57. *Gowan v. Carpenter,* 376 S.E. 2d 384 (1988).

58. *Wilsman v. Sloniewicz,* 526 N.E. 2d 645 (1988).

59. *Dohn v. Lovell,* 370 S.E. 2d 789 (1988).

60. Va. Code Ann. §§ 32-423 to 32-427; W. Va. Code Ann. §§ 16-11-1 to 16-11-2.

61. Ga. Code Ann. §§ 84-932, 84-935.2; N.C. Gen. Stat. §§ 90-271.

62. *Ponter v. Ponter,* 342 A. 2d 574 (N.J. Super. Ct. 1975).

63. 42 CFR §§ 441.250 to 441.259 (1985).

64. 22 Cal. Admin. Code §§ 70707.1 to 70707.8 [tit 22,51305.1 to 51305.6 (1980)].

65. *Downs v. Sawtelle,* 574 F. 2d 1 (1st Cir. 1978).

66. The hospital argued that, since it was being considered a "State actor," it should be entitled to a defense of qualified immunity, as is available to state officials. The circuit court of appeals decided that it was not. Other circuit courts, namely 11, 10, 8 and 5, have decided otherwise, i.e., that once characterized as state actors for purposes of Section 1983, private actors can assert a defense of qualified immunity. *See,* e.g., *Shipley v. First Federal Savings & Loan of Delaware,* Civ AN 84-521, JRR 703 F.Supp.1122. 46. 42.42 (1988).

67. Reilly, *The Surgical Solution: The Writing of Activist Physicians in the Early Days of Eugenical Sterilization,* 26 Perspect. Biological Med. 637-656 (1983); e.g., Idaho Code Ann. §§ 66-801 to 66-812, De. Code Ann. §§ 5701-5705.

68. *Buck v. Bell,* 274 U.S. 200, 47 S.Ct. 584 (1927).

69. Ala. Code Ann. 45 § 243 (1958); Ark. Stat. Ann. §§ 59-501 to 502 (1971); § 82-301 (1973); Cal. Welfare & Instit. Code Ann. § 7254 (1972); Conn. Gen. Stat. Ann. § 17-19 (1973); Del. Code Ann. 16 §§ 5701-5705 (1953); Ga. Code Ann. §§ 84-933 (1971); Idaho Code Ann. S§§ 39-3901 to 3910 (1961); Iowa Code Ann. §§ 145.1 to 145.22 (1972); Me. Rev. Stat. Ann. 34 §§ 2461-2468 (1965); Mich. Comp. Laws Ann. §§ 720.301 to 720.310 (1968); Minn. Stat. Ann. §§ 256.07-256.10 (1971); Miss. Code Ann. §§ 6957-6964, §§ 41-45-1 to -19 (1972); Mont. Rev. Stat. Ann. §§ 69-6401 to 6406 (1970); N.C. Gen Stat §§ 35-36 to -56 (1973); N.D. Cent. Code §§ 25-04.1 to 25-04.1-08 (1970); Okla. Stat. Ann. 43A §§ 341-346 (1954); Ore. Rev. Stat. §§ 436.010 to 436.150 (1973); S.C., Code Ann. §§ 32-671 to -680 (1968); Utah Code Ann. §§ 64-10-1 to -14 (1968); Vt. Stat. Ann. 18 §§ 8701-8704 (1986); Va. Code Ann. §§ 37.1-156 to -171 (1970); Wash. Rev. Code §§ 9.92.100 (1956); Wis. Stat. Ann. §§ 46.12 (1957).

70. *See,* e.g., codes for Maine, Montana, North Carolina, and Utah.

71. Statutorily required in Michigan, Oklahoma, and Virginia.

72. *Motes v. Hall City Dept. of Family & Children Services,* 306 S.E. 2d 260 (1983); *Matter of Truesdell,* 329 S.S.E. 2d 630 (1985).

73. Miss. Code Ann. §§ 41-45-1 to -19 (1972).

74. Courts failing to authorize in absence of statute include, among others, Alabama, *Hudson v. Hudson,* 373 S. 2d 310 (1979); Missouri, *Interest of MKR,* 515 S.W. 2d 467 (1974); California, *Tulley v. Tulley,* 146 Cal.

Rptr. 266 (1978), *cert. denied,* 440 US (1967); Wisconsin, *Matter of Guardianship of Eberhardy,* 294 N.W. 2d 540 (1980); Connecticut, *Ruby v. Massey,* 452 F.Supp. 361 (1978); Ohio, *Wade v. Bethesda Hosp.* 337 F.Supp. 671 (1971); and Delaware, *Matter of SCE,* 378 A. 2d 144 (1977). Courts authorizing sterilizations in absence of statute include *Stump v. Sparkman,* 436 U.S. 951 (1978); New Jersey, *In re Grady,* 426 A. 2d 567 (1981); New York, *In re Sallmuier,* 378 N.Y. A. 2d 989 (1976); Pennsylvania, *In re Terwilliger,* 450 A. 2d 1376 (1982); Colorado, *In re A.W.,* 637 P. 2d 366 (1981); and California, *Conservatorship of Valerie N.,* 219 Cal. Rptr. 387 (1985). See also West, *Parens patriae judicial authority to order sterilization of mental incompetents,* 25 J. Legal Med. 523 (1981).

75. *In re Guardianship of Matejski,* 419 N.W. 2d 576 (Iowa 1988).

76. *Sparkman v. McFarlin,* 6601 F. 2d 261 (7th Cir. 1979).

77. 50 Fertility and Sterility 519 (1988).

78. J.A. Robertson, *Ethical Issues in Preimplantation Genetic Screening,* 57 Fertil. & Steril. 1-11 (1992).

79. Ga. Code §§ 74-101.1 (1964).

80. Holding artificial insemination adulterous, e.g., *Gursky v. Gursky,* N.Y. 2d 406 (1963); *Modern view,* People v. Sorenson, 437 P. 2d 495 (1968).

81. *In re Baby Doe,* 353 S.F. 2d 877 (1987).

82. *People v. Sorenson,* 437 P.2d 495 (Cal. 1968).

83. *C.M. v. C.C.,* 377 A. 2d 821 (N.J. 1977).

84. Quigley & Andrews, *Human In Vitro Fertilization and the Law,* 42 Fertil. & Steril. 348-355, 353 (1984).

85. Uniform Laws Ann. 9A, Model Uniform Parentage Act, 1973. See 8 Family Law Quarterly 1 (1974).

86. Thatcher & DeCherney, 4 Human Reproduction, Suppl., 11-16 (1989).

87. Illinois Abortion Act of 1975, Amended 1984.

88. *Id.*

89. *Smith v. Hartigan,* 556 F.Supp. 157 (1983).

90. 55 Fertil. & Steril. 1 (1991).

91. 53 Fertil. & Steril. 225 (1990).

92. Genesis, Chapter 30, verses 1-8, *The Holy Bible* (Confraternity-Douay Version, New York 1957).

93. Winslade, *Surrogate Mothers: Right or Wrong?* 7 J. Med. Ethics 153 (1981).

94. Office of Technology Assessment Report, *Infertility: Medical and Social Choices,* 267 (1988).

95. *Id,* at 268.

96. *In re Baby M,* 537 A. 2d 1227 (1988).

97. Annas, *Protecting the Liberty of Pregnant Patients* (Editorial), 316 N. Engl. J. Med. 1213-1214 (1987).

98. *LJJ v. SAF and BFF,* 781 P. 2d 973 (1989).

99. As reported in Sec. 7, Biolaw, U:747.

100. *Australians Reject Bid to Destroy 2 Embryos,* N.Y. Times, Oct 24, 1984, at A18; Smith, *Australia's Frozen "Orphan" Embryos: A Medical, Legal, and Ethical Dilemma,* 24 J. Fam. L. 27 (1985-1986).

101. *Davis v. Davis,* W.L. 140-495 (Tenn. Cir., 1989).

102. *Commonwealth v. Cass,* 467 N.E. 2d 1324 (Mass. 1984).

103. *State v. Wickstrom,* 405 N.W. 2d 1 (Mn A. 1987).

104. *Roe v. Wade,* 410 U.S. 113, 93 S.Ct. 705 (1973).

105. *Cowe by Cowe v. Forum Group, Inc.,* 541 N.E. 2d 962 (1989).

106. *Grodin v. Grodin,* 301 N.W. 2d 869 (1987).

107. W. Chavkin, *Mandatory Treatment for Drug Use During Pregnancy,* 266 JAMA 1556-1561 (1991).

108. *Supra* note 27.

109. *Supra* note 104.

110. *Maher v. Roe,* 432 U.S. 464, 97 S.Ct. 2376 (1977); *Poelker v. Doe,* 432 U.S. 519, 97 S.Ct. 2391 (1977); and *Harris v. McRae,* 448 U.S. 297, 100 S.Ct. 2671 (1980).

111. *City of Akron v. Akron Center for Reproductive Health, Inc.,* 462 U.S. 416, 103 S.Ct. 2481 (1983).

112. *Thornburgh v. American College of Obstetricians and Gynecologists,* 471 U.S. 1014 (1986).

113. *Rust v. Sullivan,* 111 S.Ct. 1759 (1991).

114. *Webster v. Reproductive Health Services,* 109 S.Ct. 3040 (1989).

115. *Haskell v. Washington Township,* No. 87-3927, CA 6, 12/20/88.

116. *P.L.S. Partners v. City of Cranston,* 696 F.Supp. 788, D RI (1988).

117. *Akron Center for Reproductive Health, Inc. v. City of Akron,* 102 S.Ct. 2266 (1982).

118. Women's Health Center of West County v. Webster, CA 8, No. 88-1663 (Mar. 31, 1989).

119. Parental consent with judicial bypass option: *Belloti v. Baird,* 443 U.S. 622 (1979); performance in licensed facilities including outpatient clinics: *Baird v. Dept. of Public Health,* 599 F.2d 1098 (1979); presence of second physician: *Planned Parenthood v. Ashcroft,* 51 U.S.L.W. 4783 (June 15, 1983).

120. *Planned Parenthood v. Casey,* 112 S.Ct. 2791 (1992).

121. 21 Family Planning Perspectives 85 (1989).

122. *Supra* note 33.

123. *Supra* note 36.

124. *Bellotti v. Baird,* 443 U.S. 622 (1989).

125. *Jacksonville Clergy Consultation Service, Inc. v. Marinez,* 707 F.Supp. 1301 (M.D. Fla. 1989).

126. American Medical Association, *Code of Medical Ethics,* 1997.

127. *Cramer v. Morrison,* 143 Cal. Rptr. 865 (1979).

128. *Matter of the Marriage of Hodge and Hodge,* 713 P 2d 1071 (Ore. 1986).

129. *Michael H. and Victoria D. v. Gerald D.,* No. 87-746, *decided* June 15, 1989; *see* 57 U.S.L.W. 4691.

130. *Conn v. Conn,* 525 N.E .2d 612 (In App. 1988); *Doe v. Smith,* 108 S.Ct. 2136 (1988).

131. *Smith v. Doe,* 109 S.Ct. 3264 (1989), 57 U.S.L.W. 3855, *as reported by* 17 Health L. Dig. 90; *Lewis v. Lewis and Myers v. Lewis,* U.S. Sup.Ct. Nos. 88-555 and 88-683, 57 U.S.L.W. 3373.

132. *Gilbert v. General Electric Co.,* 429 U.S. 125 (1976).

133. *California Savings and Loan Association v. Guerra,* 55 L.W. 4077 (1987).

134. *International Union v. Johnson Controls,* 111 S.Ct. 1196 (1991).

135. *Hays v. Hall,* 477 S.W. 2d 402, 1972, 488 S.W. 2d 412 (1973); *Christiansen v. Thornby,* 255 N.W. 1620 (1934).

136. *Custodio v. Bauer,* 59 Cal. Rptr. 463 (Cal. 1967).

137. *Murray v. Univ. of Pennsylvania Hosp.,* 490 A. 2d 839 (1985); *Szekeres v. Robinson,* 715 P. 2d 1076 (1986).

138. *Supra* note 56.

139. *Zepeda v. Zepeda,* 190 N.E. 2d 849 (1963).

140. *Gleitman v. Cosgrove,* 227 A. 2d 689 (1967).

141. *Supra* note 5.

142. *Lininger v. Eisenbaum,* 764 P. 2d 1202 (Colo. 1988).

143. *Spencer v. Seikerl,* 742 P. 2d 1126 (Ok. 1987).

144. *Coley v. Commonwealth Edison Co.,* 703 F.Supp. 748 (ND ILL. 1989).

145. *Supra* note 104.

146. *Webster,* 109 S.Ct. 3040, No. 88-605, *decided* July 3, 1989.

147. *Hickman v. Group Health Plan, Inc.,* 396 N.W. 2d 10 (1986).

148. *In re A.C.,* 573 A. 2d 1235 (D.C. Cir. 1990).

149. *Baby Doe v. Mother Doe,* 510 U.S. 1021, 1132; 114 S.Ct. 652 (1993).

150. ABA J. 84-88 (Apr 1989).

151. Kolder, Gallagher, & Parsons, *Court Ordered Obstetrical Interventions,* 316 N. Engl. J. Med. 1192-1196 (1987).

152. C. Strong, *Court-Ordered Treatment in Obstetrics: the Ethical Views and Legal Framework,* 78 Obstet. Gynecol. 861-868 (1991).

GENERAL REFERENCES

Elias & Annas, *Reproductive Genetics & Law* (1987).

Institute of Medicine, *Medical Professional Liability and the Delivery of Obstetrical Care* (1989).

McCullough & Cherenak, *Ethics in Obstetrics and Gynecology* (1994).

Steinbock, *Life Before Birth: the Moral and Legal Status of Embryos and Fetuses* (1992).

ADDITIONAL READINGS

Barbara A. v. John G., 193 Cal. Rptr. 422 (1983).

45 C.F.R. SS46.201 (1981); SS46.204(d) (1984).

K. Benirschke, *The Placenta in the Litigation Process,* 162 Am. J. Obstet. Gynecol. 1445-1450 (1990).

C.A.M. v. R.A.W., 568 A. 2d 556 (1990).

Earl & David, *Depo-Provera an Injectable Contraceptive,* 49 Amer. Fam. Physician 891-894 (1994).

53 Fertil. & Steril. 203 (1990); *citing* 2 Lancet 790 (1988).

53 Fertil. & Steril., Suppl. 1, Appendix Z.

59 Fertil. & Steril. 956 (1993).

Freeman ed., *Prenatal and Perinatal Factors Associated with Brain Disorders,* NIH Publication No. 85-1149 (Apr. 1985).

Ikemoto, *Providing Protection for Collaborative, Noncoital Reproduction,* 40 Rutgers L. Rev. 1273, 1277 (1988).

James G. v. Casserta, 332 S.E. 2d 872 (1985).

Johnson v. Univ. Hospitals of Cleveland, 540 N.E. 2d 1370 (1989).

Jordan, *Toxicology of Depot Medroxyprogesterone Acetate,* 49 Contraception 223-230 (1994).

Karst, *The Freedom of Intimate Association,* 89 Yale L.J. 624 (1980).

K.C.K. Kuban & A. Leviton, *Cerebral Palsy,* 330 N. Engl. J. Med. 188-195 (1994).

G.S. Letterie & W.F. Fox, *Legal Aspects of Involuntary Sterilization,* 53 Fertil. & Steril. 391-398 (1990).

Louik et al., *Maternal Exposure to Spermicides in Relation to Certain Birth Defects,* 317 N. Engl. J. Med. 474-478 (1987); Warburton et al., *Lack of Association Between Spermicide Use and Trisomy,* 317 N. Engl. J. Med. 478-482 (1987); *New Studies Find No Link Between Spermicide Use and Heightened Risk of Congenital Malformations,* 20 Fam. Plan. Perspect. 42 (1988).

Malahoff v. Stiver, Newsweek, Feb 14, 1983, at 76; N.Y. Times, Feb 6, 1983.

Marciniak v. Lundborg, 433 N.W. 2d 617 (1988).

Marshall v. Univ. of Chicago Hospitals and Clinics, 520 N.E. 2d 740 (1987).

Mich. Compiled Laws, Secs. 722.853, 722.857, 722.861.

Office of Technology Assessment: *Infertility: Medical and Social Choices* (1988).

Ostergard v. United States, 677 F. Supp. 1259 (D.C. Ma 1987).

Page-Bright, *Providing Paternity: Human Leukocyte Antigen Test,* 27 J. Forensic Sci. 135-153 (1982); Joint AMA-ABA Guidelines, *Present Status of Serologic Testing in Problems of Disputed Parentage,* 10 Fam. L. Q. 247-285 (1976).

Pamela P. v. Frank S., 449 N.E. 2d 713 (1983).

Persyn, *A Survey of the Admissibility of Blood Test Results in Paternity Actions in the Fifty States and the District of Columbia,* 8 J. Legis. 301-321, 301 (1981).

Pub. L. 93-647 (1975).

Robertson, Hastings Center Report 7 (Nov/Dec 1989).

Robertson, *Procreative Liberty and the Control of Conception, Pregnancy, and Childbirth,* 69 Va. L. Rev. 405 (1983).

C.M. Salafia & A.M. Vintzileos, *Why All Placentas Should be Examined by a Pathologist in 1990,* 163 Am. J. Obstet. Gynecol. 1282-1293 (1990).

Stephen K. v. Roni L., 164 Cal. Rptr. 618 (1980).

Terrell v. Garcia, 496 S.W. 124 (Tex. 1973); *Cockrum v. Baumgartner,* 425 N.E. 2d 968 (Ill. 1981).

57 U.S.L.W. 2479 (Feb. 21, 1989).

Vol XV, Nos. 2-3 Am. J. L. & Med. 333, 356 (1989).

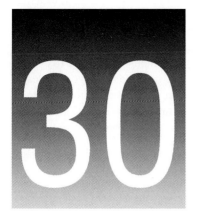

Children as patients

JOSEPH P. McMENAMIN, M.D., J.D., F.C.L.M.
JASON C. BUCKEL, J.D.

STATE INTERVENTION
CHILD ABUSE

Although much of the law governing the medical care of children is indistinguishable from that governing the medical care of adults, certain features of the former are unique. These features arise in large part because minors are seen to need special protection from others and from themselves and are generally deemed incompetent (except in specific circumstances) to grant valid consent for their own treatment. The law's solicitude for the special needs of minors sometimes gives rise to poignant conflicts between the desires and values of parents, often inviolable in other settings, and those of the child or those of the state as *parens patriae*. Resolution of these conflicts often falls to the courts.

STATE INTERVENTION

The standard of care applicable to parents obliged to provide medical attention for their children is analogous to the standard of care for physicians accused of malpractice. As the New York Court of Appeals wrote when construing a state statute, "The standard is at what time would an ordinarily prudent person, solicitous for the welfare of his child and anxious to promote its recovery, deem it necessary to call in the services of a physician."[1]

In many jurisdictions, statutes permit the state to take custody of a *neglected* or *dependent* child; these terms are variously defined[2] but have been construed to include a child deprived of medical services by the parents.[3] Examples of such deprivation include the denial of smallpox vaccination viewed by the parents as "harmful and injurious,"[4] refusal to submit to surgery necessary to save the life of a fetus,[5] refusal to permit blood transfusion required for surgery to correct congenital heart disease,[6] and withholding chemotherapy from a child suffering from malignancy.[7] Statutes finding neglect under such circumstances have been upheld against attacks under the freedom of religion clauses of federal and state constitutions and under the due process clause of the U.S. Constitution.[8] In such circumstances, however, courts may instruct state authorities to respect the religious beliefs of the parents and to accede as much as possible to their wishes without interfering with the court-ordered medical care.[9]

Although the precise limits of the requirement for the provision of medical care by parents are difficult to set, the Illinois statute construed in *Wallace v. Labrenz*[10] may be fairly typical:

[T]he statute defines a dependent or neglected child as one which "has not proper parental care." . . . Neglect, however, is the failure to exercise the care that the circumstances justly demand. It embraces willful as well as unintentional disregard of duty. It is not a term of fixed and measured meaning. It takes its content always from specific circumstances, and its meaning varies as the context of surrounding circumstances changes. . . . [I]t is of no consequence that the parents have not failed in their duty in other respects.[11]

In many jurisdictions a child treated in good faith solely by spiritual means in accordance with the tenets of a recognized religious body is exempt from the definition of a neglected child.[12] Such statutes do not necessarily prevent a court from concluding in a proper case that spiritual treatment alone is insufficient or from ordering conventional medical therapy where needed, including, if necessary, ongoing monitoring after the acute problem is rectified.[13] These statutes may, however, raise thorny equal protection, First Amendment, and other constitutional issues, because they may give preference to one group of potential offenders over others based on that group's self-proclaimed religious tenets and because they may involve the state in excessive entanglement with such questions as what a recognized religious body is, what its tenets are, and whether the accused acted in accord with such tenets.[14] Some courts, however, have no trouble finding that a parent's decision to "let God decide if the child is to live or die" is not the kind of religious belief protected under such statutes.[15]

Where medical intervention may be deemed elective, parental refusal of such intervention may be permitted if the court does not find neglect or dependency.[16] In some instances, courts have refused to intervene despite medically compelling circumstances. The Illinois Appeals Court, for example, declined to find a child neglected whose sibling had been sexually abused at home, who herself had twice gone into diabetic ketoacidosis probably because of "misuse of insulin" at home, and whose mother—suffering from a psychiatric disorder exacerbated by the stresses of child care—had a history of suicide attempts, sexual promiscuity, and placing the diabetic child in a foster home.[17]

If a parent's refusal to provide medical care is deemed egregious, however, criminal liability may be found.[18] Religious beliefs are no defense to neglect of this magnitude.[19] Significant neglect, however, even including neglect sufficient to cause death, may not necessarily be sufficient to sustain a charge of manslaughter.[20] This appears to be particularly true where the neglect is not shown to be willful.[21]

Parens patriae

The power that permits courts to intervene to mandate medical care for children whose parents fail to provide it is known as *parens patriae*.[22] This is distinct from the police power that justifies, for example, fluoridation of water:

The rationale of *parens patriae* is that the State must intervene . . . to protect an individual who is not able to make decisions in his own best interest. The decision to exercise the power of *parens patriae* must reflect the welfare of society as a whole, but mainly it must balance the individual's right to be free from interference against the individual's need to be treated, if treatment would in fact be in his best interest.[23]

The parens patriae power allows the state constitutionally to act as the "general guardian of all infants."[24] Its origins are found in antiquity:

In ancient Times the King was regarded as "Parens Patriae" of orphaned or dependent infants. . . . Under our system of government the state succeeds to the position and power of the King. Both King and State exercise this power in the interests of the people. Society has a deep interest in the preservation of the race itself. It is a natural instinct that lives of infants be preserved.[25]

Under the doctrine of parens patriae, courts are empowered to consent to treatment when the parents are unavailable to do so, as when they have abandoned the child[26] or they are just temporarily unavailable.[27] Court intervention in mandating therapy need not be predicated on an immediate threat to life or limb.[28] Although the criteria vary, one frequently invoked standard is the substituted judgment test: "In this case, the court must decide what its ward would choose, if he were in a position to make a sound judgment. Certainly, he would pick the chance for a fuller participation in life rather than a rejection of his potential as a more fully endowed human being."[29] Not only can the court overrule objections of both parent and child, but under the right circumstances it can overrule the objection of the surgeon who is to perform the procedure.[30]

A serious threat to life, however, is not per se grounds for the intervention of the court under the parens patriae doctrine. If, for example, an infant is born with myelomeningocele, microcephaly, and hydrocephalus, and failure to operate would not place the infant in imminent danger of death, surgery may not be ordered over parental objection despite its efficacy in significantly reducing the risk of infection. In *Weber v. Stony Brook Hospital* the court noted:

Successful results could also be achieved with antibiotic therapy. Further, while the mortality rate is higher where conservative medical treatment is used, in this particular case the surgical procedures also involved a great risk of depriving the infant of what little function remains in her legs, and would also result in recurring urinary tract and possibly kidney infections, skin infections, and edemas of the limbs.[31]

The court concluded that the child was not neglected even though the parents had chosen the arguably riskier of two alternatives, both of which were considered valid choices by the available expert medical testimony.

Life-threatening situations. The most commonly accepted situation in which medical therapy may be ordered for children over the wishes of their parents is where the life of the child is at stake.[32] In life-threatening situations, courts will generally find that the parents are violating state statutes concerning child neglect or endangerment if they withhold medical treatment.[33] Courts have concluded that the strong interests of the state, coupled with the best interests of the child, outweigh the parents' religious beliefs and rights.[34]

Such intervention may be ordered even when the likelihood of success is only 50%.[35] State intervention, however, may be predicated on less critical medical need. Parental objection is insufficient in most states to overcome state requirements for prophylaxis against gonococcal ophthalmia neonatorum.[36] Surgery has been ordered, despite opposition by the patient's father, to stabilize and prevent aggravation of a deformed foot, as deemed to be in the best interest of the child.[37] Even a tonsillectomy may be ordered over the objections of parents with religious reservations about the procedure, at least where the child is in the hands of a state department of social service.[38] Over parental objection a court may order medically necessitated dental attention, including plastic surgery for treatment of cleft lip and cleft palate.[39] Surgery may also be ordered if, despite the absence of a present threat to physical health, the court considers it necessary for the psychological well-being of the child.[40] Accordingly, surgery has been ordered even though it was dangerous and offered only partial correction without cure of a facial deformity.[41] In addition, an autopsy may be ordered, notwithstanding religious proscription, where state law requires the authorities to determine the cause of death.[42]

Non-life-threatening situations. Parental refusals of medical intervention are most likely to be upheld where the child's condition is not life-threatening and where the treatment itself would expose the child to great risk.[43] Such refusals are sometimes upheld even when the proposed therapy would offer great benefit to the child.[44] The court may also stay its hand if it is persuaded that the child is antagonistic to the proposed therapy and that his or her cooperation would be necessary to derive any benefit from the treatment.[45]

Usually a court will avoid intervening when the malady sought to be treated is not life-threatening.[46] As noted, however, courts sometimes fail to intervene even in the presence of disorders that are clearly life-threatening. In *In re Hofbauer* the parents of a 7-year-old boy with Hodgkin's disease did not treat him with radiotherapy or chemotherapy but rather with nutritional or metabolic therapy, including Laetrile.[47] There was expert testimony that Laetrile is effective, and the father indicated he would agree to conventional therapy if the physician prescribing the placebos advised it. Persuaded that the parents were concerned and loving and that the child was not neglected, the court held that "great deference must be accorded a parent's choice as to the mode of medical treatment to be undertaken and the physician selected to administer the same."[48] The statute at issue in *Hofbauer* allowed the following interpretation:

Adequate medical care does not require a parent to beckon the assistance of a physician for every trifling affliction that a child may suffer. . . . We believe, however, that the statute does require a parent to entrust care to that of a physician when such course would be undertaken by an ordinarily prudent and loving parent, "solicitous for the welfare of his child and anxious to promote its (sic) recovery."[49]

As a matter of law the court refused to find that the boy's parents had undertaken no reasonable efforts to ensure that acceptable medical treatment was being provided him, given the parents' concern about side effects from medical management, the alleged efficacy of the nutritional therapy and its relative lack of toxicity, and the parents' agreement that conventional treatment would be administered to the child if his condition so warranted. As long as they had provided for their child a form of treatment "recommended by their physician and not totally rejected by all responsible medical authority as, implied the court, treatment with Laetrile had been, the parents' position would be upheld."[50]

A different approach was taken in *Custody of a Minor.*[51] Applying the best interest of the child rule, the court decided that the trial court was justified in concluding that "metabolic therapy was not only medically ineffective [in the management of leukemia] but was poisoning the child . . . and, contrary to the best interests of the child."[52] This conclusion, in the court's opinion, justified the finding that the child was without necessary and proper medical care and that the parents were unwilling to provide the care required of them by the parental neglect statute.

The best interest of the child may justify intervention even when life itself is not threatened, as illustrated by *In re Kar-*

wath.[53] There, the parents had given their child up for adoption because of the mother's emotional illness and the father's unemployment and financial problems. Concern about possible hearing loss and rheumatic fever prompted the child's physician to recommend a tonsillectomy, but the father demanded that surgery be withheld unless necessary beyond the shadow of a doubt.[54] Although the court's opinion does not elaborate on the point, this position was based on the father's religious faith. The father would agree to surgery as a last resort and only after the failure of chiropractic procedures and medicine. The father also requested that the court require second and third opinions to confirm that the procedure was "necessary with reasonable medical certainty to restore and preserve the health of these wards of the State" before surgery could be undertaken.[55] Despite the father's wishes, the court ordered that the surgery be performed.[56] The fact that the parents' objection was religiously based made no difference.

Our paramount concern for the best interest and welfare of the children overrides the father's contention that absolute medical certitude of necessity and success should precede surgery. Nor is it required that a medical crisis be shown constituting an immediate threat to life and limb.[57]

Transfusions

Only flesh with its soul—its blood—YOU must not eat. And, besides that YOUR blood of YOUR souls shall I ask back. From the hand of every living creature shall I ask it back; and from the hand of man, from the hand of each one who is his brother, shall I ask back the souls of man.[58]

If anyone at all belonging to the house of Israel or the proselytes who reside among them eats any blood at all, against the person who eats blood will set my face, and I will cut him off from his people; the life of every creature is identical with its blood.[59]

These and other scriptural passages[60] provide the theological underpinning for the belief of certain religious groups, notably the Jehovah's Witnesses, that blood transfusions are contrary to the law of God. Since transfusions are a well-accepted component of the therapeutic armamentarium, many cases have examined the right of the state as parens patriae to protect the health of children with its jurisdiction as against the right of parents to raise their children according to their religious beliefs. *Parens patriae,* defined in this context as "a sovereign right and duty to care for a child and protect him from neglect, abuse and fraud during his minority," has been the basis in a number of cases for compelling transfusion of a child whose parents objected on religious grounds.[61] As seen in other instances, the courts distinguish between religious beliefs and opinions, which are held inviolable, and "religious practices inconsistent with the peace and safety of the State."[62] One court, in justifying a decision to order transfusion, wrote:

[I]t was not ordered that he eat blood, or that he cease to believe it that the taking of blood, intravenously, is equivalent of the eating of blood. It is only ordered that he may not prevent another person, a citizen of our country, from receiving medical attention necessary to preserve her life.[63]

A party seeking court intervention to authorize transfusion over parental objection is not exposed to civil liability.[64]

As in other areas where religious beliefs and children's welfare may conflict, a court may stay its hand where "the proposed treatment is dangerous to life, or there is a difference of medical opinion as to the efficacy of a proposed treatment, or where medical opinion differs as to which of two or more suggested remedies should be followed."[65] At least one court refused to order transfusions where the patient had no minor children, the patient had notified the physician and hospital of his belief that acceptance of transfusion violated the laws of God, the patient had executed documents releasing the physician and hospital from civil liability, and his refusal appeared to pose no clear and present danger to society.[66] A court may refuse to order transfusions if the child is not faced with a threat to his or her life.

If we were to describe this surgery as "required," like the Court of Appeals, our decision would conflict with the mother's religious beliefs. Aside from religious considerations, one can also question the use of that adjective on medical grounds since an orthopedic specialist testified that the operation itself was dangerous. Indeed, one can question who, other than the Creator, has the right to term certain surgery as "required." The fatal/nonfatal distinction also steers the courts of this Commonwealth away from a medical and philosophical morass: if spinal surgery can be ordered, what about a hernia or gall bladder operation or a hysterectomy? . . . [A]s between a parent and the state, the state does not have an interest of sufficient magnitude outweighing a parent's religious beliefs when the child's life is not immediately imperiled by his physical condition.[67]

A court will be most inclined to order a transfusion when life is threatened. In some situations this has been done even when the patient was an adult.[68] In general the willingness of the court to intervene increases in the case of a minor,[69] notwithstanding parents' arguments on due process[70] and free exercise grounds.[71] Courts are generally more reluctant to order transfusion for adults, but when the adult is an expectant mother, the court may well ignore the question of the right to transfuse the adult and proceed with the transfusion order based on the right to treat the child.[72]

When a child's life is in danger, the court may adopt streamlined procedures to preserve life that would not be followed or tolerated under other circumstances. For example, a transfusion can be ordered first and the hearing over the propriety of the order may be held later.[73] A hearing may be held in advance of the need for transfusion, as when a mother near term, for example, has a history of Rh incompatibility and has given birth in the past to other children with erythroblastosis fetalis requiring transfusion.[74] Even in a state where a statute provides immunity from criminal prosecution for par-

ents treating their children in accordance with their religious beliefs, the state may appoint a guardian to approve transfusions when necessary to save the life of the child.[75] This is the mechanism by which most courts enter transfusion orders. Although courts ordinarily find neglect only where parents abandon their children or otherwise fail to provide for their basic needs, such a finding can be and often is reached where, over the sincere religious objections of parents, transfusion is required. In *State v. Perricone* a child was afflicted with congenital heart disease that, from the court's description, suggested tetralogy of Fallot.[76] Transfusions were required for proper management of the condition. The parents, Jehovah's Witnesses, refused to permit such transfusions, and they were found guilty of neglect of their son even though the court found them to have "sincere parental concern and affection for the child."[77]

A group of Jehovah's Witnesses in the state of Washington brought a class action seeking to have declared unconstitutional a state statute that declared a child dependent, and thus eligible for appointment of a guardian, where transfusion was or could be vital to save the patient and the parents refused to permit it.[78] The court upheld the statute as constitutional, and the U.S. Supreme Court affirmed per curiam.[79] That the parents "have not failed in their duty to the child in other respects provides them no more shelter under such a statute than does the sincerity of their religious beliefs."[80] In analyzing the tension between the free exercise clause and statutes of this type, the court in *People v. Pierson*[81] wrote: "We place no limitations upon the power of the mind over the body, the power of faith to dispel disease, or the power of the Supreme Being to heal the sick. We merely declare the law as given us by the legislature."[82]

A threat to the very life of a child is not always deemed necessary for a court to order transfusion over parental objection. When brain damage was threatened by a rising bilirubin level in a child with erythroblastosis fetalis, the court found sufficient grounds to order transfusion, even though no mention was made of an actual threat of life.[83] In *In re Sampson* the parents did not oppose plastic surgery required for palliation of massive disfigurement of the right side of the face and neck secondary to von Recklinghausen's disease (neurofibromatosis) in a 15-year-old boy.[84] They did, however, object to the transfusions that such extensive surgery would require, although there was no threat to life and, to diminish the surgical risks, the physicians advised delay until the boy was old enough to consent. The trial court ordered surgery and was upheld on appeal. The court rejected as too restrictive the argument that it could intervene only where the life of the child is endangered by a failure to act. The court of appeals distinguished its earlier opinion in *In re Seiferth*, noting that *Seiferth* turned on the question of a court's discretion and not the existence of its power to order surgery in a case where life itself was not at stake.[85] The court had no trouble finding that religious objection to transfusion does not "present a bar at least where the transfusion is necessary to the success of the required surgery."[86]

When a child is approaching maturity and his or her life is not in imminent danger, the minor patient may have the right to express an opinion about the morality of transfusions and his or her willingness to submit to them. In *In re Green* a 16-year-old boy with scoliosis required surgery to prevent becoming bedridden.[87] His parents, Jehovah's Witnesses, opposed the use of transfusions that the surgery would necessitate. The record did not disclose whether the patient himself was a Jehovah's Witness or planned to become one. The court wrote:

Unlike *Yoder* and *Sampson,* our inquiry does not end at this point, since we believe the wishes of the sixteen-year-old boy should be ascertained; the ultimate question, in our view, is whether a parent's religious beliefs are paramount to the possibly adverse decision of the child. While the records before us give us no indication of the child's thinking, it is the child rather than the parent in this appeal who is directly involved which thereby distinguishes Yoder's decision not to discuss the beliefs of the parents vis-à-vis the children. In *Sampson* the Family Court judge decided not to "evade the responsibility for a decision now by the simple expedient of foisting upon this boy the responsibility for making a decision at some later date. . . ." While we are cognizant of the realistic problem of this approach . . . we believe that the child should be heard.[88]

More recently, however, both the Illinois and the United States Supreme Courts stopped short of imposing their authority when the unborn child's life was endangered because the mother refused, on religious grounds, to undergo a cesarean section. The Illinois Supreme Court declined to review an appellate court decision that upheld a Pentecostal's right to refuse a cesarean delivery, even though physicians deemed it essential for her unborn child's survival, and the U.S. Supreme Court, in *Baby Boy Doe v. Mother Doe,* followed suit by declining to order the lower court to convene an emergency hearing in the case.[89]

Police power

Certain public health measures are enacted pursuant to police power and upheld by the courts despite parental objection on a variety of grounds. The two best examples in health care are the vaccination of schoolchildren and fluoridation of water supplies, performed primarily for the benefit of children. *Police power* is an umbrella term not readily susceptible to precise definition:

While it is perhaps, almost impossible to frame a definition of the police power which shall accurately indicate its precise limits, so far as we are aware, all courts that have considered the subject have recognized and sanctioned the doctrine that under the police power there is general legislative authority to pass such laws as it is believed will promote the common good, or will protect or preserve the public health; and the power to determine what laws are necessary to promote or secure those objects rests primarily with the general assembly, subject to the power of the courts to decide, whether a particular enactment is adapted to that end.[90]

Often, regulations are promulgated not by the legislature but rather by a municipality, a board of public health, or some other arm of the state. In general the courts will give deference to determinations made by these bodies:

[D]etermination by the legislative body that a particular regulation is necessary for the protection or preservation of health is conclusive on the courts except only to the limitation that it must be a reasonable determination, not an abuse of discretion, and must not infringe rights secured by the Constitution.[91]

Under this standard, most such regulations such as this one will be upheld, because "abuse of discretion" is seldom found.

Vaccination

Some health professionals today may be surprised to learn that there is a long history of disputes, continuing to recent times, concerning the validity of state and local regulations that require vaccination of schoolchildren as a prerequisite for attendance in public schools.[92] A number of early decisions upheld these regulations only because an epidemic of smallpox in the patient's community warranted vaccination as an emergency measure.[93] In some cases the constitutionality of the vaccination requirement was upheld only because the court construed it to mean not that vaccination was mandated, but rather that school attendance without vaccination was not permitted.[94] More recently, it has been held that a child has no absolute right to enter school without immunization, and the school board has full authority to compel it.[95]

Questions of federal constitutionality, at least, were essentially laid to rest in the case of *Jacobson v. Massachusetts.*[96] An adult fearful of side effects because of an adverse experience with immunization as a child refused to submit to vaccination despite a compulsory vaccination law. The court upheld his conviction:

There is, of course, a sphere within which the individual may assert the supremacy of his own will, and rightfully dispute the authority of any human government . . . to interfere with the exercise of that will. But it is equally true that in every well-ordered society charged with the duty of conserving the safety of its members the rights of the individual in respect of his liberty may at times, under the pressure of great dangers, be subjected to such restraint, to be enforced by reasonable regulations as the safety of the general public may demand.[97]

The court found no violation of equal protection in the statute's exception favoring children who are medically unfit to be vaccinated, despite the absence of such an exception for adults in like condition, both because there was no reason to suspect that an unfit adult would be required to submit to vaccination and because regulations appropriate for adults are not always safely applied to children.[98] Few cases before and apparently no cases after *Jacobson* have found vaccination requirements to be unconstitutional.[99] The courts have rejected constitutional attacks on both equal protection and due process grounds.[100]

Despite the special solicitude of the courts for First Amendment rights, compulsory vaccination has been upheld even when it conflicts with the religious beliefs of citizens.[101] This is true even where, under state law, a board of education was empowered, although not required, to exempt a child whose parents object to immunization on religious grounds.[102] Personal liberty, including freedom of religion, is a relative and not an absolute right, which must be considered in the light of the general public welfare.[103] The right to practice religion freely does not include liberty to expose the community or the child to communicable diseases or the latter to ill health or death.[104] Nevertheless, some courts, generally in earlier cases only, have found it necessary to point out that vaccination requirements do not prevent children from attending schools, and children who are thereby excluded are excluded by their own consciences.[105] In other cases the courts have questioned whether the plaintiff's religious beliefs really did compel the conclusion that vaccination was immoral.[106]

Where, however, a statute provides an exemption for members of a recognized church or religious denomination whose tenets conflict with the practice of vaccination, a mother's opposition based on her personal belief in the Bible and its teachings was sufficient to entitle her and her children to the exemption.[107] A similar statute was held not applicable to a man objecting to immunization because one of his children had earlier contracted hepatitis secondary to a diphtheria shot. In so holding, the court found no violation of equal protection or due process.[108] Where exemptions are enacted for persons religiously opposed to vaccination, a local school board may not be given discretion to determine who can qualify.[109]

The vaccination regulations have been repeatedly upheld as a reasonable exercise of the police power.[110] It is no longer necessary to have evidence of an epidemic[111] or even a single case[112] to warrant imposition of the regulation. The regulation does not involve the state in the practice of medicine.[113] Evidence impugning the value of vaccination need not even be considered by the courts because such evidence is more appropriately presented to the legislature or its duly constituted agencies, such as the state board of health.[114]

Finally, there is no violation of the right to a free public education and no violation of state compulsory education laws to make vaccination a prerequisite to school attendance: "[H]ealth measures prescribed by local authorities as a condition of school attendance do not conflict with statutory provisions conferring on children of proper age the privilege of attending school, nor with compulsory education laws."[115] This is true even though it leads to the exclusion of children whose physical condition precludes vaccination.[116] It has

been held that, where a father did nothing to prevent the vaccination of his son, the child was not neglected under a regulation that barred him from school because he was unvaccinated.[117] More often, however, failure to provide for vaccination of a child may warrant a finding of parental neglect and the resultant appointment of a guardian to consent to and arrange vaccination.[118]

CHILD ABUSE

The prevalence of child abuse in the United States is alarming.[119] Estimates range from more than 1 million to as many as 4 million reported incidents per year.[120] In 1997 alone, child protective services agencies investigated an estimated 2 million reports alleging the maltreatment of approximately 3 million children and determined that just under 1 million children were victims of substantiated or reported child abuse and neglect.[121] This alarming number actually reflects a slight decrease in the number of victims of substantiated or reported child maltreatment between 1996 and 1997, from just over 1 million in 1996 (1,030,751) to just under 1 million in 1997 (984,000).[122] This was the first decline recognized in the 1990s, since the overall rate of child maltreatment increased 18% from 1990 to 1996.[123]

Child abuse is the most common cause of death of small children in the United States.[124] In fact, children age 3 and under accounted for more than three quarters of the estimated 1196 child deaths that occurred nationwide in 1997 as a result of abuse or neglect.[125] The problem has reached epidemic proportions even though abusers can be convicted of such serious crimes as assault and battery or manslaughter.[126] Also, an abuser who fatally injures a child may, in certain circumstances and jurisdictions, be sentenced to death.[127] Tragically, the perpetrators of child abuse have often been victims of child abuse themselves; the problem poses the serious threat of self-perpetuation.[128]

Perpetrators of child abuse have been characterized as psychopaths and sociopaths who are prone to alcoholism, drug abuse, sexual promiscuity, unstable marriages, and criminal activity. A 1999 study by the National Center on Addiction and Substance Abuse found children of substance-abusing parents three times more likely to be abused and four times more likely to be neglected than children of non-substance-abusing parents.[129] Abuse most often occurs at the hands of the parents. In more than 75% of the reported cases the parents are the perpetrators of the abuse, and in another 10% the perpetrators are other relatives of the victim.[130] People in other caregiving relationships to the victim, such as foster parents, account for only about 2% of all reported cases of abuse.[131] About 80% of all perpetrators are under age 40, with women more likely to be perpetrators of physical abuse and men more often perpetrators of sexual abuse.[132]

Although children from families of all income levels suffer maltreatment, some data link child abuse to socioeconomic status. The National Center on Child Abuse and Neglect found that children from families earning $15,000 or less annually were 25 times more likely to have been abused or neglected than children from families earning $30,000 or more annually.[133] Such data suggest that stress and poverty may be related to abuse and neglect.

Caffey, however, whose pioneering work in 1946 was largely responsible for the now-widespread recognition of the battered child syndrome, challenges many of the prevalent theories on causation of child abuse:

Perpetrators . . . are characteristically of normal intelligence and represent all races, creeds, in all cultural, economic, social and educational levels and are distributed proportionately in all parts of the country. As a group, with a few exceptions, they suffer from the same neuroses, the same emotional and character problems in the same range and degree as any randomly selected group of same milieu and size. Less than 10% are psychopaths.[134]

Different authors may base their conflicting conclusions on their experiences with patient populations of different socioeconomic classes. Alternatively, underreporting may be more common in middle-class and upper-class families than among the poor.[135]

Battered child syndrome

In their classic article on child abuse, Hefler and Kempe wrote that "the syndrome should be considered in any child exhibiting evidence of fracture of any bone, failure to thrive, soft tissue swellings or skin bruising, in any child who dies suddenly, or where the degree and type of injury is at variance with the history given regarding the occurrence of the trauma."[136] The authors supply additional details:

The battered-child syndrome may occur at any age but, in general, the affected children are younger than three years. . . . [T]he child's general health is below par, and he shows evidence of neglect including poor skin hygiene, multiple soft tissue injuries, and malnutrition. One often obtains a history of previous episodes suggestive of parental neglect or trauma. A marked discrepancy between clinical findings and historical data as supplied by the parents is a major diagnostic feature. . . . The fact that no new lesions . . . occur while the child is in the hospital . . . lends added weight to the diagnosis. . . . Subdural hematoma, with or without fracture of the skull, is . . . an extremely frequent finding. . . . The characteristic distribution of these multiple fractures and the observation that the lesions are in different stages of healing are of additional value in making the diagnosis.[137]

Pattern scars or bruises, such as cigarette or immersion burns; lacerations or abrasions of areas not normally so injured, such as the palate or external genitalia; and behavior changes (noncompliance, anger, isolation, destructiveness, developmental delays, excessive attention-seeking, and lack of separation anxiety) are also characteristic.[138] A physician confronted with this clinical picture would be justified in entertaining a diagnosis of child abuse.[139]

Neglect, in contrast to physical abuse, is more apt to present as malnutrition, recurrent pica, chronic fatigue or listlessness, poor hygiene, inadequate clothing for the circumstances, or lack of appropriate medical care, such as immunizations, dental care, and eyeglasses.[140] Behavioral signs, including poor school attendance, age-inappropriate responsibility for tasks such as housework, drug or alcohol abuse, and a history of repeated toxic ingestions, also may be present.[141]

Sexually abused children may have difficulty walking or sitting; thickened or hyperpigmented labial skin; torn, stained, or bloody underclothing; bruised or bleeding private parts; vaginal discharge, pruritus, or both; recurrent urinary tract infections; venereal disease; pregnancy; and lax rectal tone. It is reasonable to expect that these unfortunate children may be at increased risk for acquired immunodeficiency syndrome (AIDS), although the most common cause in children is undoubtedly maternal-fetal infection.[142] A vaginal opening greater than 4 mm in horizontal diameter is said to be characteristic of the sexual abuse of prepubescent girls.[143] Victims of sexual abuse may also have poor self-esteem, attempt suicide, display regressive behavior such as enuresis, masturbate excessively, be sexually promiscuous, withdraw from reality, express shame or guilt, and experience distortion of body image.[144]

Not all cases present in classic fashion, and typical findings are not always caused by child abuse. "Any one may coincidentally show a variety of types of physical marks (e.g., a black eye, cut lip, bruised ears, scratches, and diaper rash burns), even though their parents may be loving, concerned and reasonably careful."[145] Thus the diagnosis may not be straightforward, particularly since the history is unlikely to be easily obtained from intimidated young patients or from their guilt-ridden parents.

Reporting child abuse

In every American jurisdiction it is the legal obligation of the examining physician to report suspected cases of child abuse to authorities designated by statute.[146] Significantly, all the statutes provide immunity from civil liability for physicians reporting suspected child abuse in good faith. Typically the immunity extends to suits for slander, libel, breach of confidence, or invasion of privacy. Some statutes, such as North Dakota's, extend this protection to any reporter, other than the alleged child abuser, whether acting under statutory compulsion or not.[147] Almost all states now require professionals in other fields to report as well, including those in education, social work, child care, and law enforcement.[148] In 1997 more than 80% of all reports of child abuse that led to an investigation came from professionals in numerous areas, including educators, law enforcement and justice officials, social service workers, and medical and mental health personnel.[149]

Abusive parents have attacked these laws on a variety of grounds. In several cases the constitutionality of interrogating the suspected abusers without first issuing Miranda warnings was challenged. In all cases this argument was rejected.[150] An alleged abuser attacked as unconstitutionally vague a statute permitting an inference of neglect to be drawn where there is evidence of illness or injury to a child in the custody of a parent, guardian, or custodian who is unable to give satisfactory explanation for the illness or injury. Here, too, the statute was upheld.[151] A reporting statute was also upheld under a father's claim that it unconstitutionally infringed on his interest in seeking psychiatric help; there was no violation of his privilege against self-incrimination where the statute did not impose investigative duties on the psychiatrist and did not compel him to reveal details given by the patient.[152]

Some parents have tried to invoke the physician-patient privilege to shield themselves from the effects of disclosure. This argument has been rejected on grounds that the policy considerations underlying the reporting statutes trump those justifying the physician-patient privilege.[153] In Alaska, however, a clinical psychologist successfully invoked the privilege between himself and his child-molesting client, despite a reporting law abrogating the privilege, because the abrogation applied only to child protection proceedings instituted to identify and protect victims, not to criminal proceedings resulting from a report of abuse. (The decision neither required nor provided any answer to the question whether the psychologist's client could have invoked the privilege.[154]) In California, communication between psychotherapist and defendant-patient was privileged; the information that could be gleaned was mere repeated data already obtained from the victim.[155] Thus, with few exceptions, the courts have upheld reporting statutes.

Despite the existence and validity of these laws, many cases of child abuse go unreported. Numerous reasons have been proffered to explain this phenomenon.

Until relatively recent times the battered child syndrome was not regularly recognized even by medical specialists.[156] The common law imposed no duty to report, even when the syndrome was recognized.[157] As noted, the diagnosis is not always clear to the clinician,[158] and the legal definition may vary with the jurisdiction.[159]

Physicians knowledgeable about child abuse suspect that reporting may make the parents both more abusive and more reluctant to seek further medical care for their child in the future.[160] Therefore, unless the patient can be hospitalized long enough to ensure that a satisfactory foster home for the victim or effective counseling for the parents can be secured, the physician might be justified in concluding it is in the child's best interest not to report. The physician may anticipate that the child will remain in the parents' care, despite their abuse, as often happens in all but the most egregious cases. The physician may conclude that the best hope for serving the child is to maintain good rapport with the parents and work to prevent recurrences privately without the intervention of the authori-

ties. The physician may also hesitate to report questionable cases so as not to contribute to the undeserved guilt of blameless parents whose children's injuries are unrelated to abuse.[161]

Some physicians may be unwilling to believe that parents could willfully injure their own child.[162] Other practitioners may remain silent from a misplaced loyalty to confidentiality, failing to recognize that the patient is not the parent, but the child. Some may simply not know correct reporting procedure.[163] Some may fear the economic consequences of antagonizing the patient's parents who, if not patients themselves, are at least the minor patient's financial guarantors. Parents may also be willing and able to harm the physician's reputation in the community by claiming that he or she has made terrible and unwarranted accusations about them.[164]

Physicians may fail to report cases of abuse because of a fear of civil liability. Many may be unaware that, under the reporting statutes currently in effect in all U.S. jurisdictions, they have immunity from suit even if they misdiagnose child abuse.[165] This immunity has been upheld under state constitutional due process attack.[166] A physician may not be able to rely on such a statutory grant of immunity, however, if he or she informs some person or agency of his or her suspicions but fails to report the suspected child abuse in the manner required by law. In a 1992 California case, *Searcy v. Auerbach,* a child's mother was allowed to sue a psychologist for libel, professional negligence, and intentional as well as negligent infliction of emotional distress after he told her ex-husband in writing that he suspected her child was abused while in her custody.[167] Merely telling the father, who related the suspicions to Texas authorities, did not comply with the California statute, and therefore no immunity attached.

Similarly, a Missouri physician could not rely on the immunity granted under a child abuse reporting statute because he reported the abuse he erroneously suspected to the police, not to the Division of Family Services, as required by the statute.[168]

Even when a physician is confident of a diagnosis of child abuse, he or she may fail to report because of the threat of legal entanglement.[169] Some argue that immunity provisions are unnecessary because such causes of action as defamation, malicious prosecution, or breach of confidence are defeated by a showing of good faith.[170] However, physicians are unlikely to be aware of the effectiveness and availability of this defense, and even so, they might still dread the possible need to mount a defense.[171]

In general, physicians are probably also unaware that in at least 42 states, a failure to report child abuse can result in criminal prosecution.[172] As a rule, such failures are classified as misdemeanors,[173] and criminal penalties have been criticized because the symptoms of battered child syndrome may be subtle.[174] A search of reported state cases, however, reveals no criminal prosecutions for failure to report.[175] It is unlikely that misprision of a felony remains viable as a theory on which to ground criminal prosecution for nonreporting.[176]

On the other hand, some commentators have claimed that mandatory reporting laws are meaningless without enforcement, that sanctions make it easier for the physician to placate parents irate about mistaken reporting, and that even small penalties create a stigma physicians would seek to avoid.[177] Considering the rarity of criminal actions against nonreporting physicians, however, these arguments presently have more theoretical appeal than practical value.

Allegedly negligent failure to report

Rarely have malpractice claims been reported in which the theory of liability was negligent failure to report child abuse (as opposed to negligent diagnosis and reporting, as alleged in *Searcy v. Auerbach*[178]). In *Landeros v. Flood,* however, the California Supreme Court held that such a theory stated a cause of action under California law.[179] In *Landeros* an 11-month-old girl was brought to co-defendant hospital for diagnosis and treatment of a comminuted spiral fracture of her right tibia and fibula, for which the mother could offer no explanation. The child demonstrated numerous bruises and abrasions and, unknown to the defendant examining physician, a nondepressed linear skull fracture as well. Although the physician properly set the child's leg, he failed to diagnose and report child abuse. The patient was released to the care of her parents, who inflicted multiple subsequent injuries, including human bites and second- and third-degree burns sufficient to cause loss of use or amputation of her left hand. Later, the child's new foster parents sued both physician and hospital for negligence for failing to report the case on initial presentation, on theories of common-law negligence, noncompliance with the penal code section requiring reports of injuries related to any violation of state law, and noncompliance with the child abuse reporting statutes.[180]

The Supreme Court of California held that the plaintiff was entitled (although because of the reporting statute, not required[181]) to show by expert testimony that the standard of care at the time of the events in the case included reporting and that therefore the trial court was in error in sustaining the defendant's demurrer on this issue.[182] The court rejected the defendant's theory that the parents' later beating of the patient was a superseding cause absolving the defendant of responsibility, because if such beatings were reasonably foreseeable they would not give rise to a defense.[183] The court held further that the plaintiff was entitled to show noncompliance with the reporting statutes to raise a presumption of failure to exercise due care as an alternative legal theory to common-law negligence.[184] Thus in California a physician who negligently fails to report a suspected case of child abuse may be found liable in a civil action. The California court did indicate, however, that to establish criminal liability, it must

be shown that the physician was actually aware of the child abuse, so that the failure to report is not merely negligent but willful.[185] In at least one other unreported California case, negligence was alleged against the defendant physician for breach of statutory duty to report, but the $5 million suit was settled out of court for $600,000.[186]

The few reported cases since *Landeros* have adopted a different position on the issue of civil liability for failure to report child abuse. The Georgia and Minnesota courts of appeals have held that no private right of action is created by their respective child abuse reporting statutes. Accordingly, they have refused to allow civil suits against physicians. In *Cechman v. Travis* an administratrix sued a hospital and treating physicians on behalf of a deceased child who was killed by her abusive father after being treated at the defendant institution.[187] Although a criminal statute required that a licensed physician report suspected cases of child abuse, the court held that the statute created no private right of action in tort, in favor of an abused victim.[188] Furthermore, the physician had no common-law legal duty to protect the child from the father, and thus no common law medical malpractice claim would lie.[189]

Likewise, in *Valtakis v. Putnam,* the Minnesota Court of Appeals held that Minnesota's Child Abuse Reporting Act did not create a private right of action.[190] The case involved a suit against a psychologist and others for failure to make a proper report of a child's sexual abuse. The victim alleged that Minnesota Statute Section 626.556 created two penalties: a misdemeanor sanction and a civil suit.[191] The court disagreed. The court found that (1) the defendants had complied with the statute, (2) "no common law duty existed before the statute was enacted," and (3) a reading of the statutory language revealed that no such right of action was either expressed or implied.[192]

In *Marcelletti v. Bathani* the Michigan Court of Appeals likewise declined to extend a private right of action to an injured infant, despite clear statutory language creating civil liability for failure to report suspected child abuse.[193] In *Marcelletti* the injured infant sued a physician, Dr. Bathani, for failing to report the abuse of another unrelated child by a babysitter common to both children. The court refused to extend a right of action to the plaintiff because the statute provided an action for civil liability only to a child whose harm was proximately caused by a failure to report. The court found that the *Marcelletti* infant's injury was not proximately caused by failure of the defendant to report the abuse of another unrelated child.[194] Moreover, ruled the court, no common-law duty existed in Michigan that would support a civil action against Dr. Bathani.[195] The ability to sue, where otherwise appropriate, was a creation of statute only.

Despite *Landeros,* the more recent decisions suggest that in the absence of explicit statutory authorization, the courts may be reluctant to extend a private right of action to plaintiffs alleging harm from failure to comply with reporting statutes.

State liability

In some cases, agencies charged with responsibility for placement of foster children have been held liable under the reporting statutes for abuse by the foster parents they have selected, when the agencies knew or should have known of the abuse.[196] Some courts have found an affirmative obligation under the Fourteenth Amendment to protect or to intervene on behalf of a known or suspected child abuse victim where a special custodial relationship is created or assumed by governmental agencies.[197] Another court, ruling that a child confined to a state mental health facility has a substantive due process liberty interest in reasonably safe living conditions, found a violation of that interest when foster parents with whom the state had placed the child severely injured him and the state failed to intervene.[198] When, however, a child is abused by his father while in the father's custody, a county agency is under no duty to protect the child, even though it knew of the abuse, since the state had neither played a part in the creation of the dangers the child faced nor done anything to render the child any more vulnerable to such dangers.[199] That the state had once taken temporary custody of the child did not alter this conclusion, since in returning the child to his father's custody, it placed him in a position no worse than that in which he would have been had the state not acted at all.[200]

ENDNOTES

1. *People v. Pierson,* 68 N.E. 243, 244 (N.Y. 1903); *Owens v. State,* 116 P. 345 (Okla. Crim. App. 1911); *People v. Edwards,* 249 N.Y.S. 2d 325 (N.Y. Co. Ct. 1964); *In re Carstairs,* 115 N.Y.S. 2d 314 (N.Y. Dom. Rel. Ct. 1952).
2. Ala. Code 12-15-1(10) (2000); *Jehovah's Witnesses v. King County Hosp. Unit No. 1,* 278 F. Supp. 488 (W.D. Wash.), *aff'd,* 390 U.S. 598 (1968).
3. *Heinemann's Appeal,* 96 Pa. 112, 42 Am. Rep. 532 (Ct. App. 1880); *Mitchell v. Davis,* 205 S.W. 2d 812 (Tex. Civ. App. 1947).
4. *In re Marsh,* 14 A. 2d 368 (Pa. Super. Ct. 1940).
5. *Jefferson v. Griffin Spalding County Hosp. Auth.,* 274 S.E. 2d 457 (Ga. 1981).
6. *State v. Perricone,* 181 A. 2d 751 (N.J.), *cert. denied,* 371 U.S. 890 (1962); *In re Santos,* 227 N.Y.S. 2d 450 (N.Y.A.D. 1 Dept.), *appeal dismissed,* 185 N.E. 2d 552 (N.Y. 1962).
7. *Custody of a Minor,* 393 N.E. 2d 836, 846 (Mass. 1979); *see,* however, *Newmark v. Williams,* 588 A. 2d 1108 (Del. 1991).
8. *Supra* note 6, at 757; see also *Levitsky v. Levitsky,* 190 A. 2d 621 (Md. 1963); but *Osier v. Osier,* 410 A. 2d 1027 (Me. 1980).
9. *In re Hamilton,* 657 S.W. 2d 425 (Tenn. App. 1983).
10. *People ex rel. Wallace v. Labrenz,* 104 N.E. 2d 769 (Ill.), *cert. denied,* 344 U.S. 824 (1952).
11. *Id.* at 773.
12. *In re Eric B.,* 235 Cal. Rptr. 22 (Cal. App. 1987), *review denied.*
13. *Id.* at 26. The court need not "hold its protective power in abeyance until harm to a minor child is not only threatened but actual. The purpose of dependency proceedings is to prevent risk, not ignore it." *See also In re Ivey,* 319 So. 2d 53 (Fla. App. 1975); *In re Jensen,* 633 P. 2d 1302 (Or. App.), *review denied,* 639 P. 2d 1280 (1981).
14. *State v. Miskimens,* 490 N.E. 2d 931 (Ohio Com. Pl. 1984).
15. *In re Application of Cicero,* 421 N.Y.S. 2d 965, 966 (N.Y. Sup. 1979).
16. *Newmark v. Williams,* 588 A. 2d 1108 (Del. Super. 1991); *In re Frank,* 248 P. 2d 553 (Wash. 1952).
17. *In re Gonzales,* 323, N.E. 2d 42, 46-47 (Ill. App. 1974); *People in the Interest of D.L.E.,* 614 P. 2d 873 (Colo. 1980).
18. *State v. Chenoweth,* 71 N.E. 197 (Ind. 1904); *Stehr v. State,* 139 N.W. 676 (Neb.), *aff'd,* 142 N.W. 670 (1913); *Beck v. State,* 233 P. 495 (Okla. Crim. App. 1925); *People v. Vogel,* 242 P. 2d 969 (Cal. App. 4th Dist. 1952); *State v. Dumlao,* 491 A. 2d 404 (Conn. App. 1985); *State v. Clark,* 261 A. 2d 294 (Conn. Cir. A.D. 1969); *State v. Staples,* 148 N.W. 283 (Minn. 1914); *State v. Beach,* 329 S.W. 2d 712 (Mo. 1959); *State v. Watson,* 71 A. 1113 (N.J. Sup. 1909); *Pennsylvania v. Barnhart,* 497 A. 2d 616 (Pa. Super. 1985), *appeal denied,* 538 A. 2d 874 (Pa.), *cert. denied,* 488 U.S. 817 (1988); *New York v. Edwards,* 249 N.Y.S. 2d 325 (N.Y. Co. Ct. 1964); *State v. Barnes,* 212 S.W. 100 (Tenn. 1919); *Oakley v. Jackson,* 1 K.B. 216 (1914); *Rex. v. Lewis,* 6 Ont. L. 132 1BRC 732-CA (1903); *Nozza v. State,* 288 So. 2d 560 (Fla. App.), *cert. denied,* 295 So. 2d 301 (Fla. 1974); *Faunteroy v. U.S.,* 413 A. 2d 1294 (D.C. App. 1980); *State v. Zobel,* 134 N.W. 2d 101 (S.D.), *cert. denied,* 382 U.S. 833 (1965), *overruled on other grounds; State v. Waff,* 373 N.W. 2d 18 (S.D. 1985).
19. *Supra* note 18.
20. *Eversley v. State,* 748 So. 2d 963 (Fla. 1999); *Singleton v. State,* 35 So. 2d 375 (Ala. 1948); *Craig v. State,* 155 A. 2d 684 (Md. 1959); *New York v. Osborn,* 508 N.Y.S. 2d 746 (1986), *appeal denied,* 505 N.E. 2d 251 (N.Y. 1987); *New York v. Northrup,* 442 N.Y.S. 2d 658 (1981).
21. *State v. Watson,* 71 A. 1113, 1114 (N.J. 1909); *State v. Osmus,* 276 P. 2d 469 (Wyo. 1954); *Howell v. State,* 350 S.E. 2d 473 (Ga. App. 1986); *Justice v. State,* 42 S.E. 1013 (Ga. 1902); *Michigan v. Mankel,* 129 N.W. 2d 894 (Mich. 1964); *Missouri v. Shouse,* 186 S.W. 1064 (Mo. 1916); *In re Appeal in Cochise County,* Juvenile Action No. 5666-J, 650 P. 2d 459 (Ariz. 1981). See, however, *State v. Clark,* 261 A. 2d 294 (Conn. 1969); *Eaglen v. State,* 231 N.E.2d 147 (Ind. 1967); *State v. Williams,* 484 P.2d 1167 (Wash. Ct. App. 1971).
22. *Parens patriae* empowers the state to "care for infants within its jurisdiction and to protect them from neglect, abuse, and fraud. . . . That ancient, equitable jurisdiction was codified in our Juvenile Court Act, which expressly authorizes the court, if circumstances warrant, to remove the child from the custody of its (sic) parents and award its custody to an appointed guardian. *Supra* note 10.
23. *In re Weberlist,* 360 NY.S. 2d 783, 786 (1974).
24. *Hawaii v. Standard Oil Co.,* 405 U.S. 251, 257 (1972).
25. *Morrison v. State,* 252 S.W. 2d 97, 102 (Mo. Ct. App. 1952).
26. *Commissioner of Social Servs re D.,* 339 N.Y.S. 2d 89 (N.Y. Fam. Ct. 1972); *supra* note 23; *In re Tanner,* 549 P. 2d 703 (Utah 1976); *People v. Sorensen,* 437 P. 2d 495 (Cal. 1968); *Karin T. v. Michael T.,* 484 N.Y.S. 2d 780 (Fam. Ct. 1985); *Wener v. Wener,* 312 N.Y.S. 2d 815 (1970). See, however, *Pamela P. v. Frank S.,* 443 N.Y.S. 2d 343 (Fam. Ct.1981), *aff'd.,* 462 N.Y.S. 2d 819 (1983).
27. *Browning v. Hoffman,* 111 S.E. 492 (W. Va. 1922).
28. *Commissioner and Tanner, supra* note 26; *supra* note 23.
29. *Supra* note 23 at 783, 787.
30. *In re Sampson,* 317 NY.S. 2d 641, 658 (Fam. Ct. 1970), *aff'd,* 323 N.Y.S. 2d 253 (App. Div. 3 Dept.), *appeal denied,* 275 N.E. 2d 339 (1971).
31. *Weber v. Stoney Brook Hosp.,* 467 N.Y.S. 2d 685, 686-87 (App. Div.), *aff'd.,* 456 N.E. 2d 1186 (N.Y.), *cert. denied,* 464 U.S. 1026 (1983).
32. *In re Eric B.,* 189 Cal. App. 3d 996 (Ct. App. 1987); *People ex rel. D.L.E.,* 645 P.2d 271 (Colo. 1982); *In re Ivy,* 319 So.2d 53 (Fla. Dist. Ct. App. 1975); *People ex rel. Wallace v. Labrenz,* 104 N.E.2d 769 (Ill.), *cert. denied,* 344 U.S. 824 (1952); *Custody of a Minor,* 393 N.E. 2d 836 (Mass. 1979); *Morrison v. State,* 252 S.W.2d 97 (Mo. Ct. App. 1952); *In re Willmann,* 493 N.E.2d 1380 (Ohio Ct. App. 1986); *In re Clark,* 185 N.E. 2d 128 (Ohio Op. 2d 1962).
33. *People ex rel. D.L.E.,* 645 P.2d 271, 272-75 (Colo. 1982) (interpreting a Colorado state statute and holding that an epileptic child was neglected when her mother failed or refused to provide medical care because of her religious beliefs).
34. *In re McCauley,* 565 N.E.2d 411, 414 (Mass. 1991).
35. *In re Vasko,* 263 N.Y.S. 552 (1933).
36. Office of Attorney General, No 81-57, slip op. (Utah Dec. 14, 1981).
37. *In re Rotkowitz,* 25 N.Y.S. 2d 624 (Dom. Rel. Ct. 1941).

38. *In re Karwath,* 199 N.W. 2d 147, 150 (Iowa 1972).
39. *In re Seiferth,* 127 N.E. 2d 820 (N.Y. 1955); *In re Gregory S.,* 380 N.Y.S. 2d 620 (1976).
40. *In re Ray,* 408 N.Y.2d 737 (City Fam. Ct. 1978), *In re J.M.P.,* 669 S.W.2d 298 (Mo. App. 1984).
41. *Supra* note 30.
42. *Snyder v. Holy Cross Hosp.,* 352 A. 2d 334 (Md. App. 1976).
43. *In re Hudson,* 126 P. 2d 765 (Wash. 1942); *accord Custody of a Minor,* 379 N.E. 2d 1053 (Mass. 1978).
44. *Custody, id.* at 1062.
45. *Supra* note 39 at 820, 822.
46. *Supra* note 43 at 778; Wash. Rev. Code Ann. Sec. 26.440.020 (West Supp. 1982); Comment, *Relief for the Neglected Child: Court-Ordered Medical Treatment in Non-Emergency Situations,* 22 Santa Clara L. Rev. 471 (1982).
47. *In re Hofbauer,* 393 N.E. 2d 1009 (N.Y. 1979).
48. *Id.* at 1013.
49. *Id.,* quoting *People v. Pierson,* 68 N.E. 243 (N.Y. 1903).
50. *Id.* at 1014.
51. *Supra* note 7 at 836.
52. *Id.* at 845.
53. *Supra* note 38 at 147.
54. *Id.* at 149.
55. *Id.* at 150.
56. *Id.*
57. *Id.*
58. Genesis 9:4-5; quoted in *supra* note 6 at 756.
59. Leviticus 17:10-14; quoted in *Morrison v. State,* 252 S.W.2d 97, 99 (Mo. Ct. App. 1952).
60. Leviticus 3:17, 7:26, 27; Deuteronomy 12:23; 1 Chronicles 11:16-19; 2 Samuel 23:15-17; Acts 15:28, 29, 21:25; 1 Samuel 14:32, 33; *supra* note 30.
61. *State, supra* note 6; *Hoener v. Bertianto,* 171 A.2d 140 (N.J. Juv. & Dom. Rel. Ct. 1961).
62. *Hoener, id.* at 143.
63. *Supra* note 25.
64. *Harley v. Oliver,* 404 F.Supp. 450 (W.D. Ark. 1975), *aff'd,* 539 F.2d 1143 (8th Cir. 1976); *Staelens v. Yake,* 432 F.Supp. 834 (N.D. Ill. 1977).
65. *Supra* note 25.
66. *In re Brooks' Estate,* 205 N.E.2d 435 (Ill. 1965).
67. *In re Green,* 292 A.2d 387, 392 (Pa. 1972).
68. *Application of President & Directors of Georgetown College, Inc.,* 331 F.2d 1000, *reh'g denied,* 331 F.2d 1010 (D.C. Cit.), *cert. denied,* 377 U.S. 978 (1964); *John F. Kennedy Memorial Hosp. V. Heston,* 29 A.2d 670 (N.J. 1971).
69. *Supra* notes 6 & 10; *Application of Brooklyn Hosp.,* 258 N.Y.S.2d 621 (Sup. Ct. 1965); *In re Clark,* 185 N.E.2d 128 (Ohio C.P. 1962).
70. *In re Clark,* 148 N.E.2d 128 (Ohio C.P. 1962).
71. *Id.*
72. 377 U.S. 985 (1964).
73. *In re Clark,* 184 N.E.2d 128 (Ohio C.P. 1962).
74. *Hoenere v. Bertinato,* 171 A.2d 140, 143-44 (N.J.Jub.& Dom. Rel. Ct. 1961).
75. *State, supra* note 6.
76. *Id.*
77. *Id.* at 759.
78. *Jehovah's Witness v. King Co. Hosp.,* 278 F.Supp. 488 (W.D. Wash. 1967), *aff'd* 390 U.S. 598 (1967).
79. *Id.*
80. *Supra* note 74.
81. *People, supra* note 1.
82. *Id.* at 247.
83. *Muhlenberg Hosp. v. Patterson,* 320 A.2d 518 (N.J. Super. 1974).
84. *In re Sampson,* 317 N.Y.S.2d 641 (N.Y. Fam. Ct. 1970), *aff'd,* 323 N.Y.S.2d 253 (N.Y.A.D. 3 Dept.), *appeal denied,* 275 N.E.2d 339 (N.Y. 1971).
85. *In re Seiferth,* 127 N.E.2d 820 (N.Y. 1955).
86. *In re Sampson,* 278 N.E.2d 918 (N.Y. 1971); *Santos v. Goldstein,* 227 N.Y.S.2d 450 (N.Y.A.D. 1 Dept. 1962), *appeal dismissed,* 232 N.Y.S.2d 1026 (N.Y. 1962).
87. In re Green, 292 A.2d 387 (Pa. 1972, *appeal after remand,* 307 A.2d 279 (Pa. 1973).
88. *Id.* at 392.
89. *Baby Boy Doe v. Mother Doe,* 510 U.S. 1168 (1994).
90. *State ex rel. Milhoof v. Board of Educ.,* 81. N.E. 568, 569 (Ohio 1907).
91. *DeAryan v. Butler,* 260 P.2d 98, 102 (Cal. App. 1853), *cert. denied,* 347 U.S. 1012 (1954).
92. *McCarney v. Austin,* 293 N.Y.S.2d 188 (Sup. Ct. 1968), *aff'd,* 298 N.Y.S.2d 26 (App. Div. 1969); *In re Elwell,* 284 N.Y.S.2d 924 (Fam. Ct. 1967); *State ex rel. Mack v. Board of Educ.,* 204 N.E.2d 86 (Ohio Ct. App. 1963); *State ex rel. Dunham v. Board,* 96 N.E.2d 413 (Ohio), *cert. denied,* 341 U.S. 915 (1951).
93. *Hagler v. Larner,* 120 N.E. 575 (Ill. 1918); *Hill v. Bickers,* 188 S.W. 766 (Ky. 1916); *State ex rel. Freeman v. Zimmermann,* 90 N.W. 783 (Min. 1902); *City of New Braunfels v. Waldschmidt,* 207 S.W. 303 (Tex. 1918); *Rhea v. Board of Educ.,* 171 N.W. 103 (N.D. 1919).
94. *McSween v. Board of School Trustees,* 129 S.W. 206 (Tex. Clv. App. 1910).
95. *State ex rel. Mack v. Board of Educ.,* 204 N.E.2d 86 (Ohio Ct. App. 1963).
96. *Jacobson v. Massachusetts,* 197 U.S. 11 (1905).
97. *Id.* at 29.
98. *Id.* at 30, 39.
99. *French v. Davidson,* 77 P. 663 (Cal. 1904); *Abeel v. Clark,* 24 P. 383 (Cal. 1890); *Bissell v. Davison,* 32 A. 348 (Conn. 1894); *Hagler v. Larner,* 120 N.E. 575 (Ill. 1918); *Board of Educ. v. Maas,* 152 A.2d 394 (N.J. Super. 1959), *aff'd,* 158 A.2d 330 (N.J.), *cert. denied,* 363 U.S. 843 (1960); *Sadlock v. Board of Educ.,* 58 A.2d 218 (N.J. 1948); *State ex rel. Milhoff v. Board of Educ.,* 81 N.E. 568 (Ohio 1907); *Field v. Robinson,* 48 A. 873 (Pa. 1901); *Commonwealth v. Pear,* 66 N.E. 719 (Mass. 1903), *aff'd. sub nom. Jacobson v. Massachusetts* 197 U.S. 11 (1905); *State ex rel. Cox v. Board of Educ.,* 60 P. 1013 (Utah 1900); *Ritterbaud v. Axelrod,* 562 N.Y.S. 2d 605 (N.Y. Sup. 1990).
100. *Board of Educ. v. Maas, supra* note 99.
101. *Mosier v. Barren County Bd. of Health,* 215 S.W.3d 967 (Ky. 1948) (chiropractors); *Mannis v. State ex rel. DeWitt School Dist.,* 398 S.W.2d 206 (Ark.); *cert. denied,* 384 U.S. 972 (1966) (members of the General Assembly and Church of the First Born); *Wright v. DeWitt School Dist.,* 385 S.W.2d 644 (Ark. 1965); *State ex. rel. Dunham v. Board of Educ.,* i6 N.E.2d 413 (Ohio 1951).
102. *Supra* note 100 at 407-408.
103. *Sadlock v. Board of Educ.,* 58 A.2d 218 (N.J. 1948).
104. *People, supra* note 1; *accord In re Whittmore,* 47 N.Y.S.2d 143 (N.Y. 1944); *Wright, supra* note 101; *Cude v. State,* 377 S.W.2d 816 (Ark. 1964).
105. *Staffle v. San Antonio,* 201 S.W. 413, 415 (Tex. Civ. App. 1918).
106. *Supra* note 100; *McCartney v. Austin,* 293 N.Y.S.2d 188 (Supp. St. 1968), *aff'd,* 298 N.Y.S.2d 26 (App. Div. 1969); *In re Elwell,* 298 N.Y.S.2d 924 (Fam. Ct. 1967).
107. *Dalli v. Board of Educ.,* 267 N.E.2d 219, 223 (Mass. 1971); *accord Maier v. Besser,* 341 N.Y.S.2d 411 (N.Y. Sup. 1972); *Kolbeck v. Kramer,* 202 A.2d 889 (N.J. Super. Ct. 1964); *Davis v. State,* 451 A.2d 107 (Md. 1982); *accord Campain v. Marlboro Cent. School Dist.,* 526 N.Y.S.2d 658 (App. Div. 1988).
108. *Itz v. Penick,* 493 S.W.2d 506 Itec.); *appeal dismissed,* 412 U.S. 925, *reh'g denied* 414 U.S. 882 (1973).
109. *Avard v. Dupius,* 376 F.Supp. 479 (D.N.H. 1974).
110. *Zucht v. King,* 260 U.S. 174 (1922); *Duffield v. Williamsport School Dist.,* 29 A. 742 (Pa. 1894); *Hartman v. May,* 151 So. 737 (Miss. 1934); *State v. Hay,* 35 S.E. 459 (N.C. 1900); *supra* note 94.
111. *Supra* note 100; *Mosier v. Barren County Bd. of Health,* 215 S.W.2d 967 (Ky. 1948); *Hartman, supra* note 110.

112. *Supra* note 100 at 405; *Pierce v. Board of Educ.,* 219 N.Y.S.2d 519 (Sup. Ct. 1961).

113. *State v. Drew,* 192 A.629 (N.H. 1937).

114. *Seubold v. Fort Smith Special School Dist.,* 237 S.W.2d 884 (Ark. 1951); *Wright, supra* note 101.

115. *Supra* note 100 at 408; *accord Viemeister v. White,* 72 N.E. 97 (N.Y. 1904); *Blue v. Beach,* 56 N.E. 89 (Ind. 1900); *Hartman, supra* note 110; supra note 94; *Staffle,* 201 S.W. 413; *Zucht v. King,* 260 U.S. 174 (1922); *City of New Braunfels v. Waldschmidt,* 207 S. W. 303 (Tex. 1918); *Freeman v. Zimmerman,* 90 N.W. 783 (Minn. 1902); *State v. Hay,* 35 S.E. 459 (N.C. 1900); *Bissell v. Davison,* 32 A. 348 (Conn. 1894); *Morris v. Columbus,* 30 S.E. 850 (Ga. 1898); *Duffield v. Williamsport School Dist.,* 29 A. 742 (Pa. 1894).

116. *Hutchins v. School Committee,* 49 S.E. 46 (N.C. 1904).

117. State v. Dunham, 93 N.E.2d 286 (Ohio 1950).

118. *In re Elwell,* 284 N.Y.S.2d 924 (Fam. Ct. 1967); *Cude, supra* note 104; *In re Marsh's Case,* 14 A.2d 368, 371 (Pa. Super Ct. 1940); *Mannis v. State ex rel. DeWitt School Dist.,* 398 S.W.2d 206 (Ark.); *cert. denied,* 384 U.S. 272 (1966).

119. N.J. Mitrichen, *Child Abuse: an Annotated Bibliography* (1982), cited in Heins, "The Battered Child" Revisited, 251(19) JAMA 3295, 3298 (1984).

120. *National Briefs,* The Houston Chronicle, Oct. 28, 1993, at A4; *The Child Abuse Epidemic,* 1974, U. Ill. L. Rev. 403, 404 (1974).

121. U.S. Department of Health and Human Services, National Center on Child Abuse and Neglect, *Child Maltreatment 1997: Reports from the States of the National* Child Abuse and Neglect *Data System* (U.S. Government Printing Office, Washington, D.C. 1999).

122. *Id.*

123. *Id.*

124. *The Child Abuse Epidemic, supra* note 120.

125. *Supra* note 121.

126. *New York v. Steinberg,* 595 N.E.2d 845 (N.Y. 1992); *Massachusetts v. Gallison,* 421 N.E.2d 757 (Mass. 1981). Abusers may also be convicted for criminal negligence: *Brewer v. State,* 274 S.E.2d 817 (Ga. Ct. App. 1980); *State v. Fabritz,* 384 A.2d 275 (Md. 1975); *Pennsylvania v. Humphfreys,* 406 A.2d 1060 (Pa. Super Ct. 1979) *overruled on other grounds, Pennsylvania v. Burchard,* 503 A.2d 936 (Pa. Super Ct. 1986); *Pennsylvania v. Morrison,* 401 A.2d 1348 (Pa. Super. Ct. 1979); *Williams v. State,* 680 S.W.2d 570 (Tex. App. 1984). In homicide prosecutions, physician testimony has been held admissible to show death was caused by child-battering: *Utah v. Morgan,* 865 P.2d 1377 (Utah Ct. App. 1993); *Illinois v. Secton,* 334 N.E.2d 107 (Ill. App. 1975); *Massachusetts v. Boudreau,* 285 N.E.2d 915 (Mass. 1972); *Minnesota v. Durfee,* 322 N.W.2d 778 (Minn. 1982); North Carolina v. Wilkerson, 247 S.E.2d 905, (N.C. 1978); *Martin v. Oklahoma,* 547 P.2d 396 (Okla. Crim. App. 1976); or by nontreatment after battering: *Bergman v. State,* 486 N.E.2d 653 (Ind. App. 1985). In prosecutions for child abuse, courts may similarly receive expert physician testimony to establish that the child was battered: *California v. Jackson,* 95 Cal. Rptr. 919 (Cal. Ct. App. 1971); *California v. Ewin,* 140 Cal. Rptr. 299 (Cal. Ct. App. 1977); *Cohoon v. U.S.,* 387 A.2d 1098 (D.C. 1978); *New Jersey v. Nuniz,* 375 A.2d 1234 (N.J. Super. Ct. 1977), *cert. denied,* 391 A.2d 488 (N.J. 1978); *North Carolina v. Mapp,* 264 S.E.2d 348 (N.C. Ct. App. 1980), *North Carolina v. Fredell,* 193 S.E.2d 587 (N.C. Ct. App. 1972), *aff'd,* 195 S.E.2d 300 (N.C. 1973). *See,* generally, *Annotation, Validity and Construction of Penal Statute Prohibiting Child Abuse,* 1 A.L.R. 4th 38.

127. *House, Senate Pass Death Penalty for Child Killers,* United Press International, May 28, 1993, § Regional News (Texas Legislature); Karen Peterson, *Abuse of Children Is on the Rise,* USA Today, April 7, 1993, § Life, at 1D.

128. J. Clark, M.D. Stein, M. Sobota, et al., *Victims as victimizers: physical aggression by persons with a history of childhood abuse,* 159 Archives Int. Med. 1920 (1999).

129. J. Reid, P. Macchetto, & S. Foster, *No Safe Haven: Children of Substance-Abusing Parents* (National Center on Addition and Substance Abuse at Columbia University, New York 1999).

130. *Supra* note 121.

131. *Id.*

132. *Id.*

133. U.S. Department of Health and Human Services, National Center on Child Abuse and Neglect, *Third National Incidence Study of Child Abuse and Neglect: Final Report* (NIS-3) (U.S. Government Printing Office, Washington, D.C. 1996).

134. Caffey, *The Parent-Infant Traumatic Stress Syndrome* (Caffey-Kempe Syndrome), (Battered Baby Syndrome), 114 Am. J. Roentgenol. Radiat. Ther. & Nucl. Med. 218, 227 (1972).

135. Council on Scientific Affairs, American Medical Association, *AMA Diagnostic and Treatment Guidelines Concerning Child Abuse and Neglect,* 254 JAMA 796 at 797, 798 (1985).

136. R.E. Hefler & C.H. Kempe, *The Battered Child* 51 at 105 (1968).

137. *Id.* at 106.

138. *Supra* note 135 at 797, 798.

139. Most courts have held admissible expert testimony on the diagnosis and manifestations of child abuse. *See,* generally, *Annotation, Admissibility of Expert Medical Testimony in Battered Child Syndrome,* 98 A.L.R. 3d 306. Compare *Annotation, Admissibility at Criminal Prosecution of Expert Testimony in Battering Parent Syndrome,* 43 A.L.R. 4th 1203. *Supra* note 126.

140. *Supra* note 135 at 798.

141. *Id.*

142. *Id.*

143. *See* Cantwell, *Vaginal Inspection as it Relates to Child Sexual Abuse in Girls under Thirteen,* 7 Child Abuse & Neglect 171 (1983).

144. *Supra* note 135.

145. Ganley, *The Battered Child: Logic in Search of Law,* 8 San Diego L. Rev. 364, 365, note 2 (1971); Silver, *Child Abuse Syndrome: The "Grey Areas" in Establishing Diagnosis,* 44 Pediatrics 595 (1969); *In re Jertrude O.,* 466 A.2d 885 (Mad. App. 1983); *cert. denied,* 469 A.2d 863 (Md. 1984).

146. These laws are compiled and compared in *Physician's Liability for Noncompliance with Child Abuse Reporting Statutes,* 52 N. Dak. L. Rev. 736 (1976); Fraser, *A Pragmatic Alternative to Current Legislative Approaches to Child Abuse,* 12 Am. Cir. L. Rev. 103 (1974); Donovan, *The Legal Response to Child Abuse,* 11 Wm. & Mary L. Rev. 960 (1970). In California the reporting statute lodges substantial reports in a statewide data bank. The law does not require a professional, with no knowledge or suspicion of actual abuse, to report a minor as a victim solely because the child is under 14 years old and indicates that he or she engages in voluntary consensual sexual activity with another minor the same age. *Planned Parenthood Affiliates v. Van de Kamp,* 226 Cal. Rptr. 361 (Cal. App. 1 Dist.), *review denied* (1986). In Florida a psychiatrist treating an abusive father for emotional difficulties was not required to report the abuse under the reporting statute's mandate, which was limited to "any person . . . servicing children," since the psychiatrist had never cared for the abused child but only for the father. *Geoff. v. State,* 390 So.2d 361 (Fla. Dist. Ct. App. 1980), *aff'd after remand,* 409 So.2d 44 (Fla. Dist. Ct. App. 1981). In Minnesota, however, a man convicted of criminal sexual conduct with a 13-year-old boy was held properly convicted when the state acted on information from a crisis intake worker whom the defendant had phoned to discuss the incident; no privilege attached to the relationship between the worker and the defendant. *State v. Sandberg,* 392 N.W.2d 298 (Minn. App. 1986), *aff'd in part, reversed in part on other grounds,* 406 N.W.2d 506 (Minn. 1987). For a discussion of the consequences of reporting on parental rights, see Annotation, *Physical Abuse of Child by Parent as Ground for Termination of Parent's Right to Child,* 53 A.L.R. 3d 605, and Annotation, *Sexual Abuse of Child by Parent as Ground for Termination of Parent's Right to Child,* 58 A.L.R 3d 1074. *See also Annotation,* Validity of State Statute Providing for Termination of Parental Rights, 22 A.L.R. 4th 774, and Annotation, *Validity and Application of Statute Allowing Endangered Child to Be Temporarily Removed from Parental Custody,*

38 A.L.R. 4th 756. For a discussion of the consequences when the authorities fail to intervene on behalf of abused children, *see, generally,* Annotation, *Tort Liability of Public Authority for Failure to Remove Parentally Abused or Neglected Children from Parent's Custody,* 60 A.L.R. 4th 942.

147. *Physician's Liability, supra* note 146, at 740; *see also* ND Cert. Code § 50-25.1-09.

148. *Malpractice—Physician's Liability for Failure to Diagnose and Report Child Abuse,* 23 Wayne L Rev. 1887, 1191 (1977); Besharov, *'Doing Something' About Child Abuse: The Need to Narrow the Grounds for State Intervention,* 8 Harv. J.L. & Pub. Pol'y 539 (1988). Such laws have been criticized as too vague and thus conducive to both overreporting and underreporting, Weisberg & Wald, *Confidentiality Laws and State Efforts to Protect Abused or Neglected Children: The Need for Statutory Reform,* 18 Fam. L.Q. 143 (1984), and as self-defeating, Paulsen, *The Legal Framework for Child Protection,* 66 Colum. L. Rev. 679 (1966) ("Everyone's duty may easily become nobody's duty," *id.* at 713). The Attorney General of Texas has read his state's reporting requirements to apply even to clerics learning of abuse in their professional capacities. Op. Tex. Atty. Gen. No. JM-342 (Aug. 5, 1985). For an analysis of this position, *see* Note, *The Clergy—Penitent Privilege and the Child Abuse Reporting Statute—Is the Secret Sacred?* 19 John Marshall L. Rev. 1031 (1986). *See also Mullen v. United States,* 263 F.2d 275 (D.C. Cir. 1958).

149. *Supra* note 121.

150. *People v. Battaglia,* 203 Cal. Rprt. 370 (Cal. Ct. App. 1984); *People v. Salinas,* 182 Cal. Rptr. 683 (Cal. Ct. App. 1982); *Pennsylvania v. Anderson,* 385 A.2d 365 (Pa. Super. Ct. 1978).

151. *In re LE.J.,* 465 A.2d 374 (D.C. 1983); *Hunter v. State,* 360 N.E.2d 588 (Ind. App.), *cert. denied,* 434 U.S. 906 (1977).

152. *People v. Younghanz,* 202 Cal. Rptr. 907 (Cal. Ct. App. 1984). However, said the court, to protect the patient's expectation of privacy, the therapist should warn the patient of his or her statutory duty to testify against the patient concerning instances of child abuse; if the patient then continues therapy, he or she waives any right to challenge admissibility of the evidence later. Once a psychotherapist advised the defendant of this duty at their psychotherapeutic session, she was not required to warn him of her duty or to testify to admissions made in subsequent sessions. People v. John B., 237 Cal. Rptr. 659 (Cal. Ct. App. 1987).

153. *State v. Fagalde,* 539 P.2d 86 (Wash. 1975); *State v. Jacobus,* 348 N.Y.S.2d 907 (Sup. Ct. 1973); *Battaglia, supra* note 150; *Hunter, supra* note 151; *State v. Odenbrett,* 349 N.W.2d 265 (Minn. 1984); *Alexander v. State,* 534 P.2d 1313 (Okla. Crim. App. 1975); *State v. Anderson,* 616 P.2d 612 (Wash. 1980) *appeal after remand,* 538 P.2d 1205 (Wash.); *cert. denied,* 459 U.S. 842 (1982). *See,* however, *State v. Andring,* 342 N.W.2d 128 (Minn. 1984).

154. *State v. R.H.,* 683 P.2d 269 (Alaska Ct. App. 1984); *Daymude v. State,* 540 N.E.2d 1263 (Ind. Ct. App. 1989).

155. *People v. Stritzinger,* 668 P.2d 738 (Cal. 1983).

156. *Landeros v. Flood,* 123 Cal. Rptr. 713 (Cal. Ct. App. 1975) (in dicta), vacated on other grounds, 551 P.2d 389 (Cal. 1976).

157. *Id.* at 720.

158. *Supra* note 139.

159. 2 Am. Jur. Proof of Facts 2d 365, 390.

160. Brown, *Medical and Legal Aspects of the Battered Child Syndrome,* 50 Chi. Kent L. Rev. 45, 60 (1973).

161. Karelitz, *Maltreatment of Children,* 37 Pediatrics 377, 379 (1966).

162. Goodpasture & Angel, *Child Abuse and the Law: The California System,* 26 Hastings L.J. 1081, 1094 (1975).

163. Silver, *Child Abuse Laws—Are They Enough?* 199 JAMA 65 (1967).

164. Wolff, *Are Doctors Too Soft on Child Beaters?* 43 Med. Econ. 84, 85 (1966).

165. *Harris v. City of Montgomery,* 435 So.2d 1207, 1213 (Ala. 1983); *Brown v. Scott,* 259 S.E.2d 642 (Ga. Ct. App. 1979). In California a mandatory reporter enjoys immunity from liability even for knowingly false reports, although a voluntary reporter can be liable for a false report if he or she knew the report was false or if it was made with reckless disregard for the truth or falsity of the report. Legislation also provides state reimbursement for legal expenses incurred by mandatory reporters who successfully defend against claims resulting from reporting. *Krikorian v. Barry,* 242 Ca. Rptr. 313, 316 (Cal. Ct. App. 1987); *Storch v. Silverman,* 231 Cal. Rptr. 27 (Cal. Ct. App. 1986) (physician reporting sexual abuse of child immune from suit for negligent infliction of emotional distress brought by parents alleging defendant lacked reasonable suspicion of existence of abuse).

166. *Harris, supra* note 165 at 1213.

167. *Searcy v. Auerbach,* 980 F.2d 609 (9th Cir. 1992).

168. *Comstock v. Walsh,* 848 S.W.2d 7 (Mo. Ct. App. 1992).

169. Sussman, *Reporting Child Abuse: A Review of the Literature,* 8 Fam. L.Q. 245, 293 (1974).

170. *Id.* at 293, 294.

171. *See, generally,* Hansen, *Doctors, Lawyers and the Battered Child Law,* 5 J. Trauma 826, 827 (1965).

172. Besharov, *The Vulnerable Social Worker: Liability for Serving Children and Families* (National Association of Social Workers, 1985).

173. *Cechman v. Travis,* 414 S.E.2d 282, 284 (Ga. Ct. App. 1991) (in dicta), *cert. denied* (1992); *supra* note 169.

174. Shepherd, *The Abused Child and the Law,* 22 Wash. & Lee L. Rev. 182, 192 (1968).

175. Kohlman, *Malpractice Liability for Failure to Report Child Abuse,* 49 Ca. St. B.J. 118, 121 (1974). A search of cases since 1974 also reveals no criminal prosecutions for failure to report.

176. *Pope v. State,* 396 A.2d 1054 (Md. 1979).

177. *Supra* note 169.

178. *Supra* note 167.

179. *Landeros v. Flood,* 551 P.2d 389 (Cal. 1976).

180. *Id.* at 391-392.

181. *Id.* at 394 n. 8.

182. *Id.* at 394.

183. *Id.* at 395.

184. *Id.* at 396-397.

185. *Id.* at 397.

186. *Robinson v. Wical,* C.A. No. 37607 (Cal. Super. Ct. San Luis Obispo, filed Sept 4, 1970), cited in Note, Torts: *Civil Action Against Physician for Failure to Report Cases of Suspected Child Abuse,* 30 Okla. L. Rev. 482, 485 note 21 (1977).

187. *Cechman, supra* note 173.

188. *Id.*

189. *Id.*

190. *Valtakis v. Putnam,* 504 N.W.2d 264 (Minn. Ct. App. 1993).

191. *Id.* at 266.

192. *Id.*

193. *Marcelletti v. Bathani,* 500 N.W.2d 124 (Mich. Ct. App.) *appeal denied,* 502 N.W.2d 382 (Mich. 1993) (citing Michigan's Child Protection Law, M.C.L. § 722.621 *et seq.;* M.S.A. § 25.248(3)(1).

194. *Id.* at 126.

195. *Id.* at 129-130.

196. *Doe v. New York City Dept. of Social Servs.,* 649 F.2d 134 (2d Cir. 1981), *cert. denied sub nom., Catholic Home Bureau v. Doe,* 446 U.S. 864 (1983); *Bartels v. Westchester County,* 429 N.Y.S.2d 906 (Appl Div. 1980). See, however, *Blanca C. v. Nassau County,* 480 N.Y.S.2d 747 (App. Div. 1984), *aff'd,* 481 N.W.2d 545 (N.Y. 1985).

197. *Jensen v. Conrad,* 747 F.2d 185 (4th Cir. 1984), *cert. denied,* 470 U.S. 1052 (1985).

198. *Taylor ex rel Walker v. Ledbetter,* 818 F.2d 791 (11th Cir. 1987) *(en banc), cert. denied,* 489 U.S. 1065.

199. *DeShaney v. Winnebago County Dep't. of Soc. Serv.,* 489 U.S. 189 (1989).

200. *Id. Estate of Bailey v. County of York,* 768 F.2d 503 (3d Cir. 1985); *Doe v. Bobbitt,* 665 F. Supp. 691 (N.D. Ill. 1987), *motion granted in part and denied in part,* 682 F. Supp. 388 (N.D. Ill. 1988).

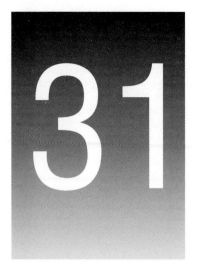

Coronary artery disease and practice guidelines

TIMOTHY E. PATERICK, M.D., J.D., M.B.A.

COMPLEXITY OF DISEASE
GUIDELINES AND STANDARDS OF CARE
MALPRACTICE LITIGATION
CONCLUSION

Coronary artery disease (CAD) is the most common disorder in cardiovascular medicine but of interest to all health care providers. It is the leading cause of death in the United States and is responsible for one in about every five deaths.[1] Malpractice allegations associated with the diagnosis and treatment of CAD occur frequently.[2-6]

This chapter focuses on one disease entity of CAD: stable angina and its standard of care in regard to the history, physical examination, risk factor analysis, electrocardiogram (EKG, ECG), chest x-ray film, probability estimate, and treadmill exercise test. Legal topics include professional liability, negligence, judicial proceedings, and the standard of care as a necessary component of a negligence case.

In a judicial proceeding, in order to prevail, the plaintiff must identify for the court the proper standard of care to which the defendant must adhere. The American College of Cardiology/American Heart Association/American College of Physicians–American Society of Internal Medicine (ACC/AHA/ACP-ASIM) *Guidelines for the Management of Patients with Chronic Stable Angina* is the model that would be used in a negligence proceeding.[7]

The AHA estimates that 6.2 million Americans have chest pain annually and that 1 million patients have myocardial infarctions (MIs).[8] Ischemic heart disease is still associated with substantial patient morbidity despite the decline in cardiovascular mortality.

COMPLEXITY OF DISEASE

The etiology of CAD is multifactorial and incompletely understood. The following key points show the complexity of managing CAD:

1. Acute CAD syndromes (unstable angina, acute MI, sudden death) result from superimposition of a coronary thrombus over an atherosclerotic plaque, resulting in a rapid increase in the severity of luminal occlusion.[9]

2. The pathological substrate for coronary thrombosis is plaque rupture (60% to 80%) and plaque erosion (20% to 40%).[10]

3. Severely stenotic plaques tend to progress to total occlusion more frequently than mildly stenotic plaques.[11]

4. Since mildly obstructive (50% diameter narrowing by angiography) plaques outnumber severe lesions 10 to one, many more cases of acute luminal occlusion result from mildly obstructive lesions.

5. Ruptured plaques and, by inference, vulnerable plaques, in contrast to intact and stable plaques, are characterized by a large lipid core, increased inflammation, thinning of fibrous cap, increased neovascularity, and reduced smooth muscle cell and collagen content.

6. Triggers of plaque rupture and thrombosis may include hemodynamic stress, physical stress, and infectious agents such as *Chlamydia pneumoniae.*[12]

7. The shoulder regions of eccentric plaques are exposed to high circumferential stress and appear to be more prone to rupture.[13]

8. Lipid-lowering drugs produce minimal change in diameter narrowing but a disproportionate reduction in the clinical event.[14]

9. Change in plaque composition with lipid-lowering drugs may contribute to "plaque stabilization," accounting for the clinical benefit of these drugs.[15]

GUIDELINES AND STANDARD OF CARE

The ACC/AHA/ACP-ASIM guidelines epitomize the reference an expert witness would utilize to determine if a physician conformed to a certain standard of conduct to protect others against unreasonable risk. The New Mexico Supreme Court articulated the standard of care for physicians; it is a duty to use "knowledge, skill and care ordinarily used by a reasonably well-qualified physician of the same field of medicine practicing under similar circumstances. . . ."[16] Medical malpractice must be shown by expert testimony on the standard of care, unless the question may be determined by the knowledge of the ordinary layman. The ACC/AHA/ACP-ASIM guidelines represent the "core in knowledge" for the treatment of chronic stable angina.

Evidence and classification of conditions

Various policy statements, care paths, and protocols are loosely referred to as "guidelines." More precisely, however, a *guideline* indicates a course to follow, which in clinical practice tends to be broad and flexible. It should be not be equated with policy, because policy is binding and typically requires disciplinary intervention for nonadherence.

The committee recommendations (guidelines) were based on available data and ranked the weight of evidence using three levels, as follows[17]:
- **A:** High; data were derived from multiple randomized clinical trials with large numbers of patients,
- **B:** Intermediate; data were derived from a limited number of randomized clinical trials with large numbers of patients, careful analysis of nonrandomized studies, or observational registries.
- **C:** Low; expert consensus was the primary basis for the recommendation.

The following ACC/AHA/ACP-ASIM classification of conditions summarizes the evidence and expert opinion and provides final recommendations for patient evaluation and therapy:
- **Class I:** Evidence or general agreement indicates that a given procedure or treatment is useful and effective against the condition.
- **Class II:** Evidence is conflicting or opinion is divergent about the usefulness or efficacy of a procedure or treatment for the condition.
  - **IIA:** Favoring usefulness
  - **IIB:** Usefulness less well established
- **Class III:** Evidence indicates that the procedure or treatment for the condition is not effective and may be harmful.

Decision-making and incomplete data

Much patient decision-making involves the perception of risk, which is subjective and variable. The diagnosis, risk stratification, and management of CAD depend on incomplete information that yields tradeoffs rather than definitive solutions. Hindsight bias is a serious problem in clinical review. Once a clinical outcome is declared "closed," the tendency is to see the events that preceded, constituted, and caused the outcome as inevitable. Outcome exerts an irresistible pressure on interpretation. Blunders with positive results are perceived as informed clinical decisions, whereas decisions that were *intelligent ex ante,* or the best that could be devised on the basis of the information available at the time, are viewed as avoidable blunders and assumed to be

negligent acts. The ACC/AHA/ACP-ASIM guidelines allow the reviewing bodies to evaluate whether the decisions were intelligent ex ante and whether the outcome was an inevitable consequence of the actions taken.[18-21]

Diagnosis: history, physical examination, and risk factors

ACC/AHA/ACP-ASIM recommendations for management of patients with chest pain include a detailed chest pain history, focused cardiovascular examination, risk factor assessment, and estimate of the probability of CAD based on this information.

The clinical history is the most important step in evaluating patients with chest pain. This information allows accurate prediction of significant CAD. The interview should address the quality, location, and duration of the pain, as well as alleviating and aggravating factors. The characterization should be precise.

The physical examination can be completely normal in patients with stable angina. Abnormalities (e.g., S3 and S4 heart sounds, mitral regurgitation, rales) that accompany the pain but disappear when the pain subsides are predictive of CAD. Evidence of noncoronary atherosclerotic disease increases the likelihood of CAD. Hypertension, xanthomas, and retinal exudates indicate the presence of CAD risk factors, including smoking, diabetes, hypertension, abnormal lipid profile, history of familial premature CAD, and history of cerebral and peripheral vascular disease.

This information is integrated to estimate the likelihood of significant CAD.

Probability estimate: treadmill test

When CAD is suspected, a probability estimate should be done to determine its likelihood. The estimate affects the utility of a common diagnostic test: treadmill exercise.[22]

The interpretation of the treadmill exercise test can be affected by varying the pretest probability of CAD from 5% to 50% to 90%. The test sensitivity is 50%, and the specificity is 90%. In the 5% group the positive predictive value of an abnormal treadmill test is only 21%. If 1000 low-probability patients are tested, 120 will have positive tests. Of these, 95 will not have significant disease. Before testing such a group, the physician must assess the value of finding CAD in 25 patients against the cost of a stress test for all 1000 patients ($1000 \times \$300 = \$30,000$). Other costs include misdiagnosis in 95 patients and the anxiety, invasive testing, unnecessary medication, and higher insurance premiums. In the 90% group a positive test raises the probability to 98%, and a negative test lowers the probability to 83%. Although the treadmill exercise test has prognostic value in this group, a negative test does not eliminate the diagnosis of CAD. For a diagnosis these patients need angiography. The 50% probability group benefits from the test results; a positive test raises the probability to 83%, and a negative test lowers the likelihood of CAD to 36%.[23]

Thus there are subsets of patients with high-probability and low-probability CAD. An accurate estimate of the likelihood of CAD is necessary for interpretation of further test results and good clinical decisions.

A clinicopathological study showed that a regression model with variables of pain type, age, and gender allows the accurate prediction of the probability of significant CAD.[24] This study was supported by angiographic data.[25] A 64-year-old man with typical angina has a 94% likelihood of CAD, and a 32-year-old woman with nonanginal pain has a 1% chance of CAD. Duke University and Stanford University carried out prospective studies that supported these data.[26]

Noninvasive testing: electrocardiogram and chest film

The ACC/AHA/ACP-ASIM guidelines address the use of the EKG and chest x-ray film in the management of chronic stable angina. A resting 12-lead EKG should be recorded in all patients with symptoms suggestive of angina. The EKG will be normal in more than 50% of patients with chronic stable angina, and therefore a normal resting EKG does not exclude CAD. EKG changes of ischemia, left ventricular hypertrophy, and Q wave infarction favor the diagnosis of angina. Rhythm disturbances during pain increase the likelihood of angina, but other forms of heart disease can cause rhythm abnormalities. Conduction disturbances have low specificity for CAD.

An EKG is abnormal in about 50% of patients with chest pain who have a normal EKG when they have no pain. ST segment elevation and depression during pain establish a high likelihood of angina. Pseudonormalization of the EKG during pain is a marker for angina. Conduction disturbances present only during pain also suggest angina.

The chest x-ray film is often normal during episodes of angina. Its usefulness as a routine test is not established. Cardiac enlargement is not specific for CAD. The chest film may be valuable in diagnosing aneurysms and pulmonary infarction or embolism.

Patient classification

The following ACC/AHA/ACP-ASIM classification of patients for the diagnosis of obstructive CAD is based on exercise testing without an imaging modality (A, B, and C indicate level of evidence):

- **Class I:** Intermediate pretest probability of CAD based on age, gender, and symptoms, including patients with complete right bundle branch block (RBBB) or less than 1 mm of ST segment depression on EKG at rest (B)
- **Class IIA:** Suspected vasospastic angina (C)
- **Class IIB**
  1: High pretest probability of CAD (B)
  2: Low pretest probability of CAD (B)
  3: Digoxin therapy and less than 1 mm of baseline ST depression (B)
  4: Left ventricular hypertrophy and less than 1 mm of ST depression (B)
- **Class III**
  1a: Wolff-Parkinson-White (WPW) syndrome (B)
  1b: Paced rhythm (B)
  1c: Greater than 1 mm of ST depression (B)
  1d: Left bundle branch block (LBBB) (B)
  2: CAD established through prior MI or angiography (B)

Exercise testing

Exercise testing is a safe procedure, with the incidence of MI or death less than one in 2500 tests performed.[27]

Absolute contraindications

1. Acute myocardial infarction within 48 hours
2. Hemodynamic instability or symptomatic rhythm disturbance
3. Severe aortic stenosis
4. Congestive heart failure that is symptomatic
5. Pulmonary infarction/emboli
6. Myocarditis/pericarditis
7. Aortic dissection

Relative contraindications

1. Left main stenosis
2. Moderate aortic stenosis
3. Electrolyte abnormality
4. Systolic hypertension greater than 200 mm Hg
5. Diastolic blood pressure (BP) greater than 110 mm Hg
6. Symptomatic bradycardia and tachycardia
7. Hypertrophic cardiomyopathy or outflow obstruction
8. Mental and physical impairment

Monitoring. An appropriately trained physician should supervise exercise testing. The EKG, heart rate, and BP should be monitored and recorded during each stage of exercise as well as during ST segment abnormalities and chest pain. The patient should be continuously monitored for EKG changes of ischemia.

Absolute indications to stop test

1. Drop in systolic BP of more than 10 mm Hg from baseline BP despite an increase in workload, when accompanied by other evidence of ischemia
2. Moderate to severe angina
3. Near syncope or ataxia
4. Sustained ventricular tachycardia
5. Technical difficulties with monitoring equipment
6. ST segment elevation greater than 1 mm in leads without diagnostic Q waves

Relative indications to stop test

1. Drop in systolic BP of more than 10 mm Hg without evidence of ischemia

2. Greater than 2 mm of horizontal or down-sloping ST depression
3. Symptomatic rhythm disturbances
4. Fatigue
5. Dyspnea
6. Claudication

Interpretation. The exercise test interpretation should include symptomatic response, exercise capacity, EKG analysis, and hemodynamic response. These variables have independent prognostic value. The most common definition for a positive exercise test is greater than 1 mm of horizontal down-sloping ST segment depression or ST segment elevation at 0.60 to 0.80 millisecond after the QRS complex, either during or after exercise.

Diagnostic characteristics. The *sensitivity* (SN) of the exercise test means the probability that a patient with obstructive CAD has a positive test, whereas the *specificity* (SP) measures the probability that a patient without obstructive CAD has a negative test. SN and SP are used to summarize the characteristics of diagnostic tests because they provide standard measures that can be used to compare different tests. SN and SP do not provide the information to interpret the results of exercise testing.

Exercise testing must be interpolated based on the positive and negative predictive value of the exercise test. The *positive predictive value* is the probability that the patient has obstructive CAD when the exercise test is positive. The *negative predictive value* is the probability that the patient does not have obstructive CAD when the exercise test is negative.[28] From the formulas for calculating the positive and negative predictive values, it is clear that the sensitivity, specificity, and pretest probability of obstructive CAD are instrumental to interpreting exercise testing.

Pretest probability. Diagnostic testing is most valuable when the pretest probability of significant CAD is intermediate (40% to 60%). The exact definition of "intermediate" is complex and a subject of debate between "Bayesians" and "Frequentists."[29] Frequentists believe pretest probability is a subjective determination that cannot be equated with a probability. There is no controversy about Bayesian analysis when the pretest probability is known.

If decision analysis is applied to this issue, pretest probability estimates are a useful clinical tool.[30] Angiographic data have shown that the pretest probability can be predicted with variables obtained from the history.[31] When the pretest probability is high, the next step is angiography; when it is low, the next step is careful follow-up. Exercise testing is most beneficial in diagnosing obstructive CAD in the intermediate group.

MALPRACTICE LITIGATION

Many health care providers are concerned that practice guidelines may lead to increased litigation if they are represented as a standard of care.[32] These worries may be ill-founded. If physi-

cians agree on a set of guidelines and use them appropriately, litigation may actually decrease. A few states have encouraged the use of guidelines in litigation, usually as a defense for physicians. Some believe that adherence to guidelines could reduce defensive medicine costs by 25% over 5 years.[33]

In fact, clinical practice guidelines are rarely used in malpractice suits. A review of litigation files from two insurance companies showed that only 17 of 259 claims involved practice guidelines. The same study surveyed 960 malpractice attorneys, who reported that guidelines are likely to be used as inculpatory evidence in 54% of cases, as exculpatory in 23%, and disputed in 23%.[34] A review of court records from 1988 to 1994 found 28 cases in which guidelines were used successfully in litigation.[35] In 22 cases the guidelines were inculpatory and in six were exculpatory. Procedural rules seem to favor defendant providers in the use of guidelines as standards of care rather than plaintiffs.

The goal of practice guidelines is systematic, scientifically derived statements of appropriate measures to be taken by physicians in the diagnosis and treatment of disease. Practice guidelines are expected to give public and private financiers of health services better tools to evaluate care. They are also being viewed as a way to ameliorate the conflict associated with the law governing medical malpractice.

Practice guidelines have emerged recently as the medical profession's way to uncover shortcomings in prevailing medical practice. In the 1980s, research produced evidence of variation in medical practice, lack of scientific underpinnings of many customary practices, and substantial overuse of many procedures.[36,37]

The movement to develop authoritative guidelines received new impetus in the budget reconciliation legislation adopted in 1989.[38] The U.S. Congress created the Agency for Health Care Policy and Research and assigned it the responsibility to evaluate medical treatments.

Some tension exists between the *professional model,* in which organized medicine is developing practice guidelines, and the *political model,* which is implicit in the federal program. Questions remain: who should set the regulatory standards, and how liberal or restrictive should they be? The guidelines can be a sword or a shield in a malpractice allegation. The medical profession should approach participation in the development of practice guidelines as an opportunity to level the playing field for all participants in the health care arena.

CONCLUSION

A reasonable, prudent physician is not expected to yield perfect outcomes but is expected to demonstrate "due diligence" when approaching clinical problems. Due diligence requires attention to the specifics of the history, physical examination, and risk factor profile. These details must be used to develop a probability estimate of the likelihood of CAD. This allows the physician to classify patients as being at low, intermediate, or high risk for significant CAD.

Practice guidelines allow reviewing bodies to judge whether the treatment was intelligent ex ante. This prevents the outcome from exerting pressure on the reviewing body to see the events as inevitable.

The practice guidelines provide the physician with a "best evidence" approach to clinical care and provide a model for the legal requisite standard of care. This permits harmony between law and medicine and resolution of potential conflict at a time when the process of conflict resolution in medical care needs attention. The complexities in law and medicine should not be seen as intractable conflicts between professionals but as a common search for caring and justice.

ENDNOTES

1. American Heart Association Committee on Emergency Cardiac Care & R.O. Cummins, *Advanced Cardiac Life Support* (The Association, Dallas 1997).

2. *Defensive Medicine,* Wall Street Journal, A18 (1997).

3. R.L. Abel, *The Real Tort Crisis: Too Few Claims,* 443 Ohio State L. J. 448 (1987).

4. P.M. Danzon, *Medical Malpractice: Theory, Evidence and Public Policy,* 22-25 (Harvard University Press, Cambridge, Mass. 1985).

5. B. McMenamin, *Don't Let Them Rush You into an HMO,* Forbes 46 (1996).

6. E. Schine & K.H. Hammonds, *In California It's, "Hell No, HMO!* Business Week 38 (1996).

7. R.J. Gibbons et al., *ACC/AHA/ACP-ASIM Guidelines for the Management of Patients with Chronic Stable Angina: a Report of the American College of Cardiology/American Heart Association Task Force on Practice Guidelines (Committee on Management of Patients with Chronic Stable Angina),* 33 J. Am. Coll. Cardiol. 2092-2197 (1999).

8. American Heart Association, *Heart and Stroke Statistical Update* (The Association, Dallas 1999).

9. E.L. Alderman et al., *Five-Year Angiographic Follow-up of Factors Associated with Progression of Coronary Artery Disease in the Coronary Artery Surgery Study (CASS),* 22 J. Am. Coll. Cardiol. 1141-1154 (1993).

10. P.K. Shah, *Plaque Size, Vessel Size and Plaque Vulnerability: Bigger May Not Be Better* (editorial), 32 J. Am. Coll. Cardiol. 663-664 (1998).

11. J.A. Ambrose et al., *Angiographic Progression of Coronary Artery Disease and the Development of Myocardial Infarction,* 12 J. Am. Coll. Cardiol. 56-62 (1988).

12. J.E. Muller et al., *Triggers, Acute Risk Factors and Vulnerable Plaques: the Lexicon of a New Frontier,* 23 J. Am. Coll. Cardiol. 809-813 (1994).

13. S.D. Gertz & W.C. Roberts, *Hemodynamic Shear Force in Rupture of Coronary Arterial Atherosclerotic Plaques* (Editorial), 66 Am. J. Cardiol. 1368-1372 (1990).

14. P. Saikku, Chlamydia pneumoniae *and Atherosclerosis: an Update,* 104 Scand. J. Infect. Dis. Suppl. 53-56 (1997).

15. B.G. Brown et al., *Lipid Lowering and Plaque Regression: New Insights into Prevention of Plaque Disruption and Clinical Events in Coronary Disease,* 87 Circulation 1781-1791 (1993).

16. *Pharmaseal Labs, Inc. v. Goffe,* 90 N.M. 753 P 2d 589, 593-594 (N.M. 1977).

17. *Supra* note 7.

18. J.K. Silver, *The Business of Medicine,* 88 (Hanley & Belfus, Philadelphia 1998).

19. W. Prosser, *The Law of Torts,* 143 (4th ed., West Publishing, St. Paul, Minn. 1971).

20. A.R. Localio et al., *Identifying Adverse Events Caused by Medical Care: Degree of Physician Agreement in a Retrospective Chart Review,* 125 Annals Int. Med. 457-464 (1996).

21. P.E. Ross, *Software as a Career Threat,* Forbes 240-246 (1995).

22. L. Campeau, *Grading of Angina Pectoris* (Letter), 54 Circulation 522-523 (1976).

23. 2 D.L. Sackeh et al., *Clinical Epidemiology: a Basic Science for Clinical Medicine,* 93-98 (Little, Brown & Co., Boston 1991).

24. G.A. Diamond & J.S. Forrester, *Analysis of Probability as an Aid in the Clinical Diagnosis of Coronary-Artery Disease,* 300 N. Engl. J. Med. 1350-1358 (1979).

25. D.B. Pryor et al., *Value of the History and Physical in Identifying Patients at Increased Risk for Coronary Artery Disease,* 118 Ann. Int. Med. 81-90 (1993).

26. H.C. Sox Jr. et al., *Using the Patient's History To Estimate the Probability of Coronary Artery Disease: a Comparison of Primary Care and Referral Practices,* 89 Am. J. Med. 7-14 (1990).

27. R.J. Stuart Jr. & M.H. Ellestad, *National Survey of Exercise Stress Testing Facilities,* 77 Chest 94-97 (1980).

28. H. Motulsky, *Intensive Biostatistics,* 145 (Oxford University Press, New York 1995).

29. H.C. Sox et al., *Medical Decision Making* (Butterworth-Heinemann, Boston 1988).

30. S.G. Pauker & J.P. Kassirer, *The Threshold Approach to Clinical Decision Making,* 302 N. Engl. J. Med. 1109-1117 (1980).

31. *Supra* note 24.

32. E.B. Hirshfeld, *From the Office of the General Counsel: Practice Parameters and the Malpractice Liability of Physicians,* 263 J.A.M.A. 1556, 1559-1562 (1990).

33. M.M. Costello & K.M. Murphy, *Clinical Guidelines: a Defense in Medical Malpractice Suits,* 21 Physician Exec. 10-12 (1995).

34. A.L. Hyams et al., *Practice Guidelines and Malpractice Litigation: a Two-way Street,* 122 Annals Int. Med. 450-455 (1995).

35. A.L. Hyams et al., *Medical Practice Guidelines in Malpractice Litigation: an Early Retrospective,* 21 J. Health Polit. Policy L. 289-313 (1996).

36. R.H. Brook et al., *Predicting the Appropriate Use of Carotid Endarterectomy, Upper Gastrointestinal Endoscopy, and Coronary Angiography,* 323 N. Engl. J. Med. 1173-1177 (1990).

37. D.M. Eddy & J. Billings, *The Quality of Medical Evidence: Implications for Quality of Care,* 7 Health Aff. (Millwood) 19-32 (1988).

38. U.S. Congress, House Committee on the Budget, *A Complete Guide to the Omnibus Budget Reconciliation Act of 1989,* 101-239 (Prentice Hall, Inc., Englewood Cliffs, N.J. 1989).

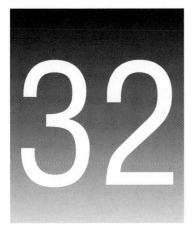

32 Domestic violence patients

JACK W. SNYDER, M.D., J.D., M.F.S., M.P.H., Ph.D.

CIVIL PROTECTION ORDERS
CRIMINAL DOMESTIC VIOLENCE PROSECUTIONS
IMPACT OF DOMESTIC VIOLENCE IN OTHER AREAS OF LAW
CONCLUSION

Domestic violence occurs when one intimate partner uses physical violence, coercion, threats, intimidation, isolation, and/or emotional, sexual, and economic abuse to maintain power and control over the other intimate partner.[1] Domestic violence is also described as a "pattern of interaction" in which one intimate partner is forced to change his or her behavior in response to the abuse or threats of the other partner.[2] Synonyms for domestic violence include partner violence, relationship violence, dating violence, teen dating violence, intimate partner abuse, spouse abuse, domestic abuse, wife abuse, wife beating, and battering.[3]

Persons most likely to experience domestic violence include (1) women who are single or who have recently separated or divorced, (2) women who have recently sought an order of protection, (3) women who are younger than 28 years of age, (4) women who abuse alcohol or other drugs, (5) women who are pregnant, (6) women whose partners are excessively jealous or possessive, (7) women who have witnessed or experienced physical or sexual abuse as children, and (8) women whose partners have witnessed or experienced physical or sexual abuse as children.[4] Domestic violence affects people from all races, religions, age groups, sexual orientations, and socioeconomic levels.[5]

Despite its widespread occurrence,[6] most domestic violence is largely unrecognized or ignored by professionals, including physicians,[7] family therapists,[8] psychotherapists,[9] and law enforcement officials.[10] Importantly, health care professionals can play a crucial role in the diagnosis, treatment, and referral of victims, helping to break the often intergenerational cycle of domestic violence.[11] Physicians can screen,[12] assess, and intervene efficiently and effectively by eliciting a history of violence,[13] asking specific questions when battering is suspected,[14] documenting the physical findings that often accompany domestic violence,[15] assessing the victim's immediate and future safety,[16] and communicating to the victim all realistic options.[17] A few states have enacted laws that specifically require medical staff to report suspected domes-

tic violence,[18] but many experts suggest that it is "absolutely contraindicated" to report cases of domestic violence to any agency or authority without the victim's direct request and consent.[19] These experts believe that mandatory reporting of domestic violence often increases the survivor's sense of powerlessness and may increase the risk of further harm, including the risk of homicide.[20] The theory that mandatory reporting may deter victims from seeking medical care is not well supported by available empirical observations.[21]

CIVIL PROTECTION ORDERS

In all U.S. jurisdictions the victim of domestic violence can obtain by statute a civil protection order (CPO).[22] Most states authorize emergency or temporary (2- to 4-week) CPOs if the victim (at an ex parte hearing) can prove immediate danger of future violence.[23] Courts also issue longer (1- to 3-year) CPOs after a full hearing, by consent, or by default.[24] Although statutes of limitation typically do not apply to persons requesting CPOs, some courts may not grant an order if the most recent threat or incident of abuse occurred several months before the filing of a petition for a CPO.[25] In most states an abused adult can file on his or her own behalf.[26] An adult also can file on behalf of a child or decision-incapable adult.[27] A few states allow minors to petition for protection on their own behalf.[28]

Basis for granting

State laws define the relationships that must exist between the parties before a CPO will be granted. Recognized targets of a CPO include current or former spouses,[29] family members who are related by blood or marriage,[30] current or former household members,[31] persons who share a child in common,[32] unmarried persons of different genders living as spouses,[33] persons in same sex relationships,[34] persons in dating or intimate relationships,[35] and persons offering refuge to victims of domestic violence.[36]

Courts and legislatures have identified several types of acts as abuse sufficient to support the issuance of a CPO.[37] Acts of abuse against the petitioner include threats,[38] interference with personal liberty,[39] harassment,[40] stalking,[41] emotional abuse,[42] attempts to inflict harm,[43] sexual assault,[44] marital rape,[45] assault and battery,[46] burglary,[47] criminal trespass,[48] kidnapping,[49] and damage to property (including pets).[50] The standards of proof for issuance or extension of a CPO include "preponderance of the evidence," "preponderance of the evidence that the petitioner is facing a clear and present or imminent danger," and "reasonable cause or grounds to believe" that abuse occurred, that there is an emergency, or that the petitioner is in immediate and present danger.[51]

Contents

CPOs typically require that the respondent shall[52] (1) not molest, assault, harass, or in any manner threaten or physically abuse the petitioner and/or his/her child(ren)[53]; (2) stay 150 yards away from the petitioner's home, person, workplace, children, place of worship, and day care provider[54]; (3) not contact petitioner and/or his/her children in any manner (personally, in writing, by mail or telephone, or through third parties)[55]; (4) vacate the residence at (location) by (date and time) (the police department shall stand by and shall give respondent 15 minutes to collect his or her personal belongings, which include clothes, toiletries, and one set of sheets and pillowcases; no other property may be removed from the premises without petitioner's permission; the police shall take all keys and garage openers from respondent, check to see that they are the right ones, and then turn keys over to the petitioner)[56]; (5) relinquish possession and/or use of the following personal property as of (date and time)[57]; (6) turn over to the police any and all weapons that the respondent owns or possesses and all licenses the respondent has authorizing the possession of or purchase of weapons[58]; (7) participate in and successfully complete a counseling program[59]; (8) relinquish custody of minor children to petitioner until further order of the court or the expiration date of the order[60]; (9) have rights of visitation with minor child(ren) under specified conditions[61]; (10) pay spousal and child support as designated[62]; and (11) pay for specified repairs, medical or health insurance costs, attorney's fees, and court costs.[63]

Enforcement

In the majority of states, violation of a CPO is a crime for which the police can arrest the offender, even if the violation did not occur in the presence of the officer.[64] The statutory trend is to augment civil or criminal contempt enforcement with misdemeanor charges and to heighten the criminal classification for violation of a CPO.[65] CPOs can and do remain in effect despite the parties' reunification or the petitioner's invitation to the abuser to enter her residence.[66]

In *United States v. Dixon*[67] the Supreme Court ruled that double jeopardy would not bar a battered woman from enforcing her CPO through criminal contempt proceedings while the state proceeds with a criminal prosecution for crimes the respondent committed against the battered woman at the time he violated the CPO, as long as the contempt proceeding and the criminal prosecution each require proof of additional elements.[68]

Consequences of violation

The sentencing of an individual after a criminal contempt conviction or a trial for crimes committed against family members has several important goals, including (1) stopping the violence; (2) protecting the victim, the children, and other family members; (3) protecting the general public; (4) holding the offender accountable for the violent conduct; (5) upholding the legislative intent to treat domestic violence as a serious crime; (6) providing restitution for the victim; and (7) rehabilitating the offender.[69] State courts have upheld a variety of sentences, including jail terms, monetary sanctions, bonds, probation, community service, electronic monitoring, and injunctions.[70]

The Violence Against Women Act

The Violence Against Women Act (VAWA), which amends various sections of the United States Code and Rule 412 of the Federal Rules of Evidence, was signed by President Clinton on September 13, 1994. This comprehensive legislation accomplished the following:

1. Established a federal civil rights cause of action for victims of gender-motivated crimes of violence[71]
2. Provided that protective orders (including ex parte orders) issued in one state are enforceable in other states as long as due process requirements are met in the issuing state[72]
3. Required that the U.S. Postal Service protect the confidentiality of addresses of domestic violence shelters and abused persons[73]
4. Permitted battered immigrant spouses and children of U.S. citizens and legal residents to self-petition the Immigration and Naturalization Service for legal resident status or to file for legal resident status even if their marriage to a U.S. citizen or lawful permanent resident is legally terminated after the petition is filed[74]
5. Permitted battered immigrant spouses and children of U.S. citizens and legal residents and parents of battered children of U.S. citizens and legal residents residing in the U.S. for at least 3 years to obtain suspension of deportation if deportation would result in extreme hardship to the alien or the alien's parent or child[75]
6. Created federal criminal penalties for crossing a state line to violate a protection order or to commit domestic violence against a spouse or intimate partner[76]
7. Mandated restitution enforceable through suspension of federal benefits, and an opportunity for the victim to inform the court regarding the danger posed by pretrial release of the defendant[77]
8. Funded a continuously operating toll-free hotline that provides the caller with names of local shelters, referrals, and domestic violence programs[78]

Regarding federal sex crimes, VAWA provides for pretrial detention,[79] payment for testing for sexually transmitted diseases,[80] and increased sentences for repeat sex offenders or where the victim of a federal sex offense is under 16 years of age.[81] VAWA also amends Federal Rule of Evidence 412 to prohibit introduction of evidence regarding the victim's sexual history.[82]

Most courts confronted with constitutional challenges to VAWA have found the act to be a valid exercise of congressional power under the Commerce Clause.[83] However, in *U.S. v. Morrison/Brzonkala v. Morrison*[84] the Fourth Circuit United States Court of Appeals held that rape and other violent crimes against women are not economic or commercial activities and are not individually connected to interstate commerce. Consequently, the court ruled that these crimes could not be regulated under the act. The Supreme Court of the United States heard oral argument in this matter on January 11, 2000.

CRIMINAL DOMESTIC VIOLENCE PROSECUTIONS

When police have probable cause to believe that domestic violence has occurred, many states mandate and others permit warrantless arrests.[85] Exigent circumstances also may give rise to constitutionally permissible warrantless searches.[86] Respondents in domestic violence cases have been criminally prosecuted for a broad range of acts.[87] Until recently, most federal cases involving domestic violence have been prosecuted under the Assimilated Crimes Act (ACA).[88] This act authorizes federal prosecutions for crimes not contained in the United States Code when a criminal offense under state law is committed within a federal enclave or in an area under the exclusive jurisdiction of the United States. Under the ACA, state substantive law is incorporated into the federal prosecution, and the federal prosecutor steps into the shoes of the state prosecutor for purposes of the charged offense.[89] Cases involving criminal racketeering also incorporate state law crimes of violence, including murder or kidnapping.[90] As of 1996, amendments to the Gun Control Act of 1968 prohibit persons convicted of domestic violence offenses from possessing firearms in or affecting commerce.[91]

In most states a defendant is justified in killing an attacker if the defendant did not provoke the attack, reasonably believed the attacker posed an imminent or immediate threat of death or serious bodily harm, and used only force proportionate to the force used or threatened against the defendant.[92] The defendant's belief that the attack was imminent and that the response was necessary for protection must have been reasonable; moreover, the defendant must have been under no duty to retreat or unable to retreat.[93]

For most of the twentieth century, victims of repeated acts of domestic violence who killed their partners could not prove self-defense because courts believed that the attack was not necessary, the use of deadly force was excessive, and the victim was the aggressor in the events immediately preceding the killing.[94] In the 1970s, however, psychologist Lenore Walker studied several hundred women in an effort to explain the psychological and behavioral patterns that commonly appear in women who have been physically and psychologically abused by an intimate partner over an extended period. Analogizing to scientific research on dogs, Walker theorized that the experience of repeated and unpreventable abuse, along with the social conditioning of women to be subservient, created in battered women a state of "psychological paralysis" that rendered them unable to seek escape or help, even when it might be available.[95] Walker coined the term *battered woman syndrome,* which soon provided the basis for expert testimony designed to convince a jury that the defendant reasonably believed she had to kill to save herself, even during an ebb in violence.[96]

Invoking the syndrome, however, may not always advance justice for battered women who kill.[97] Experts therefore have encouraged a redefinition of the "battered woman" because testimony concerning the experiences of battered women refers to more than their psychological reactions to violence and because battered women's diverse psychological realities are not limited to one particular "profile."[98] As the debate over the proper role of domestic violence expert testimony continues in the legal and scientific literature, courts have begun to admit behavioral science evidence in domestic violence cases.[99]

IMPACT OF DOMESTIC VIOLENCE IN OTHER AREAS OF LAW

The role of law in domestic violence cases extends beyond CPOs and criminal prosecutions. Children must be supported, as well as protected; the rights and benefits of employment must be maintained; tort actions may be appropriate; and the validity of prenuptial agreements may be imperiled. Policies having the potential to discriminate against victims of domestic violence may raise constitutional issues of equal protection or due process.[100]

Child custody and support

Batterers often assault their children, and the risk of child abuse and kidnapping increases when a marriage is dissolving.[101] The physical and emotional consequences for children who experience domestic violence include medical problems, substance abuse, suicide attempts, eating disorders, nightmares, fear of being hurt, loneliness, bed wetting, and delinquent behavior such as fighting, prostitution, truancy, crimes against other people, running away, dropping out of school, teenage pregnancy, cognitive disorders, and low self-esteem.[102]

To prevent the offender from using custody and support litigation as a means to extend or maintain control and authority after separation from the victim, courts have been advised to draft orders that (1) specify times of visitation, telephone calls, and participation in school or extracurricular activities; (2) designate the circumstances of exchange or transfer of the children; (3) provide for the safety of the children and the vulnerable parent, including, for example, supervised visitation, injunctions against threatening conduct, and prohibitions against asking the children about the activities of the other parent; (4) account for the current and future needs of the children and the custodial parent; (5) require the offender to participate in educational services designed for batterers; and (6) specify circumstances or conditions under which custody or visitation orders may be altered.[103] All states permit courts to consider domestic violence in relationship to "the best interest of the child."[104] Congress and some states have adopted a presumption against award of joint or sole custody to the abusive parent.[105] Judges may be required to permit testimony about domestic violence and its impact on children and the nonabusive parent.[106]

Prenuptial agreements

Domestic violence may influence prenuptial agreements in three ways. First, battering may provide a defense to the enforcement of an otherwise valid prenuptial agreement.[107] Second, domestic violence may give rise to tort claims that may offset preclusions of equitable economic distribution found in many prenuptial agreements.[108] Third, a prenuptial agreement can include a provision that the occurrence of domestic violence invalidates the terms of the contract.[109]

Employment issues

Many victims of domestic violence are harassed at work by their former or current spouses or partners.[110] Victims also may miss work because of injuries, court dates, or the need to cooperate with criminal investigations.[111] Job performance may be undermined by depression, fear, and other psychological effects of battering.[112]

Employers may incur liability if domestic violence occurs in the workplace or if they fail to respond properly.[113] Theories of liability may include the Occupational Safety and Health Administration's "general duty" clause,[114] respondeat superior, duty to warn,[115] wrongful discharge in violation of public policy[116] or an employee's privacy rights, and negligent hiring, retention, security, and/or supervision.[117] Employees who are victims of domestic violence also are protected by workers' compensation statutes,[118] unemployment insurance or benefit laws,[119] and statutes that preserve benefits for persons cooperating with the judicial process.[120] Perhaps the biggest challenge for employers dealing with domestic violence is to balance employer interests in protecting employees and ensuring workplace safety with employee interests in privacy and freedom from defamation and discrimination.[121]

CONCLUSION

All medical and legal professionals must improve their abilities to identify and confront domestic violence. Appropriate and effective recognition and intervention require vigilance, a knowledge of and a willingness to ask the right questions, and a sense of obligation to help society end this undesirable phenomenon. Knowledge of legal considerations should improve the collaboration of health care workers, legal professionals, and community programs seeking to control domestic violence—a major public health problem.

ENDNOTES

1. Valente, *Domestic Violence and the Law, in The Impact of Domestic Violence on Your Legal Practice* 1-1–1-7 (Goelman, Lehrman, & Valente eds., 1996).

2. Dutton, *The Dynamics of Domestic Violence: Understanding the Response from Battered Women,* 68 Fla. Bar J. 24 (1994). Most victims or survivors of domestic violence are women, and most batterers or perpetrators are men. *See* Bureau of Justice Statistics, U.S. Department of Justice, *Violence Between Intimates* 2-3 (1994).

3. Alpert, *Domestic Violence, in Current Diagnosis* 105-109 (9th ed., Conn, Borer, & Snyder eds., W.B. Saunders, Philadelphia, 1997).

4. *Id.* at 106.

5. *Id.* at 105.

6. National surveys estimate that at least 2 million women each year are battered by an intimate partner, and crime data from the Federal Bureau of Investigation record about 1500 murders of women by husbands or boyfriends each year. Overall, the Bureau of Justice Statistics reports that women sustained about 3.8 million assaults and 500,000 rapes a year in 1992 and 1993; more than 75% of these violent acts were committed by someone known to the victim, and 29% of them were committed by an intimate—a husband, an ex-husband, a boyfriend, or an ex-boyfriend. These figures are believed to be underestimates. *See* Panel on Research on Violence Against Women, National Research Council, *Understanding Violence Against Women* (Crowell & Burgess eds., National Academy of Sciences, 1996). *See also* Abbott et al., *Domestic Violence Against Women: Incidence and Prevalence in an Emergency Department Population,* 273 J.A.M.A. 1763 (1995).

7. *See, e.g.,* Council on Ethical and Judicial Affairs, American Medical Association, *Physicians and Domestic Violence: Ethical Considerations,* 267 J.A.M.A. 3190 (1992); Sugg & Inui, *Primary Care Physician's Response to Domestic Violence: Opening Pandora's Box,* 267 J.A.M.A. 3157 (1992); McLeer & Anwar, *A Study of Battered Women Presenting in an Emergency Department,* 79 J. Public Health 65 (1989).

8. *See, e.g.,* Avis, *Where Are All the Family Therapists? Abuse and Violence Within Families and Family Therapy's Response,* 18 J. Marital Family Ther. 225 (1992); Harway & Hansen, *Therapist Perceptions of Family Violence, in Battering and Family Therapy: A Feminist Perspective,* 42, 52 (Hansen and Harway eds., Sage Publications, Newberry Park 1993).

9. *See, e.g.,* Hansen & Harway, supra note 8, at 45-47; Sesan, *Sex Bias and Sex-Role Stereotyping in Psychotherapy with Women: Survey Results,* 25 Psychotherapy 107 (1988).

10. *See, e.g.,* L.W. Sherman, *Policing Domestic Violence: Experiments and Dilemmas* 25-27 (Free Press, New York 1992).

11. *See, e.g., supra* note 3, at 105; Warshaw, *Identification, Assessment and Intervention with Victims of Domestic Violence, in Improving the Health Care Response to Domestic Violence: A Resource Manual for Health Care Providers* 49 (Family Violence Prevention Fund, 1995).

12. A letter to the Journal of the American Medical Association reported the following experience with initiating screening protocols:

I asked eight consecutive patients who had arrived at the clinic with routine gynecologic complaints unrelated to domestic violence whether they had ever been physically abused. The results were horrifying. All eight women had been physically assaulted by their intimate partners within the past year. One patient, who had come to the office for an oral contraceptive pill refill, went directly to the district attorney's office after talking about her dangerous situation at home. Another patient started to cry as she related the details of her physical and emotional injuries. Review of the otherwise thorough charts of these women made it apparent that no physician had asked whether these patients had ever been threatened or harmed. The women were waiting for their physicians to inquire; they showed no hesitancy in talking about their experiences.

Tracy, *Domestic Violence: The Physician's Role*, 275 J.A.M.A. 1708 (1996).

13. *Supra* note 3, at 106. Appropriate questions for eliciting a history of violence include (1) Have you ever been hit, hurt, or threatened by your husband or boyfriend or partner? (2) What happens when you and your partner have a disagreement at home? (3) Have you ever been threatened, intimidated, or frightened by your partner? (4) Are you afraid for your safety or for that of your children because of anyone you live with or are close to? (5) Would you leave your partner if you could? (6) Do you feel safe in your home? (7) Have you ever needed to see a doctor or go to an emergency room because someone did something to hurt or frighten you?

14. *Id.* at 107. Appropriate additional questions when domestic violence is suspected include (1) How were you hurt? (2) Has this happened before? (3) Could you tell me about the first episode? (4) How badly have you been hurt in the past? (5) Have you ever gone to an emergency room for treatment? (6) Have you ever been threatened with a weapon, or has a weapon ever been used on you? (7) Have your children ever seen you threatened or hurt? (8) Have your children ever been threatened or hurt by your partner?

15. *Id.* at 107. Objective manifestations of domestic violence may include (1) bilateral or multiple injuries, (2) injuries in different stages of healing, (3) evidence of rape or sexual assault, (4) an explanation by the victim that is inconsistent with the type of injury, (5) delay between the time of injury and the arrival of the victim at the health care facility, and (6) prior repetitive use of emergency services for trauma.

16. *Id.* at 107. Indicators of escalating risk include an increase in the severity or frequency of assaults, increasing or new threats of homicide or suicide by the partner, the presence or availability of a firearm, and the abuser's known criminal record of violent crime.

17. *Id.* at 108. Health care professionals (HCPs) can help the victim understand that she does not deserve to be hurt or threatened by anyone under any circumstances, particularly by someone she loves. The only provocation that justifies the use of physical force against another is an initial act of violence that puts the person attacked in reasonable fear of imminent danger. In other words, only batterers are responsible for their violence.

   HCPs also can (1) convey their concern for the victim's safety; (2) advise or refer for specific medical treatment, psychological counseling, safety planning, legal assistance, support groups, or emergency shelter or funds; (3) minimize the prescription of sedating or tranquilizing medications; and (4) evaluate the need to report the violence to a governmental agency.

   See American Medical Association, *Domestic Violence: A Directory of Protocols for Healthcare Providers* (1992); American Medical Association, *Diagnostic and Treatment Guidelines on Domestic Violence* (1992); American Medical Association, *Diagnostic and Treatment Guidelines on Family Violence* (1995).

18. *See, e.g.,* Cal. Penal Code § 11161 (West 1996).

19. *Supra* note 3, at 107; Hyman, Schillinger, & Lo, *Laws Mandating Reporting of Domestic Violence: Do They Promote Patient Well-Being?* 273 J.A.M.A. 1781 (1995).

20. *Id. See also, Policy Statement of the American College of Emergency Physicians on Mandatory Reporting of Domestic Violence to Law Enforcement and Criminal Justice Agencies,* 30 Ann. Emerg. Med. 561 (1997).

21. Houry, Feldhaus, Thorson & Abbott, *Mandatory Reporting Laws Do Not Deter Patients from Seeking Medical Care,* 34 Ann. Emerg. Med. 336 (1999).

22. Klein & Orloff, *Civil Protection Orders, in The Impact of Domestic Violence on your Legal Practice* 4-1 – 4-5 (Goelman, Lehrman, & Valente eds., 1996). *See also* Keilitz, *Civil Protection Orders: A Viable Justice System Tool for Deterring Domestic Violence,* 9 Violence and Victims 79 (1994).

23. Klein & Orloff, *Providing Legal Protection for Battered Women: An Analysis of State Statutes and Case Law,* 21 Hofstra L. Rev. 801, 1031-43 and accompanying notes 1420-1509 (1993).

24. *Supra* note 22, at 4-1.

25. *Supra* note 23, at 900-905 and accompanying notes 599-632.

26. *Id.* at 842-847 and accompanying notes 204-226. For an extended discussion of efforts to improve accessibility to the courts for battered women appearing *pro se, see id.* at 1048-1065 and accompanying notes 1541-1632.

27. *Id.* at 846.

28. *Id.* at 844.

29. *Id.,* at 814-816 and accompanying notes 38-48.

30. *Id.* at 816-820 and accompanying notes 49-69.

31. *Id.* at 838-842 and accompanying notes 182-203.

32. *Id.* at 824-829 and accompanying notes 94-127.

33. *Id.* at 829-832 and accompanying notes 128-149.

34. *Id.* at 832-835 and accompanying notes 150-168.

35. *Id.* at 835-837 and accompanying notes 169-174.

36. *Id.* at 837-838 and accompanying notes 175-181.

37. *See, e.g., Knuth v. Knuth,* 1992 Minn. App. LEXIS 696 (Minn. Ct. App. June 19, 1992).

38. *Supra* note 23, at 859-863 and accompanying notes 316-353.

39. *Id.* at 858-859 and accompanying notes 308-315.

40. *Id.* at 866-869 and accompanying notes 367-406.

41. *Id.* at 874-876 and accompanying notes 445-465.

42. *Id.* at 869-873 and accompanying notes 407-437.

43. *Id.* at 864-866 and accompanying notes 354-366.

44. *Id.* at 854-858 and accompanying notes 296-307.

45. *Id.*

46. *Id.* at 849-854 and accompanying notes 237-295. Case law indicates that battery is the most common criminal ground for issuance of a CPO. Courts have issued CPOs for shoving an infant's face against a door; physically restraining, striking, kicking, punching, choking, slapping, or throwing cold water on the petitioner; yanking the petitioner by the hair; pulling out the petitioner's pubic or other hair; throwing the petitioner on the floor; bruising a child's back, legs, and buttocks; twisting the petitioner's wrist; pounding the petitioner's head on the floor; attempting to push the petitioner's face in the toilet; and ordering trained dogs to attack the petitioner.

47. *See, e.g.,* N.J. Stat. Ann. § 2C:25-19 (West 1992); Wash. Rev. Code Ann. § 10.99.020 (West 1992).

48. *See, e.g.,* Del. Code Ann. tit. 10, § 945 (1993); N.J. Stat. Ann. § 2C:25-19 (1992).

49. *Id.*

50. *Supra* note 23, at 873-874 and accompanying notes 438-444.

51. *See, e.g., id.,* at 1043-1048 and accompanying notes 1510-1540.

52. *Supra* note 22.

53. For extended discussion of "no further abuse" clauses, *see, e.g., supra* note 23, at 914-918 and accompanying notes 712-743.

54. For extended discussion of "stay away" provisions, *see, e.g. id,* at 918-925 and accompanying notes 744-782.

55. For extended discussion of "no contact" provisions, *see, e.g. id,* at 925-931 and accompanying notes 783-722.

56. For extended discussion of "orders to vacate," *see, e.g., id.,* at 931-936 and accompanying notes 823-856.

57. For extended discussion of "property rights," *see, e.g. id.* at 937-941 and accompanying notes 857-886.

58. For extended discussion of orders concerning weapons *see, e.g., id.,* at 941-944 and accompanying notes 887-909.

59. For extended discussion of treatment and counseling issues, *see, e.g., id.,* at 944-949 and accompanying notes 910-950.

60. For extended discussion of custody issues, *see, e.g., id.,* at 949-981 and accompanying notes 951-1140.

61. For extended discussion of visitation issues, *see, e.g., id.,* at 982-990 and accompanying notes 1141-1208.

62. For extended discussion of spousal and child support issues, *see, e.g., id.,* at 997-1000 and accompanying notes 1244-1263.

63. For extended discussion of other forms of monetary relief, *see, e.g., id.,* at 990-996 and accompanying notes 1209-1243. *See also id.,* at 1000-1006 and accompanying notes 1264-1300.

64. *See id.,* at 1095-1099 and accompanying notes 1828-1851.

65. *Id.* at 1097-1098 and accompanying notes 1840-1841. For extended discussion of acts constituting civil and criminal contempt, *see, e.g., id.,* at 1102-1112 and accompanying notes 1871-1939.

66. *See, e.g., Cole v. Cole,* 556 N.Y.S. 2d 217 (Fam. Ct. 1990); *City of Reynoldsburg v. Eichenberger,* No. CA-3492, 1990 Ohio App. LEXIS 1613 (Apr 18, 1990); *People v. Townsend,* 538 N.E. 2d 1297 (Ill. App. Ct. 1989); *State v. Kilponen,* 737 P. 2d 1024 (Wash. Ct. App. 1987); *supra* note 23, at 1112-1117 and accompanying notes 1940-1973.

67. 509 U.S. 688 (1993).

68. For extended discussion of the contemnor's due process rights, *see, e.g., supra* note 23, at 1120-1129 and accompanying notes 1992-2039.

69. *See* N.D. Lemon, *Domestic Violence: A Benchguide for Criminal Cases* 151 (1989).

70. For extended discussion of sentencing issues in domestic violence cases, *see, e.g., supra* note 23, at 1129-1142 and accompanying notes 2040-2105.

71. 42 U.S.C. § 13981 (1994). Victims may sue in federal or state court and seek compensatory and punitive damages, an injunction or a declaratory judgment, and attorney's fees. A prior criminal action is not required to pursue the civil remedy.

72. 18 U.S.C. § 2265 (1994).

73. 42 U.S.C. § 13951 (1994).

74. 8 U.S.C. § 1151 (1994).

75. 8 U.S.C. § 1254 (1994).

76. 18 U.S.C. §§ 2261, 2262 (1994). In *U.S. v. Page,* No. 96-4083 (6th Cir. 1998), the Sixth Circuit held that the Violence Against Women Act does not criminalize domestic violence that occurs before interstate travel. Rather the statute covers only domestic violence occurring "in the course of or as a result of" such travel. Consequently the statute criminalizes the aggravation of injuries inflicted before interstate travel only so long as the worsening of the injuries was caused by intentional violent conduct during interstate travel.

77. 18 U.S.C. §§ 2263, 2264 (1994).

78. 42 U.S.C. § 10416 (1994).

79. 18 U.S.C. §§ 2241-48 (1994).

80. 42 U.S.C. § 14011 (1994).

81. 18 U.S.C. §2245(2) (1994).

82. 28 U.S.C. § 2074 (1994).

83. *See, e.g., U.S. v. Lankford,* No. 98-10645 (5th Cir. 1999); *U.S. v. Page,* 167 F. 3d 325, 334 (6th Cir. 1999); *U.S. v. Gluzman* 154 F. 3d 49, 50 (2d Cir. 1998), *cert. denied,* 119 S.Ct. 1257 (1999).

84. *U.S. v. Morrison/Brzonkala v. Morrison,* 169 F. 3d 820 (1999).

85. *Supra* note 23, at 1148-1158 and accompanying notes 2151-2201. *See also* Wanless, *Notes: Mandatory Arrest: A Step Toward Eradicating Domestic Violence, But Is It Enough?* U. Ill. L. Rev. 533 (1996). One of the goals of mandatory arrest statutes is to change police officers' attitudes that domestic partners should be left to resolve their disputes privately and that domestic violence is not a serious crime.

86. *Supra* note 23, at 1157.

87. *See, e.g., id.,* at 1142-1148 and accompanying notes 2106-2150.

88. 18 U.S.C. § 13 (Repl. 1997).

89. *United States v. Kearney,* 750 F. 2d 787 (9th Cir. 1984).

90. 18 U.S.C. § 1961 (Repl. 1997).

91. 18 U.S.C. § 922 (g) (9). The constitutionality of these amendments has been upheld in *Gillespie v. City of Indianapolis,* No. 98-2691 (7th Cir. 1999).

92. *See, e.g., People v. Evans,* 259 Ill.App. 3d 195, 197 Ill. Dec. 278, 631 N.E. 2d 281 (1994); Stone, Defense, in *The Impact of Domestic Violence on Your Legal Practice* 7-5 – 7-8 (Goelman, Lehrman, & Valente eds., 1996); W.R. LaFave & A.W. Scott, Criminal Law, 454-463 (2d ed., West, St Paul, Minn. 1986).

93. *Id.*

94. *See, e.g., State v. Nunn,* 356 N.W. 2d 601 (Iowa App. 1984); *Commonwealth v. Grove,* 363 Pa.Super. 328, 526 A. 2d 369 (1987); *People v. Aris,* 215 Cal.App. 3d 1178, 264 Cal.Rptr. 167 (1989); *State v. Stewart,* 243 Kan. 639, 763 P. 2d 572 (1988).

95. L.E. Walker, *The Battered Woman,* 42-55 (1979); L.E. Walker, *The Battered Woman Syndrome* 95-104 (1984). Walker suggested that an abusive relationship can be described as a cycle with three phases: (1) the tension-building phase, characterized by slight instances of physical or emotional abuse; (2) the acute battering phase, characterized by more frequent and escalated instances of violence; and (3) the loving contrition phase, characterized by the offender's apologies and repeated promises to change his behavior. The term *battered spouse* refers to a woman who has been through the cycle at least twice. In phase one the woman's tendency to avoid the batterer may reinforce the pattern of abusiveness. Women in phase two tend to cope with frenzies of violence and wait for an ebb in the flow of abuse. Relief and dread are common to women in phase three; this lull in the abuse may inflict the most severe psychological trauma on the woman. *See* L.E. Walker, *Terrifying Love: Why Battered Women Kill and How Society Responds* 43-62 (1989).

96. *See, e.g., Developments in the Law: Domestic Violence,* 106 Harvard Law Review 1574 (1993); Schneider, *Describing and Changing: Womens' Self-Defense Work and the Problem of Expert Testimony on Battering,* 9 Women's Rights L. Rep. 195 (1986).

97. The profiles of battered women who kill their partners often do not fulfill the criteria of "learned helplessness" or "psychological paralysis." *See, e.g.,* Meier, *Notes From the Underground: Integrating Psychological and Legal Perspectives on Domestic Violence in Theory and Practice,* 21 Hofstra L. Rev. 1295 (1993); Allard, *Rethinking Battered Woman Syndrome: A Black Feminist Perspective,* 1 U.C.L.A. Women's L.J. 191 (1991); Schopp et al., *Battered Woman Syndrome, Expert Testimony, and the Distinction Between Justification and Excuse,* 1 U. Ill. L. Rev. 45 (1994); Stark, *Re-presenting Woman Battering: From Battered Woman Syndrome to Coercive Control,* 58 Alb. L. Rev. 973 (1995); Maguigin, *Battered Women and Self-Defense: Myths and Misconceptions in Current Reform Proposals,* 140 U. Pa. L. Rev. 379 (1991); Dutton, *Understanding Women's Response to Violence: A Redefinition of Battered Woman Syndrome,* 21 Hofstra L. Rev. 1191 (1993); Callahan, *Will the "Real" Battered Woman Please Stand Up? In Search of a Realistic Definition of Battered Woman Syndrome,* 3 Am. U.J. Gender and L. 117 (1994).

98. *See, e.g.,* Walker, *Battered Woman Syndrome and Self-Defense,* 6 Notre Dame J.L. Ethics and Pub. Policy 321 (1992) (defining battered women's syndrome as a form of posttraumatic stress disorder); Stark, *supra* note 96, at 1201 (suggesting that battered women are subject to entrapment or coercive control by the perpetrator); Dutton, supra note 96. Dutton proposes that (1) descriptive references should be made to "expert testimony concerning battered women's experiences," rather than to "battered woman syndrome" per se; (2) the scope of testimony concerning battered women's experiences should be framed within the overall social context that is essential for explaining battered women's responses to violence; and (3) evaluation and testimony concerning battered women's psychological reactions to violence should incorporate the diverse range of traumatic reactions described in the scientific literature, and should not be lim-

ited to an examination of learned helplessness, post-traumatic stress disorder, or any other single reaction or "profile."

99. *See, e.g., State v. Kelly,* 97 N.J. 178, 478 A. 2d 364 (1984); *State v. Gallegos,* 104 N.M. 247, 719 P. 2d 1268 (Ct. App. 1986); *Commonwealth v. Stonehouse,* 521 Pa. 41, 64, 555 A. 2d 772, 784 (1989); *State v. Koss,* 49 Ohio St. 3d 213, 551 N.E. 2d 970 (1990); *Arcoren v. United States,* 929 F. 2d 1235 (8th Cir. 1991) (holding that Federal Rule of Evidence 702 encompasses the use of psychiatric and psychological evidence).

100. In *Navarro v. Block,* No. 96-5569 (9th Cir. 1999), the Ninth Circuit addressed the issue of whether domestic violence crimes result in severe injury or death less frequently than nondomestic violence crimes that are considered 911 emergencies. Citing a lack of evidence supporting an assumption that domestic violence crimes are less injurious than nondomestic violence crimes, the court reversed and remanded a trial court ruling that 911 dispatcher policy equating domestic violence calls with "not-in-progress" calls, and equating nondomestic violence calls with "in-progress" calls, was rational and reasonable.

101. Bowker et al., *On the Relationship Between Wife Beating and Child Abuse, in Perspectives on Wife Abuse* 158, 164 (Yllo & Bograd eds., 1988); Pagelow, *Effects of Domestic Violence on Children and Their Consequences for Custody and Visitation Agreements,* 7 Mediation Q. 347 (1990); P.G. Jaffe et al., *Children of Battered Women* 2 (1990); Mahoney, *Legal Images of Battered Women: Redefining the Issue of Separation,* 90 Mich. L. Rev. 1, 5 (1991); G.L. Greif & R.L. Hegar, *When Parents Kidnap* 30 (1993); Edleson, *Mothers and Children: Understanding the Links Between Woman Battering and Child Abuse, in A Report of the Violence Against Women Research Strategic Planning Workshop* (Nat'l Inst. of Justice, Washington, D.C. 1995).

102. Judicial Subcommittee, Commission on Domestic Violence, American Bar Association, *Judicial Checklist, in The Impact of Domestic Violence on Your Legal Practice* 13-7 (Goelman, Lehrman, & Valente eds., 1996).

103. *See, e.g.,* Hart & Hofford, *Child Custody, in The Impact of Domestic Violence on Your Legal Practice* 5-1 – 5-6 (Goelman, Lehrman, & Valente eds., 1996). For a discussion of child support issues in the context of domestic violence, see Haynes, *Child Support, in The Impact of Domestic Violence on Your Legal Practice* 5-7 – 5-10 (Goelman, Lehrman, & Valente eds., 1996).

104. *See, e.g.,* Dakis & Karan, *Judicial Intervention, in The Impact of Domestic Violence on Your Legal Practice* 13-1 – 13-9 (Goelman, Lehrman, & Valente eds., 1996).

105. *See, e.g.,* H.R. Con. Res. 172, 101st Cong., 2d Sess. (1990); *see also* National Council on Juvenile and Family Court Judges, *Family Violence: A Model State Code* 33 (1994).

106. *Supra* note 95 at 13-1.

107. *See Foran v. Foran,* 834 P. d 1081 (Wash. Ct. App. 1992) (holding that, even where evidence of premarital domestic violence was not sufficient to support a finding that the wife was coerced into signing, it could show that it inhibited her willingness to seek independent counsel).

108. *See, e.g., Snedaker v. Snedaker,* 660 So. 2d 1070 (Fla. Dist. Ct. App. 1995) (upholding award of $125,000 for assault and battery claims despite valid prenuptial agreement that severely limited battered woman's recovery in divorce).

109. See Berner & Klaw, *Prenuptial Agreements, in The Impact of Domestic Violence on Your Legal Practice* 6-1 – 6-3 (Goelman, Lehrman, & Valente eds. 1996).

110. *See, e.g.,* New York Victim Service Agency, *The Cost of Domestic Violence: A Preliminary Investigation of the Financial Cost of Domestic Violence* (1987). In 1992 nearly 20% of the women killed in the workplace were murdered by a current or former husband or male partner. Bureau of Labor Statistics, National Census of Fatal Occupational Injuries (Aug 3, 1995).

111. *See, e.g.,* Alaska Stat. § 12.61.010(5) (1995); 18 Pa. Cons. Stat. § 4957(a).

112. *See, e.g.,* Kuperberg & Lieblein, *Corporate Liability, in The Impact of Domestic Violence on Your Legal Practice* 10-6–10-10 (Goelman, Lehrman, & Valente eds., 1996).

113. *Id.* at 10-6.

114. Occupational Safety and Health Act of 1970, § 5(a)(1), 29 U.S.C. § 651, § 654(a) (1994) (requiring an employer to "furnish each of his employees employment and a place of employment free from recognized hazards that are causing or likely to cause death or serious physical harm to his employees").

115. *See, e.g.,* 82 Am. Jur. 2d *Workers' Compensation* § 73 (1992).

116. *See, e.g., Tart v. Colonial Penn. Ins. Co.,* No. 2019 (Pa. C.C.P. Sept. 1985) (holding that a cause of action existed).

117. *Supra* note 112 at 10-7.

118. 82 Am. Jur. 2d *Workers' Compensation* §§ 358, 359 (1992 and Supp. 1995); Cal. Lab. Code § 3208.3 (Deering 1995) (holding that California's workers compensation statute encompassed compensation for a victim's psychiatric injury caused by work-related violence).

119. *See, e.g.,* Me. Rev. Stat. Ann. tit. 26, § 1193(1)(A)(4) (West 1995). Unemployment benefits may not be denied, for example, if a domestic violence victim is discharged after being absent from work due to injuries from battering, because the absence would not reflect an "intentional disregard of the employer's interests." *See Boynton Cab Co. v. Neubeck,* 296 N.W. 636 (Wis. 1941).

120. *Supra* note 104.

121. *See, e.g.,* Keller, Snell, & Wilmer, *Workplace Violence: The Employer's New Catch-22* (1995); Larson, *Employment Screening,* §§ 2.10, 3.04(1)(a), 3.04(2)(a)(b), 9.11 (1995). Also, as of 1996, at least 13 states had enacted laws designed to restrict insurance discrimination on the basis of domestic violence. These states are Arizona, California, Connecticut, Delaware, Florida, Indiana, Iowa, Maine, Massachusetts, Minnesota, New Hampshire, Pennsylvania, and Tennessee. *See* Fromson, *Insurance Discrimination Against Victims of Abuse, in The Impact of Domestic Violence on Your Legal Practice* 10-21 (Goelman, Lehrman, & Valente eds., 1996).

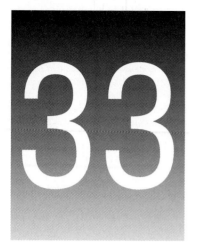

Geriatric patients

MARSHALL B. KAPP, J.D., M.P.H.

ELDER MISTREATMENT
GUARDIANSHIP AND ITS ALTERNATIVES
RESEARCH WITH OLDER HUMAN SUBJECTS
FINANCING MEDICAL CARE FOR GERIATRIC PATIENTS
ELDER LAW AS A GROWING SPECIALTY

Medical advances enable more Americans to live longer than their predecessors. In recent years the segment of our population that is older than 65 years has increased dramatically. This growth may be summarized briefly as follows.[1] Persons 65 years or older numbered 34.1 million in 1997, representing 12.7% of the U.S. population, or one in eight Americans. The number of older Americans increased by 2.8 million or 9.1% since 1990, compared with an increase of 7% for the under-65 population. About 2 million persons celebrated their 65th birthday in 1997 (5335 per day); in the same year, more than 1.7 million persons aged 65 or older died, resulting in a net increase of 214,000 (587 per day).

The older population itself is getting older. In 1997 the 65- to 74-year-old age group (18.5 million) was eight times larger than in 1990, but the 75- to 84-year-old group (11.7 million) was 16 times larger and the 85 and older group (3.9 million) was 31 times larger.

A relatively small number (1.4 million) and percentage (4%) of the over-65 population lived in nursing facilities in 1995. However, the percentage increased dramatically with age, ranging from 1% for persons aged 65 to 74 years to 5% for persons aged 75 to 84 years and 15% for persons 85 and older.

The likelihood of developing chronic health problems increases sharply with age. Most older persons have at least one chronic condition, and multiple conditions are not uncommon. The most common chronic conditions in persons aged 65 and older are arthritis, hypertension and other heart problems, sensory impairments, orthopedic impairments, and diabetes. Other problems include memory loss, dementia, and depression. Mental stress often creates serious physical complications in the aged. The major causes of death for older people are heart disease, stroke, and cancer.

Most of the generic chapters in this volume are fully pertinent to care of the elderly, although general medicolegal concepts frequently take on special meaning as applied specifically to older persons. For instance, informed consent to medical interventions is required of persons of all ages,

but when older persons are involved, special attention must be paid to issues of decisional capacity and (especially when the patient is institutionalized) the voluntariness of decisions.

This chapter does not discuss the particular application of generic concepts to older persons. Instead the purpose here is to outline several selected topics involving the intersection of law and medicine in the care of the elderly population.

ELDER MISTREATMENT

Only in the last three decades have we been willing to publicly admit, let alone begin to address, the phenomenon of serious mistreatment of older persons both within home settings and institutional environments. Unfortunately, the problem is prevalent; it is estimated that more than 2 million older adults are mistreated each year in the United States.[2] The problem is by no means limited to this country[3] or to any particular racial or ethnic group.[4]

The definition of elder abuse and neglect is a matter of state law. Each state has enacted its own statutory schema in this arena, with substantial variation among particular definitions and procedures as a consequence.[5,6]

The American Medical Association has described elder abuse and neglect as "actions or the omission of actions that result in harm or threatened harm to the health or welfare of the elderly."[7] These actions or inactions may take place in the elder's home or that of a relative, at the hands of an informal caregiver,[8] or in an institutional setting.[9] A single incident may constitute abuse or neglect in most states, although usually a repeated pattern is discovered and in some jurisdictions is necessary to meet statutory definitions of abuse and neglect. Random criminal assaults of older persons by strangers (e.g., in the context of a robbery) generally are excluded from the category of elder mistreatment as it is being considered in this chapter.

Among the different forms of elder mistreatment are physical (e.g., assault, forced sexual contact, overmedication, inappropriate physical restraints); psychological or emotional (e.g., threats); denial of basic human needs by the caregiver (e.g., withholding indicated medical care or food); deprivation of civil rights (e.g., freedom of movement and communication)[10]; and financial exploitation.[11]

One of the more alarming examples of elder mistreatment is the abandonment of older, severely cognitively impaired persons in hospital emergency departments without identification or explanation by relatives who were providing home-based care.[12] Estimates of the incidence of this practice of "Granny dumping" range up to 70,000 older persons annually.[13]

In addition, a significant proportion (up to half in some states) of reported cases of elder mistreatment fall into the category of self-neglect by older persons living alone, without any informal (i.e., unpaid family or friends) or formal (i.e., paid) caregivers.[14] Examples of self-neglect may include an individual's failure to maintain adequate nutrition, hydration, or hygiene; use physical aids such as eyeglasses, hearing aids, or false teeth; or maintain a safe environment for himself or herself. Self-neglect may be suspected in the presence of dehydration, malnourishment, decubitus ulcers, poor personal hygiene, or lack of compliance with basic medical recommendations.

A few states have enacted distinct statutes dealing with cases of institutional abuse and neglect of older residents. These statutes may apply to nursing facilities, board and care homes, and assisted living arrangements. Even without such precisely focused legislation in a particular jurisdiction, resident mistreatment by long-term care institutional staff is prohibited by federal regulations,[15] as well as by state institutional licensure statutes and common law tort standards.[16] These are significant restrictions on the use of involuntary mechanical and chemical restraints.[17] Also, several states explicitly lump together institutional and informal caregiver mistreatment in the same statutes, rather than legislatively handling them distinctly.

Every state has exercised its parens patriae power to protect those who cannot fend for themselves by enacting a statute dealing with the reporting of elder mistreatment suspicions by health care professionals to specific public welfare or law enforcement authorities.[18,19] Some state statutes single out the elderly, whereas others just use age 18 and vulnerability to mistreatment as the criteria for reporting and intervention. At least 43 states plus the District of Columbia mandate reporting of suspected elder abuse and neglect, with criminal penalties and/or civil fines specified for noncompliance in most statutory schemes. A private tort action may also be brought by a mistreatment victim whose injuries were exacerbated by the professional's failure to report in timely fashion.

The remaining jurisdictions make reporting a voluntary matter, with legislation stating that a report "may" rather than "shall" be filed. Whether reporting of mistreatment cases is required or only permitted, all of the statutes immunize the mandated or authorized reporters against any potential liability (e.g., for breach of the duty of patient confidentiality or for defamation) for making the report, as long as the report was made in good faith and without malicious intent.[20,21]

GUARDIANSHIP AND ITS ALTERNATIVES

Although the law presumes that adults are capable of making voluntary, informed, and understanding decisions that affect their lives, sometimes this presumption is not accurate.[22] A significant minority of older individuals have impaired ability to make and communicate their own choices about personal (including medical) and financial matters in a rational and authentic manner. The prevalence of dementia and other severe mental disabilities among the aged indicates the strong probability that this phenomenon will expand in the future. One important device within the legal system for dealing with the problem of cognitively incapacitated individuals, and the concomitant need for some form of surrogate decision-making on their behalf, is guardianship.

Guardianship is a legal relationship, authorized by a state court, between a ward (the person whom a court has declared to be incompetent to make decisions) and a guardian (whom the court appoints as the surrogate decision-maker for the ward). Terminology regarding this relationship varies somewhat among jurisdictions; in some states, for example, this concept is referred to as *conservatorship.*

Judicial appointment of a guardian to make decisions on behalf of a person who has been adjudicated incompetent means that the ward no longer retains the power to exercise those decisional rights that have been delegated to the guardian. The legal system historically has treated guardianship as an "all-or-nothing" proposition, global findings of incompetence being accompanied by virtually complete disenfranchisement of the ward. The trend lately, however, has been toward statutory recognition of the concept of limited or partial guardianship, which accounts for the decision-specific nature of mental capacity and the ability of some people rationally to make certain kinds of choices but not others,[23] and encouragement of judicial deference to this idea.

A number of alternatives to plenary, private guardianship exist for assisting older individuals with cognitive impairments to navigate through the vicissitudes of daily life.[24] Some of these alternatives involve advance planning, whereas others are imposed on the individual in the absence of such planning.

A variety of legal and financial strategies have evolved that enable individuals, while still mentally and physically capable of rationally making and expressing their own choices, to plan ahead for the contingency of future incapacity. These advance-planning mechanisms promote the principle of autonomy by permitting an individual to prospectively direct or shape subsequent personal decisions even if contemporaneous expression of wishes has become impossible.

Many of these devices pertain to prospective influence over monetary matters; they include joint bank accounts, automatic deposits, living trusts, personal money management services, powers of attorney, and durable powers of attorney. The chief advance planning mechanisms available for future medical decisions are the living will and the durable power of attorney for health care. These written directives[25] are discussed in depth elsewhere in this text.

Although it usually works as intended, advance financial and health care planning sometimes goes badly. The geriatric clinician may become aware, for instance, of an agent named under a now-incapacitated patient's durable power of attorney who is misusing or exploiting the patient's finances, abusing the patient, or grossly neglecting the patient's medical needs. In such circumstances, the clinician confronts ethical quandaries about whether to initiate a guardianship proceeding or otherwise request court involvement. When the clinician sees no other effective, less restrictive means of dealing with such scenarios,[26] referring the situation to the legal system, through official notification of the local adult protective services (APS) agency, is probably the best course to follow.

There also is evidence that physicians not infrequently fail to honor patients' advance medical directives.[27] A number of initiatives have been launched in a concerted effort to educate both medical professionals and the general public about the significance and expectations of advance medical planning.[28]

The majority of people who become decisionally incapacitated have failed to take advantage of the advance planning mechanisms just outlined. For this bulk of the cognitively impaired population, alternatives to standard plenary, private guardianship fall into two categories: alternative forms *of* guardianship (e.g., limited and/or temporary) and alternatives *to* guardianship.

For a growing number of older persons whose cognitive impairments would technically qualify them for guardianship—plenary or limited—the most pressing practical problem is the unavailability of family members or close friends who are willing and able to assume guardianship responsibilities. In the absence of a state public guardianship system, local volunteer guardianship program, or sufficient assets to hire a private, proprietary professional guardian, the cognitively incapacitated individual with no family or friends (the "unbefriended") often literally "falls between the cracks." Important decisions, including those involving medical treatment, may by default go without being made until an emergency has developed and the doctrine of presumed consent applies.

Even in the absence of advance planning for incapacity by the individual, some form of official guardianship for the cognitively incapacitated older person is by far the exception rather than the rule. Unplanned alternatives to guardianship include representative payees for government benefit payments, APS (including their emergency intervention powers), family consent statutes, and the informal but universally accepted practice of asking next of kin for authorization to provide or withhold specific interventions.

RESEARCH WITH OLDER HUMAN SUBJECTS

The disproportionate prevalence of dementias and other severe mental disabilities among the elderly has been noted previously. The legal, as well as ethical, Catch 22 of conducting biomedical and behavioral research using older human subjects who are severely demented or otherwise cognitively compromised presents a dilemma.[29] On the one hand, progress in developing effective treatments and cures for medical and psychological problems associated with dementia requires that research projects be done in which individuals suffering from the precise problems of interest be the basic units of study. At the same time, paradoxically, those very problems that qualify an individual for eligibility as a subject in such a research project often make it impossible for that person to engage in a rational and autonomous decision-making process about his or her own participation as a research subject.[30] This irony is exacerbated by the fact that research subjects generally are more vulnerable to possible exploitation, and hence need more protection, than patients in therapeutic situations because of, among other things, the researchers' potential conflicts of interest.

Federal regulations covering biomedical and behavioral research require that informed consent for participation be obtained from the "subject or the subject's legally authorized representative."[31] However, a subject's legally authorized representative is defined in circular fashion to mean an "individual or judicial or other body authorized under applicable [presumably state][32] law to consent on behalf of a prospective subject."[33]

A number of alternative possibilities for proxy decision-making in the research context have been identified. These devices include the durable power of attorney for research participation, reliance on family consent statutes, informal reliance on available family members as surrogate decision-makers, guardianship with specific authorization for research decisions, explicit prior court orders authorizing the incapacitated subject's participation in research protocols on a case-by-case basis, an independent patient advocate supplied by the organization sponsoring the research or by a government agency, and selection of a surrogate by the Institutional Review Board (IRB) or a long-term care facility's resident council.

Some have suggested that special procedural safeguards are necessary to protect vulnerable, cognitively impaired human subjects from injury due to research participation. These safeguards might encompass heightened IRB involvement in the protocol approval process, enhanced IRB activity in the postapproval ongoing monitoring and supervision phase of the research including serving as a forum for appeals and objections, and requiring individual subject assent (i.e., giving subjects a veto power) even when informed proxy consent to research participation has been obtained.[34] An important question, especially since the subjects of interest are mentally impaired, concerns the definition of assent to be used, namely, whether the failure to actively object to participation in a protocol is enough to be interpreted as a tacit or implied form of assent or whether some more affirmative indication of agreement is necessary.

In 1998 the National Bioethics Advisory Commission (NBAC) issued a report[35] that among other things made the following recommendations for when the potential human subjects in a research protocol are mentally impaired.

- For any protocol involving greater than minimal risk, there should be an independent assessment of each potential subject's decisional capacity.
- For any protocol involving greater than minimal risk, the IRB should require the investigator to explicitly describe to the IRB the process to be used to assess the decisional capacity of potential human subjects.
- For protocols involving greater than minimal risk and no prospect of direct benefit to that study's human subjects (a category into which most research seeking to enroll the mentally impaired elderly probably falls), the protocol should be reviewed and approved by a newly created national IRB or under guidelines established by that national IRB, and the subject's legally authorized representative must consent.

FINANCING MEDICAL CARE FOR GERIATRIC PATIENTS

Medical care (acute and chronic) for geriatric patients currently is financed through a crazy-quilt combination of personal out-of-pocket payments, Medicaid (primarily for nursing facility care), payments from private Medicare supplementary insurance policies purchased individually by the patient (i.e., "Medigap" policies), and (until recently) Medicare Parts A and B. Medicare Part C was enacted by Congress as part of the 1997 Balanced Budget Act (BBA).[36] This new program created the Medicare+Choice Program, which provides an array of private health insurance options for Medicare beneficiaries. These options include health maintenance organizations, competitive medical plans, provider-sponsored organizations, medical savings accounts, and private fee-for-service plans. Under the BBA and implementing regulations,[37] each eligible older and disabled individual now has the right to choose between remaining in federally regulated Parts A and B or enrolling in one of the Part C Medicare+Choice market-oriented options.

Explicit suggestions that certain aspects of medical care be rationed categorically according to a patient's age[38] in general have been soundly rejected in public policy debate. However, there is growing evidence that medical care is indeed rationed by age de facto, in the sense that older people in many circumstances are treated less aggressively than younger counterparts from whom they cannot be distinguished in terms of prognosis or other relevant medical criteria.[39]

ELDER LAW AS A GROWING SPECIALTY

Over the last two and a half decades, the field of elder law as a specialty of legal practice has burgeoned. Educational in-

stitutions offer specialized courses and other learning opportunities in this sphere for attorneys and other professionals, focused textbooks and practice handbooks have proliferated, journals have arisen, and national and state organizations devoted to the field have developed and grown.[40]

The content of elder law is expansive. Matters falling within this area include, at least, advice to and representation of older persons, their families, and physicians and other service providers regarding Social Security retirement and disability benefits; other federal and state benefits; Medicare and Medicaid (including asset sheltering and divestiture for eligibility purposes)[41]; housing issues, financial management (e.g., trusts), and estate planning; medical treatment decision-making and advance planning; judicial and nonjudicial forms of substitute decision-making; elder abuse and neglect; employment discrimination; and tax counseling. Elder law practice is necessarily interdisciplinary and interprofessional in nature, entailing cooperation among the attorney, physicians and other health and human services providers, governmental agencies, and nonlegal advocacy and support organizations.

ENDNOTES

1. American Association of Retired Persons, *A Profile of Older Americans* (AARP, Washington, D.C. 1998).
2. D.L. Swagerty, P.Y. Takahashi, & J.M. Evans, *Elder Mistreatment,* 59 Am. Family Physician 2804-2808 (1999).
3. M. Bradley, *Elder Abuse,* 313 Br. Med. J. 548-550 (1996).
4. T. Tatara ed., *Understanding Elder Abuse in Minority Populations* (Taylor & Francis, Philadelphia 1999).
5. L.A. Stiegel, *Recommended Guidelines for State Courts Handling Cases Involving Elder Abuse* (American Bar Association Commission on Legal Problems of the Elderly, Washington, D.C. 1995).
6. T. Tatara, *An Analysis of State Laws Addressing Elder Abuse, Neglect, and Exploitation* (National Center on Elder Abuse, Washington, D.C. 1995).
7. American Medical Association Council on Scientific Affairs, *Elder Abuse and Neglect,* 257 J.A.M.A. 966-971 (1987).
8. A.C. Homer & C. Gilleard, *Abuse of Elderly People by Their Caregivers,* 301 Br. Med. J. 1359-1362 (1990).
9. K. Pillemer & D.W. Moore, *Highlights from a Study of Abuse of Patients in Nursing Homes,* 2 J. Elder Abuse Neglect 529 (1990).
10. M.B. Kapp, *Restraining Impaired Elders in the Home Environment: Legal, Practical, and Policy Implications,* 4 J. Case Mgt. 5459 (1995).
11. American Medical Association, *Diagnostic and Treatment Guidelines on Elder Abuse and Neglect* (AMA, Chicago 1992).
12. J.R. Conrad, *Granny Dumping: The Hospital's Duty of Care to Patients Who Have Nowhere to Go,* 10 Yale L. Pol'y Rev. 463-487 (1992).
13. M. Beck & J. Gordon, *A Dumping Ground for Granny: Weary Families Drop Her in the Emergency Room,* 64 Newsweek 1991.
14. United States General Accounting Office, *Elder Abuse: Effectiveness of Reporting Laws and Other Factors,* GAO/HRD-91-74 (GAO, Washington, D.C. 1991).
15. 42 Code of Federal Regulations §§ 483.10, 483.15, 483.25.
16. P.W. Iyer ed., *Nursing Home Litigation: Investigation and Case Preparation* (Lawyers and Judges Publishing Company, Tucson, Az. 1999).
17. M.B. Kapp, *Restraint Reduction and Legal Risk Management,* 47 J. Am. Geriatric. Soc. 375-376 (1999).
18. K.C. Kleinschmidt, *Elder Abuse: A Review,* 30 Ann. Emerg. Med. 463-472 (1997).
19. M.D. Velick, *Mandatory Reporting Statutes: A Necessary Yet Underutilized Response to Elder Abuse,* 3 Elder L.J. 65-190 (1995).

20. E. Capezuti, B.L. Brush, & W.T. Lawson III, *Reporting Elder Mistreatment,* 23 J. Geront. Nurs. 24-32 (1997).

21. D.E. Rosenblatt, K.-H. Cho, & P.W. Durance, *Reporting Mistreatment of Older Adults: The Role of Physicians,* 44 J. Am. Geriatr. Soc. 65-70 (1996).

22. T. Grisso & P.S. Appelbaum, *Assessing Competence to Consent to Treatment* (Oxford University Press, New York 1998).

23. M.B. Kapp & D. Mossman, *Measuring Decisional Capacity: Cautions on the Construction of a `Capacimeter,'* 2 Psychol., Public Policy & L. 73-95 (1996).

24. M.B. Kapp, *Guardianship and its alternatives: enhanced autonomy for diminished capacity,* in *Older Adults' Decision-Making and the Law* (M. Smyer, K.W. Schaie, & M.B. Kapp eds., Springer, New York 1995).

25. N.M.P. King, *Making Sense of Advance Directives,* rev. ed. (Georgetown University Press, Washington, D.C. 1996).

26. W.C. Schmidt Jr., *Guardianship: The Court of Last Resort for the Elderly and Disabled* (Carolina Academic Press, Durham, NC 1995).

27. SUPPORT Principal Investigators, *A Controlled Trial to Improve Care for Seriously Ill Hospitalized Patients: The Study to Understand Prognoses and Preferences for Outcomes and Risks of Treatments,* 274 J.A.M.A. 1591-1598 (1995).

28. D.E. Meier & R.S. Morrison, guest eds., *Care at the End of Life: Restoring a Balance,* XXIII Generations, 198 (1999).

29. M.B. Kapp, *Decisional Capacity, Older Human Research Subjects, and IRBs: Beyond Forms and Guidelines,* 9 Stanford L. & Policy Rev. 359-371 (1998).

30. R. Dresser R, *Mentally Disabled Research Subjects: The Enduring Policy Issues,* 276 J.A.M.A. 67-72 (1996).

31. 45 Code of Federal Regulations § 46.116 and 21 Code of Federal Regulations § 50.20.

32. 45 Code of Federal Regulations § 116(e) and 21 Code of Federal Regulations § 50.25(c).

33. 45 Code of Federal Regulations § 46.102(d) and 21 Code of Federal Regulations § 50.3(m).

34. G.A. Sachs, J. Rhymes, & C.K. Cassel, *Biomedical and Behavioral Research in Nursing Homes: Guidelines for Ethical Investigations,* 41 J. Am. Geriatr. Soc. 771-777 (1993).

35. National Bioethics Advisory Commission, *Research Involving Persons with Mental Disorders that May Affect Decision-Making Capacity,* (NBAC, Washington, DC 1998).

36. Public Law No. 105-33, 1997.

37. 64 Federal Register 7968, 1999.

38. D. Callahan, *Setting Limits: Medical Goals in an Aging Society* (Simon & Schuster, New York 1987).

39. M.B. Kapp, *De Facto Health Care Rationing By Age: The Law Has No Remedy,* 19 J. Legal Med. 323-349 (1998).

40. S.J. Hemp & C.R. Nyberg, *Elder Law: A Guide to Key Resources,* 3 Elder L.J. 1-87 (1995).

41. A.D. Budish, *The All-New Avoiding the Medicaid Trap: How to Beat the Catastrophic Costs of Nursing Home Care* (Henry Holt & Company, New York 1995).

Oncology patients

MELVIN A. SHIFFMAN, M.D., J.D., F.C.L.M.

RECURRENT PROBLEMS IN LAWSUITS RESULTING FROM A FAILURE
  TO DIAGNOSE CANCER
RADIATION THERAPY
CHEMOTHERAPY
GENETICS
GENETIC COUNSELING
UNORTHODOX CANCER TREATMENTS
CONCLUSION

The oncology patient presents many medical and surgical problems for the physician that are peculiar to the cancer patient. Most lawsuits involve misdiagnosis or, more likely, late diagnosis. Legal actions can involve failure to properly treat, complications of treatment, or lack of informed consent. The statute of limitations may become an aspect of the litigation, usually in defense of the physician.

Patients alleging misdiagnosis or delayed diagnosis are basically complaining of a "loss of chance." Usually the question is whether the misdiagnosis or late diagnosis caused, to a reasonable medical probability or certainty, the patient's injury or whether the natural course of events was unchanged.

Chemotherapy is often associated with complications. There may be consent problems, including informed consent or informed refusal of care, where oncology patients are concerned. The physician may choose to use therapeutic professional discretion to keep medical facts from the patient when the physician believes disclosure would be harmful, dangerous, or injurious to the patient.

The use of radiation therapy is frequently the source of medicolegal problems. The resolution of these problems may involve invoking risk-benefit judgment, which requires comparing the anticipated benefits from therapy with its risks and weighing the consequences of no treatment.

Cancer diagnosis and therapy have been influenced by recent information obtained through genetic studies. A new frontier of possible litigation involves the privacy of genetic information, loss of employment because of a genetic abnormality, and inability to obtain or increased cost of health or life insurance because of a genetic defect. State and federal statutes have been slowly evolving to protect the rights of individuals from genetic discrimination even when there is no present observable disability and only the presumption of a disability. Because patients with cancer are often desperate, a physician must address the legal consequences of administering unorthodox treatment, particularly if the patient insists on it.

RECURRENT PROBLEMS IN LAWSUITS RESULTING FROM A FAILURE TO DIAGNOSE CANCER

Although variations in the standard of care and damage awards make generalizations imprecise, there are circumstances under which successful actions for failure to diagnose cancer have repeatedly arisen. These recurrent themes are presented here in a manner to help prevent lawsuits from failure to diagnose cancer while improving patient care and should be of value to all those physicians who treat or examine patients in various clinical settings.

Medical history

The medical history is an important part of the diagnostic workup of cancer, as well as other diseases, and is stressed in the introductory course in physical diagnosis in most medical schools. Unfortunately, many physicians neglect this important aspect of medical practice once out of medical school and either take no history at all or fail to go into depth in their patient interviews. Failure to take a medical history, or obtaining an incomplete medical history, may be a significant factor in failure to diagnose a cancer case.

As a result of a failure to obtain an adequate history, a physician may not include the diagnosis of certain cancers in the differential diagnoses or may not give proper weight to a diagnosis of possible cancer when evaluating certain clinical signs and symptoms. This inappropriately low suspicion of cancer may at times be negligent.

Example 1. Family history or racial history of certain cancers is an important factor in evaluating asymptomatic patients for cancer screening and for obtaining the proper, indicated tests in certain symptomatic patients.[1]

Example 2. Occupational exposure, such as asbestos-related occupations, or social habits, such as alcoholism or smoking, may be important factors in the medical history in evaluating a patient for pulmonary neoplasm, liver cancer, or other malignancies and, if not elicited, could be important in establishing negligence in failure to diagnose certain cancers.

Example 3. Significant x-ray exposure (e.g., breast neoplasia following tuberculosis pneumothorax collapse therapy, or thyroid cancer as a sequel to childhood radiation of benign head and neck problems), other radiation exposures (e.g., Thorotrast-induced liver cancer), or chemical exposure (e.g., benzene-induced malignancy) may be significant.

Example 4. Exposure of a patient's forebears to certain drugs or carcinogens may increase the patient's own cancer risk (e.g., vaginal clear-cell carcinoma in diethylstilbestrol [DES] daughters). Failure to inquire of this history, warn of dangers, and give guidelines to the patient herself may be considered negligent.[2]

Overreliance on certain facts obtained in taking the medical history may be just as significant in certain cases as failure to take an adequate history. Failure to detect the clues of certain symptoms as related by the patient because of a history of "cancerophobia" has been a factor in certain failures to diagnose cancer cases.[3]

Physical examination

Failure to perform a physical examination, performing an inadequate examination, overreliance on a negative examination, or failure to perform a follow-up examination may contribute to suits for failure to diagnose cancer.

Failure to perform an examination, especially after a presenting complaint referable to an organ later found cancerous, figures prominently in many failures to diagnose cancer cases, as does failure to perform follow-up examinations. In the 1985 case of *Gorman v. LaSasso,*[4] a Colorado jury awarded $1 million to a woman in her thirties who complained about the presence of a lump in her breast for six months, which was not investigated until the fourth time she complained about it.

Ordering a test in lieu of a physical examination will not necessarily protect a physician. A California jury in 1982 held for the plaintiff, who was dying of metastatic breast cancer, when her cancer was not diagnosed after her internist relied on a falsely negative mammogram report, prescribed pain medication for her breast lump, and told her to return only if the lump enlarged. An appellate court added $55,368 to the award for what the court called a frivolous appeal.[5]

Referral and testing

A physician has an affirmative duty to obtain or perform appropriate tests in the diagnosis of a suspected cancer. In

Barenbrugge v. Rich,[6] a gynecologist did not order a mammogram on his 28-year-old patient after she presented with a breast lump later proven cancerous. He contended the test was dangerous for women under age 30. His consultation with a general surgeon, who also did not order the test, did not exonerate him from blame. A 1985 Illinois jury returned a verdict for $3 million.

Failure of a physician to refer to another physician or specialist for a suspected cancer may also be a negligent act of omission. In the case of *O'Dell v. Chesney,*[7] a doctor of chiropractic treated a 63-year-old man for rectal bleeding and diabetes for two years. He was held negligent for failing to refer the patient to a medical doctor. The plaintiff died from colorectal cancer. The jury verdict of $125,000 was reduced by 40% because of the plaintiff's comparative negligence.

Failure of a physician to read the test report or consultant's recommendations or to communicate the report or recommendations to the patient may be negligent. In *Mehalik v. Morvant,*[8] a 42-year-old Louisiana woman was referred by her physician for a mammogram to evaluate a breast lump. Her physician told her that the mammogram report was negative, although the radiologist reported a suspicious mass and recommended follow-up monitoring. Relying on this report, she did not return for follow-up evaluation. A large breast cancer was confirmed later at biopsy, and the patient sued her physician for damages, with a resultant settlement.

Failure to repeat a test, perform additional studies, such as monoclonal antibody studies, or refer for biopsy when an initial test is negative may be negligent when clinical suspicion is (or should be) high that cancer may still be present.

A Massachusetts jury in the 1985 case *Brown v. Nash*[9] awarded $3 million to a woman because a surgeon failed to diagnose her breast cancer when he relied on a negative mammogram report, despite a changing physical abnormality noted in her breast. Relying on the false-negative report, he elected not to do a biopsy of an area later shown to be cancerous. The changing mass should have alerted him that a cancer was present, despite the negative report.

In *Glicklich v. Spievack,*[10] another Massachusetts court awarded $578,000 to a woman who was not referred by her primary care physician to a surgeon for a biopsy, even though he relied on a false-negative mammogram report and a negative needle biopsy of a breast lump later diagnosed as malignant.

Even where a biopsy report is negative, overreliance on that report may be negligent when clinical suspicion should be high. A federal judge in 1985, in the case of *Burke v. United States,*[11] awarded $1 million to a Maryland woman whose breast biopsy was erroneously interpreted as benign by a pathologist. Relying on this biopsy report, her surgeon dismissed her complaints of further change in her breast and did not order additional testing or perform another biopsy of the area, which later proved cancerous.

Mere reliance on a test performed by a consultant does not always mean negligence, however. A Louisiana court in

Lauro v. Travelers Insurance Co.[12] held that a surgeon was not negligent to have removed a breast for cancer when a frozen section revealed a malignancy, even though later study revealed that a nonmalignant myeloblastoma (a very rare tumor) was found on final review.

Failure to follow recommended protocol

The American Cancer Society and various professional specialty organizations have for a number of years published guidelines for physicians, suggesting schedules or protocols for early cancer detection. Although not binding in any way, these recommendations are widely disseminated through the mass media and are common public knowledge.

Failure to follow these protocols is not necessarily evidence of negligent failure to diagnose cancer. In fact, many physicians in practice do not follow these guidelines,[13,14] either because of ignorance or because they disagree with the society's educational program, which emphasizes the importance of early cancer detection.

However, it is common in litigation involving cancer diagnosis for attorneys to use compliance or noncompliance with published guidelines for health care, whether called "standards" or not, as evidence of satisfaction of the standard of care required. Box 34-1 shows the guidelines for cancer-related checkups recommended by the American Cancer Society.[15]

Delayed diagnosis of breast cancer

Delayed diagnosis of breast cancer is the most frequent cause of litigation related to cancer. Analysis of medicolegal cases shows that breast cancer is involved in 36.7% of cases of delayed diagnosis of cancer.[16] An inordinate delay in the diagnosis of breast cancer may result in a worse prognosis than if there were no delay. In legal terms, loss of chance is related to the probability (more likely than not or more than 50% chance) that there is a decrease in survival. Patients tend to perceive any delay in the diagnosis as decreasing their chance of survival.[17] Litigation is possible if a timely diagnosis is not made.

Haagenson et al.[18] found the following errors by physicians, which resulted in delay in the diagnosis of breast cancer:

1. Failure to examine a breast containing an obvious tumor while treating the patient for an unrelated disease.
2. Failure in palpation of the breast to recognize the tumor of which the patient is complaining.
3. Mistaking a cancer for a breast infection.
4. Wrongfully diagnosing a breast cancer as a benign lesion and failing to advise a biopsy or excision.
5. Disregarding a history of acute and sharp pain in the breast.
6. Disregarding a sign of retraction.
7. Failure to determine the cause of nipple discharge.
8. Relying on a normal aspiration biopsy.

Early treatment of breast cancer is sound practice because the success of treatment, such as surgery, chemotherapy, ra-

diotherapy, and immunotherapy, is predicated on minimal tumor burden.[19]

RADIATION THERAPY

More than half of all cancer patients will ultimately need radiation therapy. The physician and the patient must weigh the benefits of therapy against the possible complications. Newer techniques have been developed with the use of the electron and proton beams to allow more accurate placement of the treatment with less damage to surrounding tissues.

Principles

Ionizing radiation may be used in the treatment and palliation of malignant tumors. Radiation sources include the cobalt-60 teletherapy unit, linear accelerator, and radioactive isotopes such as iridium-192, iodine-125, and phosphorus-32.[20]

The biological effects of radiation are directly proportional to the dose. Cell death occurs from inability to reproduce, meta-

---

BOX 34-1. GUIDELINES FOR CANCER-RELATED CHECKUPS

1. Health counseling and cancer checkup to include examination for cancers of the thyroid, testicles, prostate, ovaries, lymph nodes, and skin every 3 years after the age of 20 and every year after the age of 40
2. Sigmoidoscopy after the age of 50 to include two normal examinations 1 year apart and then every 3 to 5 years
3. Stool guaiac slide test every year after the age of 50
4. Digital rectal examination every year after the age of 40
5. In women
   a. Papanicolaou test every year after age 18 or before age 18 if sexually active (After three consecutive normal examinations, test may be performed less frequently at physician's discretion.)
   b. Pelvic examination every year after age 18 or before age 18 if sexually active
   c. Endometrial tissue sample at menopause in women at high risk with a history of infertility, obesity, failure to ovulate, abnormal uterine bleeding, or estrogen therapy
   d. Breast self-examination monthly after the age of 20
   e. Breast examination every 3 years between ages 20 and 40 and every year after the age of 40
   f. Mammography every 1 to 2 years between ages 40 and 49 and every year after the age of 50

Data from American Cancer Society, *Survey of Physicians' Attitudes and Practices in Early Cancer Detection,* 35 CA 197-213 (1985); Woo, *Screening Procedures in the Asymptomatic Adult,* 254 J.A.M.A. 1480-1484 (1985); C. Metlin & C.R. Smart, *Breast Cancer Detection Guidelines for Women Ages 40 to 49 Years: Rationale for the American Cancer Society Reaffirmation of Recommendations,* CA-A Cancer J. for Clinicians 248-255 (1994); and A.M. Leitch et al., *American Cancer Society Guidelines for the Early Detection of Breast Cancer: Update 1997,* 47 CA-A Cancer J. for Clinicians 150-153 (1997).

bolic cell failure, or degeneration of the cell structure. Malignancies and normal body organs vary in their sensitivity to radiation, and therefore the dosage must be regulated in accordance with the desired results. It is possible to sensitize tissues to increase the response to radiation by the use of oxygen, nitric oxide, and metronidazole or through the use of hyperthermia.

Complications

Proper radiation may result in skin burns consisting of erythema (redness) or desquamation (dry or wet).[21] Ulceration with necrosis may be seen with prolonged healing time and scar deformity. Permanent pulmonary fibrosis in the treatment field for cancer of the breast does occur at times. Development of radiation enteritis after treatment of intraabdominal malignancies is not unknown. Excessive radiation has been one source of litigation.

In *Duke v. Morphis,*[22] radon seeds were implanted in the supraclavicular area for treatment of a malignancy. The patient suffered myelopathy and paralysis, blaming the radiation treatment plan and the manner of supervision. The plaintiff was awarded $266,700.

In *Rudman v. Beth Israel Medical Center,*[23] a similar problem of paralysis after radiation treatment of a head and neck cancer brought a $2 million settlement.

In *Barnes & Powers v. Hahnemann Medical College and Hospital,*[24] a patient with cervical cancer was treated with radiation therapy and radium implants. After a radical hysterectomy she suffered radiation cystitis, vesicovaginal fistula, radiation fibrosis of the ileum, and radiation fibrosis of the vagina. Multiple further surgeries were necessary to correct these problems. The case was settled for an undisclosed amount.

CHEMOTHERAPY

Medical oncology is a changing field, and new chemotherapeutic agents and new combinations of agents are being investigated at a rapid pace. No other medical specialty handles extremely dangerous drugs on an almost daily basis. The potential side effects of these medications can affect every organ system, and yet these drugs are helping to save or prolong more lives.

Many of the antineoplastic drugs are mutagenic, teratogenic, and carcinogenic in animals.[25] Exposure to these agents can result in the appearance of mutagenic substances in the urine.[26] There have been reports of an increased incidence of acute myelogenous leukemia in patients treated with alkylating agents,[27] and bladder cancer[28] has been associated with the use of cyclophosphamide, especially in low doses over prolonged periods.

Chemotherapeutic agents can be fetotoxic and therefore potentially dangerous to health care personnel. Drugs that have been associated with fetal malformations include folate antagonists, 6-mercaptopurine, and alkylating agents,[29] as well as the MOPP (nitrogen mustard, vincristine, procar-

bazine, prednisone) treatment for Hodgkin's disease.[30] Personnel safety guidelines have been established to protect personnel who are mixing and administering antineoplastic drugs.[31]

Many patients are aware of some of the possible physical effects of chemotherapy and are fearful of feeling sicker than they already are. This makes the oncologist's job more difficult when trying to convince patients of the potential favorable effect on their malignancy and at the same time playing down the potential dangers. Patients, however, require knowledge of the possible benefits and the possible complications, as well as any viable alternative of treatment and their potential complications.

Principles

Chemotherapeutic agents are used to kill malignant cells. Because cellular destruction occurs by the effect on reproducing cells, those cells dividing frequently are more susceptible. The drugs, however, do not discriminate between normal and malignant tissues. Therefore normal organ systems may be adversely affected.

Complications

Hypersensitive reactions may occur with edema, rash, bronchospasm, diarrhea, and hypotension.[32] Some drugs such as doxorubicin or mitoxantrone are cardiotoxic. Bleomycin may cause pulmonary fibrosis. Hair loss (alopecia), leukopenia, and anemia are accepted side effects.

In *Lefler v. Yardumian*[33] there was a leak of intravenous chemotherapy agents into the subcutaneous area of the arm. Tissue ulceration and damage to the tendons of the left hand occurred. The defense claim that the plaintiff was negligent in causing her own injuries resulted in a defense verdict.

Inadvertent overdose has been a source of litigation. In *Newman v. Geschke,*[34] a patient with throat cancer was given 12 to 15 mg of vincristine by the office nurse. This amount was nine to ten times the normal prescribed dosage. He developed neuropathies, bowel and bladder incontinence, weight loss, and alopecia and required three weeks of hospitalization. The case was settled for $450,000.

GENETICS

The recent rapid evolution of genetics in cancer research has provided physicians with the means of identifying individuals and their family members who are at high risk for developing cancer. Ethical, legal, and social implications of genetic abnormalities have become the medical community's new challenge.[35] Some of the genes associated with hereditary cancers are listed in Table 34-1.

Genetic discrimination has occurred in the past and is more likely to occur in the future without more adequate laws.[36] During the introduction of state-based screening programs for sickle cell disease during the 1970s, people were

TABLE 34-1. Genes associated with hereditary cancers

Cancer	Chromosome	Gene
Breast and ovarian cancer	BRCA1	17q21
Breast cancer	BRCA2	13q12-13
Li-Fraumeni syndrome/SBLA	p53	17p13
Lynch syndrome/HNPCC	MSH2	2p
Melanoma	MLM	9p21
Medullary thyroid	RET	10q11.2
Neurofibromatosis	NF1	17q11.2
Retinoblastoma	RB1	13q14
Turcot's syndrome		
Predominance of glioblastoma	PMS2	7p22
Multiform	MLH1	3p21.3-23
Predominance of cerebellar medulloblastoma	APC	5q21
Familial adenomatous polyposis	APC	Distal to 5´
Hereditary flat adenoma syndrome	APC	Proximal to 5´
von Hippel-Lindau disease	VIIL3	3p25
Wilms' tumor	WT1	11p13

HNPCC, Hereditary nonpolyposis colorectal cancer; *SBLA,* sarcoma, breast and brain tumors, leukemia, laryngeal and lung cancer, and adrenal cortical carcinoma.

denied health insurance and jobs simply because they were identified as carrying one copy of the gene—a trait that has no implications for their health.[37]

Four important points were made in Dr. Healy's testimony at the Hearing on the Possible Uses and Misuses of Genetic Information at a Subcommittee of the House of Representatives on October 17, 1991[38]:

1. Real benefits are expected from the use of new genetic knowledge.
2. Genetic information can be misused and abused.
3. The rights of people to determine for themselves whether to pursue genetic information about themselves must be defended even from the forced choices that discriminating social practices may create.
4. Discrimination based on genotype must be prohibited as a matter of basic civil rights.

State statutes

Before 1991, legislation addressing the genetics issues was somewhat limited to prohibition of health insurers from refusing to issue insurance or from charging higher premiums based on certain specific genetic abnormalities (i.e., sickle cell trait, hemoglobin C trait, thalassemia minor trait, and Tay-Sachs trait). In 1991 a new phase of legislation began that was directed toward prohibition of health insurers from requiring a genetic test, conditioning the provision of insurance coverage or benefits on genetic testing, or considering genetic testing in determining rates.

Laws presently in effect regarding genetic information include the following:

- Alabama Code § 27-5-13 (Michie 1982): Prohibits denial of health or disability insurance because of sickle cell anemia.
- Arizona Rev. Stat. Title 18 § 20-448 (West 1989): Prohibits refusal to consider an application for life or disability insurance on the basis of a genetic condition (a specific chromosome or single-gene genetic condition) unless applicant's medical condition and history and either claims experience or actuarial projections establish that substantial differences in claims are likely to result from the genetic condition.
- California Ann. Codes, Insurance §§ 10123.3 et seq. (West 1994): Prohibits self-insured employee welfare benefit plans from refusing to enroll a person, requiring a higher rate or charge, offering or providing different terms, conditions or benefits, or discriminating in the fees or commissions of a solicitor or solicitor firm on the basis of genetic characteristics that may under some circumstances be associated with disability in that person or that person's offspring (including, but not limited to, Tay-Sachs trait, sickle cell trait, thalassemia trait, and X-linked hemophilia A).

Prohibits life or disability insurance companies from refusing to issue, sell, or renew a policy solely on the basis of tests of a person's genetic characteristics (defined as any scientific or medically identifiable gene or chromosome or alteration thereof, which is known to be a cause of a disease, or determined to be associated with a statistically increased risk of development of a disease or disorder that is presently not associated with any symptoms of a disease or disorder).

Prohibits requiring a test of a genetic characteristic for the purpose of determining insurability other than by informed consent and privacy protection. Prohibits life disability insurer from requiring a genetic characteristic test if the results would be used exclusively or nonexclusively for the purpose of determining eligibility for hospital, medical, or surgical insurance coverage or eligibility for coverage under a nonprofit hospital service plan or health care service plan.

Prohibits negligent or willful disclosure of the results of a test for a genetic characteristic to any third party for use in a manner which identifies or provides identifying characteristics of the person to whom the test results apply except by written authorization.

- California Ann. Codes, Insurance § 11512.95 (West 1980): Prohibits nonprofit hospital service plan from refusing to enroll or accept as subscriber, requiring a higher rate or charge, or requiring any rebate, discrimination, or discount upon the amount paid of the services rendered under the plan solely by reason of the fact that the person carries a gene which may, under some circumstances, be associated with disability in that person's offspring, but which causes no adverse effects on the carrier.

- California Ann. Codes, Health and Safety § 1374.7 (West 1977): No plan shall refuse to enroll or accept, require a higher rate or charge, or make or require any rebate, discrimination, or discount upon the amount to be paid or the service to be rendered any person solely by reason that the person carries a gene which may, under some circumstances, be associated with disability in that person's offspring, but which causes no adverse effects on the carrier.
- Colorado Rev. Stat., Insurance § 10-3-1104.7 (Bradford 1994): Prohibits release of genetic testing information that identifies the person tested without specific written consent by the person tested.

Prohibits any entity that receives information derived from genetic testing from seeking, using, or keeping the information for any nontherapeutic purpose or for any underwriting purpose connected with the provisions of health care insurance, group disability insurance, or long-term care insurance coverage.

- Florida Stat. Ann., Insurance, Title 37 §§ 626.9706 & 626.9707 (West 1978): Prohibits insurer from refusing to issue, deliver, or carry a higher premium or disability insurance rate or charge for life insurance solely because the person has the sickle cell trait.
- Florida Stat. Ann. § 760.40 (West 1994): Provides for genetic testing to be performed only with the consent of the person to be tested and result may not be disclosed without the consent of the person tested.
- Iowa Code Ann. § 729.6 (West 1992): Prohibits employer, employment agency, labor organization, licensing agency, or its employees, agents, or members from soliciting, requiring, or administering a genetic test as condition of employment, preemployment application, labor organization membership, or licensure or from affecting the terms, conditions, or privileges of employment, memberships, or licensure of any person who obtains a genetic test.
- Maryland Ann. Code, Art 48A § 223 (Michie 1986): Prohibits insurer from refusing to insure or make or permit differential in ratings, premium payments, or dividends in connection with life insurance and life annuity contracts solely because the person has sickle cell trait, thalassemia minor trait, hemoglobin C trait, Tay-Sachs trait, or any genetic trait that is harmless within itself, unless there is actuarial justification for it.
- Minnesota Stat. Ann. § 144.91 (West 1977): Authorizes the state commissioner of health to develop and carry on a program to collect and interpret data, assemble, prepare, and disseminate informational material, and conduct research studies in the field of human genetics.
- Montana Code Ann. § 33-18-206 (1991): Prohibits an insurer from refusing to consider, rejecting an application, or determining rates, terms, or conditions of a life or disability contract on the basis of genetic condition unless applicant's medical condition and history and either claims experience or actuarial projections established that substantial differences in claims are likely to result from the genetic condition.
- Montana Code Ann. § 50-19-211 (1985): Establishes a voluntary genetic program to offer testing, counseling, and education to parents and prospective parents.
- New Hampshire Rev. Stat. Ann. §§ 141-H:1 141-H:6 (Michie 1996): Provides that no individual or member of the individual's family shall be required to undergo genetic testing as a condition of doing business with another person.

Prevents disclosure to any person that an individual has undergone genetic testing or disclosure of results of such testing without the prior written and informed consent of the individual.

Prohibits employer, labor organization, employment agency, or licensing agency from soliciting, requiring, or administering genetic testing as a condition of employment, labor organization membership, or licensure or from affecting the terms, conditions, or privileges of employment, membership, or licensure based on genetic testing.

Prohibits insurer, in connection with health insurance, from requiring or requesting an individual or a member of the individual's family to reveal prior genetic testing or undergo genetic testing or to condition the provision of or determine rates or any other aspect of health insurance coverage or health care benefits on whether an individual has undergone genetic testing.

- New Jersey Stat. Ann. Title 10 §§ 10:5-5 et seq. (West 1992): Prohibits employer from refusing to hire or employ or to bar or to discharge or require to retire from employment or discriminate in compensation, or in terms, conditions, or privileges of employment because of a typical hereditary cellular or blood trait (i.e., sickle cell trait, hemoglobin C trait, thalassemia trait, Tay-Sachs trait, or cystic fibrosis trait).
- Ohio Rev. Code §§ 1742.42 et seq. (Anderson 1994): Prohibits any health maintenance organization from requiring genetic testing, making inquiry to determine results of genetic screening or test, or refusing to issue or renew coverage based on results of genetic screening or testing.
- Wisconsin Stat. Ann. §§ 111.32 et seq. (West 1991): Prohibits employer, labor organization, employment agency, or licensing agency from soliciting, requiring, or administering a genetic test as a condition of employment, memberships, or licensure or affecting the terms, conditions, or privileges of employment, memberships, or licensure or terminating employment, memberships, or licensure of any person who obtains a genetic test.

• Wisconsin Stat. Ann.§ 631.89 (West 1991): Prohibits an insurer that provides health care services for individuals on a self-insured basis from requiring or requesting an individual to obtain a genetic test or reveal whether a test has been obtained and the results of the test, or conditioning the provision of or rates of insurance coverage or health care benefits on whether an individual has obtained a genetic test or what the results of the test were. This does not apply to an insurer writing life insurance coverage or income continuation insurance coverage.

Most states have general laws that prohibit unfair discrimination by both life and health insurers. These laws are too generalized to provide adequate protection for those individuals who, though presently asymptomatic, may develop future health problems as a result of a specific genetic abnormality.

Federal statutes

The only federal statute that directly relates to genetic disorders[39] establishes the ability of the government to (1) make grants and contracts with public and nonprofit private entities for projects for basic or applied research and planning; (2) establish programs for the training of genetic counselors, social and behavioral scientists, and other health professionals; (3) develop programs to educate practicing physicians, other health professionals, and the public regarding the nature and inheritance patterns of genetic diseases and the means and methods to diagnose, control, counsel, and treat genetic diseases; and (4) develop counseling and testing programs for the diagnoses, control, and treatment of genetic diseases. Under these programs there is strict confidentiality of all test results and medical records unless given informed consent by the individual. In the Public Health Service, a program is established for voluntary testing, diagnosis, counseling, and treatment of individuals with regard to genetic diseases.

The Rehabilitation Act of 1973. The Rehabilitation Act[40] prohibits discrimination on the basis of handicap by federal agencies, by any program or activity that receives federal financial assistance, and by employers having contracts of $2500 or more with the federal government. Also prohibited is discrimination in education, public housing, and eligibility for government benefits and services. "Handicap" refers to any person who (1) has a physical or mental impairment that substantially limits one or more major life activities, (2) has a record of such an impairment, or (3) is regarded as having such an impairment. Although genetic abnormality is not specifically stated, discrimination is prohibited based on an employer's fear of the employee's future real or perceived disability that may affect his or her ability to perform the job adequately or safely. In such cases, the employer must prove through expert testimony the existence of a reasonable probability of substantial risk that the employer's fear is justified and that the risk is imminent and not speculative or remote in time.[41]

Americans with Disabilities Act of 1990. One of the purposes of the Americans with Disabilities Act (ADA)[42] is to provide a clear and comprehensive mandate for eliminating discrimination against individuals with disabilities. The ADA addresses the discriminatory effects of benign actions or inaction as well as intentional discrimination.

The statute will probably be successfully invoked against various types of genetic discrimination in employment. However, there is no mention of alleviating genetic discrimination by insurance companies.

Employee Retirement Income Security Act. The Employee Retirement Income Security Act (ERISA)[43] preempts state regulation of self-insuring employers' benefit plans including health insurance. No federal laws specifically address the problem of genetic discrimination in health insurance, although many individuals are under self insured health plans not subject to state insurance laws.

Human Genome Privacy Act. The proposed Human Genome Privacy Act (HGPA) defines "genetic information" as any information that describes, analyzes, or identifies all or any part of a genome identifiable to a specific individual. HGPA would permit an individual access to his or her own genetic information with the opportunity to request correction or supplementation of that information. Disclosure of genetic information to third parties would be prohibited except by written informed authorization by the individual involved. Confidentiality is limited to safeguarding genetic information maintained by federal agencies or their contractors or grantees.

GENETIC COUNSELING

Genetic counseling is necessary before genetic testing and includes education on the natural history of genetic disorders, genetics, and surveillance. The individual and high-risk family members who have been counseled may then submit to DNA testing, if this available; the DNA test results are revealed on a one-to-one basis by the physician or genetic counselor,[44] and management recommendations are discussed. This includes methods and timing of surveillance as well as available prophylactic medical and surgical therapy.

Familial adenomatous polyposis

Colonic adenomas are likely to occur in patients with a mutant adenomatous polyposis coli (APC) gene (90% penetrance). Adenomas are manifested in 15% of gene carriers by age 10, 70% by age 20, and 90% by age 30.

Screening recommendation for patients who test negative for the APC gene in families with familial adenomatous polyposis (FAP) is flexible sigmoidoscopy at ages 18, 25, and 35 years. The lifetime risk for colon cancer is the same as for the general population (3% to 5%), and offspring will not be at risk for FAP.[45]

If testing is positive for the APC gene, annual flexible sigmoidoscopy should begin at age 10 or 11 years. When adenomatous polyposis is present, the patient is counseled to prepare for eventual colectomy, and upper gastrointestinal screening for polyposis should be performed every 1 to 3 years. Offspring will be at 50% risk for FAP.[46]

Hereditary nonpolyposis colorectal cancer

In hereditary nonpolyposis colorectal cancer (HNPCC), colonoscopy is initiated in high-risk individuals at 25 years of age and repeated biennially through age 35 and annually thereafter. If DNA testing has shown one of the HNPCC abnormalities, annual colonoscopy is started at age 20.[47]

If a patient develops colorectal cancer, subtotal colectomy is recommended because of the high incidence of multiple colorectal cancers. Women with colorectal cancer who have completed their families may submit to prophylactic hysterectomy and bilateral salpingo-oophorectomy at the same time as the colon surgery to prevent cancers that may develop under the Lynch II syndrome. Patients with DNA-proven HNPCC mutation have the option for prophylactic subtotal colectomy.[48]

Familial breast cancer syndromes

Familial breast cancer syndromes are heterogeneous and require a thorough family history (both maternal and paternal). Hereditary breast cancer is more likely in women with family members who have had early onset breast or ovarian cancer (before age 50), bilateral breast cancer, or two or more affected first-degree relatives with breast or ovarian cancer.[49] Breast cancer gene (BRCA1) predictive testing is available only under research studies, and BRCA2 testing, although cloned, is unavailable as of yet. Women at high risk for breast or ovarian cancer may have close surveillance that includes monthly breast self-examination, annual diagnostic mammograms, and physician breast examinations every 4 to 6 months.[50] The tamoxifen chemoprevention trial is currently available for high-risk women over the age of 35 years. Prophylactic bilateral mastectomy may be an option, depending on the patient's choice after adequate counseling.[51]

Women who are at high risk for breast or ovarian cancer (BRCA1) may have surveillance with transvaginal ultrasound and CA125 measurement every six months.[52] They can be offered prophylactic oophorectomy after completing childbearing following counseling.[53]

Multiple endocrine neoplasms

In affected members (chromosome 10q11.2 abnormality) of families with multiple endocrine neoplasms (MEN) 2A (and 2B) or a familial medullary carcinoma, C-cell hyperplasia (the precursor to carcinoma) occurs in 100% of patients by age 30.[54] The average age at which C-cell hyperplasia or medullary thyroid carcinoma is detected by biochemical screening (Pentagastrin and calcium stimulation tests) in at-risk subjects is 10 years.[55]

Prophylactic thyroidectomy is performed when the annual screening test becomes positive or by the age of 3 to 12 years.[56] Treating thyroxine deficiency is relatively easy.

Pheochromocytoma usually becomes evident about 10 years later than C-cell hyperplasia and medullary carcinoma. Early biochemical abnormalities include an increase in urinary epinephrine or norepinephrine. Screening should begin at the time of thyroidectomy.[57] Tumors can also be identified by computed tomography, magnetic resonance imaging, or 131 I-labeled metacodobenzylguanidine imaging, even in patients with no biochemical abnormality. However, repeated imaging studies are expensive and radiation exposure may become a hazard. Adrenalectomy is performed when a tumor is identified. Bilateral adrenalectomy is usually necessary because tumor is frequently found in the contralateral adrenal gland.

Periodic measurement of ionized serum calcium is essential to diagnose hyperparathyroidism. The involved gland should then be surgically removed. Genetic counseling is available for any hereditary cancers in which the implicated gene has been identified.

Significant cases

Hernandez v. United States.[58] The district court found for the defendant and set forth the following requirements for compliance with the standard of care in cases where a woman had a breast complaint:

1. That a history be taken to determine her age, her age at her first pregnancy, the history, if any, of breast cancer in the family, and whether or not she is using birth control pills
2. That the examination consist of visual observation of the skin and nipple and manual palpation of the breasts while she is lying down with her arms over her head.
3. That the physician, either upon finding or failing to find a lump, assess whether further diagnostic procedures or follow-up visits are indicated.

The court of appeals reversed the judgment for the defendant holding that the standard of care was different for a woman with a particular breast complaint than for a woman without a complaint and an essential element is that the physician be aware of or attempt to resolve the particular complaint presented by the patient.

Katsbee v. Blue Cross/Blue Shield of Nebraska.[59] In January 1990 the appellant, with a family history of breast and ovarian cancer, was diagnosed by her gynecologist in consultation with Dr. Henry T. Lynch (oncologist geneticist) as having a genetic condition known as breast-ovarian carcinoma syndrome. Prophylactic total abdominal hysterectomy and bilateral salpingo-oophorectomy were recommended. Preoperatively, the health insurance company refused to pay for the procedure, but the appellant proceeded with the surgery in November 1990. The appellant filed this action for breach of contract. The Supreme Court reversed the summary judgment in favor of the insurer, holding that the insured's breast-ovarian carcinoma syndrome was an "illness" defined as "bodily disorder" or "disease," within the meaning of the health insurance policy, notwithstanding the insurer's contention that the syndrome was merely predisposition to cancer.

Webster's Third International Dictionary[60] defines disease as "an impairment of the normal state of the living animal . . . . [M]any of its components . . . interrupt or modify the performance of the vital functions . . . to inherit defects of the organism or to combinations of these factors." *Dorland's Illustrated Medical Dictionary*[61] defines disease as "any deviation from or interruption of the normal structure or function of any part, organ, or system (or combination thereof) of the body that is manifested by a characteristic set of symptoms and signs and whose etiology, pathology, and prognosis may be known or unknown."

UNORTHODOX CANCER TREATMENTS

Despite persistent efforts to achieve early detection and exhaustive research aimed at developing effective treatment modalities, cancer continues to be a leading cause of death in the United States. Conventional cancer therapy includes surgery, chemotherapy, and radiation therapy in various combinations, depending on the nature and extent of disease involved in each particular case. Elaborate treatment protocols have been developed for virtually every stage of every type of cancer. These medical advances have undoubtedly resulted in increased survival or improved quality of life for some cancer patients. For many others, however, conventional cancer therapy has simply come to mean a sequence of painful, even disabling, experiences that does not in any way alter the inexorable course of the disease and does not make the patient more comfortable, productive, or fulfilled during the time that remains.

For many years, cancer victims have attempted to seek out whatever ray of hope may be offered, even in the form of treatment that the medical establishment finds to be unproven, ineffective, or even fraudulent. These include metabolic therapy, diet therapies, megavitamins, mental imagery applied for antitumor effect, and spiritual or faith healing.[62] Despite recent technological advances in orthodox medical care, unorthodox cancer treatments are increasing in popularity.[63]

Cancer victims, particularly those who are terminally ill, are vulnerable to exploitation because of their predicament. Desperate for any glimmer of hope, they are easy prey for charlatans intent on financial gain. Traditionally, the law has protected those unable to protect themselves on the basis of parens patriae. This rationale has most frequently been applied to juveniles and the developmentally disabled.

However, the state's interest in protecting its citizens must be balanced against an individual's right to have control over his or her own body and to make decisions regarding his or her own medical care. Most cancer patients are adults in full control of their mental faculties, which distinguishes them from other citizens the state seeks to protect under the parens patriae rationale.

It is this basic conflict between the state's interest in the health and welfare of its citizens and the right of the individual to make decisions affecting his or her health that has confronted legislatures and courts attempting to deal with the problem of unorthodox cancer treatments.

To date, this conflict has not been resolved uniformly. Considerable variation currently exists among the various states with regard to regulation of unorthodox cancer treatment. Interestingly, where there has been legislative action, most legislatures have granted the individual some measure of freedom in selecting cancer treatment that is unproven. In most states that have acted legislatively, however, this freedom is not unlimited. When courts have considered the subject of unorthodox cancer treatment, they have focused more on the state's right to regulate the lives of its citizens under the police power.

Legislative approaches

The overwhelming majority of legislation dealing with unorthodox cancer treatment has concerned Laetrile (amygdalin). Nineteen states have enacted legislation authorizing the manufacture, sale, and distribution of Laetrile.[64] Other unorthodox cancer treatments that have received legislative protection include DMSO (dimethyl sulfoxide),[65] Gerovital H3 (procainamide hydrochloride with preservatives and stabilizers),[66] lily plant extract,[67] and prayer.[68]

Most states that have legislatively authorized the use of Laetrile have placed concurrent restrictions on its accessibility. Twelve states require that the treatment be prescribed by a licensed physician.[69] Three states allow the use of Laetrile only as an adjunct to conventional medical therapy.[70] Many of the states that require a licensed physician's prescription of the unorthodox treatment also require that the patient first sign a consent form indicating that the physician has explained that Laetrile or DMSO has not been proved to be effective in the treatment of cancer or other human diseases, that it has not been approved by the Food and Drug Administration for the treatment of cancer, that alternative therapies exist, and that the patient requests treatment with Laetrile or DMSO.[71]

Several states have attempted to maintain a precarious balance between police power and individual rights by reserving the right to prohibit unconventional cancer treatment when it is found to be harmful as prescribed or administered in a formal hearing before the appropriate state board.[72]

The most sweeping exercise of police power has been enacted in California, where it is a crime to sell, deliver, prescribe, or administer any drug or device to be used in the diagnosis, treatment, alleviation, or cure of cancer that has not been approved by the designated federal agency or by the state board.[73] As discussed later, the statute has been upheld by the California Supreme Court against a constitutional challenge based on the right of privacy.[74]

Judicial determination regarding unorthodox cancer therapy

The lack of uniformity among the states in regulating the use of unorthodox cancer treatments has created an environment in which patients who reside in states that do not authorize the manufacture, sale, or distribution of Laetrile or other unconventional therapies have attempted to obtain those substances from other states, or even from neighboring countries.[75] In several instances, patients have resorted to legal action in attempting to obtain Laetrile.

The most extensively litigated case has been *Rutherford v. United States,* which has generated eight federal court opinions,[76] including one from the U.S. Supreme Court.[77] *Rutherford* was a class action suit brought on behalf of terminally ill cancer patients who sought to enjoin the federal government from interfering with the interstate shipment and sale of Laetrile. The district court granted the injunction and ordered the government to permit Mr. Rutherford to purchase Laetrile. The basis for the ruling was that Laetrile, in proper doses, was nontoxic and effective in curing Mr. Rutherford's cancer.[78]

On appeal, the Court of Appeals for the Tenth Circuit instructed the district court to remand the case to the Food and Drug Administration (FDA) to determine whether Laetrile was a new drug as defined in the federal Food, Drug, and Cosmetic Act,[79] and whether it was exempt from premarketing approval by the FDA under either of the Act's grandfather clauses.[80]

The FDA found that Laetrile did constitute a new drug under the applicable statutory definition because it was not generally recognized among experts as safe and effective for its prescribed use.[81] The FDA further determined that Laetrile was not exempt from premarketing approval under the applicable statute criteria.[82]

The case was then sent back to the district court, which reversed the FDA's determination and held that Laetrile was entitled to an exemption from premarketing approval and further held that denial of cancer patients' rights to use a nontoxic substance in connection with their personal health violated their constitutional right of privacy.[83]

The Court of Appeals for the Tenth Circuit subsequently approved the lower court decision allowing the plaintiffs to obtain Laetrile, but did not address the constitutional issue.[84]

The U.S. Supreme Court granted certiorari and reversed the Tenth Circuit's ruling.[85] The Supreme Court did not consider the right of privacy issue. It held that, under applicable statutory law, Laetrile was not a "safe and effective" drug, and therefore FDA approval was required before interstate distribution. The court felt that if an exception were to be made in the case of terminally ill cancer patients, that decision was for the legislature rather than the courts to make.[86]

On remand, the Tenth Circuit touched only briefly on the constitutional right of privacy issue.[87] The court simply stated that, within the context of the facts before it, a patient's selection of a particular treatment, or at least a medication, is within the area of governmental interest in protecting public health.[88]

Unfortunately, five years of litigation in the *Rutherford* case failed to yield a thorough analysis of the critical issue of whether the constitutional right of privacy affords cancer patients the right to select the treatment of their choice.

While *Rutherford* was being litigated, the California Supreme Court had occasion to consider the question of whether the state's police power could be used to restrict an individual's right of access to drugs of unproven effectiveness. *People v. Privitera*[89] involved prosecution of a physician and other individuals for conspiracy to sell and to prescribe an unapproved drug—Laetrile—intended for the alleviation or cure of cancer, in violation of applicable California statutory law.[90] The defendants appealed on the grounds that the statute was unconstitutional, and that the state and federal constitutional rights of privacy encompassed a right to obtain Laetrile.

The court, by a 5 to 2 majority, held that Laetrile was a drug of unproven efficacy and is not included in either the federal or state constitutional rights of privacy. The court further held that the statute prohibiting the prescription or administration of any drug not approved by the FDA or state board was a permissible exercise of the state's police power because it bore a reasonable relationship to the achievement of the legitimate state interest in the health and safety of its citizens.[91] The court distinguished previous cases recognizing various personal determinations as falling within the right of privacy on the ground that the prior cases were limited to such matters as marriage, procreation, contraception, family relationships, child rearing, and education, but did not include medical treatment.[92] This somewhat narrow interpretation was vigorously attacked by the dissent, which noted that the right to continue or terminate a pregnancy certainly involved medical treatment.[93] The dissent further noted that "the right to control one's own body is not restricted to the wise; it includes the foolish refusal of medical treatment."[94]

It is significant to note that none of the parties to the *Privitera* case was a cancer patient. The defendants in *Privitera* were individuals who had represented to the public that Laetrile was an effective cure for cancer and who had distributed Laetrile for profit. In some cases, the defendants neither obtained a medical history nor performed a physical examination on the patients to whom Laetrile was prescribed.[95] It is unfortunate that the court ruled on the right of privacy issue in a case in which those raising it had questionable standing to do so.

CONCLUSION

Despite a massive resource outlay directed at early detection and effective treatment of cancer, millions of cancer-related deaths are reported each year. Virtually none of the treatments labeled by orthodox medicine as ineffective has been the subject of well-controlled scientific studies.[96] The scope of research must be broadened to include all modalities in which there appears to be substantial public interest.[97] As a broader range of information becomes available, patients will be able to make more informed decisions regarding treatment.

Although some states have enacted legislation allowing patients to obtain certain types of alternative cancer therapies, the majority of state legislatures remain silent on this issue. The courts have been reluctant to affirm a cancer patient's right to select his or her own treatment as encompassed by the constitutional right of privacy. There appear to be several reasons for this: (1) An ideal fact situation, clearly defining the issue, has not yet been presented to the courts; (2) because of the rapid progression of many types of cancer, the slow justice often afforded by the court system may not be a practicable forum for terminally ill cancer patients; and (3) the courts seem disposed to defer to the state of orthodox medical knowledge as set forth in the legislative histories usually quoted in the court opinions.

Certain individual decisions regarding health care have already been recognized as falling within the constitutionally protected right of privacy. Although virtually all cancer patients can be expected, in varying degrees, to be anxious, depressed, or frightened because of their disease, the majority are still responsible, mentally sound adults. The parens patriae rationale would not seem to be applicable to such patients, as it would be in cases of juveniles or the developmentally disabled. Accordingly, the balance weighs heavily in favor of allowing cancer patients to obtain the treatment of their choice. The state's interest in protecting the health of its citizens can be adequately protected in this context by requiring an informed consent by the patient after disclosure of the nature of the proposed treatment, the fact that it has not been proved to be effective by well-controlled scientific studies, and the availability of conventional treatment.

ENDNOTES

1. Anderson, *Counseling Women on Familial Breast Cancer,* 37 Cancer Bull. 130-131 (1985).
2. Mills, *Prenatal Diethylstilbestrol and Vaginal Cancer in Offspring,* 229 J.A.M.A. 471-472 (1974).
3. *Burke v. United States,* No. M-84-425 (Md. 1984). In 1 Med. Mal. Verdicts, Settlements and Experts 9 (1985).
4. *Gorman v. LaSasso,* No. 83-CV-6311, Denver Dist. Ct. (Colo. 1983). In 1 Med. Mal. Verdicts, Settlements and Experts 17 (1985).
5. *Ok-Jae Song v. Smatko,* 208 Cal. Rptr. 300 (Cal. Ct. App. Nov 16, 1984, as corrected, Dec 11, 1984).
6. *Barenbrugge v. Rich,* No. 81L8949, Cook County Cir. Ct. (Ill. Oct 25, 1984). In 2 Med. Mal. Verdicts, Settlements and Experts 17 (1986).
7. *O'Dell v. Chesney,* No. 118-496, Riverside County Ct. (Cal. Jan 15, 1982).
8. *Mehalik v. Morvant,* No. 45173, Lafourche Parish Ct. (La. 1981) (NOTE: This case was settled on Dec 9, 1985).
9. *Brown v. Nash,* No. 63471, Suffolk Super. Ct. (Mass. June 19, 1985). In 2 Med. Mal. Verdicts, Settlements and Experts 13 (1986).
10. *Glicklich v. Spievack,* No. 80-2150, Middlesex Ct. App. (Mass. Dec 8, 1983).
11. *Burke v. United States,* No. 83-CV-6311, Denver Dist. Ct. (Colo. 1983). In 1 Med. Mal. Verdicts, Settlements and Experts 9 (1985).
12. *Lauro v. Travelers Insurance Co.,* 261 So. 2d 261 (La. 1972), *writ denied,* 262 So. 2d 787 (La. 1972).
13. American Cancer Society, *Survey of Physicians' Attitudes and Practices in Early Cancer Detection,* 35 CA 197-213 (1985).
14. Woo, *Screening Procedures in the Asymptomatic Adult,* 254 J.A.M.A. 1480-1484 (1985).
15. C. Metlin & C.R. Smart, *Breast Cancer Detection Guidelines for Women Ages 40 to 49 Years: Rationale for the American Cancer Society Reaffirmation of Recommendations,* CA-A Cancer J. Clinicians 248-255 (1994).
16. K.A. Kern, *Medicolegal Analysis of the Delayed Diagnosis of Cancer in 338 Cases in the United States,* 129 Arch. Surg. 397 (1994).
17. I.C. Henderson & D. Danner, *Legal Pitfalls in the Diagnosis and Management of Breast Cancer,* 3 Hematol. Oncol. Clin. North Am. 823 (1989).
18. C.D. Haagenson et al., *Breast Carcinoma: Risk and Detection* (1981).
19. K.A. Kern, *Historical Trends in Breast Cancer Litigation: A Clinician's Perspective,* 3(1) Surg. Oncol. Clin. North Am. 1 (1994).
20. C.M. Haskell, *Cancer Treatment* 19-27 (W.B. Saunders, Philadelphia 1980).
21. G. Fletcher, *Textbook of Radiotherapy* 284 (Lea & Febiger, Philadelphia 1980).
22. *Duke v. Morphis,* Superior Court, Tarrant County. (Tex.) No. 352-62434-80. In 4 Med. Mal. Verdicts, Settlements and Experts 43 (1988).
23. *Rudman v. Beth Israel Medical Center,* Supreme Court of the State of New York, County of New York (N.Y.) No. 4764/86. In 4 Med. Mal. Verdicts, Settlements and Experts 46 (1988).
24. *Barnes & Powers v. Hahnemann Medical College and Hosp.,* Common Pleas Court of Philadelphia (Pa.) No. 4031, 1982. In 3 Med. Mal. Verdicts, Settlements and Experts 35 (1987).
25. International Agency for Research on Cancer (WHO), 26 *IARC Monographs on the Evaluation of the Carcinogenic Risk of Chemicals to Humans* 37-384. (International Agency for Research on Cancer, Lyon, France 1981).
26. K. Falck et al., *Mutagenicity in Urine of Nurses Handling Cytostatic Drugs,* 1 Lancet 1250-1251 (1979); T.V. Nguyen et al., *Exposure of Pharmacy Personnel to Mutagenic Antineoplastic Drugs,* 42 Cancer Res. 4792-4796 (1982).
27. D.E. Bergsagel et al., *The Chemotherapy of Plasma-Cell Myeloma and the Incidence of Acute Leukemia,* 301 N. Engl. J. Med. 743-748 (1979); R.R. Reimer et al., *Acute Leukemia after Alkylating Agent Therapy of Ovarian Cancer,* 297 N. Engl. J. Med. 177-181 (1977).
28. P.H. Plotz et al., *Bladder Complications in Patients Receiving Cyclophosphamide for Systemic Lupus Erythematosus or Rheumatoid Arthritis,* 91 Ann. Intern. Med. 221-223 (1979).
29. H.O. Nicholson, *Cytotoxic Drugs in Pregnancy. Review of Reported Cases,* 75 J. Obstet. Gynaecol. Br. Commonw. 307-312 (1968).
30. M.J. Garrett, *Letter: Teratogenic Effects of Combination Chemotherapy,* 80 Ann. Intern. Med. 667 (1974).
31. R.B. Jones et al., *Safe Handling of Chemotherapeutic Agents: A Report from the Mount Sinai Medical Center,* 33 CA-A Cancer J. Clinicians 258-263 (1983).
32. R.B. Weiss & S. Bruno, *Hypersensitivity Reactions to Cancer Chemotherapy Agents,* 94 Ann. Intern. Med. 66, 71 (1981).
33. *Lefler v. Yardumian,* Superior Court, Pinellas County (IL) No. 83-14700. In 3 Med. Mal. Verdicts, Settlements and Experts 35 (1987).
34. *Newman v. Geschke,* Superior Court, Multnomah County (Ore.) No. A8609-05800. In 4 Med. Mal. Verdicts, Settlements and Experts 46 (1988).
35. E.W. Clayton, *Removing the Shadow of the Law from the Debate about Genetic Testing of Children,* 57 Am. J. Med. Genetics 630 (1995); J.H. Fanos & J.P. Johnson, *Barriers to Carrier Testing for Adult Cystic Fibro-*

sis Sibs: The Importance of Not Knowing, 59 Am. J. Med. Genetics 185 (1995); L.D. Gostin, *Genetic Privacy,* 23 J. Law Med. Ethics 320 (1995); D.E. Hoffman & E.A. Wolfsberg, *Testing Children for Genetic Predisposition: Is It in Their Best Interest?* 23 J. Law Med. Ethics 331 (1995); M. Powers, *Privacy and the Control of Genetic Information,* in *The Genetic Frontier: Ethics, Law, and Policy* 77-100 (M.S. Frankel & A.S. Teichs, eds., American Association for the Advancement of Science Press, Washington, D.C. 1994); S.M. Suter, *Whose Genes Are These Anyway? Familial Conflicts Over Access to Genetic Information,* 91 Michigan Law Rev. 1854 (1993); S.M. Wolf, *Beyond "Genetic Discrimination": Toward the Broader Harm of Geneticism,* 23 J. Law Med. Ethics 345 (1995).

36. P.R. Billings et al., *Discrimination as a Consequence of Genetic Testing,* 50 Am. J. Human Genetics 476 (1992); N.S. Jecker, *Genetic Testing and the Social Responsibility of Private Health Insurance Companies,* 21 J. Law Med. Ethics 109 (1993); J.E. McEwen & P.R. Reilly, *State Legislative Efforts to Regulate Use and Potential Misuse of Genetic Information,* 51 Am. J. Hum. Genetics 637 (1992).

37. B. Healy, *Hearing on the Possible Uses and Misuses of Genetic Information,* 3 Hum. Gene Therapy 51 (1992).

38. *Id.*

39. U.S.C.A. Title 42 §§ 300 b-1 to 300 b-6 (West 1994).

40. 29 U.S.C.§§ 791 et seq.

41. *Bentivegna v. U.S. Dept. of Labor,* 694 F. 2d 619 (9th Cir. 1982); *Mantolete v. Bolger,* 757 F. 2d 1416 (9th Cir. 1985); *School Board of Nassau County v. Airline,* 480 U.S. 273 (1987).

42. *Supra* note 33.

43. Public Law 101-336, 104 Stat 327, 42 U.S.C.S. 12101.

44. H.T. Lynch & J.F. Lynch, *The Lynch Syndrome: Melding Natural History and Molecular Genetics to Genetic Counseling and Cancer Control,* 3 Cancer Control 13 (1996).

45. G.M. Petersen & J.D. Brensinger, *Genetic Testing and Counseling in Familial Adenomatous Polyposis,* 10 Oncology 89 (1996).

46. *Id.*

47. *Supra* note 40.

48. *Supra* note 40.

49. O.I. Olopade & S. Cummings, *Genetic Counseling for Cancer: Part I.* 10(1) Principles Practice Oncology Updates 1 (1996).

50. *Supra* note 36.

51. *Supra* note 45.

52. *Supra* note 45.

53. M.C. King et al., *Inherited Breast and Ovarian Cancer: What Are the Risks? What Are the Choices?* 269 J.A.M.A. 1975 (1993).

54. D.F. Eastose et al., *The Clinical and Screening Age-at-Onset Distribution for the MEN 2 Syndrome,* 44 Am. J. Human Genetics 208 (1989).

55. R.F. Gagel, *Multiple Endocrine Neoplasia,* in *Williams Textbook of Endocrinology* 1537-1553 (J.D. Wilson et al., eds., 8th ed., W.B. Saunders, Philadelphia 1992).

56. C.J.M. Lycs et al., *Clinical Screening as Compared with DNA Analysis in Families with Multiple Endocrine Neoplasia Type 2A,* 331 N. Engl. J. Med. 828 (1994); R.D. Utiger , *Nodular Thyroid Carcinoma, Genes, and the Prevention of Cancer,* 13 N. Engl. J. Med. 870 (1994); R.F. Gagel, *Multiple Endocrine Neoplasia,* in *Williams Textbook of Endocrinology,* 1537-1553 (J.D. Wilson et al, eds.,8th ed., W.B. Saunders, Philadelphia 1992); R.L. Telalander et al., *Results of Early Thyroidectomy for Medullary Thyroid Carcinoma in Children with Multiple Endocrine Neoplasia Type 2,* 21 J. Pediatr. Surg. 1190 (1986).

57. R.D. Utiger, *Medullary Thyroid Carcinoma, Genes, and the Prevention of Cancer,* 331 N. Engl. J. Med. 870 (1994).

58. *Hernandez v. United States,* 636 F. 2d 704 (D.C. Circ. 1980).

59. *Katsbee v. Blue Cross/Blue Shield of Nebraska,* 245 Neb. 808, 515 N.W. 2d 645 (Neb. 1994).

60. *Webster's Third International Directory* (Merriam Webster Inc., Springfield, Mass. 1993).

61. *Dorland's Illustrated Medical Dictionary,* 481 (27th ed., W.B. Saunders, Philadelphia 1988).

62. Cassileth, *Contemporary Unorthodox Treatments in Cancer Medicine,* 101 Ann. Intern. Med. 105-112, 107 (1984).

63. *Id.*

64. Alaska Stat. 08.64.367; Ariz. Rev. Stat. Ann. 26-2452; Del. Code Ann. 16-4901-05; Fla. Stat. Ann. 500.1515 (West); Idaho Code 18-7301A; Ind. Code Ann. 16-8-8-1-7 (Burns); Kan. Stat. Ann. 65-6b; Ky. Rev. Stat. Ann. 311.950 (Baldwin); La. Rev. Stat. Ann. 40:676; Md. Code Ann. 18-301; Mont. Code Ann. 50-41-102; Nev. Rev. Stat. 585.495; N.J. Stat. Ann. 24:6F-1 (West); N.D. Cent. Code 23-23.1; Okla. Stat. Ann. 63-2-313; Or. Rev. Stat. 689.535; Tex. Rev. Civ. Stat. Ann. 71, article 4476-5a; Wash. Rev. Code Ann. 70.54.1310; W. Va. Code 30-5-16a.

65. Fla. Stat. Ann. 499.035 (West); Kan. Stat. Ann. 65-679a; La. Rev. Stat. Ann. 40-1060 (West); Mont. Code Ann. 42-102; Okla. Stat. Ann. 363-2-313.12; Tex. Rev. Civ. Stat. Ann. 71, article 4476.5b.

66. Nev. Rev. Stat. 585.495.

67. Okla. Stat. Ann. 63-2-313.7 (West).

68. Colo. Rev. Stat. 12-30-113(2).

69. Alaska, Delaware, Florida, Indiana, Maryland, Montana, Nevada, New Jersey, North Dakota, Oklahoma, Texas, and Washington.

70. Idaho, Indiana, and Oklahoma.

71. Arizona, Indiana, Louisiana, New Jersey, Oklahoma, Texas, and Washington.

72. Alaska, Colorado, Delaware, Louisiana, and Maryland.

73. California Health and Safety Code 1701.1 (West 1979)

74. *People v. Privitera,* 23 Cal. 3d 697, 153 Cal. Rptr. 4431, 591 P. 2d 919 (1979).

75. Marco & Laetrile, *The Statement and the Struggle,* in *Legal Medicine* 121-136 (C.H. Wecht, ed., 1980).

76. *Rutherford v. United States,* 399 F.Supp. 1208 (W.D. Okla. 1975), 542 F. 2d 1137 (10th Cir. 1976), 424 F.Supp. 105 (W.D. Okla. 1977), 429 F.Supp. 506 (W.D. Okla. 1977), 438 F.Supp. 1287 (W.D. Okla. 1977), 582 F. 2d 1234 (190th Cir. 1978), 616 F. 2d 455 (10th Cir. 1980).

77. Rutherford, 442 U.S. 544.

78. Rutherford, 399 F.Supp. 1208, 1215.

79. 21 U.S.C. 321 (P) (1) (1980).

80. Rutherford, 542 F.2d 1137.

81. 42 Fed. Reg. 39775-39787 (1977).

82. *Id.* at 39787-39795.

83. Rutherford, 438 F.Supp. 1287, at 1294-1300.

84. Rutherford, 582 F. 2d 1234.

85. Rutherford, 442 U.S. 544.

86. *Id.* at 559.

87. Rutherford, 616 F. 2d 455, 457.

88. *Id.*

89. *People v. Privitera,* 23 Cal. 3d 697, 153 Cal. Rptr. 431, 591 P. 2d 919 (1979). For a judicial decision that reached a different conclusion, see *Suenram v. Society of the Valley Hospital,* 155 N.J. Super. 593, 383 A. 2d 143 (1977). The *Suenram* court was not considering a statute, however, and in fact the New Jersey legislature authorized the use of Laetrile shortly after the court's opinion was rendered.

90. California Health and Safety Code 1707.1, which provides as follows: "The sale, offering of sale, holding for sale, delivering, giving away, prescribing or administering of any drug, medicine, compound or device to be used in the diagnosis, treatment, alleviation or cure of cancer is unlawful and prohibited unless (1) an application with respect thereto has been approved under 505 of the Federal Food, Drug and Cosmetic Act, or (2) there has been approved an application filed with the board setting forth: (a) Full reports of investigations have been made to show whether or not such a drug, medicine, compound or device is safe for such use, and whether such drug, medicine, compound or device is effective in such use; (b) A full list of the articles used as components of such drug, medicine, compound or device; (c) A full statement of the composition of such drug, medicine, compound or device; (d) A full description of the methods used in, and the facilities and controls used for,

the manufacture, processing and packaging of such drug, medicine, or compound or in the case of a device, a full statement of its composition, properties and construction and the principle or principles of its operation; (e) Such samples of such drug, medicine, compound or device and of the articles used as components of the drug, medicine, compound or device as the board may require; and (f) Specimens of the labelling to be used for such drug, medicine, compound or device and advertising proposed to be used for such drug, medicine, compound or device."

91. *People v. Privitera,* 153 Cal. Rptr. 431, 433.
92. *Id.* at 437.
93. *Id.* at 434.
94. *Id.* at 444.
95. *Id.*
96. For an example of a well-controlled study of the effect of an "unorthodox" cancer treatment, see Johnston, *Clinical Effect of Coley's Toxin: I. A Controlled Study,* 21 Cancer Chemotherapy Reports (Aug 1962).
97. *Supra* note 62.

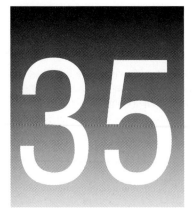

Brain-injured patients

CLARK WATTS, M.D., J.D.

PRIMARY CAUSES OF BRAIN IMPAIRMENT: DIAGNOSIS
TRAUMATIC BRAIN IMPAIRMENT
LEGAL CONSIDERATIONS

When referencing the brain, the general term *injury* should be considered in its broadest context. The brain is considered injured when it sustains pathology from whatever cause. Although this is the context in which the term will be used in this chapter, the primary focus will be on the traumatically brain-injured patient because most of the medicolegal implications of brain injury apply to this group of patients.[1]

The legal practitioner must understand how the physician will arrive at a diagnosis in these patients through the process of creating a differential diagnosis. Equally important for the legal practitioner representing brain-injured patients is an understanding of how the brain recovers, and how the injury and the recovery are quantitated. Of additional importance to the legal practitioner is an awareness of obstacles to coverage of brain injuries by insurance.

PRIMARY CAUSES OF BRAIN IMPAIRMENT: DIAGNOSIS

General considerations

Before any discussion of the differential diagnosis of primary causes of brain impairment, it is helpful to understand how one arrives at a differential diagnosis. A differential diagnosis is simply a listing, usually by probabilities (but without mathematical designations) of diseases and conditions reasonable to consider in a person suffering from brain impairment. The process of arriving at the differential diagnosis is a relatively simple one, but often poorly understood. It begins, as with all contacts between physicians and patients, with a history and a physical examination to elicit signs and symptoms from the patient. This is followed by a correlation of the signs and symptoms with the anatomy and physiology of the portion of the brain that seems to relate to those signs and symptoms. The process of time over which the signs and symptoms have been present is factored in, and the most likely disease categories, based on general pathology, are then extracted from the process. Confirmation of the conclusions at this point is obtained by laboratory tests and, finally, a differential diagnosis of specific pathology is created.

The process

Signs and symptoms. Symptoms are those complaints the patient presents to the physician. *Signs* are those findings the physician elicits by physical examination. In eliciting the signs and symptoms of a patient with suspected brain disease, it is important to keep in mind that the brain could express itself in response to disease in only a few ways. The brain may respond to disease by an alteration of the mental status of the patient. Usually an alteration of mental status is an alteration in the level of consciousness. The patient may appear conscious and be awake and alert, lethargic, or obtunded. Or the patient may present in or deteriorate into an unconscious state. An important subset of the mental status examination is a search for any derangements of intellect, orientation, self-awareness, or memory.

The patient with impaired brain function may present with motor symptoms. Most patients with this group of signs and symptoms will be noted to have certain patterns of paresis, or weakness of muscle function. Some will present, however, without significant weakness, but instead will have abnormal movements created by disorders of the nervous system such as spasticity or seizure disorders. The muscles may be flaccid, unusually rigid, or uncoordinated in action. The abnormal movements may be noted during voluntary or involuntary activity.

Pain, such as headache, is the most common form of sensory complaint. The patient may also complain of abnormal sensation, as with paresthesias, or electric-like painful phenomena, or numbness, the presence of dulled sensation. The complaint may be present spontaneously, or only when the physician, in examining the patient, obtains an admission of the symptom. Other sensory complaints may involve visual or hearing difficulties.

Disturbances of language are a common complaint of patients with brain impairment. Language disorders can be categorized in several ways, but generally they can be placed into three separate groups, called aphasias. In expressive aphasia the person has trouble expressing himself, that is, trouble making coherent, understandable sentences. The person suffering from receptive aphasia has difficulty receiving communication input and processing it into meaningful language. The verbal expressions of these individuals may appear normal, even quite articulate, but they have no relationship to input received. The person with global aphasia has elements of both and, in the worst cases, may be mute.

Finally, afflictions of the brain may present as disorders of the mind. This group of presenting signs and symptoms is mainly concerned with emotions, disturbances of reality, and alterations of self-image.

Rarely the patient has a single symptom; more often there is a constellation of symptoms. For example, a patient presenting with a tumor involving the left side of the brain may complain of lethargy, headaches, numbness and weakness of the right arm and leg, blindness in certain portions of the field of vision, expressive aphasia, and depression.

Consideration of anatomy/physiology. Groups of symptoms and signs may, with some accuracy, be related to anatomy and physiology in the process of localizing the disorder within the brain. The brain and spinal cord constitute the central nervous system. The peripheral nervous system is composed of the nerves of the body, outside the skull and spinal column. The third element of the nervous system is the autonomic nervous system, composed of the sympathetic nervous system and the parasympathetic nervous system. These two systems, as the name implies, function automatically, exclusive of voluntary control. Because of the focus of this chapter, the remainder of the discussion will be limited to the brain.

The brain resides within the skull. In the first few years of life the skull consists of a group of bony plates connected by fibrous adhesions (the sutures), which allow for expansion of the skull as the brain grows. While there is continued maturation of the brain tissue itself until approximately 16 years of age, the final weight and size of the brain and thus the skull occur before age 10. Several structures and substances support the brain inside the skull. Immediately inside the skull is a thick fibrous membrane, the dura mater, which is in reality the periosteum of the inner surface of the skull. Immediately internal to the dura is a much finer membrane, the arachnoid membrane. The arachnoid membrane contains the principal supporting substance of the brain and spinal cord, the cerebrospinal fluid. Finally, confining the substance of the brain itself is the pia mater.

The cerebrospinal fluid is formed within the ventricular system of the brain. There is one lateral ventricle in each cerebral hemisphere of the brain (see later discussion). These are joined at the midline and open into the third ventricle, which lies deep within the center of the brain where the two cerebral hemispheres join. The third ventricle is connected to the fourth ventricle by the cerebral aqueduct, a small passageway through the center of the brainstem. The fourth ventricle lies on the posterior aspect of the brainstem underneath the cerebellum. Cerebrospinal fluid is produced in all the ventricular cavities and exists from the fourth ventricle into the subarachnoid space from where it bathes the surface of the brain and the spinal cord and is eventually absorbed into the venous system over the surface of the cerebral hemispheres.

The brain consists of four elements, which are connected anatomically and physiologically. The largest mass of the brain is the *cerebrum,* composed of the two lateral cerebral hemispheres. Each has a frontal lobe anteriorly, a parietal and a temporal lobe laterally, and an occipital lobe posteriorly. The two frontal lobes in association with structures connecting the two cerebral hemispheres in the midline (portions of the limbic lobe) are functionally related to personality, emotion, and self-image. The posterior aspects of each frontal lobe provide voluntary motor function for the opposite side of the body, whereas the anterior aspects of both parietal lobes provide conscious sensory function to the opposite side of the body. Brain auditory function is served by temporal lobes, as is memory when the temporal lobes are interacting with the frontal lobes. In most individuals, voluntary and conscious speech function is located in the left frontotemporoparietal area of the left cerebral hemisphere, whereas visual-spatial orientation function is lateralized to the right cerebral hemisphere, particularly the right parietal lobe.

The second element of the brain is the *cerebellum,* located posterior, beneath the cerebrum. This paired structure is primarily responsible for involuntary actions of coordination.

Descending down from the middle of the base of the paired cerebral hemispheres, passing anterior to the cerebellum on its way into the spinal canal where it continues as the spinal cord, is the *brainstem,* the third element. It serves as a major pathway for nervous impulses to leave the brain and enter the spinal cord, and to pass from the spinal cord to the brain.

The final element of the brain is the collection of *cranial nerves,* which passes from the various other elements of the brain to structures peripheral to the skull. They conduct impulses to the brain that provide the senses of vision, smell, taste, and hearing; the voluntary functions of the face, such as mastication and sensation; and certain automatic functions of the body such as rhythmicity of the heart and autonomic bowel function.

An example of the importance of considerations regarding localization can be seen in the patient who complains of visual disturbances. If that patient were also complaining of weakness in the left hand, one would consider a lesion in the right cerebral hemisphere that is affecting the nerve fibers of vision as they pass from the eye in front to the occipital lobe in the posterior aspects of the cerebral hemisphere where vision is recognized. On the other hand, if the patient with visual disturbances were also complaining of problems with smell or taste, one might look more anterior, to the region of the eyes, as the ocular structures are more closely associated with nasal and oral mucosa from which taste emanates.

Considerations of time. In arriving at a differential diagnosis, one must not only consider the patient's signs and symptoms and anatomic/physiological correlations, but one must also factor in the time course over which the symptoms and the signs are present. For example, the patient may very well have a headache precipitated by a minor episode of head trauma. The headache would come on suddenly coincident with the trauma and persist appropriately. A headache similar in intensity and location, however, may have gradually developed over several weeks or months in a patient with a brain tumor. Likewise, a brain tumor may cause hand weakness progressively and slowly over several months, whereas a stroke, secondary to cerebral vascular embolization, may cause a sudden onset of hand weakness.

General pathologic findings. The general pathology of the underlying condition causing brain impairment may be more accurately suspected once signs and symptoms, potential location, and the dimension of time are considered. Consider an example of brainstem pathology. A collection of signs and symptoms gradually developing may suggest the development of a mass lesion such as a neoplasm or an abscess. Such a situation would rarely include the sudden onset of coma. On the other hand, consider a patient who had previously experienced over time intermittent transient numbness and weakness on one side or the other of the face and, occasionally, on both sides over time. If the patient then develops sudden onset of coma, she or he is more likely to be suffering from a cerebral vascular accident involving the brainstem than to be suffering from a tumor.

The differential diagnosis

After the physician works through the process of analysis in considering the patient's presenting signs and symptoms, the anatomic and physiological localization of the suspected lesion, the time course for the development and presentation of the suspected lesion, and the general pathological nature of the suspected lesion, the etiology of the brain impairment may preliminarily be placed into one or more categories of diseases from which a more specific differential diagnosis may be extracted. Definitions and examples of the major categories of neurological diseases are presented next. Then, the traumatic diseases are categorized in order to illustrate the process of developing a specific differential diagnosis.

Disease categories. Brain impairment may occur as a result of a disease or condition, categorized as follows: genetic, congenital/developmental, degenerative/metabolic, infectious, traumatic, neoplastic, vascular, immunological, psychogenic, and idiopathic. As with any arbitrary classification, overlapping of categories may occur, as will be apparent in the following discussion.

Most of the primary diseases of the brain associated with genetic disorders are characterized by an underlying error of metabolism. One of the earliest recognized and best understood primary brain disorders is produced by a genetic abnormality, phenylketonuria. This disorder is seen primarily in children and is highlighted by mental retardation, seizures, and imperfect hair pigmentation, and is transmitted as an au-

tosome recessive condition. The gene necessary for the activation of an enzyme, phenylalanine hydroxylase, is disturbed and the enzyme is almost completely lacking. As a result, the normal conversion of phenylalanine to tyrosine does not occur. Instead, phenylalanine is converted to phenylpyruvic acid, phenylacetic acid, and phenylacetylglutamine. With the accumulation of these metabolites in the brain, there is interference with normal maturation of the brain, neurofibers within the brain are not properly myelinated (a process of normal insulation), and other widespread and diffuse anomalies develop. Fortunately, in children born with this disorder, urine and blood levels of phenylalanine rise in the first few days and weeks of life and can be detected by a simple screening test.

In general, congenital/developmental disorders are those created by a deleterious effect of the environment, either in utero or after birth, on the developing brain. Some years ago a number of the genetic disorders were placed in this category. However, as specific abnormalities in the genome have been identified, the corresponding disorders have been removed from this category. The term *cerebral palsy* refers to a general condition caused by a number of different environmental insults to the developing brain. Although its most common presentation is a spastic weakness of all four extremities, cerebral palsy may manifest in some children as mental retardation and seizure disorders. The characteristic of this type of congenital disorder is that it is not progressive, although it may appear to be so as the child grows and becomes progressively more disabled in comparison with his or her peers. The etiological insult may occur before birth, in the perinatal period, or in the first few years of life. Cerebral palsy is believed to be caused by any number of insults including abnormal implantation of the ovum, maternal diseases, threatened but aborted miscarriages, external toxins, or metabolic insults such as maternal alcohol ingestion, which may result in hypoxia to the brain.

The category of diseases termed *degenerative metabolic disorders* is usually reserved for those conditions that develop in individuals with previously normal brain development. It is appropriate today to exclude conditions with known genetic bases, even though they express themselves later in life (such as Huntington's chorea) or conditions that are congenital or developmental and, as noted previously, appear to progress as the affected individual is compared with developing peers. Alzheimer's disease was at one time believed to be a classic condition in this category. Individuals in the prime of their senior years develop a rapid dementia much earlier than would be expected based simply on senility, associated with specific neuropathological changes in the brain of unknown etiology. Based on recent suggestions that this condition may have an underlying genetic predisposition, it may be more appropriate now to consider it as one of the genetic disorders, noting the appropriateness of genetic counseling. Aside from Alzheimer's condition, the most studied degenerative/metabolic disease of the nervous system is

Parkinson's disease. This condition is characterized by a progressive uncontrollable tremor with an associated dementia. The motor disability created by the tremor often progresses much more rapidly than the dementia, so that patients, well aware of their limitations, suffer substantial depression. For some reason certain cells within the brain are unable to manufacture an appropriate amount of dopamine, which is metabolically necessary for the function of the cells. A large number of patients infected during the influenza epidemic of 1918 developed this condition later in life. However, it is not believed that the majority of patients today have this problem secondary to viral infection.

Infectious agents have been the cause of infections of the brain. *Meningitis* is a term used to refer to infections of the coverings of the brain, whereas the term *encephalitis* is used to refer to an infection of the substance of the brain. In addition to the generalized widespread infectious processes these terms suggest, localized brain infections, or abscesses, can also occur. Management is to provide the appropriate treatment based on proper identification of the underlying etiological agent, whether bacterial, viral, fungal, or parasitic. This category of disease lends itself to a simplified discussion of how the physician might use the earlier presented scheme of analysis. A patient who has the fairly rapid development of brain impairment associated with a fever might be considered to have a disease within this category. If widespread impairment ensues that is characterized by nonfocal deficits and suppression of the mental status of the patient, one might consider meningitis or encephalitis. If, however, the disease process appears to be focal in nature, resulting in a partial paralysis (e.g., hemiparesis or weakness on one side of the body), one might consider the presence of a more focal infectious process such as a brain abscess.

The traumatic category of diseases encompasses everything associated with acute brain trauma. This includes not only diseases caused by disruption of brain tissue, but also diseases caused by systemic illnesses secondary to the traumatic episode, whether or not this trauma directly involves the head. For example, not uncommonly, after trauma to the head, the patient experiences a period of apnea, or diminished respiratory effort. If this is not corrected quickly, the patient may suffer hypoxia, or a lack of oxygen, which can damage brain cells. A more comprehensive discussion of traumatic brain disease appears later in this chapter to provide more details of the application of principles for defining a specific differential diagnosis of primary brain impairment.

The category of neoplastic diseases incubate all tumors that are progressive in development, whether benign or malignant. It includes those tumors that arise primarily within the brain and those that metastasize to the brain from extracranial sites. A benign tumor is one that grows more slowly, does not extend beyond the confines of the tumor mass itself, and does not metastasize or spread through the vascular system. The malignant tumor is a more aggressive tumor. It has a shorter time course and may spread to other parts of the brain or the body by way of the vascular stream, resulting in death in a shorter period of time than the benign tumor. However, this concept may be deceiving, in that a histologically benign tumor, placed in a critical location within the brain, may cause death quicker than a malignant tumor placed within the brain in a location that is not as critical. All tumors cause impairment by one of two mechanisms. They may produce direct pressure on the surrounding brain, or they may develop a volume that cannot be accommodated safely within the fixed cranial vault. Consequently, generalized increased intracranial pressure occurs, which adversely affects the flow of blood in sensitive areas of the brain, which may not be directly contiguous with the mass itself.

Most diseases in the vascular category affect the blood vessels directly or indirectly. Primarily congenital or developmental conditions, such as aneurysms and arteriovenous malformations, can produce sudden brain impairment by hemorrhage. Arteriosclerosis of the vessels, a degenerative/metabolic condition, may cause sudden impairment by creating an occlusion of the vessels, causing death of tissue from lack of circulating oxygen and nutrients. Occlusions may also occur with embolization of cerebral vessels by arteriosclerotic debris from other sites such as diseased heart valves.

Immunological diseases are caused by disturbances of the immune system. Multiple sclerosis is such a condition. It is characterized by repeated and progressive bouts of demyelinization of nerve cells and their axons, extensions of nerve cells that connect with other cells. These extensions ordinarily contain an insulating material called myelin. As a result of disturbances in the immune system not completely understood, the myelin is recognized by the body as a foreign substance and targeted for destruction.

The category of psychogenic diseases refers to those recognized and characterized as diseases of the mind associated with personality disorders, disturbances of emotion, and problems of self-image not placed in one of the preceding categories. Certainly, patients may be depressed as a result of head trauma or disabling conditions such as parkinsonism.

Iatrogenic diseases are those produced as a result of treatment by the physician of other conditions. A patient who develops a blood clot after surgery for a brain tumor due to inadequate hemostasis by the surgeon has developed an iatrogenic hemorrhage.

Idiopathic diseases are those for which there is no known, or reasonably suspected, etiology. As a result of dramatic recent advances in the neurosciences, especially in neuroimaging, these are so few in number that this category is presented only for completeness.

TRAUMATIC BRAIN IMPAIRMENT
Diagnosis

The process of establishing a differential neurological diagnosis has changed in the last several years. Significant technological advances in neuroradiology, especially in neuroimaging, have brought about this change. Before these advances, most differential diagnoses of brain impairment were expressed in terms of the category of diseases, with confirmation often left to surgery or autopsy. However, as the result of today's imaging technology, including computed tomography (CT), magnetic resonance imaging (MRI), and other relatively noninvasive high-resolution imaging devices, it is routine to develop a specific list of potential diseases within an individual category. This is the case with trauma.

The diagnosis of traumatic brain disease[2] usually begins with the identification of a traumatic episode resulting in either blunt or penetrating head injury. Penetrating head injuries generally produce less of a problem in the differential diagnosis because the penetrating offender, usually a bullet, will produce primary brain disruption and some hemorrhage. More challenging is the establishment of a differential diagnosis of traumatic brain disease following blunt trauma.

During blunt trauma, the brain is subjected to forces secondary to acute acceleration and deceleration of the brain within the skull, which is itself undergoing acute acceleration and deceleration. As the result of these forces, a number of pathological processes ensue. The brain may be "stunned" by relatively minor head injury without any anatomic or pathological changes, producing the so-called concussion. Renewed interest in this condition has occurred because of the exquisite detail of neuroimaging created by MRI. Some believe that through this modality previously unrecognized changes in the limbic lobe, the medial temporal lobe, and the upper brainstem may occur in concussion, accounting for the characteristic findings of transient loss of consciousness, some degree of retrograde amnesia, and difficulty with mental energy (e.g., lack of motivation), which may exist for weeks or months after the injury. Both arteries and veins may be torn, resulting in hemorrhage which may occur exterior to the brain or within the brain substance. Some portions of the brain may move through greater distances than other portions of the brain, creating shearing injuries at the interface of these moving areas—not too dissimilar from the activity at the fault line during an earthquake. Brain tissue may be disrupted. After some severe head injuries, apnea, or loss of normal respiration, may ensue, resulting in hypoxia and other metabolic changes that cause direct injury to nerve cells.

With both CT scanning and MRI scanning, intracranial hemorrhages following head trauma are easily identified. Epidural hemorrhages are arterial and are located beneath the skull but external to the most outer membrane lining the brain, the dura mater. These hemorrhages are usually associated with a skull fracture that lacerates an artery lying between the dura mater and the skull. The hemorrhage may develop rapidly over two to three hours, creating increased intracranial pressure and focal pressure on the brain. Recovery is excellent in patients who are operated on with evacuation of the hematoma before developing coma, whereas the prognosis is extremely poor in someone who develops coma before surgery.

Subdural hematomas form beneath the dura mater but external to the arachnoid membrane, which is the intermediate covering of the brain. The blood usually comes from torn veins, and develops more slowly than an epidural hematoma. It is less well localized and is often associated with other injuries to the brain because the force required to tear veins is actually greater than the force required to cut an artery following a skull fracture. As the result of the more widespread brain injury that is associated with an acute subdural hematoma, the mortality rate for subdural hematomas is higher than that for acute epidural hematomas in that more patients with acute subdural hematomas are comatose at the time of surgery. Often associated with acute subdural hematomas are intracerebral hematomas (i.e. blood clots within the substance of the brain). Although these hematomas are rarely an indication for surgery, their presence does adversely affect prognosis.

Subarachnoid hemorrhage (SAH) occurs between the arachnoid membrane and the surface of the brain (the pia mater). It may occur with minor head injuries. Although SAH, in and of itself, rarely produces primary brain impairment, it may be associated with the development, days or weeks later, of hydrocephalus, which is caused by the excessive accumulation of cerebrospinal fluid that has been normally produced within the brain but is unable to be absorbed normally because of the presence of blood in the subarachnoid space.

Injuries produced by shearing forces within the brain are rarely individually severe. However, because they may be widespread throughout the brain, collectively they can produce significant brain impairment, which is not treatable other than through the provision of primary support to the patient during the recovery and rehabilitation process. Prognosis of the patient with this condition is extremely varied depending on how widespread the problem is.

Hypoxia and other adverse metabolic stresses suffered by the brain in the posttraumatic period are a major cause of death or residual disability. When brain cells are subject to these conditions, one of three states may ensue. The brain cell continues to function relatively normally, or is one of a group of cells whose lack of functioning cannot be detected clinically. The second state the cell may move into is that of cell death. Because dead cells do not regenerate, that cell and its colleagues are removed from brain physiology and, depending on the location of the group of cells, the patient will suffer permanent deficit. The third state the cell may find itself in is "idling." In this state the cell is alive but not functioning normally. It requires time for the cell to rejuvenate itself, to recover from the insult, and to begin functioning again.

A discussion of the differential diagnosis of head injuries is not complete without some mention of posttraumatic

epilepsy. Seizure activity after trauma may be indistinguishable from nontraumatic epilepsy. The condition is due to the creation of hyperexcitable areas in the brain by the underlying disorder, or the removal of the inhibition of normally excitable brain by the disorder. Although epilepsy may be focal in presentation, it is such a generalized nonspecific response to trauma that it has little value in distinguishing for the physician the underlying brain pathology.

Putting it all together, the differential diagnosis of brain impairment begins with a history of head trauma and its attendant metabolic sequelae. The neurological status of the patient is observed over time and correlated with brain anatomy and physiology. Changes in the patient's condition are studied by neuroimaging and other laboratory technologies. Neuropsychological evaluation and response to medical and surgical treatment and rehabilitation are quantified. Through rational and objective analysis of this experience, a specific diagnosis may be made in virtually every instance.

Treatment

As alluded to previously, treatment[3] of the brain-injured patient begins with the establishment of a differential diagnosis: a general differential diagnosis based on the history and physical and a more specific differential diagnosis based on laboratory studies to include appropriate imaging studies. The general principles for the treatment of brain-injured patients are relatively uniform regardless of the etiology of the injury.

The treating physician has two primary goals from the outset. The first is to identify and treat the principal cause and result of the initial injury. The second goal of the treating physician is the prevention of secondary injury, which is that injury to the brain resulting from reaction of the brain to the initial injury.

Treatment of the initial injury may require the surgical debridement of skull fractures and brain lacerations or the evacuation of hematomas. The causes of secondary injury fall into two general categories: loss of vital metabolic substrates and compression. Failure to adequately oxygenate the patient or to maintain adequate blood pressure results in poor delivery of oxygen, glucose, and other essential nutrients to the brain, which results in further cell injury and death. Local compression by bone fragments or hematomas may cause direct injury to nervous system tissue or may impede the flow of blood to nervous system tissue. Secondary injury may result in cerebral edema or the excessive accumulation of fluid in both injured cells and the interstitial space between the cells.

The nondistensible nature of the skull may lead to an increase in intracranial pressure, which may further cause direct brain injury or injury secondary to the interference of cerebral blood flow. It is important therefore in certain patients, particularly those who are unconscious as a result of head injury or who have evidence of hematomas or cerebral edema on imaging studies, to have the intracranial pressure monitored through the use of various surgically implantable intracranial monitoring devices. Cerebral edema is usually treated with intravenous mannitol, an inert sugar that, because of its oncotic properties, causes the removal of interstitial edema during its circulation through the brain.

Other medications may be useful in the treatment of the brain-injured patient. Antibiotics may be helpful, especially if the brain has been contaminated by an open injury. There is some evidence that the prophylactic use of anticonvulsants during the first week after a disruptive brain injury may reduce the rate of seizure activity after trauma. At one time, steroids such as dexamethasone (Decadron) were routinely used in patients with traumatic brain injury, but this drug is no longer recommended for this use.

Brain recovery

It was once believed that brain cells either functioned or did not function—an all-or-none phenomenon.[4,5] It is becoming increasingly obvious that such cells may function at various levels of activity, depending on influences from surrounding cells. This is an explanation for one phenomenon seen in recovery as the result of rehabilitation. During the time period of rehabilitation, more and more brain cells move from the idling state to the active state. As they do, they exert their influence on surrounding cells, increasing the activity of the cell pool and thus improving the neurological status of the patient. A second phenomenon of rehabilitation is that of relearning. A patient's "weakness" may improve because of the increase in activity of the cell pool as mentioned earlier, or as the result of more efficient utilization of the existing cell pool through repetitive behavior during rehabilitation. It is believed, with regard to the first phenomenon, that 90% of the ultimate recovery of brain function will be seen within the first 6 months after injury, and the remaining 10% will be seen in the next 1½ years. The time frame for the second phenomenon is not understood as well and may proceed for years.

A major factor in the rehabilitation of brain-injured patients is the management of frustration and the accompanying depression. As the brain-injured patient recovers and becomes aware of his or her limitations, especially that of residual short-term memory deficit, frustration universally ensues. If this is not adequately managed, it will become institutionalized into the patient's thought and decision-making processes. The therapist and patient must confront the issue of frustration directly. They must constantly focus on ways to overcome frustration through the establishment of realistic goals. "Mental crutches" to help the patient work around mental obstructions, similar to physical impediments, may be essential. Contributing to the development of frustration is the group therapy approach to rehabilitation. Whereas the short-term costs may seemingly justify the group therapy approach, failure of an individual to be satisfactorily reha- bilitated because of the lack of individual attention may, in the long term, create greater costs.

Neuropsychological testing may be useful in defining meaningful goals and identifying mental obstructions. Al- though some believe that, through careful neuropsychologi- cal testing, it is possible to quantitate neuropsychological ab- normalities in patients with no deficits on neurological examination and neuroimage evaluation, others believe that adequate research has not been conducted to establish stan- dards for such distinctions.[6] In evaluating these matters, it is important to keep in mind the principle that the greater the lack of correlation between neuropsychological testing and neuroimaging confirmation of underlying residual brain im- pairment, the more important it is to search for preinjury ev- idence of neuropsychological abnormalities in order to un- derstand fully the problem presented by the patient in the posttraumatic period. In most cases preinjury neuropsycho- logical studies are not available on individual patients. There- fore, postinjury results must be related to preinjury perfor- mance, such as school grades, community achievement, mentor evaluations, and indirect evidence of neuropsycho- logical performance.

LEGAL CONSIDERATIONS

In general, the legal considerations for the brain-injured pa- tient vary little from those present in common and statutory law related to personal injury torts and contracts. Issues of in- formed consent generally concern the incompetent. Patients, especially elderly patients, have increasingly created advance directives, either a durable power of attorney or a living will. The laws related to these matters are generally state specific.[7] The exception is the Patient Self-Determination Act of 1990, a federal law mandating that hospitals that receive federal funds must inform patients of their right to create advance directives and to have them followed.[8]

The question often arises as to how to handle a matter of termination of treatment to include termination of life sup- port in patients who do not have advance directives. Once again, the law regarding these matters is generally state spe- cific, ranging from the permitting of a surrogate judgment maker through the use of a standard of the "best interest of the patient" to the requirement of a court-appointed guardian ad litem. The trend across the nation is to permit knowl- edgeable individuals, usually close relatives or friends, to provide evidence of what the patient would have decided. This is of particular note in situations where the patient is in a persistent vegetative state with no hope of recovery and, potentially, years of survival.

Most distressing and costly in terms of dollars and emo- tional capital is the patient in a persistent comatose state. A number of these states have been defined, but the one with the most recent exhaustive study is the persistent vegeta- tive state.[9] This patient is unconscious, is not aware of his or her environment, and cannot react appropriately to that en- vironment. The prevalence of this condition in this country is somewhere between 10,000 and 20,000 people. The per- sistent vegetative state begins clinically 1 month after in- jury. The life expectancy is 5 to 10 years, with death result- ing from medical conditions, such as pulmonary embolization caused by deep venous thrombosis or infec- tions. As would be expected, management of these patients consists of good but not necessarily skilled nursing care, maintenance of proper nutrition and hydration, and periodic evaluation for the onset of diseases secondary to the co- matose condition. Issues of termination of care often arise in brain-injured patients, particularly those in the persistent vegetative state.

Of major concern to head-injured patients and their fami- lies is denial of coverage under health insurance policies.[10] Often the portion of the policy that relates to chronic care or rehabilitation is ambiguous. As can be anticipated from the previous discussion, there are no sharp lines between acute care, rehabilitation, and custodial care. These terms and phrases are often self-defined after the fact by adjusters to provide denial. It is important that legal practitioners help medical practitioners understand the legal implications of conclusions, such as "no further medical required" or "med- ically stabilized."

ENDNOTES

1. A number of excellent treatises are available to which the reader may re- fer to expand the knowledge of the material in this chapter. Especially recommended are D.P. Becker & S.K. Gudeman, *Textbook of Head In- jury* (W.B. Saunders, Philadelphia 1989); 1-3 G. T. Tindall, P.R. Cooper, & D.L. Barrow eds., *The Practice of Neurosurgery* (Williams & Wilkins, Baltimore 1996); L.P. Roland ed., *Merritt's Textbook of Neu- rology* (9th ed., Williams & Wilkins, Baltimore 1995).

2. Space does not permit a discussion of the special circumstances sur- rounding the diagnosis and treatment of brain injury in the neonate or the very young child. A comprehensive review of this subject may be found in A. Towbin, *Brain Damage in the Newborn and its Neurologi- cal Sequels: Pathologic and Clinical Correlation* (PRM, Danvers, Mass. 1998).

3. In addition to the texts referenced (*supra* note 1), the legal practitioner might wish to review guidelines for the management of severe head in- jury published by the American Association of Neurological Surgeons, Chicago, telephone (708)692-9500.

4. For a comprehensive review of this subject, especially of the role that rehabilitation plays, see the report of the NIH Consensus Development Panel on Rehabilitation of Persons with Traumatic Brain Injury, *Reha- bilitation of Persons with Traumatic Brain Injury,* 282 J.A.M.A. 974 (1999).

5. P. Bach-y-Rita, *Recovery from Brain Damage.* 6 J. Neuro. Rehab. 191- 199 (1992).

6. As evidenced by the conflicting positions contained in the following ref- erences, it behooves any attorney representing clients with brain injuries to become familiar with the subject matter of neuropsychological testing: M.D. Lezak, *Neuropsychological Assessment* (3rd ed., Oxford University Press, New York 1995) and G.P. Prigatano, *Principles of Neuropsycho- logical Rehabilitation* (Oxford University Press, New York 1999).

7. See, A.D. Liberson, *Advance Medical Directives.* (Clark, Broadman, Callaghan, New York 1992). See also Chapter 27, this treatise.

8. Omnibus Budget Reconciliation Act of l990. Pub. L. #101-508, §4206, 4751.

9. See the publication by the Multi-Speciality Task Force, *Medical Aspects of the Persistent Vegetative State,* 330 N. Engl. J. Med. 1499, 1572 (1994).

10. See, e.g., S. McMath, *Insurance Denial for Head and Spinal Cord Injuries: Stacked Deck Requires Health Care Reform.* 10 Health Span 7-11 (July/Aug 1993); C. Rocchio, *Social Security Continued Disability Review Requires Action.* 2 TBI Challenge 4 (1998).

36

Patients with human immunodeficiency virus infection and acquired immunodeficiency syndrome

MIKE A. ROYAL, M.D., J.D., F.C.L.M.
MICHAEL A. SHIFLET, J.D.

What began as a little-noticed report of five homosexual men from Los Angeles with *Pneumocystis carinii* pneumonia in the June 4, 1981, Centers for Disease Control newsletter became an epidemic spanning the globe, killing millions, and affecting the lives of tens of millions.[1] Cases in homosexual men, intravenous drug users, hemophiliacs, and sexual partners of people in high-risk groups soon were reported across the United States. Newly absent T-helper cells seemed to be the common theme connecting these disparate groups. Lack of normal immune function left affected individuals vulnerable to opportunistic infections.

By 1984, human immunodeficiency virus (HIV) was established as the cause of this progressive T-helper cell destruction. Blood tests became widely available and presented the bad news that for every case of acquired immunodeficiency syndrome (AIDS), there were thousands of asymptomatic HIV-positive individuals who were able to transmit the virus to others. By 1988, 90,000 individuals had been diagnosed with AIDS, of whom about 50,000 had died.[2] By 1995, 500,000 had been diagnosed with AIDS, of whom more than 50% had died.[3]

In 1996, newly identified protease inhibitors (PIs) and precisely timed drug cocktails started to reverse symptoms even in seriously ill patients. In 1996 the death rate in the United States fell by 23% compared with that of 1995, and it dropped another 40% in 1997.[4] In this era of highly active antiretroviral therapy (HAART), PIs in combination with nucleoside reverse transcriptase inhibitors (nRTIs) and nonnucleoside transcriptase inhibitors (NNRTIs) have been able to reduce the amount of HIV in plasma to undetectable levels in many patients and increase life expectancy to 36 years in white men with HIV and 11 years in those with AIDS.[5] The combinations also seemed to prevent the progression to AIDS. There were 6% fewer AIDS cases in 1996, 15% fewer in 1997, and 25% fewer in 1998, leading many experts to predict a relatively normal life expectancy for those with HIV or AIDS.[6] What once was a virtual death sentence had become treatable. With new breakthroughs in antiviral therapy and transmission prevention, hopes for a cure with a vaccine are now voiced more frequently.

But to paraphrase Dickens, it has been the best of times and the worst of times in our efforts to treat HIV infection and AIDS. Because of economics (on average HAART costs $17,000 per year), only Western nations have seen the benefits. Unfortunately, AIDS-related illness is now the fourth leading cause of death worldwide.[7] An estimated 50 million individuals have been infected, of whom 33 million are still alive.[8] By November 1999 estimates, 1600 babies are born with HIV or are infected via consumption of breast milk each day.[9]

A total of 19 of 20 new cases of seroconversion and AIDS deaths occur in developing countries, with sub-Saharan Africa (particularly Botswana, Namibia, and Zimbabwe) being responsible for nearly 70% of the world's HIV infections despite representing only 10% of the population.[10] In these regions, seroconversion is almost entirely a result of heterosexual and mother-to-child transmission. In 1998 and 1999, 22 million and 23.3 million, respectively, of those positive for HIV lived in this region, compared with only 500,000 in Western Europe.[11] Life expectancy in the sub-Saharan region, which was 59 years in the 1990s, is now expected to drop to 45 years by 2005 to 2010.[12] By 2005, one of five workers in this part of the world will be HIV positive.[13]

The nations of the former Soviet Union had a greater than 30% increase in the number of HIV conversions in 1999 (estimated at 360,000), with the majority resulting from intravenous drug use.[14] In Moscow there were three times the number of cases in the first 9 months of 1999 as in all prior years combined.[15] Other regions also have been hard hit by this epidemic, with Asia now representing the fastest growing seroconversion rate, heralding a potential explosion in numbers.

The biggest problems continue to be poor access to treatment (mostly because of cost), poor understanding of basic sex education concepts, promiscuity among men who are indifferent to potential heterosexual transmission, and transmission to babies. In sub-Saharan Africa, more women than men are now HIV positive, with African girls ages 15 to 19 years five to six times more likely than boys to be seropositive.[16] This problem will cripple countries whose economies cannot match the resources of the United States or Western Europe. In 1997, for example, the United States spent $1 to $3 billion on HIV/AIDS-related illnesses, whereas sub-Saharan Africa spent only $165 million despite having almost 70% of the world's cases. For these countries the only viable option is a vaccine to prevent further transmission.

The dramatic improvements in life expectancy resulting from new drug combinations in the United States and Western Europe have created other issues of concern. Although less of a problem than in developing countries, the cost of new combination therapies may reduce access to treatment or encourage noncompliance. Adverse events from multiple drug treatments and comorbidities, such as increased susceptibility to opportunistic infections and some cancers, are greater concerns with increased life expectancy. Increasing the pool of seropositive individuals under treatment increases the potential for transmitting the virus to noninfected individuals. Failure to adhere to strict drug regimens substantially increases the chance for mutation, resistance, and tolerance.[17] Resistant strains can be passed on to others, as has been documented in 80 newly infected individuals who showed a 16.3% prevalence of HIV-1 variants with known resistance-conferring genotypes to any retroviral agent.[18] The presumption is that these cases represent transmission of treatment-resistant strains from previously treated patients.

It has been estimated that an adherence rate of 95% is necessary for optimal results.[19] This level of patient compliance is rarely achieved even in the best of situations. Noncompliance rates may approach 30%, allowing for more resistant HIV strains to emerge. Even if the cost was far less than the current $1000 to $2000 per month, other factors encourage incomplete dosing regimens. Multiple drugs must be taken at fixed times, some with food and some without, and side effects, such as malaise, nausea, and vomiting, are common.

TREATMENT

Many hoped that HIV infections could be eradicated if viral replication could be completely suppressed and chronically infected cells could be allowed to die. Using estimates of an infected cell's half-life of 10 to 14 days, it was suggested that eradication might be achievable in 2 to 3 years. These hopes dissipated in the face of newer data indicating that low-level viral replication may occur even with combination therapy at plasma HIV–ribonucleic acid (RNA) levels below detection (<50 copies/ml).[20]

As of December 1999 the consensus regarding specific antiretroviral therapy as reviewed by the International AIDS Society-U.S.A. Panel is to use initial regimens of two nRTIs and one PI, two nRTIs and one NNRTI, or two PIs and two nRTIs.[21] No definitive superiority of one regimen over another has been noted. Early treatment is recommended, but perceived benefits must be balanced against long-term adverse events. Plasma HIV-RNA levels and CD4$^+$ counts are good predictors of outcome.

Current antivirals approved by the U.S. Food and Drug Administration (FDA) include the following[22]:
- nRTIs: Zidovudine (AZT, Retrovir), didanosine (Videx), zalcitabine (Hivid), stavudine (Zerit), lamivudine (Epivir), and abacavir (Ziagen).
- NNRTIs: Nevirapine (Viramune), delavirdine (Rescriptor), and efavirenz (Sustiva).
- PIs: Saquinavir (Fortovase), ritonavir (Norvir), indinavir (Crixivan), nelfinavir (Viracept), and amprenavir (Agenerase).

HAART regimens have reduced HIV to undetectable levels in some patients, raising hopes of eradication, but recent studies have shown a swift resurgence by HIV on discontinuation with or without interleukin-2 (IL-2) added to activate resting memory cells.[23] In one study, 12 patients received HAART for a mean of 20.8 months and 14 patients received HAART for a mean of 20.1 months with IL-2 for a mean of 39 months. CD4$^+$ counts fell even before HIV could be detected, demonstrating a continual low-level "whittling away" of CD4$^+$ even during HAART.

Despite these disappointments, further research has opened doors for new approaches. Transactivator of transcription (Tat) is a small HIV protein essential for both viral replication and the progression of HIV.[24] It increases the transcription rate of viral mRNA by thousands (burst effects), helping to produce full-length transcripts of HIV genes. Tat can be excreted into plasma and enter other cells to trigger immediate transcription of all viral genes. Tat may be immunosuppressive as well by increasing susceptibility of T cells to HIV infection and making them more sensitive to apoptosis (programmed cell death). Individuals with the highest levels of anti-Tat antibodies are among those with the slowest disease progression.

Two other encouraging approaches include HIV-1 fusion inhibitors[25] and integrase inhibitors. HIV-1 fusion inhibitors are designed to block infection by preventing HIV fusion with host cells, thereby preventing insertion of viral deoxyribonucleic acid (DNA). Integrase is an enzyme crucial for insertion of HIV genetic material into the host's own DNA. In January 2000, researchers announced that two compounds, both diketo acids, blocked the enzyme's action in laboratory tests.[26]

VACCINE DEVELOPMENT

Traditional vaccine development typically involves the production of a weakened or attenuated virus that is injected into uninfected hosts to produce an immune response in hopes that, with subsequent exposure, immunological memory will bolster defenses. Unfortunately, traditional approaches have not worked well in HIV prevention. HIV has proved to be a formidable foe to vaccine research. It weakens host antibody responses and makes the cells it inhabits less noticeable to immunological surveillance by constantly changing the structure of peptide antigens (spikes) by which cytotoxic T cells recognize infected cells.[27] These spikes also can be shed into circulation, much like countermeasures released by planes or submarines to attract missiles.

The inherent limitations of current antiretroviral therapy underscore the need to develop effective vaccines, the most feasible and economical way of halting the worldwide epidemic. Several different vaccine strategies have been tested, largely in animals. These strategies include subunit vaccines, inactivated virus vaccines, attenuated live-virus vaccines, and DNA vaccines. Unfortunately, none of the vaccines tested has shown a significant effect on patients' conditions, CD4+ T cell counts, or HIV burden in the blood.[28] Because of the obvious concerns of transmission with some vaccines, the Joint United Nations Programme on HIV/AIDS (UNAIDS) has published recommendations on ethical guidelines for vaccine research.[29]

A group of prostitutes in Kenya that was thought to be immune to HIV despite numerous exposures (from which an antibody was developed) has now become infected.[30] This unfortunate turn of events has raised concerns that immunity may be reliant on continued exposure and any vaccine developed would have to be given repeatedly, certainly not a feasible approach for mass prevention programs. To help coordinate international cooperation on HIV vaccine development, the World Health Organization (WHO) and UNAIDS have created a new initiative (HIV Vaccine Initiative) to provide an independent forum for all researchers on HIV vaccines to collaborate.[31]

DISCRIMINATION

Although all 50 states offer some disability protection, discrimination against persons with HIV continues to be a major issue. Two significant disability discrimination statutes—the Vocational Rehabilitation Act of 1973[32] and the Americans with Disabilities Act of 1990 (ADA)[33]—continue to be enforced at the federal level. The ADA bars discrimination in employment,[34] government-provided services,[35] and public accommodations.[36] It applies to state and local governments, and employment provisions cover private employers with 15 or more employees.[37] Although the ADA does not specifically include HIV seropositivity, the U.S. Supreme Court has determined that it is a disability, even if the patient does not yet exhibit symptoms of AIDS.[38]

Protection from discrimination in insurance remains a great concern for HIV-positive individuals, for whom access to costly treatment regimens may become a life or death issue. Most of the legal developments that concern the financing of AIDS care involve efforts by insurers to limit or escape liability, as well as efforts by persons afflicted by AIDS to obtain coverage to which they feel entitled under their insurance plan. Although the ADA prohibits discrimination in employer-based health insurance,[39] it does allow decisions on underwriting to be based on actuarial risk.[40] Of course, the employer must show that it provides a bona fide insurance plan and demonstrate that the plan is not a "subterfuge" for disability discrimination.[41]

TESTING

The first tests for HIV antibody—enzyme immunosorbent assay (EIA) and Western blot (WB)—were developed in 1985.[42] With their development, calls for mandatory testing surfaced. But it was clear that, even ignoring the huge cost, mandatory universal testing was not a viable option. As with all diagnostic testing, the sensitivity and specificity of the test (rate of false-negative and false-positive results) must be considered. Without 100% accuracy, the emotional harm to individuals testing falsely positive and the false sense of security given those testing falsely negative outweigh any potential benefits to society. In addition, the period between infection and detectable antibody development (now about 25 days) increases potential for false-negative results.[43] Voluntary testing programs designed to encourage testing by preventing discrimination through strict confidentiality provisions and to decrease the spread of disease through awareness of HIV status and education regarding appropriate safety measures continue to be the primary testing emphasis.

Because of recent sales of home HIV tests claiming to be approved by the WHO or FDA, the FDA and Federal Trade

Commission (FTC) have sent warning letters to numerous companies.[44] The WHO does not license or approve HIV test kits, and the FDA has not approved any home-use test kit. Other than the standard tests, a rapid test (5 to 30 minutes) with sensitivity and specificity as good as EIA is the only one licensed by the FDA.[45] Saliva tests are being developed and may be available soon.

HIV transmission during medical procedures almost exclusively has been from infected patient to health care worker.[46] Prospective studies of health care workers estimate the average risk of transmission after a percutaneous exposure to HIV-infected blood is about 0.3% and after mucous membrane exposure, 0.9%.[47] The risk after skin exposure is probably less than that for mucous membrane exposure, but no data are available to better quantify the number. As of June 1997 the Centers for Disease Control and Prevention (CDC) had received 52 reports of health care workers in the United States with documented seroconversion after occupational exposure, and an additional 114 episodes were considered possible occupation transmissions.[48] Of the 52 documented episodes, 47 were exposed to HIV-infected blood, 1 to bloody body fluids, 1 to an unspecified body fluid, and 3 to concentrated virus in a laboratory setting. A total of 45 exposures were the result of needle punctures (41) or cuts with a broken glass vial (2) or other sharps (3) and 5 were mucocutaneous.

The well-recognized occupational risk has prompted the CDC to issue recommendations for postexposure prophylaxis (PEP) that include a basic 4-week regimen of two drugs (zidovudine and lamivudine) for most exposures and an expanded regimen including a PI (indinavir or nelfinavir) for exposures that pose an increased risk of transmission or where resistance to an nRTI is suspected. PEP's efficacy in reducing seroconversion has support in both animal and human studies, with some studies showing up to an 80% reduction.[49] Postexposure health care workers need not modify patient care responsibilities to prevent transmission to patients based solely on the exposure.[50] If seroconversion occurs despite PEP, the health care worker's work status should be evaluated according to published recommendations. (The 1991 CDC guidelines suggest that an expert committee could restrict a health care worker from performing "exposure prone" procedures.[51])

Despite the widely acknowledged low risk of transmission to patients from seropositive health care workers, courts have frequently upheld the decision to restrict the practice of seropositive health care workers.[52] In cases where HIV-infected health care workers have been prevented from continuing their occupations, the courts have held that the risk of harm to others must be "significant."[53] To evaluate the significance of the risk, four factors must be considered: (1) the nature of the risk, (2) the duration of the risk, (3) the severity of the risk, and (4) the probability that the disease will be transmitted.[54]

STATISTICS AND PRIVACY ISSUES

New federal guidelines published by the CDC for tracking HIV cases have raised concerns about the privacy of the patient health care records.[55] Some fear that individuals may become more afraid of being tested or that current patients may fear losing health insurance or employment.[56] The guidelines instruct states to track the number of cases and to attach the patient's name or some other identifying code to each case.[57]

Confidentiality is important if voluntary testing programs are to succeed. At the federal level, surveillance data are protected by several statutes and by removal of names and encryption of data transmitted to the CDC.[58] In addition, receipt of federal funding for state surveillance activities requires that states show an ability to guarantee security and confidentiality of reports. All states and many localities have legal safeguards for confidentiality of government-held health data that provide greater protection than laws protecting information held by private health care providers.[59] However, because the degree of protection varies from state to state, in some cases being somewhat minimal, the Model State Public Health Privacy Act[60] was developed at Georgetown University and, if enacted by states, would ensure greater confidentiality of surveillance data.

Since 1985, following CDC recommendations,[61] many states have implemented HIV case reporting as part of their comprehensive HIV/AIDS surveillance programs. As of November 1, 1999, 34 states and the Virgin Islands had done so using a confidential system for name-based case reporting for both HIV infection and AIDS.[62] Four states (Illinois, Maine, Maryland, and Massachusetts), the District of Columbia, and Puerto Rico use a coded identifier rather than the patient's name.[63] Washington state reports by patient name to enable public health follow-up and converts the name to codes after services and referrals are offered.[64] In most other states, HIV case reporting is under consideration, or laws, rules, or regulations enabling HIV surveillance should be implemented soon.

In contrast, the Department of Health and Human Services (DHHS) proposed regulations in late 1999 that aim to protect patients' electronic medical records by imposing federal regulations that would apply in any state with less protective measures for patients' electronic medical records.[65] Federal regulation would be a new approach because health care organizations have traditionally dealt primarily, if not exclusively, with the varying regulations of each state.[66] Under the new regulations, electronic (but not paper) medical records could be obtained only via a search warrant, subpoena, or other legal authorization without the patient's consent.[67] Similar protection for nonelectronic medical records would require passage of additional legislation.[68]

"SAFE NEEDLE" REGULATIONS

Intravenous drug use can be linked to nearly one of three AIDS cases and approximately half of all hepatitis C cases in the United States.[69] However, many states restrict the possession and distribution of hypodermic needles to health care workers and those who have a prescription for such devices, often on the grounds that to do otherwise would imply that drug use is acceptable.[70] Individuals and organizations that want to distribute clean needles to intravenous drug users to combat the spread of HIV often experience legal barriers, including criminal prosecution, that prevent them from doing so.[71] To address these concerns, the American Medical Association, the American Pharmaceutical Association, the Association of State and Territorial Health Officials, the National Association of Boards of Pharmacy, and the National Alliance of State and Territorial AIDS Directors have jointly urged states to coordinate efforts across professional disciplines and reduce regulatory barriers to improve access to sterile syringes and needles.[72]

In areas that allow some form of needle distribution to drug users, some groups have found innovative ways to operate. One Chicago organization, the Chicago Recovery Alliance, has instituted a paging system in which a drug user can call a pager number to obtain sterile syringes and blood testing.[73] Chicago Recovery Alliance is one of only two organizations approved under Illinois law to distribute needles to drug users and is not publicly funded, except for purposes of providing drug counseling.[74]

Approximately 600,000 to 800,000 health care workers suffer accidental needle injuries each year.[75] Health care workers often handle a patient's blood products without knowing the patient's HIV status. Even if the health care worker knows that the patient is HIV-positive, under a 1998 Supreme Court ruling, the patient cannot legally be denied health services for that reason alone.[76] To help protect health care workers from the risk of accidental injury and HIV infection by needles used in the treatment of patients, some state legislatures have recently begun implementing or considering legislation requiring the use of retractable needles.[77] California has already passed such laws, and at least 21 other states and the District of Columbia are considering similar legislation.[78] The Occupational Safety and Health Administration (OSHA)[79] and the CDC[80] also advocate the use of retractable needles by medical employers to reduce the number of needle-related injuries.

AIDS RESEARCH INVOLVING PRISON INMATES

Interest is developing in the medical community to expand AIDS research among prison inmates.[81] Despite more than a 50% drop in the number of AIDS cases in U.S. prisons from 1995 to 1997,[82] the rate of HIV infection among prisoners is still more than five times higher than that of the general population.[83] A study at Canadian correctional facilities involving face-to-face interviews in 439 men and 158 women in 1996 and 1997 points to high-risk behaviors as the reason for the prevalence of seropositivity, especially injection drug use and sexual behavior.[84] Nearly one third of the inmates had

injected drugs in the year preceding their current sentence. Among those sexually active, more than half had two or more sex partners before being incarcerated and the majority rarely used condoms.

A team at the Brown University HIV/Prison Project has developed preliminary guidelines for clinical tests involving prison inmates.[85] The idea has been met with some strong resistance because of abuses that occurred in inmate research programs during the 1950s and because some states simply outlaw inmate research altogether.[86] Advocates say the research is needed to help find treatments for AIDS and also to allow inmates access to cutting-edge treatments.[87] Administratively, such programs may be aided by a January 2000 U.S. Supreme Court decision. The court declined to review, and thus left standing, an Eleventh Circuit Court decision that allows inmates with HIV to be segregated from the rest of the prison population.[88] However, the primary concern in any research program, whether or not involving prisoners, is that it be conducted in a medically ethical manner.[89]

MEDICAL USE OF MARIJUANA TO TREAT AIDS-RELATED SYMPTOMS

Despite warnings from a recent study that support what many have long suspected, that smoking marijuana increases the risk of cancer almost as much as smoking tobacco,[90] laws have been approved in at least six states to allow the use of marijuana by seriously ill patients, including AIDS patients, to alleviate pain and other symptoms of disease.[91] Some AIDS patients report significant relief of pain and other AIDS-related symptoms from smoking marijuana—relief that they allegedly cannot obtain from taking dronabinol (Marinol) or other treatments.[92] Although some states now recognize that marijuana has some legitimate medical use, the federal government shows no signs of changing its position against the widespread use of marijuana for medical purposes.[93] The Justice Department is currently challenging the medical marijuana laws in five states,[94] and possession and distribution of marijuana remain federal crimes, outside of an approved federal trial program. The U.S. Attorney General also is challenging a federal Ninth Circuit Court of Appeals ruling that would allow a defense of "medical necessity"—a criminal act done to prevent more serious harm—as a defense to violating the federal laws prohibiting the possession of marijuana.[95] The implication of the court's decision is that the medical need to treat patient symptoms in certain cases by prescribing marijuana may be a "lesser evil" than the violation of laws against the possession and distribution of marijuana.

CONCLUSION

Medicine has come a long way in the ability to treat AIDS and HIV-related infections. New antiretroviral treatments have erased what was once a virtual death sentence. Unfortunately, the epidemic is rapidly accelerating in nonindustrialized nations that do not have the resources to cope with the problem. Vaccine research, although promising, offers only a hope for a future solution.

As more has been learned about HIV/AIDS and the infection has become treatable and is more often the result of intravenous drug use and heterosexual or mother-to-fetus transmission, the fear and hysteria bred by misunderstanding have slowly been replaced by reason and thoughtful concern over how to reduce transmission. Issues of discrimination seem to have shifted more to concerns over privacy of information and maintenance of insurance and medical treatment, but the longer life expectancy resulting from more aggressive treatment regimens provides more opportunities for individuals to suffer discrimination of some type. Moving forward into this new millennium, there is much to do, but desperation has given way to hope—hope for a cure, hope for a vaccine, and hope for greater understanding of and compassion and respect for individuals coping with HIV infection.

ENDNOTES

1. Good places for additional reading are the HIV/AIDS What's New webpage maintained by the CDC at www.cddnpin.org/hiv/whatsnew.htm, the HIV/AIDS Resources webpage maintained by the National AIDS Clearinghouse/CDC at www.cdcnpin.org/, the UNAIDS (Joint United Nations Programme on HIV/AIDS) webpage at www.Unaids.org/, and the HIV and AIDS webpage of links to other sites (including MEDLINE and AIDSline at igm.nlm.nih.gov/) maintained by the FDA at www.fda.fov/oashi/aids/other.html. The CDC's Morbidity and Mortality Weekly Report (MMWR) is available free of charge in electronic format; send an e-mail message to listserv<listserv.cdc.gov. The body content should read, "SUBscribe mmwr-toc."

2. Centers for Disease Control and Prevention, *Update: Trends in AIDS Incidence—United States, 1996*, 46 M.M.W.R. 861-867 (1997).

3. *Id.*, at 165-173.

4. UNAIDS/WHO: *HIV/AIDS Situation December 1996*, reported at www.us.unaids.org/highband/document/epidemio/situat96.html. *See also, The Status and Trends of the Global HIV/AIDS Pandemic* (Vancouver, July 5-6, 1996).

5. R. Sherer, *Summary of the 39th Interscience Conference on Antimicrobial Agents and Chemotherapy*, reported at www.ama-assn.org/special/hiv/newsline/conferen/icaac99/sherer.htm (posted Oct 25, 1999).

6. Centers for Disease Control and Prevention, *CDC Guidelines for National Human Immunodeficiency Virus Case Surveillance, Including Monitoring for Human Immunodeficiency Virus Infection and Acquired Immunodeficiency Syndrome*, 48(RR-13) M.M.W.R. 2-3 (1999); See also, P.L. Fleming, J.W. Ward, J.M. Karon et al, *Declines in AIDS Incidence and Deaths in the USA: A Signal Change in the Epidemic.* 12(Suppl A) AIDS S55-S61 (1998).

7. UNAIDS/WHO: *Press release*, www.unaids.org/whatsnew/press/eng/pressarc99/london231199.html (posted Nov 23, 1999).

8. *Id.*

9. UNAIDS/WHO: *AIDS Epidemic Update: 1999*, www.unaids.org/publications/documents/epidemiology/surveillance/wad1999/embaee.pdf.

10. UNAIDS/WHO: *Press release*, www.unaids.org/whatsnew/press/eng/ny10100.htm (posted Jan 10, 2000).

11. *Id.*

12. *Supra* note 7.

13. *Id.*

14. *Supra* note 9.

15. *Id.*

16. *Id.*

17. G. Fatkenheuer, A. Theisen, J. Rockstroh et al., *Virological Treatment Failure of Protease Inhibitor Therapy in an Unselected Cohort of HIV-1 Infected Patients*, 11 AIDS F113-F116 (1997). This study documented up to 30% to 50% resistance rates in treated individuals.

18. D. Boden, A. Harley, L. Zhang et al., *HIV-1 Drug Resistance in Newly Infected Individuals* 282 J.A.M.A. 1135-1141 (1999).

19. Panel on Clinical Practices for Treatment of HIV Infection convened by the Department of Health and Human Services, *Guidelines for the Use of Antiretroviral Agents in HIV-Infected Adults and Adolescents*, www.hivatis.org/guidelines/adult/pdf/A&ajani.pdf (posted Jan 28, 2000).

20. L. Zhang, B. Ramratnam, K. Tenner-Racz et al., *Quantifying Residual HIV-1 Replication in Patients Receiving Combination Antiretroviral Therapy*, 340 N. Engl. J. Med. 1605-1613 (1999).

21. *Updated Recommendations of the International AIDS Society-USA Panel*, 283 J.A.M.A. 381-390 (2000). *See also supra* notes 5 and 19.

22. The FDA maintains an updated list of antivirals at http://www.fda.gov/oashi/aids/virals.html. A nice overview by M. Schutz and A. Wendrow covers antivirals, side effects, mutations, resistance, and problems with drug-drug combinations, including antituberculous agents and methadone. This report can be found at http://hiv.medscape.com/updates/quickguide. A good coverage of PIs can be found in M.A. Dietrich, J.D. Butts, & R.H. Raasch, *HIV-1 Protease Inhibitors: A Review* 16 Infect Med 716-738 (1999).

23. A.S. Fauci, 5 Nat. Med. 561-565 (1999).

24. D. Blakeslee, *Tat: HIV's Achilles' Heel*, www.ama-assn.org/hiv/newsline/briefing/achilles.htm (posted Nov 16, 1999).

25. J. Stephenson, 282 J.A.M.A. 1994 (1999).

26. D.J. Hazuda, P. Felock, M. Witmer et al., *Inhibitors of Strand Transfer that Prevent Integration and Inhibit HIV-1 Replication in Cells*, Science 646-650 (2000). *See also* S. James, *Fusion Inhibitors, T-20: Chemokine Variants; Tat and Interferon Antibodies: Gallo Describes Three New Treatment Approaches.* AIDS Treatment News 4-5 (1998).

27. D. Blakeslee, *HIV and Antibodies*, www.ama-assn.org/special/hiv/newsline/briefing/antibody.htm (posted May 11, 1999).

28. P. Fast & W. Snow, *HIV Vaccine Development: An Overview*, http://www.ama-assn.org/special/hiv/treatment/vacessay.htm (posted Mar 25, 1997).

29. UNAIDS Guidance Document: *Ethical Considerations in HIV Preventive Vaccine Research*, www.unaids.org/publications/documents/vaccines/vaccines/Ethicalresearch.doc.

30. BBC News, news.bbc.co.uk/hi/english/health/newsid_619000/619316.stm (Jan 26, 2000).

31. www.unaids.org/whatsnew/press/eng/geneva2120200.html (posted Feb 21, 2000).

32. *See* 29 U.S.C.A. §§ 701-796 (West 1999).

33. *See* 42 U.S.C.A. §§ 12101-12213 (West 1999).

34. *See* 42 U.S.C.A. §§ 12111-17 (West 1999).

35. *See* 42 U.S.C.A. §§ 12131-12165 (West 1999). This prohibition includes employment discrimination. *See* 35 C.F.R. § 35.140 (1992).

36. *See* 42 U.S.C.A. §§ 12181-12189 (West 1999). Examples of public accommodations include hotels, restaurants, theaters, stadiums, convention centers, parks, museums, private schools, malls, hospitals, and health care providers.

37. *See* 42 U.S.C.A. § 12111 (West 1999).

38. *See Bragdon v. Abbott*, 524 U.S. 624 (1998).

39. *See* 42 U.S.C.A. §§ 12112(a)-(b)(2) (West 1999).

40. *See* 42 U.S.C.A. §§ 12201(c)(1)-(3) (West 1999).

41. *See* 42 U.S.C.A. § 12201(c)(2) (West 1999).

42. www.cdc.gov/nchstp/hiv_aids/hivinfo/vfax/260310.htm.

43. *See Id.*

44. www.fda.gov/oashi/aids/testwarn.html and www.ftc.gov/opa/1999/9911/cyberlink.htm.

45. www.cdc.gov/nchstp/hiv_aids/hivinfo/vfax/260310.htm.

46. K. Henry & S. Campbell, *Needle Stick/Sharps Injuries and HIV Exposure Among Health Care Workers,* 78 Minn. Med. 41-44 (1995).

47. D.M. Bell, *Occupational Risk of Human Immunodeficiency Virus Infection in Health Care Workers: An Overview.* 102(suppl 5B) Am. J. Med. 9-15 (1997).

48. *Public Health Service Guidelines for the Management of Health-Care Worker Exposures to HIV and Recommendations for Postexposure Prophylaxis.* 47(RR-7) MMWR 1-28 (1998) posted at aepo-xdv-www.epo.cdc.gov/wonder/prevguid/m0052722/m0052722.htm.

49. *Id.*

50. *Id.*

51. Centers for Disease Control and Prevention, *Recommendations for Preventing Transmission of HIV and Hepatitis B to Patients During Exposure Prone Invasive Procedures,* 40 M.M.W.R. 3-4 (1991).

52. *See, e.g., Doe v. University of Maryland Medical System Corporation,* 50 F. 3d 1261 (4th Cir. 1995) (neurosurgery resident); *Bradley v. University of Texas M.D. Anderson Cancer Center,* 3 F. 3d 922 (5th Cir. 1993), *cert. denied,* 114 S.Ct. 1071 (1994) (surgical technician); *Goetz v. Noble,* 652 So. 2d 1203 (Fla. Dist. Ct. of App., Mar 29, 1995; rehearing denied, May 2, 1995) (orthopedic surgeon).

53. *School Bd. of Nassau County, Fla. v. Arline,* 480 U.S. 273, 107 S.Ct. 1123, 94 L.Ed. 2d 307 (1987).

54. *Id.*

55. *See* Russ Bynum, *Guidelines Urge States to Collect HIV Cases with Names,* Associated Press Newswires (Dec 10, 1999), *available in* WestLaw AllNewsPlus database.

56. *See Id.*

57. *See Id.*

58. *Id* at 11.

59. L.O. Gostin, Z. Lazzarini, V.S. Neslund, & M. Osterholm, *The Public Health Information Infrastructure,* 275 J.A.M.A. 1921-1927 (1996).

60. L.O. Gostin & J.G. Hodge, *Model State Public Health Privacy Act* (Georgetown University, Washington, D.C. 1999).

61. Centers for Disease Control and Prevention, *supra* note 6 at 1-31.

62. *Id.* at 2-3.

63. *Id.*

64. *Id.*

65. See *The Coming Revolution: Proposed Patient Privacy Rules May Dramatically Change Daily Operations, Add Compliance Demands,* 10(12) Physician Manager (Nov 12, 1999), *available in* 1999 WL 13419985.

66. See *Clinton Unveils Limited Privacy Protection for Electronic Medical Records, supra* at 60.

67. *See Id.*

68. *See Id.*

69. *See* C.W. Henderson, *Groups Seek Better Access to Sterile Syringes,* Health Letter on CDC (Nov 15, 1999), *available in* WestLaw, 1999 WL 11593596.

70. *See* C. Clark, *Needle Exchange Advocates Strive Anew for County Assent,* San Diego Union & Tribune A1, *available in* WestLaw, 1999 WL 29195430 (quoting San Diego health care supervisor Dianne Jacob, responding to efforts to implement a needle exchange program, "No, no, no. A thousand times, no. It's wrong for governments to say it's OK to use illegal drugs as long as you use a clean needle. Clean needle exchanges send the wrong message to our kids.")

71. *See Medical Emergency Declaration to Be Sought for Needle Swaps,* Los Angeles Times, A33 (Dec 18, 1999); see, e.g., Cal. Bus. & Prof. Code § 4326(b) (West 2000), *available in* WestLaw, 1999 WL 26206731 (making the distribution of needles without a prescription a misdemeanor punishable by fine and/or imprisonment.)

72. *See supra* note 69.

73. See M.T. Galo, *Drug Users Have Link to Sterile Needles: Pager System Starts in Northwest,* Chicago Tribune 1 (Dec 24, 1999), *available in* WestLaw, 1999 WL 31273900.

74. *See Id.*

75. See Lauran Neergaard, *CDC Urges Use of Safer Needles to Protect Workers,* Washington Post Z07 (Nov 30, 1999), *available in* WestLaw, 1999 WL 30305865.

76. *See Bragdon v. Abbott,* 524 U.S. 624 (1998).

77. See *Scott-Levin Announces Sharp Ideas: Preventing Occupational Contamination by Needles,* Business Wire (Dec 10, 1999), *available in* WestLaw AllNewsPlus database.

78. *See Id.* California is also actively enforcing its regulations in this area by issuing fines for noncompliance. See *Fed and State OSHAs Step up Needlestick Safety Enforcement,* Business Wire (Nov 3, 1999), *available in* WestLaw AllNewsPlus database.

79. *See* M.F. Conlan, *OSHA Wants Safer Needles Used to Protect Workers,* 143(23) Drug Topics 1 (1999), *available in* WestLaw, 1999 WL 10022313.

80. *Supra* note 75.

81. *See* D. Rising, *Medical Tests on Inmates Reassessed,* AP Online (Oct 14, 1999), *available in* WestLaw 1999 WL 28128332.

82. See *AIDS Death Rate for Inmates Drops,* Los Angeles Times A31 (Nov 4, 1999), *available in* WestLaw, 1999 WL 26192733.

83. *See* S. Sternberg, *$7M to Fight AIDS, Drugs In Minorities Behind Bars,* USA Today 07D (Oct 5, 1999), *available in* WestLaw, 1999 WL 6858143.

84. L. Calzavara & A. Burchell, *HIV/AIDS in Prisons,* 5 HIV/AIDS Policy & Law 1999 posted at www.aidslaw.ca/Newsletter/FallWin99/prisons.htm.

85. *See* D. Rising, *Medical Tests on Inmates Addressed: Team Suggests Guidelines for AIDS and Hepatitis Trials for Prisoners,* Orange County Register A13 (Oct 16, 1999), *available in* WestLaw, 1999 WL 30109100.

86. *See Id.*

87. *See supra* note 81.

88. *See Onishea v. Hopper,* 171 F. 3d 1289 (11th Cir. (Ala.) 1999), *cert. denied, Davis v. Hopper,* No. 98-9663, 2000 WL 29361 (U.S., Jan 18, 2000).

89. *See supra* note 81. Rising references 1950s-era research programs in which "[i]nmates were injected with herpes, hepatitis and syphilis. Some had their testicles radiated; others were inflicted with wounds to see how they healed."

90. *See Marijuana Use Linked to Cancer,* N.Y. Times News Service D6 (Jan 14, 2000).

91. *See* H.T. George, *Medicinal Marijuana Users Wary Despite Win in Washington State,* Chicago Tribune 38 (Dec 10, 1999), *available in* WestLaw, 1999 WL 2940383.

92. See, e.g., *supra* note 90; R. George, *Gay Activist Has One Last Cause: The Right to Smoke Marijuana for Medical Reasons,* Sun-Sentinel (Ft. Lauderdale, Fla.) 1E (Oct 10, 1999), *available in* WestLaw, 1999 WL 20287971.

93. *Supra* note 91.

94. *See id.*

95. *See* B. Egelko, *Lockyer Backs "Necessity" Defense, Asks Feds to Drop Opposition,* Associated Press Newswires (Oct 14, 1999), *available in* WestLaw AllNewsPlus database; *United States v. Oakland Cannabis Buyers' Cooperative,* 190 F. 3d 1109 (9th Cir. 1999).

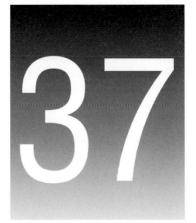

37 Pain management

BASIC CONCEPTS
DIAGNOSTIC PROCESSES
TREATMENT PROCESSES
MEDICOLEGAL AND POLITICAL ISSUES IN PAIN MANAGEMENT

Pain has challenged the human mind for recorded millennia. Pain is the single most common reason for seeking care and comfort. Although the management of pain recently became a novel discipline within the scope of medical practice, it has done so with a firm clinical and scientific foundation. Principles and standards of practice have been established using the time-tested tools of medicine—a detailed history, comprehensive physical examination, physical diagnosis, pain diagnosis, and treatment plan.[1] The obligation to relieve pain is fundamental to the physician's commitment, yet clinical surveys show that pain is generally inadequately addressed in the health care arena. Societal taboos and misconceptions regarding analgesic medications rather than lack of therapeutic options seem to be the culprits. Because pain cannot be objectively and reproducibly measured, the challenge of pain control is to balance the patient's need for relief with the physician's concern for safety and side effects.

The pain patient presents a complex amalgam of medical, emotional, social, behavioral, economic, occupational, and legal issues. This complexity makes applying the traditional disease model inadequate and inappropriate. As a result, no one medical discipline is equipped to deal effectively with complex pain syndromes.[2]

Very few human disease processes are not associated with pain. In acute presentations, most of these may be managed effectively by the application of modern medical techniques. Although pain is a common presenting complaint, its effective management remains an elusive goal. Chronic pain management in several instances is inadequate or ineffective, whereas the management of acute pain offers multiple opinions, practices, and rich clinical data. Inappropriate therapy may result in inadequate pain relief, production of iatrogenically induced debilities, or both.

In his classic text on abdominal pain, Zachary Cope (1921) observed, "If morphine be given, it is possible for a patient to die happy in the belief that he is on the road to recovery, and in some, the medical attendant may for a time be induced to share this delusive hope." As a result and despite today's improved diagnostic standards and improved dosing, many still maintain that masking a symptom may obscure its cause. Pain has been largely ignored in medical education and only recently has emerged as a subject of research. Over four decades have passed since Dr. John Bonica recognized pain as a clinical entity worthy of singular consideration as opposed to an expected accompaniment of acute trauma or the miserable complaints of neurotic individuals refusing entry into well-being.[4] In a review of more than 50 major medical textbooks of various disciplines, including surgery, general medicine, pediatrics, and oncology, Bonica found that only 54 of more than 25,000 pages addressed the issue of pain amelioration. It is because of his integrative focus that he is considered the father of modern pain theory.[5]

Formalized pain management organizations and established standards of practice evolved with ample latitude, governing quality of therapeutic services rendered. The literature of the ancients reflects pain as the universal bond of all humans, but it was not until 1953 with the publication of *The Management of Pain* by Bonica that a formal scientifically oriented treatise became available, for which the author was awarded the venerable title of "father of pain medicine." Board certification is now granted by three institutions: The American Board of Anesthesiology, a member of the American Board of Medical Specialties, and two institutions independent of the American Board of Medical Specialties. The American Academy of Pain Management (AAPM) was incorporated in 1988 and the American College of Pain Medicine established in 1992.[12] The American Pain Society, a national chapter of the International Association for the Study of Pain (IASP), was incorporated on August 8, 1978, in Washington, D.C.[13]

The Editorial Committee updated this chapter. The committtee gratefully acknowledges the past contribution of James S. Lapceuic, D.O., J.D.

The House of Delegates of the American Medical Association has recognized pain medicine as a self-designated specialty since 1994.[14]

In 1990 and 1991 an IASP task force on guidelines for desirable characteristics of pain management facilities also made recommendations for a core curriculum of professional education in pain management.[15,16] Certification standards for pain centers and comprehensive pain medicine practice programs have been established by the AAPM, the Commission on Accreditation of Rehabilitation Facilities, and the Joint Commission on Accreditation of Hospitals.[17] Of necessity, comprehensive pain treatment must encompass multidisciplinary management elements to address the complexity of the patient. In the present tumult of managed care where health care expenditures have seemingly ascended to the lodestar of in-patient care, it remains veiled whether "fungible care guidelines" can be successfully applied to the pain patient.

The International Association for the Study of Pain defines pain as "an unpleasant sensory and emotional experience associated with actual or potential tissue damage, or described in terms of such damage."[6] The definition implies that the experience of pain is subjective and always associated with nonphysical factors, yet while a patient's symptoms may be functional, the pain is real. Treatment for chronic pain (defined as pain persisting beyond the time of expected healing or arbitrarily as pain that lasts for more than three months) may also be recorded. Before Bonica's observations (see above), pain as sensation and perception was largely studied as part of the discipline of experimental psychology.

The impetus for development of this new specialty (pain management) arose out of patient protest. Those suffering acute pain as the result of injury often were accused of seeking excessive analgesic pain relief from use of "controlled analgesics." It is a well-documented fact that chronic pain patients suffered unduly because of inadequate analgesic medicinal administration. In large part because of the tenacious protests of these patients, guidelines developed encompassing multidisciplinary approaches for the management of pain and dealing with pain.[8,9]

Whereas acute pain related to illness or trauma is generally self-limited and treatable, chronic pain is the third leading health problem in the United States, affecting one third of the population.[10]

Frequently, patients with chronic pain present a dilemma to health care providers who are accustomed to treating acute pain successfully. Over the intervening years, such patients have been scourged as malingering, searching for secondary gain, psychoneurotic, hypochondriacal, or depressed.

Typically the patient's pain results from incomplete resolution of illness, injury, or operation. The pain has persisted for months to years and has presented health care providers with difficulties in identifying an organic basis for the pain to end it or validate it, arousing feelings of helplessness or hostility in the provider of care. The patient seeking help from multiple providers, including alternative sources, substantiated in the mind of the "legitimate, orthodox provider" the conclusion that no real medical disorder existed. By now, the pain has changed the patient's psychological state, and in response to the added burden of convincing providers that the pain is real, a demanding behavior develops as necessary to effect attention.

Chronic pain and the failure to diagnose and treat it are major causes of disability and excess health care expenditures. The typical patient has suffered for seven years, undergone three to five major surgeries, and expended up to $100,000 on medical bills. Further complicating the clinical scene, the risk of psychological dependence on one or more medications (often polypharmacy) exceeds 50%.[11] The chronic pain sufferer slipped through the cracks in the "health care platform" until health care finally responded with pain management as a specialty.

BASIC CONCEPTS

As noted, the new specialty of pain medicine has developed amid the radical changes in societal and professional attitudes regarding present-day physicians (health care providers), revolutionary medical technology, and the ever-growing refrain of cost containment (managed care and "less is more"). Practitioners of pain management come from multiple medical specialties with diverse backgrounds and training, and they lack the thread of a uniform base of training and experience. Although the IASP has published the *Core Curriculum for Professional Education in Pain Management,* no formal postdoctoral training program in pain medicine exists (despite the matter having been addressed by the Accreditation Counsel on Graduate Medical Education [ACGME][18,19]).

Ideally, the complete pain medicine practitioner would be physician, physical therapist, clinical psychologist, and skilled vocational rehabilitationist with board certification in anesthesiology, psychiatry, orthopedics, and neurology. That being unrealistic, the most desirable and cogent characteristics of the pain medicine specialist are an integration of the principles of these disciplines, as well as a special appreciation for the musculoskeletal and neural systems, in a disciplined, well-honed, and established physician who applies the available guidelines of pain management. With appropriate licensure to practice medicine and a documented broad and eclectic spectrum of training exposure to clinical psychology, psychiatry, physiotherapy, and vocational evaluation and rehabilitation, that physician should be further capable of wholly entertaining the pain patient's unique qualities. As Sir William Osler noted, "It is not nearly as important what illness the patient has, as what patient has the illness."

Medical training stresses adherence to a variety of standard routines of perception, decision-making, and treatment actions. Although this approach may ensure that medical practitioners tread a routine path safely within medicolegal guidelines, it is inimical to the role of the specialist in pain medicine. Here, individual requirements are especially well served by those who possess ingenuity, abstraction capability, and freedom of concept to integrate, identifying with the best elements of healing service, including but not limited to allopathy, osteopathy, homeopathy, the physical, the spiritual, knowns, and unknowns.[20-23]

Pain: epidemiology and definitions

An estimated 34 million adults in the United States suffer mild to moderate nonmalignant pain.[24] An excellent overview of the social and economic impact of pain was provided by Turk and others.[25]

As many as 50 million people are plagued with arthritic pain, 25 million suffer debilitating migraine symptoms, and 70 million suffer disabling low back pain. Current estimates indicate a yearly prevalence of symptoms in 50% of working-age adults, 15% to 20% of whom seek medical care.[26] Cancer pain affects 90% of the 8 million Americans who currently have cancer or a history of cancer; cancer is diagnosed in more than 1 million Americans annually and causes the deaths of about 1400 people every day.[27]

Pain prevalence in individuals infected with human immunodeficiency virus is estimated at 20% to 40%, and prevalence of pain increases as the disease progresses.[28]

Pain defined. The International Association for the Study of Pain defined pain as "an unpleasant sensory and emotional experience associated with actual or potential tissue damage, or described in terms of such damage."[29] In addition:

1. Pain is an unpleasant experience that may result in adverse psychosocial and politicoeconomic changes.
2. Pain is always subjective; there is no neurological or chemical test that can measure pain.
3. Pain can be generally categorized as acute or chronic (with six divisions based on temporal classifications made by Crue).[30]

Acute pain. Acute pain is a well-recognized entity that follows documented injury or illness and it generally disappears when the process heals. There are often (but not always) associated objective physical signs of autonomic nervous system activity, such as hypertension, tachycardia, pallor, diaphoresis, and mydriasis, that lend to objective documentation of the pain's etiology by laboratory methods and physical examination. In cases where cause of the acute pain is uncertain, establishing a diagnosis is paramount.

Symptomatic pain relief may be administered during the investigation. With occasional exceptions, delaying analgesia until a diagnosis is made is rarely justified. The evidence now suggests that judicious use of small opioid doses does not confound and may contribute to diagnostic accuracy in the diagnosis of abdominal pain by allaying the patient's apprehension and permitting a more thorough abdominal examination.[31] Pain is an individual, subjective perception related to mechanical and chemical alterations of body tissues. It is perceived in the cortical areas of the central nervous system and is not dependent on the precise nature or absolute amount of peripheral tissue destruction. Acute pain is usually proportional to the extent of illness or injury, although there is a potential for separation of tissue destruction from intensity of pain perception. This emphasizes the fact that pain messages may be modified at many levels of the nervous system. Acute pain is characterized by subsidence in proportion to the resolution of the causative lesion.

When a patient's pain does not resolve accordingly or persists beyond the time of expected healing, the progression to chronic pain should be suspected.

Chronic pain. Pain is a complex, subjective experience mediated through multiple components of the peripheral and central nervous systems, resulting in varying degrees of intensity, location, onset, duration, aggravating and relieving factors, and emotional responses. While acute pain sometimes serves as a protective device, pointing to onset and location of damage, chronic pain is a resultant disease state that transcends healing of the injury. By definition, chronic pain is an unremitting pain lasting six months or more, although duration per se does not represent the single criterion for diagnosis. There are many medical causes, though the physiological source may remain unclear and difficult to identify. The passage from acute to chronic pain may correlate with psychological stages similar to the stages of terminal illness.

Chronic pain syndrome is used as the descriptive for the overall debility, compromised functioning, and decompensation in all major areas of life. The following four stages of chronic pain have been synthesized for description[32]:

1. Patients in the acute pain state (0 to 2 months), as well as their health care providers, expect resolution of the pain on recovery from the precipitating event. The patient may suffer some sleep difficulties, although he or she has no new psychological difficulties (even if pain is severe).
2. Entering the subacute phase (2 to 6 months), the patient may not be depressed but is beginning to feel distressed by the enduring pain. Subtle personality or behavioral changes, such as increased irritability, insomnia or other sleep disturbances, and social isolation, may emerge. An ensuing deeper reliance on analgesics and sleep medications may begin.
3. The chronic phase (6 months to 8 years) initiates a realization by the patient that the pain might be uncontrollable and permanent, which may precipitate affective symptoms of sexual dysfunction, sleep disturbances, lowered self-esteem, guilt, hopelessness, and helplessness, which are identical to symptoms of depression. Personality inventory testing at this juncture will undoubtedly reveal elements of hysteria, depression, and hypochondriasis.

4. The subchronic phase (3 to 12 years) is characterized by the patient's adjustment and resignation to the long-suffered, persistent pain. This phase corresponds to the final stage of acceptance in patients with a terminal disease.

Patients who traverse this four-stage progression nearly always appropriately test positive for a significant degree of objective organic disease. Those who do not follow the typical progression and those who exhibit no depression at some stage are more likely to be pain exaggerators.[33] *Guides to the Evaluation of Permanent Impairment* lists the following eight criteria (the eight Ds) of chronic pain with the presence of at least four categories being adequate to establish a presumptive diagnosis of chronic pain syndrome[34]:

1. Duration: Pain exists beyond the noted occurrence of tissue healing even after prompt assessment and appropriate treatment and rehabilitation have been applied. Chronic pain syndrome can emerge within two to four weeks of injury.
2. Dramatization: Pain patients display marked verbal and nonverbal pain behaviors.
3. Diagnostic dilemma: Patients usually will have seen a large number of physicians who have performed replete, poorly coordinated diagnostic studies, many of which have failed to yield any but nebulous conclusions.
4. Drugs: Chronic pain patients frequently are taking a plethora of medications and have a history of polypharmacy.
5. Dependence: Patients become introverted and passively dependent on the health care system, their families, and the economic-political system (i.e., third-party payors) to which they may seem an appendage.
6. Depression: The chronic pain patient frequently decompensates to depression as a way of life. Such ongoing depression may exacerbate to thoughts of and attempts at suicide.
7. Disuse: Fearing movement, the patient becomes sedentary as a guard against pain, usually resulting in musculoskeletal deconditioning and perpetuation of the pain syndrome.
8. Dysfunction: Inability to negotiate the normal stresses of day-to-day existence and the resulting inadequate personality lead to a mere subsistence often accompanied by becoming ostracized. The chronic pain patient must learn how to live; the terminal patient must learn how to die.

DIAGNOSTIC PROCESSES

The pain medicine specialist must be an excellent diagnostician because early diagnosis, assessment, and treatment are the sine qua non of pain management. Delays in performing appropriate studies constitute a chief factor promoting debility from an underlying but treatable lesion simply as a result of failure to diagnose and institute appropriate therapy. It is typical of these patients to have been exposed to a random, poorly coordinated barrage of health care providers and di-

agnostic procedures. It becomes the woeful lot of the pain medicine specialist to establish a meaningful diagnosis with appropriate treatment plans for the chronic pain problem, which at first may seem undiagnosable and unmanageable. Long-standing pain, in addition to being complicated by an overlay of social and emotional factors, often seems to have no clearly available treatment options. For the physician assuming care for such a patient, there is often more of a burden than a privilege. Consequently, the first challenge is to distinguish between the objective and the exaggerating pain patient, as management and outcome expectation largely depend on these findings. It is notable that a patient who exaggerates pain is likely to have been maladjusted to some degree before the onset of pain. Unlike the management of acute pain, the management of chronic pain is multifaceted, including pharmacological therapy, lifestyle modifications, and often psychotherapy.

Practitioners should be aware of the appropriate preparation necessary to manage pain: A physician who provides care that would normally be extended by a given specialist will be held to the standard of that particular specialty.[35] Because certain specialists (e.g., orthopedists, psychiatrists, anesthesiologists, and neurologists) frequently encounter the chronic pain patient, there is the temptation to manage the patient's overall pain complaints individually, even though the patient may have progressed well into the chronic pain syndrome.

The pain medicine specialist, as diagnostician, must be attuned to the full array of differential diagnoses for each patient's complaints and must perform a comprehensive physical examination. Many syndromes—common, rare, and little known—may cause chronic pain (Box 37-1).

Comprehensive laboratory and radiological studies should be tailored to the patients' presentation so that such studies have a basis in the individualized differential diagnosis. Roentgenographic studies should be carried out when indicated, including consideration of the following procedures:

1. Computed tomography (CT) scans
2. Magnetic resonance imaging (MRI)
3. Bone scan (triple phase if complex regional pain syndrome is suspected)
4. Single photon emission computed tomography
5. Electromyography (EMG)
6. Myelography

The utility of SPECT and thermography in the diagnosis of acute or chronic pain is not uniformly agreed on.

In the interest of how best to reduce the use of diagnostic studies without detracting from patient management in both the inpatient and outpatient settings, physicians' ordering patterns are being monitored more rigorously.[36] In many instances, utilization is being modified by managed care organizations through promulgated clinical pathways, or even by policy mandates.[37]

Statistically significant levels of false-positive and false-

---

BOX 37-1. CLASSIFICATION WITH SOURCES OF PAIN

Muscle pain

    I. Myofascial pain
    II. Sprains and strains (lasting 3 to 4 weeks)
    III. Temporomandibular joint syndrome
    IV. Cancer pain
    V. Phantom limb pain
    VI. Joint and bone pain
    VII. Bursitis
    VIII. Facet joint pain
    IX. Occult fractures
    X. Osteoarthritis
    XI. Rheumatoid arthritis
    XII. Lyme disease
    XIII. Gout

Vascular pain

    I. Claudication of arteries
    II. Migraine cephalgia
    III. Cluster headache
    IV. Nerve pain
       a. Peripheral nerve entrapment
       b. Causalgia (CRPS I)
       c. Neuroma
       d. Postherpetic neuralgia
       e. Radiculopathy
       f. Reflex sympathetic dystrophy (CRPS II)
       g. Thoracic outlet syndrome
       h. Trigeminal neuralgia
       i. Tic douloureux
    V. Low back pain
       a. Congenital vertebral disorders
    VI. Degenerative disease (disk or bone source)
    VII. Intrinsic bone disease (osteoporosis)
    VIII. Metabolic disorders
       a. Diabetes mellitus
       b. Hyperthyroidism

Visceral pain

    I. Colitis
    II. Pancreatitis
    III. Chronic constipation
       a. Gallstones
       b. Hemorrhoids
       c. Polyps
       d. Ileitis
    IV. Referred visceral pain
       a. Gastrointestinal sources
       b. Genitourinary sources
    V. Psychological problems

CRPS, Complex regional pain syndrome.

negative findings exist in all studies. Conventional diagnostic studies, such as nerve conduction, radiography, EMG, and CT, may help localize but cannot measure pain. Test findings may not necessarily correlate with the patient's subjective level of pain. After appropriate psychological testing, the workup should continue to locate and identify the physical sources of pain, often a daunting task. When the source of the pain has been identified, it should be treated aggressively and appropriately to give the patient relief. A new lexicon has been suggested, comprising acute pain, chronic pain, and complicated pain.[38]

The traditional use of the Minnesota Multi-Phasic Personality Inventory (MMPI; a questionnaire of 566 items) to garner clues and attempt patient pain validation has been found inappropriate and scientifically inaccurate unless there is also a global comprehensive evaluation of the patient.[39] The MMPI results provide information about personality and may suggest whether a particular pain patient is an exaggerator, but it cannot distinguish between real and exaggerated pain. A complete patient workup may also require vocational evaluation and planning.

The initial step in pain management is careful assessment, which should lead to recognition of the need for specialty consultation, thus leading to close multidisciplinary collaboration among the entire health care team. A standard pain history may provide valuable information about the nature of the underlying process or may disclose other treatable disorders.[40] A description of the qualitative features of the pain, its time course, and any maneuvers that decrease or increase pain intensity should be sought. Pain intensity (current, average, best, and worst) should be assessed to determine analgesic needs and to serially evaluate the effectiveness of ongoing treatment. Pain descriptors (e.g., burning, shooting, sharp, or dull) may help determine the mechanism of pain and suggest the likelihood of response to various classes of conventional and adjuvant analgesics (e.g., nonsteroidal antiinflammatory drugs, opioids, antidepressants, anticonvulsants, corticosteroids).[41]

The need for ongoing reassessment of pain and documentation of clinical findings cannot be overemphasized. The four fundamental aspects of ongoing reevaluation are as follows[42] :

1. Pain intensity
2. Pain relief
3. Mood state or psychological distress
4. Pharmacological effects (side effects, abuse behavior)

The Memorial Pain Assessment Card (MPAC) is a helpful clinical tool consisting of visual analog scales that measure pain intensity, pain relief, and mood state. Patients can complete the MPAC in less than 30 seconds, providing essential information to guide ongoing pain management.

Finally, chronic pain can change a patient's level of psychological adjustment, and psychological factors can modify the subjective experience of pain, although most patients with chronic pain have an organic basis underlying their pain. The directive for the health care professional is to locate the source of the pain, determine the psychological contribution, and then treat the whole patient.[43]

TREATMENT PROCESSES

Pain management is best carried out in a multidisciplinary, multimodal approach.[44] Treatment encompasses appropriately indicated elements of physical, psychological, medical, and vocational modalities of therapy. The magnitude of a treatment center's staff may not be assumed to be determinative of its competence in treating the pain patient. Further, large multidisciplinary programs appear unlikely to be cost effective. The assembly of documentation of a pain patient's exposure to a multitude of departmental disciplines can hardly substitute for a carefully thought-out, physician-supervised program attentive to medical, psychological, vocational, and musculoskeletal reconditioning issues.

Medication

The medical management of pain presents an evolving pharmacological regimen, thoughtfully balancing maximal effective pain relief while obviating untoward effects of chronic drug regimens. As with any medical practice, the risk-benefit probabilities must be weighed. The challenge of pain control is to balance the patient's need for relief with the health care provider's concern for safety and side effects. A long-overdue modification in thinking is unfolding in the arenas of acute and chronic pain as they relate to appropriate pharmacological management. Despite the known connection between pain relief and healing, the minority of acute pain patients receives adequate analgesic therapy. There is evidence that pain control is less likely to be adequate in children, the elderly, the mentally retarded, and minorities. Patients have been denied both adequacy and frequency of analgesic dosages. For many years a disbelieving attitude pervaded and biased the health care system's approach to the patient who requested pain relief. The shrouded myth bound the following two unrealistic and unfounded beliefs: (1) patients do not hurt as much as they say they do, and (2) various medical procedures do not cause pain (a denial of reality). Coupling these unfortunate beliefs to the advent of drug crime in the United States unfortunately resulted in stringent restrictions and penalties placed by the Drug Enforcement Agency (DEA) on all uses of drugs, including legitimate applicational use by the medical profession. To avoid critical scrutiny by another physician or the DEA, a physician simply forgoes the possible risk of dealing with controlled analgesics, setting the patient adrift and alone into the grip of disabling pain. It is no longer considered illegitimate and disdainful to treat postoperative pain with adequate analgesia because the pharmacological agents are allotted for a limited time.

The *Quick Reference Guide for Clinicians* lists the following approaches for use in acute, postoperative pain management[45]:

- Cognitive behavioral interventions (e.g., relaxation, distraction, and imagery)
- Systemic opioids or nonsteroidal agents and acetaminophen
- Patient-controlled analgesia, giving the patient a sense of self-management of his or her pain (often preferable to intermittent injections)
- Spinal anesthesia (epidural opioid or local anesthetic intermittently infused versus continuously infused)
- Intermittent versus continuous local neural blockade (e.g., intercostal nerve block or local anesthetic via intrapleural catheter)
- Physiotherapy (e.g., massage and application of heat or cold)
- Transcutaneous electrical nerve stimulation

An increasing number of sources are now advocating the use of long-term opioid analgesics in selected chronic pain patients, despite the medicolegal reality of continuing heavy scrutiny by the DEA, state licensing boards, and the ever-furtive colleagues testifying to the existence of further restrictiveness. The medical literature addressing long-term opioid therapy in populations with nonmalignant pain points toward larger issues. Controlled trials suggest favorable outcomes, simply concluding that for selected groups of patients more can be done pharmacologically than is currently in vogue.[46,47] There is evidence that regulatory policies can perpetuate the undertreatment of pain by either impeding access to controlled prescription drugs or negatively influencing prescribing behavior. The latter has been suggested by recent outcomes analysis associated with multiple-copy prescription programs.[48]

Such programs, which monitor "point of sale," are strongly favored by those in regulatory and law enforcement communities and induce a marked decline in prescribing rates.[49,50] The concerns of legitimate prescribers have been affirmed in a recent nationwide survey of members of boards of medical examiners; a substantial proportion of members would potentially recommend investigation of a prescriber solely in response to the knowledge that an opioid had been administered to a patient with nonmalignant pain for more than six months.[51] Many expressed misconceptions regarding the law and regulations governing opioid prescribing in their own states. Thus available data suggest that medical decision-making regarding the use of opioids continues to be unduly influenced by fear of regulators and regulatory policies.

The chronic pain patient may have undergone the current full roster of standard treatment rendered by pain centers, including biofeedback, physiotherapy, nerve blocks, antidepressant adjunctive medications, and various philosophical applications wherein the patient supposedly will feel better if he or she does not talk about pain or display pain behaviors. Consider causalgia (which might be approximated by placing a blowtorch to a foot and leaving it there), and now imagine trying to display no change of countenance, thinking positively, making no pain gestures, breathing deeply, relaxing, and confronting the vicissitudes of daily life. Although pain medicine has made much progress, it has boundless strides yet to make.

The great stir in the realm of chronic pain is due to the increasing number of adjuvant drugs now being discovered to assist in pain management without the actual use of analgesics. This drive to use anything but analgesia induction stems in part from the previously discussed reluctance of the prescribing health care provider to use any medications outside the seemingly current fad. The following classes of medications can be considered for use without significant medicolegal risk, given appropriate patient assessment and selection as per the *Principles of Analgesic Use in the Treatment of Acute Pain and Chronic Cancer Pain*[52]:

1. Tricyclic antidepressants
2. Antihistamines
3. Benzodiazepines
4. Caffeine
5. Dextroamphetamine
6. Steroids, usually short term
7. Phenothiazines
8. Anticonvulsants

Recently, wider application in treatment of chronic pain has developed using serotonergic- specific antidepressants and calcium channel blockers. These medications are at best "adjunctive agents" from which some benefit may be derived, although no assumption can be made, even in the face of current societal thought, that these may substitute for analgesics, thus precluding all adversity. All the aforementioned "safe" medications have numerous adverse side effects (e.g., tardive dyskinesia with phenothiazines), and their probable beneficial effects result from alteration of the autonomic and central nervous systems' pain modulation perception through concomitant alteration in attentiveness.

Nerve blocks continue as a vital part of the pain management medical regimen. Among these are central and peripheral blockade, epidural steroid blocks, regional intravenous blocks, and sympathetic blocks, which should be coadministered within a multimodal therapeutic matrix so that the effectiveness of any one particular block may be augmented by the complementing effects of other therapies. In some disorders (e.g., complex regional pain syndrome) early administration of appropriate blocks (stellate ganglion or lumbar sympathetic) can be crucial. With low back pain, timeliness of certain blocks (e.g., lumbar steroid epidural) is not of major import. From a medicolegal perspective, it is the duty of the physician to order and supervise all elements of the patient's treatment program. That responsibility requires adequate medical monitoring of the continued appropriateness of the orders, patient and staff compliance with the initial orders, and competency of the staff members to carry out the orders.

The physician's responsibility, when indicated, may include formal medical impairment examinations using the guidelines of the American Medical Association. Previously the physician standard was not to comment on disability but rather to give an assessment and opinion concerning only medical impairment. It is now formally recognized that an appropriately trained physician with knowledge and insight into a patient's disorder, work setting, and familial environment can judge disability and impairment using the *Guides to the Evaluation of Permanent Impairment*.[53]

Behavioral medicine

Clinical psychology has had a major impact on the scene of pain management. The model of behavioral analysis serves as the foundation for assessment and prescription of an apt treatment program for the pain patient. In addition to medical procedures, the patient with chronic pain may be exposed to biofeedback, individual and family therapy, stress management, pain coping sessions, and bariatric and nutritional management.

Physiotherapy

Crucial to the treatment of the pain patient is musculoskeletal conditioning using physiotherapy modalities. Administration of myofascial stretching or relaxation and antiinflammatory procedures may be beneficial. The patient should receive formal education, musculoskeletal conditioning assignments, and supportive medical appliances (e.g., home use of hot and cold packs, mechanical massagers, etc.) to assist these goals. Many patients who undergo musculoskeletal conditioning before scheduled back surgery ultimately may not require the surgery. Functional capacity before and after treatment should be assessed to objectively determine the patient's ability to sustain various activities of daily living and expected work functions.

Vocational assessment and rehabilitation

When a patient's residual functional capacities and documented medical impairment preclude return to previous normal activity levels, the physician should consult the *Dictionary of Occupational Titles* (published by the U.S. Department of Labor) to accurately recommend employment placement if a return to work is feasible. At times, patients may require job readiness training to assist them in reentering the employment scene or total retraining to prepare them for an altogether different work area.

MEDICOLEGAL AND POLITICAL ISSUES IN PAIN MANAGEMENT

The chronic pain patient will eventually succumb to its control. The legal, medical, governmental, and economic sectors

that overlap at times garner the majority of attention and activity, to the detriment of the patient whose plight originally stimulated such activity. Because a patient approaches the chronic pain state through illness or injury, in many cases, unless the patient secures appropriate legal counsel, current societal machinations lay bare the question as to whether legitimate attention will be given to his or her problems. As a result, the patient may well be involved with a plaintiff's attorney, a third-party defense attorney, a rehabilitation supplier, and a state board of workers' compensation. Industry itself will maintain a vested interest in the outcome.

Sociolegal and economic principles

Patients with chronic pain and chronic pain syndrome may have varying degrees of emotional, psychological, behavioral, and environmental dysfunction marked more by subjective complaints than objective findings. These problems must be accepted as legitimate medical disorders deserving legitimate concern from society for an already complicated clinical syndrome. Alleged disability more often than not is based on the patient's evaluation and opinion of his or her ability to function. Industry as a whole, employers, and workers' compensation agencies that administer and maintain a compensation fund all stand to lose when a patient claims chronic pain-sponsored debility. Accordingly, such agencies and societal institutions, because of political and economic motives, are likely to present great resistance to legitimizing a patient's claim.

Traditional medicine holds that patient complaints without "objective findings" bespeak malingering, secondary gain, or psychological illness. Practicing attorneys within the arena of chronic pain impairment and disability face recurrent major medicolegal issues of concern revolving around the inherent difficulty in gaining legitimate recognition of such patients' problems in the absence of so-called objective findings. There seems to be a pervasive, obsessive fixation centered on some "magical test" of objectivity, absent which no legitimacy of the pain patient will be granted. That this represents current pragmatic reality is not arguable, although it should not be thus. Objective testing to measure pain does not exist. Unfortunately, more than one pain patient has been submitted to numerous medical evaluations and repetitive studies in a quest for the proverbial "provable" abnormality. The workers' compensation third-party carrier or defense attorney will insist on multiple independent medical evaluations, being fully knowledgeable that the chronic pain patient is unlikely to demonstrate hard-core test documentation of underlying etiology.

Obtaining the desired goal of ambiguity of findings, the hope then turns on the lack of "objective" results to win subsequent litigation based on the credo that there is "no identified medical disorder" to substantiate the patient's claims. Pain perception and sensation continue to defy adequate explanation through advanced medical technology and testing, which is verification of the adage, "Absence of evidence is no evidence of absence." Malingering is found infrequently.[54,55] Because of technical inadequacy and the general lack of medical understanding, a patient's complaints often lack delineation. Simply because tests do not exist to explain a patient's source of pain is no reason to conclude that no pain or complaints exist.

It is the duty of legal counsel to ensure that an accurate, comprehensive assessment is presented to the chronic pain patient, fully using the biopsychosocial model. There must be a comprehensive assessment of medical, psychological, and economic factors with adequate attentiveness to the deleterious effects of the chronic pain syndrome on the patient and family. It is the ethical duty of the attorney to ensure protection in the patient's best interest. Rapid settlement of the patient's claim to collect "quick money" is no less appalling an ethical infraction than for a physician to perform surgery without good indication.

It is unfortunately true that justice for the chronic pain patient can rarely be achieved outside the legal setting because of the motivations and dynamics of the various parties involved. In the final scene of the entrenched chronic pain syndrome, all parties, especially the patient, have suffered and will suffer unduly.

ENDNOTES

1. S.F. Brena & D.L. Koch, *A "Pain Estimate" Model for Quantification and Classification of Chronic Pain States,* 2 Anesth. Rev. 8-13 (1957).
2. W.C.V. Parris, *Common Chronic Pain Syndromes,* 6 Pain Digest 83-93 (1966).
3. American Academy of Pain Management, *Code of Ethics/Patients Bill of Rights* (The Academy).
4. J.J. Bonica, *The Management of Pain* (Lea & Febiger, New York 1953).
5. J.J. Bonica, *Biology, Pathophysiology and Treatment of Acute Pain,* in 5 *Persistent Pain: Modern Methods of Treatment* (S. Lipton & J. Miles eds., Grune and Stratton, New York, 1985).
6. H. Merskey, *Classification of Chronic Pain; Descriptions of Chronic Pain Syndromes and Definitions of Pain Terms,* International Association for the Study of Pain, Subcommittee on Taxonomy Pain 51-226 (Suppl 3, 1986).
7. D. Cohen, *Magnetic Fields of the Human Body,* 28 Physics Today 34-43 (1975).
8. R.S. Weiner ed., *Innovations in Pain Management: A Practical Guide for Clinicians* (Paul M. Deutsch Press, 1990).
9. *Acute Pain Management: Operative or Medical Procedures in Trauma* (U.S. Department of Health and Human Services, Feb 1992).
10. N. Hendler ed., *The Challenge of Pain* (MRA Publications, Greenwich, Conn. 1996).
11. N. Hendler, *How to Cope with Chronic Pain* (Cool Hand Communications, Boca Raton, Fla. 1993).
12. American Academy of Pain Medicine, 13947 Mono Way #A, Sonora, Calif. 95370.
13. American Pain Society, 5700 Old Orchard Road, First Floor, Skokie, IL 60077-1057.
14. 8 Am. Acad. of Pain Med. Newsl. (Winter 1993).
15. *Desirable Characteristics for Pain Treatment Facilities and Standards for Physician Fellowships in Pain Management* (International Association for the Study of Pain 1990).
16. *Core Curriculum for Professional Education in Pain Management* (International Association for the Study of Pain 1991).
17. W. Hodges, *Pain Center Certification Controversies and Issues* (paper presented at the Annual Conference of the American Academy of Pain Medicine, Scottsdale, Ariz. 1991).
18. *Supra* note 16.
19. 6 Am. Acad. of Pain Med. Newsl (Dec. 1991).
20. *Osteopathic Medicine: An American Reformation* (2d ed, American Osteopathic Association, 1979).
21. B.E. Jones, *Osteopathic Medicine: The Premier Profession* (Times Journal Publishing).
22. G. Vithoulkas, *The Science of Homeopathy* (Grove Press, New York 1980).
23. K.L. Pomeroy, Personal communication, *Pain Relief: A Collection of Medical and Lay Literature Testimonials* (Royal Orthopedic and Pain Rehabilitation, Scottsdale, Ariz. 1993).
24. R. Leitman et al. eds, *National Pain Survey,* (Study No. 942004, Louis Harris Assoc., New York 1994).
25. D.C. Turk et al., *Pain and Behavioral Medicine,* 73-74 (The Guilford Press, New York 1983).
26. S. Bigos et al., *Acute Low-Back Problems in Adults* (Clinical Guideline 21.5, Att. CPR, Pub. No. 95-0643, Department of Health and Human Services, Dec 1994).
27. A. Jacox et al., *Management of Cancer Pain, Clinical Practice Guideline No. 9* (AHCPR Pub. No. 04-0592, Department of Health and Human Services, March 1994.)
28. *Supra* note 26.
29. *Supra* note 6.
30. B.L. Crue Jr., *Multidisciplinary Pain Treatment Programs: Current Status,* 1 Clin. J. Pain 31 (1985).
31. P.M. Paris, *Treating the Patient in Pain,* Emergency Medicine 66-90 (Sept 1996).
32. *Supra* note 10.
33. N. Hendler, *Depression Caused by Chronic Pain,* 45 J. Clin. Psychol. 30-36 (1984).
34. *Guides to the Evaluation of Permanent Impairment* (4th ed, American Medical Association, 1993).
35. *Medicolegal Primer* 108 (1st ed., American College of Legal Medicine Foundation, 1991).
36. H.P. Forman, *Meeting of Managerial Science with Medicine,* 276 J.A.M.A. 1599-1600 (1996).
37. *Id.*
38. J. Lerner & W. Schacht, *A New Lexicon,* 6(4) A.J.P.M. 112-113 (1996).
39. E. Helmes, *What Types of Useful Information Do the MMPI and MMPI-2 Provide on Patients with Chronic Pain?* 4, No. 1 Am. Pain Soc. Bull. 1-5 (Jan/Feb 1994).
40. R.B. Patt & S.R. Reddy, Pain and the Opioid Analgesics: Alternate Routes of Administration, P.A.A.C. Notes 453-458 (1993).
41. World Health Organization, *Cancer Pain Relief* (World Health Organization, Geneva 1986).
42. K. Elliott & K.M. Foley, *Pain Syndromes in the Cancer Patient* 8 J Psychosoc. Oncol. 11-45 (1990).
43. *Supra* note 10.
44. J.J. Bonica, *The Management of Pain* (2d ed, Lea & Febiger, Philadelphia 1990).
45. *Quick Reference Guide for Clinicians: Acute Pain Management in Adults, Operative Procedures* (Department of Health and Human Services, Feb 1992).
46. W. Arkinstall et al., *Efficacy of Controlled-Release Codeine in Chronic Non-Malignant Pain: A Randomized, Placebo-Controlled Clinical Trial,* 62 Pain 169-178 (1995).
47. D.E. Moulin et al., *Randomized Trial of Oral Morphine for Chronic Non-Cancer Pain,* 347 Lancet 143-147 (1996).
48. J.R. Cooper et al., *Prescription Drug Diversion Control and Medical Practice,* 268 J.A.M.A. 1306-1310 (1992).

49. G.T. Gitchel, *Existing Methods to Identify Retail Drug Diversion in Impact of Prescription Drug Diversion Control Systems on Medical Practice and Patient Care,* 132-140 (J.R. Cooper et al. eds., National Institute on Drug Abuse Research Monograph 131, Superintendent of Documents, U.S. Government Printing Office, Washington, D.C. 1993).

50. U.S. Department of Justice, *DEA, Multiple Copy Prescription Program Resource Guide* (Superintendent of Documents, U.S. Government Printing Office, Washington D.C. 1987).

51. D.E. Joranson et al., *Opioids for Chronic Cancer and Noncancer Pain: A Survey of State Medical Board Members,* 4 Fed. Bull. 15-49 (1992).

52. *Principles of Analgesic Use in the Treatment of Acute Pain and Chronic Cancer Pain* (American Pain Society, 1992).

53. *Guides to the Evaluation of Permanent Impairment* (4th ed, American Medical Association, 1993).

54. F. Levitt & J.J. Sweet, *Characteristics and Frequency of Malingering Among Patients with Low Back Pain,* 25 Pain 357 (1986).

55. Social Security Administration, *Report of the Commissions on the Evaluation of Pain* 186 (U.S. Government Printing Office, Washington, D.C. 1986).

38

Occupational health law

CAROLYN S. LANGER, M.D., J.D., M.P.H.

THE OCCUPATIONAL SAFETY AND HEALTH ACT
KEEPING THE WORKER INFORMED
DISCRIMINATION IN THE WORKPLACE
TORT LIABILITY
LEGAL LIABILITY OF THE OCCUPATIONAL HEALTH CARE PROVIDER: MEDICAL
   MALPRACTICE
CONCLUSION

Occupational medicine is a branch of preventive medicine that "focuses on the relationship among" workers' health, "the ability to perform work, the arrangements of work, and the physical, [biological], and chemical environments of the workplace."[1]

From a medicolegal standpoint, occupational medicine is unique among the medical specialties. In no other specialty do regulatory and legislative mechanisms shape and drive the practice of medicine to the extent found in occupational health. Indeed an entire federal agency, the Occupational Safety and Health Administration (OSHA), has been established within the Department of Labor to safeguard the rights of this particular class of patients (the worker) and to specifically prevent or minimize the incidence of work-related disorders.

Providers of occupational health services also face unique challenges arising out of their dual loyalty to patients and employers. Can the occupational physician strive to uphold traditional notions of patient confidentiality, informed consent, and personal autonomy while simultaneously advancing the employer's goals of increased productivity; public goodwill; decreased workers' compensation costs; and promotion of worker, co-worker, and customer health and safety? Although dual loyalties to employer and employee create the potential for conflict and impairment of medical judgment, in reality incidents of conflict occur far less frequently than might be anticipated.[2] Occupational health care providers (whether company employees, independent contractors, or private physicians) can most effectively limit their own liability, promote the health and safety of their patients, and preserve the legal and moral rights of workers through familiarization with occupational health laws and regulations and by adherence to good medical and risk management principles.

THE OCCUPATIONAL SAFETY AND HEALTH ACT

In 1970 Congress passed the Occupational Safety and Health Act (OSH Act) "to assure so far as possible every working man and woman in the Nation safe and healthful working conditions and to preserve our human resources."[3] This legislation created OSHA, the primary functions of which are (1) to encourage employers and employees to reduce workplace hazards, (2) to promulgate and enforce standards that lessen or prevent job-related injuries and illnesses, (3) to establish separate but dependent responsibilities and rights for employers and employees with respect to achieving safe and healthful working conditions, (4) to maintain a reporting and record-keeping system of occupational injuries and illnesses, (5) to establish research and training programs in occupational safety and health, and (6) to encourage development of state occupational safety and health programs.

Coverage

The OSH Act covers all employees and all employers (defined as any person engaged in a business affecting commerce who has employees) with the following exceptions:

1. Self-employed individuals
2. Farms on which only immediate family members of the employer work
3. Working conditions or workplaces regulated by other federal agencies under other federal statutes (e.g., Mine Safety and Health Act of 1969, Atomic Energy Act of 1954, Department of Transportation regulations)
4. Government employees

Federal employees receive protection by an executive order that mandates federal compliance with OSHA regulations. State and municipal government employees may be protected if their states have OSHA-approved state plans that explicitly grant them coverage.

Standard setting

OSHA standards encompass four major categories: general industry, construction, maritime, and agriculture. In the absence of a specific OSHA standard for a particular working condition or workplace, employers must adhere to Section 5(a)(1) of the OSH Act, or the general duty clause. The general duty clause directs each employer to furnish "to each of his employees employment and a place of employment which are free from recognized hazards that are causing or are likely to cause death or serious physical harm."[4] Where OSHA has promulgated specific standards, the specific duty clause, Section 5(a)(2) of the OSH Act, mandates that employers "shall comply with occupational safety and health standards . . . promulgated under this chapter."[5]

Section 6(b) of the OSH Act authorizes the Secretary of Labor (hereinafter the Secretary) to promulgate, modify, or revoke any occupational safety and health standard. In adopting standards the Secretary must first publish a "Notice of Proposed Rulemaking" in the Federal Register and allow for a period of public response and written comments (at least 30 days, although usually 60 days or more). At the request of any interested party, OSHA will also schedule a public hearing. After the close of the comment period and public hearing, the Secretary must publish the final standard in the Federal Register.

Enforcement

The OSH Act authorizes OSHA to conduct workplace inspections. As a result of a 1978 U.S. Supreme Court decision, however, OSHA compliance officers may no longer conduct warrantless inspections without the employer's consent.[6] Because OSHA employs only about 2000 compliance officers to police more than 76.5 million workplaces, the agency has established a priority system for inspections.[7] From highest to lowest, these priorities are (1) imminent danger situations, (2) catastrophes and fatal accidents, (3) employee complaints, (4) programmed high-hazard inspections, and (5) follow-up inspections.

After an inspection, the area OSHA director may issue the employer a citation indicating the standards that have been violated and the length of time proposed for abatement of those violations. The area director also proposes penalties for these violations. The employer must post a copy of the citation in or near the cited work area for three days or until the violation is abated, whichever is longer. Table 38-1 summarizes the types of violations that OSHA may cite and the concomitant penalties that it may propose.

Employers may contest a citation, proposed penalty, or abatement period by filing a "Notice of Contest" within 15 working days of receipt of the citation and proposed penalty. The area OSHA director will forward the case to the Occupational Safety and Health Review Commission (OSHRC), an agency independent of the Department of Labor. An administrative law judge will rule on the case after a hearing. Any party may seek further review by the entire three-member OSHRC. Commission rulings in turn may be appealed to the U.S. Court of Appeals by any party.

KEEPING THE WORKER INFORMED

More than 60,000 chemicals are in commercial use today.[8] Yet the health effects of many of these substances remain unknown. It is estimated that more than 32 million workers may be exposed to toxic agents in the workplace.[9] After passage of the OSH Act, OSHA promulgated a series of regulations to provide workers with more information about the agents present in their workplaces and to enhance the detection, treatment, and prevention of occupational disorders. The following are three of these important provisions:

1. The Hazard Communication Standard[10]
2. The Recording and Reporting Occupational Injuries and Illnesses Standard[11]
3. The Access to Employee Exposure and Medical Records Standard[12]

Although employers are ultimately responsible for safeguarding the health and safety of their workers, these regulations have given employees, unions, health care providers, and governmental and nongovernmental agencies a more decisive role in the management of workplace health and safety.

TABLE 38-1. OSHA violations and penalties

Violation	Penalty*
Other than serious violation (directly related to job safety and health but unlikely to cause death or serious harm)	Discretionary penalty of up to $7000 per violation
Serious violation (substantial probability of death or serious harm, employer knew or should have known of hazard)	Mandatory penalty of up to $7000 per violation
Willful violation (employer intentionally or knowingly committed a violation or was aware of a hazardous condition and failed to take steps to eliminate it)	Minimum penalty of $5000 per violation, up to $70,000 per violation (willful violations resulting in a worker's death may lead to criminal conviction with fines up to $250,000 for an individual and $500,000 for a corporation, imprisonment, or both)
Repeat violation (violation of a previously cited violation)	Fine of up to $70,000 per violation
Failure to correct prior violation (failure to correct a violation before the abatement date)	Penalty of up to $7000 for each day beyond the abatement date

*OSHA also may issue citations and proposed penalties after conviction for falsification of records, reports, or applications; for violations of posting requirements; or for interference with a compliance officer's performance of duties.

The Hazard Communication Standard

OSHA promulgated the Hazard Communication Standard (HCS) to provide workers with the "right to know" the hazards of chemicals in their workplaces and to enable workers to take appropriate protective measures. Under the HCS, employers must (1) ensure the labeling of each container of hazardous chemicals in the workplace with appropriate identity and hazard warnings, (2) maintain and ensure employee access to Material Safety Data Sheets (MSDSs), and (3) provide employees with information and training on hazardous chemicals in their work areas. MSDSs list the chemical and physical properties of chemical substances, their health hazards, routes of exposure, emergency and first aid procedures, and protective measures for their handling and use. The HCS applies to only chemical agents. Furthermore, MSDSs are not subject to methodical review by regulatory agencies. Thus their quality and adequacy of information vary widely, and they may be of limited use to the clinician in the treatment of exposed workers

The HCS also contains important provisions for health care provider access to the identities of trade secret chemicals. When a medical emergency exists, the chemical manufacturer, distributor, or employer must immediately divulge the identity of trade secret chemicals to the treating physician or nurse if this information is requested for purposes of emergency or first aid treatment. As soon as circumstances permit, the chemical manufacturer, importer, or employer may subsequently require the physician or nurse to sign a written statement of need and a confidentiality agreement.

In nonemergency situations the chemical manufacturer, distributor, or employer must likewise disclose the identity of trade secret chemicals when requested by a health professional (defined by the regulation as a physician, occupational health nurse, industrial hygienist, toxicologist, or epidemiologist). Before disclosure, however, the health professional shall (1) submit a request in writing, (2) demonstrate an occupational health need for the information, (3) explain why disclosure of the chemical identity is essential (in lieu of other information, such as chemical properties, methods of exposure monitoring, methods of diagnosing and treating harmful exposures to the chemical, etc.), (4) enter into a written confidentiality agreement, and (5) describe procedures to maintain confidentiality of the disclosed information. The HCS is a valuable instrument for providing health professionals with information about patient exposures.

Recording and reporting requirements

Soon after passage of the OSH Act, OSHA promulgated standards to fulfill the Act's mandate for the provision of record-keeping and reporting by employers and for the development of information and a system of analysis of occupational accidents and illnesses. Under 29 C.F.R. 1904, employers with more than 10 workers must maintain a log and summary of all recordable occupational injuries and illnesses. Recordable occupational injuries and illnesses include any occupational

(1) fatality (regardless of the span between injury and death, or the duration of illness), (2) lost workday cases (other than fatalities), or (3) nonfatal cases without lost workdays that involve transfer to another job, termination of employment, medical treatment (other than first aid), loss of consciousness, or restriction of work or motion.

Employers must make entries in the log within six working days after notification of a recordable injury or illness. Generally, employers use the form OSHA No. 200 ("the OSHA log") to record this information and must retain the OSHA log for five years beyond the year of entry. Employers also often use form OSHA No. 101, workers' compensation (WC) records, or insurance reports to record supplementary information.

In addition to these record-keeping requirements, the standard further imposes a reporting requirement on working establishments. Employers must report all incidents to the nearest area OSHA office within eight hours when such accidents result in a fatality or the hospitalization of three or more employees. This requirement applies to all employers, regardless of the size of their workforce.

This standard also grants OSHA, as well as other federal and state agencies, the authority to inspect and copy these logs of recordable injuries and illnesses (although some U.S. circuit courts have upheld the need to obtain a search warrant before such inspections). The regulations also ensure employee access to all such logs in their working establishment. These provisions have proved to be a useful source of epidemiological data to employees, unions, researchers, the Bureau of Labor Statistics, and other agencies.

Access to employee exposure and medical records

Employers have no general duty to collect medical or exposure data on workers. Nonetheless, some specific OSHA standards, such as the lead standard, may require medical surveillance of workers exposed to specific agents. In other cases employers may voluntarily institute biological and environmental monitoring programs even when not mandated by OSHA. Regardless, to the extent that employers do compile medical and exposure records on workers exposed to toxic substances or harmful physical agents, they must ensure employee access to these data.

Employers shall make medical records available for examination and copying within 15 days of a request by an employee or his or her designated representative. The employer is obligated only to provide a worker with access to medical records relevant to that particular employee. Access to medical records of other employees requires the formal written consent of those other employees. Employers also must provide employees or their designated representatives with access to employee exposure records. When an employer lacks exposure records on a particular worker, the employer must provide that worker with exposure data of other employees who have similar job duties and working conditions. Under these circumstances, access to co-workers' exposure records does not require written consent. OSHA has the authority to examine and copy any medical or exposure record without formal written consent.

When medical records do exist on an employee, the employer is required to preserve and maintain these records for the duration of employment plus 30 years. Exposure records must be preserved and maintained for 30 years. Although these record retention requirements are the legal responsibility of the employer, it is recommended that independent contractor physicians who provide occupational health services to companies clarify the custodianship and disposition of medical records, specifying in advance the party to be charged with maintaining the medical records for the required duration.

The three standards discussed in this section—the HCS, the Recording and Reporting Occupational Injuries and Illnesses Standard, and the Access to Employee Exposure and Medical Records Standard—collectively keep employees informed of the nature and risks of hazardous materials in their workplaces and of any resulting exposure or health effects. By communicating these risks to workers, OSHA seeks to (1) encourage employers to select safer materials and engineering controls; (2) enable workers to use better protective measures and handling procedures; (3) familiarize workers and health care providers with valuable emergency and first aid information; and (4) minimize health hazards through earlier detection, treatment, and prevention of occupational disorders.

DISCRIMINATION IN THE WORKPLACE

Americans "with disabilities are a discrete and insular minority who have been faced with restrictions and limitations . . . resulting from stereotypic assumptions not truly indicative of the individual ability . . . to participate in, and contribute to, society."[13] The clinician functions as an important interface between disabled persons and the workplace in a variety of settings (e.g., primary care, preplacement physicals, WC and disability evaluations). It is incumbent on health care providers to make a fair and accurate assessment of workers' functional capabilities in relation to job tasks so as not to reinforce deep-rooted stereotypes about the disabled. Moreover, health care providers can play a key role in safeguarding the rights of workers and in educating employers through familiarization with recent legislative and judicial developments in the areas of employment and discrimination law.

The Americans with Disabilities Act

Congress enacted the Americans with Disabilities Act (ADA) in 1990 to eliminate discrimination against the disabled. Although the ADA addresses five separate areas, this chapter focuses exclusively on Title I, employment discrimination.[14]

Title I of the ADA prohibits discrimination against qualified individuals with disabilities in virtually all employment con-

texts (i.e., job application, hiring, discharge, promotion, compensation, job training, and other terms, conditions, and privileges of employment). The act defines disability as (1) a physical or mental impairment that substantially limits one or more of the major life activities, (2) a record of such an impairment, or (3) being regarded as having such an impairment. "Physical or mental impairment" is further defined as "any physiological disorder, or condition, cosmetic disfigurement, or anatomical loss affecting one or more . . . body systems."[15] Persons associated with individuals (e.g., family members) with disabilities also receive protection under the ADA.

Under the ADA, qualification standards, tests, or selection criteria that employers administer to job applicants must be uniformly applied, job related, and consistent with business necessity. To be consistent with business necessity, a standard must concern an essential function of the job. An employer who denies an amputee a desk job on the basis of strength testing would be in violation of the ADA if, for example, lifting were not an essential job task. Moreover, even when the qualification standards are job related, the employer must first attempt to make reasonable accommodations before excluding disabled workers on the basis of those tests. Examples of reasonable accommodations may include modified work schedules, job restructuring, equipment modification, design of wheelchair-accessible workstations, and provision of readers or interpreters.

The ADA provides the following three major defenses to employers charged with discrimination:

1. Selection criteria are job related and consistent with business necessity, and a disabled individual cannot perform essential job tasks even with reasonable accommodation.
2. Reasonable accommodation would impose an undue hardship on the employer.
3. A disabled individual poses a direct threat to himself or herself or to the health and safety of others in the workplace.

The ADA has several important implications for health professionals—whether company employees or independent contractors—who are often called on to perform employment physicals of job applicants or return-to-work assessments of injured workers. First, clinicians and employers need to recognize that the ADA bars all preemployment (preoffer) physicals. Employers may continue to administer preoffer nonmedical tests (e.g., language proficiency or strength and agility testing) that are job related, but they may require a medical examination only after extending an offer of employment. This offer may be conditioned on the results of the postoffer, preplacement physical examination provided that all applicants for a particular position are subjected to such an examination regardless of disability.

Second, clinicians should limit their role to advising employers about workers' functional abilities and limitations in performing the essential functions of the job with or without reasonable accommodation and to determining whether these workers meet the employers' health and safety requirements. To make such determinations of functional abilities and limitations, health professionals must insist that employers provide written job descriptions that accurately detail specific and essential job tasks. The employer has the responsibility to make all employment decisions and to determine the feasibility of reasonable accommodation. Nonetheless, health professionals may offer input on ways to achieve reasonable accommodation.

Third, the ADA imposes very strict limitations on the use of information from postoffer medical examinations and inquiries. Such information must be treated as confidential and must be maintained in separate medical files apart from personnel records. The employer must designate a specific person or persons to have access to the medical file. In some instances the release of confidential medical information may be allowable under the ADA, for example, to inform supervisors or first aid personnel about necessary restrictions or emergency treatment; however, a release form from the examinee is always advisable.*

Although the ADA discourages but does not explicitly prohibit clinicians from reporting actual diagnoses to employers, an action for breach of confidentiality may exist under certain state confidentiality laws if a release form is not signed by the examinee. In the absence of a release form, a clinician's best course of action is to inform the employer of functional abilities and necessary work restrictions (e.g., "no working at heights" and "no driving of company vehicles") rather than reporting actual diagnoses (e.g., "epilepsy").

Discrimination denies the disabled the many advantages of employment, including prestige, power, self-esteem, economic well-being, social outlets, and access to health insurance and other job benefits. The ADA will have far-reaching consequences in protecting the rights of the disabled and more fully integrating them into the workplace. Health professionals can play a critical role in fostering patient autonomy and educating employers while simultaneously promoting a safe and healthful workplace.

Gender discrimination, pregnancy, and fetal protection policies

As with the disabled, pregnant workers have often represented a disenfranchised group within the workplace. Although the ADA is broad sweeping, it does not shield these women from employment discrimination because "pregnancy" is not considered a physiological disorder under the Act's definition of disability. Nonetheless, pregnant workers receive ample protection under both legislative and judicial avenues.[16] The Civil Rights Act of 1964 (Title VII) prohibits

discrimination on the basis of sex and as amended through the Pregnancy Discrimination Act of 1978 further prohibits discrimination against "women affected by pregnancy, childbirth, or related medical conditions . . . for all employment related purposes."[17]

Despite the intent of these laws, a number of industries instituted fetal protection policies (FPPs) throughout the 1980s to exclude fertile or pregnant women from the workplace and to avert toxic exposures to the fetus. In some instances, companies went so far as to exclude all women, including postmenopausal women, from jobs or job tracks involving potential exposure to toxic substances unless these workers could provide documentation of surgical sterilization. These FPPs were unsound for several reasons.

1. They disregarded reproductive risks to male workers.
2. They assumed that all women in the workplace could or would become pregnant.
3. They essentially required female workers to proclaim their reproductive status to supervisors and coworkers (i.e., women remaining in the workplace were implicitly sterile).
4. They discouraged some women from applying for higher-paying jobs.
5. They encouraged other women to undergo unnecessary surgical sterilization solely to retain their jobs.
6. They overlooked the adverse health effects to the unemployed mother and child from foregone income and health benefits.

In 1991 the U.S. Supreme Court declared these FPPs to be unconstitutional in International Union, *UAW v. Johnson Controls, Inc.*[18] The court held these policies to be discriminatory because they did not apply equally to the reproductive capacity of male employees. Furthermore, the court held that "decisions about the welfare of future children must be left to the parents . . . rather than to the employers who hire those parents."[19]

There are principally only two instances in which employers may discriminate on the basis of gender or pregnancy. Employers may deny employment when gender is a bona fide occupational qualification (BFOQ) reasonably necessary to the normal operation of that particular business or enterprise. Analogous to the ADA, the qualification standards must relate to the essence of the employer's business. For example, a movie producer would be justified in claiming that male gender is a BFOQ when hiring actors for male roles. Under the safety exception, employers may discriminate on the basis of gender in those instances in which gender or pregnancy interferes with the employee's ability to perform the job. For example, airlines are permitted to lay off pregnant flight attendants at various stages of pregnancy to ensure the safety of passengers. In all other instances women should be treated equally with men in the employment setting as long as they possess the necessary job-related skills and aptitudes.

---

*Workers sometimes voluntarily disclose their diagnoses to supervisors or first aid responders on their shift to familiarize them with the signs and symptoms of their condition in the event of a medical emergency.

In light of this legislative and judicial history, the following practices that screen out individual women or the entire class of women might be construed as discriminatory:

1. Implementing FPPs or other policies that exclude women from the workplace based on gender or reproductive status
2. Applying coercion by providing female but not male workers or job applicants with information on reproductive risks or by requiring only female workers to sign waivers absolving the employer of liability in the event of an adverse reproductive outcome
3. Administering special tests or medical examinations exclusively to women
4. Using physiological parameters, such as muscle strength, as selection criteria when not a requirement for the job (For this reason, as with the ADA, job descriptions that accurately reflect job tasks are vital.)
5. Using gender as a proxy for physiological parameters even when specific physiological traits (e.g., anthropometrics and muscle strength) are a requirement for the job and a high correlation exists between gender and ability to perform the job (Employers must give each individual the opportunity to demonstrate that she meets the job parameters.)

Workers' compensation

Claims. Physicians who evaluate and treat workers with job-related injuries or illnesses must acquire a broad understanding of the workers' compensation (WC) system and an appreciation of their role in the legal disposition of WC claims.

WC systems currently exist in all 50 states and in three federal jurisdictions.[20] WC is a no-fault system that evolved in the earlier part of the twentieth century to promote expeditious resolution of work-related claims. Injured workers relinquished their rights to bring an action in torts in exchange for a rapid, fixed, and automatic payment. The quid pro quo for the employer was a limited and predictable award. WC pays for medical and rehabilitation expenses and typically up to two thirds of wage replacement.

Unlike tort actions, WC claims do not require a showing of employer negligence. Therefore even injuries or illnesses resulting from the employee's own negligence are compensable. Regardless of the cause of the injury, the worker carries the burden of proving by a preponderance of the evidence that a causal relationship exists between an occupational exposure and the resulting injury or illness; that is, the injury or illness must "arise out of or in the course of employment." Employees also are generally entitled to compensation for work-related aggravation of preexisting disorders. To qualify for WC payments, the worker must prove damages, typically by demonstrating a disability or loss in earning capacity. Even when the occupational exposure results in an injury or illness that produces no disability, the employee may still be eligible for an award if the WC laws in that jurisdiction explicitly provide for such coverage, such as

payment for scarring, disfigurement, or damage or loss of function of specific organs or body systems.

Physicians who evaluate and treat injured workers must strive to be objective when documenting physical findings and impairments. Although physicians are not discouraged from making assertions about causality, they must be prepared to support their conclusions in a deposition or courtroom should the claim lead to litigation. It is also incumbent on physicians to familiarize themselves with alternative work and transitional duty programs to minimize the length of disability.

Confidentiality. Patients will often present treating physicians with authorization forms requesting release of medical records to the patient's employer, the employer's attorney, or the employer's insurance company in support of a WC claim. By signing these release forms, patients do not waive all rights of confidentiality. It is critical that physicians disclose only information related to the disorder that forms the basis of the WC claim. Several physicians have been sued for releasing confidential information about HIV status that was unrelated to the WC claim, such as ear and sinus problems or head injury with back pain.[21,22] Patients sued these physicians under various theories, such as negligence, breach of confidentiality, breach of contract, and invasion of privacy.

TORT LIABILITY

Many WC statutes contain "exclusive remedy provisions" that hold that WC shall provide the exclusive remedy for injuries and illnesses arising out of or in the course of employment. The goals of these provisions are to foreclose litigation and to limit the employer's liability to WC. During the last few decades, however, workers have been attempting to circumvent the exclusive remedy provisions of WC laws and pursue tort suits. As in WC cases, plaintiffs in tort suits may recover for medical expenses and lost earnings, but because tort actions are more likely to take into account future promotions and job advancements, they may yield a higher award for wage replacement. Moreover, tort suits offer the additional advantage of recovery for certain types of damages unavailable under WC, such as pain and suffering, punitive damages, and loss of consortium.

Despite the greater financial incentive to bring a tort suit, the courts have been reluctant to carve out exceptions to the WC exclusive remedy provisions. The most common doctrines under which employees file tort suits are as follows[23]:

1. Third-party and product liability suits
2. Intentional harm committed by an employer
3. Injury by a coemployee (injuries by coemployee health care providers are discussed in the following section on medical malpractice)
4. Dual capacity doctrine (the employer assumes a second role or capacity sufficiently distinct from its role as employer such that workers injured by the employer while acting in this second capacity may recover outside of the WC system)

Theoretically, both WC and tort liability should provide employers with the incentive to promote a safe and healthful workplace. However, given the employer's ability to insure and to pass on some of these costs to consumers, the extent to which these goals are accomplished remains unclear.

LEGAL LIABILITY OF THE OCCUPATIONAL HEALTH CARE PROVIDER: MEDICAL MALPRACTICE

What is the legal liability of a health care provider who commits medical malpractice while under contract to provide occupational health services to a company's employees? Management hires physicians, nurses, and other health care professionals—company salaried and independently contracted—for the benefit of the company (i.e., to ensure workers' fitness for duty).

Historically, health care providers salaried by a company were considered coemployees of other workers. Consequently their negligent acts and the resulting injuries were regarded as arising out of and in the course of employment. The exclusive remedy provisions of WC laws therefore limited injured workers to recovery under the WC system. However, if the workers could establish that the health care providers were not under the control of the company but rather were functioning as independent contractors, they could avail themselves a remedy in torts.

The distinctions between coemployees and independent contractors have been problematic for the courts. Health care providers often have greater latitude than other employees in their exercise of judgment. At what point do their actions transcend the control of their employers and exceed the scope of employment? Some companies authorize and encourage occupational health care providers to furnish primary care services to employees and even to their families. At what point does the occupational health professional establish a health care provider–patient relationship, no longer acting solely for the benefit of the employer but also for the benefit of the employee?

The courts have developed two tests to determine whether an occupational health care provider is the coemployee of an injured worker (in which case the negligent act is covered by the employer's WC policy) or an independent contractor (and therefore subject to tort liability). Under the control test, health care providers are more likely to be presumed company employees when management exerts greater control over their function, operation, and judgment. For example, clinicians act under the control of the company when they must follow predetermined guidelines and protocols in conducting physical examinations (e.g., which forms to use or which laboratory tests to conduct).

Under the indicia test, the court analyzes various indices of control that normally signify employee status. For example, health care providers are more likely to be categorized as company employees rather than independent contractors if they receive a salary, health insurance, and other company benefits; fall under the company's WC and pension programs; work out of company offices; have regularly scheduled work hours; and report to the company's chain of command.[24]

Despite these two tests, the immunity of occupational health care providers continues to erode. Although the control and indicia tests provide useful guidelines concerning the potential liability of the occupational health care provider, their application results in some uncertainty because many professionals only partially meet these criteria. For example, some clinicians who have a part-time private practice may request workers to follow-up after duty hours in their private offices. Other clinicians may work out of their own offices but see exclusively company employees. Furthermore, courts appreciate that workers often rely on the results of employment physicals to their detriment and that health professionals have a high degree of skill and training and are in a better position to warn patients of harm and to insure against losses. Thus, although courts were traditionally reluctant (even in the independent contractor setting) to hold that a physician-patient relationship existed between a prospective or actual employee and the physician conducting the examination at the employer's request and for the employer's benefit, more courts are willing to recognize that the "examination creates a relationship between the examining physician and the examinee, at least to the extent of the tests conducted."[25]

Therefore the wisest approach for occupational health care providers, whether company employees or independent contractors, is to conduct examinations and treatment with due care and to disclose the results from any tests or examinations performed to the patient. Health care providers must be cautious in following up with patients because attempts to offer

---

BOX 38-1. RISK MANAGEMENT PRINCIPLES FOR OCCUPATIONAL HEALTH CARE PROVIDERS

1. Request job descriptions that reflect essential job functions.
2. For company-employed physicians, provide medical services only:
   - To employees (to employees' dependents only if company authorizes in contract and provides malpractice coverage)
   - During normal business or duty hours
   - On company premises (if available)
   - To the extent delineated in employment contract
3. Adhere to company policies.
4. Evaluate necessity and purpose of components of physical examinations and medical surveillance programs.
5. Do not order unnecessary tests.
6. Ensure that all tests are interpreted by qualified individuals.
7. Inform patients of results of all tests.
8. Ensure adequate/reasonable follow-up (appropriate to circumstances).
9. Keep good records—document, document, document.

advice or to treat may establish a health care provider–patient relationship and place their actions beyond the scope of employment. Health care providers who want to ensure that employees receive adequate follow-up without risking tort liability should consider sending certified letters to patients advising them of the results and of the need for follow-up with their own private family physicians or other specialists as appropriate. See Box 38-1 for more detailed risk management principles. Health care providers would be prudent to delineate these responsibilities in their contracts with employers. Furthermore, occupational health care providers employed by companies should not rely solely on employers' WC policies but also should be covered by malpractice insurance.

CONCLUSION

Occupational health care providers are in a unique position to ensure worker health and safety. Because they interact with injured workers at every phase of employment—preplacement, preinjury, and postinjury—they have a profound impact on the disposition of job applicants and employees in the workplace. Occupational health professionals place a strong emphasis on prevention. Familiarization with judicial, legislative, and regulatory mandates will enable them to preserve the health and uphold the rights of workers, to educate employers, and to minimize their own liability.

ENDNOTES

1. From the ACGME Special Requirements for Residency Education in Occupational Medicine, effective Jan 1, 1993.
2. J.A. Gold, *The Physician and the Corporation,* 3 Bioethics Bull. 1 (Fall 1989).
3. 29 U.S.C. §§§ 651(b) (1988).
4. 29 U.S.C. §§§ 654(a)(1) (1988).
5. 29 U.S.C. §§§ 654 (a)(2).
6. *Marshall v. Barlow's, Inc.,* 436 U.S. 307 (1978).
7. J. Miles Jr., Regional Administrator, OSHA Regional Office (Region I), Boston, private communication (Mar 14, 1994).
8. Office of Technology Assessment, *Reproductive Hazards in the Workplace* 37 (Lippincott, Philadelphia 1988).
9. OSHA 3110, Access to Medical and Exposure Records1 (1989).
10. 29 C.F.R. 1910.1200.
11. 29 C.F.R. 1904.
12. 29 C.F.R. 1910.1020.
13. 42 U.S.C. §§§ 12101 (a) (7) (Supp. IV 1992).
14. Americans with Disabilities Act of 1990: Title I, Employment; Title II, Public Service/Public Transportation; Title III, Public Accommodation & Services Operated by Private Entities; Title IV, Telecommunications; Title V, Miscellaneous Provisions.
15. Note that current drug abusers receive no protection under the ADA because illegal drug use is not considered a disability under the act. However, alcoholics and fully rehabilitated drug abusers may be protected under the ADA (unless they fail to meet productivity and other performance standards that cannot be corrected by reasonable accommodation).
16. 42 U.S.C. §§§ 2000e-2(a) (1988).
17. 42 U.S.C. §§§ 2000e(k) (1988).
18. *International Union, UAW v. Johnson Controls, Inc.,* 111 S.Ct. 1196 (1991).
19. *Id.* at 1207.
20. L.I. Boden, *Workers' Compensation, in Occupational Health: Recognizing and Preventing Work-Related Disease* 202 (B.S. Levy & D.H. Wegeman eds., Little, Brown & Company, Boston 1995).
21. *Doe v. Roe,* 190 A.D. 2d 463 (1993).
22. *Urbaniak v. Newton,* 277 Cal. Rptr. 354 (Cal.App. 1 Dist. 1991).
23. Modified from S.L. Birnbaum & B. Wrubel, *Workers' Compensation and the Employer's Immunity Shield: Recent Exceptions to Exclusivity,* 50 J. Products Liability 119 (1982).
24. See, e.g., *Garcia v. Iserson,* 33 N.Y. 2d 421, 309 N.E. 2d 420 (1970), holding that worker's exclusive remedy fell under WC law. The plaintiff could not maintain a malpractice action against a company physician because the injuries arose out of and in the course of employment since the company employed the physician at a weekly salary and took the usual payroll deductions, required the physician to work on company premises during certain scheduled hours, and included the physician in the company's medical plan and WC policy. See also *Golini v. Nachtifall,* 38 N.Y. 2d 745, 343 N.E. 2d 762 (1975), holding that WC provided the exclusive remedy to the plaintiff injured by a physician who received company salary and benefits and worked in company facilities.
25. *Green v. Walker,* 910 F. 2d 291 (5th Cir. 1990), holding that physician who was under contract to perform annual employment physicals was liable for malpractice in failing to diagnose and report cancer to examinee.

GENERAL REFERENCES

N.A. Ashford & C.C. Caldart, *Technology, Law, and the Working Environment* (Van Nostrand Reinhold, New York 1991).

B.P. Billauer, *The Legal Liability of the Occupational Health Professional,* 27 J. Occup. Med. 185-188 (1985).

J. Ladou, ed., *Occupational Medicine* (Appleton & Lange, Norwalk, Conn. 1990).

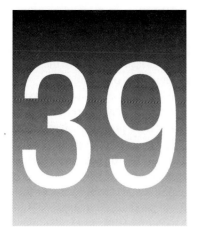

Public health law

GENIFER Y. CHAVEZ, M.D., J.D., M.P.H., M.A., F.C.L.M.

INFECTIOUS DISEASE AND IMMUNIZATION
BEHAVIORAL FACTORS AND LIFESTYLE
POLICIES OF CONTAINMENT AND PATIENTS' RIGHTS
CONCLUSION

Public health is a branch of preventive medicine that focuses on health issues in populations. These health issues include communicable diseases, noncommunicable and chronic disabling conditions, environmental health, behavioral factors affecting health, and health care planning, organization, and evaluation. Efforts to control communicable diseases include sanitation, vaccinations, and prevention of sexually transmitted diseases and diseases spread by close, personal contact. Prevention of chronic illness entails disease screening and instituting preventive programs in every setting: home, school, workplace, health care institutions, and recreational sites.[1]

Environmental health is a broad area where concerns range from the exposure of a single individual in the workplace or in the ambient environment to air, soil, and water pollution and global concerns (see Chapter 38).

Health is influenced by social factors in the environment. The prevention of disease is the major goal of public health programs. Many diseases of concern involve large numbers of people, and it is more cost-effective to prevent such diseases at an environmental level than on an individual level. It is also a more difficult challenge to motivate individuals to change their behaviors.

From a medicolegal standpoint, public health is complex because best interests for the population must be balanced against rights of the individual. Public health officials generally answer to the best interest of the community. They also must be cognizant of laws that may infringe on individuals' rights, especially in areas such as communicable diseases and state police powers. When is it legal to institute court orders to curtail the spread of a disease? Public health measures to control communicable diseases have existed in the United States since the colonial period. The courts have struggled with society's interests versus those of the individual and frequently defer decisions to other branches of government. New regard for individual liberties will be balanced both by the desire to protect society and by the social fears that once

led to strict quarantines in eugenic laws (laws that deal with the science of improving the hereditary qualities of humans) during the early 1900s.[2]

Early judicial rulings have shown considerable deference to the state's police powers to promote the public health. Strict judicial scrutiny will probably be applied to public health measures that affect liberty, autonomy, or privacy.[3] The law must protect two conflicting interests: the right of the public to be protected against disease and the right of the individual not to be unfairly restricted as a result of having or being at risk for disease.[4]

INFECTIOUS DISEASE AND IMMUNIZATION

Reporting laws that estimate morbidity, particularly those for infectious diseases, are based on a national system in effect in the United States since the 1920s. Reports from physicians, hospitals, and laboratories are sent to the Centers for Disease Control and Prevention (CDC) through health departments. This approach to surveillance has been used to characterize seasonal trends and to detect epidemics through trends and temporal relationships.[5]

Infectious agents such as human immunodeficiency virus (HIV) create other issues, such as mandatory testing. Initial state reporting requirements have expanded to help control the spread of disease. These seek to limit the activities of infected individuals by preventing them from attending school or by performing screening tests to identify carriers. Federal statutory authority has also been evoked. Now there can be liability for and compensation given to patients with acquired immunodeficiency syndrome (AIDS) who contracted the disease from blood transfusions, organ transplantation, or sexual activity. This can have a significant impact on health personnel and public health policy. The breaching of confidentiality can also result in increased bias against AIDS patients and HIV carriers, which can compound the discrimination they are experiencing in employment, housing, health care, insurance, and even in death.[6]

The requirement to receive specific immunizations for entrance into schools or the military highlights the issue of patient autonomy. To what extent can government or governmental agencies dictate to private citizens what immunizations they must receive? Amish people have tested this requirement in the courts. Recent court decisions have upheld the rights of individuals seeking exemptions from immunizations based upon religious belief.[7]

BEHAVIORAL FACTORS AND LIFESTYLE

Public health officials may infringe on patient autonomy by attempting to change behavioral factors affecting health, such as smoking, alcohol, drug abuse, and lifestyle habits.[8] Some propose that pregnant women who abuse drugs (e.g., alcohol, cocaine, marijuana) should face legal actions, such as involuntary commitment, forced treatment, or criminal sanctions. These sanctions, however, which are intended to remedy maternal-fetal conflicts, may encourage some women to avoid beneficial medical and social services or to seek abortion.[9]

Some state legislatures are proposing that patients should pay for their own lifestyle choices that negatively impact their health. Some hospitals and health care organizations are analyzing who "deserves" health care. As the need to ration health care approaches, ethics committees will lead these discussions in American society.

Public health law also affects the rights of other world citizens, especially immigrants attempting to enter the United States.

POLICIES OF CONTAINMENT AND PATIENTS' RIGHTS

A policy of containment must exclude individuals with a fatal communicable disease of public health significance to protect the public's health. This policy could be viewed as a form of racial discrimination aimed at excluding immigrants from "dangerous nations."[10] As the United States becomes more concerned with immigration problems, Congress may take more restrictive measures to limit entrance into the country. In 1993, President Clinton signed a law banning immigration by HIV-infected persons. Justification for this law is twofold: (1) to decrease the cost of caring for HIV AIDS patients and (2) to reduce the risk of spreading HIV. To avoid human rights violations, as expressed in the U.S. Constitution, the risk of a person spreading the disease in question must be real, and risk assessment must not be based on prejudice or irrational fear.[11]

Public health officials are being pressured to implement compulsory measures to check the rapid spread of AIDS. Four control measures are proposed: (1) contract tracing, (2) general isolation, (3) quarantine-modified isolation based on behavior likely to transmit AIDS, and (4) deterrents through criminal penalties. According to some, however, these measures would do little to slow the spread of AIDS. Instead, these proposals would unduly restrict the liberty, autonomy, and privacy of persons vulnerable to AIDS infection.[12]

Population and policy changes

The relationship between health and the dynamics of population change determines the need for changes in public health practice. The following four issues illustrate the relationship between public health and the community[13]:

1. Teenage pregnancy is a serious public health issue because it creates preventable health problems for both infants and mothers. These problems may interfere with education, personal development, and socioeconomic advancement for the young parents and may impact future generations.
2. Demographics are changing as the death rates continue to decline and life expectancies increase. This means more old people with more diseases and greater health care costs.
3. More than 40% of the world's populations now live in urban centers. Urbanization creates health problems related to the need for sanitation, housing, improved food supply, better transportation system, and redistribution of preventive and other health services.
4. Health care costs and services are impacted by refugees and other migrants, who may have serious public health problems, such as severe malnutrition and infections.

Tuberculosis

The resurgence of tuberculosis (TB) confronts policymakers with difficult legal and ethical questions about the proper use of state power and the resources available to protect public health.

Again, the focus must be on the limitations of government power and the obligation to balance the demands of civil liberty with the demands of public health.[14] Patients with TB who do not comply with treatment present a public health risk. Patients with active TB who do not follow their prescribed medical program pose a serious hazard to others as well as to themselves. If directly observed therapy cannot be implemented, involuntary confinement of such patients is ethically justified. Some states have created a new civil process that allows for detention of noninfectious (but persistently nonadherent) patients so that they can receive treatment.[15] A normal response to the control of TB must be sustainable and able to control the spread of the disease with minimal impact on an individual's rights.[16]

The resurgence of TB in the early 1990s with the multidrug-resistant strains led public health officials to recommend involuntary detention for persistently noncompliant patients. Once again, detention programs attempt to balance protection of the public's health with the patient's civil liberties.

In general, health departments have detained patients as a last resort and provide them with due process; however, health officials still retain great authority to bypass the "least restrictive alternatives" in certain cases and to detain noninfectious patients for months or years. As rates of TB and public attention continue to decrease, forcible confinement of sick patients should be reserved only for those individuals who truly threaten the public's health.[17]

Persons with active pulmonary TB constitute the major reservoir of infections. Since the predominant mode of infection is through inhalation of airborne tubercle bacilli in droplet nuclei, which may occur simply by talking, coughing, sneezing, or singing, this organism is highly infectious. If actively infected persons refuse treatment, the public's health is at risk because of the ubiquitous nature of disease spread.

This is the main distinction that will determine restriction of a TB patient's rights, versus not restricting an HIV patient's rights. A person with HIV or AIDS cannot infect others simply by talking, laughing, or coughing.

HIV issues

A small percentage of HIV-positive patients have a concomitant psychological or neurological disorder associated with impaired judgment. Psychoses, personality disorders, and dementias are associated with disinhibitions of impulses and diminished capacity for self-monitoring. These deficits in reasoning and judgment may prevent the patient from comprehending the significance of his or her HIV status and the consequences of sexual behavior or needle-sharing. When an HIV patient engages in high-risk sexual behavior with identifiable partners and refuses to notify them of his or her HIV status, physicians and mental health professionals may have a legal and ethical duty to warn those who are exposed.[18]

CONCLUSION

Issues of public health law are complex. Public health officials must determine the threat to the community and the preventive or modifiable factors. They also must consider the financial impact, the social cost to the community, and the impact on the individual's rights.

Many public health issues will be dealt with through the legislative and judicial processes. Many current public health problems remain to be addressed.

ENDNOTES

1. J.M. Last & R.B. Wallace, *Public Health and Preventive Medicine,* 13th ed. (Appleton & Lange, East Norwalk, Conn. 1992).
2. D.J. Merritt, *The Constitutional Balance Between Health and Liberty,* 16(6) Hastings Center Report Suppl. 2-10 (1986).
3. L. Gostin & W. Curran, *Legal Control Measures for AIDS: Reporting Requirements, Surveillance, Quantitation, and Regulations of Public Meeting Places,* 77(2) Am. J. Public Health 214-218 (1987).
4. A. Orr, *Legal AIDS: Implications of AIDS and HIV for British and American Law,* 15(2) J. Med. Ethics 61-67 (1989).
5. *Sherr and Levy v. Northport East. Northport Union Free School District,* 672 F. Suppl. 81 (E.D.N.Y., 1987).
6. G.W. Matthews & V.S. Neslund, *The Initial Impact of AIDS on Public Health Law in the United States, 1986,* 257(3) JAMA 344-351 (1987).
7. *Supra* note 1.
8. R.L. Schwartz, *Making Patients Pay for Their Lifestyle Choices,* 1(4) Cambridge Quarterly Healthcare Ethics 393-400 (1992).
9. K.A. DeVille & L.M. Kopelman, *Moral and Social Issues Regarding Pregnant Women Who Use and Abuse Drugs,* 25(1) Obstet. Gynecol. Clin. North Am. 237-254 (1998).
10. A.L. Fairchild & E.A. Tynan, *Policies of Containment: Immigration in the Era of AIDS,* 84(12) Am. J. Public Health 2011-2022 (1994).
11. G.J. Annas, *Detention of HIV-Positive Haitians at Guantanamo: Human Rights and Medical Care,* 320(8) N. Engl. J. Med. 589-592 (1993).
12. L. Gostin & W. Curran, *The Limits of Compulsion in Controlling AIDS,* 16(6) Hastings Center Report Suppl 24-29 (1986).
13. *Supra* note 1.
14. R. Bayer & L. Dupuis, *Tuberculosis, Public Health, and Civil Liberties,* 16 Annual Rev. Public Health 307-326 (1995).
15. T. Oscherwitz et al., *Detention of Persistently Nonadherent Patients with Tuberculosis,* 278(10) JAMA 843-846 (1997).
16. M.J. Booker, *Compliance, Coercion, and Compassion: Moral Dimensions of the Return of Tuberculosis,* 17(2) J. Med. Humanities 91-102 (1996).
17. B.H. Lerner, *Catching Patients: Tuberculosis and Detentions in the 1990s,* 115(1) Chest 236-241 (1999).
18. H.R. Searight & P. Pound, *The HIV-Positive Psychiatric Patient and the Duty To Protect: Ethical and Legal Issues,* 24(3) Int. J. Psychiatry Med. 259-270 (1994).

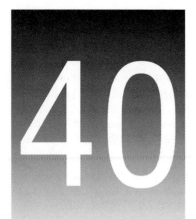

Sports medicine

RICHARD S. GOODMAN, M.D., J.D., F.A.A.O.S., F.C.L.M.

Legal aspects of sports medicine is one of the most dynamic fields in the interphase between law and medicine. *Sports medicine* can be defined as the science or practice of diagnosis, treatment, and prevention of diseases associated with a physical activity that involves exertion, is governed by rules or customs, and is often competitive. Sports medicine is accepted as a medical discipline and a medical subspecialty. Related organizations include the American Society of Sports Medicine and the American Osteopathic Academy of Sports Medicine. Publications include the American, British, and international journals of sports medicine; *Isokinetics and Exercise Science; Journal of Athletic Training; Journal of Biomechanics; Journal of Sports Medicine and Physical Fitness; Journal of Sports Traumatology and Related Research;* and *Medicine and Science in Sports and Exercise.* Other publications, such as the *American Journal of Knee Surgery, Orthopedics, and Orthopedic Review,* routinely cover sports medicine. The *Yearbook of Sports Medicine* abstracts the leading articles in the field.

Laws provide a set of rules to govern those who practice any aspect of medicine that affects participants in a sporting event. Medical law is specific for those who practice medicine that affects sports participants.

This concept—the need for a set of rules to govern medical decisions that affect an athlete—contrasts with the ruling by Judge Cardozo in the famous amusement ride case: "One who takes part in such sport accepts the dangers so far that they are obvious and necessary just as a fencer accepts the risks of a thrust by his antagonist or a spectator at a ball game the chance of contact with the ball."[1]

The courts are now being asked, "What are obvious and necessary risks?" Is the risk of contracting human immunodeficiency virus (HIV) or being exposed to HIV by competing against an opponent who is HIV positive an "obvious and necessary risk," even if it is a small or minimal risk? Is the risk of incurring a catastrophic injury, or the risk of *any* injury, an obvious risk? Is participating in a sport while handicapped or impaired and then being injured an obvious and necessary risk? Can a participant sign away his or her right to sue in response to a catastrophic injury, or to sue for *any* injury, in exchange for the right to participate? Is the risk of a catastrophic injury caused by poor coaching, poor refereeing, or poorly maintained or substandard equipment obvious and necessary?

These questions, as yet unanswered, are the province of legal aspects of sport medicine. Abrasions, bumps, bruises, contusions, and fractures may be considered part of many sports, including contact sports (e.g., football, basketball, soccer) and noncontact sports (e.g., skiing, rollerblading, gymnastics), as well as cheerleading and golf. However, catastrophic injuries, such as death, paraplegia, quadriplegia, permanent brain damage, or HIV infection, are *not* considered part of most sports and are not expected or assumed risks by the average or reasonable participant.[2-8]

One case asked whether schools can be held negligent for substantial injuries during cheerleading practice.[9] The court held that the doctrine of primary assumption of risk, as well as the failure to breach the school's duty to supervise the cheerleader and the signed release by the cheerleader's mother, barred any action.

Medical providers now include any person who acts, appears to be acting, or is assumed to be acting in the role of a health care provider, including but not limited to physicians, chiropractors, trainers, physical therapists, and physician assistants. When a participant in a sport incurs a catastrophic injury or any other injury, a question arises as to the cause of the injury or the level of treatment provided after the injury. On occasion there are reasonable grounds for the injured party to assume that the person providing or appearing to provide health care is knowledgeable in medical care or the

The author extends his appreciation to Norman Samnick of Strook, Strook, and Levan for his extensive research and for use of his facility in legal aspects of sports medicine.

need for medical care. When the care is not provided and results in a catastrophic injury, a growing tendency is to hold the responsible party liable for the lack of care or the improper care.

Among those now being held responsible for these injuries are coaches, supervisors, gym teachers, physical education instructors, trainers, the on-scene or on-call physician, and even the physician who provided the preparticipation athletic physical examination and gave clearance to participate. The providers, as well as the lessors and the maintainers of equipment (including golf carts, which can be proved to be faulty), can also be held responsible as the causal agent for the catastrophic injury.[10,11]

The field of legal aspects of sports medicine is therefore a review of the trend to expand the liability for catastrophic injuries and other injuries sustained by sports participants to those who provide equipment or maintain playing fields as well as those who are practicing sports medicine directly or indirectly. This aspect of sports law—the assignment of responsibility for any of these injuries—focuses on the potential exposure to and limits of liability of the medical and paramedical staffs; the coaching staff and the umpiring, refereeing, or officiating staff; and the suppliers of equipment and playing fields. Their potential liability has now come to the forefront in sports medicine law.

This potential liability of the coaching staff, officials, trainers, and instructors arises from their frequent role as the on-site provider of health care.[12] From a review of the cases cited, the coach is potentially liable if a catastrophic injury can be related to failure of the on-scene supervisor or health provider to do the following:

1. Provide appropriate training instruction.
2. Maintain or purchase safe equipment.
3. Hire or supervise competent and responsible personnel.
4. Give adequate warning to participants concerning dangers inherent in a sport.
5. Provide prompt and proper medical care.
6. Prevent the injured athlete from further competition that could aggravate an injury.

The coach can also be held liable if the injury can be related to the inappropriate matching of athletes with dissimilar physical capabilities and dissimilar skill levels.

Cases in which the failure to properly supervise resulted in severe injuries include the student hit by a golf club because of excessive proximity of another golf student, the wrestler injured by a teammate of much greater skill and weight, and the unpadded football player struck by a teammate's helmet.[13-16] A failure to teach proper technique to avoid injury leaves the instructor at risk. A subsequent injury (e.g., in a football game, to a cheerleader) may be related to the improper technique.[17]

Staff members also have been held responsible for improper use of or failure to insist on proper use of equipment, including golf carts, the design of paths for golf carts, and installation and maintenance of lightning warning devices. They may also be liable for subsequent injuries.[18]

Another sports medicine issue involves the responsibility for allowing an athlete to participate or the adequacy of the "release" documentation. Releases include parental "permission to participate" for minors, "clearance to participate" by physicians, "permission to allow transportation" for minors, adequacy of preparticipation medical histories and physical examinations, and allowing nonconforming athletes who have a known greater exposure to significant injuries to participate.

These aspects of liability have been tested when they conflict with (1) exculpatory agreements; (2) the concept of the sovereign immunity applied to towns, states, and governmental bodies; and (3) an individual's civil rights. Journals such as the *University of Miami Entertainment and Sports Law Review* and *Entertainment and Sports Law* cover the field of questions regarding the liability of operators or owners (e.g., indoor sports arenas, baseball parks, bowling alleys, skating rinks), proprietors (e.g., racing facilities), and promoters (e.g., boxing contests) for the safety of the patrons.[19-24]

The liability of a physician, coach, trainer, or referee who allows an athlete to participate conflicts with the other aspect of sports law—civil rights. Refusing to allow a participant to enter a sport or continue his or her participation because of the potential for a significant injury can be held as a violation of his or her civil rights or right to continue in the sport.

The legal requirement of sports medicine is to document adequately the participation or lack of participation as well as the prescribed roles of the involved parties. Any person who is a de facto provider of health care to an athlete must have a facility to document the preparticipation process, including the assumption of ordinary risks by the participant or his or her guardian; sufficient preparticipation medical clearance; adequate training in sport safety; proper equipment and playing field; and sufficient umpiring to prevent ordinary, unnecessary trauma.

ENDNOTES

1. *Murphy v. Steeplechase Amusement Co.,* 250 N.Y. 479, 482 (1929).
2. M.J. Mitten, *Amateur Athletes with Handicaps or Physical Abnormalities: Who Makes the Participation Decision?* 71 N.E.B.L. Rev. 987 (1992).
3. D.M. Weber, *When the "Magic" Rubs Off: The Legal Implications of AIDS in Professional Sports,* 2 Sports Law. 1 (1995).
4. C.J. Jones, *College Athletes: Illness or Injury and the Decision to Return to Play,* 40 Buff. L. Rev. 113 (1992).
5. P.M. Anderson, *Cautious Defense: Should I Be Afraid To Guard You? (Mandatory AIDS Testing in Professional Team Sports),* 5 Marq. Sports L. J. 279 (1995).
6. T.E. George, *Secondary Break: Dealing with AIDS in Professional Sports After the Initial Response to Magic Johnson,* U. Miami Ent. & Sports L. Rev. 215 (1992).
7. J.L. Johnston, *Is Mandatory HIV Testing of Professional Athletes Really the Solution?* 4 Health Matrix 159 (1994).
8. M.J. Mitten, *Aid-Athletes,* 2 Seaton Hall J. Sports L. 5 (1993).
9. *AARIS v. Las Virgenes Unified School Dist,* 75 Cal. Rptr. 2d 801.

10. S. Berheim, *Sports: Recreation Injuries. A Seminar For Personal Injury Lawyers, School Attorneys and General Practitioners,* Suffolk Academy of Law (Nov 1996).

11. M. Flynn, Cart 54, *Where Are You? The Liability of Golf Course Operators for Golf Cart Injuries,* 14 Ent. & Sports L. 127-151.

12. *A Guide to the Legal Liability of Coaches for a Sports Participants Injuries,* 6 Seaton Hall J. Sports L. 1, 7-127 (1996).

13. *Brahatecek v. Millard School District,* 273 N.W. 2d 680 (Neb. 1979).

14. *Stehn v. Bernard MacFadden Food,* C.A. 4398 (M.D. Tenn. (1996) 434 F. 2d 811 (6th Cir. 1970).

15. *Leahy v. School Board of Hernando County,* 450 S.D. 2d 883 (Fla. Dist. Ct. App. 1984).

16. *Massie v. Persson,* 729 S.W. 2d 448 (Ky. Ct. App. 1987).

17. *Woodson v. Irvington Board of Ed.,* Docket ESX-L-56273 (N.J. Super. Ct. Law Div., Jan 1988).

18. *Supra* note 11; *Baker v. Briarcliff,* 613 N.Y.S. 2sd 660 (N.Y. App. Div. 1994).

19. *Uline Ice, Inc. v. Sullivan,* 88 U.S. App. D.C. 104, 187 F. 2d 82.

20. *Neinstein v. Los Angeles Dodgers, Inc.* (2nd Dist.), 185 Cal. App. 3d 176.

21. *Ackerman v. Motor Sales and Services Co.,* 217 Minn. 309, 14 N.W. 2d 345.

22. *Thomas v. Studio Amusements, Inc.,* 50 Cal. App. 2d 538, 1223 p. 2d 552.

23. *Hotels El Rancho v. Pray,* 64 Nev. 591, 187 P. 2d 568,

24. *Parmentiere v McGinnis,* 157 Wis. 596, 147 N.W. 1007.

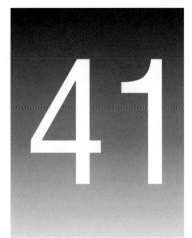

Forensic use of medical information

CYRIL H. WECHT, M.D., J.D., F.C.L.M.

BRIEF HISTORY OF FORENSIC MEDICINE
THE ADVERSARIAL PROCESS
EXPERT WITNESSES
FORENSIC PSYCHIATRY AND PSYCHOLOGY
ADMISSIBILITY OF EXPERT TESTIMONY

Forensic medicine is the area of medicine concerned with the testimony and information presented in judicial or quasijudicial settings. For example, medical information and testimony presented before hearings and trials, as well as formal legal investigations, would be considered forensic.

Forensic pathology concentrates on autopsies to be reported in legal settings. Other areas of forensic medicine, such as forensic toxicology, forensic surgery, forensic pediatrics, and other health sciences, involve presenting information in a legal forum.

BRIEF HISTORY OF FORENSIC MEDICINE

Medicine as a curiosity, superstition, science, and ultimately a form of self-preservation appears to have originated long before humans organized into communities capable of governing conduct by a legal system consisting of accepted norms. Unfortunately, historical knowledge of the interaction between law and medicine is limited by the slow development of an effective recording system. Thus the origin of forensic medicine can be traced back only 5000 or 6000 years. At that time, Imhotep, the grand vizier, chief justice, chief magician, and chief physician to King Zozer, was regarded as the god of the Egyptians. He was also the first man known to apply both medicine and law to his surroundings.[1]

In ancient Egypt, legal restrictions concerning the practice of medicine were codified and recorded on papyri. Because medicine was shrouded with mysticism, its practice was regarded as a privilege of class.[2] Despite the strong influence of superstition, definite surgical procedures and substantial information regarding the interaction of drugs indicate an awareness that humans, as opposed to gods or demons, could regulate various bodily responses.

Apparently the Code of Hammurabi (2200 BC) was the first formal code of medical law, setting forth the organization, control, duties, and liabilities of the medical profession.[3] Malpractice sanctions included monetary compensation for the victim and forcible removal of the surgeon's hand.[4]

Medicolegal principles also can be found in early Jewish laws, which distinguished mortal from nonmortal wounds and investigated questions of virginity.

Later, in the midst of substantial jurisprudential evolution, Hippocrates and his followers studied the average duration of pregnancy, the viability of children born prematurely, malingering, the possibility of superfetation, and the relative fatality of wounds in different parts of the body. Particularly noteworthy is the continuation of an interest in poisons. The Hippocratic Oath includes a promise not to use or advise the use of poisons.[5]

As in Egypt, the practice of medicine in India was restricted to members of select castes. Medical education also was regulated. Physicians formally concluded that the duration of pregnancy should be between 9 and 12 lunar months. Again, the study of poisons and their antidotes was given high priority.[6]

Although little medicolegal development occurred during the Roman era, investigations were conducted regarding the causes of suspicious deaths. This process was sufficiently sophisticated to lead one physician to report that only one of the 23 wounds sustained by Julius Caesar was fatal.[7] In addition, between 529 and 564 AD the Justinian code was enacted, regulating the practice of medicine, surgery, and midwifery. Malpractice standards, medical expert responsibilities, and the number of physicians limited to each town were clearly established. Interestingly, although it was recognized that a fair determination of the truth often necessitated the submission of expert medical testimony, such testimony was restricted to the impartial specialized knowledge of the expert.[8] Obviously this evidence was intended to aid the fact-finder, not to replace the fact-finder's independent conclusion.

Throughout the Middle Ages, issues of impotence, sterility, pregnancy, abortion, sexual deviation, poisoning, and divorce provided the backdrop for much medicolegal development. Investigatory procedures advanced as more homicide and personal injury judgments were rendered. In 925 the

English established the Office of Coroner. This office much later assumed the responsibility of the investigation of suspicious deaths.

China's contribution to forensic medicine did not surface until the first half of the thirteenth century. Apparently, medicolegal knowledge had quietly passed from one generation to another; the *Hsi Yuan Lu* ("the washing away of wrongs") was so comprehensive that its influence can be noted until fairly recently. It was a treatise detailing procedures for cause-of-death determinations and emphasized the importance of performing each step in the investigation with precision. In addition, the book noted the difficulties posed by decomposition, counterfeit wounds, and antemortem and postmortem wounds and distinguished bodies of drowned persons from those thrown into the water after death. Examination of bodies in all cases was mandatory, regardless of the unpleasant condition of the body.[9]

By the end of the fifteenth century the Justinian code was a lost relic. A new era of European forensic medicine began with the adoption of two codes of German law: the Bamberger code (Coda Bambergensis) in 1507 and the Caroline code (Constitutio Criminalis Carolina) in 1553.[10] The Caroline code, based on the Bamberger code, required that expert medical testimony be obtained for the guidance of judges in cases of murder, poisoning, wounding, hanging, drowning, infanticide, abortion, and other circumstances involving injury to the person.[11]

These works led surrounding countries to question earlier superstitious systems of legal judgment, such as trial by ordeal.[12] Legislative changes followed, particularly in France, and medicolegal volumes began to be published throughout Europe. Most noteworthy among them was Ambroise Pare's book (1575) discussing monstrous births, simulated diseases, and methods to be adopted in preparing medicolegal reports.[13] In 1602 the extent of medical information had grown such that Fortunato Fidele published four extensive volumes. Even more important, between 1621 and 1635, Paul Zacchia, physician to the Pope, contributed his extensive collection, *Questiones Medico Legales,* discussing such issues as death during delivery, feigned diseases, poisoning, resemblance of children to their parents, miracles, virginity, rape, age, impotence, superfetation, and moles.[14] Limited in accuracy by ignorance of physiology and anatomy, the book still served as an influential authority of medicolegal decisions of that time.

In 1650, Michaelis delivered the first lectures on legal medicine at Leipzig, Germany.[15] The teacher who replaced him compiled *De Officio Medici Duplici, Clinici Mimirum ac Forensis,* published in 1704.[16] This text was followed by the extraordinary *Corpus Juris Medico-Legale* by Valenti in 1722.[17] Germany significantly stimulated the spread of forensic medicine, but particularly after the French Revolution, France's system of medical education and appointment of medical experts further defined the parameters of the field.[18]

Despite these remarkable accomplishments, "witchmania," which originated in 1484 by papal edict, was still widely accepted throughout much of the eighteenth century. Thus with the blessing of the medicolegal community, thousands branded as witches were burned at the stake. Despite the repeal of British witch laws in 1736, alleged witches were murdered by mobs as late as 1760, and "witch doctors" practiced as late as 1838. France is known to have held a witch trial in 1818.[19] As Chaillé accurately stated[20]:

[W]ith the impotence of science to aid the law, it adopted miracles as explanations, suspicion as proof, confession as evidence of guilt, and torture as the chief witness, summoning the medical expert to sustain the accused until the rack forced confession.

Nevertheless, in England, medical jurisprudence pushed forward, laying the foundation for the current depth of information. In 1788 the first known book on legal medicine was published in English.[21] The following year, Professor Andrew Duncan of Edinburgh gave the first systematic instruction in medical jurisprudence in any English-speaking university. Recognition by the British Crown was evidenced in 1807, when the first Regius Chair in forensic medicine was established at the University of Edinburgh.[22] Eighty years later, the Coroner's Act defined the duties and jurisdiction of the coroner. As amended in 1926, these obligations included (1) investigation of all sudden, violent, or unnatural deaths and (2) investigation of all prisoners' deaths by inquest.[23] The 1926 amendment also set forth minimum qualifications for the position of coroner and carefully outlined its jurisdiction in criminal matters.[24] It was not until 1953 that the coroner's jurisdiction in civil matters was defined.[25]

Early American colonists brought the coroner's system, intact, to the United States in 1607.[26] Because the position was held by political appointees, most of whom lacked medical training, cause-of-death determinations could be based on little more than personal opinion. Not surprisingly, controversy concerning the validity of death investigations led Massachusetts (in 1877) to replace the coroner with a medical examiner whose jurisdiction was limited to "dead bodies of such persons only as are supposed to have come to their death by violence."[27] Eventually, New York City and other jurisdictions followed suit in an attempt to establish a profession of trained experts qualified to unravel the mysteries behind the violent deaths that increased in number each year as the population expanded. To this end, the medical examiner was given the authority to order autopsies.[28]

During the last half of the twentieth century, considerable advances were made in the area of forensic medicine. Scientific and technological improvements have provided new fabric and groundwork for jurisprudential development. The question at this point, however, is whether such development will proceed. Medicolegal teaching programs are now being offered at many universities, medical schools, and law schools, but they provide only a theoretical foundation. The forum of discussion must now proceed from the world of academia to the practitioner's realm.

THE ADVERSARIAL PROCESS

The legal system in the United States is based on the concept that there is value in the presentation of opposing points of view. The legal process is designed to provide for presentation of opposing points of view and a contest of persuasion. *Forensic medicine* is the study of all the medically related sciences in a way that concentrates on the persuasiveness of information to be presented in the adversarial process that the law applies to the determination of truth. Legal scholars and practitioners believe in the value of the process and support the concept that truth can be found best in a legal setting by allowing the parties to present conflicts regarding the facts and the law.

The concept of reasonable medical certainty is difficult for physicians to understand, but it is a purely legal concept. *Reasonable medical certainty* is a catchphrase meaning "more likely than not in a medical sense." In other words, if the likelihood of an event is more probable than not given the facts, the physician can testify with a reasonable medical certainty. Most physicians believe that "certainty" is misleading, but the legal system has no problem with the word. If a physician understands that the legal system weighs and balances the probity and veracity in terms of "more likely than not," the use of the *certainty* is more easily understood.

Methods and practice in law and medicine are widely divergent. Practitioners in law attempt to apply general principles to specific fact situations, whereas medicine is a highly individualistic and flexible application of general scientific information. Most physicians would not consider themselves empiric scientists operating within a structured environment. Medicine requires great flexibility and artistry.

In the case of law the persuasiveness of an argument always returns to generally accepted principles; therefore there is always an attempt to eliminate the uncertain and mold arguments to fall foursquare on previously accepted legal principles. As a result, when lawyers and physicians attempt to resolve conflicts, they invariably start from different places and sometimes collide before they cooperate.[29]

EXPERT WITNESSES

The layperson, judge, or jury member needs help to establish the truth. As a result, experts are allowed to provide testimony to help the fact-finder. The expert is a person who by reason of training, education, skill, experience, or observation is able to enlighten and assist the fact-finder in resolving factual issues. Experts are allowed to provide specialized information to laypersons only if the court has accepted them as experts in the first place. To be accepted properly as an expert, the court must establish that an individual fits the qualifications as stated. One can be qualified by education or experience, but one must ultimately have enough knowledge to enlighten a layperson. A judge usually makes the determination of whether an individual is an expert, and that determination sometimes is balanced against the potential for prejudice in the presentation of testimony. For example, even if a general practitioner qualifies as an expert on a neurosurgical procedure, his or her expertise must be recognizably less than the expertise of a neurosurgeon. If the judge thinks that the jury will not be able to make that distinction, the court may exclude the testimony and not qualify the expert.[30,31]

The believability and credibility of a forensic scientist are tested in the courtroom and in other legal proceedings. It is no coincidence that the term *examination* is used to describe the process of presenting testimony in a trial or hearing. Direct examination and cross-examination are ultimately a true test of an individual's knowledge of the materials presented. A good cross-examination attempts to test and disprove the assertions that are brought out in the direct examination. The effective and well-prepared attorney is more than qualified to adduce the information that will be relevant and material to the factual issues at hand. The forensic scientist must prepare adequately to present the information clearly in the most persuasive manner possible. Ultimately a forensic scientist in a legal setting is an *advocate*. The individual is tested for professional expertise, thoroughness, accuracy, and honesty.[32,33]

Opinion testimony and hypotheticals

After experts are qualified by the court and accepted to give expert testimony, they can give opinion testimony and answer hypothetical questions. Experts are allowed to give opinion testimony based on facts that are normally used by experts in forming their opinions. Such facts include text and journal information, as well as the evaluation of the facts and the gathering of evidence that is a part of the information used by experts in the field. Frequently, for example, experts can use hearsay evidence in the formation of their opinion.

In court an attorney might present a *hypothetical question* (a question based on stated assumptions) to establish an expert's opinion given certain assumed facts. If an expert is allowed to give an answer to a hypothetical question, it can be used as persuasive testimony by the opposing parties, since factual disputes often cannot be completely resolved. For example, an attorney will ask the expert to assume certain facts that are in dispute and then draw a conclusion. This kind of opinion testimony allows attorneys to advance the version of the facts that their clients offer.

Admission of evidence requires a foundation. Through the use of the witness' testimony, the validity of the physical evidence can be established. For example, a photograph must be a true and accurate representation of the situation of which the witness has knowledge. Retouched photographs and photographs that misrepresent a scene must be tested by laying the foundation so that the information can be accepted into evidence. The typical process involves the labeling of an item as an exhibit, then the foundation being laid by a witness, often the expert witness, or through a process of verification so that the exhibit can be accepted as evidence. Photographs, diagrams, demonstrations, models, slides, films, and tapes can be accepted into evidence, provided that the court finds that no attempt to misrepresent or deceive.[34]

Courts generally have a problem with accepting books, texts, journals, and treatises as evidence. The problem is that written material can be so easily abused that the courts generally recognize that in-court testimony by a witness is more easily tested and verified. On the other hand, an effective argument can be made that a journal or book, if considered authoritative, can be used because it is written in a nonadversarial context that makes it more likely to be more believable. Arguments can be made on both sides because taken out of context, a book can be misleading. In most trial courts, written materials can be used if the expert witness accepts them as authoritative. Textbooks can be used to contradict the testimony of the expert and to support that testimony.[35]

Court-appointed experts

Trial courts have the authority and in some cases have exercised the authority to appoint their own experts. Court-appointed psychiatrists, social workers, and other experts are frequently used in complex cases. This does not rule out the use of experts by opposing parties, but it does allow the court to place more weight on the testimony and evidence presented by the court-appointed expert. The credibility question ultimately still lies in the areas of persuasiveness. For example, an ineffective court-appointed expert can be overcome by an effective, believable expert for the plaintiff or defendant or for the prosecution or the defense. The forensic scientist who is appointed by the court must ultimately stand the test of the courtroom and the direct examination and cross-examination process.[36]

FORENSIC PSYCHIATRY AND PSYCHOLOGY

Psychiatric problems are frequently fraught with legal implications. Forensic psychiatry is critical to determine competence in contract actions, responsibility for torts and crimes, competence to testify, ability to give informed consent to treatment, and particularly competence to stand trial. A related area is *testamentary capacity,* which is the ability of the testator to comprehend that he or she is writing a will, is aware of the property involved and the objects of bounty, and understands to whom the property will descend at death.

The defense to a criminal charge is predicated at times on insanity. Whether the state recognizes the M'Naughton rule, the ALI rule, or the Durham or New Hampshire rule, and whether the defense is diminished responsibility or irresistible impulse, the fundamental questions are whether a mental disease or illness is present and whether it affected the accused person's behavior.

At times the granting of a divorce or annulment and the award of custody, placement, or adoption are based on the presence or absence of a psychiatric problem.

Similarly, in reproduction situations the performance of an abortion or a sterilization procedure is conditioned on the psychiatric state of the patient. Artificial insemination mandates an absence of psychiatric problems in the donor or perhaps in his or her family.

Personal injury and malpractice claims may turn on the presence of traumatic psychoneurosis. In recent years, psychiatric problems related to employment have been the basis for workers' compensation settlements. Strict product liability also has been imposed for psychiatric injury.

Inherent in the etiology and effects of alcoholism and drug habituation and abuse are psychiatric factors; physicians have been held liable for addicting patients to drugs.

Psychiatric problems are often treated along with mental retardation, juvenile delinquency, autism, and hyperactive children. Psychosurgery (i.e., prefrontal lobotomy, brain ablation, electrode implantation) and electroconvulsive therapy may be used only in indicated circumstances with proper consent.

Forensic psychiatry is critical in determining malingering, sociopathy, sexual psychopathy (rape), and other sex-related problems, such as homosexuality, transvestitism, transsexual surgery, pedophilia, and fetishism.

Suicide contemplated because of depression, if recognized, can be prevented. Depression, which can be prevented if anticipated and recognized, often is seen postoperatively, particularly after cardiac surgery, postpartum, in intensive unit care, after transplantation, and incident to dialysis.

Psychiatric malpractice claims frequently involve treatment with medications, usually undertreatment or overtreatment, and toxic reactions (e.g., tardive dyskinesia). Infrequently, misdiagnosis and delayed or erroneous treatment are alleged. Intimate therapy has only recently become a cause célèbre and cause of action.

Psychiatric implications affect patients with psychoneurosis and personality trait or character disorders, but particularly those with schizophrenia, manic-depressive psychosis, the various depressions, and paranoia. Organic brain disease can include epilepsy, cerebral arteriosclerosis, space-occupying lesions, Alzheimer's disease, and a variety of other disorders. These disorders must be distinguished from trauma, infectious metabolic chemical or electrolyte disorders, cortisone intoxication, dehydration and cerebral edema, liver and kidney failure, and other etiologies.

The credibility and qualifications of a psychiatric or psychological expert are subject to the same legal requirements as other expert testimony. Based on adequate and intense investigation and examination of the witness, the opinions of psychiatric experts are admissible for consideration by the fact-finder. There are frequently conflicting opinions about the psychological state of an individual.

The tests of admissibility for psychiatric and psychological evidence in testimony are the same as those applied to all forms of evidence. The credibility of the expert involved is one factor that complicates the admission of forensic psychiatric and psychological information. The opinions of the mental health expert about criminal and civil matters are subject to cross-examination and rebuttal by other experts.[37]

ADMISSIBILITY OF EXPERT TESTIMONY

On the last day of the U.S. Supreme Court's 1992 to 1993 term, the justices' ruling in *Daubert v. Merrell Dow Pharmaceuticals* changed the rules for the admission of testimony by scientific experts in federal courts.[38]

For nearly 70 years, most federal courts judged the admissibility of scientific expert testimony by the 1923 standard of *Frye v. United States* (i.e., Are the principles underlying the testimony "sufficiently established to have general acceptance in the field to which it belongs?").[39]

In *Daubert* the Supreme Court unanimously agreed that the *Frye* test was supplanted in 1975 when Congress adopted the Federal Rules of Evidence, which included provisions on expert testimony.

In evaluating evidence of DNA identification, medical causation, voiceprints, lie detector tests, eyewitness identification, and a host of other scientific issues, litigants and courts must now reconsider admissibility questions under *Daubert.*

The Supreme Court did not reject the *Frye* test on grounds that it was a wrong or poor judicial policy. Rather, the court simply concluded that *Frye* "was superseded by the adoption of the Federal Rules of Evidence."

Rule 702 allows opinion testimony by a qualified person concerning "scientific, technical, or other specialized knowledge that will assist the trier of fact to understand the evidence or to determine a fact in issue."

To satisfy that requirement, a court must undertake "a preliminary assessment of whether the reasoning or methodology underlying the testimony is scientifically valid and of whether that reasoning or methodology properly can be applied to the facts in issue," according to Justice Blackmun, who wrote the majority opinion.

Blackmun identified the following four factors that a court should consider in determining whether the scientific methodology underlying an expert's opinion is valid under Rule 702:

1. Whether the expert's theory or technique "can be (and has been) tested"
2. Whether the theory or technique has been "subjected to peer review and publication"
3. What the known or potential "rate of error" is for any test or scientific technique that has been employed
4. The *Frye* standard of whether the technique is generally accepted in the scientific community

Blackmun emphasized that the inquiry under Rule 702 "is a flexible one" that focuses on whether an expert's testimony "rests on a reliable foundation."

The full impact of *Daubert* may not be clear for many years, as courts apply its four-factor test to a broad range of expert evidence.

Blackmun criticized *Frye* as being "at odds with the 'liberal thrust' of the Federal Rules and their 'general approach' of relaxing the traditional barriers to 'opinion testimony.'" However, he also wrote that an expert's testimony must be "scientifically valid," which requires an independent judgment of validity by the court.

The potential impact of *Daubert* is vast, and courts will have to reconsider the admissibility of many types of scientific evidence.

The *Daubert* decision will eventually affect court rulings pertaining to such areas as polygraph testing, voiceprint analysis, questioned-documents examination, and so-called expert psychological testimony on such subjects as rape trauma syndrome and posttraumatic stress disorder.

ENDNOTES

1. Polsky, 1 Temple Law Rptr. 15, 15 (1954).
2. Smith, *The Development of Forensic Medicine and Law-Science Relations,* 3 J. Pub. L. 304, 305 (1954).
3. Harper, *The Code of Hammurabi, King of Babylon,* 77-71 (2d ed. 1904).
4. Oppenheimer, *Liability for Malpraxis in Ancient Law,* 7 Trans. Medical-Legal Soc. 98, 103-104 (1910).
5. *Supra* note 1, at 15.
6. *Supra* note 2, at 306.
7. *Id.* at 306-307.
8. *Supra* note 1, at 15.
9. Wecht, *Legal Medicine: an Historical Review and Future Perspective,* 22 N.Y. Law School L. Rev. 4, 876 (1977).
10. *Supra* note 2, at 308.
11. *Supra* note 1, at 16.
12. *Supra* note 2, at 309.
13. *Id.* at 309.
14. *Id.* at 310.
15. *Id.* at 310.
16. Chaill Aae, *Origin and Progress of Medical Jurisprudence,* 46 J. Crim. L. & Criminal 397, 399 (1949).
17. *Supra* note 1, at 16.
18. *Id.* at 17.
19. *Supra* note 16, at 400.
20. *Id.* at 400, note 24.
21. *Id.* at 402.
22. Farr, *Elements of Medical Jurisprudence* (1788). (Translated and abridged from the Elementra Medicinne Forensis of Johannes Fridericus Faselius.)
23. Polsky, 3 Medico-Legal Reader 7 (1956).
24. *An Act to Amend the Law Relating to Coroners,* 16 & 17 Geo. C. 59 (1926).
25. *Id.* at § 1.
26. Thurston, *The Coroner's Limitations,* 30 Med-Legal J. 110, 112-113 (1962).
27. Taylor, *The Evolution of Legal Medicine,* 252 Medico-Legal Bull. 5 (1974).
28. Fisher, *History of Forensic Pathology and Related Laboratory Science in Medicolegal Investigation of Death* in 4 *Guidelines of the Application of Pathology to Crime Investigation* 7 (W. Spitz, ed. 1973).
29. Wecht, *Forensic Sciences* (1984).
30. Lempert, *A Modern Approach to Evidence* (1977).
31. Curran, *Law, Medicine, and Forensic Science* (3rd ed. 1982).
32. *Supra* note 29.
33. *Supra* note 33.
34. *Supra* note 29.
35. *Supra* note 30.

36. Hirsch, *Handbook of Legal Medicine* (5th ed. 1979).
37. *Supra* note 33.
38. *Daubert v. Merrell Dow Pharmaceuticals,* 251 Fed. 2nd 1128 (9th Cir. 1991).
39. *Frye v. United States,* 293 Fed. 1013 (D.C. Cir. 1923).

ADDITIONAL READINGS

R.E.I. Roberts, *Forensic Medical Evidence in Rape and Child Sexual Abuse: Controversies and a Possible Solution,* Clin. Forensic & Legal Med. (Oct 1997).

R.D. Weber, *Malpractice Expert Witness Statute Held,* Mich. Med. (Oct 1999).

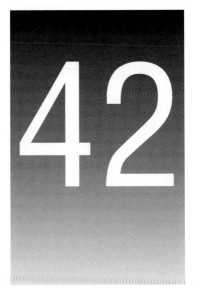

Forensic pathology

CYRIL H. WECHT, M.D., J.D., F.C.L.M.

AUTOPSIES
FORENSIC PATHOLOGY VERSUS HOSPITAL PATHOLOGY
RAPE
PATERNITY
CHILD ABUSE
DRUG ABUSE
DNA EVIDENCE
CONCLUSION

Forensic pathology is a unique and fascinating medical specialty. The training to become a forensic pathologist, as with any medical specialty, is highly specific and comprehensive, including 1 year of formal instruction in medicolegal investigation after completion of 4 years of residency training in anatomical and clinical pathology. Although scientifically specialized, the actual practice of forensic pathology cuts across a wide spectrum of everyday life, from the investigation of sudden, violent, unexplained, or medically unattended deaths (the basic jurisdiction of the forensic pathologist) to sex crimes, paternity lawsuits, child abuse, drug abuse, and a variety of public health problems. The range and diversity of such a practice provide constant intellectual stimulation and challenge.

AUTOPSIES

Autopsies should be undertaken as often as possible for many reasons, including a variety of benefits to the family of the deceased (e.g., identifying familial disorders, assisting in genetic counseling), information for insurance and other death benefits, and indirect help to assuage grief. Benefits to the public welfare include discovering contagious diseases and environmental hazards, providing a source of organs and tissues for transplantation and scientific research, and furnishing essential data for quality control and risk assessment programs in hospitals and other health care facilities. Autopsies benefit the overall field of medicine through the teaching of medical students and residents, the discovery and elucidation of new diseases (e.g., legionnaires' disease, acquired immunodeficiency syndrome [AIDS]), and the ongoing education of surgeons and other physicians regarding the efficacy of particular operations and medications. Additional benefits to the legal and judicial systems include determining when an unnatural death (accident, suicide, or homicide) has occurred and enabling trial attorneys and judges to make valid decisions pertaining to the disposition of civil and criminal cases.

In light of the significant medical contributions and substantial scientific data that have been derived directly and indirectly from postmortem examinations over the past three centuries, it is unfortunate that in the United States the Joint Commission on Accreditation of Healthcare Organizations (JCAHO), in 1970, dropped its long-standing requirement that hospitals perform autopsies in a certain percentage of patient deaths (teaching hospitals, 25%; other, 20%) to maintain JCAHO certification. Moreover, this is disturbing considering the increasing number of wrongful death cases involving medical malpractice and other personal injury and product liability claims, as well as the thousands of homicides, suicides, and drug-related deaths occurring each year, all of which require definitive and complete autopsy findings to enable individuals to pursue legitimate objectives within the civil and criminal justice systems.

Areas of concern

A surprisingly high percentage of clinicians, hospital administrators, and even pathologists have expressed a general reticence toward any new, concerted effort to increase the number of hospital autopsies performed. The reasons usually given are economic, educational, and legal. Hospital executives and other nonmedical administrative personnel are constantly seeking ways to cut costs and increase income. Postmortem examinations cost money: for the autopsy technician; for the toxicology, chemistry, and bacteriology tests on tissues and fluids; and for various supplies. Pathologists are busy with their other responsibilities and are not paid extra for performing autopsies. Attending physicians and house staff rarely attend autopsies and usually do not even seek information later concerning the autopsy results.

Attending physicians and hospital administrators are concerned that autopsies may reveal evidence of malpractice and may provide additional data for plaintiffs' attorneys in medical malpractice lawsuits. Their reasoning is that in the absence of pathological evidence, the plaintiff will have a difficult or even impossible task of proving that the death was directly and causally related to any alleged errors of omission or commission in the diagnosis and treatment of the patient (i.e., that there was any deviation from acceptable and expected standards of care on the part of the attending physicians or nurses that led to the patient's demise). In most cases, however, forensic pathologists find that autopsy results help to demonstrate that no medical negligence occurred in the patient's treatment. The objective, scientific documentation of the cause and mechanism of death can be the most important factor in dissuading a patient's family and their attorney from initiating a malpractice action or, if a lawsuit has been filed, in providing the defendant physicians and hospital with tangible evidence of an advantageous nature. Speculation and conjecture generally help plaintiffs more often than defendant physicians in medical malpractice cases in which the cause and mechanism of death are relevant issues.

The idea that new technology and improved diagnostic skills have made autopsies obsolete is incorrect and naive at best and intellectually arrogant and scientifically dangerous at worst. Although certain death cases are so well understood and unequivocally documented that it is not necessary to perform an autopsy, many clinical questions still need to be asked and answered in a majority of deaths. Regardless of the treating physician's degree of competency and experience, and despite highly sophisticated equipment such as computed tomography (CT) scans and magnetic resonance imaging (MRI), no substitute exists for examining organs and tissues at autopsy in the documentation of definitive diagnoses.

Recommendations

It would be in the best interests of society, physicians, and the advancement of medical science if more postmortem examinations were performed in appropriate cases. Economic considerations and legal trepidations should be outweighed by the need to determine accurate diagnoses and the cause and mechanism of death.

Several professional organizations have suggested that the JCAHO should assist in halting the national decline in the number of autopsies performed on patients who die in hospitals. Undoubtedly this would be a stimulus to the performance of postmortem examinations, which would enhance teaching programs and assist physicians and hospitals in peer review and risk management programs. For many years the standards have not prescribed a specific autopsy rate because the appropriate rate varies from hospital to hospital.

However, concerns have arisen that the decreased use of autopsies may have had adverse effects on medical education, research, and quality assurance programs. The JCAHO has therefore proposed standards that would require hospi-

tals to include the results of autopsies in their quality assurance programs and to develop in-house policies and guidelines that would lead to a higher rate of autopsies.

FORENSIC PATHOLOGY VERSUS HOSPITAL PATHOLOGY

Pathology as a discipline tends to conjure up conceptions in medically trained personnel that fall far short of an adequate explanation of the subspecialty of forensic pathology, although these thoughts would adequately apply to hospital pathology. Hospital pathology and forensic pathology, although sharing many training and scientific procedural factors, are significantly different in their approach to death investigation.

Hospital pathologists are charged with ascertaining pathological findings and correlating them with the existing clinical data; in other words, they find morphological changes to explain particular clinical signs and symptoms. A hospital autopsy therefore seeks to verify the diagnosis made before death and evaluate the treatment rendered pursuant to that diagnosis. The purposes of this exercise are to increase the storehouse of medical knowledge and to provide a certain degree of quality control. Philosophically, therefore, hospital pathologists tend to approach their examinations with verification and academic discovery as their objectives. This predisposition can lead the hospital pathologist to overlook subtleties that contraindicate clinical background, diagnosis, and treatment rendered.

Forensic pathology, on the other hand, approaches a death in an entirely different manner. Frequently the clinical history of the deceased does not exist or is not available so that, even if forensic pathologists were intellectually disposed to match their findings with clinical observations, diagnosis, or treatment, it often would be impossible to do so. More importantly, hospital and forensic pathology are distinguished by their jurisdictional spheres. Forensic pathology goes beyond the hospital setting and investigates any sudden, unexpected, unexplained, violent, suspicious, or medically unattended death. The term *investigation* distinguishes these two disciplines because hospital pathologists usually limit themselves to an autopsy and review of available clinical data. Forensic pathologists, however, engage in an investigation that routinely addresses the following:

1. Who is the deceased? This information, particularly in a criminal situation, is often unknown. Factors such as gender, race, age, and unique characteristics are evaluated.
2. Where did the injuries and ensuing death occur?
3. When did the death and injuries occur?
4. What injuries are present (type, distribution, pattern, cause, and direction)?
5. Which injuries are significant (major versus minor injuries, true versus artifactual or postmortem injuries)?
6. Why and how were the injuries produced? What were the mechanisms causing the injuries and the actual manner of causation?
7. What actually caused the death?

The scope of such a medicolegal investigation is necessarily broad and comprehensive. The information generated may determine whether a person is charged with a crime, is sued civilly for negligence, or receives insurance benefits. The information also may determine other critical issues. These uses depend on a general determination other than the cause of death that is alien to hospital pathology—that is, the manner of death.

The term *alien* is used because manner of death is a legal question that only forensic pathologists, armed with the results of their medicolegal investigation, are prepared to address. Hospital pathologists have little opportunity to develop a fair understanding, satisfactory appraisal, and high index of awareness of the medical, philosophical, and legal problems related to the determination of the manner of death. For them, essentially every death is natural, and even medical negligence may go undetected or may be labeled as a natural complication of disease. Drafting and signing hospital death certificates is primarily the responsibility of the attending physician, which accentuates this trend. The hospital physician often is not inclined to include in the autopsy report a specific cause of death or the full causal chain of events, especially when a possible cause for litigation might be suggested or several causes of death may be present.

None of these comparisons should be construed as an assertion that hospital pathologists are somehow incompetent. Their approach is simply different from that of a forensic pathologist. In addition, hospital pathologists are not charged with determining the answers to many of the questions that forensic pathologists must routinely address.

Also, hospital pathologists usually are not concerned with the determination of the time of death and the timing of the tissue injuries. For forensic pathologists, however, time of death and time of injuries are crucial to many civil and criminal cases and must be specifically addressed.

Forensic pathologists also focus on the crime scene and the circumstances of death in the scientific reconstruction and understanding of the autopsy findings. Unlike hospital pathologists, forensic pathologists frequently visit the scene to determine possible inconsistencies with their scientific findings.

The approach to the forensic autopsy is also different. Forensic pathologists, who are frequently exposed to the pathology of trauma, recognize the importance of a careful external examination, including the clothing, to determine the pattern of injuries and their relationship to the identification of the injurious agent. Hospital pathologists, because their subjects usually die in the hospital, generally have no need to be concerned about these factors and are satisfied with a cursory and superficial external examination. Hospital pathologists, however, are more inclined to detect and diagnose microscopic changes of rare natural diseases because of the direction of their work and the academic environment in which they function. Forensic pathologists are more familiar with subtle microscopic changes caused by poisons, noxious substances, and environmental diseases, that is, with the microscopic profile of unnatural death.

When the issue of determining the manner of death (natural versus unnatural) arises, the two disciplines dramatically diverge in application. This is a legal determination that is foreign to hospital pathologists. Since every death is natural for hospital pathologists, they rarely need to differentiate between natural and unnatural. Because of lack of experience and training, most hospital pathologists are not qualified to address this issue.

Forensic pathologists are intimately familiar with problems of causality and manner of death. Determining the manner of death is a basic responsibility they assume in every investigation, and their background and training reflect this requirement.

Identifying the deceased

An often difficult problem that initially confronts a medicolegal investigator is determination of the deceased's identity. Two relatively unknown and helpful forensic scientific disciplines, odontology and anthropology, are employed in the identification process.

Forensic dentistry. Although the application of medical and other scientific investigative techniques to the field of forensic pathology is not new, most forensic pathologists do not routinely use sophisticated dental expertise in their scientific investigations. Many techniques exist for investigation and identification in the area of odontology. Although its application in identification will never be as extensive and universal as fingerprinting, the similarities are striking. Dental structures and appliances (e.g., fillings, crowns) tend to be unique to that individual. Odontology is especially helpful in identification because dental structures do not deteriorate rapidly after death. When violence might mutilate the body either by thermal or mechanical means, the teeth are frequently still intact.

Forensic anthropology. The application of forensic anthropology to legal processes and medicolegal investigation is relatively recent. Physical anthropologists may work closely with forensic pathologists and odontologists in human identification, evaluation of injuries, and determination of gender, race, and age. Because of their special experience and background, however, physical anthropologists can make unique contributions and provide important conclusions. This is not a field of pseudoscientific guesswork. It is a complex, sophisticated, objective accumulation of hard, physical data that should properly occupy a position of top evidentiary priority in a court of law. Physical anthropologists are able to deal with purely skeletal remains (whether they are complete or fragmented), burned bodies, and semiskeletal remains that are decomposed beyond recognition and ascertain race, gender, age, and information helpful in determining the time of death, the cause of death, and more.

Time of death

Determination of time of death is primarily the province of the forensic pathologist's investigation. Determining when a death occurred can be critical in civil and especially criminal litigation. Pinpointing the time of death with unequivocal accuracy is impossible, but estimates can be made within certain parameters.

Early postmortem changes occurring hours to days after the demise include cooling of the body (algor), pooling of blood in dependent areas (livor), skin discoloration, stiffening (rigor), drying of the ocular bulbs, and fluctuations of the blood glucose levels and other body chemicals, such as the potassium concentration of the eye fluids.

Time of injury

The aging of injuries involves the determination of the interval from the infliction of the injuries to the death. This evaluation is based on (1) changes in the color and consistency of the injured areas, as revealed by macroscopic examination, and (2) alteration in the microscopic structure of the injured tissue, including inflammatory changes and evidence of repair

The gradual phases of an injury, as shown in the time-related kaleidoscopic changes of a periorbital contusion, are representative of the gross observations and information thus supplied. From an early bluish red color, the bruise changes gradually to dark violet. After 1 to 2 days it turns yellow to yellowish green, and on the fourth to fifth day it becomes slightly brown before its final absorption and disappearance. When combined with microscopic information, these changes can be helpful in aging an injury.

Normal visual observation must be supported by more refined microscopic examination; otherwise, the age of small injuries might be easily misjudged, and larger injuries with significant hemorrhaging components might appear grossly fresher because the bleeding may mask the tissue reactions. Therefore the pathologist must specifically examine microscopic sections from each of the significant areas of injury and from the tissues adjacent to the lesion. The latter requirement is essential to adequate sampling because the early tissue reaction occurs at the border between the injured and noninjured tissue.

Manner of death

The manner of death differs from the cause of death. The cause of death refers to the mechanisms that ultimately result in demise. Manner of death refers to a mechanism of death that was natural or unnatural (suicidal, accidental, or homicidal). This legal conclusion by a forensic pathologist is derived from an integration and analysis of the medicolegal investigation, including the history, the autopsy findings, and the cause of death. It can be a complicated and difficult conclusion to reach because natural and unnatural factors often intermingle and combine to cloud the ultimate cause and thus the manner of death.

Unnatural deaths can be categorized using the following general rules of thumb:

- The unnatural factor was the major precipitating factor causing death (e.g., bleeding caused by a tear of the aorta pursuant to chest impact, self-inflicted gunshot wound, or stab wound inflicted by another).
- The unnatural factor exacerbated a preexisting natural disease process (e.g., minor bleeding precipitating a fatal heart attack).
- The unnatural factor precipitated or caused a natural disease process, leading to death (e.g., pneumonia secondary to chest trauma).
- The unnatural factor, preceding or following a natural condition the deceased may have otherwise survived, contributed secondarily to the cause of death (e.g., a driver of an automobile experiences a heart attack and sustains severe blunt trauma in a crash).

When natural and unnatural causes of death intermingle, the determination of the manner of death becomes complex. The pathologist must address such difficult questions as the following:

- Was the unnatural factor of a sufficiently significant magnitude to contribute to the death?
- Was an unusual cause an inevitable result of natural conditions or a complication triggered by an unnatural (human) factor?
- What was the time element between the alleged cause and ultimate demise? (The longer the lapse, the greater the possibility of an intervening and supervening cause.)
- Was there a chain of clinical signs and symptoms between the perceived cause and the death?

Traditional autopsy findings generally do not provide the information required to reach a conclusion regarding the manner of death. A comprehensive medicolegal investigation, however, usually reveals information that, when integrated with autopsy findings, allows the pathologist to draw a reliable conclusion.

Gunshot wounds. Investigations of deaths caused by gunshot wounds are used here to illustrate some of the nontraditional means, processes, and findings employed to determine the probable manner of death. Although quite specific, the techniques discussed offer insight into the scope of any comprehensive medicolegal investigation.

Firearms account for a large proportion of unnatural deaths in the United States, most notably in homicides, but in suicides and accidents as well. Questions in such cases include the following:

1. How is the wound size or pattern related to range, direction of fire, and type of bullet?
2. Can the range of the shooting be estimated from the characteristics of the gunshot wound?
3. Can the relative positions of the victim and the source of fire be determined from the pattern and path of the wounds?

4. When several wounds are present, which was inflicted first?

Gunshot wounds are inflicted by rifled firearms, including revolvers, pistols, and rifles, that have the inside of the barrel grooved spirally to give a screwing, stabilizing motion to the ejected bullet. The pattern of the gunshot wound is produced on the target area by the elements ejected from the gun's barrel. Besides the bullet, these elements are other components of various weights and velocities, all falling behind the bullet and dissipating in the air with the increase in range. The elements ejected are the bullet, gases of combustion, primer components, soot, and burned and unburned powder.

Contact gunshot wounds, in which the firearm is actually in contact with the victim at the time of firing, are usually round or oval with abraded or contused borders surrounded by a rim of soot. The abraded borders are produced by the sides of the bullet passing through the skin. Inside the wound track, powder and soot are present. When the muzzle of the gun is pressed firmly against clothing, the hot barrel will "iron" the fabric when forcefully recoiling and thus leave on the clothing a double-ring imprint. A similar burned, brand-like mark may be left on the skin. When the contact gunshot wound is located on the skull or face, the blowing back of combustion gases rips the skin at the entrance site, producing a stellate, irregular-shaped wound. A rim of soot invariably surrounds such a wound. Distant gunshot wounds produced by ricocheting, tumbling, or deformed bullets may tear the skin and closely mimic the appearance of a contact gunshot wound. Such misleading, distant gunshot wounds, however, lack the soot and powder seen in contact gunshot wounds.

Contact gunshot wounds are most likely to be found in a suicide situation, and the presence of such a wound alerts the forensic pathologist to that possibility. Other factors to evaluate are the location of the entrance wound (e.g., a wound in the back tends to rule out suicide) and multiple wounds in vital or debilitating locations, which tends to eliminate suicide and an accident.

In a *near-contact* gunshot wound (up to 1 inch from the muzzle of the gun) the usually round entrance wound shows features similar to the contact gunshot wound except for the absence of the gun imprint and a larger rim of soot. Near-contact wounds usually are not indicative of suicide because persons committing suicide with a gun almost always press the firearm to their body. Near-contact wounds frequently are found in homicides and in accidental situations where the victim was in close contact with his or her own weapon when it misfired.

At *medium ranges* (1 to 6 inches from the muzzle of the gun) the wound is surrounded by or contains both soot and gunpowder marks. Soot is not seen around the wound when the range exceeds 6 inches, but powder marks may be seen in ranges up to 2 feet. The gunpowder marks consist of peppered, dotted bruises and abrasions called *satellites (stippling)*, which are produced by grains of burned and unburned powder striking the skin. Some of the grains of powder actually become embedded and may be observed under the microscope. The maximum range at which stippling is produced by handguns is 2 feet. The intensity of the stippling varies with the range, the kind of handgun, the ammunition, and the type of gunpowder. Medium-range wounds usually rule out suicide and are common in both accidental and homicidal situations. Making the differentiation requires evaluation of other factors.

In ranges in excess of 2 feet the satellite wounds disappear because gunpowder is not carried beyond this range by the explosive blast. The wound is usually round and surrounded by a rim of abrasion or contusion *(abrasion collar)*. In some instances the edges of the wound may show a black discoloration of dirt or grime. This discoloration should not be confused with soot; it results from bullet contaminants being wiped against the skin on entry. The grime ring consists of dirt clinging to the bullet's surface, a very thin layer of rubbed lead, or both.

A *distant* gunshot wound almost always allows the forensic pathologist to discount suicide. Self-inflicted accidental situations are likewise improbable. This leaves the possibility of an accidental wound inflicted by another or a homicide, which is the most common cause of this kind of wound.

Once inside the body, the bullet's path throughout the tissues is obviously indicative of the direction of fire. In perforation-type wounds (those entering and leaving the body), however, this determination may be more difficult and often requires correct identification of the entrance and exit wounds.

Entrance wounds on the clothing often leave soot and gunpowder residue and can be identified by visual inspection or by special techniques, such as infrared photography or microscopic examination. On the skin, entrance wounds usually can be recognized by their round or oval shape, with contused or abraded margins or with a stellate-shaped configuration if they are overlying bone. The shape of the abrasion or contusion rim should be carefully noted. This rim indicates the area where the bullet brushed against the skin and may be helpful in determining the direction of fire. A circular rim of equal width indicates a blast directed perpendicular to the skin surface, whereas in any other situation the rim is wider in the area facing the incoming direction of the bullet.

Exit wounds tend to be more atypical, irregular, or slit shaped, mimicking a stab wound or blunt trauma tears. Gunshot wounds of exit usually lack external bordering bruises because the bullet emerges from the inside. Interestingly, however, if the bullet exiting the body encounters a material tightly attached or compressed against the skin, such as a belt, the exit wound may show bruising.

The identification of the wound of entrance, the track, and the wound of exit are critical in determining the manner of death. Simply knowing the range of fire is often insufficient to rule out one or another manner of death. The direction of fire, however, can be most helpful, especially in potential suicide and self-inflicted accident situations. Angles and entry wounds that would be most difficult to attain by oneself can eliminate these possibilities and direct the pathologist's investigation toward homicide or accidental infliction by another.

RAPE

Forensic pathologists often deal with victims of violent crimes and are called on to assist the state in investigating and prosecuting such cases. Comprehension of the legal requirements for a successful prosecution makes the forensic pathologist a uniquely qualified medical expert, and a medical expert is often essential to the identification and successful prosecution of a rape case.

In the most basic medicolegal terms, rape is the penetration of a woman's genitalia by the penis of a man without the woman's consent. Ejaculation is not a necessary component, and neither is force. Rape is difficult to prosecute because it pivots on the woman's consent, and usually only the victim and the assailant are present during the commission of the crime; thus the only witness as to consent is the "prejudiced" woman herself. Thorough scientific examinations of the victim and the accused by a forensic pathologist, however, can generate substantive evidence for trial that can assist greatly in accurately determining whether a crime occurred.

Penetration

The usual circumstances of rape include the use of force by the assailant to gain access to the woman's genitalia and to effect penetration. Such violence often leaves injuries in varying degrees, depending on the struggle involved and the woman's previous coital experience. In an average-sized adult woman, life-threatening or severe injuries usually do not result from insertion of the man's penis into the vagina. A young girl who has had no previous coital experience, however, may show severe stretching or tearing of the labia and vagina from penile entry. A woman who engages in coitus frequently may show no damage at all, even in a violent situation. Injuries to the musculature or epithelium of the labia or vagina indicate penile penetration, but lack of such injuries does not rule out such penetration.

The condition of the hymen also provides evidence of penetration. Fresh injury to the hymen is usually evidenced by blood clots or hemorrhaging, but the inflammatory process that generally results from injury to other tissues is absent. Although hymenal injury may occur without penetration by way of masturbation or heterosexual sex play, fresh rupture and hemorrhaging of the hymen, especially when combined with testimony of rape, is probative evidence of rape.

The presence of seminal fluid in the woman's vagina is usually considered conclusive evidence that penetration has occurred. This finding neglects, however, the case in which ejaculation occurs while the man is in the mounting position, and the only penetration of the vagina is by the seminal fluid itself. On the other hand, the absence of ejaculatory material

at the time of examination is not unusual even when the crime of rape has occurred. Interruption of the act after penetration but before ejaculation can occur, and the rapist is often incapable of achieving ejaculation. The woman's fear of impregnation and disease frequently results in rapid washing with strong antiseptic solutions after the act. These solutions may completely remove all seminal material or introduce factors that interfere with the detection of the constituents of seminal material.

An examination of the vaginal lining sometimes generates findings indicative of penetration, such as abrasions, bruises, erosions, or vaginal vault tears. As noted, such an examination must be tempered by the knowledge that sexually active women often do not exhibit any evidence of this nature. Even virgin women may lack such findings, except that their vagina tends to be demonstrably rugose. The folds are quickly eliminated by even limited sexual intercourse, so a smooth vaginal mucosa in a purported virgin indicates penetration. Redness and swelling of the vaginal area, as well as the swelling and engorgement of the mucosa at the introitus, the clitoris, and the labia minora, strongly indicate penetration. Again, however, these conditions can result from digital manipulation and are not by themselves determinative of penile penetration.

Pathologists factor in all the evidence before reaching a conclusion of penile penetration. The emotionally charged circumstance of an allegation of rape and the resultant pressure to prosecute the rapist demand the utmost restraint and care in investigation by the pathologist to prevent a miscarriage of justice. Physiologically plausible and noncriminal explanations exist for each finding.

Consent

The next component of rape, which is much more difficult to prove, is whether the victim consented to the penetration. When the woman offered little or no resistance, the forensic pathologist is unable to offer much assistance because the investigation focuses on physical findings as opposed to mental intent. Rape, however, is usually accompanied by violence, and the evidence of violence tends to indicate that penile penetration was nonconsensual.

If force was used, there is usually evidence of this on the person or clothing of the victim. Lacerations may occur from fingernails or other objects, particularly on surface areas of the body where clothing was forcibly removed. Contusions may result from blows by fists or other objects about the face, neck, and forearms in particular. Contusions on the woman's throat caused by throttling attempts are also quite common. Bite marks on the breasts, neck, and face occur frequently, and areas on the woman's thighs may show contusions or lacerations caused by forcible spreading of the legs to achieve penile entry. Signs indicating that the woman actively resisted also may be present. The fingernails may be broken or bent from using them as defensive weapons, and debris, such as clothing fibers, hair, or skin fragments from the assailant, may be present under the nails. Beard hairs and facial epithelium are most common, but any part of the assailant's body surface may be represented.

Again, the presence of wounds does not necessarily mean that valid consent to coitus was not given. Bites, contusions, and lacerations caused by the fingernails often accompany orgasm, and sadistic or masochistic sexual responses, to which the woman gave valid consent, typically produce minor injuries and may produce severe injuries. Precoital sex play can generate lacerations on the thighs and tearing of the clothing, and postcoital fighting may occur, particularly when remuneration was expected but not forthcoming. Self-inflicted injury also has occurred in an attempt to add evidence to a spurious claim of rape.

The absence of wounds may not indicate that consent was given, as when (1) the victim offers no resistance because of fear or resignation to being raped and (2) drugs are involved. The drugs most often found on toxicological examination are alcohol and marijuana.

Gamma-hydroxybutyrate (GHB), the "date rape drug," is a potent tranquilizer that causes central nervous system (CNS) depression. It cannot be sold legally in the United States.

Flunitrazepam (Rohypnol) is a benzodiazepine available in Europe but not available in the United States. As with GHB, flunitrazepam can cause CNS depression, with the development of euphoria, hallucinations, and memory loss. It also heightens sexual desire.

Identification

In the prosecution of a rape case a critical component is the identification of the alleged assailant. The forensic pathologist accomplishes this task by employing a number of scientific analyses and common-sense observations. Surprisingly, suspects frequently are presented for examination literally teeming with evidence that they have not removed.

If penetration of the vagina by the penis was complete, there may be evidence of vaginal epithelial cells on the penis. This examination is based on the idiophilic nature of vaginal epithelium. If ejaculation occurred, seminal material may be present on the man's pubic hair, penis, or clothing. The suspect's clothing may have physiological fluids or hairs from the woman on its surface. The suspect should be examined by ultraviolet (UV) light while both clad and unclad. Semen fluoresces between 400 and 480 nm because of contamination by *Pseudomonas fluorescens.* Alternatively, an argon laser or high-intensity monochromatic light source can be used. The victim should be similarly examined. The suspect may have skin fragments or hair under his nails, and his hands or genital areas may exhibit blood or vaginal secretions from the victim.

The general body surface of the man may show signs of injuries, such as lacerations and contusions, on any part of the body as a result of being struck with fists or other objects. Bites and scratches on the hands and arms of the assailant are common in rape cases because it is often necessary to silence the woman and the arms of the assailant are placed in a vulnerable position. The face is often the first point of defensive attack by a woman, so scratches on the assailant's face and neck are also common.

Unfortunately, it is more likely that no signs are present or that explanations other than rape may have produced the evidence found. After visual examination of the alleged assailant, more scientific and definitive analyses are performed on seminal fluid, hair, and clothing to ascertain the identity of the assailant. Each of the constituents of seminal fluid is identifiable, and tests have been designed to relate results to a given man. The finding of spermatozoa allows for the examination that identifies a stain or secretion as seminal in origin. Spermatozoa can be recovered from the vaginal vault by swabbing or washing. When deposition of sperm is very recent, swabbing with direct preparation of a slide for study is usually sufficient. When more completeness is necessary, vaginal washing is done. The diluted vaginal contents then must be concentrated, usually by centrifugation, before slides are prepared. The slides are examined microscopically for motile or nonmotile spermatozoa.

Dried stains require special procedures to free the spermatozoa. The proteinaceous material present in the seminal fluid prevents good wetting by water alone. Dilute acids, bases, and detergents seldom cause spermatozoal damage and are used to free spermatozoa from dried seminal stains.

Spermatozoa adhere tenaciously to various fibers, particularly cotton, so agitation is often necessary to free them. Examination of a contaminated slide generally requires some means of visualizing the spermatozoa. Of the many histological stains that are used, the simplest and most rapid is optical staining with phase-contrast microscopy. The slides are examined for motile and nonmotile spermatozoa, as well as for malformed types. The presence of the same percentages of spermatozoa in two different samples is strong evidence of common origin.

The determination of acid phosphatase activity is widely used for identification purposes. This enzyme is present in the prostatic secretion and is especially helpful when spermatozoa cannot be found as a result of azoospermia. Similar phosphatase activity levels in samples taken from the victim and the accused tend to strongly indicate that they are the same. If the phosphatase level is low, it may have come from the woman only, since acid phosphatase is normally present in vaginal secretions. Thus a more specific test should be used to confirm the presence of semen in samples that test positive for acid phosphatase but in which no spermatozoa can be found. Prostate-specific antigen (PSA), or p30, is highly specific to semen, although trace amounts can be found in male urine and blood. The presence of PSA in blood has become a marker for prostate cancer.

Unfortunately, various chemicals may lead to incorrect results, either positive or negative. Ethanol and fluoride inhibit prostatic acid phosphatase, and certain physiological conditions, particularly fever, reduce the activity to undetectable levels. By the methods ordinarily used, phenols and acid phosphatases other than prostatic are the most important sources of positive error. Many antiseptic solutions contain free phenols, may easily contaminate the vagina, and often are found because the victims, as noted earlier, try to wash away the crime.

Hair is often transferred between the parties in the crime of rape. The species of hair and the part of human body from which the hair came can usually be determined by microscopic examination. Individual hairs may be differentiated somewhat, but a large group of hairs is more readily subject to identification. Until recently, hair was at best eliminative unless other factors were also present. The advent of neutron activation analysis, however, has led to many claims of individuality of hair samples, but as yet it is not accepted as a method of positive identification (see later discussion).

The value of clothing fibers may be limited, but when combined with other information, it can generate corroborative evidence. Frequently the assailant's clothing is stained by the blood of his victim, and this evidence is most helpful. More often, however, fibers alone are the only available sample, showing only that fibers similar to those of the accused man's clothing were found somewhere on the victim. Similarity in fibers is the strongest correlation that can be made because unlike human hairs, fibers tend to lack strong distinctions, especially when they are from synthetic material.

Investigative process

The forensic pathologist can aid in the prosecution and investigation of a case of alleged rape in many specific ways, as shown in the following step-by-step review of the investigative process:

1. Examination of the scene. The position of the victim and the state of the victim's clothing at the scene should be carefully noted. Efforts should be made to prevent contamination of the anus or vagina.
2. Photographs of the body at the scene.
3. Examination of the victim and the surrounding area at the scene using UV light or an alternate light source.
4. In fatalities, identification photographs of the body in the autopsy room.
5. Examination of the victim completely undressed using UV light or an alternate light source. Swabs are taken from any suspicious areas.
6. Large and close-up photographs of the injuries, especially of the sexual areas (mouth, vagina, anus).
7. Gentle glove examination of the mouth, vagina, and anus. To prevent contamination, gloves should be changed or washed when moving from one area to another. The physical condition of the hymen should be noted and recorded.
8. Cotton swabbing and aspirates taken from the mouth, vagina, and anus for preparation of microscopic slides, for acid phosphatase testing, and for detection of seminal fluid. A "hanging drop" slide preparation is examined immediately for motile spermatozoa.
9. Speculum examination of the vagina under adequate light to detect the presence of blood, contusions, lacerations, or presence of foreign bodies (e.g., fragments of wood sticks, glass, metal). In fatalities, microscopic sections should be taken from the areas of injury to determine their age, according to the patterns of tissue reactions.
10. Careful examination of the anus to check for presence of injuries. The presence or absence of a patulous or scarred anus indicative of chronic anal intercourse should also be noted.
11. At least 20 hairs plucked in their entirety (and not cut) from the head, axillary areas, and pubic area.
12. Fingernails cut or scraped and marked accordingly, left and right. Examination of the fingernail scrapings may reveal the presence of skin, cloth fibers, or blood that may be matched to that of the assailant.
13. Thorough external examination. Suspected bite marks should be swabbed for saliva typing and imprints lifted if possible.
14. In fatalities, a full internal autopsy, with special attention to the pelvic area, to perforation or other injuries, and to evidence of pregnancy.
15. A full toxicological examination, including analyses for alcohol, barbiturates, sedatives, and narcotics. Specific screening tests for GHB and flunitrazepam should also be included.

PATERNITY

An area peripherally related to rape in which the practicing forensic pathologist becomes involved is the identification of the father of a child. Paternity actions were once extremely charged legal actions; the only mode of proof was the testimony of the parties and their witnesses. The high emotion associated with paternity actions has not changed, but the forensic pathologist's ability to contribute to positive identification has increased greatly. The present scientific determination of paternity tends to limit or eliminate the once-common practice of the accused producing a number of men (true or false) who had sexual intercourse at or near the time of conception. Paternity, not promiscuity, is the issue, and scientific testing provides virtually positive proof of fatherhood.

Since the combination of genes peculiar to each person is found in all cells of the body (excluding the egg and sperm), an analysis of blood cells generates the information necessary to establish or exclude paternity. The first approach to scientific proof of paternity is through exclusion techniques, as follows:

- A man can be excluded when both he and the mother lack a gene that the child has, because a child cannot possess a gene lacking in both the parents.
- A man can be excluded when the child does not possess a gene that must have been inherited from the father. (A man with AB blood type cannot have a child with blood type O, because having no other blood genes to con-

tribute, either type A or type B is present in the child of a type AB father.)

Exclusion techniques are reasonably well accepted in U.S. courts because of their finality and long-standing scientific basis. Unfortunately, newer techniques to prove paternity based on both statistical probability and scientific examination are not as well accepted.

Because of the many genetic characteristics that have been identified, sampling only a few of them in the child provides a virtually positive identification index of the father. The subsequent application of mathematical techniques can statistically show whether a given man is the child's father. For example, if one identifies 20 genes in a child that have a frequency of occurrence in the general population of five, and the accused man has those same genes, it is 99.7% likely that the accused is the father.

CHILD ABUSE

The forensic pathologist enters the child abuse drama at the epilogue. The pathologist must identify the pattern of trauma and differentiate abuse from a true accident. This is a great responsibility because the decision of whether to prosecute a suspect often turns entirely on the pathologist's conclusion. A false accusation of child abuse is a traumatic experience, but it is equally distressing to free an abuser. Forensic pathologists therefore must show that the documented injuries are the result of abuse. They also must be able to exclude more natural explanations for their findings.

Recognition and categories of abusers

An association between chronic subdural hematoma and multiple limb fractures of varying ages in young children was first identified in the mid-1940s. Pathologists were unable to correlate the findings with any known disease and were looking for an exotic new disease. The medical profession was psychologically unprepared to accept that parents could seriously maim their children. Not until the mid-1950s was parental violence identified as the responsible modality for these observations. Since then, multiple studies worldwide have clarified the battered child syndrome.

Child abusers can be separated into several categories. *Intermittent child abusers* periodically batter a child but provide appropriate care between episodes. These parents do not intend to hurt their children, but they are driven by panic or compulsion and tend to be sincerely remorseful afterward. Often they are motivated to reform and can be successful in time. The child-victim of these episodes is usually grabbed by an arm or a leg and shaken forcefully, resulting in broken bones and joint dislocations.

One-time child abusers may be distinguished from the previous group, but more likely they are potential repeaters and were only restrained from further abuse by some particular circumstance.

Constant child abusers deliberately beat and mistreat the child. Their intent is to cause harm, usually with the ration-

alization that they are dispensing appropriate discipline. Such abusers are indifferent to the child's suffering. They often have personality disorders, are detached from the destructive nature of their actions, and are not inclined toward reform.

In this age of alternative lifestyles and broken families, many young mothers have live-in boyfriends. Often these men are affectionate to their girlfriend's children and contribute to their growth and well-being. Frequently, however, the child becomes the innocent victim of an emotional struggle. When resentment builds, either toward the mother or the children, men can become *intermittent habitual child abusers,* with the woman's children becoming the target of hostility.

Ignorant child abusers represent parents who mean well but whose attempts at rearing the children result in permanent injury or death. These parents are genuinely devastated by the harm they cause.

Medicolegal conflict

The difficult dilemma that faces the forensic pathologist is differentiating abuse from other causes. Abuse can be an intermittent or even a single event. In the absence of multiple unexplained or unexplainable injuries of varying ages in the child, reaching an unequivocal conclusion of child abuse can be impossible.

This situation can lead to serious conflict between medical and legal causality that hampers communication between the pathologist and the prosecutor. The physician sees an effect, such as a lacerated liver, that may result from several similar but not identical causes. The physician may be unable to determine "beyond a reasonable doubt" that abuse, to the exclusion of all other mechanisms, caused the results he or she discovers. Because physicians are legally, ethically, and morally bound not to experiment on children to determine the mechanisms, patterns, and forces involved in the creation of injuries, they can only infer from animal experiments or from retrospective studies of these victims how and with what force a specific injury is produced. The certainty of causality sought in the law is far from realized, and the pathologist's certainty is greatly diluted.

A child's life generally includes multiple bumps, bruises, lacerations, fractures, and dislocations caused by accidents, making differentiation difficult for the pathologist. Child abuse cases, however, tend to have common findings on examination or autopsy and similar perplexing problems of differentiation.

Common findings

In regard to the hemorrhage produced in the battered child, the pathologist must determine that the trauma resulted from more than one application of force. With head trauma, for example, it may be difficult to surmise that a unilateral subdural hemorrhage is not a result of a fall. If the hemorrhage is multicentric, however, associated with several external lesions (particularly contusions or lacerations) or more than one abrasion, the implication is that the child fell more than once after receiving an initial severe craniocerebral injury, was hit several times, or bounced repeatedly. The pattern and multiplicity of injury help the forensic pathologist reach a conclusion.

Typically, thoracic damage results from a combination of blows and squeezes. Multiple ribs may be fractured, either posteriorly or anteriorly, and may be displaced, resulting in perforated lungs, heart, or liver. These internal injuries can cause excessive hemorrhage into the chest cavity and, if air is sucked into the chest cavity, can produce respiratory difficulty from pneumothorax. With the exception of a pure squeeze, the chest wall contuses more easily than the abdominal wall because the skin is closer to the semirigid ribs. These contusions are common in situations involving an ignorant abuser because the injuries can result from excessive though seemingly innocent squeezing.

The internal organs can receive trauma from any direction, and an unmarked epidermis can hide extensive internal bleeding and disruption of internal organs. The areas most vulnerable are the points of attachment of an internal organ, especially at the sources of blood supply and at points at which blood vessels change direction. One such area is the middle of the superior half of the abdomen, which contains several blood vessels changing direction, particularly the vessels of the celiac trunk and their branches; the hepatic, splenic, and gastric arteries and their branches; and the accompanying veins. The loop of duodenum, the ligament of Treitz, and the pancreas are in the retroperitoneal space, and the stomach and transverse colon are in the triangle located in the peritoneal cavity. *Compression,* whether prolonged, as in a hug or squeeze, or momentary, as from a blow, is the mechanism of trauma. A stretch-stress force of sufficient acceleration and deceleration detaches the jejunum from the ligament of Treitz, lacerates the liver, contuses the intestines or stomach, or ruptures blood vessels crisscrossing the area. Other direct blows include a "kidney punch," which may lacerate the kidney from behind, with bleeding into the space around the kidney and usually surface contusion.

Final determination

The pathologist's ability to explain whether one blow or many caused the damage is more important than being able to explain all the lesions by mechanism. A child dying of multiple internal injuries and manifesting bruises over the entire body, especially if the injuries are of different ages, is more likely to have been beaten than a child with one contusion in an exposed portion of the body, with internal injuries in the same area. A problem arises when the parents allege that the child fell down a flight of steps. In this case, a careful cataloging of all lesions and an on-site study of the steps may resolve the issue.

DRUG ABUSE

Contrary to current popular opinion in the United States, drug abuse and drug-related deaths have not really abated since the advent of the sensationalized drug movement in the 1960s and 1970s; what has abated is the attention paid to this problem. The use and abuse of drugs in U.S. society, although not accepted, are no longer news. Insufficient information and education are available in relation to drug abuse and use. The forensic pathologist continues to be confronted with drug-related deaths that often may have been averted if the deceased had been more informed.

Drug excess

The forensic pathologist's task of determining the cause and manner of death is complicated by the problem of drug excess. So many drugs are available and used (illegally or legally) that a demise is often the result of drug combinations rather than the abuse and overdose of a single agent. This problem has become significant in the medical profession and on the street.

Physicians are bombarded on an almost daily basis with new, improved, and modified drugs. The volume of drugs available for use in treatment makes it virtually impossible to remain current with every agent and, more significantly, to be aware of and understand the ramifications of drug combinations. By themselves, most drugs are therapeutic, but when prescribed along with other drugs, potentially lethal combinations and synergisms can result. This is an especially insidious problem when a team of physicians orc specialists treats a patient. Although the specialists may be completely familiar with the drugs used within their narrow focus, they may be totally unfamiliar with commonly prescribed drugs for treatment outside their specialty. The result can be an adverse drug reaction or a synergistic action causing untoward effects or death.

Abused drugs and their detection

At the interface between the law and medicine, forensic pathologists are charged with the responsibility of ascertaining the existence of drugs in the systems of the deceased, determining whether these drugs caused or contributed to the demise, and rendering an opinion as to whether drugs were used or abused. Frequently abused drugs that a forensic pathologist identifies in practice include the following:

Opiates	Stimulants	Hallucinogens
Heroin	Cocaine	LSD
Morphine	Methamphetamine	Marijuana
Codeine	D-amphetamine	Mescaline
Methadone	Phenmetrazine	Psilocybin
Pethidine	Methylphenidate	Dimethyltryptamine

Depressants	Tranquilizers	Miscellaneous
Barbiturates	Thorazine	Propoxyphene
Glutethimide	Meprobamate	Pentazocine
Methyprylon	Chlordiazepoxide	Deliriants
Chloral hydrate	Diazepam	Amitriptyline
Ethchlorvynol	Oxazepam	
Paraldehyde		

Common scientific methods for detecting the presence of these drugs are gas-liquid chromatography (GLC), thin-layer chromatography (TLC), and spectrophotofluorimetry (SPF).

Drug death—or not

The frequently subtle differentiation between natural and drug-induced death, or between the death of a person undergoing legitimate medical drug treatment and death from drug abuse, may be impossible to achieve in the absence of some forewarning to the investigating pathologist. Pathological findings that could properly be attributed to natural or non-drug-related etiology may be natural medical complications arising from drug use or abuse. Unawareness of drug-related possibilities could make the forensic pathologist's opinion as to manner of death completely inaccurate. A properly conducted investigation, however, tends to reveal certain factors that alert the pathologist and usually eliminate inaccuracies in the determination.

The pathologist's first hint may come from the deceased. Unexplained coma followed by death or irrational behavior before a bizarre act resulting in death, especially in younger people, raises the possibility of a drug-related death. An investigation of the scene of death often reveals evidence such as needles, tourniquets, spoons for heating or measuring drugs, discarded plastic bags, syringes, burned matches, and other drug-related paraphernalia that may point to a drug-related demise. Even the location of the body when discovered, such as the bathroom (a common place for intravenous injection), may be helpful when combined with other information. Although the autopsy in a suspected drug-related death follows the usual scientific routine, certain findings and observations peculiar to drug users and abusers are often found.

During external examination, special care is taken to find and identify needle marks indicative of drug injection. These marks are often concealed by the abuser to reduce obvious evidence of drug use and may be found interspersed with tattoos, between the toes, in the gums, and in creases and folds of skin anywhere on the body. Abscesses, scarring, and sores are common as a result of scratching of the skin surface with contaminated paraphernalia to inject drugs intradermally (skin popping). Stains on fingertips from capsule dyes may indicate drug abuse, and the color may help identify the abused drug. Froth from the nose and mouth is a common indicator of severe pulmonary edema and congestion, which may result from death caused by depressants.

Internal examination usually generates limited information. The most common finding is pulmonary edema and congestion that, although nonspecific, is almost a constant and thus helpful in identifying drug-related death. The gastrointestinal contents may reveal traces of pills and capsules, and the dye from capsules may tinge the mucosa with an unnatural color. Examination of the nasal passages and nasopharynx may reveal irritation or even traces of drugs (usually cocaine) inhaled through the nose (snorted).

Microscopic examination tends to be nonspecific in drug deaths, but certain findings are more common in drug deaths than in other kinds of deaths. These findings include pulmonary edema, congestion, focal hemorrhage, bronchitis, and peculiarly, granulomas. Granulomas result from the intravenous injection of foreign substances such as starch, textile fibers, or talcum, either because these substances were used to dilute or cut the drug or because the injection picked up clothing fibers. Other evidence includes thrombosis, thrombophlebitis, and viral hepatitis from the use of needles.

As expected, the most significant finding is made during toxicological analysis. Using GLC, TLC, SPF, and other sophisticated techniques, the forensic toxicologist can identify the presence and concentration of drugs. The samples of choice in these analyses are blood and urine, although nasal secretions, gastric contents, bile, and tissue from the liver, kidneys, or lungs may be necessary to make a definitive determination of drug type and concentration.

DNA EVIDENCE

Analysis of deoxyribonucleic acid (DNA), the substance of the genes, has emerged as an important aid in crime detection. Hair is one of the most frequently found forms of biological evidence at crime scenes, so identification of hair through traces of DNA has considerable forensic importance. However, insufficient DNA is available in a single hair for analysis by conventional means, and the DNA from such a hair is usually degraded.

To cope with these problems, researchers use *polymerase chain reaction* (PCR) to make millions of copies of a DNA fragment, through *gene amplification,* to permit analysis. The same method can be applied to blood or semen when the sample is too small or too poorly preserved to be studied by conventional means. DNA typing with PCR can discriminate with much greater precision than blood typing. Potentially, the typing can approach the precision of a fingerprint, a degree of accuracy already possible with conventional DNA analysis, provided that a sufficient sample is available.

The typing involved in cases for evidence at a crime scene means determining which of several chemical variants of a single gene an individual has. In the research on disease susceptibility, scientists have analyzed human lymphocyte antigen (HLA) genes, which are important in human tissue typing to match recipients and organ donors. The techniques used in analyzing hairs also would be useful in choosing donor organs for transplants, in determining susceptibility to some diseases, and in performing research in other fields.

Criticism and support

Critics have stated that for both theoretical and practical reasons, DNA fingerprinting cannot determine with virtual certainty whether a person is guilty of a crime. DNA fingerprints can stretch and shift, like a design printed on rubber, making them difficult, if not impossible, to interpret. Even without these shifts, DNA patterns can be almost impossible to compare, and scientific underpinnings have not been established for determining just how unlikely it would be for DNA fingerprints from two people to match by accident.

Proponents have stated that DNA evidence can precisely identify or rule out suspects based on analyses of the genetic material in a drop of blood or in a semen stain found at the scene of a crime. Such evidence is now routinely introduced in many criminal cases. Cases have been thrown out because of laboratories' questionable methods of DNA testing. The National Academy of Sciences and Federal Office of Technology Assessment have studied DNA technology for the U.S. government.

CONCLUSION

Virtually any situation involving an interface between law and medicine may call for the expertise of a forensic pathologist. With a background in both law and medicine, forensic pathologists are uniquely qualified to stand at the nexus and serve as the necessary bridge between these two fields.

Court decisions in various jurisdictions have conferred the benefit of governmental immunity on coroners and medical examiners in lawsuits alleging administrative or professional negligence relating to the determination of cause and manner of death. These judicial rulings are based on the premise that both elected coroners and appointed medical examiners are public officers. Therefore, even if their decisions are subsequently proven to have been incorrect, as long as they were made in "good faith" with no evidence of "malice," the pathologist, acting in an official capacity as coroner or medical examiner or their agent, is entitled to governmental immunity. These decisions are consistent with long-standing concepts set forth in administrative law and common law.

The *Rosario rule* (named after a 1961 case in which it was first enunciated) states that prosecutors must give the defendant's attorney any relevant written or recorded statement made by a witness who is expected to testify in a criminal proceeding. This rule, which has been upheld on appeal, was developed to preserve constitutional guarantees of due process and the right to cross-examine an accuser.

Defense attorneys in homicide cases have appealed their clients' convictions, stating that the district attorney never turned over the medical examiner's original tape recording of the autopsy to the defense. Even if it is argued that such items are the "duplicative equivalent" of material previously given to the defense, a strict application of the Rosario rule could result in a new trial being ordered by the appellate court. Defense attorneys argue that inasmuch as a medical examiner's report is an essential component of every homicide case, that official governmental medicolegal investigative facility (coroner or medical examiner) performs a law enforcement function and has an active relationship with the prosecutor's office.

If appellate courts find that medical examiners have that kind of connection to prosecutors, the district attorney's office may eventually be responsible not only for turning over the original autopsy tape recording, but also for searching the medical examiner's entire case file for any items (e.g., notes, diagrams, sketches, memos, research material) to which defense lawyers would be entitled.

GENERAL REFERENCES

Benton et al., *Analysis of the ABAcard OneStep PSA Test for Use in the Forensic Laboratory,* Texas Department of Public Safety, Crime Laboratory Service, 1-8 (1997).

Davis & Mistry, *The Pathology Curriculum in US Medical Schools,* III Arch. Pathol. Lab. Med. 1088-1092 (1987).

DiMaio & DiMaio, *Forensic Pathology* (Elsevier Science, New York 1989).

El Sohly et al., *Prevalence of Drugs Used in Cases of Alleged Sexual Assault,* 23 J. Analytical Toxicol. 141-146 (1999).

Jachimczyk, *The Postmortem Examination,* 2 Trauma 58 (1961).

Landefeld et al., *Diagnostic Yield of the Autopsy in a University Hospital and a Community Hospital,* 318 N. Engl. J. Med. 1249-1254 (1988).

Leetsma, *Interpretation of Head Injuries in Infants and Children,* in *Forensic Neuropathology* (Raven Press, New York 1988).

Poyntz et al., *Comparison of p30 and Acid Phosphatase Levels in Post-Coital Vaginal Swabs from Donor and Caseworker Studies,* 24 Forensic Sci. Int. 17-25 (1984).

Ropero-Miller et al., *GHB and Roofies: Drugs of the 1990s,* Forensic Urine Drug Testing 1-7 (1997).

Sturner, *Sudden Unexpected Infant Death,* in 1971 *Legal Medicine Annual* (Appleton-Century-Crofts, New York 1971).

Svendsen & Hill, *Autopsy Legislation and Practice in Various Countries,* III Arch. Pathol. Lab. Med. 846-850 (1987).

Wecht, *Relationships of the Medical Examiner,* 14 Cleveland-Marshall Law Rev. 427-441 (Sept 1965).

Wecht, *The Medicolegal Autopsy Laws of the Fifty States, the District of Columbia, America Samoa, the Canal Zone, Guam, Puerto Rico, and the Virgin Islands* (rev. ed., Armed Forces Institute of Pathology 1977).

Wecht, ed., *Forensic Sciences* (5 vols., Matthew Bender & Co., New York 1982).

Wetli et al., *Practical Forensic Pathology* (Igaku-Shoin Medical Publishers, New York 1988).

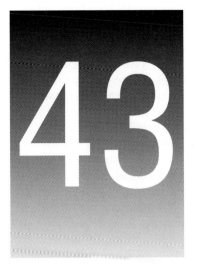

Psychiatric patients and forensic psychiatry

MARVIN H. FIRESTONE, M.D., J.D., F.C.L.M., F.A.P.A., F.A.A.F.S.

PSYCHIATRY AND CRIMINAL LAW
PSYCHIATRIC MALPRACTICE
CIVIL RIGHTS
REFUSAL OF MEDICATION

PSYCHIATRY AND CRIMINAL LAW

The purpose and rationale for the system of criminal justice in the United States are based on four fundamental concepts: isolation, retribution, deterrence, and rehabilitation.

As far back as biblical times, the issue of crime and punishment was premised on the notion of intent. The idea of wrongful or criminal guilt inherently required two elements: (1) that the wrongdoer commit an act or misdeed and, more important, (2) that the act was the product of a willing and rational intent. In other words, a crime is made up of two essential components: (1) voluntary conduct (actus rea) and (2) intent or guilty mind (mens rea).

An exception to a finding of criminal guilt historically has been reserved for minors and mentally disabled persons. In Babylonian times, for example, Jewish law held that "it is an ill thing to knock against a deaf mute, an imbecile or a minor: he that wounds them is culpable, but if they wound others they are not culpable."[1] Centuries later, a secular pronouncement was contained in the *Justinian Digest:*

There are those who are not to be held accountable, such is not a madman and a child who is not capable of malicious intention: these persons are able to suffer a wrong but not to produce one. Since a wrong is only able to exist by the intention of those who have committed it, it follows that these persons, whether they have assaulted by blows or insulted by words, are not considered to have committed a wrong.[2]

In 1265 Bracton, Chief Justice of England, wrote the first systematic treatise on English law and in it stated that neither child nor "madman" could be liable because both lacked the felonious intent necessary for an act to be considered criminal. He likened the acts of an insane person, lacking in mind and reason, to be not far removed from that of a brutish animal.[3] Other notable jurists, including Lord Hale, Chief Justice Mansfield, and Chief Justice Holmes in the United States, have all recognized the need to excuse from criminal responsibility any person incapable of forming the requisite criminal intent.[4]

Competency to stand trial

Society's sense of morality dictates that an individual who is unable to comprehend the nature and the object of the proceedings against him or her, to confer with counsel, and to assist in the preparation of his or her own defense may not be subjected to a criminal trial. The oft-quoted legal theorist, Blackstone, in defining this common law rule said:

If a man in his sound memory commits a capital offense, and before arraignment for it, he becomes mad, he ought not be arraigned for it; because he is not able to plead to it with that advice and caution that he ought. And if, after he has pleaded, the prisoner becomes mad, he shall not be tried; for how can he make his defense?[5]

Borrowing from this common-law principle, one of the fundamental tenets of American jurisprudence is the entitlement of every defendant to be afforded a fair and adequate hearing. For this requirement of fairness to be effectuated, the individual litigant must be capable of meaningful participation in the ongoing events of the legal process. The requirement that a litigant be competent to stand trial is of such moral and philosophical importance to the system of justice that it is considered a fundamental element and recognized as a constitutional right. In *Pate v. Robinson* the Supreme Court held "that the failure to observe a defendant's right not to be tried or convicted while incompetent to stand trial deprives him of his due process right to a fair trial."[6]

Despite the constitutional recognition that a defendant must be competent at the time of the trial, the determination and parameters of this fundamental principle have been the source of continued ambiguity. For example, such common mental status criteria as orientation to time and place and the

469

capacity to recollect past events have been found to be insufficient in determining trial competency. Various states have established standards by which to measure a defendant's competency to stand trial. At a bare minimum, it is sufficient to say that the fundamental fairness of law requires at least a finding of competency consistent with the test developed in *Dusky v. United States:* "[T]he test must be whether he has sufficient present ability to consult with his lawyer with a reasonable degree of rational as well as factual understanding of the proceedings against him."[7]

As seen from the general nature of this test, dispute and controversy are not uncommon in a case where a defendant's capacity is at issue. Although numerous federal and state decisions have sought to devise a more objective test, none has been totally successful. As a rule, any substantial impairment that interferes with a defendant's capacity to communicate, testify coherently, or follow the proceedings of the trial with a "reasonable degree of rational understanding" leads to a determination of incompetency.

The determination of competency is essentially a threefold procedural process. The first step can be characterized as the *trigger stage.* Both the prosecution and the defense, as well as the court, may raise or trigger the issue of incompetency whenever there is a suggestion that the defendant may not be competent to stand trial. In fact, the trial court is under constitutional obligation to recognize and respond to any evidence that the defendant may not be mentally fit for trial. Once the issue has been raised, neither the defendant nor counsel can waive the issue and have the case brought to trial. Fundamental fairness of law requires that a defendant be competent throughout a trial.[8]

After the issue of a defendant's competency is raised, common procedure is for the court to appoint one or more independent experts to conduct a psychiatric examination. Two issues, one procedural and one substantive, are important to note. Although in most jurisdictions a question of competency automatically triggers an impartial psychiatric examination, a defendant has no constitutional right to one. Also, the function of a competency evaluation, as opposed to an insanity defense evaluation, is that the sole issue to be decided is whether the defendant is sufficiently competent "at that time" to proceed in his or her own defense during the trial. Evidence of incompetency, insanity, or other forms of incapacity during the commission of the crime is not germane to the question of competency to stand trial.

After the question of competency is raised, the court then determines whether there is *sufficient evidence* to justify a formal hearing. At this second stage the role of a psychiatrist is vital. Often the results of a psychiatrist's examination are persuasive in the court's determination of competency. For example, in the federal court system and in some states, if a psychiatric examiner concludes that the defendant is likely to be incompetent, a judicial hearing on the issue is required. Although neither the U.S. Supreme Court nor any state has articulated clearly how

much evidence of incompetency is necessary to compel a hearing, as a rule, evidence sufficient to raise a bona fide doubt will suffice the constitutional standards.[9]

At a separate and distinct legal proceeding, the third stage, the *competency hearing,* takes place. The importance of competency to participate in one's own defense is so fundamental to the system of justice that a competency hearing can be held at any time during a trial proceeding. Typically, the psychiatric expert who initially evaluated the defendant is the prime witness at this proceeding. A competency hearing is similar to and different from a normal trial in several respects. It is similar in that it is adversarial in nature. In addition to the findings of the court-ordered psychiatric expert, both the state and the defense may produce their own witnesses (lay and expert) regarding the defendant's competency, along with any other evidence. Also, the defendant has a right to counsel and is permitted to cross-examine the other side's witnesses. However, unlike a normal trial, the defendant has no options regarding adjudication before a judge or jury. A competency hearing is typically before a judge. Also, in most states the defendant must prove incompetency by at least a preponderance of the evidence, although in the federal courts the prosecutor must carry the burden. In another important distinction, because of the special circumstances in which a competency hearing is carried out, the defendant's right to invoke the privilege against self-incrimination is narrowed. The U.S. Supreme Court in *Estelle v. Smith* concluded that a defendant may not claim the privilege against self-incrimination to prevent the examining psychiatrist from testifying about the defendant's competency.[10] However, the court did rule that the privilege against self-incrimination (Fifth Amendment) may bar the disclosure of statements or any resulting psychiatric conclusions from those statements if they were made during the pretrial competency hearing or a subsequent sentencing proceeding.

Although the involvement of the psychiatric expert in this situation might appear to be curtailed, the contribution that expert findings and testimony make in a competency proceeding is invaluable to a system of fundamental justice.

The disposition of persons found incompetent to stand trial is procedurally uniform in the United States. However, differences in state statutes provide for a variety of rights and limitations. Traditionally, defendants found mentally incompetent to be tried were automatically referred to a state institution until they were found to be competent. In effect, a defendant's stay in a mental hospital, often an institution for the criminally insane, could drag on indefinitely and often did. Release could be effectuated only if either the defendant was found to be competent, at which time trial proceedings would then be initiated, or the prosecution dropped the charges. In 1972 the landmark case *Jackson v. Indiana* addressed this traditional practice of indefinite commitment of defendants found incompetent to stand trial.[11] First, the court held that although automatic commitment in and of itself is not prohibited, the length of commitment could not exceed a "reasonable period of time necessary to determine whether there is a substantial probability that he will attain that capacity in the foreseeable future." Also, the court determined that the state would bear the burden of demonstrating progress in the attainment of competency, so that a defendant whose competency does not appear reasonably foreseeable must be either formally committed pursuant to standard civil commitment procedures or released.

Insanity defense

Probably no single issue in the annals of criminal law has stirred more controversy, debate, and comparison among laypersons, as well as jurists, than the insanity defense. The 1982 jury decision finding John Hinckley not guilty by reason of insanity for the shootings of President Reagan and three other persons stunned the nation, and this decision thrust back into the public consciousness questions regarding the viability and fundamental morality surrounding the defense.

By the mid-eighteenth century a significant attempt was made to apply some form of cognizable formula for determining insanity. Judge Tracy in *Rex v. Arnold* suggested that one of the essential requisites for determining criminal responsibility was whether the accused was able to distinguish "good from evil" at the time of the offense.[12]

Later in the century, Hawkins wrote an important treatise on the subject that revised this moralistic standard to the more cognitively based question of "right and wrong."[13] Despite what appeared to be an improvement in providing some form of rule for evaluating insanity, the right-wrong test was short lived.

In 1800 the interpretation of legal insanity broadened significantly with the inclusion of insane delusions as an acceptable ground for the defense. In *Hadfield's Case* the addition of delusions, or false beliefs that are firmly held despite incontrovertible evidence to the contrary, was first accepted by the common-law court.[14] Hadfield, a soldier who had suffered severe head trauma during the French wars, attempted to shoot King George III to attain martyrdom, which he was convinced was his destiny. Despite the lack of a "frenzy or raving madness," his counsel contended that the delusion was the true character of insanity:

These are the cases which frequently mock the wisdom of the wisest in judicial trials: because such persons often reason with a subtlety which puts in the shade the ordinary conceptions of mankind; their conclusions are just and frequently profound; but the premises from which they reason, when within the range of the malady, are uniformly false—not false from any defect of knowledge or judgment; but, because a delusive image, the inseparable companion of real insanity, is thrust upon the subjugated understanding, incapable of resistance, because unconscious of the attack."[15]

Following counsel's argument, the court practically preempted the proceeding by ordering an acquittal. Some 40

years later a similar attempt was made on the lives of Queen Victoria and Prince Albert by Edward Oxford. Oxford, like Hadfield, suffered from the delusion of martyrdom and was also acquitted.[16] Despite the notoriety of these two cases, the application of the insanity defense based on delusional beliefs was not widely successful.

In 1843 a significant change in the legal rule used to determine insanity was created. In the trial of Daniel M'Naughton[17] the defendant expressed feelings of great persecution by the pope and Tories, the political party in power at that time. To rid himself of this torment, M'Naughton decided to kill Sir Robert Peel, the prime minister. Not knowing Peel by sight, M'Naughton lay in wait at his residence and mistakenly shot his secretary, Henry Drummond, who was leaving the prime minister's home. In addition to the numerous medical experts who all testified to M'Naughton's insanity, the court also summoned two physicians who were simply observing the trial. Because neither physician was partisan to the proceedings, both were afforded a special degree of credence. On their unanimous conclusion that the defendant was indeed insane, Chief Justice Tindal halted the proceedings, and the jury promptly found M'Naughton "not guilty by reason of insanity." Several days after the verdict, Queen Victoria, herself the target of assassination by the insanity acquittee Edward Oxford, summoned the House of Lords to a special session. The Lords were instructed to clarify and more strictly define the standards by which a defendant could be acquitted by reason of insanity. Out of this session the so-called M'Naughton rule was developed.[18] This rule provides the following:

The jurors ought to be told in all cases that every man is presumed to be sane and to possess a sufficient degree of reason to be responsible for his crimes, until the contrary can be proved to their satisfaction; and that, to establish a defense on the ground of insanity, it must be clearly proved, that, at the time of the committing of the act, the party accused was labouring under such a defect of reason, from disease of the mind, as not to know the nature and quality of the act he was doing or, if he did know it, that he did not know he was doing what was wrong.[19]

In essence, the M'Naughton rule, often referred to as the "right-wrong" test, has three elements that must be proven to establish insanity. The accused, at the time of the crime, must be suffering from some mental illness that caused a defect of reason such that he lacked the ability to understand the nature and quality of his actions or their wrongfulness.

Thus passed the eighteenth-century "good-evil" standard into the right-wrong test of the nineteenth century. Moreover, the M'Naughton decision marked the advent of the psychiatric expert witness as the key figure in defenses based on insanity. Henceforth, psychiatrists would be afforded special latitude in offering retrospective opinions regarding the defendant's state of mind at the time of the offense, whether his or her conduct emanated from some form of mental disease, and whether the defendant was cognizant of the wrongfulness of his or her conduct.

For more than a century the M'Naughton test served as the basic standard by which the insanity defense was judged in the United States and Great Britain. Even today a significant minority of states still apply it in its original form. Despite its extensive utility, it was later criticized. Even with its fairly broad language, the M'Naughton test was often narrowly construed as an evaluation of a defendant's cognitive capacity to distinguish right from wrong. Furthermore, its scope of application was greatly influenced by the perception of many psychiatrists that the concept of disease of the mind encompassed only psychosis, to the exclusion of other pathologies.

As advances in psychiatric theory were made, the M'Naughton rule came under increasing attack as being antiquated. The major argument was that some forms of mental illness affect a person's volition or power to act without impairing cognitive functioning. In other words, although many mentally ill individuals might be able to distinguish between right and wrong, they could not control their wrongful actions. To rectify this perceived deficiency, a number of states broadened the M'Naughton rule to include an additional element known as the "irresistible impulse" test.[20] The irresistible impulse test in essence stated that even though an individual might understand the nature and quality of his or her act and the fact that it is wrong or unlawful, he or she is nonetheless compelled to commit the act because of mental illness. This test basically rests on four assumptions:

[F]irst . . . there are mental diseases which impair volition or self control, even while cognition remains relatively unimpaired; second . . . the use of M'Naughton rule alone results in findings that persons suffering from such diseases are not insane; third . . . the law should make the insanity defense available to persons who are unable to control their action, just as it does to those who fit M'Naughton; fourth, no matter how broadly M'Naughton is construed there will remain areas of serious disorders which it will not reach.[21]

Regardless of whether the irresistible impulse test was developed by state statute or case law, it was never used as a sole standard but as a modification of the M'Naughton test.

Despite the addition of the irresistible impulse concept to the determination of insanity, this too was believed to be too narrow in light of contemporary psychiatry. In 1954 Judge Bazelon, writing for the U.S. Court of Appeals for the District of Columbia in the decision on *Durham v. United States,* rejected the M'Naughton rule as too limited and held the following:

We find as an exclusion criterion the right-wrong test is inadequate in that (a) it does not take sufficient account of psychic realities and scientific knowledge, and (b) it is based upon one symptom and so cannot validly be applied in all circumstances. We find that the "irresistible impulse" test is also inadequate in that it gives no

recognition to mental illness characterized by brooding and reflection and so delegated acts caused by such illness to the application of the inadequate right-wrong test. We conclude that a broader test should be adopted.[22]

Accordingly, the court articulated a broader standard that provided that "[a]n accused is not criminally responsible if his unlawful act was the product of a mental disease or defect." Apparently, the purpose of the Durham rule,[23] with the description of mental disease or defect deliberately vague, was to afford greater flexibility to psychiatric testimony to circumvent narrow or psychiatrically inapposite legal inquiries.[24,25] As expected, the Durham rule, or New Hampshire rule as it was sometimes called, created considerable controversy because of its ambiguity and semantically indefinite meaning. It was never widely accepted in the legal system and was adopted in only three jurisdictions: New Hampshire, Maine, and the District of Columbia. Ultimately, the same Court of Appeals for the District of Columbia that created it abolished the Durham rule in 1972.

In the early 1960s the American Law Institute (ALI) drafted a model provision intended to reasonably bridge the narrowness of the M'Naughton rule and the expansiveness of the Durham rule. Incorporated in its Model Penal Code, the ALI standard stated the following:

A person is not responsible for criminal conduct if at the time of such conduct as a result of mental disease or defect he lacks substantial capacity either to appreciate the criminality of his conduct or to conform his conduct to the requirements of the law.[26]

The ALI test differs from the M'Naughton standard in three ways. First, it incorporates a volitional element to insanity, thereby providing an independent criterion, the ability (or inability) to control one's conduct. Second, the ALI substitutes with the phrase, "lacks substantial capacity to appreciate the wrongfulness of conduct," which in effect takes into account a defendant's affective or emotional state instead of simply cognitive comprehension. Finally, the ALI standard does not require a total lack of appreciation of the nature of the defendant's conduct but instead that only "substantial capacity" is lacking. Arguably, the ALI test embraces a broader spectrum of psychiatric disorders sufficient to trigger the insanity defense because it contemplates mental defects as well as diseases.

The ALI test is accepted in a majority of jurisdictions and has been frequently cited as being considerably more applicable than its predecessors. For example, its incorporation of both a cognitive and a volitional element of impairment is viewed as more consistent with the contemporary conceptualization of mental illness in general. Its move away from total (e.g., M'Naughton) to substantial incapacity also appears to be realistic in terms of modern psychiatry. It broadens the role of the psychiatric expert by providing additional questions to be addressed, while leaving the responsibility of the ultimate decision up to the jury.

The ALI standard, despite its improvements in incorporating language indicative of advances in modern psychiatry, leaves the interpretation of "mental disease or defect" wide open. To address this ambiguity, most courts have relied on the definition provided in the case *McDonald v. United States.*[27] In *McDonald* the court defined mental disease or defect as "any abnormal condition of the mind which substantially affects mental or emotional processes and substantially impairs behavior controls."[28] This definition was created to help clarify the Durham standard but turned out to provide guidance for courts using the ALI rule. It is important to keep in mind that the insanity defense under the ALI standard is a two-pronged test. In addition to providing the existence of a mental disease or defect, the defendant then had to show that the disease or defect so impaired judgment that he or she was not able to conform conduct to the requirements of the law (volition element).

In 1984, Congress enacted its first legislation addressing the insanity defense:

(a) Affirmative Defense. It is an affirmative defense to a prosecution under any Federal statute that, at the time of the commission of the acts constituting the offense, the defendant, as a result of a severe mental disease or defect, was unable to appreciate the nature and quality of the wrongfulness of his acts. Mental disease or defect does not otherwise constitute a defense.

(b) Burden of Proof. The defendant has the burden of proving the defense of insanity by clear and convincing evidence.

Diminished capacity. In response to the narrowness and seemingly severe restriction imposed by the M'Naughton standard, the California Supreme Court introduced the concept of diminished capacity in the 1949 case *People v. Wells.*[29] The defense affords the court the opportunity to consider an individual's mental state as a mitigating factor in certain situations. Typically, the diminished capacity defense is used when a defendant is charged with first-degree murder. In effect it permits psychiatric testimony regarding a defendant's mental condition at the time of the commission of the crime in order to address the issue of the defendant's ability to form the requisite intent (mens rea) to commit the offense. Thus in a first-degree murder trial, the defense would attempt to put on psychiatric testimony to demonstrate the accused person's lack of capacity to appreciate the nature and quality of his or her conduct. Diminished capacity, unlike the insanity defense, is not a complete bar to criminal responsibility. If successfully established, its effect is to mitigate or reduce the criminality of the offense from first-degree murder to second-degree murder, or manslaughter, which would result in a lesser sentence.

At one point at least 15 states recognized some variation of the concept of diminished capacity. Because of difficulties in definition, application, and administration, however, it has often been criticized as producing inconsistent and unfair decisions. Today the diminished capacity defense is used by only a small number of states and has failed to generate the support or fill the gap that its creators had intended. The concept was abandoned in California in 1981 after the successful but highly controversial use of the concept by defense counsel for Dan White, who had a finding of murder for the killing of the mayor and county supervisor of San Francisco mitigated to manslaughter.[30] This case stirred nationwide sentiment because of White's successful use of the "Twinkie defense," in which it was argued that the defendant's heavy consumption of junk food caused an impairment in his mental condition.

Other defenses. The development of the two-pronged ALI test, in addition to broadening the range of behavior that would excuse a defendant from criminal responsibility as compared with the M'Naughton test, also has opened the door to other forms of "illnesses" that could be considered to form the basis of an insanity defense.

Posttraumatic stress disorder (PTSD) is a form of mental condition that develops as a result of some traumatic event, such as combat war experience, plane or car crashes, and natural disasters. The most salient symptoms manifested by an individual with PTSD include recurrent elements and phases of the past trauma in dreams, uncontrollable and emotionally intrusive images, dissociative states of consciousness, and unconscious behavioral reenactments of the traumatic situation.

PTSD has been raised most frequently in criminal cases by Vietnam veterans as a form of insanity defense. Typically, the argument is made that the defendant's criminal behavior resulted from combat in Vietnam. Arguably, situations in which the defendant's criminal actions appeared to suggest some causal connection with a reenactment of a former war experience, in the absence of any other plausible explanation, is the most apropos time to raise a PTSD insanity defense. For example, the two murder trials of Vietnam veteran Charles Heads poignantly illustrate this defense. After his return from Vietnam, Heads frequently complained of depression, incessant nightmares, and flashbacks. One day in 1977, Heads, reacting to a fog-laden mist that surrounded a field adjacent to his brother-in-law's home in Louisiana, grabbed a rifle from his car and attacked the house. In the ensuing moments, he fatally shot his brother-in-law. Heads claimed that for an instant he was reliving combat. In his first trial in 1978, however, the jury rejected this temporary insanity claim.[31]

Because of a serious error by the trial judge, the Supreme Court suspended his life sentence and ordered a new trial. In 1981 a second jury heard his characterization of that fateful day and heard testimony from several veterans regarding their experiences of stress emanating from the war. This jury found Heads not guilty by reason of temporary insanity stemming from his past combat experiences.[32] This was the first PTSD defense successfully used in a capital case.

Even when the defendant displays clear signs of PTSD, however, there is no guarantee the defense will be accepted. In addition to demonstrating the existence of the illness, it must also be shown that it so impaired the defendant that it directly caused the criminal act. Although a majority of PTSD criminal cases involve war veterans, the defense is certainly not confined to this group.

Another illness now being asserted as a basis for the insanity defense is *pathological gambling.* As recognized by the American Psychiatric Association in its mental health diagnostic guide, the *Diagnostic and Statistical Manual of Mental Disorders* (DSM IV), pathological gambling is classified as an extreme impulse control disorder. A person is considered a pathological gambler if evidence shows a persistent and recurrent inability to resist the impulse to gamble and the gambling compromises, disrupts, or damages family, personal, and vocational pursuits.[33] Pathological gambling has had only limited success as a form of insanity defense in light of the conflict between psychiatric experts regarding whether it is a true mental disorder. Also, jurisdictions that have dropped the volitional elements from the insanity standard have completely cut out the most salient feature of this disorder. Similarly, courts that apply a somewhat strict view of the "mental disease or defect" part of the ALI rule have tended to conclude that pathological gambling does not meet the cognitive standard. As a result, fewer defendants are expected to be able to successfully raise pathological gambling as a defense.

Addressing the issue of *premenstrual syndrome* (PMS), researchers, although far from uniform in their description and determination of etiology, appear to have generally accepted the following as requisite criteria for a PMS diagnosis: (1) symptoms occur cyclically each month; (2) emotional symptoms must be primary symptoms; (3) symptomatic relief coincides with or shortly follows full flow of menses; (4) symptoms must be present during every premenstrual phase for at least a year; and (5) symptom severity must be moderate to severe.[34] Women report a wide variety of symptoms or changes in relation to the premenstruum.[35] Among the most common symptoms cited are hot flashes, changes in libido, acne, changes in energy level (e.g., hypomanic behavior), diminished self-esteem, mood swings, suicidal feelings, irritability, impulsivity, insomnia, and difficulty concentrating. Because of conflict in the medical community regarding PMS, it generally has not proved to be an accepted defense in limiting criminal responsibility. In only a handful of cases in England has PMS been successfully pled to reduce the seriousness of criminal charges. For example, in one case a woman pled that she suffered from a temporary hormonal imbalance during the commission of a murder, and her charge was reduced to manslaughter by reason of diminished responsibility.[36]

In light of the difficulty of establishing PMS as a recognizable mental illness at this time, the likelihood of a successful defense based on it is considered minimal.

Abolition of the insanity defense. Before 1930, Washington, Mississippi, and Louisiana had tried without success to do away with the insanity defense. Even before then, as well as after, numerous commentators had sought to abolish the defense.[37,38]

In 1979, Montana became the first state to constructively limit the use of an insanity plea. It amended its Code of Criminal Procedure to delete the section recognizing the insanity defense, which was substantially consistent with the ALI standard. The legislature substituted a new section that limited the relevancy of mental disease to the determination of mens rea of criminal intent. The Montana section stated: "Evidence that defendant suffered from a mental disease or defect is admissible whenever it is relevant to prove that the defendant did or did not have a state of mind which is an element of the offense."[39]

Three years later Idaho explicitly abolished the use of insanity as a separate defense to charges of criminal acts. As in Montana, however, the Idaho statute recognized that a defendant's mental state may be relevant to the issue of criminal intent[40]: "[N]othing herein is intended to prevent the admission of expert evidence on the issue of mens rea or any state of mind which is an element of the offense, subject to the rules of evidence."[41] Alabama and Utah have followed similar courses in either restricting a plea of insanity to the question of criminal intent or abolishing it altogether.

As alluded to earlier, the change in Montana and Utah to a mens rea approach in effect is a constructive abolition of the use of insanity as a defense because a person must be found so impaired that he or she is incapable of forming the intent to commit the act. For example, if a defendant purposefully shoots and kills a person, the defendant will not avoid criminal responsibility by claiming that his or her conduct was the result of a hallucination, delusion, or some form of thought disorder. A mens rea statute would only relieve persons of responsibility if they were unable to form the requisite intent to commit the crime. To establish the lack of intent, it would be necessary to demonstrate that the defendant was completely unaware of what he or she was doing or did not believe the act being committed (shooting a gun at victim) was actually taking place. A common illustration is that the defendant believed the gun was a banana and that he or she wasn't trying to kill the victim but instead was only squirting the victim with banana seeds.

This degree of impairment indicates the narrowness of the mens rea approach. For any more than a handful of all insanity acquittees each year to be found nonresponsible under this standard is highly doubtful. John Hinckley, Monte Durham, Daniel M'Naughton, Hadfield, and any number of other notable defendants whose insanity trials helped shape the insanity law in this area certainly would not qualify.

Despite this fact, proponents for abolishing the insanity defense argue that there is no constitutional requirement that a defense of mental illness exist at all.[42] Furthermore, allowances for the lack of mens rea comport with the historically held tenet that fundamental morality requires exculpation when a person truly does not know what he or she is doing. It is also argued that the mens rea standard is much easier to administer, thereby reducing the likelihood of confusion and complications frequently arising from contradictory expert testimony. Similarly, abolitionists and proponents of the mens rea test contend that an individual's mental state at the time of the crime still would be considered with regard to treatment, rather than penal alternatives.

NARROWING THE STANDARD. In 1983 the American Bar Association's (ABA's) House of Delegates passed a resolution to cut back the standard to be used for pleading insanity. This resolution stated: "The ABA approves, in principle, a defense of nonresponsibility for crime(s) which focuses solely on whether the defendant as a result of mental disease or defect was unable to appreciate the wrongfulness of his or her conduct at the time of the offense charged."[43]

In effect the ABA was dropping the volition or irresistible impulse prong from the ALI standard in favor of a strictly cognitive formulation. The reason for this change was basically twofold. Rejecting, but recognizing, certain state efforts to either completely or constructively abolish the defense, the ABA's proposal sought to diminish some of the ambiguity that many had claimed had infected the defense, while still maintaining its moral integrity and foundation. By dropping the volition element and applying the word "appreciate," the standard would be broad enough to encompass cases of severe reality impairment and would avoid the often difficult and controversial task of addressing compulsion. Also, commentary supporting this change suggests that this standard is consistent with contemporary psychiatric expertise and avoids the problem of vague or overinclusive interpretations of mental disease.

The American Psychiatric Association (APA) also supported a modification of the ALI standard. Carefully considering the evidence that various commentators have advanced regarding the present standards (principally M'Naughton and ALI) and other widely circulated alternatives (e.g., the mens rea approach, guilty but insane plea, complete abolition), the APA concluded that a more limited retention of the defense was required. Cognizant of the long history of difficulty that jurists and experts have had in defining mental disease and defect, the APA proposed a standard that would encompass only individuals with serious disorders and permit relevant psychiatric testimony on the majority of cases in which criminal responsibility was an issue. The APA proposed the following:

A person charged with a criminal offense should be found not guilty by reason of insanity if it is shown that as a result of mental disease or mental retardation he was unable to appreciate the wrongfulness of his conduct at the time of the offense. As used in this standard, the terms mental disease or mental retardation include only those severely abnormal mental conditions that grossly and demonstrably impair a person's perception or understanding of reality and that are not attributable primarily to the voluntary ingestion of alcohol or other psychoactive substances.[44]

As with the ABA, the APA's proposal has dropped the volition element in favor of a solely cognitive standard. The only difference between the two organizations' proposals is the APA's specificity regarding the nature and severity of the mental disease or defect to be considered.

The federal government and the American Medical Association (AMA) favored much greater limitations that approximate the mens rea alternative. Numerous bills in Congress have urged various legislation, ranging from complete abolition (use of a mens rea standard) to the creation of a new plea, "not guilty only by reason of insanity." Other proposed legislation included shifting the burden of proof to the defendant to prove he or she was insane at the time of the offense (e.g., in the Hinckley trial the government had the difficult task of proving Hinckley sane beyond a reasonable doubt) and abolishing the insanity defense in prosecutions of assassination attempts on the president.

The U.S. Justice Department recommended a comprehensive set of changes affecting a variety of areas in criminal justice. Entitled the Comprehensive Crime Control Act of 1984, several provisions pertaining to the insanity defense were included[45]: (1) limiting the (insanity) defense to those who are unable to appreciate the nature or wrongfulness of their acts, (2) placing the burden (of proof) on the defendant to establish the defense by clear and convincing evidence, (3) preventing expert testimony on the ultimate issue of whether the defendant had a particular mental state or condition, and (4) establishing procedures for federal civil commitment of a person found not guilty by reason of insanity if no state will commit defendant.

GUILTY BUT MENTALLY ILL. In 1975 Michigan became the first state to adopt the alternative plea "guilty but mentally ill" (GBMI) or "guilty but insane" (GBI). Presumably dissatisfied with the definitional and procedural problems of the insanity defense and the belief that its abolition was not constitutionally sound, Michigan sought a compromise. Also, Michigan sought to decrease the number of successful insanity pleas in its courts, since a 1974 court held that insanity acquittees must be treated the same as civil committees.[46] In effect this 1974 ruling permitted a significant number of insanity acquittees to be released from hospitalization fairly quickly, which raised a concern for public safety. To date, 11 other states have enacted similar GBMI legislation, many because of the Hinckley decision.[47]

Because it is at the forefront of this alternative defense plea, Michigan's law has served as a model for other states. Therefore there is sufficient procedural commonality to permit generalization. When an insanity plea is entered, a psychiatric evaluation is required. At the conclusion of the trial, a jury is presented with four possible verdicts: (1) not guilty, (2) guilty, (3) not guilty by reason of insanity, or (4) guilty but mentally ill. The GBMI verdict requires a finding of three factors: the accused was (1) guilty of the crime, (2) mentally ill at the time the offense was committed, and (3) not legally insane at the time of the offense.[48] Most states adopting the GBMI plea require that these factors be proved by a preponderance standard (e.g., 51 out of 100 chances). After a finding of guilty but mentally ill, the court has the discretion to impose any sentence within the statutorily prescribed limits of the crime committed. Typically, sentencing is geared toward psychiatric care within the confines of a prison. If no treatment is available in prison, probation contingent on outpatient treatment is always an option.

Despite the appearance of a novel alternative incorporating both rehabilitative and retributive aspects, the GBMI plea has been heavily criticized, even in its home state.[49] Opponents of the plea state that it is exceedingly difficult to discriminate between a finding of guilty but mentally ill and not guilty by reason of insanity (NGRI) in light of the similarity in definition. A similar concern is that juries will misuse the GBMI plea out of ignorance, thereby finding a defendant guilty when an NGRI finding was more appropriate. Also, the title "guilty but mentally ill" is considered deceptive because it implies some form of mitigation but actually provides no special allowance.

Proponents who tout this alternative on humanitarian grounds because of the treatment element are often confronted by the fact that treatment is not guaranteed, but only part of a criminal sentence.

In effect then, despite a change in name and arguably greater choice of alternatives, a jury's verdict of GBMI is basically no different for a defendant than a verdict of guilty.

PSYCHIATRIC MALPRACTICE

The development and emergence of malpractice lawsuits against psychiatrists have been very gradual and seemingly of recent occurrence. Before 1970, civil actions for psychiatric-related injuries were relatively rare. As a medical specialty, psychiatry was considered almost immune from lawsuits because it was a difficult area to build a case against a practitioner.

An early study of malpractice claims against psychiatrists occurring between the years 1946 and 1962 cited only 18 cases of negligent or civilly liable conduct.[50] Although this study was restricted to cases that had been appealed and reported, thus not accounting for cases settled out of court or unreported, the number was still remarkably low. In these early lawsuits, the defendant psychiatrists rarely lost, and when they did the judgment was generally small. Until the 1970s the incidence of lawsuits against psychiatrists remained quite low. Because of the intimate nature of the psychiatrist-patient relationship, patients were likely to be reluctant to acknowledge or expose their psychiatric history. Other obstacles included (1) the lack of an accepted method of practice within the profession, which made it difficult to

establish a breach of standard of care; (2) the reluctance of other psychiatrists to testify as experts against another colleague; (3) the adeptness of psychiatrists in dealing with a patient's negative experience, thereby avoiding litigation; (4) the difficulty in proving patient injury, in the absence of actual physical harm; and (5) the possible reluctance of the legal profession to delve into an area (of medicine) in which there are few consistent answers.

Malpractice actions against psychiatrists have steadily increased since the early 1970s, but this fact must be seen in context. The incidence of claims against psychiatrists still remains much lower than against other physicians,[51] and most claims do not result in successful verdicts against the psychiatrist.

Along with the incidence of malpractice actions, the variety of claims against psychiatrists has also increased. Some causes of action reflect acts of negligence or substandard care for which any physician may be found liable. These malpractice areas include negligent diagnosis, abandonment from treatment, various intentional and quasi-intentional torts (assault and battery, fraud, defamation, invasion of privacy), failure to obtain informed consent, and breach of contract. Areas of liability specific to psychiatry include harm caused by organic therapies (electroconvulsive therapy [ECT], psychotropic medication, psychosurgery), breach of confidentiality, sexual exploitation of patients, failure to control or supervise a dangerous patient or negligent release, failure to protect third parties from potentially dangerous patients, false imprisonment, and negligent infliction of mental distress. These claims represent the major causes of action that may be brought against a psychiatrist.

Malpractice actions based on a psychiatrist's use of psychotropic drugs have been fairly infrequent considering the widespread use of this form of treatment during the past 20 years. However, a study of claims filed between 1972 and 1983 against psychiatrists showed that 20% of the actions were related to medication.[52] With managed care, more frequent utilization of the psychiatrist as the prescriber of medication with the psychotherapy, and primary care parceled out to psychologists and other nonmedical therapists, more actions based on medication can be expected.

A psychiatrist's failure to adequately monitor or provide sufficient warnings and instructions about a drug's side effects provides an opportunity for several different allegations of negligence. In *Duvall v. Goldin* a psychiatrist was sued by a third party who was struck in a car accident by an epileptic patient having a seizure while driving.[53] The plaintiff alleged that the psychiatrist had a duty to inform the patient of the effects of his medication when driving to protect other individuals possibly endangered by the patient's conduct. The Michigan Court of Appeals reversed the trial court's dismissal of the case and held that there were reasonable facts raised by the complaint to void summary judgment for the psychiatrist.

Relatives of patients who have committed suicide by taking an overdose of medication often file suit, claiming that the psychiatrist was negligent in prescribing the drugs. In the treatment of suicidal patients a delicate balance exists between providing clinical treatment, which involves certain risks, and applying protective, less therapeutic measures. In recognition of this balance, a psychiatrist will not automatically be found liable if a patient commits suicide with medication provided for treatment. Negligence is likely to be found in high-risk situations in which either the psychiatrist's choice of intervention (e.g., medication) or manner of supervision was unreasonable under the circumstances.

Another area of concern with regard to liability involving drug treatment is *tardive dyskinesia* (TD). Despite limited cases, the frequency and dangerousness of the side effects and the amounts of the damages awarded have created considerable interest within the psychiatric profession, particularly among clinicians who prescribe antipsychotic medication.

Claims of negligence in cases involving TD are fairly similar to those in other drug-treatment lawsuits. Liability can result from the lack of an adequate examination (e.g., patient history, physical examination, or laboratory tests; failure to closely monitor or treat side effects; failure to obtain the patient's informed consent; failure to project and control drug reactions). The *Clites v. Iowa* case is one of the first decisions specifically dealing with TD and aptly illustrates some of the liability considerations inherent in the issue of drug therapy.[54] The plaintiff was a mentally retarded man, who had been institutionalized since age 11 and treated with major tranquilizers from age 18 to 23. TD was diagnosed at age 23, and the plaintiff subsequently sued. He claimed that the defendants had negligently prescribed medication, failed to monitor its effects, and had not obtained his informed consent. A damage award of $760,165 was returned and affirmed on appeal. The court ruled that the defendants were negligent because they deviated from the standards of the "industry." Specifically, the court cited a failure to administer regular physical examinations and tests; failure to intervene at the first sign of TD; the inappropriate use of drugs in combinations, in light of the patient's particular condition and the drugs used; the use of drugs for the convenience of controlling behavior rather than therapy; and the failure to obtain informed consent.

Informed consent and refusal

A major consideration regarding treatment of the mentally disabled patient is the competence to consent to treatment. For mentally retarded patients, the degree and ability to understand treatment information are relatively fixed, given the nature of their disability. Therefore, if the patient's retardation impairs his or her ability to understand the information disclosed, consent must be obtained from the patient's legal guardian or from the court. The problems encountered with patients with other mental disorders are far less predictable and finite. Questions such as, "Is the information being un-

derstood clearly or is it distorted?" or "Can all information be properly assimilated and does the patient have the capacity to express his or her decision?" are important considerations. Certainly if a patient is psychotic or hallucinating and cannot assimilate information about a proposed procedure, he does not have the capacity to reach a decision about the matter in question. Some patients are incapable of evaluating information in what most people would call a "rational manner." A treatment decision might ordinarily be based on perceived personal objectives or long-term versus short-term risks and benefits. Some patients, however, accept or reject a treatment without considering "factual information." Further, a patient's refusal to give consent to a procedure may only be a manifestation of the illness, not the patient's wishes.[55]

Another problem confronting the psychiatrist is some patients' fluctuating periods of lucidity. As a rule, for a psychiatrist or any other physician treating a patient of questionable competency, liability is limited if a reasonable effort was made to determine a patient's competency at the time of consent. If the patient provides consent to treatment (e.g., initiation of psychotropic medication) and then later claims not to understand what was disclosed, the question of competency is evaluated on the reasonableness of the physician's basis for the conclusion of competency. If the patient is not competent, a psychiatrist or physician generally is required to seek the consent of the patient's guardian. Consistent with other common-law concepts regarding consent (e.g., forming a contract, executing a will), the law does not recognize an agreement that is not the product of a person's free will.

Freedom from coercion, fraud, or duress is the pivotal requisite to ensuring that a patient's consent is voluntary. Any act, subtle or overt, that impinges on a patient's decision-making process may be sufficient to invalidate a patient's consent, for example, a patient who is threatened by the hospital staff, restricted from engaging in favored activities, or forced to do irksome tasks unless consenting to treatment. More subtle but equally coercive is the physician who emphasizes the consequences of not having a particular treatment and downplays the risks. The courts are particularly sensitive to the manner, content, and conditions in which information is given and consent is provided when vulnerable patients such as the mentally disabled, elderly, or physically weak are involved.

Exceptions. Under certain circumstances, disclosing risks to the patient and obtaining consent may not be necessary. Psychiatrists and physicians should be wary, however, about relying on an exception if it can be avoided, since support by the courts is inconsistent.

Four exceptions to obtaining informed consent are commonly recognized, although all four might not necessarily be available in a particular state. In the first exception, which applies in a situation involving a threat of serious injury or loss of life when it is impossible to obtain the consent from a patient or other authorized persons on the patient's behalf, the law will imply a consent. Referred to as the "emergency exception," two considerations must be heeded to avoid potential liability. First, the patient's condition must be so serious that treatment could not be delayed without risking serious injury. Second, the patient's condition, not the surrounding circumstances, must determine the existence of the emergency.

The second exception occurs in certain circumstances in which information is withheld when disclosure of risks and alternatives might have a significant detrimental effect on a patient's physical or psychological condition. The privilege may apply when disclosure might enhance the risk of the treatment itself or interfere with the patient's ability to make a rational decision. However, the privilege will not be upheld simply because a physician believes a patient would refuse the treatment if informed of the risks.

A third exception to the requirement of informed consent is recognized when the patient is incompetent and the procedure contemplated is a routine remedial measure (e.g., daily custodial care of incompetent institutionalized psychiatric patients). However, if informed consent is required for a specific treatment (e.g., ECT), the consent of a guardian or appointed substitute decision-maker is required.

Finally, a patient may knowingly and voluntarily waive the right to give an informed consent. In other words, no disclosure of the risks of a treatment is necessary when a patient specifically requests that he or she not be told the risks.

Breach of confidentiality

The duty to safeguard the confidentiality of any communication in the course of psychiatric treatment is the cornerstone of the profession. This obligation of confidentiality is fundamental, but none is more keenly sensitive to its importance than mental health professionals. This point is aptly reflected in the ethical codes of the various mental health organizations. For example, Section 4 of the *Principles of Medical Ethics with Annotations Especially Applicable to Psychiatry* reads in part as follows:

A physician shall respect the rights of patients, of colleagues and of other health professionals, and shall safeguard patient confidences within the constraints of the law. . . . confidentiality is essential to psychiatric treatment. This is based in part on the special nature of psychiatric therapy as well as on the traditional ethical relationship between physician and patient. . . . Because of the sensitive and private nature of the information with which the psychiatrist deals, he/she must be circumspect in the information that he/she chooses to disclose to others about the patient. The welfare of the patient must be a continuing consideration.[56]

In essence, confidentiality refers to the right of a person (e.g., patient) not to have communications revealed without authorization to outside parties. The issue of confidentiality in a psychiatric perspective embodies two fundamental rationales. First, a patient has a right to privacy that should not be violated except in certain legally prescribed circum-

stances. Second, physicians have historically been enjoined (on an ethical basis) to maintain the confidences of their patients. In doing so, patients should feel more comfortable revealing information, which would enhance their treatment.

Psychiatrists have always been susceptible to ethical sanctions if they breach patient confidentiality, but liability for monetary damages is a relatively recent development. Several legal theories allow a patient plaintiff recovery for breach of confidentiality. Besides statutory bases, some courts have upheld a cause of action based on breach of confidentiality on a contract theory.[57] Accordingly, a psychiatrist is considered to have implicitly agreed to keep any information received from a patient confidential, and when he or she has failed to do so, there is a breach of that implied contract term by the psychiatrist. In cases based on this theory, damages typically have been restricted to economic losses flowing directly from the breach, but compensation based on any residual harm (e.g., emotional distress, marital discord, loss of employment) is precluded.[58]

Theories based on invasion of privacy have supported recovery involving breach of confidentiality. The law defines invasion of privacy as an "unwarranted publication of a person's private affairs with which the public has no legitimate concern, such as to cause outrage, mental suffering, shame, or humiliation to a person of ordinary sensibilities."[59] This theory has limited appeal to plaintiffs in jurisdictions requiring a public disclosure of personal facts as opposed to disclosure to a single person or a small group.

A minority of courts has upheld claims for breach of confidentiality based on breach of fiduciary duty of the psychiatrist.[60] Similarly, claims based on violations of medical licensing statutes and physician-patient privilege statutes have provided remedies for unconsented disclosures of confidential information,[61] although with limited success. Such actions, when successful, are presumably based on public policy grounds.

In many states the legal duty to maintain patient confidentiality is governed by mental health confidentiality statutes. These statutes outline the legal requirements covering confidentiality. For example, the Illinois Mental Health and Developmental Disabilities Confidentiality Statute contains 17 sections covering the duty of confidentiality, exceptions to it, rules and procedures for authorizing disclosures, patient and third-party access rules, penalties or violations, and provisions for civil actions by parties injured by unauthorized disclosures.[62]

Failure to warn or protect

Confidentiality was considered sacrosanct by the psychiatric profession until the Supreme Court of California heard the case *Tarasoff v. Regents of the University of California* in 1976.[63] *Tarasoff* involved a university student from India who became obsessed with a young woman (Tatiana Tarasoff) he met at a dance. She clearly indicated that she had no interest in the young man. Following this rejection, he began individual therapy at the university counseling center. After several sessions the treating psychologist concluded that his patient might try to harm Ms. Tarasoff. The psychologist enlisted the aid of the campus police to detain the patient to ascertain his eligibility for civil commitment. The police interviewed the patient and concluded that he was rational. Based on his assurances that he had no desire to harm Ms. Tarasoff and would refrain from seeing her, they decided not to detain him. The supervising psychiatrist for the case reviewed the facts to that point and concluded there was no basis for commitment. The patient terminated treatment, and 2 months later killed Tatiana Tarasoff.

Tatiana's parents filed a wrongful death action against the university, the treating psychologist, the supervising psychiatrist, and the campus police. The plaintiffs asserted that the defendants owed a "duty to warn" Tatiana of the impending danger that the patient posed to her. The California Supreme Court agreed. In affirming but modifying their earlier holding (1974) the court held the following:

[W]hen a therapist determines, or pursuant to the standards of his profession should determine, that his patient presents a serious danger of violence to another, he incurs an obligation to use reasonable care to protect the intended victim against such danger. . . . Thus [the discharge of this duty] may call for [the therapist] to warn the intended victim or others likely to apprise the victim of the danger, to notify the police, or take whatever other steps are reasonably necessary under the circumstances.

The reaction to both decisions, referred to as *Tarasoff I* and *Tarasoff II*, was immediate, forceful, and frequently vehement. The majority of the early commentary, especially from the psychiatric profession, was critical of the numerous unanswered questions left by the California court. This new theory of liability imposed questions such as the following: Was a duty owed if the threat of danger was not aimed at anyone in particular? What steps did a psychiatrist or therapist have to take to discharge the duty? Was a duty to warn still owed if the potential victim was already aware of the patient's threat or dangerous propensities? How was a therapist's determination of dangerousness to be judged if the profession itself disclaimed the ability to accurately predict future behavior? In some cases these and other questions have been addressed in piecemeal fashion by the numerous "duty to warn/protect" decisions since *Tarasoff*.

The response by the courts following the 1976 California decision has been inconsistent and at times, confusing. Several courts have followed the holding of *Tarasoff,* concluding that a therapist was liable for not warning an identifiable victim. For example, courts in Kansas and Michigan have ruled that the duty to warn was restricted only to readily identifiable victims.[64] A slightly broader but analogous limitation has been fashioned by decisions in Maryland and Pennsylvania, where the courts have recognized a duty to warn only when the victim is "foreseeable."[65]

The second case to apply the *Tarasoff* ruling, *McIntosh v. Milano,* added a slightly broader twist to the duty-to-warn theory.[66] In *McIntosh* a 17-year-old patient fatally shot a young neighborhood woman. Evidence revealed that the patient had disclosed to the defendant psychiatrist feelings of inadequacy, fantasies of being a hero or important villain, and using a knife (which he brought to therapy one session) to intimidate people. The patient also shared that he had once fired a BB gun at a car in which he thought the victim was riding with her boyfriend. However, the psychiatrist denied that the patient had ever expressed any feelings of violence or made any threats to harm the victim. The parents of the victim claimed that the psychiatrist knew the patient was dangerous and owed a duty to protect the victim. The New Jersey court, in denying a motion for summary judgment, agreed and held that *Tarasoff* applied, based on the therapist-patient relationship. The court found a more general duty to protect society that was analogous to a physician's duty to warn others (in the general public) of persons carrying contagious disease.

Representing the broadest expansion of the *Tarasoff* duty-to-warn theory was a Nebraska decision of *Lipari v. Sears, Roebuck and Co.*[67] A patient, who recently had dropped out of the Veterans Administration (VA) day treatment program, purchased a shotgun from Sears. He resumed treatment, only to drop out against medical advice approximately 3 weeks later. A month after the second termination he walked into a crowded nightclub and randomly discharged the shotgun, injuring the plaintiff and killing her husband. The plaintiff claimed that the VA should have known the patient was dangerous and that the VA was negligent for not committing him. The court held that Nebraska law recognized a duty to protect society, following the holdings of *Tarasoff II* and *McIntosh.* More significantly, they held that foreseeable violence was not limited to identified, specific victims but may involve a class of victims (e.g., the general public at large).

Two other cases, one in Washington State[68] and another in California, have expanded the duty to warn to include victims who were not specified or readily identifiable. In *Hedlund v. Orange County* the victim was a woman in couples therapy with a man with whom she lived.[69] During a session when she was not present, the man told the therapist that he planned to harm her. While in a car with her son next to her, the man shot at her. The woman sought damages for herself and her son, who, she claimed, suffered emotional harm. Rejecting the defendant's argument that they owed no duty of care to the young boy, the California court extended the duty to warn to foreseeable persons in close relationship to the specifically threatened victim.

Fifteen days before the *Hedlund* decision, the U.S. District Court in Colorado decided the case *Brady v. Hopper.*[70] The plaintiffs were all men who had been shot by John Hinckley during his attempted assassination of President Reagan. The plaintiffs alleged that the defendant's psychiatrist, John

Hopper, knew or should have known that Hinckley was dangerous. Relying heavily on the *Lipari* decision, the plaintiffs claimed that the defendant should have known that the president was Hinckley's intended victim and that they were a class of people reasonably foreseeable to be at risk because of this danger. The court focused its decision on the issue of foreseeability of the risk to the specific plaintiffs involved. While affirming the duty of therapists to protect third parties, the court's conclusion was prefaced with the admission: "[T]he existence of a special relationship does not necessarily mean that the duties created by that relationship are owed to the world at large." In rejecting the plaintiffs' claims that the defendant was liable to them, the court concluded: "In my opinion, the specific threats to specific victims rule states a workable, reasonable, and fair boundary upon the sphere of a therapist's liability to third persons for the acts of their patients." Therefore, under *Brady,* a determination of dangerousness, in general, will not create a duty to protect without a specific threat to a specific victim. In December 1984 the Court of Appeals for the Tenth Circuit, in a three-page opinion, affirmed the district court's opinion in *Brady.*[71] In essence, it deferred to the discretion of the lower court, stating reversal only could be found if a gross error in the application of the law had occurred.

Cases to date involving some form of the duty-to-warn theory can be viewed as falling somewhere on a continuum based on two common factors: (1) a threat (or potential for harm) and (2) a potential victim. At one end is the *Brady* decision with its "specific threat specific victim" rule, and at the other end is *Lipari,* which held that "foreseeable violence" created a duty to protect "others," regardless of whether the victim was identified or specified. In addition, decisions in Maryland, California, Pennsylvania, and Iowa have refused to apply the theory by either rejecting it outright or finding no liability based on the facts of the case.[72]

At present, most courts have held that in the absence of a foreseeable victim, no duty to warn or protect will be found. Reviewing the cases, a few facts stand out. Most notable is the relative absence of litigation that most commentators thought would occur after the *Tarasoff* decision in 1974.[73]

Whatever the extent of the duty imposed by the *Tarasoff* decision and its progeny, a psychiatrist or therapist cannot be held liable for a patient's violent acts unless it is found that (1) the psychiatrist determined (or by professional standards reasonably should have determined) that the patient posed a danger to a third party (identified or unidentified) and that (2) the psychiatrist failed to take reasonable steps to prevent the violence.

The liability considerations that underlie the treatment and care of the dangerous patient generally differ according to the amount of control a psychiatrist, therapist, or institution has over the patient. As a general rule, psychiatrists who treat dangerous or potentially dangerous patients have a duty of care, which includes controlling that individual from harming other persons inside and outside the facility as well as himself or herself. On the other hand, the outpatient who presents a possible risk of danger to others creates a duty of care, which may include warning or somehow protecting potential third-party victims. Although some facts may require an expansion of the duty of care in one or the other setting (in-patient, outpatient), this general distinction is important to more clearly understand the legal issues and preventive considerations that the dangerous patient presents.

The duty of care owed to dangerous or potentially dangerous patients in an in-patient setting is very similar in principle to those duties governing the treatment of suicidal patients. Causes of action alleged by third parties injured by the dangerous or violent acts of an inpatient generally involve one of two situations. In one situation the inpatient is discharged and shortly thereafter harms a third party. The plaintiff sues whoever made the decision to discharge the patient, claiming that he or she was negligently released. In the second general situation an inpatient escapes from the hospital and then harms someone. The claim in this scenario is typically that the physician or facility in charge of the patient's care was negligent in either supervision or control of the patient.

In both general scenarios the analysis for determining liability is similar. As in cases involving suicide, a treating psychiatrist or other practitioner cannot be held liable for harms committed after a patient's discharge (e.g., negligent release) unless the court determines (1) that the psychiatrist knew or should have known that the patient was likely to commit a dangerous or violent act and (2) that in light of this knowledge, the psychiatrist failed to take adequate steps to evaluate the patient when considering discharge. Similarly, in cases involving third parties injured by a dangerous patient who has escaped, the court evaluates (1) whether the psychiatrist knew or should have known that the patient presented a risk of elopement and (2) in light of that knowledge, whether the psychiatrist took reasonable steps to supervise or control the patient. The actions of a psychiatrist in a negligent discharge or negligent control or supervision claim are scrutinized based on the reasonableness of the actions and the standards of the profession.

Sexual exploitation

From a legal standpoint, the courts have consistently held that a physician or therapist who engages in sexual activity with a patient is subject to civil liability and in some cases to criminal sanctions. The reason for this overwhelming condemnation rests in the exploitative and often deceptive practice that sex between a health care professional (e.g., psychiatrist, physician, therapist) and patient represents. The fundamental basis of the psychiatrist-patient relationship is the unconditional trust and confidence patients have in the therapist. This trust permits patients to share their most intimate secrets, thoughts, and feelings. As therapy progresses, unconscious feelings of conflict, fears, and desires originating from important relations in the patient's past are said to be "transferred" to the therapist in the present. This *transference phenomenon* is a common occurrence in psychotherapy and often provides a therapist valuable information to analyze and interpret. The transference phenomenon makes a patient vulnerable to the emotions being experienced, such as feelings of love. Therefore the therapist must conduct the treatment with sensitivity and care. A similar phenomenon, *countertransference,* occurs when a therapist experiences unconscious conflicts and feelings toward a patient. As with patient transferences, countertransference feelings should be recognized as important therapeutic information and analyzed to gain insight into how to better understand the patient.

When psychiatrists or other practitioners engage in sexual activity with a patient, they have exploited the vulnerability created by the therapeutic relationship and breached their legal and ethical duty of exercising due care. From a legal perspective, this breach of duty is probably best described in the landmark case *Roy v. Hartogs.*[74] The plaintiff alleged that the defendant had engaged in sexual relations with her for approximately 13 months. This relationship eventually caused her extreme emotional and physical deterioration and resulted in two separate hospitalizations. The defendant initially claimed that a New York statute relating to interference with the marital relation prevented sexual activity from being the basis of a malpractice action. The court rejected this claim, stating that not all actions involving sexual activity were barred by the statute. Reinforcing this conclusion, the court stated:

[T]here is a public policy to protect a patient from the deliberate and malicious abuse of power and breach of trust by a psychiatrist when that patient entrusts to him her body and mind in the hope that he will use his best efforts to effect a cure. The right is protected by permitting the victim to pursue civil remedies, not only to vindicate a wrong against her but to vindicate the public interest as well.

In addition to sexual activity, other types of behavior that demonstrate a manipulation of the transference phenomenon or therapeutic relation may be subject to civil liability. For example, a Florida court found a psychiatrist guilty of "conduct below acceptable psychiatric and medical standards" when it was discovered that he had told a patient that he loved her and would divorce his wife to marry her.[75] In the widely cited case *Zipkin v. Freeman* the defendant psychiatrist was found guilty of a blatant mishandling of the therapy transference when it was shown that he had manipulated his patient to leave her husband and children, invest in ventures controlled by him, and become his mistress and travel companion.[76]

In addition to civil sanctions, a practitioner may face criminal liability if there is evidence that some form of coercion, usually in the form of tranquilizing medication, was used to induce compliance or reduce resistance to the initiation of the sexual activity. A psychiatrist or other practitioner may be charged criminally if the sexual activity involves a child or adolescent patient. In a situation involving a minor, no evidence of force or coercion needs to be demonstrated to support a finding of criminal liability.

In the landmark case *Roy v. Hartogs,* expert testimony concluded that "there are absolutely no circumstances which permit a psychiatrist to engage in sex with his patient."[77]

However, some therapists do attempt to rationalize their actions. Some of the most common defenses, all of which to date have been rejected by the courts, include that the patient consented to having sex, that the sexual relation was not a part of treatment, or that the treatment ended before the sexual relations began.

Abandonment

Once an agreement (explicit or implicit) to provide medical services has been established, the physician is legally and ethically bound to render those services until the relationship has been appropriately terminated. If a physician terminates treatment prematurely and the patient is harmed by the termination, a cause of action based on "abandonment of treatment" may be brought. Generally, in the absence of an emergency or crisis situation, treatment can be concluded safely if a patient is provided reasonable notice of the termination and is assisted in transferring the care to a new physician. Proper transfer of care typically implies that the original psychiatrist or physician prepares and makes available the patient's records as needed by the new physician. It is also prudent for the original care provider to give the patient written and verbal notice to avoid any possible questions regarding the nature, timing, or extent of the announcement of termination. This is particularly important when treating psychiatric patients or persons who are psychologically vulnerable because there may be a tendency to misconstrue or deny a verbal notice.

The issue of abandonment frequently arises when either no notice of termination has been given or the extent of this notice has been insufficient in some way. Although there are no rules or guidelines per se regarding sufficiency of the notice, a therapist who decides to terminate treatment is expected to act reasonably. For example, if few therapists are available in the area to accept transfer of the patient's case, the treating therapist should afford the patient a longer notice period to locate a replacement. If a patient refuses or is unable to locate another therapist, however, the treating psychiatrist or therapist has no obligation to treat the patient indefinitely. The reasonableness of a therapist's notice therefore is judged on the totality of the relevant circumstances.

Patients who are experiencing some sort of crisis or emergency situation require special consideration. For example, a therapist who is treating a patient who is suicidal or presents a possible danger to some third party is not likely to be considered to be acting reasonably if he or she terminates treatment. From a clinical perspective, such a move may exacerbate a patient's already vulnerable feelings and prompt the patient to do something that he or she might not have otherwise done.

Legally, the courts are not likely to consider a therapist's decision to terminate treatment reasonable during a time when care is required. Therefore a therapist should be wary of ending therapy during a period of emergency and instead should hold off termination until a more appropriate time.

Patient control and supervision

The treatment of patients who pose a risk of danger to themselves or others presents a unique clinical and legal challenge to the mental health profession.

A lawsuit for patient suicide or attempted suicide is often brought by a patient's family or relatives claiming that the attending psychiatrist, therapist, or facility was negligent in some aspect of the treatment process. Specifically, there are three broad categories of claims that encompass actions stemming from patient suicide. The first is when an outpatient commits suicide or is injured in a suicide attempt. Plaintiffs in this situation claim that the psychiatrist or therapist was negligent in failing to diagnose the patient's suicidal condition and provide adequate treatment, which is typically hospitalization. The second situation is when an inpatient is given inadequate treatment and commits or attempts suicide. Typically, the essence of a negligence claim involving inadequate treatment is that the patient was suicidal and the psychiatrist failed to provide adequate supervision. The last general situation is when a patient is discharged from the hospital and shortly thereafter attempts or commits suicide. Family members, or the injured patient, frequently claim that the decision to release the patient was negligent.

The treatment of suicidal or potentially suicidal patients inherently requires a psychiatrist or other practitioner to make predictions regarding future behavior. The mental health profession has frequently disclaimed ability to predict future behavior with any degree of accuracy. As a result, the law has tempered its expectation of clinicians in identifying future dangerous behavior. Instead of a strict standard requiring 100% accuracy, the law requires professionals to exercise reasonable care in their diagnosis and treatment of patients at risk.[78] Accordingly, a court will not hold a practitioner liable for a patient's death or injury resulting from suicide if the treatment or discharge decision was reasonably based on the information available.

In an attempt to enhance the recovery of patients at risk of suicide, some hospitals use what is known as an *open ward policy*. This policy permits a patient considerable freedom of movement within the hospital and minimizes procedures that are constraining, such as seclusion, physical and chemical restraints, and constant observation. In some cases the courts have recognized the therapeutic value of this procedure and concluded that the professional is in the best position to balance the risks and benefits of increased patient freedom. In doing so, the courts have basically deferred to the judgment of the professional, even though the professional's decision may later prove to be wrong. This deferment to professional judgment is as much an acknowledgment of the difficulties psychiatrists face in attempting to predict future behavior as it is an acceptance of certain practices and procedures of modern psychiatry. A 1981 federal district court decision sums up its conclusion as follows:

[M]odern psychiatry has recognized the importance of making every effort to return a patient to an active and productive life. Thus the patient is encouraged to develop her self-confidence by adjusting to the demands of everyday existence. Particularly because the prediction of danger is difficult, undue reliance on hospitalization might lead to prolonged incarceration of potentially useful members of society.[79]

A few courts have refused to make such a deferment and instead have kept to the more traditional evaluation of the reasonableness of the precautions provided.[80] The issue of reasonableness, whether involving the diagnosis, supervision, or discharge of a patient, is usually measured in terms of the accepted standards of the profession. Expert testimony is needed to establish or disprove that the defendant psychiatrist failed to exercise the reasonable care other psychiatrists would have used in that or similar circumstances. The risk of liability is greatly enhanced when it can be demonstrated that a practitioner or institution failed to follow its own usual practices and procedures for treating a patient at risk for suicide.

Unusual and experimental therapies. The etiologies of many mental disorders (e.g., schizophrenia, depression) remain among the most perplexing mysteries to social scientists, biological psychiatrists, and researchers. As a result, psychiatrists have less definitive diagnostic and treatment methodologies than most other medical specialists. Therefore a greater opportunity exists for variance in treating mental disorders.

Treatments considered unusual or experimental may range from the use of certain lesser known or infrequently administered medication to a method of treatment that is completely unorthodox or unique to the individual applying it. Although the majority of practitioners in a particular locale may treat a certain psychopathology in the same manner or with the same type of medication, a treatment is not necessarily negligent simply because it is different. In the few cases that have addressed claims alleging negligence stemming from unusual or experimental treatments, the courts have typically applied the respectable minority standard. This standard states that if a particular treatment or procedure is recognized by a respectable minority in the profession, there will be no finding of a breach of due care.

However, unusual or experimental procedures that involve physical contact that inflict some form of pain on a patient may be malpractice per se, either in terms of negligence or as an intentional tort (e.g., assault and battery). In *Abraham v. Zaslow,* for example, a female patient was subjected to a procedure known as rage reduction of Z-therapy.[81] This experimental procedure involved restraining the patient and tickling and poking her while she was being interviewed by a psychotherapist. There was no evidence to demonstrate any recognition of acceptance of this technique within the psychotherapy profession. The court held that this manner of treatment was an intentional and harmful contact that resulted in the patient suffering severe emotional distress, physical bruising, and internal bodily damage.

CIVIL RIGHTS
Voluntary hospitalization

Mentally ill persons can be admitted to a psychiatric hospital or institution in essentially two ways. The first is to be involuntarily committed. The other and more common means is for the individual to sign in voluntarily, which is similar to a patient entering a general medical facility. In other words, admission is effected through what is legally and clinically presumed to be a free and voluntary action on the part of the patient.

Voluntary or consensual hospitalization of the mentally ill person is a relatively new idea. Massachusetts enacted the first voluntary admission statute in 1881, but other states were slow to follow. By 1949, only 10% of all mental patients were voluntary admissions. For about the next 20 years, states struggled to amend and revise their commitment laws to define and establish realistic procedures for voluntary admission. By 1972 most psychiatric admissions were voluntary.

The purpose of voluntary hospitalization for mentally ill persons is to dispel the coercion, trauma, and stigma normally associated with involuntary hospitalization and to afford the same opportunity for treatment to mentally ill patients that is available to those with physical illness.

The majority of states now provide for two forms of consensual admission: informal voluntary hospitalization (pure) and formal voluntary hospitalization (conditional). The distinction between these two forms has to do with the regulations governing discharge. In the case of informal voluntary admission, the patient must be released on request. By law or policy, some states limit the scope of this form of admission due to the potential for patient manipulation. The more formal or conditional form of voluntary admission permits the hospital to detain a patient for a specified time after a request for discharge. For example, South Dakota permits "release within at least five days—excluding Saturday, Sunday and holidays—from request."[82] The conditional release is designed to provide institutions adequate time to evaluate a patient with respect to need for initiating involuntary commitment proceedings. Initiation of these proceedings thus allows a hospital to detain a patient for the statutorily mandated time or, in some cases, for as long as it takes to convene a commitment hearing. The rationale behind the allotment of additional time for possible commitment is therapeutic in that it provides patients who may be angry, impulsive, or manipulative an opportunity to reconsider their request for discharge.

This extra time also affords the clinical staff a chance to develop outpatient treatment plans if the patient remains undeterred in the desire to leave the hospital.

One issue of increasing importance in relation to the idea of voluntary hospitalization of the mentally ill person is the question of competency to consent. Presumably, the act of voluntarily entering a psychiatric hospital requires the patient to be legally competent to make such a decision. Many of the first statutes authorizing voluntary commitment made the requirement of competency a specific element. The rationale for such a strict requirement was, at least in part, to prevent clearly incompetent patients from being improperly manipulated by psychiatrists and mental hospitals. This concern is clearly elaborated in the case of *Application for William R.*:

I have previously called to the attention of the organized Bar (see N.U.L.J. Editorial 1/29/58) that the pink form is being increasingly used by the Department of Mental Hygiene for the transfer and admission to state mental institutions, without judicial consideration, of most of the senile aged who do not make positive objection, and that it accounted for more than 1,000 such transfers within a period of nine months in 1957 from Kings County Hospital alone. I pointed out that this is a development of recent date, conceived as a technique for circumventing judicial sanction, due to much criticism by judges and doctors alike of certification procedures of aged seniles to state mental institutions as being morally wrong. This newly used technique effectively shunts seniles into involuntary confinement without awareness by them of their plight and without their actual approval or judicial surveillance. These unwanted seniles may not even hope to escape factually involuntary confinement because the possibility of private care, often provided at a judicial hearing, is denied to them and of course, they cannot thereafter effect their own release.[83]

More recent laws, however, designed to encourage voluntary admission and based on a theory that it ensures needed treatment, omit such requirements in most states. The dilemma regarding the issue of a patient's competency to be hospitalized voluntarily remains unresolved. To date, the question of whether a patient by voluntary admission must be competent to exercise an informed consent has not been authoritatively addressed by any court. This lack of judicial scrutiny is largely a consequence of present-day voluntary admission procedures. A person who has been coerced into voluntarily signing in or lacks the capacity to fully comprehend the consequences of the application for admission is unlikely to have any grounds on which to raise either issue since, at any time, a request for discharge can be made. Such an individual would then be either released pursuant to that request or committed pursuant to state involuntary commitment statutes. In either event, at least in theory, the issue of invalid or improper voluntary admission would have been negated, thereby preventing any court from hearing the significant issues surrounding this aspect of the voluntary admission process.

Rights of the voluntary patient. The rights of the voluntary psychiatric patient are unclear in most cases and at best, inconsistently applied in courts that have addressed this issue. Primarily, the question of "rights" revolves around three areas: (1) access to inpatient treatment, (2) the legal right to refuse unwanted treatment, and (3) the ability to be discharged when so desired.

To date, no reported cases have squarely addressed the question of whether there is a "right to in-patient treatment" for the voluntary patient under state or federal law. Individual states have been left to develop their own laws regarding the acceptance and discharge of voluntary patients. For example, a Missouri voluntary discharge statute reads: "He may discharge any voluntary patient if to do so would, in the judgment of the head of the hospital, contribute to the most effective use of the hospital in the care and treatment of the mentally ill."[84]

This seemingly arbitrary basis for discharge is quite similar to statutory language common in admission statutes. The issue of a patient's right to admission is as much a social question as it is clinical in that it undoubtedly encompasses the question of whether individuals unable to afford inpatient psychiatric services may be denied access to such treatment on the basis of economic status. This question remains unresolved.

Similarly, the right to immediate discharge is the subject of much debate. From a practical perspective, most voluntary admissions are accepted on a conditional basis because informal admissions tend to be more costly in terms of staff time and resources (e.g., administrative paperwork must be completed every time a patient chooses to leave). Therefore the majority of patients are subject to mandatory detention, a provision that greatly limits the patient's freedom to decide when he or she wishes to be released.

The question of whether a voluntary patient has the right to refuse treatment (e.g., psychotropic medication) and remain as a patient has been rejected by at least one appellate court. In *Rogers v. Okin* the court rejected a lower court's finding of such a right to refuse treatment and instead concluded that applicable state statutes (Massachusetts) provided no such guarantee that voluntary patients had a choice of treatment.[85] Instead, it concluded that state law left decisions regarding the treatment of patients to the judgment and discretion of the hospital physicians and staff. Despite this holding, the issue of the rights of voluntary patients remains far from settled.

Involuntary hospitalization

Basis and rationale. Involuntary hospitalization or civil commitment refers to state-imposed involuntary detention or restrictions of personal freedom based on a determination that a person is mentally ill and dangerous to self or others or is gravely disabled.

The institution of the civil commitment process is based on two fundamental common-law principles. The first relates to the right of the government, provided by the U.S. Constitution to the individual states, to take whatever actions are necessary to ensure the safety of its citizens. Referred to as the *police power,* this authority is limited by the states' constitutions and by the Fourteenth Amendment of the U.S. Constitution.

The other rationale used to justify the involuntary commitment of mentally ill persons is the *parens patriae* doctrine. This concept, which denotes that the state is acting in place of the parent, prescribes that the "sovereign has both the right and the duty to protect the person and the property of those who are unable to care [for] themselves because of minority or mental illness."[86] From a practical perspective, numerous state statutes and case law, in an attempt to cut back the broadness of certain state commitment provisions, have either abolished the parens patriae rationale or made it contingent on a finding of dangerousness (e.g., thereby invoking the salient purpose of the police power).

Commitment standards. The civil commitment process can be viewed in terms of (1) the criteria or standards governing whether someone is committable and (2) the procedural rules regulating the process.

In most jurisdictions the basic criteria for involuntary civil commitment are the product of a statute. The wording and interpretation of the various commitment laws differ from state to state, but the standards for commitment are similar.

Typically, all states require an individual to demonstrate clear and convincing evidence of at least two separate and distinct elements. The first pertains to the individual's mental condition. Nearly every state requires a threshold finding that a person suffers from some mental illness, disorder, or disease. The second and often more critical requirement is a determination that some "specific adverse consequence" will ensue, as a result of the mental illness, if the person is not confined. Commonly couched in language such as "likely to harm self or others," "poses a real and present threat of substantial harm to self or others," or "dangerous to himself or others," this element is frequently referred to in references as simply the "danger to self or others" requirement. In some states, such as Delaware and Hawaii, this element is extended to harm to property as well as persons.

Closely related to both the mental illness and dangerousness requirements is the standard of "gravely disabled." This standard is somewhat similar to the mental condition requirement in that it typically applies to a person's ability to provide self-care. This is not a uniform standard as are the other two criteria but represents an attempt by a minority of states to provide a broader description of the kind of manifest behavior that may prompt commitment. An example of a state statute applying the gravely disabled standard is the following:

Gravely disabled means that a person, as a result of mental or emotional impairment, is in danger of serious harm as a result of an inability or failure to provide for his or her own basic human needs such as essential food, clothing, shelter or safety and that hospital care is necessary and available and that such person is mentally incapable of determining whether or not to accept treatment because his judgment is impaired by his mental illness.[87]

Commitment procedures. Nearly all states provide two basic methods or procedures by which an individual can be taken against his or her will and transferred to a psychiatric facility for detention and examination. The first procedure is referred to as the *emergency commitment,* which under appropriate circumstances permits the commitment of an individual without any prior formal due process hearing. The second procedure is based on a court order that follows a formal hearing, held before the individual's confinement.

The emergency commitment procedure can generally be initiated by any adult who signs a petition under oath, asserting that immediate treatment is needed for the safety of an individual. This petition is typically accompanied by at least one and sometimes two certificates of examination by a qualified examiner. These certificates attest that the examiner (usually a psychiatrist, physician, or clinical psychologist) has concluded that the individual is in need of immediate treatment and is likely to pose a threat of danger to self or others. The executed petition and certificates then are presented to either the police or a mental health facility to effectuate the taking into custody and transportation of the individual to a psychiatric facility. In many states the police are permitted to take a person they believe requires immediate hospitalization into custody and to a psychiatric facility without certification by a qualified examiner. However, this form of abbreviated commitment is usually valid for only 1 day unless a certificate is subsequently executed. In any event, all individuals involuntarily committed under emergency procedures must be provided a judicial-type hearing to ascertain further need for commitment within a statutorily prescribed time, which may vary from 1 to 6 weeks.

In the absence of an emergency, most states permit the involuntary commitment of an individual after a more formal admission process. Referred to as *commitment by court order,* this procedure may also be initiated by any adult who has reason to believe an individual is in need of hospitalization. A petition is filed with the court and in some cases accompanied by at least one certificate executed by a qualified examiner. Pursuant to the submitted petition, regardless of certification, the court is then authorized to order the individual to undergo a psychiatric evaluation. On confirmation that the individual needs hospitalization, a formal hearing is scheduled to adjudicate the individual's need for commitment. The hearing serves to determine whether the statutory conditions for commitment are met.

In essence, the basic difference between the two procedures for commitment is the timing of the formal hearing: before court-ordered commitment or after emergency commitment. The procedures described reflect the general form of the two methods used in most jurisdictions, but the precise requirements, procedural safeguards, and time requirements differ greatly from state to state. Therefore any clinician, attorney, or advocate involved in this area of law should become thoroughly familiar with the particular state's statutory requirements.

Least restrictive alternative. Up to the late 1960s, a patient civilly committed to a state institution could expect to remain there for a major portion, if not the duration, of his or her life. Often criticized as mere human warehousing, the majority of mental institutions in America failed at achieving anything remotely therapeutic. Usually, the best that a civilly committed patient could hope for was bare-minimum custodial care. The thought of ever leaving the institution was a fleeting fantasy for many patients, and those who were discharged were rarely any better off than when they were admitted.

Patients legitimately committed due to mental illness and posing risk of danger might remain hospitalized long after the time when one or both of these conditions no longer existed. Because states rarely required the periodic evaluation of those civilly committed, however, a patient could literally waste away in the hospital despite no longer qualifying for detention. This situation represented a serious abridgment of the civil liberties of patients with mental illness and spurred considerable concern by libertarians, scholars, and civil rights activists.

In 1966 the case *Lake v. Cameron* (applying D.C. law) signaled a significant advancement in the recognition of civil rights of mentally disabled persons.[88] *Lake* involved the involuntary commitment of a 60-year-old woman diagnosed as senile but not considered a danger to herself or others. Writing for the majority, Chief Judge Bazelon held that a person could not be involuntarily committed to a psychiatric hospital if alternative placements could be found that were less restrictive on a patient's constitutional right to liberty. From this opinion the doctrine of the "least restrictive alternative" (LRA) was developed which, at least in theory, recognized and sought to protect the rights to liberty of patients who were so routinely ignored in the past.

After the *Lake* decision, numerous states adopted legislation requiring courts to consider less restrictive alternatives whenever appropriate. In the absence of statutory authority, several lower federal courts upheld the validity of the LRA doctrine based on implied constitutional grounds. This implied reasoning was addressed in the seminal case *Lessard v. Schmidt:*

Even if the standards for an adjudication of mental illness and potential dangerousness are satisfied, a court should order full-time involuntary hospitalization only as a last resort. A basic concept in American justice is the principle that "even though the governmental purpose be legitimate and substantial, that purpose cannot be pursued by means that broadly stifle fundamental personal liberties when the end can be more narrowly achieved. The breadth of legislative abridgment must be viewed in light of less drastic means for achieving the same basic purpose."[89]

The LRA doctrine has been applied to numerous other forms of restraining a patient's liberty within the hospitalization process (e.g., the use of physical restraints and seclusion rooms). In extending the scope of the doctrine to other treatment procedures, respect for a patient's civil rights is acknowledged, the hospitalization experience becomes less stigmatizing, and positive patient-staff relations are fostered.

Despite the social, therapeutic, and psychological value of the LRA doctrine, its application is subject to severe limitations. As Chief Judge Bazelon held in *Lake,* a less restrictive alternative must actually exist in order for the doctrine to apply.

From a practical standpoint this requirement presents a major setback in most cases because such less restrictive alternatives rarely are available. The practical value of the LRA doctrine therefore is limited unless the courts take the initiative to create, or order, alternative placements. In the absence of legislative authority, this development is unlikely.

Rights of the civilly committed patient. The right to treatment and habilitation, to the basic necessities of life, to refusal of treatment, and to treatment in the least restrictive environment have all been litigated and afforded varying degrees of protection.

The concept of a right to treatment was first articulated in 1960 when Dr. Morton Birnbaum proposed that:

The courts, under their traditional powers to protect the constitutional rights of our citizens begin to consider the problem of whether or not a person who has been institutionalized solely because he is sufficiently mentally ill to require institutionalization for care and treatment actually does receive adequate medical treatment so that he may regain his health, and therefore his liberty, as soon as possible; that the courts do this by means of *recognizing and enforcing the right to treatment;* and, that the courts do this, independent of any action by any legislature, as a necessary and overdue development of our present concept of due process of law. [emphasis in original][90]

A constitutional right to treatment, or to "habilitation," was held to apply to mentally disabled individuals in the landmark case *Wyatt v. Stickney.*[91] The court held that in the absence of the opportunity to receive treatment, mentally disabled individuals in institutions were not patients but were residents with indefinite sentences. Further, the court stated that basic custodial care or punishment was not the purpose of involuntary hospitalization. The purpose, they concluded, was treatment. In its subsequent opinions the court developed an extensive remedial plan that was intended to establish minimum constitutional standards for adequate treatment and habilitation of mentally disabled persons.

A second basic constitutional right, the right to liberty, was addressed in the Supreme Court decision *O'Connor v. Donaldson.*[92] Donaldson had been involuntarily confined in a state mental institution for almost 15 years and was suing the state for depriving him of his constitutional right to liberty. In the first award granted to a mentally ill patient based on a violation of constitutional rights, Donaldson received $20,000 in damages. In addressing the deprivation of liberty that involuntary confinement imposed, the court concluded that three conditions had to be met to justify release: (1) the institution was not offering proper treatment; (2) the patient did not present a danger to self or others; and (3) the person was capable of living in the community with the assistance of family or friends. Although these narrow conditions were illuminated in later litigation, *Donaldson* laid the foundation for future constitutional litigation regarding the rights of the mentally ill.

The U.S. Supreme Court has not yet squarely addressed the issue of the right to refuse treatment. The issue of whether an involuntarily committed patient has a constitutional right to refuse treatment (antipsychotic medication) was before the high court in 1982 in *Mills v. Rogers,*[93] but it was sidestepped and sent back to a lower federal court for reconsideration.

Despite the Supreme Court's refusal to decide *Mills,* several lower federal courts have sought to resolve the issue of right to refuse treatment. In one of the most noted cases, *Rennie v. Klein,* the Court of Appeals for the Third Circuit affirmed the finding that a constitutional right to refuse treatment existed.[94] However, the appeals court differed from the lower court when it adopted a "least intrusive means analysis." Under this analysis, antipsychotic drugs could be forcibly administered in a nonemergency situation to patients who had never been adjudicated incompetent, only if such treatment was the least restrictive mode of treatment available.

A year after *Rennie* the U.S. Supreme Court held in the landmark case of *Youngberg v. Romeo* that mentally retarded residents of state institutions had a constitutional right to the basic necessities of life, reasonably safe living conditions, freedom from undue restraints, and the minimally adequate training needed to enhance or further their abilities to exercise other constitutional rights.[95] Of significant importance to future civil rights cases involving mentally disabled persons was the court's deference to the judgment of qualified professionals to establish minimal adequate training and to safeguard a patient's liberty interests. In seeking to minimize judicial interference in the daily administration of institutions, the court held that "liability may be imposed only when the decision is such a substantial departure from accepted professional judgment, practice or standards as to demonstrate that the person responsible actually did not base the decision on such a judgment."[96]

The full impact of *Youngberg* has yet to be determined, but at least one significant civil rights case, *Rennie v. Klein,* has been redefined because of it. In 1983 the Third Circuit Court of Appeals rejected the "least intrusive means analysis" and adopted the standard of "whether the patient constitutes a danger to himself or others" in determining whether medication can be forcibly administered.[97]

REFUSAL OF MEDICATION

In a suit involving constitutional rights, patients at a state mental institution filed suit challenging conditions at their institution. Among the conditions they challenged was the use of psychotropic drugs. The court noted that the drugs cause a number of adverse reactions, the most serious being tardive dyskinesia, which interferes with all motor activity, making speech incomprehensible and breathing and swallowing extremely difficult.

Whatever the constitutional basis for the foregoing decision, a federal district court in Ohio found that the guarantee of due process gives a mental patient the right to refuse psychotropic drugs. The court said that a patient is being deprived of liberty without due process if forced to accept these medications (unless the patient is a danger to self or others). Because the inviolability of one's body is one of the oldest rights recognized in the law, the court related that informed consent is essential before treatment, except in emergencies. Even with mentally ill patients, an unwilling patient lessens the prospects for successful drug therapy. According to the judge, hospital efficiency is no justification for ignoring constitutional rights. The court suggested that an impartial decision-maker from outside the hospital conduct a hearing before any involuntary treatment with psychotropic drugs.

The court acknowledged that mental patients had a constitutional right to refuse treatment, at least in some situations. As a constitutional minimum, the state must have at least probable cause to believe that a patient was in a state of mental health that could not justify forced drugging, the court said. The high court ruled that the state had no interest that could override the need for patients' consent to treatment unless they were dangerous to themselves or others. The state must follow a due-process procedure, including some kind of hearing before an impartial decision-maker, before it can involuntarily treat a patient. The court set out constitutionally required safeguards to be followed in treating mentally ill patients. The use of psychotropic drugs to physically restrain patients violated their right to treatment in a humane, therapeutic environment.[98]

A federal appellate court for New Jersey ruled that involuntarily committed patients have a constitutional right to refuse administration of antipsychotic drugs. A patient in a state mental institution filed suit during his twelfth hospitalization after an involuntary commitment proceeding. A federal trial court recognized a constitutional right to refuse treatment. The appellate court modified the trial court's injunction and incorporated the rules of a state administrative bulletin. The Supreme Court reversed and remanded for reconsideration in light of its decision in a related case. On remand, the federal appellate court said that the proper standard for determining whether drugs can be administered against the patient's will was based on accepted professional judgment. The procedures outlined in the state administrative bulletin satisfied the due-process requirements for applying the professional judgment standard. The bulletin required a physician to explain the reasons for the medication and to specify risks and benefits, to have procedures for patient consultation with family members, and to provide for a review by other professional staff and meetings with the treatment team.[99]

In *Guardianship of Richard Roe III* a noninstitutionalized patient was found to be incompetent and his father was appointed guardian.[100] The father then sought contingent authority to consent to the forcible administration of antipsychotic medication. The Massachusetts Supreme Judicial Court denied this request, holding that except in an emergency, in cases of forced medication, the "substituted judgment" of an incompetent person must be exercised by a judge, not a guardian. If the judge determines that the patient would consent to antipsychotic medication, it should be ordered; if the judge determines that the patient would refuse, then he or she must weigh those state interests that can override the right to refuse. Only an "overwhelming" state interest will suffice. The protection of third parties was seen as a potentially overriding interest in this case, but the court cautioned that a bona fide "likelihood of violence" must be established. The Massachusetts court emphasized that its holding was limited to noninstitutionalized, incompetent individuals and did not apply to patients in state hospitals.

Several involuntarily committed patients brought a class action suit in a federal court against officials and staff of a Massachusetts state hospital. They had been forcibly administered antipsychotic drugs during their hospitalization. The drugs administered (Thorazine, Mellaril, Prolixin, Haldol) had significant adverse reactions that could be disabling, such as TD. The patients claimed that forcible administration of the drugs violated their constitutional rights. A federal trial court agreed and said that patients must consent before the administration of drugs except in an emergency. An appellate court agreed in part but said that a hospital's professional staff should have substantial discretion in deciding when an emergency required involuntary administration of medication. The U.S. Court of Appeals for the First Circuit has delineated the circumstances whereby patients at state mental hospitals may be forcibly administered antipsychotic drugs. The opinion deals with the balancing of the state's police powers and parens patriae powers with the rights of the institutionalized patient.[101]

The court first addressed the situation in which the state in exercising its police power may forcibly medicate a mentally ill patient. The district court said, "A committed mental patient may be forcibly medicated in an emergency situation in which a failure to do so would result in a substantial likelihood of physical harm to that patient, other patients, or to staff members of the institution." Addressing the difficulty in setting a "clear-cut unitary standard of quantitative likelihood that violence would occur," the court of appeals said, "The professional judgment call required in balancing these varying interests and determining whether a patient should be subjected to forcible administering of antipsychotic drugs demands an individualized estimation of the possibility and type of violence, the likely effects of particular drugs on a particular individual, and an appraisal of the alternative, less restrictive forces of action." Remanding the case to the district court, the court of appeals summarized its holding on this issue as follows:

The district court should not attempt to fashion a single "more-likely-than-not" standard as a substitute for an individualized balancing of the varying interests of particular patients in refusing antipsychotic medication against the equally varying interests of patients—and the state—in preventing violence. . . . [The] court should leave this typical, necessarily *ad hoc* balancing to state physicians and limit its own role to designing procedures for ensuring that the patients' interests in refusing antipsychotics are taken into consideration and that antipsychotics are not forcibly administered absent a finding by a qualified physician that those interests are outweighed in a particular situation and less restrictive alternatives are unavailable.

As for the use of the parens patriae power to justify forcible medication, the court said, "The *sine qua non* for the state's use of its parens patriae power as justification for the forcible administration of mind-affecting drugs is a determination that the individual to whom the drugs are to be administered lacks the capacity to decide for himself whether he should take the drugs." However, "the commitment decision itself is an inadequate predicate to the forcible administration of drugs to an individual where the purported justifications for that action is the state's parens patriae power." The court ruled that "absent an emergency, a judicial determination of incapacity to make treatment decisions must be made before the state may rely on its parens patriae powers to forcibly medicate a patient, but as a constitutional matter the state is not required to seek individualized guardian approval for decisions to treat incompetent patients with antipsychotic drugs. What procedural safeguards might be required, short of individualized guardian review, we leave for the present to the district court." The case was remanded to the district court for further proceedings. The U.S. Supreme Court, nevertheless, believed the case applicable to the patients in *Rogers v. Commissioner of the Department of Mental Health,* who were citizens of Massachusetts. Because state law had changed and may have provided broader protection to the patient than required under the U.S. Constitution, the court remanded the case for reconsideration. The Massachusetts Supreme Judicial Court held the opinion that an involuntarily committed patient is competent to make treatment decisions. Incompetence must be determined by a judge, and only after a patient is judged incompetent can he or she be forcibly administered antipsychotic drugs. There is no state interest great enough to permit involuntary administration of drugs in a nonemergency situation. Forcible treatment is permissible in an emergency and to prevent the immediate, substantial, and irreversible deterioration of a serious mental illness, the court said.[102]

In *Rogers v. Okin* the U.S. Supreme Court ruled that some psychiatric patients have a qualified right to refuse psychotropic, or mind-altering, medication and that some form of administrative review of this kind of treatment should be instituted. However, the court did not set definitive guidelines and left it to the states to establish right-to-refuse policies.[103]

A *qualified right* implies that a patient may exercise the right to refuse medication only if he or she does not present some special condition such as incompetency or dangerousness. If a patient has such a condition and refuses medication, he or she may be forcibly treated. In all the judicial opinions issued thus far, the existence of an emergency also serves as justification for overriding patients' refusals. All the states that recognize the right to refuse medication also have procedures to override the right in emergencies, and a majority of states permit overriding patients' refusals in nonemergencies. The exact procedures used to override patients' refusals vary considerably from one hospital to another. In the states where the right to refuse is qualified by more than the existence of an emergency, competency and commitment standards are used to determine which patients may refuse medication. Most states that have officially initiated a procedure to implement the right to refuse treatment have provided more than one method; often, more formal methods such as statutes and litigation are followed by the development of more detailed administrative rules and departmental policies.

Despite the existence of these policies, many people "are frustrated about the confused status of this issue." Some are trying to approach the problem in innovative ways, for example, by instituting a multidisciplinary panel to review all medication refusals. Nevertheless, an apparently common approach is to have "written procedures representing official guidelines, but in practice to fail to extend to patients a meaningful right to refuse medication."[104]

ENDNOTES

1. J. Quen, *Anglo-American Criminal Insanity: an Historical Perspective,* 10 J Hist. Behavioral Sci. 313 (1974).
2. *Justinian Digest* 48, 8.2 (Dec 533).
3. S. Grey, *The Insanity Defense: Historical Development and Contemporary Relevance,* 10 Am. Crim. Law Rev. 555 (1972).
4. *Id.*
5. 4 W. Blackstone, *Commentaries* 24 (Clarendon Press, Oxford 1769).
6. *Pate v. Robinson,* 383 U.S. 375, 86 S.Ct. 836, 15 L.Ed. 2d 815 (1966).
7. *Dusky v. United States,* 362 U.S. 402, 80 S.Ct. 788, 4 L.Ed. 2d 824 (1960).
8. *Drope v. Missouri,* 420 U.S. 162, 95 S.Ct. 896, 43 L.Ed. 2d 103 (1975).
9. *Id.*
10. *Estelle v. Smith,* 451 U.S. 454, 101 S. Ct. 1866, 68 L.Ed. 2d 359 (1981).
11. *Jackson v. Indiana,* 406 U.S. 715, 32 L. Ed. 2d 434, 92 S. Ct. 1845 (1972).
12. *Rex v. Arnold,* 16 How. Sr. Tr. 695 (C.P. 1742).
13. 1 Hawkins, *Pleas of the Crown* 1 (1824).
14. *Hadfield's Case,* 27 State Trial 1281 (1800).
15. *Id.*
16. R. Reisner, *Law and The Mental Health System* 564 (West 1985).
17. 4 State Tr. N.S. 847, 8 Eng. Rep. 718 (1843).
18. American Psychiatric Association, *Statement on the Insanity Defense* 3 (Dec 1982).

19. *M'Naughton's Case,* 4 State Tr. N.S. 847, 8 Eng. Rep. 718, 721-22 (H.L. 1843) (per Lord Chief Justice Tindal).
20. A. Goldstein, *The Insanity Defense* 67 (Yale University Press, New Haven 1967).
21. *Id.*
22. *Durham v. United States,* 214 F. 2d 862, 874 (D.C. Cir. 1954).
23. *Id.* at 874-875.
24. D. Weschler, *The Criteria for Criminal Responsibility,* 22 Univ. Chi. Law Rev. 367 (1955).
25. *Supra* note 20.
26. Model Penal Code § 4.01 (1962).
27. *McDonald v. United States,* 312 F. 2d 847 (D.C. Cir. 1962).
28. *Id.* at 851.
29. *People v. Wells,* 203 P. 2d 53 (Cal. 1949).
30. Cal. Penal Code § 28(b) (1981); *People v. White* 117 Cal. App. 3d 270, 172 Cal. Rptr. 612 (1981).
31. *Heads v. Louisiana,* 370 S. 2d 564 (La. 1979), *remanded for further consideration* 444 U.S. 1008 (1980).
32. *State v. Head,* No. 106, 126 (1st Jud. Dist. Ct., Caddo Parrish, Oct 1981).
33. *DSM IV* 615-618 (4th ed. 1994).
34. R. Haskett & J. Abplanalp, *Premenstrual Tension Syndrome: Diagnostic Criteria and the Selection of Research Subjects,* 9 Psychiatry Res. 125 (1983).
35. R. Haskett & M. Steiner, *Diagnosing Premenstrual Tension Syndrome,* 37 Hosp. Community Psychiatry 33-34 (1986).
36. *British Legal Debate: Premenstrual Tension and Criminal Behavior,* 17 New York Times (Dec 29, 1981).
37. M. Guttmacher, *The Role of Psychiatry in Law* (Thomas, Springfield, Ill. 1965).
38. B. Wooten, *Crime and Criminal Law* (Stevens, London 1963).
39. Mont. Code Ann. § 46-14-102 (1979).
40. 4 Idaho Code § 18-207 Cumm. Supp. (1986).
41. *Id.* at § 18-207c.
42. *Supra* note 32.
43. American Bar Association, Standing Committee on Association Standards for Criminal Justice, *Proposed Criminal Justice Mental Health Standards* (ABA, Chicago 1984).
44. 7 Mental Disability L. Rep. 136 (1983).
45. Comprehensive Crime Control Act of 1984 (Government Printing Office, Washington, D.C. 1984).
46. *People v. McQuillan,* 221 N.W. 2d 569 (Mich. 1974).
47. L. Blunt & H. Harley, *Guilty but Mentally Ill: an Alternative Verdict,* 3 Beh. Sci. & Law 49 (1985) [citing Alaska, Delaware, Georgia, Illinois, Indiana, Kentucky, New Mexico, Pennsylvania, South Dakota, Michigan & Utah].
48. Mich. Comp. Laws Ann. 768.36(1), *enacted in* Public Act 1980 of 1975.
49. R. Petrella et al., *Examining the Application of the Guilty but Mentally Ill Verdict in Michigan,* 36 Hosp. and Community Psychiatry 254 (1985).
50. W. Bellamy, *Malpractice in Psychiatry,* 118 Am. J. Psychiatry 769 (1962).
51. P. Slawson, *Psychiatric Malpractice: A California Statewide Survey,* 6 Bull. Am. Acad. Psychiatry & L. 58 (1978).
52. Clin. Psychiatric News 1 (Oct 1983).
53. *Duvall v. Goldin,* 362 N.W. 2d 275 (Mich. App. 1984).
54. *Clites v. Iowa,* 322 N.W. 2d 917 (Iowa Ct. App. 1981).
55. G. Annas et al., *Informed Consent to Human Experimentation: the Subject's Dilemma* (Ballinger, Cambridge, Mass. 1977).
56. American Psychiatric Association, *Principles of Medical Ethics with Annotations Especially Applicable to Psychiatry* (APA Press, Washington, D.C. 1985).
57. *Doe v. Roe,* 93 Misc. 2d 201, 400 N.Y. S.Z. 668 (1977); *Clayman v. Bernstein,* 38 Pa. D&C 543 (1940); *Spring v. Geriatric Authority,* 394 Mass, 274, 475 N.E. 2d 727 (1985).
58. *Spring, supra* note 57.
59. *Doe, supra* note 57.
60. *MacDonald v. Clinger,* 84 A.D. 2d 482, 446 N.Y. S. 2d 801 (1982).
61. *Clark v. Geraci,* 29 Misc. 2d 791, 208 N.Y.S. 2d 564 (1960).
62. Illinois Mental Health and Developmental Disabilities Confidentiality Act S.H.A. Ch. 91, § 801 (1987).
63. *Tarasoff v. Regents of the University of California,* 17 Cal. 3d 425, 529 P. 2d 334, 131 Cal. Rptr. 14, 551 P. 2d 334 (1976).
64. *Durflinger v. Artiles,* 563 F. Supp. 322 (D. Kan. 1981), *ques. cert.* 234 Kan. 484, 673 P. 2d 86 (1983), *aff'd* 727 F.2d 889 (10th Cir. 1984); *Davis v. Lhim,* 335 N.W. 2d 481 (Mich. App. 1983), *remanded on other grounds* 422 Mich. App. 8, 366 N.W.2d 73 (1985), *on remand* 147 Mich. App. 8, 382 N.W. 2d 195 (1985), *on appeal* N.W.2d (Mich. July 1986).
65. *Shaw v. Glickman,* 415 A.2d 625 (Md. App. 1985); *Leedy v. Hartnett,* 510 F. Supp. 1125 (N.D. Pa. 1981) (interpreting Pa. law).
66. *McIntosh v. Milano,* 168 N.J. Super. 466, 403 A. 2d 500 (1979).
67. *Lipari v. Sears, Roebuck and Co.,* 497 F. Supp. 185 (D. Neb. 1980).
68. *Peterson v. State,* 100 Wash. 2d 421, 671 P. 2d 230 (1983).
69. *Hedlund v. Orange County,* 34 Cal. 3d 695, 194 Cal. Rptr. 805 (1983); *(Bluebook,* p. 179)
70. *Brady v. Hopper,* 570 F. Supp. 1333 (D. Colo. 1983).
71. *Brady v. Hopper,* 751 F. 2d 329 (10th Cir. 1984).
72. *Shaw v. Glickman,* 45 Md. App. 718, 415 A. 2d 625 (1980); *Thompson v. County of Alameda,* 27 Cal. 3d 741, 167 Cal.Rptr. 70 (1980).
73. F. Buckner & M.H. Firestone, *Where the Public Peril Begins: 25 years after Tarasoff,* J. Legal Med. (Sept 2000).
74. *Roy v. Hartogs,* 31 Misc. 2d 350, 366 N.Y. S. 2d 297 (Civ. Ct. N.Y. 1975), *aff'd* 85 Misc. 2d 891, 381 N.Y. S. 2d 587 (App. Term 1976).
75. *Anclote Manor Foundations v. Wilkison,* 263 So. 2d 256 (Fla. Dist. Ct. App. 1972).
76. *Zipkin v. Freeman,* 436 S.W. 2d 753 (Mo. 1968).
77. *Supra* note 73.
78. *Brown v. Kowlizakis,* 331 S.E. 2d 440 (Va. 1985).
79. *Johnson v. United States,* 409 F. Supp. 1283 (M.D. Fla. 1981).
80. J. Smith, *Medical Malpractice: Psychiatric Care* 504-505 (1986); *Lange v. United States,* 179 F. Supp. 777 (N.D., N.Y. 1960).
81. *Abraham v. Zaslow,* No. 245862 (Santa Clara City Super. Ct. Cal., Oct 20, 1970).
82. 94 S.D. Codified Laws Ann.,§§ 27 A-8-10 & 11 (1984).
83. *Application for William R.,* 9 Misc. 2d 1984, 172 N.Y. S. 2d 869 (1958).
84. *Goodman v. Parwatkar,* 570 F. 2d 801 (8th Cir. 1978).
85. *Rogers v. Okin,* 478 F. Supp. 1342 (D. Mass. 1979), *aff'd in part, revised in part,* 634 F. 2d 650 (1st Cir. 1980), *vacated & remanded* sub nom *Mills v. Rogers,* 457 U.S. 291 (1982), *remanded* 738 F. 2d 1 (1st Cir. 1984); *Rogers v. Commissioner of the Department of Mental Health,* 458 N.E. 2d 308 (Mass. Sup. Jd. Ct. 1983), *following the holding of In re Roe III,* 421 N.E. 2d 40 (Mass 1981).
86. H. Ross, *Commitment of the Mentally Ill: Problems of Law and Policy,* 57 Mich. L. Rev. 945 (1959).
87. Conn. Gen. Stat. Ann. § 17-176 (West 1976).
88. *Lake v. Cameron,* 364 F. 2d 657 (D.C. Cir. 1966).
89. *Lessard v. Schmidt,* 349 F. Supp. 1078 (E.D. Wisc. 1972).
90. Birnbaum, *The Right to Treatment,* 46 A.B.A.J. 499 (1960).
91. *Wyatt v. Stickney,* 325 F. Supp. 781 (M.D. Ala.), *enforced* 334 F. Supp. 1341 (M.D. Ala. 1971), *orders entered* 344 F. Supp. 373 344 F. Supp. 387 (M.D. Ala. 1972), *aff'd in part, rev'd and remanded in part* sub nom. *Wyatt v. Aderholt,* 503 F. 2d 1305 (5th Cir. 1974).
92. *O'Connor v. Donaldson,* 422 U.S. 563 (1975).
93. *Mills v. Rogers,* 457 U.S. 1119 (1982).
94. *Rennie v. Klein,* 653 F. 2d 836 (3d Cir. 1981).
95. *Youngberg v. Romeo,* 457 U.S. 307 (1982).
96. *Id.*
97. *Rennie v. Klein,* 720 F. 2d 266, 269 (3d Cir. 1983).

98. *Davis v. Hubbard,* 506 F. Supp. 915 (D.C. Ohio 1980).
99. *Rennie v. Klein,* 720 F. 2d 266 (N.J. 1983).
100. *Guardianship of Richard Roe III.*
101. *Rogers v. Okin,* 634 F. 2d 650 (C.Al 1980).
102. *Rogers, supra* note 85.
103. *Supra* note 100.

104. *Anderson v. Anzoak,* 663 P. 2d 570 (Ariz. App. 1982); *Goedecke v. State of Colorado, Department of Institutions,* 603 P. 2d 123 (Colo. Sup. Ct. 1979) (*modified on denial of rehearing,* 1979); *In re the Mental Health of K-K-B,* No. 51, 467 (Okla. Sup. Ct. 1980); *A.E. v. Mitchell,* 724 F. 2d 864 (Utah 1983); *Rivers v. Katz,* No. 191, N.Y. App. (June 1986).

IV

Legislative and Business Aspects of Medicine

Practice organizations and joint ventures

MARK E. RUST, J.D.
ELLEN L. LUEPKE, J.D.

PRACTICE ORGANIZATIONS AMONG PHYSICIANS
MANAGED HEALTH CARE
JOINT VENTURES
ANTITRUST CONSIDERATIONS
REGULATORY AND RELATED CONSIDERATIONS
CONCLUSION

Throughout much of the twentieth century, fee-for-service solo practice characterized the medical delivery system in the United States.[1] At the dawn of the twenty-first century, this type of medical practice had diminished in importance, replaced primarily by health care delivery systems that emphasize large, physician contracting groups or the "vertical integration" of physicians, hospitals, other health facilities, and related health care providers.[2] Managed care, the dominant method for financing and delivering care, is largely driving this change, prompted by technological advances, the glut of specialist physicians, and health care costs, which soared through the 1970s and 1980s but seemed to subside in the mid-1990s coincident with high managed care penetration.[3] Meanwhile, increased educational debt and an inability to participate adequately in managed care on an equitable basis have made it more difficult for the individual practitioner to enter or maintain the solo practice.

In the 1970s and 1980s the insurance industry responded to employer demands for manageable health benefit costs by developing new products and introducing methods of controlling costs for services covered under conventional insurance plans. These included discounted fee-for-service organizations, such as preferred provider organizations (PPOs), and payer devices, such as prospective payment, concurrent review, and second opinions. The 1990s saw an explosion in managed care as delivered through health maintenance organizations (HMOs), particularly in response to the Health Security Act proposed by President Clinton in 1993.[4] Federal and state governments acted to limit their financial liability under Medicare and Medicaid by limiting fee increases and increasing utilization and quality assurance reviews. In response to these forces, physicians are organizing, along with other providers, in arrangements designed to help profitably deliver high-tech, quality health care at funding levels now forcefully controlled by government and employers.

To participate in these new arrangements, physicians have restructured the way they practice. In addition to using partnerships, sharing arrangements, group practices, and multiple specialty groups, physicians are developing joint venture contracting arrangements, joining physician-hospital organizations, or forming practice management companies. Grouping physicians in large practices, whether fully integrated for all practice purposes or in joint ventures for some limited purposes, often leads to economies of scale not achieved by a solo practice. Technology has permitted the development of out-patient surgery, imaging, lithotripsy, mammography, laser, and walk-in medical centers. Joint ventures between those who have the ability and willingness to fund such facilities and those who know how to manage them have played a key role. Physicians have banded together and invested in various types of outpatient centers, although such activity has been sharply circumscribed by federal legislation in the 1990s, limiting the types of investments referring physicians can make in such ventures.[5] The resulting physician practice arrangements are designed to maximize delivery and price efficiency in the managed care environment.

PRACTICE ORGANIZATIONS AMONG PHYSICIANS

The physician may be an owner, shareholder, employee, or independent contractor of a practice. The form such practice takes is designed to accommodate physician and business needs.

Solo practice, sole proprietor

The simplest form of physician practice, although increasingly rare, is the solo practitioner, sole proprietor form.

Advantages. The physician is free to establish professional relationships as necessary to create a practice environment.

Disadvantages. As with any other proprietorship, the owner is personally responsible for the liabilities of the business on a personal level. This includes liability for local, state, and federal medical regulations (e.g., occupancy and use, medical licensing, tax, provider reimbursement requirements), as well as all regulations controlling a regular business. The legal disadvantage of the sole proprietorship is the personal liability of the owner for business losses, debt, and negligence. The practical disadvantage to the sole proprietorship form is the difficulties inherent in coverage and participating with any degree of control in sophisticated managed care contracting arrangements.

Sharing arrangements

Sharing arrangements are associations between two or more physicians in which they share office space, equipment, and possibly employees. They may also share coverage of hospital and office patients on a rotating basis or when one or the other is not available.

Advantages. Sharing arrangements permit shared overhead expenses, allowing the participants to attain economies not available in a solo practice. Depending on the arrangement, it may permit shared capital expenditures and relative savings in rent, salaries, fixed costs such as utilities, and assured coverage. A sharing arrangement can exist between solo practitioners who are incorporated or unincorporated. The physicians involved may be partners in ventures that provide services to their individual practices, such as real estate and computer equipment. It has much of the advantages of solo practice while diluting the disadvantages.

Disadvantages. The practices may become so interlocked that to the general public the physicians are regarded as partners and not as solo practitioners. Legally, this means expanded liability for what may be deemed a de facto partnership. Failure to maintain separate employees, records, and billing may be introduced as evidence that there was no separation of medical practices. Liability may not only be extended from one practice to another for day-to-day business dealings but also in the event of medical negligence.[6] In addition, poor planning of the arrangement at its inception, as well as the lack of a clear and comprehensive agreement, will lead to trouble. The ground rules of the sharing arrangement must be established at the time of its creation and be reflected in a contract. Purchases (if jointly made), employee benefits (if shared), lease responsibilities, and other aspects of the arrangement must be defined.

Any employee sharing arrangement may lead to complex benefit plan questions. For example, it may not be possible for one physician with a generous retirement plan to share an employee with a second physician, when neither the second physician nor the employee has any retirement plan benefits.

Partnership

As defined in the Uniform Partnership Act now adopted in various forms by 49 states, a partnership is an association for two or more persons to carry on, as co-owners, a business for profit.[7] The "partner" may be a legal entity such as a corporation. A partnership is contractual in nature but is regulated and controlled by the partnership statute of a given state. Being contractual, the parties may structure the relationship to suit their specific needs. The partnership agreement should spell out the relative duties and obligations of the partners. The agreement should cover the right to manage, operate, and share profits and losses.

Partners have several fundamental rights unless specifically otherwise stated in the agreement: (1) equal participation in the management of the partnership business and (2) majority voting rules. Other than in a limited partnership, or by agreement of the parties, profits and losses are shared equally and, theoretically, no partner can draw a salary. Salary is, in reality, profit.

If not created for a specific period, any partner can terminate a partnership at any time. The death of a partner terminates the partnership unless arrangements have been made to carry on the business in surviving partners' names. Loss of a partner can be chaotic to the business, and the partnership agreement should foresee this eventuality.

Advantages. A partnership provides the device for sharing overhead, arranging formally among the partners to share comprehensively all aspects of their business, and pooling capital. Other advantages include equal management, control, and shared profits.

Disadvantages. The tax consequences, rights and obligations, and liability of a partnership should be assessed before its formation. Being a partner in a general partnership carries certain rights but also creates obligations and liabilities. A general partner is personally responsible for the actions of his or her partners if those acts were made within the scope of partnership business. This extends to professional negligence, as well as commitments for equipment and loans. The partners are also personally responsible for business losses. For these reasons, it is important to determine the reliability of potential partners before entering this type of business arrangement.[8]

Corporation

Unlike a partnership, which can be maintained even without a formal agreement or filing, a corporation is strictly a creation of statute. It is an entity with a defined business purpose that comes into being only after a formal filing. It is created by one or more individuals pursuant to statute to act as the legal representative of those individuals who contribute to its formation or become shareholders in the entity. Most states allow the formation of a *professional corporation*. This subspecies of corporation permits a licensed professional to form a corporation to engage in the business of practicing medicine in those states that would otherwise forbid such practices by regular business corporations. The definition of a professional or description of who can incorporate this type of business is contained within the appropriate state statute.[9] Professionals who incorporate generally form professional corporations, which may also be designated as *professional associations* or *service corporations* (SCs). One or more physicians can form professional corporations.

The major difference between a corporation and a partnership is the degree to which a participant may suffer personal liability for the acts of colleagues. A partner has unlimited personal liability for all partnership losses whether he or she individually incurred them or not. In a corporation, losses are limited to the extent of investment; only rarely can personal assets be touched. A professional corporation is equally liable for the acts of its physician employees in the event of medical negligence, just as any company is liable for the acts of its employees. For this reason, professional liability policies are written in the name of the individual physician with supplemental coverage for the corporation. Thus in the event of a suit for medical negligence, both physician and corporate assets may be at risk if the award or settlement exceeds insurance policy limits, but not the personal assets of fellow physician shareholders.

The physicians should explore asset management at the time of corporate inception. A shareholder is not responsible for the ordinary business losses of a corporation, and a corporation may be dissolved when liability exceeds assets without prejudice to its shareholders. Tax treatment is another major difference between a partnership and a corporation. Partnership profits and losses accrue to the personal tax returns of partners, but, unless a corporation elects Subchapter S status (now available[10] to corporations with fewer than 75 shareholders who have only one class of stock), the corporation will pay a tax on profits before distribution of dividends. Those professional corporations usually define all net revenue as salary paid out by the corporation, not profit, to avoid this result on a normal yearly basis.

The corporate form does not offer all the technical "loophole" protections that it is often thought to offer. At one time, corporations could deposit a greater percentage of salary into a pension plan than could an individual. This anomaly was rectified by the Tax Reform Act of 1986. Separate corporations cannot be maintained and controlled by physician owners that would have the effect of cutting off rank-and-file employees from the employee benefits, such as the pension plan, enjoyed by the physician owners.[11]

Advantages. Limited personal liability, possible benefit plans, certain tax breaks, and continuity in the event of the death of a shareholder are some advantages of incorporation. The practice is also more saleable if it possesses a corporate name and life outside its existing individual physician founder.

Disadvantages. Forming a corporation involves double taxation and significant difficulties in a tax-advantaged sale of the physician practice (unless the corporation has elected Subchapter S status) and in the maintenance of the corporate entity (e.g., minute books, records, attorney fees).

Limited liability company

Starting in 1994, physicians in many states had the opportunity of forming their practice as a limited liability company (LLC). LLCs are recognized in virtually every state, but not all states recognize the right of an LLC to perform medical services.

The LLC was specifically designed to take advantage of the type of tax treatment available to partnerships (where profits and losses flow directly through to the owners) while providing the type of liability shelter that is typically identified only with corporations. This type of entity, by the late 1990s, was rapidly becoming the entity of choice for physician joint ventures formed for the purpose of managed care contracting.

Advantages. The LLC offers the advantage of a single level of tax at the owner level with the highest degree of protection from liability for the acts of fellow owners. Further, these taxation benefits can be obtained, unlike in the S corporation, regardless of the number of owners or classes of ownership.

Disadvantages. Case law is not well developed with respect to LLC disputes. LLC formation is more involved, and the governance mechanism is less familiar to most physicians. Costs are generally higher for the maintenance of an LLC than for a corporation. Also, if an LLC decides for business purposes to retain capital in a particular year instead of distributing it to the owners, the owners will still be credited with the receipt of such monies and will be taxed accordingly.

Independent contractor

A physician may choose to provide services as an independent contractor to an individual physician, a professional corporation, health care institution, urgent care center, or any other practice setting available. This is a contractual relationship in which the physician generally has no equity interest. The services may be provided on a continuous or temporary basis.

Advantages. No commitment to office space or overhead mobility, a fixed work schedule, and fixed income on an hourly, daily, or weekly basis are some of the advantages of being an independent contractor.

Disadvantages. The independent contractor may be expendable, may be uninsured, and has no permanency to his or her practice situation. The relationship is strictly a matter of contract between the parties, so lack of a written agreement clarifying the parties' intention is a serious mistake. The issue of medical negligence insurance should also be examined carefully. The agreement should specify who will provide and pay for the insurance. Generally, if one is engaged as an independent contractor by a *locum tenens* agency, malpractice insurance will be provided. If an independent contractor appears to operate in a manner more often associated with employees, the Internal Revenue Service (IRS) may characterize the physician as an employee, triggering a series of negative tax consequences for both parties. A series of common-law tests are available to make this determination.[12]

Employee

Increasingly, physicians are starting or remaining in practice as the employee of an institution, another physician, medical group, or other practice setting. The key part of this relationship is the contract between the parties, which should address salary and benefits, incentives, liability insurance (and prior acts or "tail" coverage), termination, requirements for hospital privileges, and restrictive or noncompete covenants.

Advantages. The employment relationship is often strengthened by rights spelled out in a contract. A contract is a written expression of the agreement between two parties. Both independent contractors and employee physicians are sometimes faced with the same problem. Because they lack an equity position in the practice, clinic, office, or other health institution, such physicians may have a difficult time negotiating language sufficient to protect their position in the community, as well as liability and income. Such physicians must understand, however, that the contract is the ultimate definition of the working relationship between the parties and that generally, oral understandings not expressed in the contract's "four corners" will not be taken into account. Before starting a long-term relationship, an employee can test the good faith of his or her employer by seeking clarification of a number of issues. The contract should at a minimum specify responsibility for insurance coverage, tail insurances, and termination. The individual employee's objective should be to protect himself or herself from termination, just or unjust, without malpractice tail insurance coverage.

The written agreement may also include a noncompete clause or restrictive covenant, which restricts a departing physician from seeing patients he or she previously saw through the employer. The validity of these covenants varies with the jurisdiction. From the employed physician's viewpoint, if inclusion can be avoided, it should be omitted, although from the employer's viewpoint, it may be a nonnegotiable part of the deal. For an employed physician, if inclusion cannot be avoided, it should be limited as to when it will apply, and a cash buyout formula should be defined in the agreement.

MANAGED HEALTH CARE

Provider services were traditionally delivered to the health care consumer on a direct fee-for-service basis. Even physicians who were hospital based or employed generally billed the consumer directly. With the advent of the federal government as payer through Medicare, for patients 65 and over, and with the expansion of third-party insurance coverage to employees as part of a negotiated pension and benefit package, the traditional financial relationship of provider and patient evolved.

For many decades, from the 1930s and 1940s through the 1970s, insurance simply paid the lion's share of the physician's charge directly to the physician on a claim assigned to him by the patient, and the patient paid the remainder. By the late 1970s and 1980s, however, government and employers stepped in to create an alternative system, one where they could manage the product to reduce costs rather than allowing consumers to choose and pay directly for services. The pervasiveness of these alternative delivery methods, spurred largely by the payers and, most significantly, HMOs, PPOs, and their progeny, gradually eroded the ability of the physician to control what was paid for his or her services and where those services were performed. It even changed, in many cases, whether the patient could continue to see his or her own physician. What used to be called "alternate and managed health care delivery systems," because it was the alternative to the standard indemnity approach, has become the standard itself and today is simply known as "managed health care."

The dominant forms of managed health care are HMOs and PPOs. These organizations introduced prepayment and negotiated fees for service as an alternative to traditional fee for service. The HMO is generally a prepaid plan whereby primary care providers are paid on a monthly capitated basis for each enrollee, who in turn pays a relatively nominal coinsurance payment for medical service. The PPO is a provider group, traditionally assembled by an insurance company but today increasingly organized by physicians or entrepreneurs, that provides services on a discounted basis to the consumer.[13]

Health maintenance organizations

The term *health maintenance organization* was first coined by Dr. Paul Ellwood in the mid-1960s.[14] The Nixon administration pushed federal legislation and financing during the late 1960s and early 1970s, which enabled HMOs to gain a national foothold.[15] National membership in HMOs has grown to approximately one quarter of the population.[16]

An HMO is an integrated health care delivery system that combines the traditional financial risk of a health insurer with the hospital and physician service delivery responsibilities of a provider network. The HMO presumes it can contain costs by limiting hospitalizations, specialty referrals, and procedures and shifting some financial risk to the provider. It sells insurance coverage to consumers on a premium basis and attempts to create a provider network that is both competent and cost conscious. The goal in assuming the financial risk is the delivery of quality health care to the enrolled consumer at a controlled and predictable price. To do so, the HMO usually contracts with providers on a per capita basis for primary care and a discounted basis for diagnostic and specialty referrals. To enforce the system, many plans use a "gatekeeper" concept in which the primary care provider determines whether specialty or diagnostic referral is needed. Consumer self-referral is generally excluded from coverage.

HMOs generally structure themselves on one of five models for delivery of physician services: staff, independent practice association (IPA), group, network, and mixed.

Staff model. HMO-owned clinics staffed by physician employees are known as staff model HMOs. Such models are increasingly rare. Cost savings in this model are achieved by fixed provider costs and HMO ownership of hospitals and ancillary service centers. Control of these cost centers increases profitability for the plan as a whole by decreasing referred, in-patient, emergency department, and diagnostic costs.

Independent practice association. This model has two categories. In the first category the IPA may consist of providers, such as primary care and specialist physicians, assembled as a provider group by the plan, who contract individually or by group to provide services. These services may be paid on a fee-for-service or discounted basis but increasingly are paid on a per capita, or capitation, basis. In *capitation* the provider is paid on a per member, per month basis in advance of delivering care. The IPA in this case consists of a physician panel that is assembled by the HMO.

The second category, provider-created IPAs, represent and negotiate contracts for the group as a whole with HMOs. The IPA is composed of individual practitioners and group practices. Physician-controlled HMOs and IPAs raise significant issues under antitrust law. These providers may substantially control the market, as reflected by their large market share. Even when such groups are small, they may have been seen as an illegitimate joint venture of physicians that attempts collectively to set a fee-for-service price for its physicians without benefit of any form of clinical integration; this is a criminal violation of the antitrust laws (see later section on joint ventures).

Group model. In this model an HMO contracts for services with independent practice groups; the basis for the contract may be either discounted fees or capitation in exchange for exclusivity. Hospitals, diagnostic centers, surgicenters, and urgent care centers may be arranged on a similar basis for services not provided by the group. Although price fixing within an independent group is not possible and therefore not an issue, size can be, particularly where the HMO is primarily controlled by its relationship with a single group.

Network (primary care) model. In this form, primary care providers are assembled in a network that serves as the provider panel. The primary care physicians serve as gatekeepers paid on a capitation basis who limit referrals to hospitals, specialists, and diagnostic centers. The HMO sometimes contracts for specialty services, and sometimes transfers "full medical risk" for medical service delivery to the group, which in turn subcontracts with specialists. Less commonly, the HMO may contract through such a group for "full risk," including hospital services, and the group will subcontract for both specialist and hospital services.

Mixed models. The mixed model may be any combination of the preceding systems. This system is more complex to assemble, but it may allow an HMO to tailor services to a specific market need.

HMOs employ various methods to control costs. The first method limits covered services for enrollees to a specific provider network. The second method requires a copayment, which is usually nominal. The third method limits services to the primary care physicians, the so-called gatekeepers who determine whether specialty referral and diagnostic testing are necessary. The HMO contract with patients or "subscribers" denies these individuals the right of self-referral. Additionally, the contract between the HMO and providers tends to put the providers at financial risk for overutilization of services. These services may be diagnostic tests, specialty referrals, or hospitalizations. In some cases the contract creates a holdback amount of about 10% to 20% of the capitation, discounted, or fee-for-service rate. Often the HMO will also create a pool or budgeted account for diagnostic testing and hospitalizations. If the primary care physician has a low referral or utilization rate at the end of each quarter or year, the HMO may share a portion of savings from this budgeted account in a bonus to the provider.

Preferred provider organizations

PPOs evolved as another form of managed health care. An HMO is considered an integrated managed health care system in that it assumes risk for patient care. It integrates the financial aspects of an insurance company and the health delivery dimension of a provider network. In contrast, the PPO deals only with health care delivery; it is not an insurance company. This permits the PPO to escape most of the state, federal, and insurance regulations that apply to an HMO. The PPO contracts with physicians who deliver services on a discounted basis. The employer or administrator of the PPO is able to offer financial incentives to enrollees in the form of lower health care costs. The physicians, in turn, agree to abide by the utilization and quality assurance controls implemented by the PPO. The beneficiary is responsible for a deductible and coinsurance fee for services rendered. If the beneficiary sees a physician or obtains a service outside the panel, financial disincentives are imposed in the form of higher deductibles and coinsurance payment.

Non–hospital-based facilities

As coverage plans evolved and facilities providing care morphed from the one-dimensional world of the hospital to the multidimensional world of urgent care centers (walk-in medical centers), ambulatory surgical centers, diagnostic imaging centers, and freestanding laboratories, opportunities for physicians to be employees, independent contractors, or investors have increased. The advantage of being an investor, where not prohibited by law, is that the return on equity is related to the investment and thus generates passive income. An employee owner shares in profit in the facility as an investor, while also earning income on a fee-for-service or salary basis as a professional who provides services.

The issue of ownership and self-referral, however, is a problem for the health care industry, especially for the provider. The temptations for overutilization and overcharging are great. A physician-run laboratory is utilized about 30% to 40% more than a commercial non-provider-owned entity.[17] As a result, a number of states[18] have passed laws that prohibit referrals by a physician to a facility in which he or she has an interest, variously defined narrowly as an "ownership" interest or broadly as any "financial" interest (sweeping in debt, rentals, indirect ownership by relatives, and the like).

Most significantly, federal law now circumscribes a large variety of the types of ventures referring physicians may participate in as owners or, indeed, on any basis. The 1992 federal ban on physician referrals to clinical laboratories in which the referring physician has a financial interest outside their own office *(Stark I)* was expanded in 1994 to prohibit referrals for 12 designated health care services, including hospital in-patient and out-patient services, diagnostic services, and physical therapy *(Stark II).*[19] For the definition of what constitutes a "referral" and what constitutes a "financial interest" in such arrangements, Congress chose the broadest language possible.[20] As a result, Stark I and Stark II cast a large number of previously legal physician-related ventures into either clear illegality or the shadows of legal uncertainty. Before participating in any of these ventures, legal counsel intimately familiar with physician practices and the subtleties of the federal anti–self-referral ban must be consulted.

Legal considerations

PPOs and HMOs, as well as entities formed for the operation of a facility that provides an alternative to hospital-based care, have diverse ownership structures. They range from large, publicly held corporations to small, physician/investor-owned companies. To understand why these structures are chosen, it is essential to understand three related areas of law: the law of joint ventures, the antitrust law, and the general regulatory controls on the delivery and corporate practice of medicine.

JOINT VENTURES

Changing patterns of health care utilization and reimbursement, along with increasing competitive pressures, have led to declining revenues and market share for both physicians and institutions. In an attempt to compensate for these declines in both patient and cash flow, physicians, hospitals, and other types of health care providers have joined forces to prevent or reverse such losses through joint ventures. In recent years the joint venture has become a common method to capitalize on new opportunities in the health care market. Hospitals and physicians may need one another to form HMOs, PPOs, physician hospital organizations (PHOs), and other associations that compete with commercial models. Hospitals often need physicians to be partners in out-patient ventures, including out-patient diagnostic facilities (e.g., magnetic resonance imaging [MRI] centers, mammography centers, other imaging services), urgent care centers, freestanding surgicenters, and freestanding rehabilitation centers, although the federal and state anti–self-referral laws have severely curtailed the numbers and types of such ventures. Because these types of ventures primarily need capital for construction and equipment, they could be built by hospitals, alone, without the joint ventures cooperation of physicians. However, the need for active physician participation in and commitment to providing services in the evolving health care delivery system often forces hospitals to reach out to physicians as partners.

Joint ventures among physicians, health care providers, institutions, and businesspersons are a growing phenomenon. The legality of these ventures depends on federal and state policies that regulate referral relationships and commercial competition generally. Each venture requires that both federal and state law be researched as to the venture's legality. Unfortunately, no clear law can be found and applied. Rather, extrapolations and analogies may have to be drawn from vague or loosely related statutes and cases. Ultimately, the joint venture may be forced to proceed on the basis of a series of educated guesses. A syndicated real estate venture might be legitimate, whereas a physician-owned MRI center may not, even though the venture involves the same two parties. Variations in state law make it extremely difficult to apply one type of experience to another state without adequate research into that jurisdiction's laws and regulations.

Rather than giving specific legal advice, which is impossible without reviewing all the facts of a particular venture, this section provides a primer for the creation of a joint venture.

Definition and characteristics

A joint venture is an association of two or more persons or entities that combine their resources to carry out a business enterprise for profit. This suggests creation of a new entity having managerial, financial, and productive capacity to enter or serve a new market. The agreement between the parties may establish a completely new entity or utilize preexisting entities to serve new markets or provide a new product. Creation of a completely new venture having independent management, facilities, and autonomy is generally advisable to avoid unnecessary legal and tax complications. The degree of independence enjoyed by the joint venture from either party is important in determining whether the enterprise is a bona fide business. The bona fides of the business are important in determining the existence of fraud, individual liability, or corporate liability.

Joint ventures are created to meet hospital, physician, and business goals. Their main purpose may not be solely for capital formation. The reason why two parties may joint venture together, when these two parties have a referral relationship, is always subject to close scrutiny under the federal anti-kickback law, a criminal statute.

In addition to raising capital, hospitals may develop relationships with physicians, insurance companies, and others (1) to develop "new profit centers" within the hospital or in an out-patient setting; (2) to create alternative delivery systems to satisfy third-party payers; (3) to increase and enhance market penetration of the physicians and hospital; (4) to alter hospital-patient mix, limit debt financing, and increase community support for the hospital; and (5) to cement the relationship with physicians and other providers who support the institution. This list could be extended, but the goal is increased profitability by controlling costs, penetrating the patient care market on both an in-patient and out-patient basis, and securing the support of the local community and health providers.

Physician goals for entering joint venture agreements with one another or with hospitals include (1) entering new service areas, (2) creating out-patient facilities, (3) increasing or maintaining market share, (4) controlling costs, (5) sharing financial risk, and (6) participating in investment opportunities and acquiring capital management and marketing skills that might otherwise be more expensive to acquire. Joint ventures also allow physicians to invest and profit in areas that might otherwise be closed to them.

Joint venture permutations include physician-physician, physician-hospital, and realtor-physician. They range from life retirement centers to physician-owned laboratories and surgicenters. Because these ventures have increased in such numbers, the federal government, mostly through regulation of Medicaid and Medicare, has had the effect of limiting the access of physician referrers to certain investment vehicles. Increased capital requirements created by new equipment and treatment modalities have forced providers and institutions to reassess their relationship.

The six basic legal models for establishing joint ventures are (1) contract, (2) corporate (the traditional choice), (3) partnership (limited and general), (4) LLC (the form most often used in recent years because of its tax flexibility), (5) franchise, and (6) venture capital.

Contract model

The contract model is simplest, because the entire joint venture is contained within the four corners of a contract between the parties.[21] This could involve a service agreement lease, for example, in which physicians lease land from a hospital for the construction of a building that they then lease back to the hospital. In that example, the hospital does not have to contribute capital, and the builders have a leased building with a guaranteed rate of return. No separate legal entity would be formed. Instead, the relationship is defined by the contract itself and is negotiated on the relative power of the joint venture partners.

The advantages to this form of joint venture are that it is simple to organize and understand, and it requires no new corporations or infrastructure. The contractual relationship is between preexisting entities. The disadvantage is that the contractual relationship creates new liabilities for the parties while lacking the near-permanence and additional protection that grow from the creation of an entity.

Corporate model

This model requires a corporate entity to be formed by the joint venturers, who will become shareholders. The joint venturers may be physicians, hospitals, or other investors. Individuals, corporations, or partnerships may own shares. Ownership need not be limited to physicians or hospitals.

The corporation acts through its board of directors. These joint ventures begin with a preincorporation agreement establishing terms of participation. The board has the day-to-day authority to run the business and set policy. The preincorporation agreement might describe the business plan, but it would not be incorporated into the bylaws of the corporation.

The corporation model results in a distinct legal entity that may expand on its own without further joint venturer participation or increased risk. The corporation will protect the investors from legal responsibility that exceeds their capital investment. The disadvantage to the corporation form, unless formed as a nonprofit organization, is that it is generally subject to double taxation. In addition, compliance with state and federal securities laws may be necessary before capitalization, increasing start-up costs.

General partnership model

A general partnership is the association of two or more entities or persons who act as co-owners of a for-profit business. Profits and losses are equally shared unless otherwise agreed in the partnership agreement. The partnership agreement states the rights and duties of the partners. The partnership agreement specifies any arrangement the partners may wish to institute. The partnership is subject to the specific statutes of the state in which it is created.

The advantages of the partnership are single taxation and joint ownership and management. The major disadvantage is that each general partner is legally obligated to third parties for 100% of the losses, debts, and liability of the business as a whole.

Limited partnership model

A limited partnership consists of at least one general partner with unlimited liability who is responsible for the management of the business. There can be one or more limited partner investors who have equity ownership with a liability potential limited to the amount of their investment, but who are not involved in the management.

The advantages are similar to a general partnership; however, limited partners are not responsible for losses in excess of their contributions. General partners in a limited partnership may be incorporated, thus limiting liability to their corporate assets. Limited partners gain security and limit their losses but are barred from exerting day-to-day control over the business. Management participation of a limited partner may expose them to the liability of the general partner.

Limited liability company

The LLC is the preferred choice for joint ventures among physicians, often seen in the development of physician networks formed for managed care contracting purposes.[22] An LLC protects participants from liability, just as a corporation does, but allows all revenues and expenses associated with the enterprise to be treated, from a tax perspective, as though the entity is a partnership.[23] Thus an LLC is usually regarded as closer to a partnership than a corporation.

This tax advantage is important. Particularly in an evolving health care market, where consolidation is rampant and where the likelihood of the LLC being subsumed or acquired by another entity is high, negative tax consequences from such sales must be anticipated.

Within an LLC, physicians may retain earnings, declare profits (and losses), or reap the benefits of sales proceeds without the double-taxation penalty. They may also create different classes of ownership interests and avoid any limitation on the size of membership. Further, a network of physicians could preserve its option of offering memberships to individual physician participants, as opposed to their professional corporations, without fear of exposing these personal participants to the liabilities of the entity.

An LLC may also be the choice of physicians and hospitals that co-venture certain projects, and this leads to one disadvantage when physicians venture with hospitals exempt from federal taxation. From a business perspective, there may be good reasons to retain LLC earnings in the venture for new costs or infrastructure. To a tax-exempt organization, there is no impact. To the tax-paying physician, however, those retained monies are deemed income on which tax is owed, even though the physician never actually received a distribution. This is the subject of ongoing tension in such ventures.

Venture capital model

The most common venture capital approach to joint venturing among physicians, hospitals, and commercial interests currently may be found in management services organizations (MSOs), generally associated with hospitals but sometimes privately held, and physician practice management companies (PPMCs), usually associated with commercial investors or publicly traded companies. In both cases the management company purchases the assets of a physician's practice, including furniture, fixtures and equipment, and accounts receivable. It also purchases the obligation of the physician group and its individual physicians not to practice elsewhere in competition with the venture. A physician's professional corporation remains intact, possessing only its employment relationships with its physician shareholders and physician employees, and their ongoing relationships and contracts to provide medical services. The management company then contracts with the professional corporation on a long-term basis (usually 20 to 40 years) to manage the professional corporation in exchange for some percentage of revenues, usually calculated in a specific formula designed to comply with state corporate practice of medicine and fee splitting rules.

Because the management company does not practice medicine but solely maintains assets and purchases accounts receivable from the professional corporation on a regular basis through its management agreement, it is largely free of a wide range of state and federal regulations that might otherwise apply to a medical practice limiting opportunities for investor participation. As a result, everyone from hospitals to commercial financial houses to Wall Street may participate as a joint venture with physicians in their effort to become a larger and more sophisticated player in the evolving health care marketplace.

Financing considerations

State and federal interest in the nature of joint ventures and referral patterns may affect the type of venture and finance arrangements selected by the joint ventures. Stark I, Stark II,[24] and evolving tax law (particularly where a venture with a tax-exempt entity is concerned) have subjected physician joint venture to increasing governmental review. Arrangements where physicians "self-refer" to a service or facility where they have a financial interest are suspect. As a result, these laws may play a role in the way in which a venture is financed.

Conventional debt financing. Debt financing takes the form of a loan payable in a specific term, a revolving line of credit, or a demand line of credit. In general, a loan involves a set amount, for a certain term with a specified rate of interest. It may be for interest only with a balloon payment or amortized over a set time. The interest may be specified or may vary according to a specified formula (e.g., prime rate).

Bonds. Tax-exempt bonds issued by a state or a political subdivision of a state may be exempted from federal taxation. They generally are not tax free in the state issued unless the state waives the right to tax the bonds. At least 75% of the bonds issued by the state or a political subdivision must be used in a tax-exempt trade or business, as specified in Section 501-C-3 of the IRS code.

Industrial development bonds are bonds issued to create nonexempt businesses, which are defined as entities with more than 25% of the proceeds used to finance nonexempt businesses. Tax-exempt status is determined on a case-by-case basis.

Public and private equity and debt offering. Securities registration statements for a public offering must be filed, and the requirements are time consuming and costly. Exemptions to the filing and disclosure requirements include insurers of securities, incorporators of businesses, and all offers of sales in which 80% of the sales, proceeds, revenues, and assets remain in one state for the first 6 months. Resales must be made within the same state 9 months after the sale. The aggregate offering price must be less than $1.5 million, and the Securities and Exchange Commission (SEC) must clear the offering 10 days before the offer of sale.

Qualified private equity offerings are exempted from requirements to file a security statement. The requirements to qualify for the exemption are precise and statutorily mandated. The dollar amount must be less than $500,000, regardless of the number of investors. Alternatively, the offering can be for less than $5 million to 35 or fewer unaccredited investors and an unlimited number of accredited investors. An accredited investor must have a net worth exceeding $2 million or a net income in excess of $200,000 for the last 2 years. In some states an offering limited to less than 50 or 35 investors, depending on the state, may be exempt under state blue-sky laws.

Venture capital. Venture capitalists are risk takers who gamble that a gain will be achieved by private or public sale of a newly established business. Venture capitalists only recently entered the physician segment of the health care industry in significant numbers, largely as a result of development of PPMCs. Previously, venture capitalists have assisted in starting up ambulatory health care companies in the 1980s. In return for their capital, they often assume a large degree of control and a preferred percentage of profits.

Equipment lease financing. Equipment may be acquired for the purpose of leasing to a health care facility or medical practice. The facility may be a hospital, ambulatory care center, or physician's office or clinic. The advantages may be accelerated depreciation, guaranteed rent, and capital conservation for the lessee.

The terms of the lease financial arrangements, maintenance agreements, sublease, replacement, or acquisition by the lessee are all subject to negotiation as part of the contract, but may be subject to fair market value limitations when executed between referring parties.

ANTITRUST CONSIDERATIONS

Antitrust law distinguishes between impediments to competition that are "horizontal" (i.e., between competitors) and those that are "vertical" (i.e., impede competition because a product has been tied up through a relationship between the various players that produce the product's components, such as the primary care physicians, specialists, and hospitals that, together, produce the in-patient hospital product). This section focuses primarily on horizontal issues, which most often arise in the development of the new physician organizations that are responding to the evolution in managed care.

The key distinction between types of physician organizations pivots on the degree to which the organizations are "integrated" on the one end of the spectrum or "nonintegrated" on the other end, with degrees of integration or "partial integration" in between. A medical clinic that is a single professional corporation with multiple specialty physicians as employees is fully integrated. On the other end of the spectrum, an IPA that engages only in fee-for-service contracts and does not attempt to build any sort of joint clinical data operation is completely nonintegrated. Network joint ventures that negotiate fees with clinical integration; network joint ventures that negotiate risk-based contracts, such as capitation; PPMCs that manage a variety of professional corporations; and PPMCs that manage a single professional corporation provide increasingly greater, but not full, integration along the integration scale.

The key elements in determining the degree of integration are the extent to which previously separate organizations have combined their assets and the extent to which the previously separate organizations will combine their liabilities in the future. Certain specific attributes of integration may be important, such as the degree to which the parties share defined liabilities (e.g., risk under a capitation contract) or the degree to which the parties share defined assets, which may grow or evaporate depending on their collective performance (e.g., fee withholds under contracts performed by the group). Also important are the degree to which the participants in the combination have invested their own capital and the degree to which the venture participants intend to create new efficiencies through clinical integration (i.e., tracking information on all participants and using that information to reduce utilization, reduce costs, and increase profits or revenues to venture participants).

No horizontal entity can negotiate contracts on behalf of its members without first achieving the degree of integration required to avoid triggering the antitrust laws. Section 1 of the Sherman Antitrust Act prohibits contracts, combinations, or conspiracy in restraint of trade.[25] Physicians who are independent actors and who collectively negotiate for fees are engaged in a *per se violation* of Section 1, meaning that no further argument regarding the rationale for such behavior will be entertained by a court that is considering either the criminal or civil penalties for such behavior. These principles exclude traditional IPA fee-for-service agreements from collective negotiation.[26] Approaches have been developed to allow individual IPA members to opt into or out of such agreements, which are generally referred to as *messenger model* devices.[27]

However, physician joint ventures such as IPAs and networks that seek to negotiate non-fee-based contracts (capitation, global arrangements, substantial withholds), or such ventures that have sufficient clinical integration and desire to negotiate fee-based contracts, will not be subject to per se treatment but rather will be permitted to collectively negotiate such contracts if such collective negotiations are reasonable under the economic circumstances. This important development arose from the joint statements of the U.S. Department of Justice and the Federal Trade Commission (FTC) issued in August 1996.[28] The most significant and subtle development in those joint statements is the groundbreaking acknowledgment by the enforcement agencies that even fee-based contracts can be jointly negotiated by a physician group if the group is legitimate in its desire to integrate clinically and is not a sham group simply designed to maintain or increase utilization and prices. Finally, when all physicians are contained in a single, fully integrated group, there can be no fee negotiation difficulty under the antitrust laws. The group is a single actor, and violations of Section 1 can occur only when two or more parties or entities combine or conspire to violate it.

Even fully integrated groups, however, could violate the antitrust laws if they are large enough to exert market power. For example, physician mergers in which "all the doctors in town" are involved might be prohibited if their effect "may be substantially to lessen competition or tend to create a monopoly" under another important antitrust law, the Clayton Act.[29] Even joint ventures, such as physician networks, are subject to this prohibition. As a result, the FTC and the Justice Department identified market shares of physicians that, in joint ventures, will never create a cause for concern. If physicians formed groups that include a larger percentage of physicians than those identified in the joint statements (30% of the physicians in a particular specialty in nonexclusive groups), a "rule of reason" analysis would have to be conducted to determine whether such a venture was lawful.

Because of the imprecise nature of determining when a group has "market power," the group's "percentage of market share" is used as a rough rule of thumb for whether the group will have market power. This is a presumption that may, and should in the case of physicians, be rebutted. Commentators have consistently pointed out that market share is only one factor requiring consideration when determining market power.[30] Enforcement agencies have extensively refined their view of market percentages as an indicator of possible anticompetitive effects.

Enforcement agencies have stated that exclusive physician networks consisting of 20% or fewer of the physicians in each specialty with active hospital staff privileges who practice in the relevant geographic market and share substantial financial risk, or nonexclusive physician networks consisting of no more than 30% of such physicians, will not, absent extraordinary circumstances, be challenged by the agencies. To show that they do not believe networks should be limited to 30% of physicians, however, they have issued a series of advisory opinions and business review letters that have "blessed" networks with significantly greater than 30% market share.[31] As an important limit to the agencies' willingness to bless sizeable networks, they are particularly reluctant to bless networks where they believe that it is difficult, if not impossible, for competitors to enter the market.[32]

REGULATORY AND RELATED CONSIDERATIONS

Joint ventures and medical delivery arrangement are affected by a wide variety of regulations. This section focuses on those unique to medicine.

Licensure

Joint ventures may be organized between physicians and hospitals or by physicians alone. Freestanding urgent care centers or surgicenters may be organized and run solely by and for the benefit of the physicians who provide services, or they may be open to physician and nonphysician investors. These permutations may be determined by state licensing requirements.

A hospital-run facility may fall under the general licensing and certificate-of-need regulations (if any) of the particular state; each state's statutes must be reviewed. In most states freestanding surgicenters, HMOs, and diagnostic facilities are highly regulated, whereas an urgent care center may be treated as a physician's office, with little or no regulation imposed.

Regardless of the specific state regulations that regulate these centers, generally accepted legal precepts will apply. Each facility must be able to deliver the type and quality of services it advertises. The appropriate staff, equipment, and ancillary support services must be provided to maintain acceptable standards of care. Failure to maintain these standards opens the door to litigation not only with the physicians and entity but also with the investors.

The Joint Commission on Accreditation of Healthcare Organizations (JCAHO) has approved standards applicable to freestanding urgent care centers. Its *Accreditation Manual*, generally updated yearly, contains these standards. The National Association of Freestanding Emergency Centers has established the Accreditation Association for Ambulatory Care. This voluntary association provides an *Accreditation Handbook* that should be used as a guide to the establishment and management of freestanding urgent care centers. Standards are suggested concerning medical records, patient rights, and services provided by the facility.

Insurance regulations

Joint ventures may create insurance companies. Since the advent of HMOs, physicians, hospitals, and other joint venturers have joined forces, in many combinations, to provide health insurance plans to consumers. The HMO was the first and probably the most popular method of uniting physicians. By accepting the economic burden of the patients, the HMO falls under the jurisdiction of both federal HMO and state insurance regulations, and PPOs may also fall under the purview of the state insurance statutes. Regulation of PPOs is generally much less onerous than that applicable to HMOs and other types of insurance companies.

Although an HMO must comply with federal HMO legislation if it intends to become "federally qualified," state law generally controls HMOs and PPOs. These laws impose reserve requirements, regulatory approval of the text of policies, reinsurance, and frequent and regular reporting to state agencies. The joint ventures may be unable to sell the product even if the business is in compliance with all regulations. As investors, the physicians and other providers have to maintain an arm's-length relationship to avoid any questions of price fixing. The plan itself, whatever the product mix, may be compelled to offer certain types of benefit packages and may not be allowed to exclude or rate insured clients.

Tort liability for the enterprise

There is a growing trend in the United States to hold organizations independently responsible for their acts. The concept of corporate negligence has begun to permeate the medical arena. As a result, PPOs, HMOs, hospitals, and other entities (e.g., laboratory services, urgent care centers, diagnostic centers) are potentially liable for negligence, regardless of provider affiliation.[33]

Additionally, there is the potential for employers and the insurance network to be liable, because patients in prepaid plans are forced to select physicians from the panel chosen by the plan and indirectly by the purchaser of the insurance.[34] This expanded liability imposes on the joint venturers an obligation to follow through with credentialing, peer review, quality assurance, and risk management where required.

A further component of the problem is the limitation of care provided. The HMO and PPO tend to try to limit referrals and laboratory testing. Under the guidelines established by the joint venture, this may indicate a breach in the standard of care. As physicians, hospitals, health care providers, and venture capitalists enter the health care arena, their liability exposure mushrooms. In considering a joint venture with diversified services, the investor should explore the potential for personal liability. One way to limit loss exposure is to institute risk management programs. Florida was one of the first states to initiate mandatory risk management as a component of health delivery systems.[35]

The integration of internal utilization review, quality assurance, and risk management programs may decrease potential loss exposure. The Health Care Quality Insurance Act of 1986 created a national data bank for reporting physicians and providing data to certain organizations to credential physicians.[36] Failure to properly credential an individual could open the way for civil litigation based on failure to report or failure to query the data bank for information.[37]

Fraud, abuse, and ethical considerations

Medicare has prohibited the solicitation, receipt, or payment of any fee directly, indirectly, overtly, or covertly for the referral of a Medicare or Medicaid beneficiary for a covered item of service, whether it be for goods, services, facilities, or other benefits.[38] The advent of physician-owned ventures has opened an area of potential abuse.

The Judicial Council of the American Medical Association has ruled that physicians can engage in commercial ventures, but they should be aware of potential conflicts of interest. If the physician's commercial interest conflicts with patient care, alternative arrangements should be made.[39]

Stark I/II is designed to deal with the issue of physician self referral. It reverses the burden of the fraud and abuse statutes, which require the government to prove illegal intent to refer or receive referrals for remuneration. Instead, it prohibits all referrals between financially interested parties unless they meet narrow exceptions, and it requires the physician to prove an exception has been met.

Legislation enacted in 1987 allows the inspector general of the Department of Health and Human Services (DHHS) to exclude a person from Medicare participation if he or she engages in a prohibited remuneration scheme. The act also required the secretary of DHHS to promulgate "safe harbor" regulations, which give physicians comfort that their referral relationships are legal. Legislation enacted in 1996 extends the reach of federal law into fraudulent health care billing in the commercial sector, making such activities a federal crime.[40] The growing use of "Qui Tam" actions, or whistle-blower lawsuits, has generated a new growth industry in litigation involving schemes for overbilling.[41]

In addition to the federal statutory prohibition on "fraud and abuse," the careful planner of health care ventures must also consider the statutory and common-law prohibitions on fraud that might be applied to any industry. Schemes to "kick back" money to a referrer of services or to seek payment without providing service outside the Medicare payment system might constitute fraud under a state statute.[42]

Corporate practice of medicine

Corporations are generally prohibited from practicing medicine.[43] The standards established by a facility or other type of venture must reflect standards promulgated by health care providers and not by the partnership, corporation, or any other type of entity. The goal is to provide quality care while avoiding interference with the provider-physician relationship. The JCAHO and state, federal, and voluntary accrediting agencies strive to maintain provider control over standards of care.

Joint ventures may create managed health care entities, diagnostic facilities, treatment centers, or other types of health care delivery mechanisms. In each of these cases the role of the nonprovider manager and investor should be kept separate from the care delivered. To avoid pitfalls, the organization should structure the relationship of the providers, specify the type of facility, and delineate the responsibilities of the nonprovider managers and owners.

Ethical considerations

The medical literature, legislative subcommittees, insurance carriers, and the public all question the entrepreneurial aspects of joint ventures among physicians, hospitals, diagnostic facilities, and treatment centers. The suspicion is that a system of self-referral will lead to overutilization with concomitant increases in health care costs.

The ethical and legal issue of fee-for-service medicine for patients at facilities owned by the referring physicians alone or in conjunction with another institution has been raised as a result of increasing health care costs.

CONCLUSION

Increasing market competition and capital requirements have brought together different combinations of providers, hospitals, and business persons; however, their interests are not always the same.

The formation of a joint venture can subject investors to antitrust investigation, private litigation, state and federal enforcement activity, and increased exposure to negligence, both medical and corporate. In addition, investors may have ethical conflicts within their investor groups.

Increasing governmental intrusion affects the methods used to create a joint venture, with regard to both legal requirements and capital contributions. Nevertheless, the promotion of integrated services, the exploitation of new markets, and the provision of new and valuable services for the health care consumer present exciting challenges for physicians and hospitals.

ENDNOTES

1. P. Starr, *The Social Transformation of American Medicine* (Basic Books, New York 1982).
2. Hermann et al., *Integrated Delivery Systems in a Changing Healthcare Environment: New Legal Challenges,* Monograph No. 1 (Forum on Healthcare Law of the American Bar Association, Nov 1994).
3. Levit et al., *Health Care Spending in 1994,* 15 Health Affairs 130-144 (Summer 1996).
4. Health Security Act, H.R. 3600/S1757, Report No. 773, *Medicare and Medicaid Guide* (Commerce Clearing House, Chicago 1993).
5. 42 U.S.C. 1395nn.
6. *Insiga v. LaBella,* 14 Fla. L. Weekly 214 (Apr 21, 1989).
7. Uniform Partnership Act, Am. Jur. 2D.
8. Uniform Partnership Act §18.
9. Fla. Stat. § 607, Professional Service Corporations 766.101, 1988 (Florida); 805 ILCS 15/1 *et seq.* (Illinois).
10. Pursuant to the Small Business Administration Act of 1996, the number of eligible shareholders has increased from 35 to 75. In addition, certain charitable and other organizations can now be S corporation shareholders (the law used to limit shareholders to individuals only).
11. Internal Revenue Code, § 414M.
12. Internal Revenue Code, § 530, as modified by the Small Business Job Protection Act of 1996; *Riverbend Country Club v. Patterson,* 399 S.W. 2d 382 (Tex. Civ. App. 1965). The IRS, under its Audit Guidelines for agents, has also set forth a checklist of 20.
13. For a comprehensive listing of such organizations, see *Health Network and Alliance Sourcebook* (Faulkner & Gray, Inc., New York, http:\www.FaulknerGray.com\healthcare).
14. *The Flowering of Managed Care,* Med. Economics (March 1990).
15. *Supra* note 1.
16. Pear, *Congress Weighs More Regulation of Managed Care,* New York Times 1 (March 10, 1997).
17. Mitchell et al., *New Evidence of the Prevalence and Scope of Physician Joint Ventures,* 268 J.A.M.A. 80 (1992).
18. For a detailed listing of current state law relating to physician self-referral prohibitions, *see* Mayo, *State Illegal Remuneration and Self-Referral Laws,* NHLA Monograph Series (National Health Lawyers Association, Washington, D.C. 1997).
19. Omnibus Budget Reconciliation Act of 1993, Pub. L. No. 103-66, 107 Stat. 312 (1993). The designated services are physical therapy services; occupational therapy services; radiology, including magnetic resonance imaging, computed tomography scans, and ultrasound services; radiation therapy services and supplies; durable medical equipment and supplies; parenteral and enteral nutrients, equipment, and supplies; orthotic and prosthetic devices; home health services and supplies; out-patient prescription drugs; and in-patient and out-patient hospital services.
20. "Referral" is defined as, in the case of an item or service for which payment may be made under Part B of Medicare, the request by a physician for the item or service, including a consultation by another physician and any test or procedure ordered by, or to be performed by, that other physician (or someone under his or her supervision). Additionally, *the request or establishment of a plan of care* by a physician that includes the provision of a designated health service constitutes a referral. 42 U.S.C. § 1395nn(h)(5)(A)(B). (Emphasis added.)
21. Rosenfeld, *Joint Venture Organizational Models,* Twelve Topics in Healthcare Financing 38-44 (Winter 1985).
22. Rust, *Advice for the Doctor: the Formation of Single Specialty Networks,* 42 Practical Lawyer (Oct 1996).
23. The authority for treating limited liability companies as partnerships for tax purposes comes from U.S. Treasury regulations that state that the classification of an entity as a partnership or an association taxable as a corporation depends on whether the entity has more corporate characteristics than noncorporate characteristics. The four relevant corporate characteristics are (1) continuity of life, (2) centralization of management, (3) limited liability, and (4) free transferability of interests. To be taxable as a "partnership," an entity must lack at least two of the four factors. See *Philip G. Larson,* 66 T.C. 159 (1976); *George Zuckman,* 524 F. 2d 729 (Ct. Cl. 1975).
24. Racketeer Influenced and Corrupt Organizations Act, 18 U.S.C. 1961.
25. 15 U.S.C. § 1.
26. *Arizona v. Maricopa County Medical Society,* 457 U.S. 332 (1982).
27. *United States of America v. Healthcare Partners, Inc., Danbury Area IPA, Inc., and Danbury Health Systems,* Civil Action No. 395-CV-01945 RNC, Sept 995 (definition of messenger model in final judgment action against independent physician association).
28. United States Department of Justice, Federal Trade Commission, *Statement of Antitrust Enforcement Policy and Healthcare* (Aug 1996).
29. 15 U.S.C. § 12-27.
30. Landes & Posner, *Market Power in Antitrust Cases,* 94 Harv. L. Rev. 937 (1981).
31. Letter from Ann K. Bingaman, Department of Justice, to J.F. Fischer (Jan 1996) ("substantially more" than 30% of several specialties in a number of local markets, including more than 50% in one specialty); letter from Ann K. Bingaman to M.J. Fields (Dec 1995) (44% of board-certified dermatologists); letter from Ann K. Bingaman to D. Hartzog (Oct 1994) (up to 50% of chiropractors).

32. Department of Justice Business Review letter to Ted R. Callister (March 1996) finding that the Orange Los Angeles Medical Group, Inc. (ORLA) operating with in excess of 30% of the anesthesiologists in the defined market, may be challenged by the Department of Justice.

33. *Darling v. Charleston Memorial Hospital,* 211 N.E. 2d 253 (1966); *Pedrosa v. Bryant,* 677 P. 2d 166 (1984).

34. *Harrell v. Total Healthcare, Inc.,* 781 S.W. 2d 58 (1989). Court stated that an IPA model HMO owed a duty to its participants to investigate the competence of its panel members and to exclude physicians who pose a "foreseeable risk of harm."

35. Fla. Stat. 766.110, 395.041, 641.55, 624.501.

36. Pub. L. 99-660 (Nov 1986); 42 U.S.C. 11101 *et seq.*

37. 42 U.S.C. 11135 Section 425(b).

38. 42 U.S.C. 1320a-7(b)(b).

39. *Report of the Judicial Council of the American Medical Association,* J.A.M.A. 2425 (Dec 1984).

40. Health Insurance Portability and Accountability Act of 1996, Pub. L. 104-191, 110 Stat. 1936 (1996). Subtitle E, Section 241 adds: "Federal health care offense" defining a new federal health care offense in the criminal code to mean a violation of, or conspiracy to violate, a number of provisions in the federal criminal code if the violation or conspiracy relates to a "health care benefit program."

41. Relief includes injunctive actions and the seizure of assets, 18 U.S.C. § 1345(a)(1), (2).

42. *Supra* note 22.

43. Chase-Lubitz, *The Corporate Practice of Medicine Doctrine: an Anachronism in the Modern Healthcare Industry,* 40 Vanderbilt Law Rev. 445 (1987); *Berlin v. Sarah Bush Lincoln Health Center,* 279 Ill. App. 3d 447 (1996).

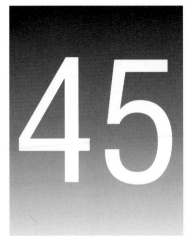

Coproviders and institutional practice

EDWARD E. HOLLOWELL, J.D., F.C.L.M.
BARRY H. BLOCH, J.D.

COPROVIDERS
INSTITUTIONAL PRACTICE

COPROVIDERS

Physicians do not practice alone. That fact is unalterable in our complex medical care system. Physicians depend on the expertise and competence of technicians, nurses, nurse practitioners, physician assistants, paramedics, administrators, nurse's aides, orderlies, medical records personnel, and even maintenance and repair staff, just to name a few coproviders. In addition, it is important to recognize that the relationships of coproviders are necessarily bilateral. The competence of the individuals working together is additive rather than independent. It is obvious that the observations and efforts of all those who provide care for a patient affect the outcome; as a result the legal interdependence of coproviders is unavoidable. The more complex that health care becomes and the more technical the capabilities of health care providers, the greater the interdependence of coproviders. Further, when coproviders work together smoothly and professionally, it is evident to the patient; this instills trust and facilitates communication, which, in turn, tends to minimize malpractice and malpractice claims. It is often the feeling or perception that something was wrong that influences a patient to seek an attorney and file a claim. Good teamwork catches errors before untoward results occur. It also creates the perception in the patient that he or she is receiving competent, efficient, and high-quality health care.

The definition of coproviders in the context of the health care system can be greatly expanded. For example, the competence of the line worker involved in the manufacturing process of a piece of medical equipment could, in the most extreme assessment of the nature of "coproviders," affect the performance of nurses and physicians who use that particular piece of equipment.

The authors gratefully acknowledge the past contributions of John Dale Dunn, M.D., F.C.L.M.; James B. Couch, M.D., J.D., F.C.L.M.; Marvin Firestone, M.D., J.D., F.C.L.M.; Gary N. Hagerman, LL.B., F.C.L.M.; and William Goebert, Jr., M.D., J.D., F.C.L.M.

The first part of this chapter focuses on the health care providers who are directly involved with the patient and who have some form of professional licensure or responsibility for patient care. These providers include physicians, nurses, nurse practitioners, physician assistants, dentists, podiatrists, licensed psychologists, vocational nurses, registered technicians, and other personnel who work in the health care system and directly affect the provision of care to the patient. In addition, the nature of relationships that create coexisting responsibilities and duties among these providers is discussed.

The second part of the chapter explores legal aspects concerning the hospital, the institution in which these health care providers work together. It focuses primarily on the hospital's legal relationship to its patients and to the physicians who serve on its staff and committees.

State licensure

Licensed professionals are obligated not only to act within the authority and parameters set out by their own licensure act, but also, in most states, are required to report other professionals if they know that those professionals were acting in violation of the licensure acts. For example, state laws require that physicians report the incompetence of another physician if it has the potential to harm a patient. Physicians are also required to report the incompetence or impairment of a nurse or any other health care provider. In this respect, licensure creates a public duty that, at times, can override the natural instinct not to be a "tattletale."

Once a physician has been reported to his or her licensing board, the board will meet with the physician if the board believes the problem can be remedied informally. The licensing board may even ask the physician to voluntarily surrender his or her license if it is necessary to protect the public. Whether the license is surrendered or not, the physician can be diverted to a supportive program if he or she acknowledges the existence of a problem. If the physician refuses to acknowledge the problem, the board can formally charge the physician with violating the state's licensing act and order the physician's appearance before it at a formal hearing. In some states, under some conditions, the board may suspend the physician's license or impose less severe limitations on his or her practice privileges if doing so is deemed to be in the public's interest.

At such a hearing, the board usually receives evidence and testimony. It then makes findings of fact and forms conclusions of law as to the charges and appropriate action or sanction. Most states permit a sanctioned physician to request a stay of the sanction and to bring an appeal of the board's decision before a court of law. Of course, if the board finds insufficient proof (usually according to a preponderance of the credible evidence) in the facts to support an order or sanction, the matter is dismissed and, if necessary, the license and privileges are restored.

Practice in a health care institution

Apart from the responsibility created by state licensure laws to report professional impairment or incompetence or other acts in violation of licensing law, institutional environments may create an additional burden and duty for professionals: monitoring the competence and performance of coproviders with whom they work. The interdependence of professionals within a particular institutional environment is best exemplified by the hospital, but it exists in other health care settings such as nursing homes, mental health institutions, and outpatient settings. Obvious examples would be the responsibilities of the medical staff to the institution to monitor the quality of health care in the hospital as outlined by state licensure laws, voluntary accreditation standards, and common sense, as well as the common law.

In many cases institutions, which normally depend on the quality of the peer review conducted by their medical staffs, have been found liable for failure to discover or for choosing to ignore an individual health care provider's incompetence where that individual is practicing within that institution.[1] This well-established common-law rule receives additional support as a reasonable interpretation of the Standards of Accreditation of the Joint Commission on Accreditation of Healthcare Organizations (JCAHO), which are voluntary. In addition, the common law reflects the interpretation of state licensure laws requiring effective quality assurance programs in hospitals, medical association standards, and medical society standards. Further, the institutional duty to provide quality care ultimately rests with the hospital's governing body.

Thus health care providers find themselves obligated and responsible for the competence and quality of their peers' performance and for discovering and preventing the incompetence or impairment of professionals at other levels— either above or below their own—from harming the public in general or an individual patient. Thus nurses are obligated to report an impaired, incompetent, or otherwise deficient physician; but they would also be required to report a technician who fails to function at an acceptable level.

Peer review

Quality assurance programs in hospitals depend on the process of peer review because coproviders with the same professional training are the best judges of the competence and capabilities of their peers and colleagues. The quality assurance process is described best in terms of problem solving and the promotion of desired levels of patient care. Although it is easy to talk in generalities about the importance of quality, the actual process of quality assurance is difficult in the health care setting. However, the duty to provide good and effective peer review is clear.

Quality assurance programs. All health care institutions, health care provider groups, health maintenance organizations (HMOs) and managed care programs, and others directly or indirectly responsible for patient care necessarily deal with the developing field of quality assurance (QA) in health care. Small area analysis, comparison of health care practices, and widespread inconsistencies in approaches to various disease processes and surgical problems have created great concern and even governmental intervention in attempts to standardize approaches to health care problems. The unfortunate by-product of this concern and resulting standardization is that it is difficult to be certain of the relative benefits of the various approaches to problems. It is clear that many management approaches are effective, and diversity in health care should not be discarded for a theoretical and unproven cost or quality benefit. In medicine as well as in other "arts," there are many ways to "skin a cat."

The *Journal of the American Medical Association* has a regular column on clinical decision-making. The editor's specific objective is the ongoing study of the problems of variation in clinical approaches to medical problems.[2]

In QA programs, it is important to eliminate deviations below and outside of acceptable medical practice, particularly those deviations that put patients at risk. Therefore the JCAHO, medical societies, medical professional organizations, and others are actively involved in attempting to establish standards for practice. The American Medical Association has also studied standards in cooperation with Rand Corporation, and 20 medical specialty societies have published some form of standards.

Standards of care. Quality assurance, peer review, and coprovider relationships are dependent on the personal perceptions of those providing the care together, regarding what are considered to be appropriate standards of care. Unfortunately, the legal system and professional liability litigation in particular have confused how such standards are considered and applied in a way not easily explained. This can cause "defensive medicine."

This does not mean that it is impossible to reconcile institutional practice with understanding these standards. What is necessary is the acknowledgment that quality assurance and risk management must work in tandem, with each complementing the other to ensure that medical care is provided that meets the patient's needs and interests. An understanding of those needs is the first step. The legal system defines the duty a health care provider owes to the patient in terms of what is in the patient's interest:

1. To use his or her best judgment in care and treatment
2. To exercise reasonable care and diligence in the application of his or her knowledge and skills
3. To act in compliance with the standard of health care required by law[3]

Thus risk management and quality assurance programs must be used to constantly educate the institution's staff regarding how to fulfill these duties during the day-to-day provision of health care.

Normative versus actual standards of care. Elsewhere in this text the issues regarding standards of care are defined more completely. However, it is important to recognize that, generally, courts define a standard of care in terms of that degree of skill and expertise normally possessed and exercised by a reasonable and prudent practitioner with the same level of training in the same or similar circumstances. What this means in a courtroom can become quite different from what the health care provider contemplates while treating the patient. Too often, medical testimony presented in a courtroom deals with issues as they relate to "normative" standards rather than "actual" standards. In reality, physicians hope to perform at one level but actually perform at another level. For example, John Holbrook, M.D. (personal communication), an emergency physician interested in risk management in Massachusetts, reviewed more than 100,000 emergency department records and found that fewer than 5% of patients treated at the emergency department for a headache actually received a funduscopic examination. Whether this would be an actual standard that is acceptable is subject to debate, but it cannot be ignored as a reality. In a courtroom, the normative standard is described for the benefit of the judge or jury as expected performance recited by a "medical expert" adequately and sometimes superlatively qualified to discuss a particular area of professional expertise. It may not be an actual standard but rather a "normative" standard defined as the degree of skill and expertise that we strive to achieve rather than actually achieve as average prudent practitioners. Of course, states can and often do define who is a "medical expert" and what, generally, is the standard of care, as statutory definitions, for application in the courtroom.

In the quality assurance setting, it is important for those involved in the definitions of standards and practices to recognize the difficulties of defining appropriate standards of care and evaluating coproviders. Within those parameters it is still possible to define unacceptable deviance and deal with it appropriately as part of the peer review mechanism. However, difficulty can arise, especially in evaluating coproviders, when disparity exists among researchers, instructors, and various schools and institutions that train the coproviders. Such disparities need to be considered in both individual evaluations and coprovider training. Such continuing training can be a useful tool for establishing the "normative" standard an institution adheres to, in order to avoid any conflicts and unnecessary disputes over adherence. It is possible that a significant number of investigations and staff disciplinary actions arise not from actual lack of knowledge or personal dedication to high quality of care but from differences in training among coproviders.

Normally quality assurance programs are described in terms of the "controlled loop" process of identification of a problem, discussion, and evaluation resulting in proposed action, real action, and then reevaluation to determine whether the problem has been properly managed. Every professional organization that assumes responsibility for patient care, including hospital medical staffs, managed care organizations, and medical practice groups, must establish a quality assurance program. Without such a program, these patient care organizations will not be able to efficiently monitor the health care their coproviders provide.

There has been an increasing interest in and use of guidelines for comparing actual performance with the applicable standard of care. Some institutions prepare internal guidelines for the most commonly encountered or performed conditions or situations, basing them on academic research. Other institutions make use of external sources, such as The National Guideline Clearinghouse (NGC). The NGC maintains a comprehensive database of evidence-based clinical practice guidelines and related documents produced by the Agency for Healthcare Research and Quality (AHRQ). It works with the American Medical Association and the American Association of Health Plans. Its stated mission is to provide physicians, nurses, and other health professionals with a source of objective, detailed information on clinical practice guidelines. By doing so, it is promoting the dissemination, implementation, and use of such guidelines. The NGC's database is available on the Internet at http://www.guideline.gov/.

Disciplinary activities in peer review. Practicing with coproviders necessarily results in disciplinary peer review actions when unacceptable and incurable deviance is identified. It is important for those involved in peer review and quality assurance matters that have a direct impact on an individual practitioner to be aware of the concept of due process and the laws of the state and nation that govern disciplinary and peer review activities in the health care setting. The Health Care Quality Improvement Act of 1986[4] is a federal statute that provides guidance for establishment of due process within peer review through specific requirement:

1. The subject physician must be notified of an organization's intent to bring disciplinary action.

2. The subject physician must have an opportunity to respond, request a hearing if he or she desires, and prepare a defense.
3. The subject physician must have adequate notice of the nature of the charges.
4. The subject physician must receive the right to advice and counsel of the physician's choice, including an attorney, in any hearing conducted as part of peer review.
5. The subject physician must receive a fair hearing with an impartial panel of noncompeting peers for consideration of the proposed action to be taken.
6. The subject physician must be given an opportunity to examine the evidence against him or her, prepare a defense, cross-examine witnesses, and present arguments in his or her favor.
7. A written opinion must be provided by the hearing panel if disciplinary action is recommended, along with the written decision of the health care governing body or final arbitrator.

The importance of these guidelines lies in the statutory establishment of bilateral protection. The organization that is conducting peer review and following these guidelines ultimately derives as much benefit from them as the physician who is at risk. If a physician who has been disciplined under a peer review proceeding decides to sue individuals who participated in the process or the institution for having imposed the discipline, and if the defendants can show that the disciplinary action was undertaken in the "reasonable belief" that it was for the furtherance of good health care and with no malice or inappropriate motivations, this federal law provides "qualified immunity" from the civil claim. Further, if the defendants prove that the sanctioned physician's suit was brought inappropriately, they can collect damages for defense expenses and court costs. The federal law provides this remedy to encourage physicians to participate in peer review. However, failure to conduct peer review can create potential liability under the common-law theories described earlier.

Supervisory liability

Physicians supervise nurses, technicians, assistants, paramedics, and, at times, other physicians. This supervision can be direct, but it is often done by telephone, radio, or written communications. Generally, a physician's responsibility and potential liability for such injuries and mistakes resulting from the care given under such supervision are directly proportional to the degree of control held over the coproviders' actions and the supervisor's knowledge of such actions.

Physicians who are supervising their own employees bear special responsibilities because direct vicarious liability exists for any employees' negligent actions. Likewise, where a state's laws grant special status to nurse practitioners and physician's assistants, authorizing expanded delegated duties, such laws generally require that physicians formally report to the state the supervisory relationship's existence. Fur-

ther, such reports or applications for approval often formally create delegated standard orders and other protocols to provide for proper guidelines. In addition, many states have established definite limits on the nature of the supervision that might be provided. For example, most states require the supervising physician to be physically available to the nurse practitioner or physician's assistant for consultation and assistance. However, in many states these coproviders can act, within their standing orders, in a relatively liberal manner, sometimes even using signed prescription pads. Some state medical practice acts provide that a physician can delegate any responsibility to a properly trained person; thus the basic issue in determining vicarious liability can center on the physician's judgment of that coprovider's qualifications. Of course, one would not expect to find a physician delegating performance of a neurosurgical procedure to a physician's assistant; it is far more common to find less critical responsibilities delegated to the coprovider, such as when a nurse harvests veins for cardiovascular surgeons.

Vicarious liability is that liability arising from an employer-employee relationship. Employee physicians, nurses, technicians, and others can create liability for their employer through their negligence, if such negligence causes an injury. One should also be aware of the "borrowed servant" doctrine; a physician using employees of another to carry out the borrower's activities can be held liable for the "borrowed" employee's negligence. One's liability when borrowing another's "servant" is proportional to the amount of control one exercised. For example, in the health care setting, the "captain of the ship" theory at one time was used to resolve the issue of liability for the acts of nurses and others in the operating room. However, the courts have recognized that surgeons do not directly control the administrative duties of others in the operating room. Scrub technicians, circulating nurses, anesthesiologists, and others are working there, although they must defer to the judgment and authority of the surgeon on the case. Obviously, they have separate and independent duties and responsibilities proportional to their professional competence. It is therefore unreasonable to make the surgeon liable for an improper sponge, needle, or instrument count, just as it would be inappropriate for a surgeon to be responsible for the conduct of an anesthesiologist who fails to properly intubate the patient. If the problem comes to the surgeon's attention and he or she fails to act in the patient's interest, liability increases proportionately, but the primary responsibility still lies with that person who acts independently regardless of the level of professional expertise and who has separate and independent ministerial duties and authority.

Radio control and prehospital care

An interesting and important area of medical care involving delegation of medical practice to a remote person is the use of radio control for prehospital care. Separate and independent duties and responsibilities are created for licensed prehospital care personnel. In addition, it is important to recognize that prehospital care services are required by law to have a medical director who establishes proper medical care/prehospital care protocols and monitors the competence of the prehospital care personnel through a functioning quality assurance program.

The physician who either directs or controls the paramedic at the scene has the same liability as a physician who would direct or control a nurse and has ultimate responsibility for the patient. In the case of radio control, the physician has a responsibility proportional to his or her knowledge of the situation, recognizing that the physician is dependent on the eyes, ears, and observational skills of the paramedic or emergency medical technician (EMT).

Appropriate prehospital care protocols still vary widely throughout the United States. Variations easily result from the diverse qualifications of persons working in prehospital care settings, from personal opinions of medical directors, and from different state laws. State law specifically designates levels of skill in terms of basic care providers, special skill care providers, and full paramedic level providers. National and state registry and licensure are a part of the definition of these various levels of skill. The control of prehospital care personnel is similar to the type of remote control that exists when patients are in the hospital and nurses are used as observers reporting to physicians the condition of a patient and then carrying out appropriate therapeutic and diagnostic orders.

Ultimately, the health care professional who delegates responsibilities to others or controls others by providing care directly and in person or remotely by phone or radio is still responsible to act in a professional manner and within acceptable standards of care. A professional duty to monitor the coprovider's professional competence and ability, above or below one's level of licensure or professional skill, is a controlling factor and a legal principle that must be accepted by all professionals. In the institutional setting, coproviders are codependent and coresponsible. Even though direct responsibility may not exist, indirect responsibility for general considerations of quality assurance requires vigilance and appropriate action when problems and an incompetent coprovider are identified.

Independent contractors

Whether a health care provider is an independent contractor is a question implicating labor, employment, and tax law, as well as a consideration that affects professional liability. If a person works as an employee, the employer's vicarious liability is direct, but if that person is an independent contractor, the liability would be in proportion to the amount of control exercised. For example, many physicians function as independent contractors in various settings, but they exercise independent judgment over their professional practice. The independent contractor concept is one that properly suits a professional role because professionals are licensed as individuals and are responsible for making personal professional decisions about patient care. However, hospitals, health care facilities, and professional individuals are still responsible for monitoring the competence of the independent practitioner.

Ostensible agency

In most states, certain independent contractor relationships have been found to be ineffective to deflect liability from the party contracting for the services. For example, in a hospital situation, an independent physician contractor may be the only one available to the patient; therefore the hospital may automatically be considered to be vicariously liable through ostensible agency. It has used the agent physician for carrying out some of its institutional responsibilities.[5] When the patient has no way of knowing that the physician is not an employee or when the hospital uses the physician just as the hospital would use an employee, many states accept the concept that the hospital is therefore vicariously liable for the physician's actions. This area has not been as well defined outside the hospital-based physician situation, because other members of the medical staff are more independent. The concept generally has widespread support in the case of hospital-based physicians when patients come to a hospital and have no choice as to which physician to pick.[6]

Independent contractors working within a hospital setting or in a medical group are still subject to the same basic peer review and quality assurance controls, and therefore the institution or the professional organization can be considered liable if it fails to properly conduct the following: (1) proper credentialing and application; (2) adequate peer review and quality assurance review; (3) monitoring of physicians for ongoing appropriateness of care, continued education if indicated, and proper recertification, relicensure, and other matters related to ongoing practice requirements; and (4) proper corrective and disciplinary action when a physician performs inappropriately or below the standard of care.

Under the common law propounded by most states, the hospital may be considered liable for poor peer review. This liability of a health care institution as outlined in the common law has been extended to the medical staff when the medical staff knows that a physician has become incompetent and fails to take corrective action.[7]

Consultants and referring physicians

A consultant and the referring physician share responsibility for the patient's care based on their respective proportion of knowledge and control and the foreseeability for potential harm. For example, if the general practitioner refers the patient to a neurosurgeon for a neurosurgical problem, then his or her responsibility for the case decreases in proportion to his or her knowledge of the problem, control over the care given the patient, and actions taken in response to any problems identified. Failure to choose an appropriate consultant can occasionally create liability for the referring physician, particularly if the choice of consultant is based not on the competence of the consultant, but on other financial or personal relationships. If the consultant is known to be incompetent and it can be proven that the referring physician used that consultant anyway, then liability would revert to the referring physician.

Substitutes and sharing on-call time can create some liability if one shares call or chooses a substitute who is incompetent. This would generally depend on the facts and circumstances. For example, if a physician going on vacation is not careful in his or her choice of a competent substitute, the patient could easily consider this as failure to take proper care in choosing a substitute. In the case of sharing call with another physician, the responsibility is less because the other physician is independent. However, if a physician using shared call knows that another physician sharing call is incompetent or impaired, he or she exposes the patients in his or her practice to that physician and would be considered liable in proportion to his or her knowledge of the incompetence or impairment of the call-sharing physician.

Nursing and other technical practices in the hospital

State nurse practice acts are the laws that define the proper scope of nursing practice. These laws and hospital protocols and procedures control the scope of nurses' professional activities. The physician is not responsible for designing protocols and policies, although the medical staff is generally responsible for the quality of care in the hospital.[8] In the case of a hospital setting or other health care institutional setting, the administration generally includes nursing administration and therefore sets policy for the nursing practices within that institution. The medical staff provides oversight for the governing body on the quality of care provided in the institution, but depends on the nursing administration to develop policies and protocols for nursing care. The physician would be responsible for incompetence or impairment of a nurse or an inappropriate nursing action.

The physician should either intervene to prevent harm to the patient or deterioration of the patient's condition or report the events so that actions can be taken by the health care institution. Failure to do so, to ensure that the professional staff of the hospital is functioning in a way that provides quality patient care, could result in liability for the physician. The same responsibilities exist for nurses toward other nurses or technicians and for technicians with regard to other professional personnel in the hospital.

Professionals within a hospital or health care institutional setting assume liability in proportion to their knowledge of the problem and their ability to effect change. Within the institution, following protocol and procedure for registering complaints and attempting to provide for corrective action satisfy the responsibilities of the individual. The failure of the institution to act after being informed would create a separate institutional liability.

State medical practice acts and nurse practice acts as well as federal law[9] provide immunity for people who report in good faith the incompetence, impairment, or inappropriate practice of another professional.

Conclusion

The health care environment requires cooperation and teamwork. Physicians are dependent on many other health care professionals in a health care institution to ensure good patient care. These interdependencies are unavoidable and are increasing in magnitude and complexity; therefore it is important to understand that, generally, the team members' potential liability and legal responsibility are easy to analyze. The degree of duty and responsibility is in proportion to the amount of control and knowledge of potential for foreseeable harm. The health care professional is obligated to take actions to protect the interests of patients, who are innocent parties in the health care environment. A failure to act in the interest of good patient care or in the protection of the public welfare creates liability. Apart from concern about becoming a codefendant because of a failure to discipline or supervise, health care professionals should consider the fact that there are many different ways to fail the patient, including allowing another to harm the patient. The public responsibility of licensed health care professionals is the "brother's keeper" responsibility. Health care institutions, on the other hand, have a separate and independent corporate responsibility to ensure quality of care within their organizations. Failure to require proper credentials, inappropriate hiring practices, and failure to develop proper quality assurance and peer review within the institution place the governing body and the institution at great risk if patient harm results from that failure.

INSTITUTIONAL PRACTICE
Historical origins

Hospitals evolved in this country during the eighteenth, nineteenth, and early twentieth centuries along the lines of the European (particularly the British) model as charitable institutions and, in some cases, as almshouses for the poor. Because of this focus, many hospitals were affiliated with or originated from various religious orders. To foster and support these institutions, the law developed the doctrine of charitable immunity of hospitals from legal liability.[10] The cases recognizing this doctrine represented a natural outgrowth of their community's origins and the interest in providing services primarily to the downtrodden in society.

It was not until the 1870s, when university teaching hospitals and municipal hospitals began to appear, that secular institutions began to flourish. Despite this shift away from religious affiliations, hospitals continued to enjoy insulation from legal liability, retaining charitable immunity, primarily because of their origins.

Evolution of functional hospital organization and management (1914 to 1984). Early in this century, hospital organizations began to evolve into bipartite and tripartite institutions. The leading case to perpetuate this separation was *Schloendorff v. New York Hosp.,* a New York Court of Appeals decision issued in 1914.[11] The administrative staff was regarded as the governing body responsible for the overall administration of the hospital, while the medical staff was in charge of rendering patient care. The artificial separation was promulgated in the courts by their erecting a distinction between the "purely ministerial acts" performed by the hospital administration contrasted with medical acts performed by members of the hospital medical staff:

It is true, I think, of nurses, as of physicians, that in treating a patient, they are not acting as servants of the hospital. But nurses are employed to carry out the orders of the physicians, to whose authority they are subject. . . . If there are duties performed by nurses foreign to their duties in carrying out the physician's orders, and having relationship to the administrative conduct of the hospital, the fact is not established by the record.[12]

This medical/ministerial dichotomy continued after *Schloendorff,* although the functional distinction between hospital administration and medical staffs became increasingly blurred. The forces behind this blurring were the increasing use of professional management and business practices, and the increased professionalism of hospital-employed ancillary health care providers. Physicians are expected to understand, appreciate, and direct multifaceted teams, which often specialize within their own fields in very complex procedures, such as organ transplantation or treatment of specific communicable diseases. Thus, the difference between medical and administrative acts is often decided based on all of the surrounding circumstances, making for limited consistency and predictability. For example, it was held that administering the right blood by transfusion to the wrong patient was a "ministerial act" in *Necolaff v. Genesee Hosp.,*[13] while administering the wrong blood to the right patient was a "medical act" in *Berg v. N.Y. Society for the Relief of the Ruptured and Crippled.*[14]

This distinction was finally abrogated in 1957, in *Bing v. Thunig.*[15] The New York Court of Appeals overturned *Schloendorff.* Since *Bing,* both regulatory and common law in the health care field have evolved to reflect the interrelationships and interdependencies of the hospital and its medical staff. The JCAHO guidelines also reinforce this corporate relationship.[16] This view of the medical staff as an integral component of the hospital corporation has been confirmed in the decision of *Johnson v. Misericordia County Hosp.*[17] The antitrust case of *Weiss v. York Hosp.*[18] may have muddied the water somewhat by referring to the medical staff as being independent to the extent that it may be the "sole decision maker." Nevertheless, in terms of more practical economic realities, for both hospitals and their medical staffs to survive and, perhaps, thrive in the increasingly competitive health care marketplace, each must emphasize its common

directives and capitalize on them in forming new partnerships. To paraphrase Benjamin Franklin, we must hang together or, surely, we shall hang separately.

Evolution of the legal responsibilities for quality assurance in the hospital

THE MOVEMENT AWAY FROM CAPTAIN OF THE SHIP DOCTRINE. The evolution of the legal responsibilities for quality assurance within the hospital paralleled to a great extent the organizational changes throughout this period. A major development in establishing the legal view that the hospital is more than just a physician's workshop, but with independent responsibilities of its own, arose from the decision of *Tonsic v. Wagner.*[19] In that decision, the Supreme Court of Pennsylvania overturned their "captain of the ship" holding (from *McConnell v. Williams,* in which a hospital might escape liability for the negligent acts of employees temporarily under the direction of independently contracting physicians): "But such an employee can be temporarily detached, in whole or in part, from the hospital's general control."[20] Thus the *Tonsic* decision firmly established the principle that a hospital should be held liable for the negligent act of any of its employees even if under the supervision of a nonemployee at the time.

THE EXTENSION OF HOSPITAL LIABILITY TO THE ACTS OF INDEPENDENT CONTRACTORS: APPARENT AGENCY. The doctrine of apparent agency has substantially contributed to the demise of the hospital's independent contractor defense. One of the most important judicial pronouncements of this doctrine came again from the Superior Court of Pennsylvania in the case of *Capan v. Divine Providence Hosp.*[21] First, the hospital's changing role creates a likelihood that patients will look to the institution rather than the individual physician for care. Thus patients commonly enter the hospital seeking a wide range of hospital services rather than personal treatment by a particular physician. This is especially true for patients who have no family practitioner. It would be absurd to require such a patient to be familiar with the law of respondeat superior, meaning the patient would have to ask each health care provider whether he or she is an employee of the hospital or an independent contractor. . . . Similarly, it would be unfair to allow this secret limitation on liability contained in a physician's contract with the hospital to bind the unknowing patient.

Liability of hospitals and medical staff physicians
Hospital admissions

NONEMERGENCY. In general, a hospital has no duty to admit a patient. However, it must not discriminate because of race, color, or creed. Under limited circumstances, based on statutory (governmental hospitals), contractual (subscribes to an HMO or other similar arrangement), or common-law principles (injury caused by the hospital), the hospital may have a duty to admit. In hospitals engaged in clinical research mandated by the government, the institution is usually allowed discretion to refuse admission, even if the patient may meet criteria for admission. A teaching hospital, however, may not admit a patient contingent on the patient's participation in the teaching program. Otherwise, the patient's constitutional right of privacy would be invaded.

Even if a patient otherwise has a right to be admitted, if there is no medical necessity or if the hospital does not possess the services needed, the hospital need not admit the non-emergency patient.[22] The principle of no duty to admit reflects judicial restraint in dictating how a hospital should allocate scarce medical resources. Although many of the cases supporting this common-law principle date back to the turn of the century, the majority of the courts continue to apply this doctrine today.[23]

Special circumstances may exist that obligate a hospital under common-law doctrines to admit a patient if a prior relationship existed between the hospital and patient or where the hospital was the cause of patient injury (i.e., has placed the person in a position of peril). Such circumstances exist if the original injury or complication of treatment occurred as the result of the hospital's acts or omissions or the hospital begins to provide care to the patient. The hospital may be liable for abandonment if admission is denied under such circumstances.

EMERGENCY. The national trend of the law is to impose liability on hospitals for refusal to treat emergencies or if negligent care is provided in their emergency departments. Theories supporting such liability include the following: (1) reliance, (2) agency (respondeat superior), (3) apparent authority ("holding" self out), (4) corporate negligence, and (5) nondelegable duty. These theories are discussed next.

Reliance theory. If the patient relies on a hospital's well-established custom to render aid in an emergency situation, then the hospital may be found liable for refusing to provide the necessary care or for providing negligent care. In *Wilmington General Hosp. v. Manlove,*[24] the hospital was found liable under this theory. A child needing emergency care was not admitted to the hospital after the child's private pediatrician could not be reached to approve the admission. In *Stanturf v. Sipes,*[25] the hospital was held liable when the administrator refused to approve the admission because of the patient's inability to pay. The court stated:

The members of the public . . . had reason to rely on the [hospital], and . . . that plaintiff's condition was caused to be worsened by the delay resulting from the futile efforts to obtain treatment from the . . . [hospital].[26]

Agency theory. If the emergency department personnel who deviate from the applicable standard of care and cause harm to the plaintiff are considered "servants" of the hospital, then the hospital is vicariously liable under the doctrine of respondeat superior. A servant is defined as "a person employed to perform services in the affairs of another and who

with respect to the physical conduct in the performance of the service is subject to the other's control or right to control."[27] Other than house staff, staff physicians are usually considered "independent contractors" rather than "servants." Courts must determine that an agency relationship exists based on an analysis of the facts of the case before holding a hospital liable under this theory.[28]

In *Thomas v. Corso,*[29] the hospital was found liable when the emergency room nurse failed to contact the on-call physician. *Citizens Hosp. Ass'n. v. Schoulin*[30] is a similar case. The claim was based on nursing negligence in failing to report all the patient's symptoms to the on-call physician, failing to conduct a proper examination, and failing to follow the physician's directions. The court found the hospital liable under respondeat superior.

Apparent authority. A hospital may be found vicariously liable for an emergency room physician's negligence even if the physician is considered an independent contractor. The facts would have to establish apparent authority (also referred to as "ostensible agency" or "agency by estoppel"). This theory of liability exists because the hospital is "holding itself out." The hospital will be found liable when it permits or encourages patients to believe that independent contractor physicians are the hospital's authorized agents. The "holding out" must come from the hospital, not the physician.

The landmark case on which this theory is based is *Gizzi v. Texaco, Inc.*[31] In Gizzi, Texaco was held liable for its representations to the public, "You can trust your car to the man who wears the star." This advertisement was sufficient to support the jury's finding against Texaco for the apparent authority it vested in an independent contractor/dealer. The contractor had sold a used car in which the brakes failed, injuring the purchaser. Texaco did not profit from the sale but was aware that the dealer was engaged in this collateral activity.

Corporate negligence. The doctrine of corporate negligence asserts that there exists an independent duty of the hospital for the medical care rendered in its institution. Like the apparent agency theory, it holds the hospital liable for an independent contractor/physician's negligence. However, a corporate negligence claim is based on the hospital's independent negligence in allowing an incompetent physician to practice on its premise.

Nondelegable duty. The main reason for employers to use independent contractors is to "farm out" services that may be of benefit to the employers but that they may not be willing or able to provide themselves. They also may wish to avoid legal liability for such services. The immunity from liability may be misused or abused. The independent contractor immunity is therefore riddled with exceptions.[32]

For public policy reasons, certain duties delegated to an independent contractor have been determined not to confer immunity on the employer. These exceptions have been termed nondelegable duties. They usually represent situations wherein the employer's duty is important, urgent, or imperative. Employers who have such responsibilities cannot avoid liability by delegating those responsibilities to an independent contractor.

In *Marek v. Professional Health Services, Inc.,*[33] the health service was held liable even though it entrusted the reading of a patient's chest x-ray film to a competent independent contractor/radiologist. The theory of liability was that reading the film was a nondelegable duty.

In another case, the Alaska Supreme Court ruled that the defendant hospital was vicariously liable for negligence in its emergency department.[34] Such a duty "may be imposed by statute, by contract, by franchise or by charter, or by common law."[35] As discussed in this landmark case, the hospital had a nondelegable duty to provide nonnegligent care in its emergency department, based on its state license as a general acute care hospital, JCAHO standards, and its own bylaws.

Statutory bases for hospital liability for emergency room care. Negligence through the provision of substandard care is not the only source of liability. In the last three decades, the law has made denial of emergency care grounds for liability. In *Guerro v. Copper Queen Hosp.,*[36] a privately owned hospital operated only for employees of one company was held liable for refusing treatment to an illegal alien who sought care. The Arizona Supreme Court reasoned that the state licensing statute precluded the hospital from denying emergency care to a patient.

A federal law, the Emergency Medical Treatment and Active Labor Act, commonly referred to as the *antidumping statute,* is contained in the miscellaneous provisions of the Budget Reconciliation Act (COBRA) of the Ninety-ninth Congress.[37] This statute is a codification of common law theories of liability and emergency department duties. It applies to all hospitals that participate in Medicare and other government medical assistance programs created by the Social Security Act.

The law has had a significant impact on emergency medical care in hospitals. It has improved the plaintiff's chances of recovering damages from hospitals because it eliminates the requirement of proving some of the elements of medical negligence. It governs hospitals with an emergency department wherein a patient with an emergency medical condition or a woman in active labor seeks medical care. If such a patient is "transferred" from the health care facility to another facility or is discharged, the patient may recover damages for "personal harm" if the condition worsens during or after such transfer or discharge. The patient must prove only that the condition was not "stabilized" at the time of transfer and that the condition deteriorated because of the transfer. To avoid liability, the attending physician or other medical personnel at the hospital must sign "a certification that, based upon the information available at the time, the medical benefits reasonably expected from the provision of appropriate medical treatment at another facility outweigh the increased risks" of transfer.

In addition to the certification requirement, the transfer must also be an "appropriate transfer." Although the signed certification is a simple enough procedure for the hospital to incorporate within its medical record forms, the requirements that will satisfy the transfer include all the following: (1) the receiving facility . . . has available space and qualified personnel . . . has agreed to accept transfer . . . and to provide appropriate medical treatment; (2) the transferring hospital provides . . . appropriate medical records of examination and treatment; (3) transfer is effected through qualified personnel and transportation equipment; and (4) such other requirements as the Secretary [of Health and Human Services] may find necessary.

Presumably the physician or other medical personnel who transfer the patient have the requisite knowledge of the staffing and competence of the receiving facility and have sought agreement for acceptance by the receiving facility before transfer. These requirements seem applicable whether the receiving facility is an outpatient clinic, nursing home, day care program, or a more intensive treatment center.

Although the physician must be acting as an employee or under contract with the hospital and the hospital must be a participating Medicare provider for the penalty provisions of this law to apply, these are not required for recovery of damages under state law. In addition, the hospital will be liable for damages under this statute or state law whether or not the involved physician is considered an independent contractor under state law.

This federal law seems to preempt state law that "directly conflicts with any of its requirements." It further provides for federal jurisdiction and allows the injured individual to obtain "such equitable relief as is appropriate," giving the federal court discretion to award damages it considers to be warranted. Legal action may be brought up to 2 years after the violation.

A patient who suffers "personal harm" resulting from violation of provisions of this law will be entitled to those damages allowed under the state's substantive law of personal injury and wrongful death statutes. In addition to these damages, penalties of up to $50,000 per violation against the hospital and involved physician alike are applicable to provider hospitals and their employed or contracted physicians. The hospital receiving the transferred patient is also indemnified against any financial losses by the transferring hospital if the transferring hospital has violated the statute.

Clearly, hospitals are no longer to be considered the "physician's workshop." Thus the modern hospital is an integrated center for delivery of health care services, possessing in-house staff and independent contractor/physicians with an array of staff privileges. The hospital can farm out professional services; however, based on public policy and other legal considerations, the trend of the law is to hold the hospital liable for harm resulting from negligence in handling admissions and transfers of patients in its emergency department. As hospitals have become more profitable and business oriented, the adversarial relationship and the law governing hospitals, patients, and physicians have changed. Although there is no duty for nonemergency admissions by hospitals, under emergency circumstances, the trend of the law is for hospital liability if the patient is harmed as a result of denial of admission or improper care.

Corporate liability of hospitals. No doctrine exemplifies the notion of a hospital as a corporate entity with subsidiary components functioning interdependently to deliver a health care product better than the judicially pronounced theory holding a hospital corporately liable for the quality of care delivered by its medical staff. Under this doctrine, it does not matter whether the staff members are employees or purely independent contractors. Under corporate liability, the hospital may be held directly liable for its own negligence in ensuring the quality of health care delivered within its walls.

This doctrine of direct corporate liability of hospitals is traceable to the famous case of *Darling v. Charleston Memorial Hosp.*[38] In the *Darling* case, a patient was admitted for treatment of a broken leg through the emergency room of a private, nonprofit hospital, and was attended by a hospital staff physician who was rotating on emergency duty. The attending physician was not skilled in orthopedic work, and a cast was improperly applied so that circulation to the leg was blocked. Although the patient subsequently complained about the leg, and the nurses involved in his care observed the discoloration of his toes, nothing was done. When he was finally examined by another physician, the leg required amputation. The court's decision against the hospital could have been based on a finding of apparent agency on the grounds that the plaintiff had no reason to think that the hospital's attending physician was not employed by the hospital. However, the court went further in holding the hospital itself directly liable for breaching its own duty of care to the patient in failing to "require consultation" with a member of the hospital surgical staff skilled in such treatment or to review the treatment rendered to the plaintiff, and to require consultants to be called in as needed.

The court recognized the hospital's own central role in the overall treatment of the patient, thereby requiring the hospital itself to become directly involved in the health care delivery process. Hospitals could be held directly liable for their own corporate negligence in providing health care services. Before this case, the corporate duties of hospitals were limited to three areas, unrelated to direct patient care:

1. The duty of reasonable care in the maintenance and use of equipment
2. The availability of equipment and services
3. The duty of reasonable care in the selection and retention of employees

Since Darling and its progeny, hospitals must be much more mindful of their selection and retention of staff physicians.[39-43]

Medical staff credentialing

Evolution of the basic hospital-physician relationship. The rights, duties, and protections afforded to the hospital and its medical staff have traditionally been analyzed by reference to the quality and quantity of the delivery of patient care. The law recognizes that the hospital's governing body must assess the qualifications of physicians who request admission to the hospital staff and must monitor the quality of medical care delivered to hospital patients.

The hospital is generally protected under the law when its decision whether to appoint or reappoint is based on considerations related to the quality of medical care rendered within the hospital or to a physician's professional conduct. Such considerations may involve an assessment of the physician's technical and clinical competence, as well as other relevant factors, such as his or her ability to cooperate with co-workers and support staff.

Although the hospital governing body has the duty to ensure the quality of patient care in the hospital, it has neither the expertise nor the proximity to specific situations to monitor adequately the actual delivery of medical services. Accordingly, the typical hospital governing body delegates much of its quality assurance responsibilities to the medical staff, and the governing body retains the ultimate monitoring or oversight responsibility. The medical staff organization usually uses its committee structure to provide the actual quality assurance mechanism by which the institution's quality of care may be maintained. This structure is formalized through the hospital and medical staff's bylaws, rules and regulations, standards of performance, and procedures for peer review.

The professional and economic significance of hospital staff privileges. The hospital, with its special care facilities and interaction of experts and trained professionals, has been the major centralized provider of medical services in the United States for over a century. However, more and more treatment procedures are becoming decentralized with establishment of ambulatory surgery centers, less invasive treatments, and home health care. However, it remains true that a physician who is denied access to a hospital facility may be severely hampered in his or her practice. Gaining and retaining clinical privileges in at least one hospital has become practically essential for most physicians to practice medicine.

Still, staff privileges are just that—privileges. There is no fundamental or constitutional right to practice at a particular hospital.[44] In some jurisdictions, however, the profession of a valid license may create a right to appointment in the absence of actual incompetence.[45] The current revolution in health care financing and competition is adding yet another layer of complexity to this decision-making process. As physicians seek to attain or retain clinical privileges on the one hand, hospitals and medical staffs are becoming more selective with respect to whom they grant clinical privileges.

In some cases, as part of long-term strategic planning, whole departments of clinical services may be eliminated or curtailed substantially because of economics, an adverse reimbursement climate, and patient population needs. All of these developments have brought the dilemma of hospital corporate liability versus physician staff privileges disputes into bold relief. These issues are discussed in more detail later in this chapter. The remainder of this part deals with the various types of staff privileges available, the process involved in obtaining and retaining them, and the protections, theories of liability, and remedies available in the denial, deferral, limitation, or withdrawal of these staff privileges.

Nature and type of staff membership

Active medical staff. In most hospitals the active medical staff consists of practitioners who meet certain basic educational, training, and background experience requirements. Typically, they are either board certified or board eligible in their area of specialty. They may regularly admit patients to the hospital, or are otherwise involved in the care of hospital patients, or participate in a teaching or research program of the hospital. They are normally required to actively participate in the staff's patient care audit and quality assurance activities. It is not unusual for active staff members to be required to provide care within their area of specialty to those "unassigned" patients who are admitted through the emergency room. Each active medical staff member retains responsibility within his or her area of professional competence (as prescribed by clinical privilege delineation determinations) for the daily care and supervision of each patient in the hospital for whom he or she provides services.

Consulting staff. Typically the consulting staff consists of practitioners who are members of the active staff of another hospital where they actively participate in the patient care audit and other quality assurance activities, who are of recognized professional ability in a specialized field, and who are not members of another category of the medical staff. Consulting staff members cannot admit patients, and their clinical privileges are limited to their particular area of expertise.

Courtesy staff. The courtesy staff consists of practitioners who admit a limited number of patients per year and who are members of another hospital's active medical staff, where they actively participate in patient care audit and other quality assurance activities.

Affiliate staff. The affiliate staff group consists of practitioners who are not active but have a long-standing relationship with the hospital. Typically, these practitioners may not admit patients or be eligible to hold office or vote in general staff and special meetings.

Outpatient staff. The outpatient staff consists of practitioners who are regularly engaged in the care of outpatients on behalf of the hospital or in a program sponsored by or associated with the hospital, who do not wish to assume all the responsibilities incumbent on active staff membership.

Each outpatient staff member retains responsibility within his or her area of professional competence for the daily care and supervision of patients under his or her care, while actively participating in the patient care audit or other quality assurance activities required of the staff.

Honorary or emeritus staff. Members of the honorary or emeritus staff are practitioners who are not active in the hospital but are being honored for their outstanding accomplishments or reputation. These members may also be former members of the active staff who have retained and may retain admitting and clinical privileges to the extent recommended by the medical board and board of directors.

House staff. Members of the house staff group are either fully licensed physicians or physicians who have received appropriate certification from the state medical board authorizing them to enter postgraduate study in a particular hospital. They may admit patients within the specialty department to which they are assigned with the approval of an active staff member in that department who is responsible for the care of that patient, and they may exercise clinical privileges as established within the residency training program.

Allied health professional staff. Allied health professionals represent a group of nonphysician coproviders, including podiatrists, nurses, psychologists, and so forth, who may provide specified patient care services under the supervision or direction of a physician member of the medical staff. They may write orders to the extent established in the rules of the staff and department to which they are assigned, but not beyond the scope of their licenses, certificates, or other legal credentials. The 1990 JCAHO Accreditation Manual for Hospitals accommodates the entry of these nonphysician providers into the hospital's health care delivery system.

Staff application and renewal

The public/private hospital distinction. Constitutional and statutory protections typically have imposed more restrictions on public hospitals in the area of staff privileges decisions. Increasingly, however, acts of formerly private hospitals have come under a level of scrutiny similar to that for public hospitals.

The two most common theories of medical staff guarantees advanced by physicians have been (1) that the hospital has a fiduciary relationship with the public because of its tax-exempt status, as well as its health and charitable activities, and (2) that by virtue of the hospital's receipt of certain public monies (e.g., Hill-Burton funds), its acts amount to "state action." Such hospital acts were therefore claimed to be subject to the Fifth and Fourteenth Amendments to the Constitution, requiring due process of law for the benefit of persons otherwise being deprived of life, liberty, or property rights. This justification finds its specific application to the physician appointment and reappointment process through the analysis of staff privileges as a necessary means of guaranteeing the liberty right of practicing one's profession.

Delegation of credentialing decisions to the medical staff. The governing body of the hospital (although ultimately responsible for the quality of care delivered) delegates to the medical staff the decision-making process for physician credentialing. The medical staff ordinarily then delegates these specific functions to a select credentials or peer review committee to make these determinations. Initial appellate decision-making authority for these determinations is usually passed to a medical executive committee. The composition of this committee is variable, but it usually consists of clinical department and division chiefs or service and section heads, as well as medical and hospital administrative personnel.

The process. A current or aspiring member to a medical staff submits a completed application including proof of medical education, licensure, board eligibility or certification, supporting materials including recommendations concerning current clinical competence and ethical practice, recent (5 years) ongoing as well as adverse claim experience, and a completed privileges delineation request form to the secretary of the medical staff or the hospital administrator. After this, the physician may be interviewed by the department chair, who prepares a written report and recommendation concerning staff appointment and clinical privileges, which is then transmitted to the credentials committee.

After initial processing, the application for past record is reviewed by the credentials committee. The credentials committee then transmits to the medical executive committee (sometimes known as the medical board) a written report and recommendation as to staff appointment, category, department, and clinical privileges delineation, including special conditions.

The medical executive committee then forwards to the executive director for transmittal to the board of directors a written report and recommendation for clinical privileges to be granted with any special conditions to be attached to the appointment. Physicians receiving adverse determinations may follow an appellate procedure roughly paralleling the foregoing process.

Considerations for acceptance or rejection

The following represent general criteria considered in the staff privileges decision-making process:

1. Education, training, background, and experience
2. Need in the department
3. Ability to work with others
4. Ability to meet eligibility or other requirements specified in bylaws
5. Freedom from conflict of interest
6. Utilization of hospital experience facilities
7. Maintenance of professional liability insurance
8. Willingness to make a full-time commitment to the institution
9. Whether the hospital is the physician's primary inpatient facility
10. Status of medical record-keeping and risk management experience
11. Freedom from false or misleading information
12. Current clinical competence, ethical practice, and health status
13. A willingness to comply with bylaws and regulations
14. Continuing medical education as required
15. Evidence of previous or current action taken in licensure or privilege matters.

Several of the preceding criteria might carry potential antitrust implications if applied to deny or limit clinical privileges in some contexts. Curtailment, based on these criteria, should specify with considerable particularity why privileges were denied, deferred, or limited.

Legal protections available to the physician

Hospital and medical staff bylaws. It is well settled under the law that hospitals acting through their medical staffs must comply with their own internal procedural rules (i.e., bylaws). Failure to do so, at the very least, will invite judicial review. On finding a significant failure, a court could nullify the whole process and require the hospital to review the physician's qualifications again in accordance with all internal policies, procedures, and bylaws. Examples of particular procedural rules that should appear in bylaws include (but are not limited to) the following:

1. Adequate notice to the physician of the adverse decision
2. Making available a fair hearing process for aggrieved physicians
3. Communicating adequately to physicians the factors governing the credentialing decision
4. Allocating properly the burden of proof during the hearings

Contract theory of medical staff bylaws. In Pennsylvania and some other states, the medical staff bylaws may be viewed as part of a contractual relationship between the hospital and members of its medical staff, so that modifications may only be made pursuant to amendment procedures established in the bylaws themselves. In Pennsylvania, as well as other states adopting this approach, it may be considered a breach of contract for a hospital to violate procedural protections afforded under its medical staff bylaws in the physician credentialing process.

There may have been an inadequate number of court decisions to make it clear whether any such breach would make available to aggrieved physicians the whole panoply of common-law contractual remedies. It is also unclear whether this contractual analogy may apply to the situation of an applicant who is not yet a member of the medical staff.

Protection from economic harm. There may be some protection from tortious interference with a physician's ability to practice his or her profession. In many jurisdictions (e.g., New Jersey), this has been recognized as a valid claim under tort law. In general the intent to deny privileges without legal justification is sufficient to permit this type of claim to go forward in litigation. In addition, interference with trade or business may be alleged as a violation of the federal or state constitution, if the hospital is considered to be a public institution as discussed earlier. If two or more individual staff members or other persons conspire to deny privileges wrongfully, then a "restraint of trade" claim may also be possible (i.e., a Sherman Act Section 1 violation as discussed later in the antitrust subsection). In addition to possible claims under federal antitrust laws, some state courts (notably New Jersey) also permit these suits.

Protection from defamation. Physicians involved in the credentialing process are usually seen to be protected from defamation, or "the holding of a person up to ridicule, in a respectable and considerable part of the community." Typically, the hospital and medical staff may have available several defenses to the claim by physicians that they have been defamed during the credentialing process.

First, no liability from defamation will attach to the hospital or its staff if the allegedly defamatory statements are true. Second, the physician applicant consents to the making of these statements by voluntarily going through the credentialing process. Third, public policy requires that persons who are asked to give statements to assist in the credentialing process should be protected by the law for such statements, to ensure that they are given without fear of reprisal and to ensure that the best possible decisions are made to ensure patient safety and welfare. In most contexts, this is a qualified privilege. In the absence of malice, this privilege applies to physicians and others involved in credentialing decision— physicians, in making comments, must make them in a proper setting for statements to be protected.

Due process protection. In the case of hospitals owned or controlled by public agencies or private hospitals acting under the color of state law by having a fiduciary relationship with the public, substantive and due process safeguards may become available to physicians seeking to attain or retain staff privileges.

Substantive due process requires that the reasons behind the denial of a physician's staff privileges must be rational and not arbitrary or capricious. Claims based on an alleged violation of substantive due process may involve, for example, challenges to per se rules imposed by the hospital, such as minimum educational requirements (beyond those required for licensure) or board certification in a clinical specialty.

Procedural due process requires that the physician receive adequate safeguards concerning the process itself in determining whether he or she should be granted staff privileges at a particular hospital. A significant number of federal court decisions have held that denial of privileges by a private health care provider is not sufficiently regulated or controlled by the state to invoke federal jurisdiction.[46,47] However, it is now becoming clear that regardless of whether the hospital concerned is public or private, a physician has a federally protected right to due process.[48,49] These procedural safeguards may include (but are not limited to) the following:

1. Notification of the adverse determination[50]
2. If the physician requests a hearing, written notice of the charges with sufficient specificity to give the physician adequate notice with sufficient specificity of the reason for an adverse ruling[51]
3. Adequate time to prepare a defense[52]
4. Opportunity for prehearing discovery[53]
5. A hearing panel composed of impartial, fair-minded physicians[54]
6. Appearance before the decision-making panel
7. Assistance of legal counsel during the hearing
8. Cross-examination of witnesses
9. Presentation of witnesses and evidence in defense[55]
10. Transcript of panel hearing available for review before appellate hearing[56]
11. Written decision from the panel for judicial review

Employment practices discrimination. A newer possible theory that physicians might be able to assert comes under the umbrella of employment practices discrimination. Although this cause of action historically arose in occupations other than medicine, it may be available, at least, to employed physicians. Another type of action might become available to physicians who have lost or failed to obtain staff privileges as a result of their having made prior written or oral statements critical of peers or of the policies of the hospital at which they have lost privileges. A relevant court decision in this connection is *Novosel v. Nationwide Insurance Co.*[57] There the federal appeals court in Philadelphia upheld an employee's right to sue his employer, where he may have been wrongfully discharged for having asserted a right protected by an important public policy, namely, freedom of speech and political association.

Antitrust safeguards. Approximately 26% of this country's physicians are involved in exclusive contracts with hospitals. These contracts with radiologists, pathologists, anesthesiologists, and sometimes cardiologists or emergency physicians have become the subject of Sherman Act antitrust challenges in recent years. To invoke a violation of Section 1 of this act, a plaintiff must assert the following:

1. That the parties against whom the antitrust action is brought have agreed among or between themselves (i.e., conspired) to engage in activities that restrain trade
2. That the effect of this conspiracy is to restrain trade and is anticompetitive in nature
3. That these anticompetitive practices affect consumer choice of services in a relevant market population covered by the agreement or conspiracy
4. That these anticompetitive practices have a substantial and adverse impact on interstate commerce

Aggrieved parties have also alleged violation of Section 2 of the Sherman Antitrust Act. Section 2 prohibits the willful acquisition or maintenance of monopoly power in a relevant geographic market within which the provider of services operates, and as a practical matter to which the purchaser of those services may turn for these services. Acquiring or maintaining the power to control market prices and exclude competition in such an area could amount to a Section 2 violation involving monopolistic practice. Section 2 violations do not require a conspiratorial agreement. Assuming that federal jurisdiction may be established by showing that anticompetitive practices have a substantial adverse impact on interstate commerce, an analysis of the merits of an antitrust claim in a credentialing case may proceed.[58] In the most famous recent case analyzing the merits of an antitrust claim concerning the staff privileges of an unsuccessful applicant to a closed medical staff of anesthesiologists, the U.S. Supreme Court held that this type of exclusive contract did not violate Section 1 of the Sherman Antitrust Act.[59]

The theory of liability was that, through the vehicle of this exclusive contract, consumer choice was limited because the anesthetic services of the hospital were illegally tied to its surgical services (i.e., if you went to a hospital to undergo surgery, then you had to accept the exclusive panel of anesthesiologists). The Supreme Court, however, held that there was no shortage of other hospitals with comparable services in the New Orleans area from which patient/consumers could choose other surgeons and anesthesiologists for their operations.

Justice O'Connor and three other justices concurred in the result, but stated that this type of practice should have been sustained because it was justified by matters of medical and administrative efficiency (i.e., it satisfied rules of reason while not constituting an illegal practice according to federal antitrust laws). This decision (although not finding an antitrust violation) may be most significant to the health care industry by confirming that relationships among hospitals, physicians, and their patients are subject to the same antitrust principles that apply to others involved in commercial activities.

This decision may be just as notable for what it does not say. For example, exclusive contracts in the areas with only one hospital near state borders, which involve services with independent markets, may well violate Section 1 of the Sherman Act. Clearly, now that the courts regard health care as a commercial activity, the range of antitrust violations may well increase depending on the specific facts and circumstances in each case.

In 1984 the Third Circuit United States Court of Appeals reconfirmed the applicability of traditional commercial analysis to the activities of hospitals and their medical staffs in excluding certain groups from staff membership.

In *Weiss v. York Hosp.*,[60] Dr. Malcom Weiss had filed a Sherman Act antitrust action as a member of a group (osteopathic physicians) who had been excluded from membership on the hospital's medical staff. The lower court had found that this group boycott by York Hospital and its medical staff violated Sections 1 and 2 of the Sherman Act. The Third Circuit Court of Appeals in Philadelphia, while reversing the Section 2 violation finding, concurred with the lower court that this practice violated Section 1 of the Sherman Act. The appellate court found that regardless of whether or not the medical staff was acting as an agent or independently of the hospital in this practice, there was a conspiracy among individual staff physicians to exclude osteopathic physicians.

This case confirmed that regardless of whether or not the medical staff is an entity separate from the hospital, individual physicians compete with each other and thus may conspire to limit competition in violation of Section 1 of the Sherman Act. With the dramatically increasing numbers of M.D.s, D.O.s, D.D.S.s, D.P.M.s, D.C.s, M.S.N.s, P.A.s, and other health care professionals, the impact that this case should have on future efforts by M.D.s to boycott certain non-M.D. groups cannot be overstated.

Available remedies to aggrieved physicians

A physician denied clinical privileges may be entitled to a variety of remedies if he or she prevails in litigation against the hospital. The remedy usually depends on the infraction. An injunction may be available. The court may prevent the hospital from denying or curtailing staff privileges (permanently or at least until a full hearing and final decision is made by the hospital concerning appointment or reappointment).

To obtain injunctive relief, a physician must show that he or she could be harmed irreparably if the injunction is not granted. However, even if a physician can show this and gets an injunction, this finding will not act to prevent the hospital from denying staff privileges based on subsequent events. Furthermore, injunctive relief is inappropriate if internal hospital administrative remedies have not been exhausted or are still available as prescribed by hospital and medical staff bylaws. In appropriate circumstances (usually limited to federal cases involving public institutions), a court may order a hospital to appoint or reappoint a physician or at least to grant a hearing or other procedural safeguards during the credentialing process.

Another remedy is monetary damages—compensatory or punitive. Compensatory (or civil) damages may be justified if the court finds that the hospital or its medical staff interfered with the physician's right to practice his or her profession, or that the denial of privileges was part of a conspiracy to violate the applicant's civil rights. Such damages must be proven by the physician, based on (1) his or her inability to admit patients to the hospital, (2) the denial of privileges at other hospitals because of the bad publicity generated by this adverse decision, (3) the physician's loss of patients or income because of the denial, or (4) the loss of the physician's professional standing or reputation in the community.

Punitive damages are unlikely to be imposed except when the denial of privileges was the result of legally willful, wanton conduct that the court seeks to prevent in the future by making an example of the defendants.

A group or even an entire class of physicians or nonphysician medical personnel may seek any of these remedies. A class action may be brought in which the allegation concerns discriminatory exclusion of minorities, osteopathic physicians, dentists, nurse practitioners, physician assistants, chiropractors, podiatrists, or others.

Guidelines for hospital and medical staff credentialing

Hospital and medical staff bylaws. There are many key people primarily responsible for staff privileges decisions. These department chairs and members of the medical executive and credentials committees must be well versed in the procedural and substantive safeguards provided to physicians by law and by the hospital and medical staff bylaws, rules, and regulations.

In determining whether to appoint or reappoint a physician, the decision-makers should identify the specific reason or reasons for restricting staff privileges. The medical executive and credentialing committee should specify as many reasonable grounds for denial as possible and, whenever appropriate or relevant, should reference these grounds to medical staff bylaw provisions.

Grounds for denial or limitation of privileges should be adequately documented. They must be reasonably related to a legitimate purpose or purposes, preferably in furtherance of the hospital's overall mission. Moreover, the hospital, through its medical staff and executive committee, should be sure that its actions demonstrate that it applies these grounds in a nondiscriminatory fashion, using principles of fair play and due process as established in its hospital and medical staff bylaws.

Specific measures to minimize liability. There are other, more specific measures a hospital can and should take to minimize its potential liability exposure in credentialing matters.

First, the hospital must ensure that it complies with the various statutes, regulations, and informal requirements governing the conduct of the hospital and its medical staff. This crucial goal should be achieved by drafting the hospital and medical staff bylaws carefully and clearly in accordance with the guidelines of the state department of health, the JCAHO, and the Department of Health and Human Services. Further, if the hospital accepts Medicaid patients, its bylaws should comply with the guidelines of the state department of public welfare. Of particular importance, the medical staff bylaws must comply with state department of health regulations and JCAHO guidelines regarding the classification and delineation of privileges. They should provide mechanisms for review of decisions affecting clinical privileges, including guarantees that physicians may be heard at each step of the process. Even when the medical staff sets out to adopt by-

laws that are as straightforward as possible, it should ensure that credentialing and hearing procedures are fully and clearly set forth and followed.

Second, the hospital should implement measures during the application and reapplication process that will reduce the likelihood that a rejected physician will have a basis for subsequent legal action. For example, during the initial evaluation or reevaluation of a physician, an interview between the physician and the chairman of the department of service is advisable. This interview should be more than cursory; it should be designed to determine the extent of the physician's commitment to the hospital and to identify any problems that might arise during the credentialing process.

The hospital should verify the applicant's credentials and solicit written recommendations. The facility must also query the National Practitioner Data Bank to check for reports of privilege actions or malpractice settlements on the applicant. For physicians just out of training, professors and program directors should be asked to submit evaluations. The hospital should specify that it will use the comments to assist in evaluating the physician's suitability for clinical privileges in the hospital, and may communicate the substance of the comments to the physician. After it has cleared this with the commentators, it should scrutinize all solicited and unsolicited information for bias.

Third, the hospital should notify in writing all physicians whose requested privileges are denied or restricted. The notice should sufficiently detail the reasons, supported by adequate documentation. The decision should be communicated as being irrevocable and mandated by an interrelated combination of factors, rather than because of one or another specific reasons. This reduces the likelihood that the applicant will attempt to challenge the decision by challenging one of its bases. The hospital must scrupulously avoid irrelevant or potentially prejudicial considerations (such as "the hospital already has enough female obstetricians"). Physicians involved in the decision-making process for a potential competitor may be advised to excuse themselves or to abstain in the voting process. It should base its decision primarily on its need to maintain high-quality medical care. The hospital must communicate the reasons to the physician with appropriately chosen language. Hospital counsel may assist in this drafting.

Fourth, the hospital should maintain thorough documentation throughout the evaluation period. This provides protection to the hospital, medical staff, and individual members of the credentials and executive committee in the event of subsequent litigation by rejected physicians. The hospital, through its medical staff and various committees, should also take steps to enable applicants to withdraw gracefully before a formal denial of privileges, if that would be the likely outcome of a full review.

Minimizing due process claims

PROCEDURAL DUE PROCESS. Hospitals should satisfy procedural safeguards during the credentialing process to avoid claims by rejected physicians that they were not treated fairly or had an inadequate opportunity to be heard. At a minimum, the hospital should provide timely notice to physicians concerning the restriction of privileges, or of adverse decisions by the credentialing or executive committee or the governing body. Additional safeguards may include the following:

1. Independent legal counsel for the physician during the formal hearing process (although this may not extend to representation during the hearing itself)
2. Liberal discovery by the physician and his or her attorney before formal hearing
3. The right to cross-examine evaluators
4. Right of appeal to the governing board
5. Notification in writing of all adverse decisions and the reasons for them

SUBSTANTIVE DUE PROCESS. Courts have recognized that there are many permissible justifications for denying or restricting clinical privileges. One such justification is the physician's inability to meet the legitimate eligibility requirements specified in the bylaws. These eligibility requirements may relate to the physician's education, the length or nature of the physician's residency, the amount or nature of the physician's professional liability insurance coverage, or other specifics regarding the physician's training, experience or competence, ethical practice, or adherence to professional standards.

Another legitimate reason for denying or restricting privileges is the perceived inability of the physician to make a full-time or otherwise adequate commitment to the responsibilities expected of staff members. This inability may be due to the physician's conflicting commitments at other hospitals, or simply because the physician does not choose to commit to the hospital's operational and administrative needs. If the physician would be a particular asset to the staff, however, then the hospital may wish to extend to him or her courtesy or consulting privileges. It is similarly appropriate to deny clinical privileges to a physician who fails to meet any other requirements imposed by the hospital or medical staff bylaws, such as the failure to submit the necessary references or to attend a sufficient number of meetings or pay dues.

As a final example, the hospital may base its denial on "interaction considerations." These may include the physician's poor patient relations, his or her uncooperative or disruptive behavior, or any similar perceived inability to contribute to the supportive atmosphere of trust and cooperation essential to the successful administration of the hospital and the delivery of high-quality health care.

Many other substantive criteria have been legitimately used by hospitals to justify restrictions or denials of clinical privileges. Some criteria, however, may have anticompetitive overtones. In the current procompetitive health care climate, these criteria should be evaluated carefully before being used as a basis for justifying the restrictions of a physician's clinical privileges, regardless of their legitimacy.

Some of these suspect criteria may include, under appropriate circumstances, the services in the department, the lack of need for the physician's specific services, or any other alleged overburdening of the hospital's facilities.

Medical staff peer review

The Patrick decision. On May 17, 1988, the U.S. Supreme Court decided one of the most important cases affecting the medical staff peer review process in this century. In *Patrick v. Burget,*[61] the court held that where medical staff peer review was not actively administered or supervised by the state, physicians sitting on peer review committees were not entitled to absolute immunity from federal antitrust actions, if their actions to exclude other physicians from staff membership were for anticompetitive or other reasons not directly related to improving the overall quality of care.

The *Patrick* decision established constraints on physician peer review, the reasons for excluding physicians from medical staffs, and the procedures used in achieving this. Following *Patrick,* physicians may not be excluded primarily for economic, as opposed to quality of care, considerations. Moreover, to escape federal antitrust liability, the peer review must allow physicians undergoing evaluation full fair hearing protection to ensure adequate procedural due process. Medical staff physicians and their hospitals can use a number of approaches to limit their federal antitrust liability. Specifically, some of these include (but are not limited to) the following:

1. Rewrite medical staff bylaws to ensure that all requisite procedural due process safeguards protecting the evaluated physician are in place and are enforced fairly
2. Have each medical staff peer review member establish his or her freedom from economic conflicts of interest before making recommendations that could adversely affect the staff privileges of another potentially competing physician
3. Have physician peer reviewers subject their own requests for continuing staff membership and clinical privileges to review bodies constituted by professionals not sitting on the same committees or departments that are chaired by the physician being evaluated to avoid possible claims of undue influence
4. Have as chairs of credentialing committees and other sensitive medical care review committees salaried physician executives who are not dependent on referrals from physicians being evaluated

As instructed by the U.S. Supreme Court, if physician peer reviewers are still not satisfied with the protections afforded by the *Patrick* decision, then they may look to Congress—specifically to the protections from federal antitrust immunity following from compliance with the Health Care Quality Improvement Act of 1986.[62]

The Health Care Quality Improvement Act of 1986. In an attempt to minimize the problem of unqualified physicians hopping from state to state and to improve the process of physician credentialing in general, Congress, on November 14, 1986, passed the Health Care Quality Improvement Act. This act, in conjunction with the Medicare and Medicaid Patient Protection Act of 1987 and the Social Security Amendments of 1987, created a National Practitioner Data Bank, which will collect, store, and release information on the nation's six million health care practitioners, including the following:

1. The details of any professional liability actions filed against them following the implementation of the bank
2. The circumstances behind any licensure restrictions
3. Whether they have had their staff or clinical privileges restricted for a period of more than 30 days at any hospital or other health care entity
4. The facts behind any professional society membership loss or restriction

Hospitals and other health care entities must access this information concerning all physicians and nonphysician health care practitioners whenever these persons are subject to credentialing or recredentialing. Failure to do so will result in the hospital or health care entity losing the act's limited federal antitrust immunity provisions. In any corporate liability or similar action it will be presumed that the hospital or other health care entity has knowledge of these practitioners' credentials (or relative lack thereof).

The hospital must also request information from the clearinghouse routinely, every 2 years, concerning all licensed health care practitioners with medical staff membership or clinical privileges at the hospital.

The act allows the Secretary of Health and Human Services by regulation to provide for disclosure of clearinghouse information affecting a particular physician or health care practitioner, to that person. Procedures would also be established for disputing the accuracy of such information. The act enables parties involved in medical malpractice actions, including plaintiffs' attorneys, to obtain access to information held by the clearinghouse.

Risk management principles

One area in which risk management is particularly necessary involves exclusive contracts between hospitals and physicians. They are usually permissible; however, they must have rational reasons to support their existence. Legitimate reasons for exclusive contracts include (but are not limited to) the following:

1. Controlling the efficient administration of a specific type of medical service
2. Limiting the department's size to cope with bed limitations and the hospital's overall mission
3. Maintaining the economics of hospital operations
4. Optimizing the effective use of personnel and technologies by having such controlled by only one physician group

5. Promoting uniform teaching and research methodologies
6. Limiting the utilization of certain technological equipment to those most qualified

When negotiating exclusive contracts, it is usually unwise to specify too narrowly in the contract language the reasons for entering into the exclusive arrangement. Overspecification might restrict the hospital's maneuverability in the event that the exclusive contract is challenged on specific antitrust grounds. The exclusive contract should delineate reasons for its existence, but it is better to frame these reasons in general terms, such as those specified in the previous paragraph. Similarly, it is better to specify several reasons for the exclusive arrangement rather than merely one reason. Some attorneys believe it may be best simply to use broad language supporting the hospital's goal of optimal medical care within the limitations of the facilities and resources available.

Hospitals and their staff physicians have become more economically interdependent than ever. Both must be continually conscious of how their present health care practice styles may economically affect their ability to continue to provide high-quality care in the future. A hospital's ability to compete effectively will soon be related directly to its ability to influence the economic aspects of its physicians' medical practice styles. Similarly, a physician's ability to compete effectively will soon depend on his or her ability to gain ready access to the extensive resources of at least one economically viable hospital with state-of-the-art technology and high-quality personnel.

Hospitals have a legal right and duty to maximize the quality of care provided on the one hand, but they also must afford certain safeguards to physicians in the appointment and reappointment process. The key to minimizing litigation is to strike a delicate balance between the private rights of physicians to practice medicine and the public rights of patients to reasonable medical care.

Hospitals (and physicians) face unprecedented economic pressures to compete effectively in a buyer's market. Exclusive arrangements between hospitals and physicians in an attempt to insulate themselves from this free market competition may subject them to the risk of treble damages arising from Sherman Act Section 1 or 2 violations. These arrangements must be reasonable in light of the practices of comparable institutions, local market conditions, and the medical as opposed to the economic motivations behind such agreements.

The practice of medicine in America is in the midst of an unprecedented economic transformation. This metamorphosis will carry into the next century. The traditional providers, including inpatient hospitals and fee-for-service private practitioners, must take the lead to respond to this changing environment. These providers have the unique skills and resources that permit them to compete effectively with virtually any new alternative health care delivery system, without compromising the quality of care or the integrity of the medical profession.

*Hospital privileges and due process**

Because of the increasing number of practicing physicians[63] and expanding theories of liability against hospitals based on the granting of privileges[64] or the failure to restrict or revoke privileges,[65] there are now a significant number of judicial decisions dealing with the entire privileging process. What follows discusses the legal issues involved with special emphasis on the due process rights that must be accorded to a physician when his or her[66] privileges are denied, reduced, or revoked.

The nature of a physician's interest in hospital privileges. As mentioned, the great majority of physicians need hospital facilities for the pursuit of their profession.[67] Although a physician does not have a constitutional right to practice medicine in a hospital,[68] the obtaining of a medical degree and a license to practice medicine does give the physician a property interest that is given certain constitutional protection. In *Anton v. San Antonio Community Hospital,*[69] the court described this interest as follows: "The essential nature of a qualified physician's right to use the facilities of the hospital is a property interest which directly relates to the pursuit of his livelihood."[70] The court in *Unterhiner v. Desert Hospital District of Palm Springs*[71] stated: "A doctor who has been licensed by the state to practice medicine has a vested right to practice his profession and it cannot be said that there are no elements of a right to be admitted to a hospital."[72] Because the states and their subdivisions are prohibited by the United States Constitution from depriving any person of property without due process of law,[73] a hospital must afford a physician substantive and procedural due process when it acts with regard to his or her hospital privileges.[74]

PRIVATE VERSUS PUBLIC HOSPITALS. Numerous decisions have dealt with the distinction between private and public hospitals.[75] When a public hospital is involved there is no question that the hospital is acting as an agency of the state.[76] In cases involving a private hospital there usually must be a finding that the hospital's actions constituted state action or were done under color of state law.[77] This requirement of state action has been found where the hospital receives substantial federal or state funds,[78] licensing by the state,[79] or even contributions from the public during the hospital's annual fund drive.[80] Some courts have chosen to focus on the responsibilities of the hospital rather than the rights of the physicians and have held that a private hospital occupies a fiduciary trust relationship between itself, the medical staff, and the public, and the actions of the hospital are, therefore, subject to judicial review.[81] In cases involving judicial review of hospital decisions regarding privileges, California has done away with the distinction between private and public hospitals altogether.[82]

A significant number of federal court decisions hold that denial of privileges by a private health care provider is not sufficiently regulated or controlled by the state to invoke federal jurisdiction.[83] Nevertheless, it is becoming clear that regardless of whether the hospital concerned is public or private, a physician has a federally protected right to due process[84] and the right to be free from arbitrary action on the part of a hospital.[85]

INITIAL PRIVILEGES VERSUS EXISTING PRIVILEGES. The majority of decided cases dealing with hospital privileges involve a physician whose previously granted privileges are revoked or reduced.[86] Some cases, however, deal with the physician's rights on initial application for privileges.[87] It has been pointed out that a physician who has had privileges has more of a "vested interest than one who is newly applying."[88] In California, the extent and nature of judicial review depend on whether the decision of the hospital involved an initial application or existing privileges. In cases involving existing privileges, the court is to make an independent judgment review in determining whether the decision of the hospital is supported by the weight of the evidence. In cases involving new applications, the court is to make a substantial evidence review to determine whether the decision of the hospital is supported by substantial evidence in light of the whole record.[89] Even though a physician applying for new privileges may have less of a vested interest than one who has already been granted privileges, the physician must be afforded due process that is adequate to safeguard the physician's interest in pursuing his or her profession, and the hospital cannot act arbitrarily or discriminatorily with regard to his or her application.[90]

The physician's due process rights in hospital proceedings. Hospital proceedings that affect a physician's privileges usually occur on four different levels. At the first level there may be a complaint brought against a physician who already has privileges by a patient, another physician, the administrator of the hospital, or the board of directors.[91] At the second level a committee of the hospital, usually the credentials committee when a new application for privileges is involved, or the executive committee of the medical staff where existing privileges are involved, conducts an inquiry into whether the subject physician's privileges should be granted, denied, restricted, or revoked. No reported cases have been found that give the physician any due process rights at these two levels. Once a decision has been made by a committee or other authority within the hospital that may adversely affect the physician's present or requested privileges, the physician should be given the following due process rights.

NOTIFICATION OF THE ADVERSE RECOMMENDATION. Once an adverse recommendation has been made that, if approved by higher authority, will result in denial, revocation, or restriction of a physician's privileges, the physician must be

---

*From Hagerman, 13 L.A.M.P. 51 (July 1985).

notified and informed of his or her right to request a hearing before a panel established to review his or her privileges or application for privileges.[92]

WRITTEN NOTICE OF THE CHARGES. If the physician requests a hearing, then he or she must be given written notice of the charges that will be presented against him or her at the hearing.[93] The charges must be sufficiently specific to give the physician adequate notice of the nature of the charges.[94] A few courts have noted with apparent approval the practice of providing the physician with the hospital chart numbers of those cases that substantiate the charges against him or her.[95] Although this may be sufficient in view of the reasonable assumption that the physician can read his or her own charts, one court has said that the charges must state "in reasonable fullness the nature of the criticism in each case."[96]

ADEQUATE TIME TO PREPARE A DEFENSE. After the physician has been advised of the charges, he or she must be given adequate time to prepare a defense.[97] The time interval between notification and the hearing date will necessarily vary somewhat according to the circumstances and the extent and complexity of the charges that the physician must defend against.

PREHEARING DISCOVERY. The physician or the physician's attorney sometimes wishes to conduct discovery before the hearing before the panel. Courts have reached different decisions on this issue depending on the nature of the discovery sought. In *Garrow v. Elizabeth General Hospital,*[98] the court held that the information that was relied on in making the adverse recommendation should be made available to the physician before the hearing so as to enable the physician to make adequate preparations for a defense. Similarly, in *Suckle v. Madison General Hospital,*[99] the court held that the physician had a right to access all relevant hospital and medical records during the period in which he was preparing a response to the charges. In cases where the discovery sought is more formal in nature, however, it has not been allowed.[100] This is in keeping with the often made statement that, in hospital due process proceedings, the physician is "not entitled to a full blown judicial trial."[101] In *Woodbury v. McKinnon,*[102] the physician involved was not allowed to conduct discovery by means of depositions and interrogatories to obtain evidence to support his contention that other members of the medical staff were not as good as he was.

A HEARING PANEL COMPOSED OF IMPARTIAL, FAIR-MINDED PHYSICIANS. The panel charged with the responsibility of giving the physician his or her due process hearing must be composed of physicians who are impartial and fair minded.[103] If any physician on the panel actively participated in the investigation of the subject physician or made the original adverse recommendation, then he or she will be subject to challenge on the grounds of bias or lack of impartiality.[104] In other words, if the functions of investigator, prosecutor, and judge are being carried out by the same person, then a fair hearing will be presumed to be unavailable and actual bias need not be shown.[105] Courts have recognized, however, that prior involvement by a hearing panel member on some other level will not disqualify that person from sitting on the panel if the involvement was not substantial and did not bring about the adverse recommendation under review.[106] The following additional factors have been identified as having a high probability of destroying impartiality: (1) the panel member has a direct pecuniary interest in the outcome; (2) the member has been personally involved in a dispute with the subject physician or has been the target of his criticism; or (3) the panel member is embroiled in other matters involving the physician whose rights he or she is determining.[107] As stated in *Applebaum v. Board of Directors:* "Biased decision makers are constitutionally impermissible and even the probability of unfairness is to be avoided."[108] If the hospital is a small one and the matter has been particularly vitriolic and disruptive, then consideration should be given to having physicians from outside the immediate hospital area sit on the hearing panel. It has been said, however, that the physician under review is "not entitled to a panel made up of outsiders or of physicians who had never heard of the case and who knew nothing about the facts of it or what they supposed the facts to be."[109]

In some instances the physician or his or her attorney has sought to *voir dire* the panel members to discover any bias or lack of impartiality. In *Duffield v. Charleston Area Medical Center, Inc.,*[110] the subject physician asked for and received permission to examine all members of the panel before the hearing began. The trial court in *Hackethal v. California Medical Association and San Bernadino County Medical Society*[111] concluded that the subject physician's *voir dire* of the panel members was unduly restricted, and this was found to be a denial of procedural due process. Because a physician has a vital interest in having a fair and impartial panel, it appears that he or she should have a reasonable opportunity to question the panel regarding any matters that may affect their objectivity or lack thereof.

APPEARANCE BEFORE THE PANEL. The right to personally appear before the decision-making panel and be heard has been held to be essential.[112] As stated in *Grannis v. Ordean:* "The fundamental requisite of due process of law is the opportunity to be heard."[113] The opportunity to speak on one's behalf must also be given at a time when it will be effective. As the court said in *Lew v. Kona Hospital,* "The fundamental requirement of due process is the opportunity to be heard at a meaningful time and in a meaningful manner."[114] Thus, in a case where all the proceedings leading up to a letter of termination of privileges were done in secret and without any opportunity to be heard, it was found that the physician had not received due process and his privileges were reinstated.[115]

ASSISTANCE OF LEGAL COUNSEL DURING HEARING. To date only one jurisdiction has recognized the right of a physician to be assisted by legal counsel in a hospital due process hearing. In *Garrow v. Elizabeth General Hospital*,[116] the Supreme Court of New Jersey examined the issue and found that in view of the physician's substantial interest in such proceedings, the ability of an attorney to marshal the evidence, counter adverse testimony, and present argument on the physician's behalf tipped the balance in favor of allowing the physician the right to an attorney at mandated hospital hearings.[117] The court also pointed out that the attorney would be subject to the control of the person in charge of the hearings.[118] A few courts have held that it should be within the discretion of the hearing panel as to whether legal counsel may attend the hearing and actively participate.[119] Other courts have noted the participation of counsel for the physician without indicating whether the allowance of counsel in such proceedings is required in order to satisfy due process.[120]

CROSS-EXAMINATION OF WITNESSES. Although some courts have held that a physician is not constitutionally entitled to cross-examine witnesses who testify against him or her at the hearing,[121] the better rule clearly appears to be that a physician does have the right to confront and cross-examine any witnesses who appear and testify against him or her.[122] Due process means fair procedure,[123] and to allow a witness to testify against the physician without being subject to cross-examination would certainly seem to violate the rules of fair play.

PRESENTATION OF WITNESSES AND EVIDENCE IN DEFENSE. The right of a physician to present witnesses and evidence in his or her own behalf has been clearly recognized.[124] This is an integral part of fundamental fairness that has been equated with procedural due process.[125]

TRANSCRIPT OF PANEL HEARING. It is advisable to have an accurate record made of the due process hearing so that any objections raised by the subject physician can be reviewed in a hospital appellate review of the panel's decision.[126] In addition, without an accurate record it may be difficult for a court to determine whether the physician was accorded due process at the hearing.

WRITTEN DECISION FROM PANEL. The decision of the panel should be written so that it can provide a record for hospital and judicial review.[127] A copy should be given to the physician.[128] In reaching its decision the panel must not rely on *ex parte* communications that were not made known to the physician in question, and the decision must be based on evidence that was presented at the hearing and to which the physician had an opportunity to respond.[129] The decision of the panel should be based on substantial evidence.[130]

The fourth level of hospital proceedings concerning a physician's privileges is appellate review of the decision of the hearing panel and a final decision by the governing authority. Hospital bylaws normally provide a mechanism whereby the physician can obtain review of the panel decision by an appellate review committee.[131] The physician is usually allowed to submit a written statement of his or her position to the committee, but the right to make an oral statement is within the discretion of the appellate review body.[132] New or additional evidence not raised during the due process hearing or otherwise reflected in the record will be allowed to be introduced at the appellate review level only under unusual circumstances.[133] After the appellate review committee issues its decision, the final decision must be made by the highest governing authority of the hospital. The final hospital decision is transmitted to the physician concerned, and the hospital proceedings are then complete.[134]

The scope of judicial review of hospital decisions. It is now well established that courts have jurisdiction to review hospital decisions that adversely affect a physician's privileges.[135] In addition to jurisdiction based on alleged violations of rights guaranteed by the Fifth and Fourteenth Amendments, federal courts often find jurisdiction under 42 U.S.C. § 1983[136] in conjunction with 28 U.S.C. § 1343(3).[137] However, the extent of judicial review in such cases is limited.[138] If the court finds that the physician was afforded due process in the hospital proceedings[139] and the hospital neither violated its bylaws[140] nor acted in an arbitrary or capricious manner,[141] the decision of the hospital will be upheld. This limited review is necessitated by the court's lack of medical expertise, as was pointed out in *Laje v. R.E. Thomason General Hospital:*

Judicial intervention must be limited to an assessment of those factors which are within the court's expertise to review. For this reason, our cases have gone no further than to require that the procedures employed by the hospital are fair, that the standards set by the hospital are reasonable, and that they have been applied without arbitrariness and capriciousness.[142]

It has also been said that "the decision of a hospital's governing body concerning the granting of hospital privileges is to be accorded great deference."[143] Therefore once the court has determined that the decision of the hospital is "supported by substantial evidence and was made using proper criteria, after a satisfactory hearing, on a rational basis, and without irrelevant, discriminatory and arbitrary influences, the work of the court comes to an end."[144]

Conclusion. In light of current judicial concepts of due process, it appears that the distinction between public and private hospitals will continue to lose viability where physicians' hospital privileges are concerned. It is also expected that more jurisdictions will follow New Jersey in allowing the physician to be represented by counsel at the due process hearing. Because the panel hearing is by far the most important proceeding for the physician, this seems both sensible and fair.

Although a physician applying for privileges may be seen as having less of a vested interest than one who has previously enjoyed them, it is apparent that both are equally entitled to due process. In every case the hospital must be guided by fundamental fairness; keep in mind the words of the U.S.

Supreme Court in *Hannah v. Larche:* "Due process is an elusive concept. Its exact boundaries are undefinable, and its content varies according to specific factual contexts."[145]

Hospital-required malpractice insurance*

The increased number of suits against health care providers, the increased number of health care providers in each suit, and the increased amount of awards and settlements have created unrest, tension, and distrust between hospitals and their medical staff. Physicians have a decerebrate posturing response to being named in a malpractice suit. They have a lesser "knee-jerk" response when having to pay malpractice insurance premiums. Hospitals are developing the same responses because of escalating malpractice premiums and claims. Their corporate assets are being threatened. Their costs continue to escalate. The inevitable government regulation that results has added to their problems. When the hospital requires insurance for staff privileges, the effect is similar to adding sodium to water. The resulting explosion not only damages the hospital and its medical staff, but also involves the legal community, the state and federal legislature, and ultimately, as always, the public.

The National Association of Insurance Companies' 1975 to 1978 study showed that more than 70% of paid claims are a result of physician activity occurring in the hospital.[146] Hospitals have increasing legal "corporate responsibility" for physician activities. The trustees of hospitals have "fiduciary responsibility" to maintain corporate assets. Joint and several liability makes hospitals the "deep pocket" for uninsured or poorly insured physician staff members.

Physicians have not only patient care requirements, but also hospital-related functions such as teaching, emergency care, emergency coverage, and committee functioning, especially in credentialing and policy making. The line between physician patient care activity and hospital patient care activity becomes more and more indistinct. Hospitals and their physician staff look to each other for support but once sued, look to each other for money. This is a major problem that is frequently solved by hospitals paying more than their fair share to the injured patient.

Is mandatory fiscal responsibility as a requirement for staff privileges a viable answer? In some states hospitals require this, and in some states the requirement is linked with licensure. We shall discuss what happens with the two approaches. In the mid-1970s in response to the "malpractice crisis," Alaska, Hawaii, Idaho, Kansas, Kentucky, North Dakota, and Pennsylvania all required physicians to carry professional liability insurance as a condition of obtaining and maintaining licensure. In Hawaii, the Hawaii Medical Association sought to enjoin the state from enforcing the malpractice insurance requirement against them by a preliminary injunction.[147] This suit was dismissed but the licensing board did not enforce

*From Goebert, 13 L.A.M.P. 1 (Nov 1985).

the requirement, so the next year Hawaii legislatively deleted it. Also, Alaska repealed the requirement in 1978.[148] Now individual hospitals are reacting by requiring financial responsibility as a condition for staff privileges.

Kentucky and North Dakota ruled the requirement unconstitutional. Kentucky found the statute a violation of due process.[149] The legislature had arbitrarily imposed and restricted the practice of medicine, mainly because all health care providers were being considered inherently negligent or financially irresponsible. There had not been a legislative finding that such was the case. On the other hand, in North Dakota the State Supreme Court found all statutory malpractice changes unconstitutional.[150] When addressing the mandatory insurance provision, the court specifically withheld a final decision but did have serious doubts as to the constitutionality of requiring malpractice insurance for all physicians without regard to their ability to pay when the law was silent on the effect of some physicians' inability to pay the premiums.

On the other hand, Pennsylvania, Idaho, and Kansas courts ruled in favor of the law. Pennsylvania stated that there existed a rational relationship between requiring insurance and the public interest in ensuring compensability.[151] There is no unconstitutional denial of equal protection nor a prohibition against pursuing one's occupation. The Idaho Supreme Court remanded the malpractice statutes back to the lower courts for further investigation, but they had no problem stating that protection to patients who may be injured as a result of medical malpractice is in the public welfare and compulsory insurance is constitutional.[152] The Kansas Supreme Court also found its statute constitutional.

These cases are important because they give the legal arguments both pro and con for allowing a state to specifically regulate the medical profession by requiring insurance. They address the right to engage in a lawful occupation, the police power of the state, and substantive due process of individuals guaranteed by the constitution. Some courts required only a rational reason for the legislature to require insurance. Other states require a more serious constitutional scrutiny than the rational basis analysis, because the regulation is not truly related to competence and places some burden on the individual's right to engage in a lawful profession. Close scrutiny will balance the respective interest of both the physician and the public.[153]

Can hospitals require malpractice insurance as a condition of privileges? Yes, but in the absence of a statute, state hospitals would have the same type of scrutiny placed on them as state statutes had in the preceding paragraphs. In an earlier case, a California hospital that required malpractice insurance as a condition of admission was challenged successfully. The rule was arbitrary and not related to the state's regulation of physicians.[154] Following this case, the California legislature passed a law allowing hospitals to require malpractice insurance, and this was found constitutional.[155] In 1977, a survey of U.S. community hospitals showed that out of 4478 hospitals, 26.4% required physicians to have a minimum amount of malpractice insurance.[156]

When private hospitals require malpractice insurance for staff privileges, physicians present a number of arguments.[157] First is "state action" because the private hospital is receiving either state or federal funds; therefore the court has jurisdiction to determine whether an impermissible imposition infringed on constitutional rights of the physicians' civil rights.[158] The physicians will allege a breach of contract action because hospital privileges were given for a longer length of time. The hospital is taking away privileges without showing that the physician is unqualified or unskilled. Many of the physicians have been members of hospital committees and have been on the teaching staffs of universities, and all have state licensure. Some arguments show a violation of the antitrust provisions of the Sherman Act if any of the deciding physicians involved with denying privileges are in competition with the physician being restricted.[159]

A number of cases have addressed the question of a hospital acting under the color of state law. These have found that the specific activity complained of by the physician being denied privileges must be related to the way that the state is acting on the private hospital. There must be a nexus between state action and denial of privileges. These cases show that the granting of funds from Hill-Burton monies, Medicaid, Medicare payments, training of residents from state institutional programs, use of tax-free bonds, hospital licensure and inspection by the state, and reporting of privileges revocations to a state board all are state actions or federal actions; but none have a required nexus. The restricted physician must show that those state actions have something to do with a denial of privileges when the physician does not have insurance.[160-162] The due process hearings required in civil rights actions under U.S.C. §§ 1983 have not been upheld, but state courts have said that hospitals need to show or need to give due process to physicians before a revocation of privileges.[163] The test in these cases is whether a hospital acts arbitrarily and capriciously or denies the physician due process. Physicians have also argued that they are unable to afford the insurance, that they do not have a big enough practice, or that they have an indigent patient population in their practice and therefore the public will suffer.[164-166]

Hospitals argue, on the other hand, that this is not arbitrary and capricious. It is rational policy supported by good fiscal management and preservation of the hospital resources.[167] The requirement is not excessively burdensome and can be met by providing insurance or fiscal responsibility. The hospital must be able to show that it has done everything necessary to obtain facts supporting the policy. Meetings with concerned individuals, a review by the medical staff executive committee, surveys of the physicians, letters to other hospitals and to insurance people finding out the costs and alternatives, and attempts at legislative tort reform are all things that would be helpful to a hospital initiating these actions.

The courts have supported and allowed the hospitals to initiate such action. Florida,[168] Arizona,[169] Louisiana,[170] and Indiana[171] have all heard arguments both pro and con and ruled in favor of the hospital and against the restricted physician as long as procedural due process and prior notice was afforded to the physician. Physicians scream, but the courts have not listened.[172,173]

Courts have addressed the California legislative policy of allowing a hospital to require malpractice insurance, and they have stated that the interests of society that are served by such insurance requirement are not so arbitrary that it would be considered unreasonable. The amount of insurance established by the hospital and the requirement that the insurance company must be admitted to do business in California were reasonable.[174]

The final argument in favor of this policy is that the real reason for such a policy is the requirement that the hospital pay its fair share of liability and the physician pay his or her fair share of liability. In Holmes, the situation is summarized as follows:

We cannot ignore the realities of modern procedural practice. If a patient is injured while in the hospital regardless of who is at fault, the hospital will almost always be joined as a codefendant. Despite the outcome of such an action, the hospital must expend valuable financial resources in its own defense, and will, if innocent of wrongdoing, be more likely to recover its expenses from the tortfeasor physician if that physician is insured. If, indeed, some conscientious lawyer decides not to include the hospital in an action where the finger of negligence points directly and solely to the doctor, we can be certain it will only be because the physician does indeed have malpractice insurance.[175]

The hospital has the right to take reasonable measures to protect itself and the patient it serves. We cannot say, as a matter of law, that the hospital board's attention to its medical staff's malpractice insurance is unlawful, arbitrary, or capricious. As a practical matter, we cannot say it is irrational or unreasonable. In Pollack, the court states:

We find the plaintiff (physician) has no liberty or property interest sufficient to invoke the due process requirements of the Fourteenth Amendment. While the right to practice an occupation is a liberty interest protected by the Fourteenth Amendment, . . . plaintiff is not precluded from exercising that right by the insurance requirements in order to continue his membership on the hospital staff. . . . Requiring its staff physicians to carry insurance and to submit proof to the hospital of that fact is surely a reasonable exercise of financial responsibility on the part of the hospital.[176]

Basically, the hospital has three alternatives regarding malpractice insurance:

1. To use the information regarding the physician's malpractice as one of the criteria to decide on appointment or reappointment

2. To require malpractice coverage as a condition of appointment or reappointment

3. To take no policy position

The first two of these alternatives are legally permitted. The last does not solve the problem. The hospital can avoid much internal stress by recognizing that this problem is a shared or joint problem with the medical staff. The hospital should involve the staff in trying to solve the problem. Alternatives can be searched for and harmony fostered.

ENDNOTES

1. *Darling v. Charleston Community Hosp.,* 200 N.E. 2d 149 (Ill. Sup. Ct. 1965); *Elam v. College Park Hosp.,* 183 Cal. Rptr. 156 (1982); *Corletto v. Shore Memorial Hosp.,* 350 A. 2d 534 (N.J. Sup. Ct. 1975).

2. D. M. Eddy, *Clinical Decision Making: From Theory to Practice—The Challenge,* 1 J.A.M.A. 287-290 (1990).

3. *See* e.g., *Wall v. Stout,* 310 N.C. 184, 192, 311 S.E. 2d 571 (1984); also see *Physicians, Surgeons, Etc.,* 61 Am. Jur. 2d §167, 298-299 (1981).

4. Pub. L. 99-660, part IV; 42 U.S.C. § 11111 et seq.

5. *Brownsville Medical Center v. Garcia,* 704 S.W. 2d 68 (Tex. App. Corpus Christi 1985).

6. *Smith v. Baptist Memorial Hosp. System,* 720 S.W. 2d 618 (Tex. App. San Antonio 1986, writ ref. n.r.e.).

7. *Corletto, supra note 1*

8. Joint Commission on Accreditation of Healthcare Organizations, *Accreditation Manual for Hospitals,* Standard M.S. 6 et seq. (JCAHO, Chicago 1990).

9. *Supra* note 4.

10. *McDonald v. Massachusetts General Hosp.,* 120 Mass. 432, 21 A. 529 (1876).

11. *Schloendorff v. New York Hosp.,* 211 N.Y. 125, 105 N.E. 92 (1914).

12. *Id.* at 132 and 194.

13. *Necolaff v. Genessee Hosp.,* 296 N.Y.S. 936, 73 N.E. 2d 117 (1947).

14. *Berg v. N.Y. Society for the Relief of the Ruptured and Crippled,* 154 N.Y.S. 455, 456 (1956).

15. *Bing v. Thunig,* 2 N.Y. 2d 656, 143 N.E. 2d 3 (1957). But see *Weiss v. Rubin,* 9 N.Y. 2d 230, 173 N.E. 2d 791, (1961) in which the Court of Appeals found that the surgeon had a duty to inquire into details of how the hospital performed its duty (providing blood for transfusion) as part of his duty of reasonable care. Justice Van Voorhis' dissent called for strict application of *Bing.*

16. Cf. generally, *supra* note 8, at Medical Staff Section.

17. *Johnson v. Misericordia County Hosp.,* 99 Wis. 2d 708, 301 N.W. 2d 156 (1981), *aff'd,* 99 Wis. 2d 78, 301 N.W. 2d 156 (1981). The Wisconsin Supreme Court also held that a hospital has a legal duty to its patients to exercise reasonable care in selecting its medical staff and in granting privileges but, in *Humana Medical Corp v. Peyer,* 456 N.W.2d 355 (1990) declined to find or establish an ancillary duty requiring a hospital to disclose credentialing information to a third party.

18. *Weiss v. York Hosp.,* 745 F. 2d 786 (1984).

19. *Tonsic v. Wagner,* 329 A. 2d 497 (Pa. 1974).

20. *McConnell v. Williams,* 361 Pa. 355, 65 A. 2d 243 (1949). But see J. Jones' dissent, in *Yorston v. Pennell,* 153 A. 2d 255 (1959), which would have circumscribed application of this rule to matters only within the directing physician's responsibility.

21. *Capan v. Divine Providence Hosp.,* 410 A. 2d 1282 (Pa. Super. Ct. 1979).

22. *People v. Flushing Hosp. and Medical Center,* 471 N.Y.S. 2d 745 (N.Y. Cir. Ct. 1983), where the hospital was charged with a misdemeanor when it refused emergency care because the hospital was full; *People ex rel. M.B.,* 312 N.W. 2d 714 (S.D. 1981), where the South Dakota Supreme Court ruled that a lower court exceeded its jurisdiction by ordering an admission when no space was available; *contra, see Pierce*

County Office of Involuntary Commitment v. Western State Hosp., 97 Wash. 2d 264, 644 P. 2d 131 (1982), where the Washington Supreme Court interpreted a state mental health statute to require admission of all patients who sought treatment at the hospital, despite a lack of space.

23. *See,* e.g., *Fabian v. Matzko,* 236 Pa. Super. 267, 344 A. 2d 569 (1975).

24. *Wilmington General Hosp. v. Manlove,* 54 Del. 15, 174 A. 2d 135 (1961).

25. *Stanturf v. Sipes,* 447 S.W. 2d 558 (Mo. 1969).

26. *Id.* 4475.W. 2d, at 562.

27. Restatement (Second) of Agency §220 (1958).

28. *See,* e.g., *Smith v. St. Francis Hosp.,* 676 P. 2d 279 (Okla. App. 1983). However, Oklahoma's Supreme Court extended this reasoning, applying the patient's perception of whether the hospital merely served as the physician's work site, to avoid finding respondeat superior was applicable. *See Weldon v. Seminole Muni.,* Hospital, 709 P. 2d 1058 (Okla. 1985).

29. *Thomas v. Corso,* 265 Md. 84, 288 A. 2d 379 (1972).

30. *Citizens Hosp. Ass'n. v. Schoulin,* 48 Ala. App. 101, 262 So. 2d 303 (1972).

31. *Gizzi v. Texaco, Inc.,* 437 F. 2d 308 (3d Cir. 1971).

32. *See* F. Harper, F. James, Jr., & O. Gray, Law of Torts 26.11, 60-94 (2d ed. 1986) for a discussion of the immunity rule and its exception.

33. *Marek v. Professional Health Services, Inc.,* 179 N.J. Super. 433, 437 A. 2d 538 (1981).

34. *Jackson v. Power,* 743 P. 2d 1376 (Alaska 1987). In a comparison case, *Harding v. Sisters of Providence,* no. 371 (Alaska, Oct 16, 1987), liability was extended to an independent contractor/radiologist's negligence on the basis of a nondelegable duty owed by the hospital to its patients. Distinguished: *Miltiron v. Franke,* 793 P. 2d 824 (1990).

35. W. Prosser & W. Keeton, Law of Torts §71 at 511-512 (5th ed. 1984).

36. *Guerro v. Copper Queen Hosp.,* 112 Ariz. 104, 537 P. 2d 1329 (1975). *Thompson v. Sun City Community Hospital,* 688 P. 2d 647, (1983).

37. 42 U.S.C. §1395dd (Apr. 7, 1986).

38. *Darling v. Charleston Memorial Hosp.,* 33 Ill. 2d 326, 211 N.E. 2d 253 (1965); *cert. denied* 383 U.S. 946 (1966). Distinguish this situation from that in *Weldon, supra* note 28, wherein the patient's care "was never within the discretion of the hospital."

39. *Fiorentino v. Wagner,* 227 N.E. 2d. 296 (1967).

40. *Moore v. Board of Trustees of Carson City Hosp.,* 495 P. 2d 605 (Nev. 1972).

41. *Mitchell City Hosp. Authority v. Joiner,* 229 Ga. 140, 109 S.E. 2d 413 (1972). *Butler v. South Fenton Med. Center,* 215 Ga. App. 809, 452 S.E. 2d 768 (1994).

42. *Purcell v. Zimbleman,* 18 Ariz. App. 75, 500 P. 2d 335 (1972).

43. *Corletto v. Shore Memorial Hospital,* 138 N.J. Super. 302, 350 A. 2d 534 (1975).

44. *Hayman v. Galveston,* 273 U.S. 414, (1927).

45. *Porter Memorial Hosp. v. Harvy,* 279 N.E. 2d 583 (1972).

46. *Lubin v. Crittenden Hosp. Ass'n.,* 713 F. 2d 414 (8th Cir. 1983).

47. *Cardiomedical Assoc. v. Crozier-Chester Med. Ctr.,* 536 F. Supp. 1065 (E.D. Pa. 1982).

48. *Northeast Georgia Radiological Assoc. v. Tidwell,* 670 F. 2d 507 (5th Cir. 1982). In *Bellam v. Clayton County Hospital* the U.S. District Court limited this principle to instances in which the privilege was terminated or withdrawn, declining to apply it where a privilege was just restricted. But see *Bloom v. Hennepin County,* 783 F. Supp. 418 (D. Minn. 1992), in which the court determined that there was no right to due process arising out of revocation of privileges, when the plaintiff held the privileges pursuant to the bylaws and a contract with the hospital, which was terminated.

49. *Klinge v. Lutheran Charities Ass'n. of St. Louis,* 523 F. 2d 56 (8th Cir. 1975).

50. *Silver v. Castle Memorial Hosp.,* 53 Haw. 475, 497 P. 2d 564, *cert. denied* 409 U.S. 1048 (1972).

51. *Christhilf v. Annapolis Emergency Hosp. Ass'n., Inc.,* 496 F. 2d 174 (4th Cir. 1974).

52. *Id.*

53. *Garrow v. Elizabeth General Hosp.,* 79 N.J. 549, 401 A. 2d 533 (1979).

54. *Supra* note 49, at 60.

55. *Branch v. Hempstead County Memorial Hosp.,* 539 F. Suppl. 908 (W.D. Ark. 1982).

56. California Medical Association-California Hospital Association, Uniform Code of Hearing and Appeal Procedures §3(e).

57. *Novosel v. Nationwide Insurance Co.,* 721 F. 2d 894 (1983).

58. *Cardiomedical Association, Ltd., v. Crozier-Chester Med. Ctr.,* 721 F. 2d 68 (1983).

59. *Jefferson Parish Hosp. District No. 2 v. Hyde, M.D.,* 466 U.S. 2 (1984).

60. *Supra* note 18.

61. *Patrick v. Burget,* 486 U.S. 94 (1988).

62. Health Care Quality Improvement Act of 1986 (Pub. L. 99-660, as amended by Pub. L. 100-93 and 100-177).

63. Tarlov, *Special Report, Shattuck Lecture: The Increasing Supply of Physicians—The Changing Structure of the Health-Services System and the Future Practice of Medicine,* 308 N. Engl. J. Med. 1235 (1983).

64. *Supra* note 17; Annot. 51 A.L.R. 3d 981 (1973).

65. *Supra* note 42; *Elam v. College Park Hosp.,* 132 Cal. App. 3d 332, 183 Cal. Rptr. 156, *modified,* 133 Cal. App. 3d 94 (1982).

66. Hereinafter "his" refers to members of either sex.

67. *See Falcone v. Middlesex County Medical Society,* 34 N.J. 582, 170 A. 2d 791 (1961).

68. *Supra* note 44; *Sosa v. Bd. of Managers of Val Verde Memorial Hosp.,* 437 F. 2d 173 (5th Cir. 1971).

69. *Anton v. San Antonio Comm. Hosp.,* 19 Cal. 3d 802, 140 Cal. Rptr. 442, 567 P. 2d 1162 (1977).

70. *Id.* at 814, 140 Cal. Rptr. at 454, 567 P. 2d at 1174.

71. *Unterthiner v. Desert Hosp. Dist. of Palm Springs,* 33 Cal. 3d 285. 188 Cal. Rptr. 590, 656 P. 2d 554 (1983).

72. *Id.* at 297, 188 Cal. Rptr. at 598, 656 P. 2d at 562.

73. U.S. Constitution, amend. V, XIV.

74. *Supra* notes 49 and 51; *Woodbury v. McKinnon,* 447 F. 2d 839 (5th Cir. 1971).

75. *See,* e.g., *supra* note 50 and cases cited therein; *The Physician's Right to Hospital Staff Membership: The Public-Private Dichotomy,* 485 Wash. U.L.Q. (1966).

76. *Foster v. Mobile County Hosp. Bd.,* 398 F. 2d 227 (5th Cir. 1938).

77. *See,* e.g., *Suckle v. Madison Gen. Hosp.,* 362 F.Supp. 1196 (W.D. Wis 1973), *aff'd,* 499 F. 2d 1364 (7th Cir. 1974).

78. *Supra* note 51.

79. *Schlein v. Milford Hosp.,* 423 F. Supp. 541 (D. Conn. 1976). The Second Circuit United States Court of Appeals declined to adopt this case because it applies to the reasoning that clinical privileges do not create property interests. *See Greenwood v. New York,* 163 F. 3d 119 (2d Cir. 1998).

80. *Sussman v. Overlook Hosp. Ass'n.,* 231 A. 2d 389, 95 N.J. Super. 418 (1967).

81. *Supra* notes 50 and 53; *Greisman v. Newcomb Hosp.,* 40 N.J. 389, 192 A. 2d 817 (1963).

82. *Supra* note 69; *Ascherman v. St. Francis Memorial Hosp.,* 45 Cal. App. 3d 507, 119 Cal. Rptr. 507 (1975).

83. *Supra* notes 46 and 47, and cases cited therein.

84. *Supra* notes 48 and 49.

85. *Citta v. Delaware Valley Hosp.,* 313 F.Supp. 301 (E.D. Pa. 1970); *Avol v. Hawthrone Comm. Hosp. Inc.,* 135 Cal. App. 3d 101, 184 Cal. Rptr. 914 (1982); *Kelly v. St. Vincent Hosp.,* 102 N.M. 201, 692 P. 2d 1350 (1984).

86. *See generally,* Comment, *Hospital Medical Staff Privileges: Recent Developments in Procedural Due Process Requirements,* 12 Willamette L.J. 137 (1975).

87. Sosa, *supra* note 68; *supra* notes 71, 76, 79, and 80.

88. *Supra* note 71.

89. *Supra* notes 69 and 71.

90. *Supra* notes 71, 76, 79, and 80.

91. Avol, *supra* note 85.

92. *Supra* note 50; *see* JCAHO, *Accreditation Manual for Hospitals,* Standards for Medical Staff, standard III, 104 (JCAHO, Chicago 1995); California Medical Association-California Hospital Association, *Uniform Code of Hearing and Appeal Procedures,* 32 (1972).

93. *Supra* notes 51 and 53.

94. *Supra* notes 50 and 77. However, specificity that amounts to pleading of evidence is not constitutionally required. *Truly v. Madison Gen. Hosp.,* 673 F. 2d 763 (5th Cir. 1982).

95. *Supra* note 74; *Branch v. Hempstead County Memorial Hosp.,* 539 F.Supp. 908 (W.D. Ark. 1982); *supra* note 69.

96. Woodbury, *supra* note 77, at 1211.

97. *Supra* note 51; *Miller v. Eisenhower Med. Ctr.,* 27 Cal. 3d 614, 166 Cal. Rptr. 826, 614 P. 2d 258 (1980); *supra* note 50.

98. *Supra* note 53.

99. *Supra* note 77.

100. Woodbury, *supra* note 74; *Hackethal v. California Med. Ass'n. and San Bernardino County Medical Society,* 138 Cal. App. 3d 435, 187 Cal. Rptr. 811 (1982).

101. *Supra* note 49, at 60.

102. Woodbury, *supra* note 74.

103. *Supra* note 49; *Citta, supra* note 85; *Hackenthal, supra* note 100; *Applebaum v. Board of Directors,* 104 Cal. App. 3d 648, 163 Cal. Rptr. 831 (1980).

104. *See, e.g.,* Applebaum, *supra* note 103.

105. Citta, *supra* note 85.

106. *Duffield v. Charleston Area Med. Ctr., Inc.,* 503 F. 2d 512 (4th Cir. 1974); *Hoberman v. Lock Haven Hosp.,* 377 F. Supp. 1178 (M.D. Pa. 1974).

107. Hackethal, *supra* note 100; Applebaum, *supra* note 103.

108. Applebaum, *supra* note 103, at 104 Ca. App. 3d at 657, 163 Cal. Rptr., at 840.

109. *Supra* note 49, at 63.

110. Duffield, *supra* note 106.

111. Hackethal, *supra* note 100.

112. *Supra* note 51; *Poe v. Charlotte Memorial Hosp., Inc.,* 374 F. Supp. 1302 (W.D. N.C. 1974).

113. *Grannis v. Ordean,* 234 U.S. 385, 394, 34 S.Ct. 779, 783, 58 L.Ed. 1363, 1369 (1914).

114. *Lew v. Kona Hosp.,* 754 F. 2d 1420 at 1424 (9th Cir. 1985).

115. *Poe, supra* note 112.

116. *Supra* note 53.

117. *Id.*

118. *Id.*

119. *Supra* notes 50 and 69.

120. *Laje v. R.E. Thomason Gen. Hosp.,* 564 F. 2d 1159 (5th Cir. 1977); Citta, *supra* note 85; Miller, *supra* note 97.

121. Woodbury, *supra* note 74; *Kaplan v. Carney,* 404 F. Supp. 161 (E.D. Mo. 1975); *supra* note 80; in *Woodbury* and *Kaplan* no witnesses testified.

122. *Supra* notes 50, 51, 55; Poe, *supra* note 112; Hackethal, *supra* note 100.

123. Poe, *supra* note 112.

124. *Supra* notes 50 and 55; Hackethal, *supra* note 100.

125. *Supra* note 53.

126. Section 3(e) of the California Medical Association-California Hospital Association *Uniform Code of Hearing and Appeal Procedures* provides: "Record of Hearing. The judicial review committee may maintain a record of the hearing by one of the following methods: a shorthand reporter present to make a record of the hearing, a recording, or minutes of the proceedings. The cost of such shorthand reporter shall be borne by the party requesting same."

127. *Supra* note 50.

128. See *supra* note 49, at 60.

129. Duffield, *supra* note 106; Suckle, *supra* note 94; *supra* note 50.

130. *Storrs v. Lutheran Hosp. & Homes Society of America,* 661 P. 2d 632 (Alaska 1983); *see* Laje, *supra* note 120; Sosa, *supra* note 87; Kaplan, *supra* note 121.

131. *See* Hershey & Purtell, Medical Staff Bylaws. Art. XVI (1985).

132. *Id.* at §16.6-2.

133. *Id.* at §16.6-5.

134. *See generally, supra* note 49.

135. *See,* e.g., *supra* notes 50, 51, and 53.

136. "Every person who, under color of any statute, ordinance, regulation, custom, or usage, of any state or territory, subjects, or causes to be subjected, any citizen of the United States or other person within the jurisdiction thereof to the deprivation of any rights, privileges, or immunities secured by the Constitution and laws, shall be liable to the party injured in an action at law, suit in equity, or other proper proceeding for redress."

137. *See,* e.g., *Daly v. Sprague,* 675 F. 2d 716 (5th Cir. 1982).

138. *Supra* notes 49, 50, and 114.

139. *See,* e.g., Woodbury, *supra* note 74.

140. *See,* e.g., *supra* note 48; *In re Murphy v. St. Agnes Hosp.,* 484 N.Y.S. 2d 40 (App Div 1985); however, failure to strictly comply with the by-laws will not be fatal if due process if given. Kaplan, *supra* note 121; Avol, *supra* note 85.

141. *See,* e.g., *supra* note 76.

142. Laje, *supra* note 120, at 1162.

143. *Id.; see* Hollowell, *Decisions about Hospital Staff Privileges: A Case for Judicial Deference,* 11 Law Med. and Health Care 118 (1983).

144. Woodbury, *supra* note 74, at 846.

145. *Hannah v. Larche,* 363 U.S. 420, 442, 80 S. Ct. 1502, 1514, 4 L. Ed. 2d 1307, 1321 (1960).

146. Bulletin of the American College of Surgeons (Mar. 1982).

147. *Hawaii Medical Ass'n. v. State of Hawaii,* No. 49777 (Hawaii, 1st Cir. Feb. 4, 1977): Haw. Rev. Stat. §§4538, 67136 (1976); Haw. Rev. Stat. §§4538, (1977).

148. Alaska Stat. §§08.64.215a (1976); repealed 1978 Alaska Sess. Laws §§40 ch. 177.

149. *McGuffy v. Hall,* 557 S.W. 2d 401 (Ky. 1977).

150. *Arenson v. Olson,* 270 N.W. 2d 125 (N.D. 1977).

151. *McCoy v. Commonwealth Board of Medical Education and Licensure,* 37 Pa. Comwlth. 530, 391 A. 2d 723.

152. *Jones v. State Board of Medicine,* 97 Idaho 859, *cert. denied* (1976).

153. These constitutional issues are thoroughly discussed in Muranaka, *Compulsory Medical Malpractice Insurance Statutes: An Approach in Determining Constitutionally,* 12 U.S.F.L. Rev. 599 (Summer 1978).

154. *Rosner v. Peninsula Hospital District,* 224 Cal. App. 2d 115 (1964).

155. *Wilklerson v. Madera Community Hosp.,* 192 Cal. Rptr. 593 (Cal. App. 1983).

156. Unpublished results prepared by D.L. Matthews, Projects Director, American Hospital Association Hospital Data Center, in Association with Andrew J. Korsak and Ross Mullner.

157. Propriety of Hospitals' Conditioning Physicians' Staff Privileges on his Carrying Professional Liability or Malpractice Insurance, 7 A.L.R. 4th 1238 (1981).

158. Action of Private Hospital as State Action under 42 U.S.C.S. §§1983 or Fourteenth Amendment, 42 A.L.R. Fed. 463.

159. *Watkins v. Mercy Hosp. Medical Center,* 520 F. 2d 894 (9th Cir. 1975).

160. *Pollack v. Methodist Hosp.,* 392 F.Supp. 393 (E.D. La. 1975).

161. *Kavka v. Edgewater Hosp., Inc.,* 586 F. 2d 59, *cert. denied* (7th Cir. 1978. reported sub nom, *Musso v. Suriano*).

162. *Asherman v. Presbyterian Hosp. of Pacific Medical Center, Inc.,* 507 F. 2d 1103 (9th Cir. 1974).

163. *Supra* note 50; *Silver v. Queen's Hosp.,* 63 Haw. 430, 629 P. 2d 1116 (1981).

164. Laird, *Requiring Liability Insurance Is Unfair,* Am. Med. News 20 (Apr 24, 1981).

165. Lufton, *Hospital Privileges Revoked: Malpractice Insurance Ruling Awaited,* Am. Med. News (Sept 4, 1981).

166. *Hospital Privileges, Restraint of Trade, and Professional Liability,* 10 Neurosurgery 285 (1982).

167. Sosa, *supra* note 68.

168. *Maxie v. Martin Memorial Hosp. Ass'n., Inc.,* No. 82330Ca (Fla. Cir. Ct. May 24, 1983).

169. *Holmes v. Maricopa,* 473 P. 2d 477 (Ariz. 1977).

170. *Supra* note 160.

171. *Renforth v. Fayette Memorial Hosp. Ass'n., Inc.,* 383 N.E. 2d 368 (Ind. Ct. App. 1978).

172. Doudera, *Can or Should a Hospital Require Its Medical Staff to Obtain Malpractice Insurance,* 6 Med. Legal News 16 (Summer 1978).

173. *Professional Liability Insurance as a Requirement for Medical Staff Privileges,* 10 Neurosurgery 788 (1982); *Professional Liability Insurance as a Condition for Staff Membership,* 80 J. Med. Soc. N.J. 334 (May 1983).

174. *Supra* note 155.

175. *Holmes v. Hoemaku Hosp.,* 573 P. 2d 477, (Ariz. 1977).

176. *Supra* note 160.

GENERAL REFERENCES

J. Couch & N. Caesar, *Physician Staff Privileges Disputes: A Risk Management Guide for Hospitals and Medical Staffs,* 81 Philadelphia Med. (Sept 1985).

J. Couch & N. Caesar, *Cooperation between Hospitals and Physicians for Better Cost Effective Medical Care Delivery: The Health Care Joint Venture,* 81 Philadelphia Med. (Oct 1985).

J. Couch, N. Caesar, & W. Steigman, *The Legal and Economic Significance of Hospital Medical Staff Appointments and Exclusions,* 81 Philadelphia Med. (Feb 1984).

J. Couch, N. Caesar, & W. Steigman, *The Effect of Some Recent Antitrust Decisions Regarding Hospital Medical Staff Privileges,* 81 Philadelphia Med. (June 1985).

C.D. Creech, *The Medical Review Committee Privilege: A Jurisdictional Survey,* 67 N.C.L. Rev. 179 (Nov 1988).

Furrow, *The Changing Role of the Law in Promoting Quality in Health Care: From Sanctioning Outlaws to Managing Outcomes,* 26 Hous. L. Rev. 147 (1989).

Gnessin, *Liability in the Managed Care Setting,* in *Practicing Law Institute Handbook Series: Managed Health Care in 1988—Legal and Operational Issues,* 471 PLI/Comm 405 (Sept 1, 1988).

Hall, *Institutional Control of Physician Behavior: Legal Barriers to Health Care Cost Containment,* 137 Pa. L. Rev. 431 (1988).

Harvard Law Review Association, *Antitrust-State Action-Private Parties Immune from Liability When Acting in an Official Capacity: Sandcrest Outpatient Services v. Cumberland County Hospital System,* 853 F. 2d 1139 (4th Cir. 1988), 102 Harv. L. Rev. 1080 (Mar 1989).

E. Hollowell, *The Medical Staff: An Integral Part of the Hospital or a Legal Entity Separate from the Hospital?* Presented at the Twenty-fifth Annual International Conference on Legal Medicine, New Orleans, La. (May 1985).

Joy, *The Health Care Quality Improvement Act of 1986: A Proposal for Interpretation of Its Protection,* 20 St. Mary's L.J. 955 (Oct. 1, 1989).

Rosenberg, *Independent Practice Associations: Moving toward an Integrated Medical Group Model,* 471 PLI/Comm 197.

A. Southwick, *Hospital Liability: Two Theories Have Been Merged,* 4 J. Legal Med. 1 (1983).

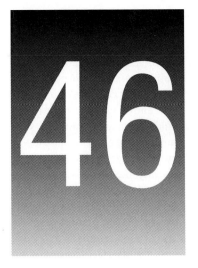

46 Liability exposure facing managed care organizations

MILES J. ZAREMSKI, J.D., F.C.L.M.
BRUCE C. NELSON, J.D., A.L.C.M.

THEORIES OF LIABILITY
ERISA PREEMPTION
CONCLUSION

The emergence and prevalence of managed care as a delivery system for medical care and treatment have given rise to various forms of liability exposure that face all forms of managed care organizations (MCOs). Health maintenance organizations (HMOs), preferred provider organizations (PPOs), preferred provider arrangements (PPAs), point-of-service plans (POSs), and other forms of MCOs encounter direct liability exposure in lawsuits initiated against them by their plan enrollees and affiliated physicians alike. With today's newfound prevalence of managed care, it is incumbent on an MCO to understand the extent of its own liability exposure.

The benefit to an MCO of understanding the potential exposure is perhaps obvious—the organization's financial viability can depend on it. Legal liability in the field of health care poses potentially significant economic consequences to each and every organization, institution, and individual involved in the health care business as a result of the very nature of that business. Wrongful conduct in the provision of medical care and treatment can translate into significant injury or death, and consequently the degree of liability imposed in those circumstances through legal proceedings can be enormous. Therefore understanding liability exposure is not only economically prudent, it will better enable an MCO to develop an internal structure and a way of doing business that minimizes its liability risks. Furthermore, public outcry against MCOs is on the rise, and, as a result, the states as well as Congress have endeavored to stem this tide through legislative efforts. Several states have already enacted managed care legislation, some of which provides yet another source of potential liability to MCOs. And while the federal government is yet to enact federal laws on the subject, such legislation is under consideration—laws that would affect managed care liability.

The key to minimizing an MCO's liability exposure is to understand both the various types of legal claims that have been asserted against MCOs and the particular conduct that gave rise to those claims. Furthermore, it is worthwhile to become familiar with some of the claimants' successes and failures in lawsuits against MCOs and, particularly in successful cases, to note the extent of financial liability imposed against MCOs.

To facilitate understanding, this chapter (1) sets forth and explains various legal theories under which MCOs' enrollees and affiliated physicians have asserted claims directly against MCOs, (2) describes the particular allegedly wrongful conduct that has given rise to claims under each of these legal theories, and (3) presents an in-depth review of lawsuits and resulting case law that has developed under these respective theories. This chapter then addresses the impact on managed care liability of a federal legal doctrine known as ERISA Preemption.

THEORIES OF LIABILITY

Although managed care remains an evolving concept of health care delivery, plaintiff-patients and physicians have sued MCOs under an increasingly wide array of legal theories, including both common law and statute-based theories. The following discussion analyzes the types of claims against MCOs that have arisen most frequently and that have led to the most significant liability exposure to MCOs. The types of claims addressed herein, however, should not be viewed as an exhaustive list of legal theories of liability under which an MCO is subject to risk. Because of the emergence of various forms of MCOs, case law in this area is limited at best. Moreover, there is little doubt that the evolution of managed care will allow for novel theories of liability to be asserted against MCOs. Notwithstanding, MCOs can and should be alert to those types of claims that have arisen and those that expose the organization to the most significant risk.

The case law reviewed in this chapter analyzes claims asserted by plaintiffs against MCOs under each of the following legal theories: vicarious liability, ostensible agency theory, medical malpractice, bad-faith denial of benefits, negligent utilization review, breach of contract, negligent credentialing, corporate negligence, fraud, misrepresentation, antitrust violations, and statutory claims. Although this imposing list implicates many different forms of allegedly wrongful conduct, it is important to note that in many cases, two or more of these theories have been asserted to redress a particular allegedly wrongful act. For example, in some cases alleged negligence on the part of an affiliated physician has led to a claim against the MCO under the theory of vicarious liability, whereas in other cases a charge of physician negligence is asserted against the MCO in the form of a claim for medical malpractice. Likewise, in some lawsuits an MCO's determination to deny a request to provide a particular form of care or treatment to an enrollee has given rise to a claim for bad-faith denial of benefits; in others the same conduct is labeled negligent utilization review. Furthermore, the ambitious plaintiff (or perhaps more accurately stated, the ambitious plaintiff's attorney) may assert claims under several different theories against an MCO—all within the same lawsuit—to redress to the same allegedly wrongful act. It is nevertheless beneficial for MCO management to understand each of these legal theories to minimize its liability exposure as effectively as possible.

Vicarious liability

One of the more commonly asserted claims against MCOs is made under the legal theory of vicarious liability. Vicarious liability, also known as respondeat superior, imputes liability to an employer or principal for the wrongful acts of its employee or agent. In the MCO context, plaintiff enrollees assert vicarious liability claims directly against MCOs for the allegedly wrongful acts of its employees or agents. To establish MCO liability, a plaintiff must demonstrate that the allegedly negligent individual was either directly employed by the MCO or, alternatively, was controlled by the MCO to the extent of being the MCO's agent.

Although vicarious liability claims against MCOs have arisen in several contexts, such a claim is most typically asserted with respect to the allegedly negligent acts of a physician affiliated with the MCO; that is, the enrollee who believes a physician has committed malpractice may assert against the MCO a claim for vicarious liability, attempting to hold the organization liable for the acts of its affiliated physician. Typically, however, the physician is not a direct employee of the MCO, and accordingly, an initial issue becomes whether a contracting physician is an agent of the MCO. Case law on this subject (discussed later) has turned primarily on the issue of the MCO's degree of control over medical decision-making by that physician and on whether the MCO holds out that physician to its plan enrollees as an employee or agent of the MCO: The greater the degree of control, or the more an enrollee is led to believe the physician

to be under the MCO's control, the more likely an enrollee will prevail in demonstrating the agency relationship. If, however, this agency test is not satisfied, then the MCO cannot be found liable under a vicarious liability theory.

Although most vicarious liability claims against MCOs seem to derive from allegedly negligent conduct of its affiliated physicians, MCOs, like any entity, must be alert to the fact that any of its employees and agents are potentially subject to a negligence claim (simple negligence as opposed to medical malpractice) in the course of that person's duties on behalf of the MCO, and consequently, the MCO is potentially subject to a vicarious liability claim. For example, an enrollee may seek to hold an MCO vicariously liable because of an allegedly negligent decision by that MCO's employees or agents to deny certain medical care or treatment to an enrollee. The point is that vicarious liability can arise out of the acts of every individual employee or agent of the MCO. But, as stated, most typically such claims are associated with charges of physician malpractice.

Case law. Most courts consistently hold that where the MCO directly employs its physician members, the MCO can be held vicariously liable for the negligent acts of that physician. For example, in *Sloan v. Metropolitan Health Council of Indianapolis Inc.*[1] an Indiana appellate court reversed the trial court's dismissal of an HMO in a malpractice lawsuit, holding that the HMO could be vicariously liable for the negligence of a physician under its direct employ. The Sloan court premised its ruling on the facts that (1) the physician was employed by the HMO, (2) the HMO paid the physician's salary, (3) the physician practiced under the direction of HMO personnel, and (4) the physician was prohibited under his employment contract from engaging in outside employment.

Likewise, in *Robbins v. HIP of New Jersey*[2] a New Jersey court held that an HMO could be held vicariously liable for the professional negligence of its employed physicians. The Robbins court rejected the HMO's argument that a New Jersey statute precluding HMOs from practicing medicine provided the HMO with immunity from vicarious liability.

Case law, however, is less clear involving independent contracting physicians, where the question arises as to whether an agency relationship exists between the independent physician and the MCO. To answer this question, courts have looked both to the degree of control exercised by the MCO over the independent contractor and also to the MCO's representations to its enrollees with respect to the status of contracting physicians. These cases reflect relative uncertainty of an MCO's potential risk with negligent contracting physicians. Interestingly, marketing materials are often the culprits that bolster a plaintiff's allegation of an agency relationship between the contracting physician and the MCO, thereby supporting the enrollee's vicarious liability claim.

In *Schleier v. Kaiser Foundation Health Plan*[3] the federal Court of Appeals for the District of Columbia held an MCO liable for the negligence of an independent contracting physician brought into the patient's care by an MCO member-physician. *Schleier* is particularly significant because the court applied the theory of vicarious liability even though the independent physician merely consulted with respect to the plaintiff's care and treatment. In holding the MCO liable for the acts of the physician in question, the court considered the following factors: (1) The MCO selected and engaged the physician, (2) the MCO paid the physician, (3) the MCO had the power to terminate its relationship with the physician, (4) the MCO had the authority to control the physician's conduct, and (5) it was a common business practice of the MCO to engage the participation of consultants in the care and treatment of its enrollees. (Although the *Schleier* court vacated the trial court's award of $825,000, it did so only for a recalculation of damages.)

More recently, a New Jersey court made a more detailed analysis of whether a negligent physician was an agent of an MCO for purposes of vicarious liability. In *Dunn v. Praiss*[4] the plaintiff sued the MCO where it had a referral contract with a urologist who, the plaintiff alleged, negligently delayed a diagnosis of testicular cancer. In determining that the urologist in fact was an agent of the MCO, the court relied on the facts that (1) the MCO used a capitation fee payment basis, (2) the urologist had no freedom to accept or reject a particular patient, (3) examinations by the urologist occurred at the MCO's office, (4) the MCO's contract with the urologist extended for a prolonged period (3 years), (5) literature given to patients by the MCO listed the subject urologist, and (6) the patients were not notified of the independent status of any of the MCO's affiliated specialists. The court concluded that MCO "controlled" the urologist and therefore upheld the plaintiff's claim against the MCO under vicarious liability. The *Dunn* opinion suggests that if the MCO had sufficiently represented to its enrollees that the subject physician was an independent consultant, the MCO may not have been found vicariously liable. (Similar to *Schleier*, the *Dunn* court vacated the trial court's judgment on damages [$2,904,240] but only for purposes of recalculation.)

By contrast, the Michigan court used a rather simplistic and very broad analysis to hold an MCO vicariously liable. In *Decker v. Saini*[5] the court held that the plaintiff had stated a claim for vicarious liability against both a member physician and a nonmember, independent contracting physician. The court reasoned that the trier of fact was free to determine from the trial that both the member physician and nonmember physician were agents of the defendant HMO. The *Decker* court summarily acknowledged that the member physician could be found vicariously liable; however, the court cautioned that whether an HMO is vicariously liable per se for the negligent acts of a nonmember physician should depend on the circumstances of each case.

Courts finding an MCO not to be vicariously liable for the negligence of contracting physicians have used a variety of tests and have considered an array of factors in reaching that conclusion. In *Chase v. Independent Practice Association*[6] a Massachusetts court focused on the degree of control an independent practice association (IPA) had over an allegedly negligent physician with respect to medical decisions. In *Chase* an HMO contracted with an IPA to provide medical services to HMO enrollees. The IPA in turn entered into an agreement with an obstetrics and gynecology (OB/GYN) group to provide services. This contract included language emphasizing that "each party is and shall continue to be an independent entity. Neither party is the agent or representative of the other. . . ."[7] A patient allegedly injured by the negligence of a physician from the OB/GYN group sued the physician, the HMO, and the IPA. The Massachusetts court upheld summary judgment in favor of the IPA, emphasizing the independent contractor status of the physician and the IPA's lack of control over that physician's medical decision-making. The *Chase* court also rejected the plaintiff's claim that she believed the allegedly negligent physician to be an employee of the IPA. The court held that the plaintiff failed to show a reliance on representations by the IPA that the physician (or the physician group) was an employee of the IPA.

In *Mitts v. HIP of Greater New York*[8] a New York court reached the same result, relying on the facts that the allegedly negligent physician was clearly an independent contractor and that the HMO did not directly provide care and treatment for its enrollees. In *Williams v. Good Health Plus, Inc.*[9] a Texas court came to the same conclusion in relation to an HMO, based on the latter of the two factors relied on in *Mitts*. The *Williams* court held that the HMO could not be vicariously liable because under a Texas statute, HMOs were prohibited from practicing medicine; therefore there could be no agency between the HMO and its affiliated physicians.

In *Raglin v. HMO Illinois, Inc.*[10] an Illinois court rejected a claim of vicarious liability against an HMO, focusing on whether the MCO "practiced medicine." The court found that there was insufficient evidence of the type of control by the HMO over the physician necessary to impute an agency relationship, where the HMO's subscriber certificate specifically stated that the HMO did not furnish medical care and could not render medical judgments. The court further rejected the plaintiff's agency assertion because she failed to demonstrate that she relied on any representation of the HMO that implied the subject physician was the HMO's agent.

Six years after *Raglin*, another Illinois appellate court reaffirmed and reiterated *Raglin's* holding, and, arguably, expanded the scope of an HMO's potential liability in Illinois to a patient injured through malpractice. In *Petrovich v. Share Health Plan of Illinois*[11] an HMO member patient sued her HMO for injuries allegedly resulting from negligent medical treatment, arguing that the HMO was vicariously liable (under apparent agency theory) for the physician's negligence. The subject physician was one of the HMO's "participating physicians" who allegedly failed to timely diagnose the plaintiff's squamous cell carcinoma. The *Petrovich* court held that the HMO could be liable under apparent agency theory if "the HMO, by its actions or statements, led a third party, who may have been unaware of the independent contractor relationship, to believe that the physicians were controlled by the HMO."[12]

More recently, however, in November 1998, another Illinois appellate court seemed inclined to curtail the trend of *Raglin* and *Petrovich*. In *Jones v. Chicago HMO Ltd. of Illinois*[13] a mother, whose child sustained brain damage from meningitis, filed suit against her HMO, asserting claims for institutional negligence, vicarious liability, and breach of contract. In first considering the institutional (or corporate) negligence claim, the *Jones* court labeled the language quoted previously from *Raglin* as mere dicta and further interpreted that language to limit corporate negligence claims against HMOs to claims of negligent utilization review (UR) and negligent selection of physicians (despite the fact that *Raglin* clearly lists negligent UR as *an example,* not the only type, of an independent act of corporate negligence). Because *Jones* involved claims based on neither physician selection nor UR, the court upheld summary judgment for the HMO on the institutional negligence count. On the vicarious liability count based on apparent authority, the court held the claim viable under *Petrovich* and found that there was an issue of fact as to whether the HMO held out the physician as its agent, thereby precluding summary judgment on that claim. Finally, regarding the plaintiff's contract claim, the *Jones* court held that there were two germane contracts related to the defendant HMO—one between it and the subject physician, and the other between it and the Illinois Department of Public Aid (a contract to provide health care services to Medicaid recipients). Because the *Jones* plaintiff was not a party to either and because she disavowed any third-party beneficiary claims she might assert, the court dismissed the contract action.

Jones, however, does not necessarily indicate that Illinois courts are easing legal pressure on HMOs. In March 1999, another Illinois appellate court established the viability of a common law action, this time not against an HMO but a physician for his failure to disclose to the patient certain financial incentives contained in his contract with an HMO—a decision, however, ripe with implications regarding claims against MCOs. In *Neade v. Portes*[14] a patient with classic symptoms of coronary artery blockage saw the defendant physician at his family clinic. The physician ordered a thallium stress test and an electrocardiogram (EKG or ECG) and concluded from those tests that the patient did not suffer from coronary artery disease. Also, the defendant physician allegedly disregarded another physician's recommendation that the patient undergo an angiogram. Three months later, the patient died of a massive myocardial infarction caused by artery blockage. The patient's estate sued the physician and his family clinic for medical negligence and breach of fiduciary duty. The fiduciary duty claim was based in part on the physician's failure to disclose to the patient a financial incentive provided by the HMO to minimize patient referrals and diagnostic testing, such as an angiogram.

The *Neade* court reversed the lower court's dismissal of the fiduciary duty claim, based in part on the fact that Illinois recognizes a fiduciary relationship between physician and patient. Although Illinois courts have refused to allow a breach of fiduciary duty claim that is based entirely on the same allegations as a parallel claim for medical malpractice and further have failed to allow allegations of physician motive to support a malpractice claim, the court found that the allegations supporting the *Neade* plaintiff's fiduciary duty claim—undisclosed financial incentives—did not mirror the allegations establishing his malpractice claim (i.e., failure to perform the appropriate diagnostic tests and to diagnose the plaintiff's condition). Furthermore, the motive issue underlying the fiduciary duty claim was *not* the basis of the negligence action. Based on this reasoning, the court held that the defendant physician's failure to disclose the subject financial incentives, together with the plaintiff's injury, stated a claim for breach of fiduciary duty.

The significance of *Neade* with respect to direct HMO liability exposure derives from the fact that many HMOs contractually bind or at least pressure their affiliated physicians not to disclose to patient enrollees financial incentives to minimize referrals and treatment. It is certainly plausible, if not likely, that if a physician can incur liability for concealing such incentives, the HMO may face liability as well, if not directly from the patient, then, arguably, indirectly in a contribution or indemnity claim asserted by a physician.

As shown by the following examples, jury verdicts against MCOs resulting from the malpractice of an affiliated physician can be substantial. In 1995, in *Ching v. Gaines* a California jury ruled against an HMO, awarding a plaintiff $3 million for the negligence of a member physician to timely refer the plaintiff to a specialist.[15] Also, in 1995 in *McLellan v. Long Beach Community Hosp,* another California jury imposed a $5.8 million verdict against an HMO for a member physician's negligence in causing brain damage to an infant during delivery.[16] California does not present an isolated situation. In a 1994 Missouri case, *Lowe v. Prime Health Kansas City,* a plaintiff sued an HMO and the physician to which it referred the plaintiff for medical negligence resulting in paraplegia. The HMO settled, paying the plaintiff $1.2 million.[17]

Conclusion. Clearly, physician negligence creates exposure to the MCO and to the physician. With today's prevalence of malpractice claims, coupled with the monetary size of the claims involved, physician negligence presents one of the most significant risks facing MCOs. There is also little question from the foregoing case law that an MCO that directly employs its physician members is subject to greater exposure based on vicarious liability than the MCO that affiliates itself with independent contracting physicians. Regarding independent contractors, an MCO can reduce its vicarious liability risk by emphasizing to its enrollees through its contracts, promotional literature, and direct communications that the contracting physicians are not employees or agents of the organization. Although conflicting at times, case law demonstrates that it is unlikely to wholly eliminate vicarious liability exposure.

Ostensible agency theory

The theory of ostensible agency is related to vicarious liability. Whereas vicarious liability is premised on the existence of an agency relationship, ostensible agency (also called "apparent agency") implies an agency relationship resulting from the conduct of the principal and/or the agent and, specifically, conduct from which a third party is reasonably led to believe that an agency relationship exists.

The relationship between these theories is seen in *Decker*, where the court held that the plaintiff had stated a cause of action against the MCO under vicarious liability because the allegedly negligent physician was the ostensible agent of the defendant MCO.[18] Clearly, these legal theories can arise in tandem.

Several courts, though, have allowed claims of ostensible agency to proceed against MCOs labeled as such without reference to vicarious liability. In those cases, courts have held that the MCO was liable for its contracting physician's negligence because the MCO created the appearance that the physician was in its employ, was its agent, or depicted the physician as one of its employees and because the patient detrimentally relied on this appearance.

Case law. In *McClellan v. Health Maintenance Organization of Pennsylvania*[19] the plaintiff sued an HMO, alleging, among other things, that the negligent physician was the ostensible agent of the HMO. The trial court granted the HMO's motion to dismiss, but on appeal the Pennsylvania Superior Court reversed, holding that the plaintiff had sufficiently pled her cause of action based on ostensible agency. Regarding that claim, the plaintiff had alleged that the HMO held the physician out as its agent; that the HMO represented to the plaintiff that the contracting physician was qualified, competent, and had been carefully screened by the HMO; and that the physician was negligent in administering care and treatment.

The appellate court in *Boyd v. Albert Einstein Medical Center*[20] relied on similar factors in overturning summary judgment in favor of an HMO. The court held that there was a genuine issue of material fact as to whether the allegedly negligent physician was the ostensible agent of the HMO. The court considered the following facts: (1) medical fees were paid directly to the HMO rather than to the contracting physician; (2) the patient was required to choose his primary care physicians from a limited list, (3) the allegedly negligent physician was screened by the HMO and required to follow HMO rules and regulations, (4) the plaintiff could not see specialists without a referral from an HMO-affiliated physician, and (5) primary care physicians could only refer patients to specialists who were on a prescribed list chosen by the HMO. From these facts, the *Boyd* court remanded the case to the trial court to determine whether the HMO held itself out as the defendant-physician's employer. As seen in *Dukes v. United States Health Care Systems of Pennsylvania, Inc.*,[21] to sustain a claim under a theory of ostensible agency, a plaintiff must show that he looked to the HMO for medical care and that the HMO held out the allegedly negligent physician as its employee.

Conclusion. It appears from the foregoing case law that whether an allegedly negligent, contracting physician can subject an MCO to direct liability under ostensible agency theory depends principally on how an MCO presents its contracting physicians to its enrollees. These cases suggest that an MCO can minimize liability exposure under this theory by emphasizing to its enrollees—through promotional materials, contracts, and personal communications—that contracting physicians are independent contractors and that they are not employees or agents of the MCO.

Medical malpractice

A cause of action for medical malpractice in the managed care context is encompassed within claims under vicarious liability and ostensible agency theory. Typically, a medical malpractice claim is directed specifically against the allegedly negligent physician who actually provided care and treatment to the enrollee. Technically, where an enrollee seeks to hold an MCO liable for that negligent conduct, the enrollee's cause of action should be couched under the theories of vicarious liability or ostensible agency because ultimately, it was not the MCO itself that perpetrated the conduct in question. However, where an enrollee asserts a claim arising out of alleged malpractice by a physician, under the theory of either vicarious liability or ostensible agency, the MCO faces potential liability to the same extent as would the allegedly negligent physician. Obviously, the degree of financial exposure will vary in each case, but the history of medical malpractice lawsuits demonstrates that in cases of severe adverse consequences resulting from physician negligence, the potential liability facing any and all responsible parties can be very substantial. Although no MCO can eliminate the risk of claims arising out of physician conduct, an MCO can reduce this risk by taking steps to ensure that it affiliates only with highly competent physicians who have not been the subject of many malpractice claims—particularly, many successful malpractice claims.

Negligent utilization review and bad-faith denial of benefits

Another legal theory commonly asserted against MCOs pertains to a determination by the MCO not to provide certain care or treatment. MCOs face exposure based on these determinations where the enrollee suffers adverse medical consequences that are allegedly the result of the MCO's decision to deny treatment. Enrollees of an MCO plan have asserted claims on this issue under several different legal theories. Most typically, the enrollee's cause of action is phrased as a claim for bad-faith denial of benefits or, alternatively, for negligent utilization review—utilization review being the process by which an MCO renders a determination as to whether to afford an enrollee particular care or treatment. Where specific care and treatment are denied by the MCO, enrollees have also asserted claims under corporate negligence theory and breach of contract. These latter two theories of liability are addressed separately later in this chapter.

An MCO's potential liability exposure under claims for bad-faith denial of benefits and negligent utilization review is as substantial as it is under the professional liability theories discussed previously. Just as negligent care and treatment by a physician can cause significant injury to an enrollee and thus potentially significant liability to an MCO, a decision to deny treatment that is later proven to have been medically appropriate or necessary can create significant injury to the patient and, hence, significant liability exposure to the MCO. In fact, the potential exists for greater exposure to the MCO from wrongful denial of benefits than from vicarious liability resulting from malpractice for this reason: Under malpractice-related claims, the MCO, if held liable, is ultimately liable for the conduct of another, whereas, with respect to the denial of benefits, the MCO itself is specifically making that determination. A jury, through its verdict, may be more inclined to punish the actual "wrongdoer" more severely than it would a party that is legally responsible for the wrongful conduct of another.

Although the process of utilization review varies from one MCO to another, reported cases arising out of this process reveal the principal contexts in which a decision on benefits under a health plan leads to a lawsuit. Specifically, MCOs often require physicians to obtain approval from the MCO, for instance, before ordering diagnostic tests, referring an enrollee to specialists, and extending the duration of an enrollee's inpatient hospitalization. As the case law in this area demonstrates, a decision by an MCO, the effect of which is to deny an enrollee treatment, is ripe with risk. Should subsequent events prove that the denied treatment should have been provided, the MCO is a likely target of litigation.

Case law. Arguably the most startling case regarding MCO liability for its utilization review process is *Fox v. Health Net,* in which a California jury awarded a health plan enrollee damages against an HMO totaling $89 million ($12 million in compensatory damages and $77 million in punitive damages).[22] The *Fox* plaintiff alleged that the HMO was liable for her emotional distress and ultimate death as a result of the organization's bad-faith refusal to authorize cancer treatment. Significantly, the case included allegations that the HMO's decision to deny Ms. Fox the cancer treatment she desired was motivated ultimately by financial concerns, which may well explain the overwhelming punitive damage award. Although the *Fox* case was settled for an undisclosed amount after the verdict was issued, the jury's damage award should alert MCOs and physicians alike that denial of benefit determinations can create enormous liability exposure.

Wickline v. State of California[23] is particularly instructive regarding MCO liability arising out of a decision to deny medical benefits. In this case a physician determined that a patient should remain in the hospital for a longer time than authorized by an HMO. The HMO, however, authorized only half of the amount of time requested by the physician. Although the HMO was not found liable in that particular case, the California appellate court stated:

The patient who required treatment and who is harmed when care which should have been provided is not provided should recover for the injuries suffered from all those responsible for the deprivation of such care, including, when appropriate, health care payors. Third party payors of health care services can be held legally accountable when medically inappropriate decisions result from defects in the design or implementation of cost containment mechanisms as, for example, when appeals made on a patient's behalf for medical or hospital care are arbitrarily ignored or unreasonably disregarded or overridden. However, the physician who complies without protest with the limitations imposed by a third-party payor, when his medical judgment dictated otherwise, cannot avoid his ultimate responsibility for his patient's care. He cannot point to the health care payor as the liability scapegoat when the consequences of his own determinative medical decisions go sour.

Similarly, in *Wilson v. Blue Cross of Southern California*[24] the court reversed a trial court's dismissal of an enrollee's suit against an MCO arising out of its utilization review. In *Wilson* the defendant MCO, through its utilization review process, denied the plaintiff—a psychiatric patient—further hospitalization. (At trial there was evidence that the enrollee's physician did not agree with the MCO's determination on hospitalization, but he failed to appeal that decision under the MCO's utilization review appeals procedures.) The patient was discharged and shortly thereafter committed suicide. The *Wilson* court remanded the case, holding that the defendant MCO could be held liable for the death of the patient if its utilization review decision was a "substantial factor" in causing that death.

Although the *Fox* verdict is an unusually high jury verdict, other cases reflect the fact that liability exposure resulting from the wrongful denial of benefits can be nevertheless substantial. In *Goodman v. California Physician's Service,* a jury awarded a plaintiff $1.25 million for the defendant-MCO's bad-faith failure to authorize benefits for treatment of multiple sclerosis, which resulted in the progression of the plaintiff's disease and emotional distress. The jury obviously ignored the MCO's contention that the desired treatment was too experimental to be covered under the plan.[25]

In *Gitterman v. Health Net* an arbitrator awarded the plaintiff $245,000 against an MCO for its bad-faith failure to preauthorize benefits for a lung transplant. The damage award was based on the plaintiff's emotional distress and eventual death.[26] Similarly, in *de Meurers v. Health Net* an arbitrator awarded the plaintiff $1 million against an HMO that failed to authorize an autologous bone marrow transplant. Noteworthy in that case was the arbitrator's finding that Health Net had engaged "in extreme and outrageous behavior exceeding all bounds usually tolerated in a 'civilized'" society in refusing to fund the plaintiff's transplant. The arbitrators also criticized the HMO's "heavy-handed" tactics in pressuring the plaintiff's oncologist to reverse his support for the transplant.[27]

This discussion contains many examples of extraordinarily high jury verdicts and settlements in cases in which insurance carriers are sued for denial to approve and fund certain health care treatments. It is reasonable to believe that with the increasing prevalence of managed care, these verdicts and settlements could become equally common in the managed care context.

Understandably, the most significant liability exposure results where the enrollee is denied medical treatment and as a consequence suffers irreparable injury before resorting to litigation. In some situations, however, the plaintiff has used the courts to obtain certain benefits before irreparable harm resulted. In *Hughley v. Rocky Mountain Health Maintenance Organization, Inc.*[28] an HMO enrollee sued his HMO for refusing to approve his claim for high-dose chemotherapy for breast cancer. While the parties were arbitrating the propriety of the HMO's decision to deny the desired chemotherapy treatment, the Colorado Supreme Court upheld a lower court injunction ordering the HMO to approve and fund the treatment, but under the condition that the plaintiff post a bond that would ensure that the HMO would be repaid should its decision to deny benefits be found proper.

In other situations an enrollee who has been denied treatment by an MCO but then obtained that denied treatment outside the MCO's network has filed a claim simply for reimbursement of the expense of the treatment. If an enrollee in that situation proves an entitlement to the denied treatment, the MCO will be found liable, but the liability of simply reimbursing the enrollee is likely to be substantially less significant than being found liable for adverse health consequences resulting from the enrollee never obtaining the treatment.

MCOs are also subject to liability related to the denial of benefits through fines levied by state agencies. In *FHP, Inc. v. Mendoza* an HMO was fined $500,000 by the State of California for failing to pay a bill for surgery performed on a child suffering from a rare form of cancer. After the cancer diagnosis had been made, the HMO proposed that the patient's surgery be performed by a surgeon who worked within the HMO network but who, according to the plaintiff, lacked the surgical skills to operate on the plaintiff's rare tumor. On their own initiative, the patient's parents were able to find a surgeon experienced with their daughter's cancer, and this physician operated on the patient at Stanford University. The HMO, however, refused to pay the bill, which exceeded $50,000, contending that the patient went outside the HMO network to find a specialist without prior approval from the HMO. Not only did the state fine the HMO, an arbitrator ordered the HMO to reimburse the plaintiff for her expenses.[29]

Likewise, in *Rhode Island v. United Behavioral Systems* the State of Rhode Island fined an MCO for improperly restricting patients' access to mental health care. The MCO agreed to pay a consent judgment in the amount of $75,000, which comprised a $25,000 fine and $50,000 to be invested in the study of industry practices regarding the provision of mental health care.[30]

Conclusion. Clearly, MCO liability exposure related to decisions on approving and denying medical care and treatment has been one of the most significant sources of financial risk facing MCOs. That risk is predicated essentially on erroneous medical decisions being made in the utilization review process. To minimize this risk as much as possible, it is incumbent on each MCO to optimize quality assurance in its internal utilization review processes and procedures.

However, there is reason to believe that liability exposure related to utilization review and the denial of benefits may be reduced in the future by applying the legal doctrine of "ERISA preemption" to enrollees' claims arising out of MCOs' benefits decisions. (See section on ERISA Preemption.)

Breach of contract

Another theory of liability asserted against MCOs is breach of contract. The MCO is typically a party to two separate forms of contracts, both of which expose it to potential liability under claims of breach. One such contract is with its employee or contracting physician. Claims under this contract could include allegations that a contracted physician is deselected (or terminated) in violation of the contract or alternatively, that the MCO has failed to pay the physician for medical services rendered.

The other such contract is between the MCO and its enrollee. In most cases an enrollee's affiliation with the MCO is premised exclusively on that contract, so it is not unusual for any type of alleged misconduct on the part of the MCO to appear in a claim for breach of contract. Arguably, an enrollee's cause of action for professional negligence, wrongful denial of benefits, failure to provide competent physicians (member, contracting, or consulting), and those under other theories could each be labeled a claim for breach of contract. Because it is a commonly used litigation strategy to assert each and every applicable cause of action, even where two or more such claims seek to redress the very same conduct, many lawsuits include, among other claims, a cause of action for breach of conduct.

Case law. Most often, MCOs have contractual relationships with their affiliated physicians (member-employees or independent contractors), and breach claims have arisen regarding various provisions in such contracts. One of the more common claims made by a physician against an MCO is that the organization wrongfully terminated its relationship with the physician in breach of their agreement.

In *Harper v. Healthsource New Hampshire, Inc.*[31] an HMO terminated an employee-member physician, allegedly because he failed to satisfy the organization's recredentialing criteria. After the physician sued, the HMO was successful in having the case dismissed based on its argument that the plaintiff-physician was an at-will employee who could be fired without cause. The New Hampshire Supreme Court reversed the decision, holding that the HMO's termination of its affiliation with the plaintiff violated a term of his at-will employment contract, that is, the implied term of good faith and fair dealing. The *Harper* court reasoned that firing the plaintiff-physician impacted not only his own individual interests, but also the community's interests, because of the unique relationship between physicians and the public; accordingly, the court stated, public policy concerns were implicated. The *Harper* court concluded that whether the plaintiff was terminated with or without cause, he was nevertheless entitled to a determination at trial as to whether he was terminated in breach of the covenant of good faith and fair dealing—a term implied in his employment contract.

Enrollees' claims for breach of contract, by contrast, are substantially more diverse and cover the spectrum of allegedly wrongful acts in which an MCO might engage. Because such claims often seek to redress physical injury suffered as a result of allegedly negligent treatment or the wrongful denial of benefits, breach claims filed by enrollees, on balance, create a substantially greater liability risk to MCOs than breach claims filed by physicians. However, enrollees' lawsuits against their MCOs are rarely driven by a breach-of-contract claim; this claim often seems tagged on as an additional cause of action. For example, *McClellan v. Health Maintenance Organization of Pennsylvania*[32] and *de Meurers v. Health Net*[33] both included multiple causes of action, including a breach of contract claim, to redress the same alleged injury.

An exception to that rule is the 1995 Oregon case of *Thomas v. Sisters of Providence Good Health Plan of Oregon.*[34] In *Thomas* the plaintiff sought to hold the defendant HMO liable for his injuries and did so by posturing his claim as one for breach of contract. Specifically, the plaintiff alleged that the HMO breached its contract with the plaintiff by failing to timely authorize a neurological procedure, the delay from which allegedly caused permanent nerve damage. Although *Thomas* never went to trial, the case reportedly settled through a payment by the HMO to the plaintiff in the amount of $1 million.

Conclusion. Case law under these contractual theories of liability is not particularly elucidating because with respect to lawsuits filed by physicians, the breach claim is premised on the particular terms of the MCO's agreement with its affiliated physicians; with regard to lawsuits filed by enrollees, the breach claim generally appears to be a "throw-in" in a lawsuit driven by a vicarious liability claim, wrongful denial of benefits claims, and so on. Nevertheless, MCOs must be aware that each term set forth in both of those contracts may be a future source of liability. Not only is the patient a potential adversary, but so, too, is the physician (or physician group).

Corporate negligence and negligent credentialing

The application of the legal theory known as corporate negligence (also called "corporate liability theory") is a relatively recent phenomenon in the managed care arena. Corporate negligence theory:

> . . . imposes liability on an entity for the negligent acts of an individual because of the entity's control over the individual. In the health care context this theory of liability is typically applied in cases involving hospitals and their staff physicians. It is also applied in cases involving HMOs and their staff or contract physicians. In these cases, courts have found hospitals and HMOs have an independent duty to their patients to investigate adequately and review the competence of staff physicians and panel providers. This theory of liability is often based on a public policy observation that hospitals and HMOs are in a far better position than their patients to supervise a physician's performance and provide quality control.[35]

Not unlike vicarious liability, this theory is premised on the organization's responsibility for the performance of those individuals under its control; therefore it can be applied to any employee or agent of the MCO. In practice, however, at least in the managed care context, this legal theory has been used to attack the allegedly negligent selection, retention, or supervision of its participating physicians, that is, negligent credentialing.

Case law. The Illinois Supreme Court first applied the theory of corporate negligence in the health care context. In *Darling v. Charleston Community Hospital*[36] a hospital was held to be negligent as a corporate entity for failing to adequately investigate and verify the references and other credentialing information of a physician. Because many forms of MCOs engage in the same type of credentialing performed by hospitals, it was not surprising that the theory of corporate negligence would apply in the managed care setting; however, it took more than 20 years.

In 1989 the Missouri Appellate Court in *Harrell v. Total Health Care, Inc.*[37] held that an HMO could be held liable under corporate negligence theory for its failure to properly investigate the qualifications of the physicians contracted to serve on its panel of providers. The *Harrell* court reasoned that, because of the HMO's restrictions on which physicians enrollees could engage, enrollees were subject to an unreasonable risk of harm if the HMO's panel included incompetent physicians. Although the Missouri Supreme Court, on further appeal,[38] held that a state statute granted immunity from liability to the HMO, the court nevertheless found that an HMO could be held liable for the negligent credentialing of its physicians.

Similarly, in 1992 the Pennsylvania Supreme Court in *McClellan v. Health Maintenance Organization of Pennsylvania*[39] held that an HMO has a nondelegable duty to select and retain competent physicians and may be liable for a breach of its duty to use reasonable care in selecting physicians. The *McClellan* court reinstated the plaintiff patient's complaint against an MCO, finding that the plaintiff could, and did, state a claim against the MCO for negligent selection, retention, and evaluation of the plaintiff's primary care physician.

Conclusion. An MCO's potential exposure for claims of negligence arising out of its credentialing processes is actually more easily minimized than other forms of liability exposure. An MCO must consistently exercise diligence in evaluating affiliated physicians, for purposes of initial selection and retention. Where an MCO fails to do so, it is potentially at risk of being targeted under a claim for corporate negligence.

Fraud and misrepresentation

To prove fraud or misrepresentation, a plaintiff must show that the defendant made false representations about or concealed material facts for the purpose of deceiving another into acting or remaining passive, as desired by the party misrepresenting or concealing the facts. Proving fraud or intentional misrepresentation requires a showing of intent by the defendant, although negligent misrepresentation is actionable in most if not all states.

Fraud and misrepresentation claims can arise in the managed care context—as in most any context—to redress a variety of allegedly wrongful conduct, and such claims have been filed by physicians and enrollees alike. The following examples demonstrate the breadth of conduct attacked through claims of this nature.

Case law. In *Deutsch v. Health Ins. Plan of Greater New York*[40] the plaintiff physician asserted a claim for fraudulent misrepresentation against the defendant HMO for failing to disclose information material to his contract with the HMO. The plaintiff's contract granted him the exclusive right to treat all HMO enrollees, as well as all enrollees in affiliates of the defendant HMO, who required audiological care and treatment. The plaintiff alleged that just before entry into his contract with the HMO, the HMO learned that one of its affiliates would not agree to refer its audiological patients to the plaintiff. The HMO entered into the contract with plaintiff anyway, aware of its affiliate's position but without disclosing that fact to plaintiff. The plaintiff learned of this fact and then subsequently allowed his contract to automatically

renew—all before he filed suit. The *Deutsch* court dismissed the fraud claim, but only because the plaintiff had waived his right to bring it by allowing the contract to renew without protest.

By contrast, in *Pulvers v. Kaiser Foundation Health Plan*[41] the plaintiffs who brought a fraud claim were enrollees in an MCO plan. The plaintiffs alleged fraud based on the fact that the MCO had represented itself in its promotional literature to be a nonprofit organization, without disclosing the fact that it offered a system of financial incentives to affiliated physicians. Under that system, physicians were paid a bonus for not ordering "unnecessary" tests and treatments. Plaintiffs claimed that the nondisclosure amounted to fraud because they had been led to believe that they would receive the "best quality" care and treatment. The *Pulvers* court rejected the plaintiffs' fraud claim, holding that such financial incentive systems are common throughout the managed care industry and, arguably, are worthwhile; nondisclosure of such a system did not constitute fraud on plan enrollees.

Similarly, *Teti v. U.S. Healthcare*[42] involved an HMO's failure to disclose to enrollees a financial incentive plan offered to affiliated physicians. *Teti* was a class action suit filed by enrollees in the defendant HMO. Although not premised exclusively on common-law fraud, plaintiffs alleged that their HMO violated the federal Racketeering Influenced and Corrupt Organizations Act (RICO) by its fraudulent failure to disclose to its enrollees its "Compensation Referral Fund," a financial incentive program offered to the HMO's affiliated physicians. Although the federal district court dismissed the case, it did so principally because the plaintiffs failed to allege how they were damaged by the HMO's nondisclosure. Arguably, if plaintiffs had incurred damage (and perhaps if they premised their claim as one for common-law fraud, which is easier to support than a RICO claim), the defendant HMO would have encountered a greater risk of exposure.

The issue of the nondisclosure of financial incentives—the issue in both *Pulvers* and *Teti*—has been the subject of an increasing amount of litigation. Many of these lawsuits arise because MCOs, in their contracts with affiliated physicians, contain what has been referred to as a "gag clause," that is, a clause requiring a physician not to disclose to an MCO's enrollees any financial incentives offered to the physician to limit the amount of care provided. To avoid such disputes and in fairness to enrollees, as of November 1996, 16 states had enacted and 12 more states were considering laws requiring MCOs to disclose to its enrollees certain health plan information, including financial incentives to limit care. Moreover, even where gag clauses are not prohibited, several major MCOs around the country have opted to remove them from their contracts with affiliated physicians.[43]

A variety of other actions by an MCO have induced enrollees to file fraud claims against it. In *HealthAmerica v. Menton*[44] a plaintiff charged fraud when his HMO agreed to pay his physical therapy expenses only for a period of 60 days, after it had induced him to enroll in the HMO and terminate his previous health plan. The plaintiff's previous plan would have covered his physical therapy expenses indefinitely.

In *Fink v. Delaware Valley HMO*[45] the plaintiff's fraud claim (along with other causes of action) arose out of the defendant HMO's alleged failure to approve a surgery on the plaintiff's shoulder, failure to obtain informed consent to certain other treatment, and failure to supervise medical performance of its physicians and staff.

Conclusion. It is difficult to draw conclusions from the fraud and misrepresentation claims brought against MCOs because such claims have been asserted both by physicians and enrollees, and more importantly, because there is a wide array of conduct by MCOs that has given rise to these lawsuits. The foregoing examples should be viewed merely as a glimpse of the types of conduct that may create liability exposure under the theories of fraud and misrepresentation.

Antitrust violations

Lawsuits have also been filed against MCOs alleging violations of federal and state antitrust laws. Although these are less common than the theories of liability discussed earlier, it is nevertheless worthwhile for an MCO to have a sense of its antitrust obligations.

In *Levine v. Central Florida Medical Affiliates, Inc.*[46] a physician brought federal and state antitrust claims against a PPO, a hospital affiliated with that PPO, and several other entities, premised on the physician's loss of staff privileges at the defendant-hospital and his denial of membership in the defendant PPO. The federal district court found in favor of the defendants, holding that (1) their agreement to establish certain rates for medical treatment did not constitute illegal price fixing, and (2) their agreement to restrict the size of their provider panel and discourage providers from referring PPO enrollees to non-PPO-affiliated physicians did not have an unlawfully anticompetitive effect on the plaintiff. The Eleventh Circuit Court of Appeals affirmed the district court ruling.

However, there have been instances where an MCO has been held liable in an antitrust claim. In *Brokerage Concepts, Inc. v. U.S. Healthcare, Inc.*[47] the plaintiff asserted federal antitrust violations (along with RICO and fraud claims) against U.S. Healthcare, two of its subsidiaries (a third-party administrator [TPA] and an HMO), and several individual corporate officers for requiring pharmacies seeking membership in U.S. Healthcare's pharmacy network to purchase the services of the defendant TPA for all of their claims. The jury delivered a verdict against the defendants in the amount of $1.6 million plus attorneys' fees.

In *Blue Cross & Blue Shield United of Wisconsin v. The Marshfield Clinic*[48] the plaintiff health insurer brought claims against an HMO under federal antitrust laws, alleging a conspiracy to divide and monopolize markets and fix prices. The jury awarded the plaintiff $48 million. (That verdict was reduced to $20 million by the trial court and later reversed, in large part, by the appellate court, which ordered a new trial on damages.[49])

Although antitrust claims are much less frequently asserted against MCOs than other types of claims, clearly, MCOs must keep in mind that antitrust liability exposure can be enormous.

Statutory claims. Claims against MCOs based on *common law* dominated the legal landscape throughout the first decades of the managed care era. More recently, however, statute-based claims against MCOs are becoming increasingly prevalent as states endeavor to stem the tide of anti-MCO sentiment through laws providing for direct claims against MCOs. Consider the following:

One of the more popular sources of public dissatisfaction with the managed care industry is a perception that MCO administrators, rather than physicians, are dictating medical care and treatment decisions. Although, ultimately, a physician renders the care and treatment, managed care plans often explicitly do not cover certain types of treatment. When a patient obtains such a "claim denial" from the MCO, the patient, who is dependent upon managed care coverage in order to financially afford the desired or even prescribed treatment, may not be able to receive that treatment. Moreover, MCOs frequently maintain contractual relationships with their affiliated physicians which influence or even curtail the physicians' ultimate independence to render treatment decisions. For example, most MCOs employ cost-containment mechanisms that discourage certain more expensive treatment. One such prevalent mechanism is a cash bonus system that rewards physicians for not prescribing certain treatments. Patients have alleged that such mechanisms to be cash rewards for minimizing care and treatment, and, arguably, infringing upon the physicians' duty of loyalty to the patient.

Consequently, several state legislatures have enacted "managed care reform" statutes, many of which explicitly provide for a cause of action directly against an MCO for "imposing" improper care and treatment. In 1997, for example, Texas—one of the first states to address legislatively the public's outcry against the managed care industry—enacted managed care reform legislation that provides three principal patient rights vis-à-vis managed care organizations (MCOs).[50] First, the law establishes a statutory cause of action against MCOs that impose on patients negligent treatment decisions (i.e., the law permits malpractice claims to be filed against MCOs). Second, the statute bars retaliation by MCOs against affiliated physicians who, against the wishes of the MCO, advocate to their patients a particular course of treatment. Finally, the law provides patients a right of independent review of medical treatment determinations rendered by MCOs as to whether a particular treatment is "medically necessary."[51]

Subsequently, quite a few states, including California, Georgia, New Mexico, and Oklahoma have followed the lead of Texas, with managed care reform legislation of their own. Notably, though, just how each state has addressed the issue has varied. In California the state legislature has imposed a statutory duty of ordinary care on MCOs in the provision of "covered" medically necessary treatment, and has afforded a statutory right to MCO enrollees to sue the MCO for damages arising out of a failure to exercise that level of care.[52] Georgia has enacted a comparable provision, pursuant to which:

Any claim administrator, health care advisor, private review agent, or other person or entity which administers benefits or reviews or adjusts claims under a managed care plan shall exercise ordinary diligence to do so in a timely and appropriate manner in accordance with the practices and standards of the provision of the health care provider generally. . . . [A]ny injury or death to an enrollee resulting from a want of such ordinary diligence shall be a tort for which a recovery may be had against the managed care entity offering such a plan.[53]

New Mexico also allows direct lawsuits against MCOs, but does so through its consumer protection laws rather than as part of its general healthcare statutes.[54] Notwithstanding that fact, however, New Mexico's consumer protections for MCO enrollees are so broad in scope that New Mexico arguably imposes one of the greatest risks of statutory liability on MCO's of any state that has enacted patient protection legislation. Significantly, New Mexico offers patients an explicit right to *actual* damages for any loss arising out of any failure by an MCO to satisfy these statutory duties to its enrollees. Oklahoma also provides a direct cause of action against an MCO for breach of a duty to exercise ordinary care in the provision of medical care and treatment.[55]

Conclusion. There seems little doubt that this trend toward opening a statute-based door to direct claims against MCOs will not stop in these nine states. At present, New York, Tennessee, Connecticut, Massachusetts, Florida, Virginia, Wisconsin, Michigan, and Illinois are each contemplating managed care reform legislation, designed to strengthen patients' hand over their MCO. More significantly, Congress, too, has leapt aboard this same bandwagon. The leading federal bill impacting managed care liability seeks to retract the shield so often wielded by MCOs—the shield known as ERISA Preemption.

ERISA PREEMPTION
Background of ERISA

MCO liability is affected and complicated to a profound degree by the legal doctrine known as ERISA Preemption. ERISA Preemption works to bar state law–based claims that infringe on the scope of the federal statute known as ERISA.

In 1974 Congress enacted ERISA, the Employee Retirement Income Security Act,[56] which, among other things, established standards of conduct for fiduciaries of employee pension plans to protect the financial interests of participants. ERISA was enacted to "replace a patchwork scheme of state regulations with a uniform set of federal regulations."[57] ERISA preemption functions to preempt, or supersede, any claim based on state law and provides in its place a claim asserted directly under the provisions of ERISA.

ERISA preemption comes into play in the context of MCOs only with respect to health care plans that are provided through an employer, and usually only with respect to plans that are self-insured. A health benefit plan that is insured through outside insurance is generally subject to state insurance law and hence not preempted, and such a plan that is not offered through employment is simply outside the scope of ERISA and, likewise, not preempted. ERISA preemption has the effect of reducing liability risk to MCOs because where it applies, the doctrine bars state-law claims against MCOs, enforcing instead only the much less stringent restrictions imposed on plan fiduciaries under ERISA.

Whether any particular state law claim asserted against an MCO is preempted by ERISA depends essentially on whether the claim is deemed to "relate to" an employee benefit plan.[58] The exceptions to the preemption doctrine are claims under state laws that regulate the fields of insurance, banking, and securities, which are not preempted by ERISA.[59] In *Pilot Life Inc. Co. v. Dedeaux*[60] the U.S. Supreme Court held that ERISA's preemption provisions are "deliberately expansive" and that the phrase "relates to" should be defined very broadly. Because the Supreme Court did not set forth any rules clarifying the meaning of the phrase "relates to," federal and state courts have been left to grapple with ERISA's application to managed care, reaching varying, and at times conflicting, results.[61] Notwithstanding, case law, particularly recent case law, has established some general criteria for determining whether any particular claim against an MCO is preempted by ERISA.

From 1974 through 1994, American courts were increasingly preempting state-law claims, including those against MCOs, under the position that most state laws that regulate health benefits do relate to employee benefit plans. Two significant cases from the early 1990s reflect this trend.

In *Corcoran v. United Healthcare, Inc.*[62] the plaintiff brought a medical malpractice and wrongful death lawsuit against United Healthcare, an organization that performed utilization review under contract with the plaintiff's employer's pension plan. The plaintiff's physician had sought approval of United Healthcare for inpatient hospital care because of complications in the plaintiff's pregnancy. United Healthcare denied the request as medically unnecessary. Soon thereafter, while the plaintiff was at home, the fetus went into distress and died. The plaintiff alleged that her fetus' death resulted from the health plan's negligence in denying her inpatient hospitalization.

In *Corcoran* the Fifth Circuit affirmed the district court's finding that the plaintiff's tort claims were preempted by ERISA. The appellate court reasoned that even though the defendant's utilization review decision amounted to a medical decision, that decision was made only in the context of determining whether certain benefits were available under the employer's benefits plan—a determination falling under the purview of ERISA—and accordingly, the plaintiff's claims were preempted.

A case decided shortly after *Corcoran, Elsesser v. Hospital of the Philadelphia College of Osteopathic Medicine,*[63] began to establish a general outline of what types of claims are preempted. *Elsesser* is particularly instructive in this sense because it involved various claims arising out of an array of allegedly wrongful conduct. The *Elsesser* plaintiff sued her HMO, asserting claims for (1) vicarious liability and ostensible agency arising out of physician negligence, (2) corporate negligence resulting from the MCO's direction to the plaintiff's physician to cease providing a particular type of treatment, and (3) breach of contract and fraudulent misrepresentation for erroneously stating in its contracts and promotional literature that its affiliated physicians had gone through a vigorous credentialing process. The *Elsesser* court decided that Congress never contemplated having professional liability claims proceed as ERISA claims, and accordingly, the court ruled that the plaintiff's malpractice-related claims (i.e., claims under the theories of vicarious liability and ostensible agency) were not preempted and should proceed under state law. The *Elsesser* court, however, preempted the plaintiff's claims for corporate negligence, breach of contract, and misrepresentation, reasoning that each arose out of the plaintiff's alleged inability to obtain the health benefits for which she paid. Claims of that nature, the court held, indeed are implicated by ERISA because they relate to the provision of employee health benefits.

Recent developments

In April 1995 the U.S. Supreme Court appears to have reversed the trend toward preemption, addressing this issue in *New York State Conf. of Blue Cross & Blue Shield Plans v. Travelers Ins. Co.*[64] In this case several HMOs challenged a New York statute imposing hospital surcharges, arguing that these fees unlawfully penalize patients covered by commercial insurers and self-insured plans. The Second Circuit Court of Appeals held that the subject surcharges were meant to increase the costs of certain insurance and HMO health care and that this purposeful interference with the choices that ERISA plans make for health care coverage constitutes a "connection with" ERISA plans triggering preemption. The Second Circuits Court's opinion was squarely based in then-recent Supreme Court precedent, in which the high court held that ERISA's preemption clause must be read broadly to reach any state law having a connection with, or reference to, covered benefit plans [65]

The Supreme Court, however, rendered a somewhat surprising decision limiting that long-applied principle. The Supreme Court ruled that New York's surcharge laws bore only on the costs of benefits and the relative costs of competing insurance to provide them. The court found that because uniformity in the costs of health benefits is not an ob-

jective of preemption, New York's surcharge laws had only an indirect economic impact on ERISA plans and accordingly, did not have the requisite connection with ERISA plans to trigger preemption.

Even years later, it is impossible to gauge the entire impact of *Travelers,* particularly because that decision has allowed lower courts more latitude in determining which types of claims relate to benefits plans and which do not, and those lower courts have not all been consistent in this regard. The establishing trend is to draw a distinction between those types of claims that arise out of the quantity of benefits provided versus those that pertain to the quality of health benefits. Specifically, claims related to malpractice (including claims stated under the theories of vicarious liability and ostensible agency) pertain to the quality of health care received by a plan enrollee; as stated in *Elsesser,* ERISA was never intended to supplant state law–based claims for professional negligence. Claims challenging an MCO's decision to deny benefits, on the other hand, pertain to the quantity of health care benefits an enrollee receives, and these claims, courts are holding, fit squarely within the purview of ERISA. Accordingly, such claims are preempted. The following cases, which were decided after the Supreme Court's decision in *Travelers,* reflect this position.

In June 1995 the Third Circuit Court of Appeals rendered its decision in two consolidated cases: *Dukes v. U.S. Healthcare, Inc.,* and *Visconti v. U.S. Healthcare.*[66] The plaintiffs in these two cases filed suit in state court against their respective HMOs—formed by defendant U.S. Healthcare—claiming damages under various theories for injuries arising from the medical malpractice of HMO-affiliated physicians and hospitals. Specifically, the *Dukes* plaintiffs alleged that (1) the HMO was liable under the doctrine of ostensible agency for the negligence of the HMO's physicians, and (2) the HMO was liable under the doctrine of corporate liability theory for its negligence in the selection, retention, and monitoring of its affiliated physicians. Likewise, in *Visconti* the plaintiffs asserted claims against their HMO for vicarious liability (arising out of physician negligence) and direct liability (related to the administration or management of the benefit plan). U.S. Healthcare removed the cases to federal court and sought to have them dismissed as preempted by ERISA. The respective federal district courts indeed dismissed each case.

On appeal, the Third Circuit stated that the plaintiffs' claims were properly preempted if they were asserted "to recover benefits due . . . under the terms of [the] plan, to enforce . . . rights under the terms of the plan, or to clarify . . . rights to future benefits under the terms of the plan."[67] The Third Circuit concluded, however, that none of the plaintiffs' claims could be defined this way:

We find nothing in the legislative history suggesting that . . . [ERISA] . . . was intended as a part of the federal scheme to control . . . the quality of benefits received by plan participants. Quality control of benefits, such as the health care benefits provided here, is a field traditionally occupied by state regulation, and we interpret the silence of Congress as reflecting an intent that it remains such.[68]

Several months later, the Tenth Circuit Court of Appeals broached this subject in *Pacificare of Oklahoma, Inc. v. Burrage.*[69] *Pacificare* considered whether ERISA preempted a vicarious liability claim against an HMO arising out of physician malpractice. The Tenth Circuit identified the following four categories of laws that relate to an employee benefit plan and therefore are preempted: (1) laws that regulate the type of benefits or terms of ERISA plans; (2) laws that create reporting, disclosure, funding, or vesting requirements for ERISA plans; (3) laws that provide rules for the calculation of the amount of benefits to be paid under ERISA plans; and (4) laws and common-law rules that provide remedies for misconduct growing out of the administration of the ERISA plan.[70]

The *Pacificare* court concluded that the plaintiff's claims arising out of the alleged malpractice of an HMO-affiliated physician did not fall under any of these four categories, and therefore it ruled that the plaintiff's claims were not preempted by ERISA.

In September 1995 the Seventh Circuit heard a case similar to *Pacificare* and reaffirmed the developing rule that malpractice-related claims against MCOs are not preempted by ERISA. In *Rice v. Panchal*[71] the plaintiff alleged that the defendant was liable for the medical malpractice under the theory of respondeat superior. The Seventh Circuit held that the plaintiff's malpractice claim did not rest on the terms of the ERISA plan in question, nor did it require construction or interpretation of the terms of the ERISA plan and therefore was not subject to the preemption clause.

More recently, in February 1997 the Eighth Circuit Court of Appeals applied this developing principle to a state-law claim for fraudulent misrepresentation. In *Shea v. Esensten*[72] the plaintiffs asserted a fraudulent misrepresentation claim based on the defendant HMO's failure to disclose to its enrollees the organization's practice of providing primary care physicians with financial incentives to minimize referrals to medical specialists. The plaintiff alleged that the primary care physician's failure to refer her husband to a cardiologist caused his death from heart failure. The Eighth Circuit held that the plaintiff's claims were preempted under ERISA.

Despite reaching a result contrary to the results reached in the Third, Seventh, and Tenth Circuit cases, the Eighth Circuit appears to have applied the same principles relied on in those cases and reached a conclusion that is consistent with those holdings. Unlike the malpractice-related claims against MCOs at issue in *Dukes, Pacificare,* and *Rice,* the claim in *Shea* pertained to the administration of the benefits plan. Failing to disclose aspects of the plan to the plaintiff in *Shea* led to the denial of health care benefits in the form of treatment from a cardiologist. This denial affected on the quantity of benefits, not the quality of benefits, and accordingly, pre-empting the *Shea* claim appears in line with the Third Circuit's reasoning in *Dukes.*

Similarly, the fraud claim in *Shea* relates directly to the type of benefits or terms of an ERISA plan, relates directly to disclosure requirements for an ERISA plan, and arguably, arises under common-law rules that provide remedies for misconduct growing out of the administration of the ERISA plan. The *Shea* holding is therefore consistent with the test applied by the Tenth Circuit in *Pacificare.*

Most recently, the impact of the doctrine of ERISA preemption in a claim against an HMO reached the United States Supreme Court, in what is arguably one of the more significant holdings in this area of the law. In *Pegram v. Herdrich*[73] the court decided that an HMO's financial incentive scheme that rewards its affiliated physicians for minimizing medical care and treatment does not per se violate ERISA. The court premised its holding on its conclusion that the HMO is not acting as an ERISA fiduciary when it uses any particular physician compensation scheme.

The impact of ERISA on a damages claim is aptly illustrated by the procedural history of this case. *Herdrich* involved a patient who went to her HMO-affiliated physician for pain in the middle area of her groin. The physician discovered a 6 × 8 cm inflamed mass in the patient's abdomen but decided to hold off ordering an ultrasound to investigate the mass. During the waiting period, the patient's appendix ruptured, causing peritonitis.

Herdrich sued the physician and the HMO in Illinois state court, alleging high-damage malpractice and fraud. Defendants asserted that the fraud counts were preempted by ERISA and removed those claims to federal court. Although the federal district court dismissed the patient's fraud counts, it granted her leave to amend one of those counts. The plaintiff's amended count, brought under ERISA and solely against the HMO, alleged a breach of fiduciary duty arising out of the HMO's implementation of a physician compensation scheme that financially rewarded affiliated physicians for minimizing medical care and treatment. The federal district court dismissed that amended count, and the patient appealed to the Seventh Circuit Court of Appeals. The Seventh Circuit reversed the district court, reinstating the plaintiff's ERISA claim against the HMO. With a scathing attack on the managed care industry, the Seventh Circuit Court held that, although financial incentive schemes do not per se constitute a breach of fiduciary duty, the one at issue in *Herdrich* stated a claim for breach of fiduciary duty under ERISA, because the claim alleged that the HMO's incentive plan destroyed the fiduciary trust between health plan participants and health plan providers where the HMO rewarded physicians for minimizing treatment to the detriment of the plan participant. The HMO appealed that decision to the U.S. Supreme Court, which agreed to hear the case.

On appeal, the significance of this issue led to a barrage of *amicus* briefs supporting each side on the issue, including briefs by the American College of Legal Medicine, the American Medical Association, and the federal government. The defendant HMO argued that it was not an ERISA fiduciary and that, even if it was, its incentive plan did not fall within the ambit of ERISA prohibitions. The patient plaintiff argued, of course, for affirmance of the Seventh Circuit's ruling.

On June 12, 2000, the Supreme Court issued a unanimous opinion, holding that the *Herdrich* HMO was not acting as an ERISA fiduciary when it used its financial incentive scheme, and, therefore, it did not implicate an ERISA fiduciary duty in using such a compensation mechanism. Perhaps in response to the Seventh Circuit's blistering opinion, the *Herdrich* court began its decision with a discussion of financial incentives in the managed care industry. The court found managed care, by its very nature, to be a system that rations health care, and that managed care organizations (MCOs) use, as they must, various mechanisms to manage that rationing process. Cash rewards to physicians for not providing what is believed to be unnecessary treatment, the court found, is pervasive throughout the industry, and, accordingly, a finding for the plaintiff would render the vast majority of MCOs ERISA violators. The court acknowledged that the rationing process in *Herdrich* led to a bad result, but that such a result opens the door to a state malpractice claim, and does not necessitate the availability of the federal court system.

Herdrich also addressed the generally recognized concept that decisions governing the quantity of health care provided (i.e., whether a patient is plan-eligible for a particular treatment) *do* implicate ERISA, whereas decisions as to the quality of health care (i.e., whether a patient is the victim of malpractice) *do not* implicate ERISA. The court found that the decision to use the financial incentive plan at issue in *Herdrich* was in certain respects a mixed decision pertaining both to the quantity of health care (i.e., whether certain treatment was provided), and qualitative decision-making by the plaintiff's physician (i.e., whether certain treatment was appropriate at the time). *Herdrich* concluded that these "mixed" decisions do not fall within the scope of the fiduciary duties encompassed by ERISA.

The immediate impact of *Herdrich* may be limited to the conclusion that an MCO does not per se violate ERISA by using a financial incentive scheme to reward physicians for minimizing care and treatment; but the decision has possible implications that both favor MCOs and patients. Note that the *Herdrich* ERISA claim was *not* premised on an allegation of failure to disclose such a cost-containment mechanism to the plaintiff plan participant, which has been a more commonly asserted claim against MCOs. Nevertheless, lower courts may read *Herdrich* to bar ERISA claims in these nondisclosure suits. In the other direction the court's decision seems to indicate that financial incentive schemes, and perhaps cost-containment mechanisms generally, do not at all fall within the scope of ERISA. This interpretation could open the door to more patient high-damage state court law-

suits against MCOs, because arguably MCOs may not rely on the ERISA preemption shield that, to date, has protected them in great measure. The ultimate impact of *Herdrich,* therefore, is yet to be seen.

State and federal legislation: the impact of ERISA preemption

That many state jurisdictions now permit direct statute-based patient claims against MCOs does not vitiate the potential application and impact of ERISA preemption on such statutory claims. As noted previously, the doctrine of preemption bars a state law–based claim where the subject matter is covered (i.e., preempted, by federal law). This doctrine is no less applicable to state statutory claims than it is to state common law claims. Accordingly, a state statutory claim against an MCO that relates to the quantity of health care benefits provided by the MCO is, or at least should be, every bit as preempted by ERISA as a state common claim based of the same nature.

This fact is particularly evident with respect to a challenge asserted to the Texas managed care statute. As noted previously, the Texas law essentially creates three general patient rights. First, it establishes a statutory cause of action against MCOs that impose on patients negligent treatment decisions (i.e., the law permits malpractice claims to be filed against MCOs—the "liability provision"). Second, the statute bars retaliation by MCOs against affiliated physicians who, against the wishes of the MCO, advocate to their patients a particular course of treatment (the "antiretaliation provision"). Finally, the law provides patients a right of independent review of medical treatment determinations rendered by MCOs as to whether a particular treatment is "medically necessary" (the "independent review provision").

Promptly after enactment of this Texas legislation, several HMOs and health insurers—including three affiliates of Aetna, which together provide managed care services to about one million Texas residents—filed suit, alleging that all three principal aspects of the law are preempted by ERISA. In 1999 the federal district court found that ERISA did not preempt the liability provision in the statute, but did preempt both the antiretaliation and independent review provisions in the act. Plaintiffs and the State of Texas appealed.

In June 2000 the Fifth Circuit Court of Appeals issued its decision in *Corporate Health Ins., Inc. v. Texas Dept. of Ins.,* affirming in part and reversing in part. With respect to the liability provision, the appellate court upheld the district court's determination that ERISA did *not* preempt the statutory creation of a malpractice claim against MCOs. The court based this conclusion on the fact that the law did not create a coverage claim premised on an MCO's denial of coverage for medical service recommended by a treating physician, which likely would have been preempted, but rather created a medical malpractice claim, an area traditionally governed by state law. Likewise, the Fifth Circuit concluded that the antiretaliation provision is *not* preempted by ERISA, this time, however, reversing the district court's decision. The appellate court reasoned that the antiretaliation provision is related to quality of care, an area governed by state law, in the sense that the provision realigns the interests of physicians and their patients with respect to treatment decisions. Finally, with respect to the independent review provision, the Fifth Circuit distinguished between the various determinations subject to independent review under the statute. The court found that a statutory right to independent review of the medical treatment decisions deals solely with quality of care determinations, and thus is *not* preempted by ERISA. By contrast, a statutory right to independent review of coverage decisions, according to the court, falls squarely within the ambit of ERISA, and thus *is* preempted. *Corporate Health* severs those portions of the Texas statute held preempted, leaving the balance of the act in force.

Corporate Health makes clear that federal courts will hold state statutory claims against MCOs, and the state statutes on which those claims are based, to the same degree of ERISA Preemption scrutiny that has become commonplace with state common law claims. Moreover, preemption issues may well overwhelm the legal landscape in this area of the law, because, for very practical reasons, state statutes affording direct claims against MCOs and such claims themselves are simply more likely to be preempted than state common law claims against MCOs. With common law claims, many were filed, and many were preempted while the law in this area evolved. However, as federal ERISA preemption doctrine has seemingly stabilized with the "quantity versus quality" distinction addressed previously, plaintiffs' attorneys are simply less likely to file the sort of state common law claims that are routinely preempted. On the other hand, legislators, in enacting managed care reform, are more likely influenced by public sentiment than the possibility that the laws they create may be nullified through preemption. Where a constituency is crying out for managed care reform and the right to hold MCOs responsible essentially for medical malpractice, it would seem that almost any state legislator is simply inclined to pay heed to that outcry, regardless of the preemptive possibilities of ERISA.

One form of legislative action—federal legislation—is immune to ERISA preemption. ERISA preempts only state law claims in favor of federal law, but new federal law cannot be preempted by another federal statute. However, Congress is ill-advised to passage contradictory legislation, and, therefore, the most effective way to address the ERISA preemption issue through federal legislation is through amendment to ERISA itself. Congress is currently contemplating such legislation.

Of the various bills that have flourished and floundered in Congress, arguably the most publicized and successful to date is House Resolution 2723, better known as the Norwood-Dingell Bill. Norwood-Dingell amends ERISA to allow, under certain circumstances, direct state law claims against MCOs, regardless of the whether the claim arises out of a complaint over the quality or quantity of health care benefits provided. In 1999 the U.S. House of Representatives passed Norwood-Dingell by an overwhelming majority of the House vote. The moved on to the United States Senate, where it currently remains in conference (and is now known as H.R. 2990).

Norwood-Dingell, if enacted, completely alters the scope of liability faced by MCOs. MCOs for decades have received profound protection from ERISA—protection that could, arguably, evaporate through passage of Norwood-Dingell or any similar alternative bill. The significance of this legislation warrants the inclusion of its relevant provisions in Appendix 46-1.

In essence, Norwood-Dingell appears to wholly eliminate ERISA preemption in the context of patient lawsuits against any type of MCO. To be clear, this bill is not a clarification of when ERISA preempts a state law claim, nor is it an endorsement of the federal courts' "quantity versus quality" distinction. Rather, it opens the door for an injured patient to sue her MCO directly, provided she can establish some reasonable causal connection between the actions of the MCO and the resulting injury. Arguably, proving such a causal connection may not be particularly difficult, considering that, under the doctrine of *respondeat superior* and the various agencies theories discussed previously, the MCO may be held vicariously liable for any action of an affiliated physician. Indeed, Norwood-Dingell, if it becomes law, will represent a fundamental change in the existing laws regarding managed care liability.

One other piece of federal legislation has garnered a fair amount of publicity and consternation. In June 2000 a bill (actually an amendment to a prior bill) was introduced in the U.S. Senate, a bill known as the Nickles Amendment. This proposed legislation appears to offer an alternative to Norwood-Dingell, but a much more narrowly tailored alternative. Nickles affords some limited remedial relief for patients whose claims are denied, but offers little with respect to recovering actual monetary damages. Moreover, Nickles is afflicted by the fact that it essentially requires a plaintiff to pursue her medical treatment-based claims in two forums—her negligence-related claims in state court and her MCO plans in federal court. Because managed care reform legislation has arisen as a result of the public's outcry against what they perceive to be the inequities in the managed care industry, it seems unlikely that the members of Congress will assuage their constituents that Nickles, which represents only a marginal change from existing law, will adequately remedy their concerns.

Summary

It is difficult to predict if the two-decade trend toward preempting most all claims against MCOs has ended with the clear lines drawn in the recent federal appellate cases discussed earlier. The "quality of benefits" versus "quantity of benefits" distinction relied on by many courts not only renders the application of ERISA preemption more consistent and predictable but also appears to follow the actual statutory language of ERISA. Significantly, the U.S. Supreme Court's decision in *Pegram v. Herdrich* appears, effectively, to endorse that distinction.

Assuming that the quality-versus-quantity distinction prevails as the law of the land, determining which theories of liability are likely to be preempted becomes an easier task. The clear principle established by the federal appellate courts in *Dukes, Pacificare,* and *Rice* is that malpractice-related claims against MCOs (i.e., claims under the theories of vicarious liability and ostensible agency) are not preempted by ERISA.

Although the law of preemption regarding other types of claims is not entirely clear, the quality-versus-quantity distinction provides a sound basis on which to predict whether ERISA applies. For example, claims alleging the wrongful denial of benefits or negligent utilization review appear to implicate the quantity of benefits received; therefore it seems likely that all such claims are preempted. As evidenced by the *Shea* case, fraud and misrepresentation claims pertaining to the administration of disbursement of benefits likewise are preempted. Predicting whether a breach of contract claim will be preempted is nearly impossible because breach claims attack such an array of conduct by an MCO; sometimes the issue is "quality of benefits," whereas in other cases the issue is "quantity of benefits." Breach claims, therefore, must be analyzed on a case-by-case basis.

Finally, perhaps the most difficult preemption prediction pertains to claims for negligent credentialing. On the one hand, credentialing involves the administration of personnel that will service a plan's enrollees, which suggests that such a claim would be preempted. On the other hand, credentialing determines the quality of health care received by plan enrollees through the screening of physicians to better ensure quality health care delivery, which suggests that such a claim would not be preempted. Unfortunately, there is a dearth of case law on this subject, particularly recent case law, making it nearly impossible to draw any conclusions.

Of course, all the distinctions on when ERISA preemption does and does not apply in the managed care context could be rendered moot, if Congress amends ERISA to eliminate its preemptive effect in this context. Only time will tell. In the meantime, however, ERISA preemption continues to dominate the law regarding lawsuits against MCOs; consideration of this issue remains essential to MCOs in addressing strategies designed to minimize their liability exposure.

CONCLUSION

The various common law and statutory theories of liability discussed throughout this chapter demonstrate that MCOs face liability exposure not only from different sources, but also arising from a wide array of conduct. It is incumbent on the MCO to understand these liability risks and to develop an internal structure designed to minimize those risks without reducing the level of quality in the health care they provide.

ENDNOTES

1. *Sloan v. Metropolitan Health Council of Indianapolis, Inc.,* 516 N.E. 2d 1104 (Ind.App. 1987).2.
2. *Robbins v. HIP of New Jersey,* 625 A. 2d 45 (N.J. Super. 1993).
3. *Schleier v. Kaiser Foundation Health Plan,* 876 F. 2d 174 (D.C. Cir. 1989).
4. *Dunn v. Praiss,* 606 A. 2d 862 (N.J. Super.Ct. 1992).
5. *Decker v. Saini,* 1991 WL 277590 (Mich.Cir.Crt. Sept 17, 1991).
6. *Chase v. Independent Practice Association,* 583 N.E. 2d 251 (Mass. App. 1991).
7. *Id.* at 253.
8. *Mitts v. HIP of Greater New York,* 478 N.Y.S. 2d 910 (N.Y. 1984).
9. *Williams v. Good Health Plus, Inc.,* 743 S.W. 2d 373 (Tex. 1987).
10. *Raglin v. HMO Illinois, Inc.,* 595 N.E. 2d 153 (Ill.App. 1992).
11. *Petrovich v. Share Health Plan of Illinois,* 296 Ill.App. 3d 849, 696 N.E. 2d 456 (1st Dist. 1998).
12. *Id.* at 361.
13. *Jones v. Chicago HMO Ltd. of Illinois,* 301 Ill.App. 3d 103, 703 N.E.2d 502 (1st Dist 1998).
14. *Neade v. Portes,* 303 Ill.App. 3d 799, 710 N.E. 2d 418 (2d Dist. 1999).
15. Sedgwick et al., *Healthcare Liability Deskbook: Managed Care Organizations and Their Liability Exposures* (Clark Boardman Callaghan 1996).
16. *Id.*
17. *Id.*
18. *Supra* note 5.
19. *McClellan v. Health Maintenance Organization of Pennsylvania,* 604 A. 2d 1053 (Pa. 1992).
20. *Boyd v. Albert Einstein Medical Center,* 547 A. 2d 1229 (Pa.Super.Ct. 1988).
21. *Dukes v. United States Health Care Systems of Pennsylvania, Inc.,* 848 F.Supp. 39 (E.D.Pa. 1994).
22. *Supra* note 15.
23. *Wickline v. State of California,* 192 Cal.App. 3d 1630, 239 Cal.Rptr. 810 (1986).
24. *Wilson v. Blue Cross of Southern California,* 222 Cal.App. 3d 660, 271 Cal.Rptr. 876 (1990).
25. *Supra* note 15.
26. *Id.*
27. *Id.;* see also Zaremski et al., *Reengineering Healthcare Liability Litigation,* in I.S. Rothschild, *Liability of Managed Care Organizations* (Michie Co. 1997).
28. *Hughley v. Rocky Mountain Health Maintenance Organization, Inc.,* 927 P. 2d 1325 (Colo. 1996).
29. *Supra* notes 15 and 27.
30. *Supra* note 15.
31. *Harper v. Healthsource New Hampshire, Inc.,* 674 A. 2d 962 (N.H. 1996).
32. *McClellan v. Health Maintenance Organization of Pennsylvania,* 604 A. 2d 1053 (Pa. 1992).
33. *Supra* note 15.
34. *Id.*
35. American Academy of Hospital Attorneys of the American Hospital Association, *Hospital-Affiliated Integrated Delivery Systems: Formation, Operation, and Contract Handbook* (1995) at 243-244.
36. *Darling v. Charleston Community Hospital,* 200 N.E. 2d 149 (Ill.App. 1964), *aff'd,* 211 N.E. 2d 253 (Ill. 1965), *cert. denied,* 383 U.S. 946 (1966).
37. *Harrell v. Total Health Care Inc.,* 1989 WL 153066, *aff'd,* 781 S.W. 2d 58 (Mo. 1989).

38. *Harrell v. Total Health Care, Inc.,* 781 S.W. 2d 58 (Mo. 1989).
39. *McClellan v. Health Maintenance Organization of Pennsylvania,* 604 A. 2d 1053 (Pa. 1992).
40. *Deutsch v. Health Ins. Plan of Greater New York,* 573 F.Supp. 1433 (S.D.N.Y. 1983).
41. *Pulvers v. Kaiser Foundation Health Plan,* 99 Cal.App. 3d 560, 160 Cal.Rptr. 392 (1979).
42. *Teti v. U.S. Healthcare,* 1989 U.S.Dist. LEXIS 14041 (E.D.Pa., 11/21/89), *aff'd,* 904 F. 2d 694 (3rd Cir. 1990).
43. *See* 43 American Medical News, 39(American Medical Association, Nov 18, 1996).
44. *HealthAmerica v. Menton,* 551 So. 2d 235 (Ala. 1989).
45. *Fink v. Delaware Valley HMO,* 612 A. 2d 485 (Pa.Super. 1992).
46. *Levine v. Central Florida Medical Affiliates, Inc.,* 72 F. 3d 1538 (11th Cir. 1996).
47. *Supra* note 15.
48. *Blue Cross & Blue Shield United of Wisconsin v. The Marshfield Clinic,* 883 F.Supp. 1247 (W.D.Wis. 1995).
49. *Blue Cross & Blue Shield United of Wisconsin v. The Marshfield Clinic,* 65 F. 3d 1406 (7th Cir. 1995).
50. Tex. Civ. Prac. & Rem. Code, §88.001 et. seq. (2000).
51. *Id.*
52. Cal. Civ. Code §2438 (West 2000).
53. Ga. Code Ann. §51-1-48 (1999).
54. N.M. Stat. Ann. §59A-57-1 et. seq. (2000).
55. Okla. Stat. Tit. 63, §2525 et. seq. (2000).
56. 29 U.S.C.§1001 et seq.
57. Gabriel Minc, *ERISA Preemption of Medical Negligence Claims Against Managed Care Providers: The Search for an Effective Theory and an Appropriate Remedy,* 29 Journal of Health and Hospital Law 97 (1996).
58. 29 U.S.C. §1144(a).
59. 29 U.S.C. §1144(b)(2)(A).
60. *Pilot Life Inc. Co. v. Dedeaux,* 481 U.S. 41 (1987).
61. *See* Zaremski et al., *supra* note 27.
62. *Corcoran v. United Healthcare, Inc.* 965 F. 2d 1321 (5th Cir), *cert. denied,* 113 S.Ct. 812 (1992).
63. *Elsesser v. Hospital of the Philadelphia College of Osteopathic Medicine,* 802 F.Supp. 1286 (E.D. Pa.1992).
64. *New York State Conf. of Blue Cross & Blue Shield Plans v. Travelers Ins. Co.,* 514 U.S. 645 (1995).
65. *See e.g., District of Columbia v. Greater Washington Board of Trade,* 506 U.S. 125 (1992).
66. *Dukes v. United States Health Care System Inc.,* 57 F. 3d 350 (3rd Cir. 1995), *cert. denied,* 116 S.Ct. 1063 (1996).
67. *Id.* at 356.
68. *Id.* at 350 (emphasis added). *See also Rice v. Panchal,* 65 F. 3d 637 (7th Cir. 1995), which followed *Dukes,* holding that a lawsuit, based on respondeat superior, brought against Prudential health plan was not preempted by ERISA. The court held that the claims against the subject HMO did not fall under the gambit of the terms of the plan, but rather were based on state law of respondeat superior.
69. *Pacificare of Oklahoma, Inc. v. Burrage,* 59 F. 3d 151 (10th Cir.1995).
70. *Id.* at 154, quoting *Airparts Co. v. Custom Benefit Servs.* of Austin, Inc., 28 F. 3d 1062, 1064 (10th Cir. 1994).
71. *Rice v. Panchal,* 65 F. 3d 637 (7th Cir. 1995).
72. *Shea v. Esensten,* 107 F. 3d 625 (8th Cir. 1997).
73. *Pegram v. Herdrich,* __ U.S. __ (June 12, 2000).
74. *Corporate Health Ins., Inc. v. Texas Dept. of Ins.,* __ F.3d __ (5th Cir. June 20, 2000), aff'd on panel rehrg., __ F.3d __ (5th Cir. July 27, 2000).

Appendix 46-1 **Relevant ERISA provisions**

SECTION 1302. ERISA PREEMPTION NOT TO APPLY TO CERTAIN ACTIONS INVOLVING HEALTH INSURANCE POLICYHOLDERS

IN GENERAL.—Section 514 of the Employee Retirement Income Security Act of 1974 (29 U.S.C. 1144) (as amended by section 301(b)) is amended further by adding at the end the following subsections:

(f) PREEMPTION NOT TO APPLY TO CERTAIN ACTIONS ARISING OUT OF PROVISION OF HEALTH BENEFITS.

  (1) NON-PREEMPTION OF CERTAIN CAUSES OF ACTION.

    (A) IN GENERAL.—Except as provided in this subsection, nothing in this title shall be construed to invalidate, impair, or supersede any cause of action by a participant or beneficiary (or the estate of a participant or beneficiary) under State law to recover damages resulting from personal injury or for wrongful death against any person

      (i) in connection with the provision of insurance, administrative services, or medical services by such person to or for a group health plan as defined in section 733, or

      (ii) that arises out of the arrangement by such person for the provision of such insurance, administrative services, or medical services by other persons.

    (B) LIMITATION ON PUNITIVE DAMAGES.

      (i) IN GENERAL.—No person shall be liable for any punitive, exemplary, or similar damages in the case of a cause of action brought under subparagraph (A) if

        (I) it relates to an externally appealable decision (as defined in subsection (a)(2) of section 1103 of the Bipartisan Consensus Managed Care Improvement Act of 1999);

        (II) an external appeal with respect to such decision was completed under such section 1103;

        (III) in the case such external appeal was initiated by the plan or issuer filing the request for the external appeal, the request was filed on a timely basis before the date the action was brought or, if later, within 30 days after the date the externally appealable decision was made; and

(IV) the plan or issuer complied with the determination of the external appeal entity upon receipt of the determination of the external appeal entity.

The provisions of this clause supersede any State law or common law to the contrary.

(ii) EXCEPTION.—Clause (i) shall not apply with respect to damages in the case of a cause of action for wrongful death if the applicable State law provides (or has been construed to provide) for damages in such a cause of action which are only punitive or exemplary in nature.

(C) PERSONAL INJURY DEFINED.—For purposes of this subsection, the term 'personal injury' means a physical injury and includes an injury arising out of the treatment (or failure to treat) a mental illness or disease.

(2) EXCEPTION FOR GROUP HEALTH PLANS, EMPLOYERS, AND OTHER PLAN SPONSORS.

(A) IN GENERAL.—Subject to subparagraph (B), paragraph (1) does not authorize

(i) any cause of action against a group health plan or an employer or other plan sponsor maintaining the plan (or against an employee of such a plan, employer, or sponsor acting within the scope of employment), or

(ii) a right of recovery, indemnity, or contribution by a person against a group health plan or an employer or other plan sponsor (or such an employee) for damages assessed against the person pursuant to a cause of action under paragraph (1).

(B) SPECIAL RULE.—Subparagraph (A) shall not preclude any cause of action described in paragraph (1) against group health plan or an employer or other plan sponsor (or against an employee of such a plan, employer, or sponsor acting within the scope of employment) if

(i) such action is based on the exercise by the plan, employer, or sponsor (or employee) of discretionary authority to make a decision on a claim for benefits covered under the plan or health insurance coverage in the case at issue; and

(ii) the exercise by the plan, employer, or sponsor (or employee) of such authority resulted in personal injury or wrongful death.

(C) EXCEPTION.—The exercise of discretionary authority described in subparagraph (B)(i) shall not be construed to include

(i) the decision to include or exclude from the plan any specific benefit;

(ii) any decision to provide extra-contractual benefits; or

(iii) any decision not to consider the provision of a benefit while internal or external review is being conducted.

(3) FUTILITY OF EXHAUSTION.—An individual bringing an action under this subsection is required to exhaust administrative processes under sections 1102 and 1103 of the Bipartisan Consensus Managed Care Improvement Act of 1999, unless the injury to or death of such individual has occurred before the completion of such processes.

(4) CONSTRUCTION.—Nothing in this subsection shall be construed as

(A) permitting a cause of action under State law for the failure to provide an item or service which is specifically excluded under the group health plan involved;

(B) as preempting a State law which requires an affidavit or certificate of merit in a civil action; or

(C) permitting a cause of action or remedy under State law in connection with the provision or arrangement of excepted benefits (as defined in section 733(c)), other than those described in section 733(c)(2)(A).

(g) RULES OF CONSTRUCTION RELATING TO HEALTH CARE.—Nothing in this title shall be construed as

(1) permitting the application of State laws that are otherwise superseded by this title and that mandate the provision of specific benefits by a group health plan (as defined in section 733(a)) or a multiple employer welfare arrangement (as defined in section 3(40)), or

(2) affecting any State law which regulates the practice of medicine or provision of medical care, or affecting any action based upon such a State law.

EFFECTIVE DATE.—The amendment made by subsection (a) shall apply to acts and omissions occurring on or after the date of the enactment of this Act from which a cause of action arises.

SEC. 1303. LIMITATIONS ON ACTIONS.

Section 502 of the Employee Retirement Income Security Act of 1974 (29 U.S.C. 1132) (as amended by section 304(b)) is amended further by adding at the end the following new subsection:

(o)(1) Except as provided in this subsection, no action may be brought under subsection (a)(1)(B), (a)(2), or (a)(3) by a participant or beneficiary seeking relief based on the application of any provision in section 1101, subtitle B, or subtitle D of title XI of the Bipartisan Consensus Managed Care Improvement Act of 1999 (as incorporated under section 714).

(2) An action may be brought under subsection (a)(1)(B), (a)(2), or (a)(3) by a participant or beneficiary seeking relief based on the application of section 1101, 1113, 1114, 1115, 1116, 1117, 1119, or 1118(3) of the Bipartisan Consensus Managed Care Improvement Act of 1999 (as incorporated under section 714) to the individual circumstances of that participant or beneficiary, except that

(A) such an action may not be brought or maintained as a class action; and

(B) in such an action, relief may only provide for the provision of (or payment of) benefits, items, or services denied to the individual participant or beneficiary involved (and for attorney's fees and the costs of the action, at the discretion of the court) and shall not provide for any other relief to the participant or beneficiary or for any relief to any other person.

(3) Nothing in this subsection shall be construed as affecting any action brought by the Secretary.

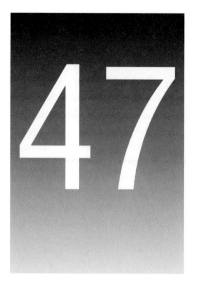

Physician as an employer

CHARLES G. HESS, M.S., M.D.

HAZARD COMMUNICATION STANDARD
AMERICANS WITH DISABILITIES ACT
BLOOD-BORNE PATHOGENS STANDARD
CLINICAL LABORATORY IMPROVEMENT AMENDMENTS
FAMILY AND MEDICAL LEAVE ACT
TUBERCULOSIS CONTROL GUIDELINES
HEALTH INSURANCE PORTABILITY AND ACCOUNTABILITY ACT

Physicians, acting as employers, must satisfy certain financial obligations, including withholding taxes, FICA, Medicare, and unemployment insurance. Several federal laws—the Equal Pay Act of 1963, Civil Rights Act of 1964 (title VII), the amended Age Discrimination in Employment Act of 1967, and the Equal Opportunity Act of 1972—passed in the United States since 1963 have profoundly affected the practice of medicine. Laws passed since 1980, however, have given the government unprecedented control over the practice of medicine. This chapter deals with the changing responsibilities of the physician, in his or her role as an employer, under recent federal regulations.

HAZARD COMMUNICATION STANDARD

Noncompliance with the Hazard Communication Standard by physician-employers can result in substantial monetary penalties (per violation). There are almost 600,000 chemical products in existence in the United States, with new ones being introduced each year.[1] Some of these chemicals pose serious problems for exposed employees. In 1983 the Occupational Safety and Health Administration (OSHA) issued a regulation called *hazard communication* that applied to employers in the manufacturing sector. Under the Hazard Communication Standard (HCS), the employee is required to be informed of the contents of the law, the hazardous properties of chemicals encountered in the workplace, and measures (such as safe handling procedures) needed to protect employees from these chemicals. The law was expanded in 1988 to include employers in the nonmanufacturing sector such as the physician-employer; thus HCS became the first regulation to concern itself specifically with the health and safety of medical employees.[2] The HCS was revised in February 1994.

Under the general duty clause of this law, the physician-employer "shall furnish a place of employment which is free from recognized hazards that are causing or are likely to cause death or serious physical harm to his or her employees." The physician-employer is required to post the Job Safety and Health Protection Poster (OSHA Form 2203) in his or her office or clinic. Any fatal accident or accident that results in the hospitalization of three or more employees must be reported to the nearest OSHA office within 8 hours.

Hazard communication plan

Under HCS, each physician-employer who has one or more employees exposed to a hazard is required to develop a written program to protect those individuals. This hazard communication plan (HCP) must outline those health and safety policies and procedures placed into effect by the employer to protect his or her workers. The stated purpose of the HCP is to reduce the occurrence of illnesses, injuries, and fatalities in the workplace.

Hazardous chemicals. A complete inventory must be taken once a year of all products in the office or clinic. The HCS requires that all chemicals imported, produced, or used in a workplace undergo a "hazard determination." This evaluation, which may be delegated to an employee, should include not only medical supplies (such as isopropyl alcohol and bleach), but also office supplies (such as copier toner and correction fluid).[3] OSHA considers products to be hazardous when a hazardous chemical makes up 1% or more of the product or a carcinogen makes up 0.1% or more of the product. There are essentially two ways to determine whether a product is considered hazardous. One way involves writing the product's manufacturer or distributor for a material safety data sheet; the other involves comparing chemicals in office products with those on one of four lists recommended by OSHA.

Most consumer products containing hazardous chemicals that are used in the office are cleansers.[4] Medications that are dispensed by a pharmacist to a health care provider for direct administration to a patient are exempt.[5] Drugs in solid form (pills or tablets) are also considered exempt; until recently, most injectables and other medications used in an office were also considered exempt from HCS.

Material safety data sheets. A material safety data sheet (MSDS) is an informational sheet furnished by a product's manufacturer to the user in order to identify the hazardous characteristics of the product. Every hazardous product must have an MSDS, provided by the manufacturer or distributor on written request. In 1986 OSHA developed Form 174 to provide a universal form that would meet the HCS requirements. Use of the form is not mandatory, but OSHA requires all the information on the form.

Once a year, requests should be made for MSDSs on all hazardous products that have been changed or are new to the office. Such sheets should be kept for 5 years.[6] Under the revised HCS, MSDSs may be kept on a computer disk or microfiche (rather than paper) as long as there are "no barriers to employee access."[7] Under the present rule, drug package inserts cannot be accepted in lieu of MSDSs for "less than solid" drugs (creams, ointments, liquids, and injectables).[8] Drug samples, if not used in the office, do not require MSDSs. After MSDSs are obtained, they have to be "rated" in order to create hazard labels. If the MSDSs received by the office have not already been rated by the manufacturer, this is best done using a modification of the method suggested by Suchocki.[9]

Hazard labels. Under HCS, the physician-employer is required to label, tag, or mark hazardous chemicals in the office or clinic. The purpose of the label is to serve as an "immediate warning" and as a "reminder of more detailed information" in the MSDS. Instead of labeling specific containers, OSHA also permits the posting of proper information on the front or back sides of cabinet doors where hazardous materials are stored.[10] The label must show the identity of its hazardous chemical or chemicals and any appropriate hazard warnings. There is no single labeling system recommended by OSHA. The most widely used label is an adaptation of one developed by the National Fire Protection Agency (NFPA 704 Standard). The NFPA label is a diamond-shaped, color-coded label, with a different color for each represented hazard.

Training program. The HCS requires employers to provide a training program for all employees exposed to hazards in the routine performance of their duties. As with training programs under other standards, employees must be trained at scheduled staff meetings, with each session documented on a training log.

AMERICANS WITH DISABILITIES ACT

In 1990 the Americans with Disabilities Act (ADA) was passed to prevent unfair discrimination against disabled persons with visual, hearing, and other physical and mental impairments. This law prohibits discrimination on the basis of disability and protects qualified applicants, employees, and the general public with disabilities from discrimination in all aspects of employment and public access to services and facilities.[11] All sorts of disabilities are covered, including persons with cancer, human immunodeficiency syndrome (HIV), blindness, deafness, attention deficit disorder, learning disabilities, mental retardation, and mental illness. Individuals who are former drug or alcohol abusers are also covered under ADA. The law requires the physician-employer to place a poster in his or her office describing the provisions of ADA.

Titles

As a five-part regulation, ADA requires several different aspects of compliance. Only titles I and III, however, are applicable to medical practices.

Title I. The original law prohibited job discrimination in offices with 25 or more employees after July 26, 1992. The present law, however, exempts only those employers with fewer than 15 employees. Under Title I, the employer must use the same employment standards in all hiring, paying, training, promoting, and firing decisions. Neither the physician-employer nor any of his or her office staff may engage in any illegal job-recruiting or job-interviewing practices. For example, during a job interview, the employer cannot inquire about a history of disability, illness, absenteeism, or workers' compensation benefits. The employer cannot ask the applicant about the presence of a disability but can ask about the applicant's ability to perform certain tasks. Also, a physical examination cannot be performed until an offer of employment has been made. Although the applicant can be excluded for his or her inability to perform "essential" tasks, the applicant cannot be excluded for an inability to perform "marginal" tasks. If a disabled person applying for a job is judged to be the best-qualified applicant (without consideration of the applicant's disability), ADA requires the employer to hire that individual. Also, a physician-employer cannot decide against hiring a disabled person because employment of that individual would require "reasonable accommodation," that is, "one that does not cause significant difficulty or expense in relation to the employer's operations, financial resources or facilities."[12] Additional stipulations in this section require employers to make certain accommodations for disabled persons already employed.

Title III. Under Title III, the physician-employer is responsible for making his or her practice accessible to persons with disabilities. As of January 26, 1992, persons owning, leasing, or operating places of public accommodation must reasonably change their policies, procedures, and practices to promote equal opportunities for all individuals.[13] All existing health care facilities must make their common use areas "accessible" if removal of structural barriers is "readily achievable," that is, "easily accomplished and able to be executed without much difficulty or expense."[14]

Access. Accessibility guidelines for new construction and alteration of existing structures have been developed for ADA. For example, an adequate number of "accessible" parking spaces should be provided—at least one accessible space for every 25 parking spaces. Furthermore, one of every eight accessible spaces must be van accessible and must be so marked.[15] Total compliance is required only for new construction and alterations. Tax incentives are available for the removal of architectural barriers.

Auxiliary services. The ADA requires the physician-employer to provide (and pay) for those auxiliary aids and services necessary to ensure effective communication with individuals "unless an undue burden or fundamental alteration of services would result."[16] In some cases, office policies and procedures may have to be altered. For example, an office or clinic may need to allow the entry of guide dogs for blind patients. With regard to auxiliary aids, the needs of the patient must be considered in deciding whether to use a notepad, Brailled materials, other formats (e.g., audiotape), or an interpreter.

Does the physician have to hire a sign-language interpreter? The area of concern to most physicians is how to deal with hearing-impaired patients. The answer to the question is "maybe." Although the intent of the law is to require appropriate auxiliary aids and services "when necessary," the service must not cause "significant difficulty or expense."[17] The law does not impose on a physician the requirement that primary consideration be given to a disabled person's requests. In most cases, an interpreter should not be needed if a patient can read questions and write answers. Another alternative to the use of a notepad is a computer terminal on which the physician and patient can exchange typewritten messages. The Justice Department cites situations in which it believes the services of an interpreter are needed.[18] One example is when a hearing-impaired person needs to undergo major surgery. Other areas besides health include financial, legal, and personal matters. The end result, however, is that "in those situations requiring an interpreter, the public accommodation (such as a physician's office or clinic) must secure the services of a qualified interpreter, unless an undue burden would result."[19]

BLOOD-BORNE PATHOGENS STANDARD

The second federal law to concern itself with the safety of medical employees was the Blood-Borne Pathogens Standard (BBP) of 1991, by OSHA. The intent of this law is to reduce exposure in the health care workplace to all blood-borne pathogens, particularly the hepatitis B virus (HBV) and HIV. Hepatitis B virus infection is considered the major infectious blood-borne occupational hazard to health care workers; the Centers for Disease Control and Prevention (CDC) estimate that there are approximately 8700 such infections in health care workers in the United States each year, causing approximately 200 deaths.[20] With regard to HIV, CDC estimates that about one million Americans are infected with the virus; as of September 1, 1993, CDC had logged nearly 400,000 AIDS cases, with about 200,000 deaths.[21] There are reports of at least 46 workers who apparently were infected with HIV through occupational exposure to blood or other potentially infectious materials.[22]

Exposure control plan

Any employer having at least one employee with occupational exposure is required to have a written exposure control plan (ECP). The stated purpose of the plan is to eliminate or minimize occupational exposure to blood and other potentially infectious materials. The employer is required to make a copy of this plan available to all employees and any OSHA representative. It must be reviewed and updated at least once a year.

Exposure determination

Each employer who has one or more employees with occupational exposure is required to perform an exposure determination. The exposure determination list consists of the following:

1. A list of job titles in which all employees have occupational exposure
2. A list of job titles in which some employees have occupational exposure
3. A list of all tasks (or groups of closely related tasks and procedures) that identify certain employees within a job classification where some, but not all, employees have occupational exposure

Exposure incident

The ECP must also explain how the employer will evaluate the circumstances surrounding exposure incidents. This evaluation should include the circumstances of the incident, synopsis of present controls, and evaluation of present "failures."

Exposure control

The BBP was drafted so that employees will be protected by performance-oriented standards. The specific provisions of the ECP are an effort to make clear "what is necessary" to protect employees. It is the responsibility of the physician-employer to limit worker exposure through implementation of the following categories of control:

1. Universal precautions
2. Workplace controls
3. Personal protective equipment
4. Housekeeping policies
5. Hazard communication policies
6. Hepatitis B program
7. Training program

Universal precautions. OSHA's method for reducing worker exposure to blood-borne pathogens is based on the adoption of universal precautions as the foundation for a plan of infection control. Under the BBP, workers are required to exercise universal precautions to prevent contact with blood or other potentially infectious materials.

Workplace controls. Workplace controls are of two types: engineering controls and work practice controls. Engineering controls reduce employee exposure by either removing the worker from the hazard or removing the hazard itself. Examples of engineering controls are sharps containers, biosafety cabinets, and self-sheathing needles.

Work practice controls reduce employee exposure by altering the manner in which a procedure is performed. The employer is required to incorporate the following work practice controls into the ECP:

1. Washing hands: Employers are required to provide hand-washing facilities that are readily accessible to employees.
2. Handling blood: Mouth pipetting or suctioning of blood or other potentially infectious materials is prohibited.
3. Handling equipment: Equipment used for diagnosis or treatment must be examined before servicing or shipping and must be decontaminated unless the employer can demonstrate that decontamination of such equipment is not feasible.
4. Handling personal items: Employees must not keep food and drink either in refrigerators, freezers, shelves, or cabinets or on countertops or benchtops where blood or other potentially infectious materials are present.
5. Handling sharps: Employees must not bend, break, or shear contaminated needles and other contaminated sharps. Contaminated needles and other contaminated sharps cannot be recapped or removed unless it can be demonstrated that no alternative is feasible or that such action is required by a specific medical procedure. At the close of 1999, four states (California, New Jersey, Maryland, and Tennessee) had passed laws requiring the use of "safe" sharps.[23] Needle safety legislation was pending in 19 other states. These safety devices are defined as "needleless systems or needle devices with engineered sharps injury protection." A new interpretation of this standard by OSHA requires proof of a facility's review of such technology to determine whether or not these new devices are needed to reduce exposure incidents in a specific workplace.

Personal protective equipment. When engineering and work practice controls are insufficient to eliminate exposure, personal protective equipment (PPE) must be used "to prevent or minimize the entry of materials into the worker's body."[24] The BBP states that "when there is occupational exposure, the employer shall provide, at no cost to the employee, appropriate personal protective equipment such as, but not limited to, gloves, gowns, lab coats, face shields or masks and eye protection, and mouthpieces, resuscitation bags, pocket masks, or other ventilation devices." OSHA places the responsibility of protecting employees directly on the employer. The employer must not only provide appropriate PPE but also make sure that it is used "when necessary."

Housekeeping policies. The BBP requires employers to keep workplaces "in a clean and sanitary condition." Under housekeeping policies, the employer is required to schedule, and then to implement, a written agenda for cleaning and decontaminating the office, including the following:

1. Cleaning of surfaces
2. Cleaning of equipment
3. Cleaning of linens
4. Discarding of regulated waste

Hazard communication policies. BBP requires the use of hazard communication through labels or signs to ensure that employees receive adequate warning in order to eliminate or minimize their exposure to blood-borne pathogens. Such labels are to be affixed to refrigerators and freezers containing blood or other potentially infectious material, as well as other containers used to store, transport, or ship blood or other potentially infectious materials. Red bags or red containers may be substituted for labels.

Hepatitis B program. The employer is required to make the hepatitis B vaccine available to all employees who have occupational exposure. Ordinarily, the hepatitis B vaccination series has to be offered within 10 working days of the initial assignment at no cost to the employee. Those who decline to accept the vaccination must sign a statement to that effect. For those who have had an exposure incident, the employer is also required to obtain a postexposure evaluation and a medical follow-up examination. After an exposure incident, the employer is required to provide the employee with the following information:

1. The route and circumstances of exposure
2. The name of the source individual (unless impossible)
3. The results of the source individual's blood test, if available

The employer is required to furnish the employee with a copy of the evaluating physician's written opinion within 15 days of receipt of his or her report. As part of the medical follow-up examination, the employee is entitled to prophylactic medications (if recommended by the U.S. Public Health Service), counseling sessions, and medical evaluation of postexposure illnesses. Medical records for each employee with regard to hepatitis B vaccination and occupational exposure must be kept for the duration of employment plus 30 years.

Training program. Training about the hazards associated with blood and other potentially infectious materials must be provided by the employer to all employees with occupational exposure. The employer is required to keep training records for all employees with occupational exposure for 3 years from the date on which the training occurred. The same rules that apply to medical records also apply to training records.

CLINICAL LABORATORY IMPROVEMENT AMENDMENTS

The Clinical Laboratory Improvement Amendments (CLIA) were passed in 1988 to ensure the accuracy of laboratory tests performed on human specimens. Most of the regulations became effective on September 1, 1992. The physician is no longer able to perform tests on patients in his or her office without legal permission from the federal government.

Certification

This law requires all laboratories, including physician office laboratories (POLs), to obtain one of five certificates: a registration certificate, a certificate of waiver, a certificate of provider-performed microscopy, a certificate of compliance, or a certificate of accreditation. Even if only one test is performed (and even if no charge is made for that test), the Health Care Financing Administration (HCFA) requires the physician-employer to obtain a certificate. Once an application is received, HCFA may issue a registration certificate, together with a CLIA number (for requests for laboratory testing reimbursement made to Medicare or Medicaid third-party payers after January 1, 1994).

A registration certificate permits a laboratory to continue operations for 2 years or until a determination of compliance can be made, whichever is shorter. The certificate of accreditation can be issued by the Commission on Office Laboratory Assessment (COLA) to those laboratories (including POLs) desiring an alternative to federal inspections under CLIA. Also, a laboratory in a state with a federally approved licensure program may choose to receive a state license in place of a CLIA certificate, provided it complies with the regulations of that state.

Categories of tests

Present laboratory tests, numbering about 10,000, have been classified according to the degree of difficulty in the performance of the test.[25] This ranking initially resulted in a three-tier organization of tests into categories called *waived, moderate complexity,* and *high complexity,* to which a fourth category (now called provider-performed microscopy) was added in February 1993. Depending on its certification, a laboratory can perform tests in one or all four categories.

A laboratory that limits itself to performing waived tests is essentially exempt (except for manufacturers' instructions) from CLIA requirements. Procedures classified under provider-performed microscopy must be performed by either the physician or a health care provider, in conjunction with an examination of the patient in the office. As of December 1999, 42 analytes had at least one test system classified as waived, and another 6 fell in the provider-performed category. Laboratories performing waived and provider-performed microscopy tests are not subject to routine inspections, but are subject to random compliance and complaint investigations.

Nonwaived tests

Those laboratories performing provider-performed microscopy, moderate-complexity tests, and high-complexity tests must fulfill certain requirements for personnel standards, patient test management, quality control, proficiency testing, and quality assurance.

Personnel standards

Each laboratory performing nonwaived tests must meet certain personnel standards (PS), which are tied to the complexity of the testing process. The rules, which differ for moderate-complexity testing and high-complexity testing, list detailed personnel responsibilities and qualifications; qualifications are based on formal education, laboratory experience, and/or laboratory training. Laboratories performing tests in the moderate-complexity category must employ a laboratory director, technical consultant, clinical consultant, and testing personnel. Laboratories performing tests in the high-complexity category must employ a laboratory director, technical supervisor, clinical consultant, general supervisor, and testing personnel.

Patient test management

Each laboratory performing nonwaived tests is required to have in place a system ensuring the correct performance of the entire testing process, beginning with the preparation of the patient and ending with the distribution of test results. Patient test management (PTM) consists of two parts: (1) written policies and (2) documentation (to verify the former).[26] The regulations require written policies for the following:
1. Preparing patients
2. Processing (collecting, preparing, identifying, storing, transporting, and discarding) specimens
3. Reporting results

With regard to test results, normal or reference ranges must be available, but they do not have to be printed on reports. The laboratory is also required to develop a written policy (or protocol) to follow when a life-threatening or "panic" value occurs. The protocol demands that the individual ordering the test or the individual responsible for utilizing the test results be notified immediately when any test result indicates an immediate danger to a person's life.

With the second part of PTM, three documents are required: the test requisition, the test record (patient log), and the test report, all of which must be kept for a minimum of 2 years. Tests can be performed only on the oral, written, or electronic (computer) order of an "authorized person." That authorized person will usually be the physician (or another state-authorized individual). The authorized person must sign written requests; oral orders are permitted as long as written orders are obtained within 30 days. The "three Rs" of PTM allow a laboratory to track and positively identify patient specimens as they move through the complete testing process. Specific information must be contained in these three documents to comply with the law.

Quality control

Manufacturers of instruments, kits, and test systems usually provide guidelines for quality control (QC) of their products. One kind of internal QC procedure involves the use of QC samples; these samples, similar to patient specimens, have known test results. QC samples, when run at the same time as patient specimens, can provide the operator with a "within run" check to confirm test results.[27] Each laboratory performing nonwaived tests is required to develop and follow written QC procedures that monitor the quality of the analytic testing process of each test method. Of the two sections on QC, one contains general requirements, and the other contains special requirements for specialties or subspecialties.

Laboratories using uncleared tests must follow the full QC rules. Full QC rules are also required for all tests of moderate complexity that have been cleared but modified or developed in-house and for all tests of high complexity.

Proficiency testing

One way of making sure a particular laboratory's performance is in line with that of other laboratories performing the same analysis involves the testing of unknown samples from an outside source. Just as QC samples provide a type of internal QC, proficiency testing (PT) offers a kind of external QC. Each laboratory performing tests of moderate or high complexity must enroll in an approved PT program for all specialties or subspecialties in which it desires to be certified. The PT provider must be either a private, nonprofit organization or a federal or state entity.

Once the laboratory has been enrolled, the PT provider will send samples to its subscriber three times a year; each shipment includes five samples for that "event." The samples, whose values are not known, are run along with the laboratory's regular workload of patient specimens. It is unlawful to send portions of PT samples to other laboratories for "comparison" studies. The final results are sent to the PT provider, together with an attestation form signed by both the operator and the laboratory director. For most tests, the minimum passing score is 80%.[28] Any laboratory failing two consecutive or two out of three testing events will be subject to sanctions (including cancellation for that specialty, subspecialty, or test).

Quality assurance

Every laboratory performing nonwaived tests must implement and follow written policies and procedures for a quality assurance (QA) program designed to monitor and evaluate the quality of the total testing process. CLIA is the first standard to require a QA program as part of the law. It is the responsibility of the employer, as laboratory director, to ensure the accuracy of test results and the adequacy of laboratory services. In a POL, laboratory testing may be done by two workers or one worker and the director; in such cases, all members should make up the QA committee. The QA committee is responsible for making sure that "quality" evaluations take place and that corrective actions take place whenever problems are identified. To reach this goal, at least seven key elements must be addressed. A QA audit checklist should include the following[29]:

1. Procedure manual
2. Personnel standards
3. Patient test management
4. Quality control
5. Proficiency testing
6. Complaint investigations
7. Quality assurance review

FAMILY AND MEDICAL LEAVE ACT

The Family and Medical Leave Act (FMLA), which became effective on August 5, 1993, requires any physician-employer of 50 or more employees to grant up to 12 weeks of unpaid leave for certain family and medical reasons each "benefit" year. For most businesses, the benefit year begins on September 1 and ends on August 31. If a medical practice is incorporated, this law also includes any physician-employees.[30] To qualify for this leave, employees must have worked at least one full year and at least 1250 hours during the year.

Under some circumstances, employees may take FMLA leave intermittently—that is, take leave in blocks of time or in reduced normal or weekly schedules. Also, in some cases, employees may be able to couple accrued paid leave (such as sick leave, vacation time, or personal time off) to cover some or all of unpaid FMLA leave. Unpaid family and medical leave can be used to take care of any of the following circumstances:

- A birth, adoption, or foster care placement of a child of an employee
- A serious health condition of an employee's child, parent, or spouse
- A serious health condition of the employee (making the employee unable to perform his or her duties)

The physician-employer is ordinarily required to grant medical leave for the following treatments[31]:

- Radiotherapy for cancer
- Chemotherapy for cancer
- Medical therapy for complications from pregnancy
- Medical therapy (inpatient hospital care) for cosmetic surgery
- Medical therapy for substance abuse

When a physician-employer is notified of the need for a medical leave, he or she must furnish the employee a written explanation of the employee's rights and responsibilities under FMLA. The information provided should detail such requirements as whether medical approval (certification) for the leave is required, whether the leave is to be counted against authorized leave, and whether the same or equivalent position will be available on the employee's return to work.

Under the FMLA, employees returning to work are entitled to their old job or an equivalent job with the same pay, benefits, and conditions of employment. If insurance was provided to the employee before his or her leave, the employer is required to maintain health benefits coverage on the same terms as if the employee had continued to work. Under this law, the physician-employer is allowed to designate certain employees as "key employees"; a key employee may not be allowed to return after FMLA leave.

TUBERCULOSIS CONTROL GUIDELINES

It was estimated that by the year 2000, there would have been 250,000 cases of active TB and 20,000 deaths.[32] Tuberculosis has long been recognized as a potential hazard to workers in health care facilities. Final guidelines for TB control, published in October 1994, are recommended for all inpatient health care facilities, regardless of size, including medical offices. The recommendations cover all employees who have exposure to *Mycobacterium tuberculosis.* Although the guidelines use the term *recommended,* the interpretation is that these "guidelines" are required by OSHA. A final TB standard was scheduled to be published during the year 2000.[33]

Risk assessment

A risk assessment must be performed for all medical practices. The physician-employer should assign this responsibility to one individual (the TB control officer) or a committee (the TB committee). The appointed individual or committee must determine the probability for risk to health care workers in the practice. To complete the baseline risk assessment, the incidence of reported TB cases in the community during the previous year must be known; this information can be obtained from the local or county health department. Also, medical records of the practice must be reviewed to determine whether any employees or patients were diagnosed with TB during the previous year. With this and other information, an initial risk assessment can be performed. After the initial baseline assessment, periodic reassessments are required of all practices.

Levels of risk

A risk assessment will place the practice in one of five "risk" categories. Placement of a practice in a risk category enables the employer to determine what further actions (and their frequency) are required by the guidelines. Levels of risk are classified as follows: minimal, very low, low, intermediate, or high.

1. Minimal risk
   a. No reported cases in the TB community profile, and no TB patients treated in the previous 12 months
   b. PPD skin testing not required
   c. Risk assessment repeated in 12 months

2. Very low risk
   a. Reported cases in the TB community profile
   b. Employee skin test conversion rate no greater than before
   c. Fewer than two positive employee skin test conversions during a 3-month period
   d. No evidence of person-to-person transmission
   e. No TB patients treated in the previous 12 months ("refers" all patients with TB)
   f. PPD skin testing required
   g. Risk assessment repeated in 12 months

3. Low risk
   a. Reported cases in the TB community profile
   b. Employee skin test conversion rate no greater than before
   c. Fewer than two positive employee skin test conversions during a 3-month period
   d. No evidence of person-to-person transmission
   e. One to five TB patients treated in the previous 12 months
   f. PPD skin testing required
   g. Risk assessment repeated in 12 months

4. Intermediate risk
   a. Reported cases in the TB community profile
   b. Fewer than two positive employee skin test conversions during a 3-month period
   c. Suggestive evidence of person-to-person transmission
   d. Six or more TB patients treated in the previous 12 months
   e. PPD skin testing required
   f. Risk assessment repeated in 6 months

5. High risk
   a. Reported cases in the TB community profile
   b. Employee skin test conversion rate greater than before
   c. Two or more positive employee skin test conversions during a 3-month period
   d. Evidence of person-to-person transmission
   e. PPD skin testing required every 3 months
   f. Risk assessment repeated in 3 months

Tuberculosis control plan

After the initial risk assessment, a written TB control plan should be developed, implemented, and maintained by the TB control officer or TB committee. This individual or committee should be familiar with the current recommendations of the CDC and other authorities concerning TB control. The plan should be reviewed after each risk assessment to make sure it meets the practice's current needs.

Practice precautions

In general, the practice should follow certain precautions while evaluating or treating patients with suspected or confirmed cases of TB. At the least, these patients should be separated as much as possible from other patients. Minimal precautions with respect to the suspected TB patient should consist of the following:

- Giving health care workers masks (to protect employees from becoming contaminated)
- Giving the patient a separate waiting area (such as a separate waiting room, designated examination room, or isolation room)
- Giving the patient tissues to cover his or her nose and mouth (when sneezing or coughing)
- Medical offices.

Medical offices. Although no engineering control requirements are presently in effect, suggestions have been made with regard to ventilation precautions. For practices with TB patients, an air filtration system should be used to reduce the risk of transmitting TB. Recommended air-cleaning units include units that recirculate the air through high-efficiency particulate air (HEPA) filters. If the practice has a portable room filtration unit with an HEPA filter, it should be used in waiting areas or rooms where suspected TB patients are placed.

Employee precautions. Use of PPE for respiratory protection is optional for a minimal risk practice; variable for a very low risk practice; and required for low, intermediate, and high risk practices. At a minimum, the practice should provide a facemask for the exposed worker to protect him or her from becoming contaminated by the patient. If a patient exhibits signs or symptoms of TB, the worker should use an HEPA filter mask to reduce risk of exposure. The exposed employee should use only certified devices with specified capabilities (such as HEPA filter masks) when present in rooms where cough-inducing procedures are performed.

Patient management

Employees should familiarize themselves with the protocol for identifying and evaluating patients who may have active TB. Practices that both evaluate and treat TB patients should follow the published recommendations for handling TB patients in outpatient facilities.

Management of patients with suspected active TB. The management of patients with suspected active TB always begins by asking patients about a previous history of TB or symptoms suggestive of TB. Diagnostic workup for TB infection should include, in addition to a PPD skin test, a complete history and physical examination, a chest x-ray, and perhaps microscopic examination and culture of sputum or other body fluids. For diagnostic workup and treatment, the practice may choose to perform these itself or refer the patient to a practice in a facility capable of handling TB patients.

Management of patients with active TB. Patients considered to have active TB should be started on treatment according to currently recommended guidelines. Again, the practice may choose to have the patient treated elsewhere even if the practice itself makes the diagnosis.

Employee management

Health care workers in offices or clinics in which there is a likelihood of exposure to patients who have infectious TB should be screened (skin tested), counseled, and trained. Any employee who has a persistent cough for three weeks or more associated with signs or symptoms suggestive of active TB (fever, anorexia, weight loss, bloody sputum, or night sweats) must be evaluated promptly for active disease. A worker with such signs and symptoms should not be allowed to return to work unless the worker is determined not to have TB or the worker is determined not to be infectious (i.e., through screening or receiving therapy).

Screening. As part of the risk assessment process, employees should be screened for TB infection with the Mantoux form of purified protein derivative (PPD). The PPD skin test should be conducted annually at no cost to the employee (unless the practice is at an intermediate or high risk level). All employees must have PPD skin testing when there has been an exposure to an infectious patient without appropriate infection-control precautions at the time of exposure. Office staff with signs or symptoms suggestive of active TB should also be skin tested. Whenever an employee has a positive PPD skin test or PPD conversion, he or she should be further evaluated for active TB. A worker who has a past history of a positive skin test should so notify the physician-employer so that the worker can be screened with a chest x-ray. Otherwise, a false-positive test will raise the risk level of the practice. Such workers should be excluded from further skin tests unless they develop signs or symptoms of TB or become exposed to an infectious patient.[34]

Counseling. An employee with a positive PPD skin test should receive counseling regarding the significance of the positive skin test. Counseling helps the worker understand the difference between latent TB infection ("the infection") and active TB infection ("the disease"). Health care workers should be particularly aware of the need for preventing TB transmission in facilities where HIV-infected individuals receive care. Latent TB infection progresses rapidly to active TB in HIV-positive individuals. Employees who work in facilities treating multidrug-resistant TB (MDR-TB) patients should know their HIV status to protect themselves.

Training. The purpose of the training is to educate employees with regard to risk assignment levels, the TB control plan, and methods used to recognize the signs and symptoms of TB. All members of the office staff should be trained in treating TB disease initially (before their first assignments) and thereafter periodically (usually annually). Employees should also be retrained whenever the practice's risk level changes to a higher level.

Case investigations of employees

A stepwise plan must be developed for investigating those employees who experience positive skin test results or PPD conversions. For those employees suspected of having active TB, an investigation should be conducted in the following manner[35]:

1. The employee should be promptly evaluated for active TB with a complete history, physical examination, chest x-ray, and possibly other diagnostic tests.
2. If a diagnosis of either latent TB or active TB ("the disease") has been made, the employee should be treated with either preventive or curative therapy.
3. Other employees with possible exposure should receive PPD tests to determine whether the practice has experienced any further transmission of the disease. Case investigations should also include any patients or other individuals who may have had significant exposure.
4. After treatment of the employee has begun, an effort should be made to discover (by history) the source of the employee's TB exposure. The Public Health Department must be consulted to allow contact investigation of possible community contacts.
5. An effort should also be made to determine whether problems exist with work practice controls (such as detection of TB patients) or engineering controls (such as portable HEPA filtration units). If such problems are suspected, the practice must follow the high risk protocol (with PPD screening) until there have been two consecutive 3-month periods without evidence of transmission of TB.

Any positive skin test result or confirmation of active TB must be recorded on the employee's medical record. Any treatment of that employee must also be documented on the record. If a practice has 11 or more employees, this becomes a reportable incident on OSHA Form 200. The physician-employer may also be required to provide information to other agencies such as OSHA, CDC, and the Public Health Department.

HEALTH INSURANCE PORTABILITY AND ACCOUNTABILITY ACT

The Health Insurance Portability and Accountability Act (HIPA) of 1996 helps eligible employees maintain insurance coverage when changing jobs or policies. The law prohibits insurance carriers or other entities from denying insurance coverage to employers of between 2 and 50 employees. Unfortunately, it does not apply to all previously covered employees.

HIPA prevents employers and insurers from raising premiums or limiting coverage to employees based on medical history, genetic information, health status, disability, receipt of health care, claims experience, or evidence of insurability. Under Title I, employers and insurers are no longer able to limit coverage of a preexisting condition to longer than 12 months (or 18 months in the case of a late enrollee). A waiting period may be imposed for a preexisting condition diagnosed or treated with 6 months of the insured's enrollment date if the enrollee has had no prior coverage for more than 12 consecutive months.

After the waiting period of 12 or 18 months, an insurer cannot deny coverage for any previously treated medical condition. However, time-limited exclusions restrict employees who are presently receiving medical treatment under an insurance plan (and have been covered for less than 12 consecutive months) from moving to another job or insurance company without first suspending medical treatment or personally financing medical expenses.[36] Furthermore, the preexisting condition protections apply only to employees who have incurred less than a 63-day loss in insurance coverage while changing jobs or policies.[37]

Since July 1, 1996, the physician-employer (or his plan broker or health insurer) has been obligated to provide a certificate of coverage to any insured employee leaving the practice.[38] It is the physician-employer's responsibility to notify employees leaving a practice that they either (1) remain covered under the present plan for a designated period or (2) become covered under a new plan after a designated waiting period.[39]

ENDNOTES

1. A. McLaughlin & J. Pendergrass, *Hazard Communication: A Compliance Kit* A-1 (U.S. Government Printing Office, Washington, D.C. 1988).
2. L. Traverse, *The Generator's Guide to Hazardous Materials/Waste Management* 119 (Van Nostrand Reinhold, New York 1991).
3. Program notes, Eagle Associates seminar, presented by Joseph Suchocki (Apr 1990).
4. J. Suchocki et al., *The Safety Resource Guide for OSHA Compliance,* 12 (Eagle Associates, Ann Arbor, Mich. 1990).
5. *Hazard Communication Changes,* Am. Prac. Adv. 116 (1994).
6. *The Illusive Material Safety Data Sheet,* Am. Prac. Adv. 120 (1993).
7. *Supra* note 5, at 117.
8. *Alert for Material Safety Data Sheets,* Am. Prac. Adv. 77 (1993).
9. *Supra* note 4, at 17.
10. *Questions and Answers,* Am. Prac. Adv. 10 (1992).
11. *The Americans with Disabilities Act of 1990,* Am. Prac. Adv. 43 (1995).
12. *Reviewing the Americans with Disabilities Act,* Am. Prac. Adv. 43 (1995).
13. *The Americans with Disabilities Act of 1990,* Am. Prac. Adv. 47 (1992).
14. *Id.*
15. *Supra* note 13, at 49.
16. *What Every Doctor Needs to Know (Americans with Disabilities Act)* [information sheet] (American Medical Association 1990).
17. H. Barton, *Physicians Discover Maze of Regulations under ADA,* 88(11) Tex. Med. 55 (1992).
18. *Id.* at 56.
19. *Id.*
20. S. Dunn, *Needle Safety Laws Loom on the Horizon,* Physicians Marketplace 44 (1999).
21. *Id.*
22. *Id.*
23. *Id.* at 6
24. Occupational Exposure to Bloodborne Pathogens (summary), 29 C.F.R. Part 1910.1030 at 64124.
25. *CLIA 1988 Compliance (information sheet)* 4 (American Proficiency Institute 1993).
26. *Patient Test Management System Trilogy,* Am. Pract. Adv. 61 (1992).
27. *Supra* note 25, at 9.
28. *Regulations for Implementing Clinical Laboratory Improvement Amendments of 1988: A Summary,* 267 J.A.M.A. 1731 (1992).

29. C. Hess, *Office Compliance Manual* 91(All-Med Press, Houston 1995).

30. *Family Leave Law,* Am. Pract. Adv. 7 (1993).

31. *Practice Growth Means Revisiting Personnel Issues,* Am. Med. News 18 (Jul 17, 1995).

32. J. Starke, *Tuberculosis: What the Pediatrician Really Needs to Know (and Do),* program notes, Infectious Diseases in Children Symposium (Nov 1996).

33. *Updating Your TB Control Plan,* Am. Pract. Adv. 123 (1995).

34. *Inside Training: TB Infection Control Plan—Part I,* Am. Pract. Adv. 201 (1996).

35. *Tuberculosis and Airborne Guidelines,* Am. Pract. Adv. 138-140 (1994).

36. *Health Insurance Portability and Accountability Act of 1996: A Tempered Victory,* 24 J. Law, Med. & Ethics 381 (1996).

37. *Id.*

38. *A New Health Insurance Law Enacted,* Am. Pract. Adv. 34 (1997).

39. *Id.*

48

Health professionals and the regulated industry: the laws and regulations enforced by the U.S. Food and Drug Administration

FREDDIE ANN HOFFMAN, M.D.

PETER H. RHEINSTEIN, M.D., J.D., M.S.

No textbook in legal medicine would be complete without a discussion of the U.S. Food and Drug Administration (FDA) and the regulation of products for the U.S. marketplace. The U.S. market is almost unique in that the number and type of products available to the practicing health professional are based on marketability and competitiveness rather than on preselection by a national governmental body. With the recent advent of managed care, however, this marketplace is changing.

Many federal agencies have an impact on product development. For example, the United States Department of Agriculture (USDA) regulates meat, poultry, veterinary biologics, and grain products (Fig. 48-1). The Federal Trade Commission (FTC) is responsible for nonprescription drug, device, and food advertising and promotion. The FDA, however, is by and large the most important agency with respect to products used in the practice of medicine. It is responsible for the regulation of $1141 billion, approximately one fourth of the gross national product, of which 57% represents foods, 10% drugs and biologics, 30% medical devices (including energy-emitting products such as cathode ray tubes and microwave ovens), and 3% cosmetics. Although foods represent the largest category of consumer purchases, the FDA spends almost twice as much in the regulation of drugs and biologics (Figs. 48-2 and 48-3).

This chapter provides an overview of the current laws and regulations that govern the manufacturing, packaging, import and export, and approval of products for the U.S. marketplace. Also discussed are the requirements for the development of new products and the responsibilities of clinical investigators, manufacturers, and health professionals in the use of both investigational and approved products, as well as for products for which approval is not required.

HISTORICAL PERSPECTIVE

Most food and drug regulation has been an outgrowth of consumer concern with safety of products. In the United States the earliest federal legislation to address this issue dates back to the Drug Importation Act passed by Congress in 1848, which required U.S. Customs inspection to stop entry of adulterated drugs from overseas. However, it was not until the twentieth century that product regulation by the federal government was truly established. In 1902 the Biologics Control Act ensured the purity and safety of serums, vaccines, and similar products used to prevent or treat diseases in humans. At this time Congress also authorized the federal government to establish food standards and to study the effects of chemicals on digestion and health. On June 30, 1906, the first comprehensive Food and Drugs Act was enacted,

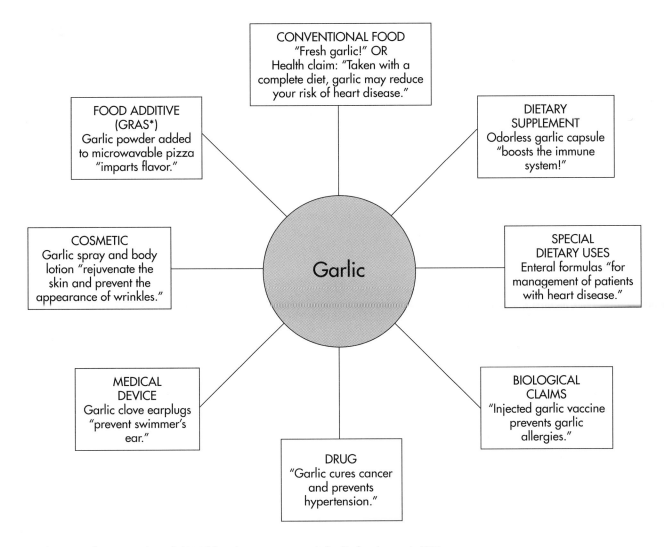

*Garlic is generally recognized as safe (GRAS) based on its common use in food before January 1, 1958.
21 CFR 57 0.30(a)(1).

Fig. 48-1. The U.S. Regulatory Classification (e.g., claims for garlic products). (Courtesy Freddie Ann Hoffman, M.D., and Thomas Garvey IV, J.D.)

which was signed into law by President Theodore Roosevelt. The new law prohibited interstate commerce in misbranded and adulterated foods, drinks, and drugs, and it required ingredients to be listed on the labels of drugs. On the same day, the Meat Inspection Act was passed. These actions by Congress were the result of disclosures of unsanitary conditions in meat packing plants, the use of poisonous preservatives and dyes in foods, and exaggerated claims for unproven and dangerous patent medicines.

These new laws were under the jurisdiction of the USDA until 1927, when a separate regulatory agency was formed. First known as the Food, Drug and Insecticide Administration, it was renamed the Food and Drug Administration in 1930. Although many had tried and failed to revise the now outdated

1906 statute, it was not until 1937 when a major disaster occurred (the death of 107 people, mostly children, after ingestion of an "elixir of sulfanilamide" containing a poisonous solvent) that the need to establish drug safety before marketing and to enact the pending food and drug law was fully realized. The Federal Food, Drug, and Cosmetic Act (FDCA) (21 United States Code [U.S.C.] 321 to 394) was passed in 1938 and contained many new and important provisions, the most monumental of which was the requirement that new drugs be shown to be safe before marketing. This authority initiated a new direction in drug regulation in the United States.

Following this major legislation, many new laws were passed in the ensuing years, refining the law and expanding the responsibilities of the nascent agency. The Insulin

$1,141 billion

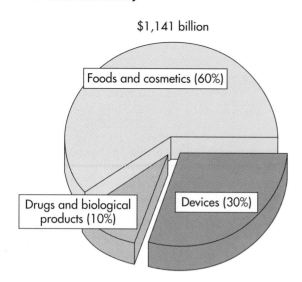

Fig. 48-2. U.S. consumer expenditures on regulated industry. (From the U.S. Food and Drug Administration.)

Total $916 million

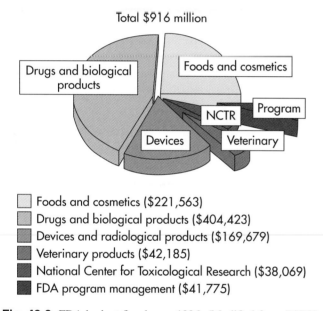

Foods and cosmetics ($221,563)

Drugs and biological products ($404,423)

Devices and radiological products ($169,679)

Veterinary products ($42,185)

National Center for Toxicological Research ($38,069)

FDA program management ($41,775)

Fig. 48-3. FDA budget fiscal year 1996. (Modified from DHHS, PHS, FDA, *FDA Almanac, FY 1996*, DHHS Publication No. [FDA] 96 1254.)

Amendment was passed in 1941, requiring the FDA to test and certify purity and potency of insulin. In 1945 the Penicillin Amendment required the FDA's testing and certification of safety and effectiveness of all penicillin products. Later amendments extended this requirement to all antibiotics up until 1983, when such control was found no longer to be needed and was abolished. In 1962 a new drug, thalidomide, had been approved in Europe to induce sleep and was reported to have caused birth defects in thousands of babies born to women who took the drug during pregnancy. The

FDA was able to prevent this disaster from occurring in the United States and through many public hearings raised awareness and support for even stronger drug regulation. These events culminated in the passage of the Kefauver-Harris Drug Amendments of 1962, adding yet another major component to modern drug regulation in the United States. Not only did drug manufacturers need to demonstrate the safety of a drug to the FDA before marketing it, but they also had to prove its effectiveness for the intended indication. Shortly thereafter the Fair Packaging and Labeling Act (15 U.S.C. Sections 1451 1461) of 1966 added the requirements that all consumer products in interstate commerce be honestly and informatively labeled, bearing a legible, prominent statement of net quantity of contents in terms of weight, measure, or numerical count. The FDA enforces its provisions on foods, drugs, cosmetics, and medical devices.

In response to the mandate set forth by the 1962 Kefauver-Harris Drug Amendments, the FDA established the Drug Efficacy Study Implementation (DESI) program to examine the effectiveness of those new drugs that were approved before these amendments, solely on the basis of safety under provisions of the 1938 act. Similar and related drugs for which "new drug applications" had never been filed were also examined. Exempted from the review were drugs, such as phenobarbital, that had been marketed before the 1938 statute. In 1966, at the agency's request, the National Research Council of the National Academy of Sciences assembled 30 panels of experts to determine whether the information submitted by manufacturers would stand up to the test for "substantial evidence" of effectiveness, as required by the new law. The panels reviewed 3443 drugs with 16,000 separate therapeutic claims. About 60% of the claims were rejected on this review. Although 60% of the drugs had at least one claim that was found to be acceptable, only 12% of the drugs were found effective for all of the claimed indications.

Over the last 30 years, Congress has continued to expand the FDA's regulatory responsibilities, necessitating frequent reorganization. The 1968 Radiation Control for Health and Safety Act extended its scope to protect consumers against unnecessary exposure to radiation from electronic products, and in 1971 the Bureau of Radiological Health was transferred to the FDA. In addition, sections of the Public Health Service (PHS) Act of 1944, relating to biological products for human use (42 U.S.C. 262 to 263), mammography (42 U.S.C. 263b), and control of communicable diseases (42 U.S.C. 264) were also added to the list of the FDA's responsibilities in 1972.

The FDA's regulatory history is represented in its various programs. Currently the FDA has five major regulatory centers: the Center for Biologics Evaluation and Research, the Center for Drug Evaluation and Research, the Center for Devices and Radiological Health, the Center for Food Safety and Applied Nutrition, and the Center for Veterinary Medicine. Another center, the National Center for Toxicological Research located in Arkansas, was founded to examine the effects of chemicals in the environment, extrapolating data from experimental animals to human health. Besides these centers, the agency maintains an Office of External Affairs, which serves as a liaison to consumers, health professionals, the media, legislators, other organizations, and foreign governments, and an Office of Regulatory Affairs, which oversees the local FDA offices, coordinates with the States, and conducts compliance activities for the agency as a whole.

The mission of the FDA is to enforce laws enacted by the U.S. Congress and to establish and enforce regulations to protect the health, safety, and pocketbook of the consumer.[1] In general, the FDCA is intended to assure the consumer that foods are pure and wholesome, safe to eat, and produced under sanitary conditions; that drugs and devices are safe and effective for their intended uses; that cosmetics are safe and made from appropriate ingredients; and that all labeling and packaging are truthful, informative, and not deceptive.

The agency conducts its functions from its headquarters in the Washington, D.C., metropolitan area and its field offices located throughout the nation. More than half of the agency's 9000 employees are scientists and professionals, including physicians, dentists, veterinarians, pharmacists, nurses, chemists, microbiologists, engineers, and attorneys. To enforce the FDCA and other laws under its jurisdiction, the FDA uses modern scientific methods. Actions taken by the agency staff must be based on scientific facts that can be supported in court. The principal authorities relied on for laboratory methods are the Official Methods of Analysis of the Association of Official Analytical Chemists and the United States Pharmacopeia/National Formulary.[2] These compendia of tested, analytical methods are the leading, internationally recognized guides to analytical procedures for law enforcement in the United States. In addition, as part of their new drug applications (discussed later), manufacturers frequently establish analytical methods for newly marketed products.

Premarket testing and approval

The FDCA and the PHS Act require manufacturers of certain consumer products to establish, before marketing, that such products meet the requirements of the law and are properly labeled. New drugs, biological drugs, and certain devices (including their labeling) must be approved for safety and effectiveness. Substances added to food must be approved as safe, "generally recognized as safe," or "prior sanctioned." Color additives used in foods, drugs, cosmetics, and medical devices must be approved as safe and suitable, or approved as safe by specific FDA regulations based on scientific data. Samples of color additives and insulin drugs must be tested and certified by FDA laboratories. Residues of pesticide chemicals in foods must not exceed safe tolerances set by the Environmental Protection Agency and enforced by the FDA. Such premarketing clearances are based on scientific data provided by manufacturers, subject to review and acceptance by government scientists for scope and adequacy.

FDA regulations prescribe the type and extent of premarket testing that must be conducted, depending on the legal requirements applicable to the particular product and on the technology available to fulfill those requirements. Testing may include physical and chemical studies, nonclinical laboratory studies, animal tests, and clinical trials on humans. The importance of the toxicological and other data derived from such investigations demands that they be conducted according to scientifically sound protocols and procedures. The FDA has published regulations in Title 21, Code of Federal Regulations, Part 58 (21 CFR 58) prescribing good laboratory practices (GLPs) for conducting nonclinical research.

For each product category, the FDA has published a set of current good manufacturing practices (GMPs). GMPs stipulate what kinds of buildings, facilities, equipment, and maintenance are needed, as well as the errors to avoid, to ensure sanitation. They also deal with such matters as toilet and washing facilities, cleaning of equipment, materials handling, and vermin control. GMPs for drugs, biologics, and devices differ and are far stricter in their requirements than are GMPs for food. Within the food category, GMPs for food products differ depending on the product. For example, the GMPs for conventional foods are different from those of dietary supplements. GMPs emphasize written records documenting compliance within process controls for every step of the production process.

Current good clinical practices

Sponsors, clinical investigators, and clinical trial monitors are responsible for knowing their respective responsibilities when it comes to clinical evaluation of products. The FDA's proposed policy, titled "The Obligations of Sponsors and Monitors of Clinical Investigations," was published in the Federal Register on September 27, 1977. Parts 312 (drugs, biologics) and 812 (medical devices) contain the current regulations that apply to investigational use of products. The proposed policy was more comprehensive than the final negotiation of the regulations, "General Responsibilities of Investigators" (Sections 312, Subpart D, and 812, Subparts E and G). These regulations are concerned primarily with the selection and qualifications of the clinical investigators and the documented commitment of the investigator to supervise and to assume responsibility for those involved in the clinical studies; to prepare and follow a scientifically sound protocol; to maintain control over the disposition of all test articles; to obtain appropriate human subject protection assurances; and to monitor, record, and report clinical events and adverse events to the product sponsor, to the Institutional Review Board(s) (IRBs), and to the FDA. The FDA has made publicly available information regarding IRBs and human subject protections, which can be accessed from the FDA Web-site or by telephone. (HYPERLINK http://www.fda.gov/oc/oha/default.htmhttp://www.fda.gov/oc/oha/default.htm ; telephone: 301-827-1685.)

Enforcement actions against clinical investigators

Failure to comply with the regulatory responsibilities may result in the agency taking enforcement action. Submission of false data to secure approval is a criminal violation of the laws that prohibit giving false information to the government. Two enforcement tools are used by the FDA to protect the integrity of the product approval process: debarment and disqualification. Sponsors or investigators that are convicted of criminal actions or who are found to have engaged in activities to undermine the drug approval process can be prevented from obtaining or participating in subsequent drug approvals or from providing any services to a drug product applicant. This procedure, called *debarment,* extends to persons working for applicants of human, animal, and biological drug products. The FDA is authorized to conduct debarment procedures by the Generic Drug Enforcement Act of 1992 through amendments to the FDCA (Sections 306 to 308). Fines may range from $250,000 for an individual who commits a prohibited act under Section 307 and up to $1 million for any corporation, partnership, or association found guilty. Debarment actions are published in the Federal Register.

Clinical investigators who violate FDA regulations can be "disqualified" through informal hearings conducted by the FDA (21 CFR 16). Disqualification prevents the investigator from receiving investigational products.[3] In the past the regulation applied only to drugs, biologics, and intraocular lenses. As of March 14, 1997, the agency published its Final Rule, which now includes all investigational devices.[4] Although fewer than 20 physicians have been convicted of crimes involving tests of new drugs since 1978, more than 110 clinical investigators have been sanctioned for actions not prosecuted as criminal or have signed consent agreements.

Sponsors are also required to certify that they did not and will not use the services of a debarred individual or firm in any capacity in connection with the application. Section 306(k) further requires that applicants for approval of certain generic drugs provide information concerning criminal convictions of individuals and firms involved in the applications. Lists of clinical investigators who have been disqualified, of those who have signed consent agreements, and of debarred investigators are available from the FDA, along with information about reinstatement.

GENERAL CONSIDERATIONS FOR REGULATED PRODUCTS
Adulteration and misbranding

The FDCA prohibits distribution within the United States or importation of articles that are adulterated or misbranded. The term *adulterated* includes products that are defective, unsafe, filthy, or produced under unsanitary conditions (Sections 402, 501, 601, codified at 21 U.S.C. 342, 351, 361). The term *misbranded* includes statements, designs, or pictures in labeling that are false or misleading, as well as the failure of the manufacturer to provide required information in labeling (Sections 403, 502, 602, codified at 21 U.S.C. 343, 352, 362). Detailed definitions of adulteration and misbranding are in the law itself, and hundreds of court decisions have interpreted them. The law also prohibits the distribution of any article required to be approved by the FDA, if such approval has not been given, the refusal to provide required reports, and the refusal to allow inspection of regulated facilities pursuant to Section 704 (21 U.S.C. 374).

Product recall and reporting systems

Although the GMP requirements are stringent for drugs, biologics, and devices, defective products may reach the market. Under the FDCA, the FDA has the authority to remove violative products from the market. Removal, or recall, of products is a major means by which the FDA fulfills its mandate of consumer protection. Voluntary recall may be initiated by the manufacturer or shipper of the product, or at the request of the FDA, and is the quickest way to remove the product from the market. In situations involving imminent hazards to health associated with the use of a product, the FDA may order the recall, or the notification to product users, or both. For medical device recalls, manufacturers are required to notify health professionals by issuing a Medical Device Notification at the FDA's request and to report to the FDA actions undertaken to remove or correct violative devices in commerce. Voluntary Safety Alerts can also be issued. Recall actions undertaken by industry are reported weekly in the FDA Enforcement Report.

There are three categories of product recall. Class I designation signifies an imminent health hazard, for which the consequences may be serious illness or death (e.g., incorrect dose, contamination with a pathogenic organism). Class II designation is assigned when the product may cause temporary or reversible adverse health consequences, or where the probability of serious consequences is remote (e.g., potency assay does not meet specifications). A Class III recall is designated when it is unlikely that the product will produce adverse health consequences. Class III recalls are often administrative in nature (e.g., label printing errors) and may have little or no impact on the product's use.

Accurate and complete production and shipping records are vital to the success of a product recall. Although cooperation in a recall may make court proceedings unnecessary to remove the product from the market, it does not relieve a person or firm from possible civil or criminal liability for violations. The FDA prefers, when possible, to promote compliance by means other than going into court. The FDA has the authority to observe conditions or practices of a manufacturer, and during inspections when conditions are noted that may result in violations, a written report (FDA Form 483) of the observations is left with management. By correcting these conditions or practices promptly, manufacturers may bring their operations into compliance. FDA inspectors will also report any voluntary corrective action they witness during an inspection, or that which management may bring to their attention. Copies of these reports are available to the public through the FDA's Freedom of Information office.

Product seizures

Also within the FDA's authority is the right to seize products. Seizure is a civil court action against goods to remove them from the channels of commerce. After seizure, the goods may not be altered, used, or moved, except by permission of the court. The owner or claimant of the seized merchandise is usually given about 30 days by the court to decide on a course of action. The claimant may do nothing, in which case the goods will be disposed of by the court; decide to contest the government's charges by filing a claim and answering the charges, and the case will be scheduled for trial; or consent to condemnation of the goods, while requesting permission of the court to bring the goods into compliance with the law. To bring the goods into compliance, the owner of the goods is required to provide a bond (money deposit) to assure the court that the orders will be carried out and must pay for FDA supervision of any compliance procedure.

Drug quality reporting system

From 1971 to 1982 the FDA contracted with the U.S. Pharmacopeial Convention to receive and process reports of poor quality pharmaceuticals. As a result of the rapid growth in the pharmaceutical industry, the FDA has subsequently established the in house Drug Quality Reporting System (DQRS), a voluntary system to monitor the quality of drugs and devices. The FDA is encouraging health professionals to participate in reporting product problems through the agency's toll free hotline (1 888 INFO-FDA (1-888-4630-332). Reportable problems include improper labeling, defects, performance failures, poor packaging, and incomplete or confusing instructions.

Drug and device listing and establishment registration

Listing of all drugs, biologics (including blood products), device products, veterinary drugs, and medicated premixed animal feeds and registration of the establishments where they are either manufactured or processed is required under Section 510 of the FDCA (21 U.S.C. 360; also see 21 CFR 207). The authority to require registration and listing of blood banks is from the PHS Act (see 21 CFR 607.20 607.21). "Establishments" include facilities to repackage or otherwise change the container, wrapper, or labeling of a product, and the law applies to both bulk and finish dosage forms, as well as products for export. Failure to register and list is a violation of the law at Section 301(p).

The FDA uses the National Drug Code numbering system in assigning a number. The first five numeric characters of the 10 character code identify the manufacturer or distributor

and are known as the Labeler Code. The FDA will expand the Labeler Code from five to six numeric characters when the available five character coded combinations are exhausted. The last five numeric characters of the 10 character code identify the drug and trade package size and type. The segment that identifies the drug formulation is known as the Product Code, and the segment that identifies the trade package size and type is known as the Package Code.

Device registration differs from drug registration. A drug establishment owner or operator must register within 5 days of initiating operations and submit a list of every drug product in commercial distribution at that time. Devices for human use proposed for commercial distribution must undergo not only registration, but also premarket notification (Section 510(k), codified at 21 U.S.C. 360(k)) of the FDA at least 90 days before beginning such distribution (21 CFR 807), unless specifically exempted by regulation (Section 514, codified at 21 U.S.C. 360d). This allows the FDA to determine if premarket approval is necessary. Establishment registration must be updated annually and product listing submissions updated each June and December where material changes have occurred in the listings.

Color additives

A color additive is a dye, pigment, or other substance, whether synthetic or derived from a vegetable, animal, mineral, or other source, that imparts a color when added or applied to a food, drug, cosmetic, or the human body (Section 201(t), codified at 21 U.S.C. 321(t)). Under the FDCA, foods, drugs, cosmetics, and some medical devices are adulterated if they contain color additives that have not been proven safe to the satisfaction of the FDA for the particular use. Regulations (21 CFR 73, 74, and 81) list the approved color additives and the conditions under which they may be safely used, including the amounts that may be used when limitations are necessary. Separate lists are provided for color additives for use in or on foods, drugs, medical devices, and cosmetics. Some colors may appear on more than one list.

Orphan products: regulation and promotion of products for rare diseases and conditions

In 1983 the Orphan Drug Act (Pub. L. 97 414, 96 Stat. 2049) amended the FDCA to promote the development of drugs and biological products for "rare" diseases or conditions. The amendment provides manufacturers with economic incentives. Revisions have been made in the original legislation in each succeeding Congressional session. A rare disease or condition is taken to mean one that affects fewer than 200,000 persons in the United States, or affects more than 200,000 persons in the United States and for which there is no reasonable expectation that the development cost will be retrieved in the domestic sales of the product. In 1988 the Act was amended to establish that the filing of an application for "Orphan Drug Designation" must be made before the filing of a marketing application (new drug application or product license application). Designation of a product does not in any way alter the standard regulatory requirements for marketing approval. However, it does permit tax credits (26 U.S.C. 44H) for clinical research undertaken by a sponsor to generate required data and the granting of exclusive approval for 7 years for a designated drug or biological product. The FDA has a limited program to fund clinical and preclinical studies for the development of such products. Occasionally this funding has also been extended to medical device and medical food studies. Although funding authorization has been regularly extended by Congress, separate funds have not been appropriated under the Orphan Drug Act. The FDA's Office of Orphan Product Development funds both grants and cooperative agreements through its general appropriation.

In 1996 regulations were added to 21 CFR 814 Subpart H that allow for the development of Humanitarian Use Devices (HUDs), that is, devices for which the use population would be less than 4000 persons annually in the United States.[5] The new regulations delineate the requirements for the designation of HUDs, which include "temporary" marketing approval for the designated device "notwithstanding the absence of reasonable effectiveness that would otherwise be required under sections 514 and 515 of the act." "HUD" designation is also administered through the Office of Orphan Product Development (see Section 814.100).

FOODS

Foods are defined as (1) articles used for food or drink for humans or other animals, (2) chewing gum, and (3) articles used for components of any such article (FDCA, Section 201(f), codified at 21 U.S.C. 321(f)). Foods are regulated by the Center for Food Safety and Applied Nutrition and include products classified as conventional foods, food additives, spices, dietary supplements, and foods for special dietary use.

In general, sanitation is a major focus of food regulation. A food is considered adulterated, and therefore illegal, if it contains harmful substances that are either added, or occur naturally, that may render it injurious to health; if it has been prepared, packed, or held under unsanitary conditions; or if any part of it is unfit for consumption (see Section 402(a), codified at 21 U.S.C. 342(a)). Raw agricultural products are illegal if they contain residues of pesticides not authorized by, or in excess of, tolerances established by regulations of the Environmental Protection Agency (Section 402(a)(2)(b) and Section 408).

Labeling

Foods are subject to required labeling under both the FDCA (Section 403(f), codified at 21 U.S.C. 343(f)) and the Fair Packaging and Labeling Act (FPLA) (Pub. L. 80 1296, codified at 15 U.S.C. 1451 61), the details of which may be found in the regulations (21 CFR 101). However, in anticipation of changes to the metric system, the FPLA, which pertains only to consumer commodities, was amended by Public Law 102 329 to require that labels printed on or after February 14, 1994, bear a statement of the quantity of the contents in terms of the SI metric system, as well as in terms of the customary inch/pound system of measure.

The Nutrition Labeling and Education Act (NLEA) of 1990 (Pub. L. 101 535, 104 Stat. 2353) has led to significant changes in food labeling regulations, addressing three primary areas: the nutrition label, nutrient content claims, and health claims. The regulations specify the nutrition information that must be on the label and the format in which it is to be presented (Fig. 48-4). The regulations also identify those instances in which a food product is exempt from all or certain requirements for nutrition labeling (21 CFR 101.9). The regulations further specify the display of which nutrients are required and their order. In addition to these mandatory nutrients, manufacturers may voluntarily choose to include other information, such as other vitamins and minerals for which Recommended Daily Intakes (RDIs) have been established. In addition to nutrients, the NLEA requires standards to define serving sizes (21 CFR 101.12). Nutrient content claims are those that describe the amount of a nutrient in the food (such as "sodium free" or "low fat") and are defined by FDA regulation (21 CFR 101.13). Food additives and colors are required to be listed as ingredients.

Infant formulas

The Infant Formula Act of 1980 (Pub. L. 94 1190) establishes nutrient requirements (Section 201(z)) and provides FDA authority to establish GMPs and requirements for nutrient quantity, nutrient quality control, and record-keeping, and for reporting and recalling infant formulas that pose a potential hazard to health. In addition, the manufacturer must notify the FDA 90 days before any charitable or commercial distribution of any new infant formula or any product that has had a major change in its formulation or processing. Quality control procedures for ensuring nutrient content are also specified in the regulations (21 CFR 106), and additional regulations in response to amendments are being promulgated.

Dietary Supplement Health and Education Act of 1994

On October 25, 1994, President Clinton signed into law the Dietary Supplement Health and Education Act (DSHEA) (Pub. L. 103 417, 108 Stat. 4325), which amended the FDCA to include several provisions that apply only to dietary supplements and dietary ingredients of these supplements. As a result of these provisions, dietary ingredients used in dietary supplements are no longer subject to the premarket safety evaluations required of other new food ingredients or for new uses of old food ingredients. However, they must meet the requirements of other safety provisions.

DSHEA amends the adulteration provisions of the FDCA. Under DSHEA a dietary supplement is adulterated if it or one

The new food label will carry an up-to-date, easier-to-use nutrition information guide, to be required on almost all packaged foods (compared to about 60 percent of products up till now). The guide will serve as a key to help in planning a healthy diet.*

Serving sizes are now more consistent across product lines, are stated in both household and metric measures, and reflect the amounts people actually eat.

The **list of nutrients** covers those most important to the health of today's consumers, most of whom need to worry about getting <u>too much</u> of certain nutrients (fat, for example), rather than too few vitamins or minerals, as in the past.

The label of larger packages may now tell the number of calories per gram of fat, carbohydrate, and protein.

Nutrition Facts

Serving Size 1 cup (228g)
Servings Per Container 2

Amount Per Serving

Calories 260   Calories from Fat 120

	% Daily Value*
Total Fat 13g	**20%**
Saturated Fat 5g	**25%**
Cholesterol 30mg	**10%**
Sodium 660mg	**28%**
Total Carbohydrate 31g	**10%**
Dietary Fiber 0g	**0%**
Sugars 5g	
Protein 5g	

Vitamin A 4%	•	Vitamin C 2%
Calcium 15%	•	Iron 4%

* Percent Daily Values are based on a 2,000 calorie diet. Your daily values may be higher or lower depending on your calorie needs:

		Calories:	2,000	2,500
Total Fat	Less than		65g	80g
Sat Fat	Less than		20g	25g
Cholesterol	Less than		300mg	300mg
Sodium	Less than		2,400mg	2,400mg
Total Carbohydrate			300g	375g
Dietary Fiber			25g	30g

Calories per gram:
Fat 9 • Carbohydrate 4 • Protein 4

New title signals that the label contains the newly required information.

Calories from fat are now shown on the label to help consumers meet dietary guidelines that recommend people get no more than 30 percent of the calories in their overall diet from fat.

% Daily Value shows how a food fits into the overall daily diet.

Daily Values are also something new. Some are maximums, as with fat (65 grams <u>or less</u>); others are minimums, as with carbohydrate (300 grams <u>or more</u>). The daily values for a 2,000- and 2,500-calorie diet must be listed on the label of larger packages.

* This label is only a sample. Exact specifications are in the final rules.
Source: Food and Drug Administration, 1994

Fig. 48-4. The new food label at a glance. (From DHHS, FDA, *Focus on Food Labeling: Read the Label, Set a Healthy Table.* An FDA Consumer Special Report. May 1993, DHHS Publication No. 93 2262.)

of its ingredients presents "a significant or unreasonable risk of illness or injury" when used as directed on the label or under normal conditions of use. A dietary supplement that contains a new dietary ingredient (i.e., an ingredient not marketed for dietary supplement use in the United States before October 15, 1994) may be adulterated when there is inadequate information to provide reasonable assurance that the ingredient will not present a significant or unreasonable risk of illness or injury. Supplement manufacturers must notify the FDA at least 75 days before marketing products containing new dietary ingredients by providing the agency with the documentation of safety. Any interested party, including a manufacturer of a dietary supplement, may petition the FDA to issue an order prescribing the conditions of use under which a new dietary ingredient will reasonably be expected to be safe. The Secretary of the Department of Health and Human Services (DHHS) may also declare that a dietary supplement or dietary ingredient poses an imminent hazard to public health or safety. However, as with any other foods, it is a manufacturer's responsibility to ensure that its products are safe and properly labeled before marketing. The agency is in the process of promulgating regulations for dietary supplements, including GMPs, which will revise 21 CFR 101.36.

The DSHEA provides that retail outlets may make available "third party" materials to help inform consumers about any health-related benefits of dietary supplements. These materials, which include articles, book chapters, scientific abstracts, or other third party publications, cannot be false or misleading, cannot promote a specific brand of supplement, and must be displayed with other similar materials to present a balanced view. The literature must be displayed separately from the dietary supplements themselves and may not have other information attached, such as product promotional literature.

Dietary supplement claims

The new legislation allows for four types of claims to be made for dietary supplements: health, nutrients, structure and function, or well-being. Health claims, such as the claim that folic acid may reduce the risk of developing neural tube birth defects in infants born to mothers taking the supplement, must be preapproved by FDA. They can be approved only if the product qualifies to bear the claim. Statements about classical nutrient deficiency diseases, such as vitamin C preventing scurvy, are permissible as long as these statements disclose the prevalence of the disease in the United States. DSHEA also allows manufacturers to describe the product's effects on structure or function of the body or the well-being achieved by consuming the dietary ingredient. To use these claims, manufacturers must have substantiation that the statements are truthful and not misleading, and the product label must bear the statement: "This statement has not been evaluated by the Food and Drug Administration. This product is not intended to diagnose, treat, cure, or prevent any disease." Unlike health claims, nutritional support statements need not be approved by the FDA before marketing products; however, the agency must be notified no later than 30 days after a product that bears the claim is first marketed.

Like other foods, dietary supplement products must bear ingredient labeling. If a supplement is covered by specifications in an official compendium and is represented as conforming, it is misbranded if it does not conform to those specifications. If not covered by a compendium, a dietary supplement must be the product identified on the label and have the strength it is represented as having. Nutrition labeling is also required.

Food additives

Food additives are substances that by their intended uses may become components of food, either directly or indirectly (such as plastic or vinyl packaging materials; Section 409, codified at 21 U.S.C. 348)), or that may otherwise affect the characteristics of the food (Section 201(s), codified at 21 U.S.C. 321(s)). Food additives come to the U.S. market through petition (21 CFR 171). If the FDA concludes from the evidence submitted that the additive will be safe, a regulation permitting its use is issued, specifying the amount of the substance that may be present in or on the foods, the foods in which it is permitted, the manner of use, and any special labeling required.

In the law, the Delaney clause (Section 409(c)(3), codified at 21 U.S.C. 348(c)(3)) provides that no food additive may be found safe if it produces cancer when ingested by humans or animals. On August 3, 1996, President Clinton signed the Food Quality Protection Act into law (Pub. L. 104 170), administered by the Environmental Protection Agency, which resolves what has been called the Delaney paradox. Under the Delaney clause, paradoxically the FDCA had prohibited the EPA from setting a tolerance level for processed foods, which were allowed to contain greater levels than the tolerance for the same pesticide in the raw agricultural commodity, if the risk were not a cancer risk. The new law provides that tolerances for pesticide residues in all types of foods (raw or processed) will be set under the same provisions of law and that the standards apply to all risks, not just cancer risks.

Although food packaging materials are subject to regulation as food additives, the FDA has generally not enforced the food additive provisions on ordinary housewares, such as dishes, flatware, cooking utensils, and electrical appliances. Housewares, however, are not exempt from the general safety provisions of the FDCA. Regulatory actions have been taken against cookware and ceramic dinnerware containing leachable lead or cadmium.

Artificial sweeteners

The Saccharin Study and Labeling Act (Pub. L. 91 1451), passed November 23, 1977, prohibited for 18 months any new regulations restricting or banning the sale of saccharin or products containing it. Congress has extended the legislation several times and as of August 6, 1996, extended the Act to May 1, 2002 (Pub. L. 104 180). It requires further scientific evaluation of the carcinogenic potential of saccharin and a label warning: "Use of this product may be hazardous to your health. This product contains saccharin which has been determined to cause cancer in laboratory animals." Artificially sweetened products are required to be labeled as Special Dietary Foods (21 CFR 105.66, see later discussion). The foods permitted to contain such sweeteners, and the amounts, are specified in the food additive regulations.

Sulfiting agents

Some individuals have severe reactions (e.g., asthma, anaphylaxis) to sulfiting agents. Although sulfiting agents are permitted for use in food under 21 CFR 182.3616, 182.3637, 182.3739, 182.3766, 182.3798, and 182.3862, their use is prohibited on fruits and vegetables intended to be served or sold raw to consumers, or to be presented as fresh; in meats; and on foods that are a significant source of vitamin B_1. When a sulfiting agent is present in a detectable amount (10 parts per million) in a finished food, regardless of whether it has been directly added or indirectly added, it must be declared on the label of the food. If the sulfiting agent is added directly to the food and has a technical or functional effect in the finished food, it must be declared on the label, irrespective of the amount present in the finished food.

Alcoholic beverages

Beer, wine, liquor, liqueur, and other alcoholic beverages are specifically subject to the FDCA, which is enforced by the Bureau of Alcohol, Tobacco and Firearms (BATF) of the U.S. Treasury Department. Accordingly, questions of labeling and composition should be taken up with the Bureau. This is not the case for cooking wines or for certain other wine beverages, such as diluted wine beverages and cider beverages having less than 7% alcohol by volume, which are solely within the jurisdiction of the FDA. The importation of absinth and any other liquors or liqueurs that contain an excess of *Artemisia absinthium* is prohibited.

Foods for special dietary uses and foods used as drugs

Foods for special dietary uses are another class of foods under the law (FDCA Section 411(c)(3), codified at 21 U.S.C. 350(c)(3)). These foods may supply a special dietary need that exists because of a physical, physiological, pathological, or other condition, including but not limited to the conditions of disease, convalescence, pregnancy, lactation, infancy, allergic hypersensitivity to food, underweight, overweight, or the need to control the intake of sodium. An example might be the foods used in phenylketonuria diets.

When a food for special dietary use, or for that matter, any food or dietary supplement, is labeled, advertised, or promoted with claims of disease prevention, treatment, mitigation, cure, or diagnosis, the FDA regards these claims as *drug claims.* Such products must comply with the drug provisions of the FDCA, unless the claim is a *health claim* authorized by regulation. Also, if a food product is recognized in an *official compendium,* such as the United States Pharmacopeia (USP), the product is considered to be both a drug and a food (see later discussion). For example, cod liver oil is recognized in the USP, and products offered for sale as cod liver oil must comply with the identity standard prescribed by the USP and conform to the other specifications set forth in that official compendium.

Many herbs and other botanical products once thought to have medicinal value continue to be marketed for various purposes. If no therapeutic claims are made or implied in the labeling or other promotional material, such products are regarded as foods and subject only to the food provisions of the law. For example, the herb ginseng is permitted to be sold as a tea. Contrary to popular belief, however, botanical products are not necessarily harmless. Plant products can be toxic, and some may be extremely dangerous. Natural constituents of botanical products are sensitive to the conditions of growth (e.g., soil, light, water), as well as processing conditions. To maintain identity, characterization, and integrity of active components of botanical products, emphasis should be placed on harvesting, storing, handling, packaging, and shipping under conditions that will prevent contamination or deterioration. Attention to these parameters is of particular importance when the botanical is being marketed as a drug.

Food standards

Without standards, different foods could have the same names, or the same foods could have different names. Both situations would be confusing and misleading to consumers and create unfair competition. FDA regulations include a "general standard of identity" (21 CFR 130.10) for modified versions of traditional standardized foods (the standards for traditional foods are contained in 21 CFR 131 through 169). Such modified versions (e.g., reduced fat or reduced calorie versions of traditional standardized foods) must comply with the provisions of 21 CFR 130.10. Standards of quality established under the FDCA must not be confused with standards for "grades" that are published by the U.S. Department of Agriculture for meat and other agricultural products and the U.S. Department of the Interior for fishery products.

Under the FDCA, a standard of quality is only a minimum standard (21 CFR 130.14). International food standards (the Codex Alimentarius) have been developed by committees of the World Health Organization and the Food and Agriculture Organization of the United Nations, of which the United States is a member. The U.S. government may adopt Codex standards in whole or in part, in accordance with the procedures outlined in the preceding paragraph. The purpose of these regulations is to ensure safety from harmful bacteria or their toxins, especially the deadly *Clostridium botulinum.* This can be accomplished only by adequate processing controls and appropriate processing methods, such as cooking the food at the proper temperatures for a sufficient time, adequately acidifying the food, or controlling water activity. The regulations were first adopted in 1973 and revised in 1979 (21 CFR 108.25 and 108.35).

Bioengineered foods

New technologies have made it possible to insert or delete genetic material from plants that are used in the production of food and animal feed products. To date, the FDA is unaware of information that would distinguish genetically engineered foods as a class from foods developed through other methods of plant breeding. Unlike European countries, the United States does not currently require that foods be labeled if they contain ingredients made through genetic modification or bioengineering. Based on the current law, although the FDCA requires that all labeling be truthful and not misleading, it does not require disclosure of information solely on the basis of consumers' desire to know. The FDA will require specific labeling if the composition of a food developed through genetic engineering or any other method differs significantly from its conventional counterpart. In the United States, however, there are currently no specific requirements for manufacturers to disclose the method of development.

Trade agreements and harmonization efforts have brought this issue to the forefront. To address the issue of the safety and labeling of genetically modified food ingredients, the FDA held three public meetings to discuss these topics in the fall of 1999. On May 3, 2000 the agency announced in a departmental news release that it intends to refine its regulatory approach to foods derived from biotechnology. The agency is planning to publish a proposed rule mandating that the developers of bioengineered foods and animal feeds notify the agency before marketing these products. Specific information will be required to be submitted to help the FDA determine whether there are any potential safety, labeling, or adulteration issues.

DRUGS FOR HUMAN USE

Drugs for human use are regulated through the FDA's Center for Drug Evaluation and Research (CDER). The FDCA defines drugs as "articles intended for use in the diagnosis, cure, mitigation, treatment, or prevention of disease in man or other animals" and "articles (other than food) intended to affect the structure or any function of the body of man or other animals" (e.g., articles intended for weight reduction). See FDCA Section 201(g), codified at 21 U.S.C. 321(g). The manufacturer's intended use determines whether an article is a drug. Intended use is provided by the product's labeling, or it may be inferred from advertisements or promotional activities carried out on behalf of the manufacturer. Thus foods and cosmetics may also be subject to the drug requirements of the law if therapeutic claims are made for them.

Drug manufacturers are required to operate in conformity with current GMPs (discussed earlier), which include adequately equipped manufacturing facilities, adequately trained personnel, stringent control over the manufacturing processes, reliable and secure computerized operations, and appropriate finished product examination and testing (21 CFR 210 and 211). The FDCA prohibits the adulteration or misbranding of any drug and requires that new drugs be reviewed and approved by the FDA before entering the market. The definitions of drug adulteration, misbranding, and

new drug appear in Sections 501, 502, and 201(p) of the Act, codified at 21 U.S.C. 351, 352 and 321(p), respectively.

Official drugs

The FDCA designates the USP, the Homeopathic Pharmacopeia of the United States (HPUS), and the National Formulary (NF) as official compendia (Section 201(j)). Since 1980, the USP and the NF have been published in a single volume by the USP Convention. USP monographs provide standards, specifications, and methods of analysis for approximately 3200 drugs. NF monographs contain standards for some 250 other pharmaceutical materials. All drugs named in the compendia are required by the FDCA to meet the standards of strength, quality, or purity set forth in such compendia and must be packaged and labeled in the manner prescribed by the official compendia.

If a drug differs from or falls outside the limits specified in an official compendium, the nature and extent of its difference from such standard must be plainly stated on the label (Section 501(b), codified at 21 U.S.C. 351(b)). A drug not recognized in an official compendium is adulterated if its strength differs from or its purity or quality falls below that which it purports to have or is represented to possess (Section 501(c), codified at 21 U.S.C. 351(c)). For example, any drug intended for use by injection and any ophthalmic ointment or solution must be sterile; if such a product is contaminated with microorganisms, it is adulterated. Also, a drug is adulterated under the FDCA if any substance has been mixed with it so as to reduce the quality or strength of the product or to constitute a substitute of the product (Section 501(d), codified at 21 U.S.C. 351(d)).

New drugs

The largest category of drugs from a regulatory standpoint is that defined as "new drugs" (Section 201(p), codified at 21 U.S.C. 321(p)). A drug may be new for many reasons, including the following: (1) it contains a newly developed chemical; (2) it contains a chemical or substance not previously used in medicine; (3) the drug has previously been used in medicine, but not in the dosages or for the conditions for which the sponsor now recommends its use; or (4) the drug has become recognized by qualified experts as "safe and effective" for its intended uses as a result of investigational studies, but has not otherwise been used to a material extent or for a material time.

About 90% of the drugs marketed since the 1938 FDCA was passed are new in a medical and legal sense. A new drug may not be commercially marketed in, imported to, or exported from the United States, unless it has been approved as safe and effective by the FDA. Such approval is based on a new drug application (NDA) (21 CFR 314) submitted by the sponsor of the drug (usually, but not always, its manufacturer), containing acceptable scientific data, including the results of tests to evaluate its safety, and "substantial evidence" of effectiveness for the conditions for which the drug is to be offered (Section 505, codified at 21 U.S.C. 355). For exceptions concerning exported drugs, see later discussion. Substantial evidence is defined by the law as "evidence consisting of adequate and well controlled investigations, including clinical investigations, by experts qualified by scientific training and experience to evaluate the effectiveness of the drug involved, on the basis of which it could fairly and responsibly be concluded by such experts that the drug will have the effect it purports or is represented to have under the conditions of use prescribed, recommended, or suggested in the labeling or proposed labeling thereof" (Section 505(d)).

After a drug is approved, its formula, manufacturing process, labeling, packaging, dosage, and methods of testing generally may not be changed from those stated in the NDA, unless a supplemental application has first been filed and approved (21 CFR 314.70). However, changes to increase assurance of safety and effectiveness are to be put into effect at the earliest possible time, without waiting for approval (21 CFR 314.70(c)(2)). Detailed instructions are given in the regulations. Drugs that are not new are not subject to the new drug procedure, but they must comply with all other drug requirements, including registration, labeling, and manufacturing practices.

Investigational drugs

To establish safety and efficacy, a new drug that is not yet approved must be studied. New drugs under study are considered *investigational* (Section 505(i), codified at 21 U.S.C. 355(i)). Drug development in the United States usually proceeds in an orderly fashion from discovery, through preclinical studies (in vitro and animal studies), through clinical studies, to the filing of the NDA. Investigational drugs may not be distributed or imported for trial on humans, unless the sponsor has filed an acceptable investigational new drug (IND) application, as specified by the regulations (21 CFR 50 and 312). A product being studied under an IND may not be promoted or advertised for the indications being studied in the IND investigation or otherwise commercialized before it is approved for commercial marketing (21 CFR 312). Clinical trials are usually conducted in stages, called *phases* (Fig. 48-5). Initial studies in humans are generally called Phase I, the objective of which is to describe safety and establish initial doses for study. Further studies to discover activity in humans, called Phase II, are often controlled trials in which safety and efficacy can be evaluated. Although not delineated by regulation, Phase III trials are usually considered pivotal to confirm the results for an NDA. Additional postmarketing studies after approval are often termed Phase IV by the industry. Such studies are sometimes required by the FDA at the time of marketing approval to establish safety further in a broader population.

The design of the clinical protocol should be supported by information already known about the product. This includes information about the pharmacology, toxicity, and

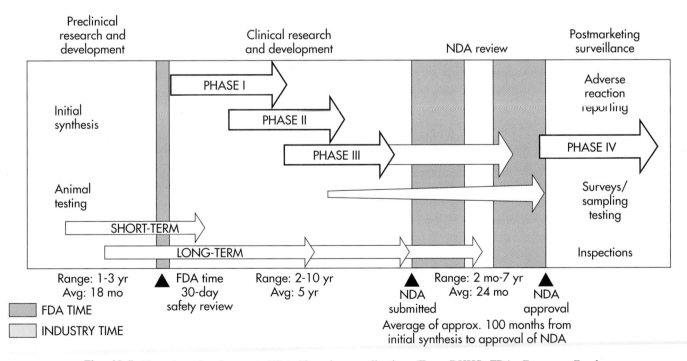

Fig. 48-5. New drug development. *NDA,* New drug application. (From DHHS, FDA, *Focus on Food Labeling: Read the Label, Set a Healthy Table.* An FDA Consumer Special Report. May 1993, DHHS Publication No. 93 2262.)

effects observed in preclinical studies, as well as any previous human use that supports the safety of the dose, route, and schedule. Protocols must contain essential elements, including objectives, a description of the study population, subject selection criteria, product information, monitoring plan, end point determination, and analyses to be performed. The protocol must also be accompanied by an informed consent form that meets the requirements under 21 CFR 50.20 and 50.25. The FDA is continually evaluating the risk to benefit ratio in permitting trials to proceed and in approving drugs for the U.S. market. The FDA publishes *Guidance* documents on clinical drug development, as well as on other parts of the approval process.

Accelerated approvals and expanded access to investigational products

Procedures governing the development of new drugs, antibiotics, and biologics (discussed later) for the treatment of serious or life-threatening illnesses have been updated and revised. Under Subpart E of the regulations (21 CFR 312.80 to 312.88),[6] the FDA seeks to accelerate the development of such products by encouraging early consultation with the agency by sponsors and, if expanded access is needed, the development of a Treatment IND during the later phases of product development and approval with appropriate postmarketing surveillance and additional studies, if necessary, based on a risk/benefit analysis.

The Treatment IND permits the wider use of promising agents when four criteria exist: (1) the product is intended to treat serious or immediately life-threatening disease; (2) there is no comparable or satisfactory alternative drug or other therapy; (3) the drug is under investigation in a controlled (Phase II or III) clinical trial or all clinical trials have been completed; and (4) the sponsor of the controlled clinical trial is actively pursuing marketing approval with due diligence (21 CFR 312.34). Treatment IND proposals may include cost recovery proposals that must be reviewed and approved by the agency.[7] The agency has added an additional policy, called *Parallel Track,* that currently addresses only products designed to treat human immunodeficiency virus (HIV)-positive populations. According to this policy, promising products in very early stages of development (promising preclinical or Phase I data) are made available to those patients who cannot participate in the controlled clinical trials because of severe disease or geographic considerations or because the controlled trials are fully enrolled.[8]

The accelerated approval regulation[9] allows the FDA to grant marketing approval for a new drug product for serious or life-threatening disease, on the basis of clinical trials establishing that the drug product has an effect on a surrogate end point that is likely to predict clinical benefit. Such approval is subject to the requirement that the sponsor studies the drug further to verify and describe its clinical benefit. The regulation also permits the FDA to restrict distribution to certain facilities with special training or experience, or it may be conditioned on the performance of specified medical procedures. Approval granted under this regulation may be withdrawn if a postmarketing clinical study fails to verify clinical benefit, if the sponsor fails to perform the required postmarketing study with due diligence, if use after marketing demonstrates that postmarketing restrictions are inadequate to ensure safe use of the drug product, if the sponsor fails to adhere to the postmarketing restrictions agreed on, if the promotional materials are false or misleading, or if other evidence demonstrates that the drug product is not shown to be safe or effective under its conditions of use.

Prescription and nonprescription drugs

Drugs are also categorized by the law on the basis of dispensing requirements. Prescription drugs may be dispensed only by or on the prescription of a licensed practitioner, such as a physician, dentist, or veterinarian. However, the definition of a licensed practitioner is a matter of state law and varies from state to state. Prescription drugs are required to be labeled with the legend: "Caution: Federal law prohibits dispensing without prescription" (Section 503(b)(4), added in 1951 by Pub. L. 65 648, codified at 21 U.S.C. 353(b)(4)). In general, a drug is restricted to the prescription class if it is not safe for use except under professional supervision. Under the FDCA, this includes habit-forming drugs and any drug that is unsafe "because of its toxicity or other potentiality for harmful effect, or the method of its use, or the collateral measures necessary to its use . . ." (Section 503(b)(1)). Most prescription drugs are new drugs.

The Prescription Drug Marketing Act, which was enacted in 1988, amended Section 503 of the FDCA, codified at 21 U.S.C. 353, to prohibit reimportation of domestically produced prescription drugs. Prescription drugs may legally be shipped by the manufacturer or distributor only to persons and firms who are regularly and lawfully engaged in the wholesale or retail distribution of prescription drugs and to hospitals, clinics, physicians, and others licensed to prescribe. Consumers may receive prescription drugs only through a licensed practitioner or, on his or her order, by a registered pharmacist. Under certain limited circumstances, a limited supply of drugs may be shipped directly to a consumer, for personal use only from a foreign source, in accordance with the personal importation guidance policy.

Over-the-counter drugs

Nonprescription drugs, commonly called over-the-counter (OTC) drugs, are those generally regarded as safe for the consumer to use by following the required directions and warnings on the label. OTC drugs carry indications for conditions that are generally self-limiting or can be recognized and successfully treated by consumers. Most OTC drugs have undergone a monograph process as described in 37 F.R. 85 (January 5, 1972).

In 1972 the FDA began a review of OTC drug products as part of the mandate of the 1962 drug amendments.[10] Because there are more than 300,000 marketed OTC drug products, the FDA is reviewing the active ingredients and the labeling of more than 80 therapeutic classes of drugs, instead of individual drug products, as in the prescription Drug Efficacy Study Implementation (DESI) review. Ingredients reviewed are classified in one of three ways: Category I generally recognized as safe and effective and not misbranded, Category II not generally recognized as safe and effective or misbranded, and Category III insufficient data available to permit classification. *Misbranded* products are those whose labeling is false or misleading.

The OTC review is a three-phase rule-making process, which includes an advance notice of proposed rule-making (advisory panel recommendations), a proposed rule (tentative final monograph), and a final rule (final monograph) for each therapeutic class of drugs under consideration. The first phase was accomplished by advisory review panels, which considered the drugs by class (e.g., analgesics, antacids) and presented their recommendations to the FDA. The agency then published these recommendations in the Federal Register and requested public comment on them. Panel reports have been published on all drug classes.

During the second phase, the FDA presents its tentative conclusions, which are based on the panel's findings, on public comments, and on new data that may have become available. The FDA publishes a proposed rule in the Federal Register, and this proposed rule allows time for public comment or in some cases, a hearing before the Commissioner, and for submission of new data. Most of the proposed rules have also been published.

The FDA's final monograph, the third phase, identifies those active ingredients that are generally recognized as safe and effective for specified uses and that may be marketed as OTC drug products. The monograph also identifies those labeling claims that may appear on the products. OTC drug products containing any active ingredient or labeling claim that is not so recognized must be removed from the market. Some products can be reformulated or appropriately relabeled. For ingredients or claims not included in the monograph, a manufacturer has the option of filing an NDA. A manufacturer may also petition to amend a final monograph to include additional ingredients or to modify labeling. However, the firm may neither market the drug nor use the labeling claim until the NDA is approved or the final monograph is amended. The FDA expects to complete the OTC review by publishing final rules within the next few years.

Some drugs are switched from prescription to OTC status through a supplemental NDA, which may demonstrate a new OTC dose that is lower than prescription strength, or may cite a track record of outstanding safety as a prescription drug to justify switching to OTC sale. OTC drugs must also comply with the requirements of the Fair Packaging and Labeling Act (21 CFR 201.60).

Prescription drug user fees

To augment the FDA's resources to reduce the time to approval, in 1992 Congress passed the Prescription Drug User Fee Act (PDUFA; Pub. L. 102 571, Title I). This law authorizes the FDA to collect user fees for certain applications for approval of human drug and biological products, on establishments where the products are made, and on such products that are on the market. User fees are devoted entirely to the review of human drug applications. The FDA Modernization and Accountability Act of 1997 reauthorized PDUFA through September 30, 2002. Products covered by PDUFA include most human prescription drugs, including those of a biological origin, and OTC drugs that are marketed under an approved NDA. Products that are not covered are generic drugs, OTC drugs that are monographed, whole blood and blood components used for transfusion, some large volume parenterals, allergenic extract products, in vitro diagnostic biological products, and certain drugs derived from bovine blood. When specific conditions are met, the FDA may waive, reduce, or delay payment of the fees.

The label and "labeling" of drugs

The FDCA defines label to mean the written, printed, or graphic matter on the immediate container (Section 201(k), codified at 21 U.S.C. 321(k)) and the outer carton or wrapper of the package. Labeling includes all labels and other written, printed, or graphic matter accompanying the product. The word *accompanying* is interpreted very broadly; therefore labeling may include material that does not physically accompany the product, if it serves to identify the article, tell its uses, give directions, and so on. How a drug is labeled is determined by its classification, that is, whether it is an investigational drug, a new drug, a prescription only drug, or an OTC drug. Each of these has special labeling requirements.

The label itself must bear identifying information, such as the dosage strength and the quantity of content, active ingredients, expiration date, name and quantity or proportions of any habit forming substance with appropriate statements (e.g., "Warning: May be habit forming," as stated in Section 502(d), codified at 21 U.S.C. 352(d)). An important provision states that a drug is misbranded if its labeling is false or misleading in any particular (Section 502(a), codified at 21 U.S.C. 352(a)). Prescription drugs must state the legend (mentioned earlier). The package insert should contain the following sections: description, clinical pharmacology, indications and usage, contraindications, warnings, precautions, adverse reactions, drug abuse and dependence, overdosage (where applicable), dosage and administration, and how supplied (21 CFR 201.50 through 201.57). For OTC preparations, the principal display panel must bear similar information, as required under 21 CFR 201.61 to

201.62. Additionally, most OTC drug products are required to have tamper resistant packaging and labeling (21 CFR 211.132). Drugs that are dispensed by a licensed practitioner are exempted from the need to use the labeling required in the manufacturer's package if the dispensed products have the pharmacist's label containing the legally required elements, such as the names and addresses of the prescriber and patient, directions for use, and so on (Section 503(b)(2), codified at 21 U.S.C. 353(b)(2)). In addition to the requirements listed, a drug must not imitate another drug or be offered for sale under the name of another drug (Sections 301(I) and 502(I)(2)).

Advertisements for prescription drugs

Whereas advertisements for OTC drugs are regulated by the Federal Trade Commission, advertisements for drugs sold by prescription are regulated by the FDA (Section 502(n), codified at 21 U.S.C. 352(n)).[11] Generally, such advertising is directed to health professionals, although there is no prohibition on advertisements to consumers. The regulations for prescription drug advertisements are specific in the kinds of information that is necessary to be included (21 CFR 202). These regulations apply regardless of whether the advertisement is directed to health professionals or consumers. Dissemination of prescription drug advertisements that are not in compliance with the regulations constitutes misbranding. Advertisements may be submitted to the FDA for comment before publication. A drug can be advertised for only those conditions that the FDA has approved an NDA or an appropriate supplement. These conditions are listed in the approved package insert. By including the term *Physicians' Desk Reference* (PDR) in the definition of labeling, FDA regulations (21 CFR Section 202.1) require that, if a manufacturer chooses to list a product in the PDR, the listing must be in the same words as the package insert. Testimonials of users constitute misbranding if they give the impression that a preparation is effective for a condition for which it could not otherwise be promoted.

Statements by sales representatives

The objective intent of the persons legally responsible for the labeling of drugs is determined by their expressions or may be shown by the circumstances surrounding distribution of a product. For example, the objective intent may be shown by labeling claims, advertising matter, or oral or written statements by such persons or their representatives. The circumstances may show that the article is misbranded because such persons or their representatives know that the drug is offered for a purpose for which it is neither labeled nor advertised (21 CFR Section 201.128). The FDA maintains a Medical Advertising Information Line (1 8800 23 USFDA or 1 800 238 7332) for health professionals wishing to report questionable promotional activities. A toll free fax line (1-800-344-3332) is also available.

Industry supported continuing medical education

Scientific and educational activities on therapeutic and diagnostic products (human and animal drugs, biological products, and medical devices) for health care professionals that are performed by or on behalf of the companies that market the products have traditionally been viewed by the FDA as subject to regulation under the labeling and advertising provisions of the FDCA. On November 27, 1992, the FDA published a draft policy statement (57 F.R. 56412)[12] to distinguish between those activities supported by companies that are otherwise independent from the promotional influence of the supporting company and those that are not. That statement describes the circumstances under which companies can support educational programs involving their products without being subjected to the legal constraints that govern product advertising and promotion.

An important element of the policy is a written agreement between the supporting company and the provider of an educational program, stating that the activity is to be nonpromotional and educational and that the company is to play no role in the design or conduct of the program that might bias the treatment of the topic. The policy statement was the product of extensive consultation with scientific and health care professionals, regulated industry, consumer groups, and other government agencies. This policy, which speaks to FDA-regulated companies that support continuing medical education (CME), reflects documents issued by the Accreditation Council for Continuing Medical Education speaking to accredited providers, the Association of American Medical Colleges speaking to CME faculty members, and the American Medical Association speaking to physicians.

Sales and samples

Section 503 of the FDCA (codified at 21 U.S.C. 353), as amended by the Prescription Drug Marketing Act, prohibits the sale, purchase, or trade of prescription drug samples and drug coupons. A drug sample is a unit of a prescription drug that is not intended to be sold, but is intended to promote the sale of the drug product. A coupon is a form that may be redeemed at no cost or at a reduced cost for a prescription drug, and counterfeiting of drug coupons is prohibited. The law also prohibits resale of prescription drugs purchased by hospitals or other health care entities, or donated or supplied at reduced cost to charitable organizations. Exceptions for group purchasing organizations, nonprofit affiliates, and entities under common control are provided in the FDCA. Additional exceptions provide for medical emergencies and for dispensing of drugs pursuant to a prescription. Under Section 503 a manufacturer or distributor is also permitted to distribute drug samples to a licensed practitioner or pharmacy of a health care entity by mail or by other means on written request. Records must be maintained by manufacturers and distributors and made available to the FDA on request.

Federal Anti Tampering Act

The Federal Anti Tampering Act (Pub. L. 98 127), signed into law in 1983, amends Title 18 of the U.S. Code to establish graduated penalties for tampering with intent to cause injury or death. The penalties range from a maximum of $25,000 and 10 years imprisonment in the case of an attempt to tamper to a maximum of $100,000 and life imprisonment in a case where death results from the tampering. The law also establishes penalties for tampering with or mislabeling consumer products with intent to injure a business; for knowingly communicating false information that a consumer product has been tainted and if such tainting had occurred, would create a risk of death or bodily injury; and for threatening and conspiracy to tamper with a consumer product. *Consumer product* is defined as including any articles subject to the FDCA, and the FDA is designated as having authority to investigate violations.

Drugs with special requirements: antibiotics, insulin, and drugs of abuse

Until recently, two classes of drugs had special requirements for testing: insulin and penicillin. The Insulin Amendment of 1941 required insulin—both the crystals and the finished dosage form—to be batch tested and certified by the FDA. Approval of an NDA is a prerequisite for acceptance of samples for certification by the FDA. Such samples are selectively tested by the agency for conformance to standards published in the insulin regulations. Fees are charged to defray the testing and administrative costs of the insulin certification program. The Penicillin Amendment of 1945 also had required the FDA to test and certify the safety and effectiveness of all penicillin products, and later amendments extended this requirement to all antibiotics. However, in 1983 such control was found to be no longer needed and was abolished. New products may now require the equivalent of an approved NDA or an abbreviated new drug application (ANDA) in order to be marketed. An ANDA is an application to market a generic equivalent to a drug product previously approved under an NDA. Safety and efficacy are demonstrated through a bioequivalence study showing that the generic delivers its active ingredients to the same extent and at the same rate as the previously approved product.

The Anti Drug Abuse Act of 1988 amended the FDCA by providing severe criminal penalties for the distribution of anabolic steroids and human growth hormones without a physician's prescription. Persons convicted of illegally distributing anabolic steroids may be imprisoned up to 6 years and may be fined (Section 303(e)), and persons convicted of illegally distributing human growth hormones may be imprisoned for up to 10 years and may be fined (Section 303(f)). Moreover, any person convicted of illegally distributing human growth hormones will also be subject to the asset forfeiture provisions of the Controlled Substances Act and will be subject to criminal forfeiture of property (e.g., cars, boats, homes) used to support the illegal distribution and property purchased with the proceeds of the illegal distribution.

Homeopathic drugs

Homeopathy is a system of medicine that was popularized in the 1700s by Samuel Hahnemann in Germany. It is based on the Law of Similars, which contends that "like treats like." For this reason, when a product that produces symptoms, such as fever or nausea, at higher (pharmacological) concentrations is diluted and shaken (succussed) to very low concentrations below which any of the active substance may be reasonably assured to be present, the product is considered to treat the symptom that it produced. Any product that is labeled as homeopathic must, by definition, be a drug. This includes products that might otherwise be regulated as biologics or foods at higher concentrations. Official homeopathic drug products are recognized by the HPUS. Homeopathic drugs, although not approved as safe or effective through the IND/NDA process, still must meet drug GMPs and labeling requirements under FDCA. The majority of homeopathic drugs currently sold in the United States today are OTC drugs given by the oral route. The agency is reviewing its policies with respect to homeopathic drugs at this time.

BIOLOGICAL PRODUCTS

The FDA Center for Biologics Evaluation and Research (CBER) is responsible for biological products. The regulation of biologics has a different legislative history and regulatory approach from that of drugs. Since 1902, federal law has required that special premarket controls apply to biological products, as well as the licensing of both the product and the establishment. The legislation of 1902 was introduced and enacted following the deaths of 12 children resulting from their having received improperly prepared diphtheria antitoxin. Biological drugs for animals are regulated under the Animal Virus, Serum, and Toxin Act of 1913 administered by the U.S. Department of Agriculture (see later discussion under Animal Products), whereas human biologics are regulated by the FDA, under the 1944 Public Health Service (PHS) Act (42 U.S.C. 262). Biological products are legally defined also as drugs or devices and therefore are subject to all of the adulteration, misbranding, and registration provisions of the FDCA.

Section 351(a) of the PHS Act defines a biological product as ". . . any virus, therapeutic serum, toxin, antitoxin, vaccine, blood, blood component or derivative, allergenic product, or analogous product . . . applicable to the prevention, treatment, or cure of diseases or injuries of man. . . ." Biologics include such vitally important products as polio and measles vaccines, diphtheria and tetanus toxoids, and skin test substances, as well as whole blood and blood components for transfusion. More recently, biological products include the monoclonal antibodies, cytokines, growth factors, and genetically engineered products that have come about through new biotechnology. Because many biological products are derived from human sources, or from living organisms, they are by nature potentially dangerous if improperly prepared or tested.

Unlike most drugs, the regulation of biological products is largely achieved through control of the manufacturing process. Biological products are required to demonstrate potency, sterility, purity, and identity (see 21 CFR Part 610). In addition, such products must undergo a "general safety" test, which is conducted in animals to determine if there is an unsafe batch (Section 610.11). Close surveillance of biologics production, batch testing, and research toward improving the quality of biologics are activities conducted by CBER staff, and the development of standards for these products and proper control procedures are backed by the center's research program.

In addition to the traditional biological products described in the PHS Act, CBER has jurisdiction over selected medical devices, drug products, and banked human tissue intended for transplantation. The devices are primarily articles used in blood banks or plasmapheresis centers, such as containers for collecting and processing blood components, blood storage refrigeration units, and blood bank supplies. The drug products and devices are regulated under the provisions of the FDCA. Banked human tissue intended for transplantation is regulated under the authority of the PHS Act to prevent the spread of communicable disease (21 CFR 1270).

On December 14, 1993, the FDA issued an interim Final Rule, which was finalized July 29, 1997,[13] establishing a requirement for certain infectious disease testing, donor screening, and record-keeping for heterologous human tissue transplantation. The requirements would apply to human tissues (bone, ligaments, tendons, cartilage, skin, fascia, and corneas) but not to vascularized organs (livers, hearts, or kidneys), bone marrow, semen, human milk, or any other tissue currently regulated by the FDA as a device or biological (blood and blood products, heart valves, corneal lenticules, and dura mater). The new rule requires testing of donors for HIV and hepatitis B and C viruses only at facilities and with individuals engaged in the procurement, processing, storage, or distribution of human tissues intended for transplantation. Individual physicians who are not engaged in these activities or firms only engaged in storage of tissues are not subject to the requirements. Tissues intended for uses other than transplantation, such as in research, are also exempt. Records of donor screening and testing must be kept for 10 years, and all transplanted tissues must be accompanied by the appropriate records. The FDA may order the retention and recall and destruction of tissue that is not in compliance with the interim rule.

Licensing

Under the PHS Act, a manufacturer wishing to ship a biological product in interstate commerce, or for import or export, must obtain a U.S. license. These licenses are granted following a showing that the establishment and product meet specific standards (21 CFR Parts 600 through 680 and Part 211). These regulations are designed to ensure continued safety, purity, potency, and effectiveness. To apply for licensing, the manufacturer must submit information in a product license application (PLA), which demonstrates that the manufactured product meets the specified standards, and must successfully complete a prelicensing inspection by FDA investigators. Once licensed, the FDA inspects most establishments at least once every 2 years (see 21 CFR 600.20, 600.21, and 600.22).

Batch samples and lot release protocols

Before a licensed biological product is released for commercial sale or use, specified materials must be submitted to and cleared by CBER. These materials include a sample of the product and detailed records, that is, the lot release protocols of the manufacture of each lot of the product, including all results of each test for which results are requested. CBER reviews the protocols and may conduct its own safety, purity, and potency tests on the samples. The manufacturer cannot issue a product subject to lot release procedures until notification of official release is received from the agency. The FDA supplies standard reference preparations for potency tests of certain licensed products, including antitoxins, bacterial and viral vaccines, and skin tests. Manufacturers are required to obtain and use these preparations in their testing of licensed products.

Labeling

The PHS Act specifies that biologics be plainly labeled with the proper name of the article; the name, address, and license number of the manufacturer; and the appropriate expiration date of the product. CBER reviews all labeling for biologics before their licensing. In addition, all important changes in approved labeling must be submitted for approval. For prescription biological drugs, the manufacturer must also comply with FDA regulations in 21 CFR 201.56 and 201.57.

Blood banks

Interstate shipment of blood and blood components requires the issuance of U.S. product and establishment licenses, in accordance with the PHS Act. A licensed blood bank must comply with appropriate federal standards in preparing and testing the products being shipped. In accordance with FDA regulations (21 CFR 607.20 and 607.21), every blood bank collecting units of blood must register with the FDA within 5 days after commencing operations and must submit a list of blood products prepared. All blood banks must operate in compliance with the FDA's current GMP regulations for blood and blood components (21 CFR 606) and are by law subject to FDA inspection once every 2 years. As with other products, blood and blood components must undergo registration and

product listing. Establishment registration and product listing do not permit a blood bank to ship blood or blood components in interstate commerce unless the blood bank also holds valid U.S. establishment and product licenses.

Investigational new biologics and biological drugs

The requirements for filing an IND application for a biological product are essentially the same as for drugs (see earlier discussion on investigational drugs) except that the application should be sent to the office that is responsible for handling the particular biological (e.g., blood, vaccines, therapeutics).

COSMETICS

Cosmetics are under the jurisdiction of the Center for Food Safety and Applied Nutrition (CFSAN) at the FDA. Cosmetics marketed in the United States, whether made here or imported, must comply with the FDCA, as well as the Fair Packaging and Labeling Act, and the regulations issued under the authority of these laws (21 CFR Parts 700 to 740). The color additive regulations applicable to cosmetics are in 21 CFR Parts 73, 74, 81, and 82. Section 201(I)(1) of the FDCA defines cosmetics as articles intended to be applied to the human body for cleansing, beautifying, promoting attractiveness, or altering the appearance without affecting the body's structure or functions. Included in this definition are products such as skin creams, lotions, perfumes, lipsticks, fingernail polishes, eye and facial makeup preparations, shampoos, permanent waves, hair colors, toothpastes, deodorants, and any ingredient intended for use as a component of a cosmetic product. Soap products consisting primarily of an alkali salt of fatty acid and making no label claim other than cleansing of the human body are not considered cosmetics under the law.

Cosmetics that are also drugs

Products that are cosmetics but are also intended to treat or prevent disease, or affect the structure or function of the human body, are considered both drugs and cosmetics, and these must comply with both the drug and cosmetic provisions of the law. Examples include fluoride toothpastes, sun tanning preparations intended to protect against sunburn, antiperspirants that are also deodorants, and antidandruff shampoos. Most cosmetics that are also drugs are OTC drugs. Some are new drugs for which safety and effectiveness had to be proved to the agency before they could be marketed.

As with other regulated products, the FDCA prohibits the distribution of cosmetics that are adulterated or misbranded (Section 602). With the exception of color additives and a few prohibited ingredients, cosmetic manufacturers may, on their own responsibility, use essentially any raw material as a cosmetic ingredient and market the product without prior FDA approval. However, a cosmetic containing an unlisted color additive (i.e., one not approved by the FDA for its intended use) is considered adulterated and subject to regulatory action (21 CFR Parts 73, 74, 81 and 82). If the safety of a cosmetic is not adequately substantiated, the product may be considered misbranded and may be subject to regulatory action unless the label bears the following statement: "Warning: The safety of this product has not been determined." Although the FDCA does not require that cosmetic manufacturers or marketers test their products for safety, the FDA strongly urges cosmetic manufacturers to conduct whatever toxicological or other tests are appropriate to substantiate the safety of the cosmetics.

Although there is no mandatory registration for cosmetic products, firms may voluntarily make available safety data or other information before a product is marketed in the United States. However, voluntary registration and assignment of a registration number by the agency do not denote approval of a firm, raw material, or product by the FDA. Any representation in labeling or advertising that creates an impression of official approval because of registration or possession of a registration number will be considered misleading (21 CFR Parts 710, 720, and 730).

Cosmetic labeling

Cosmetics distributed in the United States must comply with the labeling regulations published by the FDA under the FDCA and the Fair Packaging and Labeling Act. As mentioned earlier, labeling means all labels and other written, printed, or graphic matter on or accompanying a product, and the label statements required by the FDCA must appear on the inside and any outside container or wrapper. Fair Packaging and Labeling Act requirements (e.g., ingredient labeling) only apply to the label of the outer container. The labeling requirements are codified at 21 CFR 701 and 740. Cosmetics bearing false or misleading label statements or otherwise not labeled in accordance with these requirements may be considered misbranded and may be subject to regulatory action.

Declaration of ingredients is only required for cosmetics produced or distributed for retail sale to consumers for their personal care (21 CFR 701.3). Cosmetics that are also drugs must first identify the active drug ingredient(s) before listing the cosmetic ingredients (21 CFR 701.3(d)).

Some cosmetics must bear label warnings or cautions prescribed by regulation (21 CFR 740). Cosmetics in self-pressurized containers (aerosol products), feminine deodorant sprays, and children's bubble bath products are examples of products requiring such statements. Some products must also be sold in tamper-resistant packaging. For example, liquid oral hygiene products (e.g., mouthwashes, fresheners) and all cosmetic vaginal products (e.g., douches, tablets) must be packaged in tamper-resistant packages when sold at retail (21 CFR 700.25).

ANIMAL PRODUCTS

The Center for Veterinary Medicine (CVM) at the FDA regulates the drugs, devices, feeds, pet foods, and the color and food additives intended for animals under the FDCA. Animal biologics (e.g., vaccines) are regulated under a separate act, the Animal Virus, Serum, and Toxin Act (AVSTA) of 1913 (21 U.S.C. Sections 151 et seq.), which has been subsequently amended. The AVSTA is administered by the Veterinary Biologics Staff at USDA. Many of the requirements for veterinary products are similar to those for the comparable human products.

Products administered or used by food-producing animals are evaluated for not only their effect on the animal, but also for their residues in food tissues, such as meat, milk, and eggs. To protect the national food supply, the FDCA requires the approval of applications for use of new animal drugs in the manufacture of animal feeds. Food additives that have been found to induce cancer may be used in feed for food-producing animals if no harm comes to the animal and there is no residue of the substance or its metabolites in edible tissues reaching the consumer (Section 409(c)(3) (A)). Such substances may not be added to other animal or pet foods. As with human food, animal feeds and pet food may not be adulterated or misbranded, and labeling may not be false or misleading.

Medical devices for animals, although subject to the same prohibitions against misbranding and adulteration as human medical devices, are not subject to premarket approval as is required of some classes of human medical devices. Cosmetics for animals are considered grooming aids and are not subject to the FDCA, provided no therapeutic claims are made. Pet foods are also subject to the labeling requirements of the Fair Packaging and Labeling Act. The Association of American Feed Control Officials is currently developing definitions for nutrient content claims, such as "lite," as consistent with those developed for human foods.

Animal prescription drugs may be dispensed only by a licensed veterinarian or on the prescription or other order of a licensed veterinarian (Section 503(f) and 21 CFR 201.105). The label must bear the statement: "Caution: Federal law restricts this drug to use by or on the order of a licensed veterinarian." As with human products, a "new animal drug" may not be commercially marketed or imported for commercial marketing unless it has been approved as safe and effective in the United States. The data must be specific for each species of animal for which the drug is intended. Antibiotic drugs for animal use are also new animal drugs under the law (Section 201(v)). The regulations now exempt all antibiotic drugs for animal use from the requirements of batch certification (Section 507(c)), but not from meeting specified quality characteristics. The Generic Animal Drug and Patent Term Restoration Act (GADPTRA) of 1988 provides for the approval of generic copies of previously approved animal drugs.

More recently, on October 9, 1996, President Clinton signed into law the Animal Drug Availability Act. The new law amends the FDCA to increase the availability of animal drug products by modifying the current definition of "sub-stantial effectiveness"; creating a new category of drugs called the *Veterinary Feeds Directive Drugs,* allowing for the approval and use of sophisticated new animal drugs in the feed of food-producing animals without compromising animal or human safety; and supporting flexible labeling, broadening the drug approval process to make more drugs available to treat minor species.

Pesticidal drugs

Depending on the claims made, animal products that are pesticidal preparations, such as rodenticides, fungicides, and insecticides, may be subject to both the Federal Insecticide, Fungicide and Rodenticide Act (7 U.S.C., Sections 136 et seq.), administered by the Pesticide Registration Division of the Environmental Protection Agency, and the FDCA, administered by the FDA. A Memorandum of Understanding between the two agencies specifies which agency will process petitions for products subject to dual jurisdiction. Petitions may be submitted to either agency and will be referred, if necessary.

MEDICAL DEVICES

Medical devices, administered through the Center for Devices and Radiological Health (CDRH) at the FDA, include several thousand health care products, from simple articles such as tongue depressors and heating pads to in vitro test kits, contraceptive devices, anesthesia machines, and heart valves. Under the FDCA, a device is defined as any health care product that does not achieve its principal, intended purposes by chemical action in or on the body or by being metabolized. Products that work by such chemical or metabolic action are regulated as drugs. The Medical Device Amendments of 1976 revised and extended the device requirements of the 1938 FDCA, resulting in significant new authority to ensure safe and effective devices. Later the Safe Medical Devices Act (SMDA) of 1990 and the Medical Device Amendments of 1992 enhanced premarket and postmarket controls and provided for additional regulatory authority.

Classification

The 1976 Medical Devices Amendments required devices to be categorized into one of three regulatory classes. Devices that were marketed in the United States before passage of the Act were considered "preamendment devices" (Section 513). Preamendment devices were classified based on recommendations of expert panels, concerning safety issues. Class I devices (e.g., tongue blades) are subject to "general controls" that apply to all devices, irrespective of class. General controls include the registration of manufacturers, record-keeping requirements, labeling requirements, and compliance with GMP regulations. Class II devices (e.g., catheters) are subject to "special controls" where general controls are insufficient to ensure safety and effectiveness, and for which enough information exists to develop special controls to provide such assurance, including performance standards, post-market surveillance, patient registries, guidelines, recommendations, and other appropriate actions. In the case of life-supporting or life-sustaining devices, special controls shall be identified, if any, that are necessary to provide adequate assurance of the safety and efficacy of such devices. Class III devices, which include implanted and life-supporting or life-sustaining devices, must undergo premarket approval through the filing of an investigational device exemption (IDE) application and a premarketing application (PMA). Such devices must have FDA approval for safety and effectiveness before they can be marketed, unless the FDA determines that premarket approval is unnecessary. The FDA cannot require PMAs until 30 months after a product is classified or until 90 days after a regulation calling for the application, whichever comes later. Premarket approval can be required of other devices if general controls are insufficient to ensure safety and effectiveness and insufficient information is available to establish special controls.

Devices marketed after the passage of the 1976 amendments are considered either "substantially equivalent" to a preamendment device, or not. Substantially equivalent devices are in the same regulatory class as the preamendment device to which they are comparable. Any new device that has not been shown to be substantially equivalent is automatically in Class III. A group of preamendment and post-amendment devices that were previously regarded as new drugs are also categorized as Class III by the 1976 amendments. These particular devices are known as *transitional products.* Regulations on classification of devices are in 21 CFR 860 and in Parts 862 through 892.

Reclassification

The class of a device product may be changed through a formal Citizen's Petition process made to the agency, or the agency may initiate the process. For example, acupuncture needles, which were not marketed for human use in the United States before May 1976, were therefore classified as Class III devices. In 1994 the agency received five Citizen's Petitions to reclassify the needles. On April 1, 1996, the agency ruled that indeed sufficient information was presented about the manufacturing and safety of the product to support a reclassification from a Class III to a Class II device.[14]

Premarket notification for new devices

Unless specifically exempted by regulation, before marketing, all manufacturers are required to give the FDA 90 days notice by submitting a premarket notification (Section 510(k)). During the 90-day period, the FDA will determine whether the device is "substantially equivalent" to a preamendment device. A device may not be marketed until the firm receives a notice from the agency, acknowledging that it is equivalent to a device that does not require a PMA. Those firms submitting premarket notifications, called *510(k)* no-

tices of equivalency to a Class III preamendment device, must certify that a reasonable search has been conducted of all known information about the predicate device. The FDA should receive a summary of all adverse safety and efficacy data, and the firm should submit the information on request. Those firms submitting premarket notifications to the FDA for Class I and II devices must provide an adequate summary of safety and efficacy data that is available to the FDA on request and made available to the public within 30 days of any request once the device has been found to be substantially equivalent.

Unless and until the FDA determines that the device is substantially equivalent to a device that does not require premarket approval, the device is Class III. For Class III devices, a PMA will need to be filed that contains evidence substantiating the safety and effectiveness of the device for the indication sought for marketing.

Notification of defective devices

Repair, replacement, or refund. The FDA can order manufacturers to notify the public of any product defect that represents a health hazard and can order manufacturers to repair, replace, or refund the cost of these defective devices. In situations in which there is a reasonable probability that continued use of a device would cause serious injury or death, the FDA can issue an order to cease further distribution and notify consignees of the agency's concerns. After an opportunity for a hearing, the FDA may amend the order to vacate it, order the modification of the device to eliminate the risk, or order the recall of the device (Section 518, codified at 21 U.S.C. 360h) (see also 21 CFR Part 810).

Mandatory recall and tracking. For devices that may have serious health consequences (i.e., life-supporting or life-sustaining or permanently implantable devices), a tracking method is required to be in place at the time the device is marketed. The tracking methods should be able to locate expeditiously the devices while in distribution channels, as well as those distributed to patients. Firms must conduct audits to ensure their system is effective and capable of locating possibly defective devices in case of a recall situation (21 CFR Parts 810 and 821).

Investigational devices

Class III and, in some cases, Class II devices may require clinical studies for marketing. While studies are ongoing to determine their safety and effectiveness, the devices are considered *investigational devices* (Section 520(g)). Similar to the drug and biologics regulations, sponsors who wish to conduct these investigations can be granted exemptions from certain requirements of the FDCA, which would otherwise impede these studies, by filing an IDE application 21 CFR 812 (general) and 813 (intraocular lenses). Unlike the drug regulations, if a study is reviewed and found by an Institutional Review Board to be of nonsignificant risk to the subjects, the trial may be conducted without filing an IDE. However, the FDA may require an IDE to be filed at a later date if the manufacturer needs to submit a marketing application (e.g., PMA). Consultation with the agency staff is recommended.

Custom devices

Medical devices ordered by health professionals to conform to their own special needs or to those of their patients (e.g., certain dental devices and specially designed orthopedic footwear) are considered *custom devices* and are exempt from registration and otherwise applicable performance standards or premarket approval requirements (Section 520(b)). The exemption applies only to devices not generally available to or used by other health professionals. Custom devices are not exempt from other provisions of the FDCA and regulations.

Electronic products and radiation control

Electronic products and radiation control are also under the purview of the Center for Devices and Radiological Health. Electronic products include all products or equipment capable of emitting ionizing or nonionizing radiation or sonic, infrasonic, or ultrasonic waves (21 CFR Parts 1000 to 1050). The comprehensive Radiation Control for Health and Safety Act was enacted in 1968 to protect the public from unnecessary exposure to radiation from electronic products (Sections 531 to 542).

The FDA sets and enforces performance standards to limit radiation emissions. The standards apply to products offered for sale or use in the United States, whether or not they are manufactured domestically. Performance standards are prescribed for the protection of the public health and safety. The standards (21 CFR 1020 to 1050) prescribe maximum allowable radiation levels and other approaches to control radiation emissions without specifying design features. Federal electronic product and radiation safety performance standards are in effect, regardless of whether the products are used for medical purposes. As with other devices, electronic products that fail to meet performance standards and defective products must be repaired, replaced, or refunded to the purchaser (21 CFR 1003 and 1004). Dealers and distributors of electronic products must maintain records of products for which performance standards are available to facilitate the location of purchasers for notification or recall (21 CFR 1002).

Mammography Quality Standards Act

The Mammography Quality Standards Act (MQSA) of 1992 was enacted to establish uniform, national quality standards for mammography. The MQSA amends the PHS Act (Section 354, codified at 42 U.S.C. 263b) by requiring certification and inspection of all mammography facilities. Covered under the law are all facilities producing, processing, or initially interpreting mammograms in the United States, whether for screening or diagnostic purposes, except for fa-

cilities of the Department of Veterans Affairs (DVA), which are exempt from the Act.

At this time, the DVA has voluntarily agreed to conform to the MQSA requirements, and through an intra-agency agreement, the FDA has agreed to inspect the DVA facilities. The FDA has published regulations to establish requirements and standards for accrediting bodies and application procedures for such bodies, as well as the quality standards for mammography facilities and procedures for facility certification (21 CFR 900).

ADVERSE EVENT REPORTING

Any product can conceivably have toxic or undesired effects. Numerous studies of the incidence of adverse effects from regulated products that resulted in hospital admissions are estimated at 3% to 11% annually, many of which could have been avoided. Prompt reporting and adequate documentation are essential for the FDA to evaluate the seriousness of adverse events associated with regulated products. An *adverse drug experience* is defined by the regulations (21 CFR 310.305(b)(2)) as ". . . any adverse event associated with the use of a drug in humans, whether or not considered drug related." This includes adverse events occurring in the course of the use of a drug product in professional practice; as a result of an overdose, whether accidental or intentional; as a result of abuse or recreational use; from withdrawal; and as any reaction that occurs because of a failure to produce an expected pharmacological or biological action. Adverse experiences that result in death, hospitalization, or permanent disability are always considered serious. Cancer, congenital anomalies, and overdose are adverse drug experiences that are also considered serious.

A large portion of adverse event reports reach the FDA through product manufacturers. Such reports originate largely as voluntary communications from physicians, pharmacists, or other health professionals. Although reporting by health professionals remains voluntary, product sponsors are required to keep the FDA informed regarding any developments that may affect the safety and effectiveness of their products, whether under clinical study or after FDA approval for marketing. (See FDCA, Sections 505(i), (j), and (k), and 21 CFR 310.303, 310.304, 310.305, 312.32, and 314.)

MedWATCH (FDA form 3500)

To promote the voluntary reporting of adverse events by health professionals, the FDA simplified its reporting process. In 1993 the MedWATCH (FDA form 3500) was developed to encompass the reporting of all FDA-regulated products (except vaccines, which are discussed later). Within the following 8 months, the FDA received more than 6700 reports: 65% from drugs, 20% from medical devices, 11% from drug quality problems, 4% from biologics, 1% from foods, and less than 1% from veterinary products. Pharmacists represented 55% of the reporters, with 16% of the reports made by physicians, 8% by nurses, 1% by dentists, and 6% by other health professionals. The MedWATCH form is designed to represent a case history report on a single patient for which the names of both the patient and the reporter are protected from disclosure. The FDA reviews the reports as a signal for new or unexpected effects. It assists the agency in determining whether a change in the product's labeling is required, such as cautions, warnings, further dose modifications, or revision of instructions for use. It may also result in improvement of the product's manufacture, or in some cases where necessary, recall of the product from the market.

Adverse effects arising from a drug product can range from mild side effects to severe reactions, including death. Events may be predictable or unpredictable. Predictable events are most often expected extensions of an individual drug's known pharmacological properties and are responsible for the majority of events encountered. Unpredictable events, however, include idiosyncratic reactions, immunological or allergic reactions, and carcinogenic or teratogenic events. Unlike predictable events, these events are usually not associated with the known pharmacological activity of the product. They seem to be more a function of patient susceptibility than the intrinsic toxicity of the drug. They are rarely avoidable and are generally independent of dose, route, or schedule of administration. Unpredictable events are often among the most serious and potentially life-threatening of all adverse events and are the major cause of important drug-induced disease.

A MedWATCH reporting form may be found in every issue of the FDA Medical Bulletin, which is distributed at no cost to licensed physicians and pharmacists and is also available in the PDR and on the FDA's Website. Reporting may be done by mail, telephone (1-800-FDA-1088), modem (1-800-FDA-7737), or facsimile (1-800-FDA-0178).

Adverse events during investigational studies

The FDA specifies which individuals involved with the investigation, control, or manufacture of products are required to report adverse drug experiences. Adverse events that occur during clinical studies are to be reported to the FDA, as specified in the regulations for Investigational New Drugs for drug and biologics or Investigational Device Exemption for devices. For example, sponsors of clinical studies being conducted under the exemption of an IND application, holders of approved new and abbreviated new drug applications, and manufacturers, packers, and distributors of certain marketed prescription drugs must report adverse drug experiences to the FDA.

Medical device reporting

In accordance with the Medical Device Reporting (MDR) requirements, manufacturers shall notify the FDA's Center for Devices and Radiological Health as soon as possible, but no later than 5 calendar days after receipt of information, concerning any device that has been responsible for, or is as-

sociated with, a death or serious injury. A device malfunction that would be likely to cause or contribute to a death or serious injury, if the malfunction were to recur, shall be reported by the manufacturer to the FDA within 15 working days (21 CFR 803). Although physicians' offices are exempt, facilities using devices must report deaths associated with the use of a device to the FDA and the manufacturer. Those incidents involving serious injury must be reported to the manufacturer of the device. Distributors of medical devices are required to report to the FDA any deaths, serious illnesses, and serious injuries that are attributed to medical devices. Distributors are also required to report certain device malfunctions to the manufacturer and to submit an annual report to the agency that certifies the number of medical device reports filed during the preceding year or that no reports were filed (21 CFR 804).

Vaccine adverse event reporting system

Under the National Childhood Vaccine Injury Act of 1986, the FDA manages a joint surveillance program for human vaccine products with the Centers for Disease Control and Prevention, located in Atlanta, Georgia. Reports of adverse events can come from any source, including health professionals, patients, parents of patients, or manufacturers. Although vaccine problems are intensely sought after during the developmental process, the Vaccine Adverse Event Reporting System (VAERS) program is designed to identify new problems that may arise after marketing a vaccine.

According to the 1994 report, Research Strategies for Assessing Adverse Events Associated with Vaccines by the Institute of Medicine, VAERS is designed to detect signals or warnings that there might be a problem rather than to answer questions about the causal association of the event. However, such signals can generate hypotheses about causality, which can be tested through other methods, such as epidemiological or laboratory studies.[15] (To obtain a VAERS reporting form, call 1-800-822-7967.)

Cosmetic adverse reaction monitoring

Consumer reporting of adverse reactions is the principal mechanism for the FDA to learn about harmful cosmetics in the marketplace. The Cosmetics Adverse Reaction Monitoring (CARM) program monitors and reviews consumer adverse reaction reports to determine the nature of the injury and any appropriate action that should be taken to protect public health. Although most adverse reactions to cosmetics are relatively mild and are not reported by consumers to the FDA, even a mild adverse reaction can mean that a cosmetic product contains a harmful ingredient that should not be used in some cosmetic products. (Consumers may report events directly to the nearest FDA field office, by telephone to the CARM program 202-205-4706, or by mail to FDA, Complaint Coordinator, Office of Cosmetics and Colors [HFS 106], 200 C Street, S.W., Washington, D.C. 20204.)

FDA'S ROLE IN THE "PRACTICE OF MEDICINE"

Although the FDA regulates most products used in the practice of the healing arts (e.g., medicine, dentistry, acupuncture), it does not directly regulate the practices themselves. Where applicable, the approvals and licensing of health professionals are left as issues of the state (see Chapter 8). In addition, the FDA does not regulate procedures, techniques, or lifestyle interventions (e.g., exercise or diet). Procedures such as bone marrow transplantation are considered *technologies* that are evaluated by both federal and private organizations. Such *technology assessments* can have a major impact on whether insurance carriers or health management organizations will allow or reimburse for the procedures. In the past the Agency for Health Care Policy and Research has conducted federal evaluations of product classes and technologies to determine if the federal carriers, such as Medicare, Medicaid, and Civilian Health & Medical Program of the Uniformed Services (CHAMPUS) will provide coverage. The process by which evaluations are made differs from the FDA's review process in many ways. The information used to make the evaluation for coverage is most often based on publicly available data and relies on the FDA's determination not only that a product has been approved as "safe and effective" for the indication but also that the product or technology is "reasonable," "necessary," and "cost effective." These latter criteria do not bear on the FDA's current approval process.

Unlabeled uses of FDA-approved products

Although the FDCA prohibits a manufacturer or distributor of an approved drug from labeling, advertising, or promoting the product for uses other than those approved by the FDA, the FDCA does not prohibit the manner of use by a health professional in the management of his or her own patients. Once a product has been approved for marketing, a practitioner may prescribe the drug for *unapproved* or, more accurately, *unlabeled* uses, which may be appropriate under certain circumstances and may in fact reflect approaches that have been extensively reported in the medical literature.[16] Indeed, valid new uses for marketed products are often first discovered by innovative approaches taken by health professionals, which are later confirmed by well-controlled clinical trials. Before the product's label may be revised to include new indications, the substantiating data must be submitted to the FDA for review and approval. This process takes time, and without the cooperation of the manufacturer whose product is involved, it may never occur. For this reason, accepted medical practice often includes unlabeled uses that are not reflected in the product's current labeling.

The FDA has taken a similar stance with respect to medical devices. In 1994, after a number of inquiries regarding the safety and effectiveness of surgical screws commonly used in the pedicles of the spine, the FDA issued a Talk Paper to clarify the regulatory status of this unlabeled use.[17] Although a variety of bone screws have been approved by the

FDA for posterior fixation of the sacral spine and for anterior fixation of the cervical, thoracic, and lumbar spine, no screws have been approved for placement in the vertebral pedicles as part of a spinal fixation system. Devices that the FDA has cleared for spinal fixation are wires, hooks, and rods. The use of the screws was considered to be an unlabeled use. FDA-approved clinical trials are required to generate adequate data for a complete evaluation of this new use. The agency subsequently took action to stop seven manufacturers from illegally promoting the use of the screws as pedicle screws, for which they were not approved.

For veterinary practice, two new laws have amended the FDCA, expanding the ability of veterinarians to prescribe unlabeled uses to animals. The Animal Medicinal Drug Use Clarification Act of 1994 allows veterinarians to prescribe extralabel use of not only veterinary drugs, but also approved human drugs for animals under specific circumstances. The Animal Drug Availability Act of 1996 allows the FDA to modify its current definition of "substantial effectiveness" and supports flexible labeling, by broadening the drug approval process to extrapolate information to "minor" species—those animals that are too few in number to allow cost recovery from the development of indications for these species.

Alternative or complementary medical practices

Although the FDA has no legal or regulatory definition for alternative or complementary medicine, it does regulate the products used in such practices. As in the conventional practice of medicine, the FDA does not regulate the use of massage, light or music therapy, meditation, or prayer per se. However, when any product is used and promoted for the purpose of diagnosing, preventing, treating, curing, or mitigating human or animal illness, by definition in the FDCA it becomes a drug or device. Products are regulated based on their intended use, as determined by their label and labeling (see earlier discussion). The FDA does not comment on the source or historical controversies that may surround a use of a particular product, and many useful and well accepted approved drugs and devices were derived from unusual and unexpected sources.

Since 1992, when Congress appropriated funding to the National Institutes of Health (NIH) to establish an Office of Complementary and Alternative Medicine (now the National Center for Complementary and Alternative Medicine), there has been a marked increase in the research conducted into the uses and roles of previously unaccepted interventions. As the result of an interest in conducting a clinical investigation with such products, the FDA has also experienced the need generated by the public to examine not only the uses, but also potential harmful effects of such products. Certain classes of products deemed *complementary* or *alternative* by the NIH have given rise to new issues that the FDA has had to address. For example, needles used in the practice of acupuncture, once Class III devices and therefore investigational (since they were unapproved postamendment devices), have now been reclassified and are legally marketed Class II devices today. The botanical products (containing plants or plant constituents as a finished product), which to date have largely been marketed as conventional foods, teas, spices, and dietary supplements, are now being evaluated in many cases for their pharmaceutical properties as potential drugs under INDs. From 1994 to the present, the FDA has been involved in several workshops sponsored by the Drug Information Association and the NIH to determine the scientific basis for using these unpurified products as drugs.[18] In August 2000, the CDER published a draft guidance document on botanical drug development. This document outlines general principles that should be addressed by sponsors who are intending to file INDs and NDAs with the FDA.

MOVEMENT OF PRODUCTS
Imports

The FDA implements a Memorandum of Understanding with foreign government counterpart authorities to help ensure the safety, efficacy, and quality of FDA-regulated products exported to the United States. For a product to enter the United States, foreign food products, drugs, biologics, cosmetics, medical devices, and electronic products that emit radiation, as defined in the FDCA and related laws, are subject to the same standards as domestic goods, with the exception of most meat and poultry. In addition, all products must contain informative and truthful labeling in English. With a few exceptions, if the label bears representations in a foreign language, it must have all of the required statements in the foreign language, as well as in English. The Tariff Act of 1930 (19 U.S.C. 130461) requires that all imported articles be marked with the English name of the country of origin.

Importers must file an entry notice and acquire a bond to cover their goods for release with the U.S. Customs Service (Customs). The FDA is notified by Customs of the entry and makes a decision as to the article's admissibility. To make a determination of compliance with FDA law, the FDA may sample the entry and have it analyzed in an FDA laboratory. If there is a violation, the product is refused admission. Before the product is refused admission, however, the importer is provided an opportunity to challenge the detention by proving that the product complies with the law. Alternatively, the importer can submit an application to the FDA to recondition the product to bring it into compliance (see FDCA Section 801). The FDA may automatically detain some products under an FDA Import Alert. This procedure is an administrative act of detaining a product without physical examination and is generally based on past history or other information indicating the product may be a violation. Once a product is placed on automatic detention, normal entry may not resume until the shipper or importer proves that the product meets FDA standards.

Personal imports

There has always been a market in the United States for some foreign-made products that are not available domestically. For example, individuals of differing ethnic backgrounds sometimes prefer products from their homeland or products labeled in their native language. Others seek medical treatments that are not available in this country. Drugs are sometimes mailed to this country to allow continuation of a therapy initiated abroad. FDA personnel do not routinely inspect mail or personal baggage. U.S. Customs brings items to the FDA's attention. Importation is generally permitted for those products representing a supply for 3 months or less of therapy and that are personally carried, shipped by a personal noncommercial representative of the consignee, or shipped from a foreign medical facility where a person has undergone treatment. Generally denied entries are large shipments of which the quantity suggests commercial distribution and small shipments solicited by traditional mail order promotions.[19]

Exports

FDA-regulated products produced by U.S. firms for export usually do not need to meet the same standards as products for the domestic market. Under Section 801(e) of the FDCA, if the item is intended for export only, meets the specifications of the foreign purchaser, is not in conflict with the laws of the country to which it is being shipped, and is properly labeled, it is exempt from the adulteration and misbranding provisions.

Additional statutory provisions are imposed on the export of new drugs for human or animal use and biological products. Although in general, such products must be approved as being safe and effective before export from the United States, exceptions do exist. Under the Drug Export Amendments Act of 1986 (Pub. L. 99 660), unapproved drugs and biologics may be exported to any of 21 countries listed in the Act. These countries have premarket approval systems comparable to that of the United States. To be exported, the drug must be approved for use in the importing country. In addition, the drug must be the subject of an IND, and the drug manufacturer must be actively pursuing marketing approval in the United States. In addition, if an unapproved drug is intended for the treatment or prevention of tropical diseases, it may be exported if the FDA finds that the drug is safe and effective for use in the country to which it is being exported. A partially processed biological product, which requires further manufacture before it becomes a finished product, may also be exported to any of the listed countries, if the finished product is approved in the importing country or if that approval is being sought. In all cases, the product must be properly labeled, not be contrary to the public health interest of the United States or that of the importing country, and meet GMPs. Similar provisions for devices are also described in the law (see Sections 514 to 516 and Section 520(g)).

Foreign trade zones

While awaiting a favorable market in the United States or nearby countries, products may be held in *foreign trade zones.* These are areas within the United States as designated by Customs, to hold or otherwise manipulate goods for an unlimited period of time without being subject to Customs entry, payment of duty, tax, or bond. These areas are considered outside the Customs territory of the United States for purposes of Customs importing procedures. However, the location of an establishment in a foreign trade zone has no bearing on the jurisdiction of the FDA or the applicability of the laws it administers. Foreign trade zones are part of the United States, and the movement of regulated products into or out of such zones, including exports, constitutes interstate commerce. Therefore regulated products in foreign trade zones must comply with those laws administered by the FDA.

Interstate shipments

Within the United States, compliance with the FDCA is monitored through periodic inspections of facilities and products, analyses of samples, educational activities, and legal proceedings. When violations are discovered, there are many regulatory procedures available. Adulterated or misbranded products may be voluntarily destroyed or recalled from the market by the shipper or may be seized by U.S. Marshals on orders obtained by the FDA from federal district courts. Sponsors or individuals responsible for violations may be prosecuted in the federal courts, and if found guilty, they may be fined, imprisoned or both. Continued violations may be prohibited by federal court injunctions. Violation of an injunction is punishable as contempt of court. Civil money penalties may be pursued for certain specific violations. Any or all types of regulatory procedures may be employed, depending on the circumstances.

ENDNOTES

1. DHHS, PHS, FDA, Requirements of Laws and Regulations Enforced by the U.S. Food and Drug Administration. DHHS Publication No. (FDA) 89-1115 (Revised 1997).
2. The Committee of Revision of the United States Pharmacopeial Convention, Inc., *USP 23 The United States Pharmacopeia NF 18 the National Formulary* (The United States Pharmacopeial Convention, Inc., Rockville, MD 1995).
3. S. L. Nightingale & G. Bagley, *FDA Sanctions for Practitioners for Violations of Clinical Trial Regulations and Other Misconduct,* 81(1) Federation Bulletin 7-13 (1994).
4. DHHS, FDA, *21 CFR Part 812. Investigational Device Exemptions; Disqualification of Clinical Investigators, final rule,* 62(50) Federal Register 12087-12096 (Friday, March 14, 1997).
5. DHHS, FDA, *21 CFR Parts 20 and 814. Medical Devices; Humanitarian Use Devices, final rule,* 61(124) Federal Register 33232-33248 (Wednesday, June 26, 1996).
6. DHHS, FDA, *21 CFR Parts 312 and 314. Investigational New Drug, Antibiotic, and Biological Drug Product Regulations; Procedures for Drugs Intended to Treat Life-Threatening and Severely Debilitating Illnesses, interim rule,* 53(204) Federal Register 41516-41524, Part VI (Friday, October 21, 1988).
7. DHHS, FDA, *21 CFR Part 312. Investigational New Drug, Antibiotic, and Biological Drug Product Regulations, treatment use and sale final rule,* 52(99) Federal Register 19466-19477, Part IV (Friday, May 22, 1987).
8. DHHS, FDA, *PHS, 21 CFR Parts 312. Investigational New Drug, Antibiotic, and Biological Drug Product Applications, clinical hold and termination, final rule; Expanded Availability of Investigational New Drugs through Parallel Track Mechanism for People with AIDS and Other HIV Related Disease,* notice 57(73) Federal Register 13250-13259, Part V (Wednesday, April 15, 1992).
9. DHHS, FDA, *CFR Parts 314.500 314.560 and 601.40 46. New Drug, Antibiotic, and Biological Drug Product Regulations, accelerated approval final rule,* 57(239) Federal Register 58942 58960, Part VIII (Friday, December 11, 1992).
10. DHHS, PHS, FDA, *An Introduction to FDA Drug Regulation: A Manual for Pharmacists* (DHHS, PHS, FDA Center for Drug Evaluation and Research and Office of Regulatory Affairs, May 1990).
11. DHHS, *Office of the Inspector General, Prescription Drug Advertisements in Medical Journals* (June 1992), OEI 01 90 00482.
12. DHHS, FDA, *Draft Policy Statement on Industry Supported Scientific and Educational Activities, Notice,* Federal Register, 56412-56414 (Friday, November 27, 1992).
13. DHHS, FDA, *21 CFR Parts 16 and 1270. Human Tissue Intended for Transplantation, final rule, 62(145)* Federal Register 40429-40447 (Tuesday, July 29, 1997).
14. FDA, *Acupuncture Needle Status Changes,* FDA Talk Paper, T96 21 (April 1, 1996).
15. I.B. Stehlin, *How FDA Works to Ensure Vaccine Safety,* 29(10) FDA Consumer Magazine 6 10 (1995).
16. FDA, Use of Approved Drugs for Unlabeled Indications, 12(1) FDA Drug Bulletin 4-5 1982).
17. FDA, *Pedicle Screws,* 24(1) FDA Medical Bulletin 10-11 (1994).
18. F.A. Hoffman & D. Eskinazi, NIH Office of Alternative Medicine conference: Federal Agencies Explore the Potential Role of Botanicals in US Health Care, 1(3) J Alternative Complementary Medicine 303-308 (1995).
19. FDA, Chapter 9 71 Coverage of Personal Importations, FDA Regulatory Procedures Manual, Part 9, Import Procedures (1988).

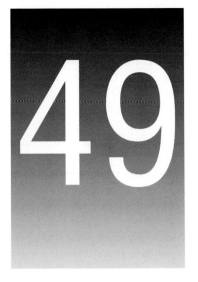

Telemedicine and electronic mail

FILLMORE BUCKNER, M.D., J.D.

A SIMPLE EXPLANATION
ADVANTAGES
AS A TOOL IN PHYSICIAN-PATIENT COMMUNICATION
DISADVANTAGES
GUIDELINES FOR USE IN PHYSICIAN-PATIENT COMMUNICATIONS
ADMISSIBILITY IN COURT
CONCLUSION

Electronic mail (e-mail) occupies a singular position in health care law. It is part of telemedicine law, is part of medical records law, and has many of the legal attributes of the telephone in health care law. It mimics the evidentiary issues involving traditional mail. It is important at the outset of any discussion of e-mail to distinguish between the two categories of e-mail, internal, based on a closed internal network, and external, based on the Internet. For all practical purposes, internal e-mail is a secure and integral part of a telemedicine network. Security can be assured by access restrictions, authentication procedures, and network encryption. The access restrictions currently preclude patients' e-mail accounts on internal networks. Internal e-mail therefore needs no discussion beyond that already given with regard to telemedicine. This discussion concerns external e-mail, or that e-mail common to the majority of providers and patients, which is based on modem, wireless, or cable access to the Internet and transmitted from one user to another via the Internet. It is by far the fastest growing means of communication worldwide. The speed, ease, and low cost of sending information over the Internet have made it the communication medium of choice of industry and commerce, and it is rapidly becoming the patient's method of accessing health care information.

A SIMPLE EXPLANATION

The computer has become an essential tool in the practice of both medicine and law. The presence of this tool on the provider's desktop has given rise to a new mode of communication, e-mail. E-mail is an electronic message generated on a computer addressed to one or a number of recipients. There is no practical limit to the number of recipients or the location of the recipients. The message may contain text, word-processing documents, spreadsheets, graphics, or data files. The message is then sent by a wireless, cable, or more commonly telephone connection to an Internet service provider (ISP). A standard header is applied to the e-mail, identifying the sender's ISP. All Internet addresses consist of a series of four groups of digits separated by dots. The digits are a code, indicating the network, subnetwork, and local address. In addition, custom dictates that a standard message heading, consisting of the sender's name and address, recipient's name and address, date, list of those receiving a copy of the message, list of attached documents or graphics, and subject line, be included.

The message then travels, via the Internet, to the ISP of the recipient or recipients. The Internet is best thought of as a vast spider web of interconnecting users and networks. There are multiple connections and routes to any single destination. Information sent from one user to another on the Internet usually passes through any number of routers and subsets of networks. To ensure efficient transmission, messages may be broken up and portions sent by entirely different routes to be reassembled when they reach the recipients' ISPs. None of this routing is under the control of either the sender or the receiver. The message is bound to be intact at only two points in its travels, when it reaches the sender's ISP and when it reaches the recipient's ISP. The message will probably be stored and archived at the sender's ISP and is certain to be stored and archived at the recipient's ISP. The recipients access the message from their computer screens on command. Messages may be stored on the computer, printed, forwarded, replied to, or deleted, without recopying.

ISPs function as electronic mail boxes or more aptly postal services. In this way e-mail differs from regular mail (known as *snail mail* in e-mail parlance). ISPs are provided by private commercial, organizational, or educational institutions, as well as local, state, and federal government agencies but not by the U.S. Postal Service. Therefore e-mail is not subject to postal laws.

ISPs usually are known by their domain names. Domain names consist of two levels of identification. The upper level indicates the type of entity operating the provider (e.g., net for network, com for commercial, edu for educational, org for organization, and gov for government), and the lower level indicates the entity's name. ISPs may be large for-profit corporations, such as America Online (AOL) or AT&T Net; professional organizations providing Internet access for their members, such as the American Trial Lawyers Association's online service (ATLA NET); or educational institutions providing online services for their faculty and students, such as the University of Washington (u.washington.edu).

Regardless of the ISP, at the time of registration, users must agree to a terms of service agreement, or a set of operating rules. These operating rules govern the user's communications and the contents therein. They frequently forbid the transmission of communications containing pornography, mass solicitations, chain letters, pyramid schemes, messages for "illegal purposes," or "offensive material"; the ISP normally reserves the right not to transmit forbidden material. Such regulations, which may or may not be explicitly expressed, imply that the ISP reserves the right to inspect traffic in and out of its site. The ISP has the legal right to do so. The Electronic Communications Privacy Act of 1986[1] specifically covers e-mail and provides criminal and civil penalties for the interception of electronic data. However, it carefully spells out an exception for providers of electronic communications services, such as ISPs.[21]* Thus an external e-mail communication has a built-in gap to guarantee confidentiality.

A number of commercial e-mail software programs are available for the personal computer. Many of these programs allow messages to be prioritized or can filter out messages from a designated source. Almost all e-mail programs allow special handling of messages with certain letter or digit sequences in specific locations. Some of the more sophisticated programs allow several levels of triage, with a set order of application. A well-organized e-mail message triage program can be set up on any state-of-the-art personal computer using any of the leading e-mail software packages.

ADVANTAGES

E-mail is an often under-appreciated technology. It has the advantage of extremely low cost. The e-mail user pays either a low monthly fee to an ISP or elects to use an organizational, institutional, or commercial ISP that offers free Internet access. Thus sending an e-mail message is less expensive than sending an overnight letter or a fax. Messages can be sent to any location on the globe with no surcharge per message.

Like the telephone, e-mail is fast. Messages travel thousands of miles in milliseconds rather than the days required by the Postal Service. E-mail is more convenient than the telephone. It is easily typed on the computer keyboard at any time; there is never a busy signal. It is asynchronous, requiring neither the recipient's presence nor availability; therefore it completely eliminates the time-consuming "telephone tag" that plagues communication by phone. The user is never left "on hold," listening to elevator music or repeated messages that his or her call is "valuable." E-mail messages also are tagged on the recipient's screen, indicating what action has been taken with regard to the message. Therefore an e-mail message is less likely than a telephone message to be lost, ignored, or forgotten. In addition, unlike the telephone, it is a written, not spoken, message. Thus it is edited, more formal, and probably more carefully crafted than a phone conversation or voice-mail message.

E-mail is particularly well suited for transmitting to the patient anything the patient would have to write out if it were transmitted orally. E-mail also provides a ready-made permanent record that can be printed to become part of a patient's paper medical record or be exported electronically to the patient's electronic medical record without manual recopying. As mentioned, the message also may be forwarded to other interested parties without retyping. Because it is a typed message, illegibility is eliminated. E-mail also allows the sender to embed links to applicable or educational sites on the Internet.

AS A TOOL IN PHYSICIAN-PATIENT COMMUNICATION

Besides its obvious uses to facilitate committee activities and other communications, including curbside consultations between clinic staff and remote providers,[3] e-mail has taken on a distinctive role in physician-patient communications. With the expanding use of computers by the public, many patients now own computers. It is estimated that approximately 135 million Americans use e-mail and send more than 500 million messages per day.[4] Of the patients who own computers or are planning to purchase one within 6 months, a substantial majority would like to use e-mail to interact with their physician.[5] Only a small minority of physicians has exploited this interest to improve communications with patients. However, among the various physician-patient interactions via e-mail that have been advocated or adopted are the following:

- Postoperative checks on patients[6]
- Directions and educational materials to patients[7]
- Prescription refill requests[8]
- Appointment requests, reminders, and changes[9]
- Referral requests[10]
- Medication questions[11]
- Adverse drug reaction reports[12]
- Laboratory and diagnostic test results[13]
- Insurance information[14]
- Home-generated test results (glucose levels, urine volumes, blood pressures, etc.)[15]
- Get well cards or birthday greetings[16]

---

*This holds equally true for employers who act as their own ISPs.

In addition, e-mail allows the physician to send a series of standardized letters, such as thank you letters for referrals, notices of office hour changes, holiday greetings, notices of holiday-related office closures, information regarding changes in coverage, new phone numbers, and a myriad of similar notifications, to both patients and colleagues.

DISADVANTAGES

E-mail is a marvelous communication tool but is marked by security defects with no currently known solution. E-mail differs from regular mail in that it is not sent in an envelope. It resembles a postcard rather than a letter because it is open to its carrier or carriers. The message is sent through many connections and networks during transmission. The message usually is fragmented and, although it is theoretically possible for it to be seized and read anywhere in the milliseconds along the way, its practical vulnerability lies in the ISP or ISPs of the sender and recipient. There, it is intact and stored and may be easily and legally accessed by ISP personnel. At this point it is also most vulnerable to "hackers." Personal information may be read, copied, altered, or forwarded without the sender or recipient ever knowing of the intrusion. E-mail also is infinitely easier to forge than is regular mail. There is no handwriting or scriptive signature to compare, and rare type fonts and graphic identifiers may be readily scanned and duplicated on a computer.

Encryption or secure socket layer-hypertext transfer protocol (SSL-HTTP)[17] ensures security, but neither method is practical in the communication between physician and patient.*[18] In addition, it is inherently easier to send material to the wrong address when using e-mail. To send e-mail, the sender usually clicks on a name on a list and the letter is automatically addressed. All computer users have experienced the frustration of discovering that the cursor was one line up or one line down from the intended item on a menu. Therefore e-mail is more frequently misaddressed than is regular mail. The recipient, with little more than the push of a button, may forward the message to any individual or individuals anywhere in the world without recopying or securing the sender's permission. Another potential problem results from the fact that ISPs routinely make backup copies of all messages. These backup copies may remain in the system long after the message has been erased from both the sender's and recipient's computer memories. Finally, there is a measure of social inequality in the distribution of e-mail capability. E-mail service is directly correlated to income and distributed unevenly across racial and ethnic groups.[19]

---

*In addition to their lack of practicality, neither technique may be necessary to preserve the physician-patient privilege or a fiduciary duty of confidentiality. Recent court cases indicate that an e-mail message, like a telephone conversation, reserves the attorney-client privilege and is considered ethical practice. See also ABA Standing Committee on http://www.abnet.org/cpr/ethicopinions.html

GUIDELINES FOR USE IN PHYSICIAN-PATIENT COMMUNICATIONS

Every mode of communication carries some risk of unauthorized interception and disclosure. There is a reasonable expectation of privacy in communicating via e-mail even though security is not guaranteed.[20] Adequate informed consent must be obtained from the patient, and carefully crafted guidelines must be adhered to.

American Medical Informatics Association guidelines

In 1997 the American Medical Informatics Association (AMIA) adopted the guidelines proposed by its task force on clinical use of electronic mail with patients. The guidelines, called *White Paper: Guidelines for the Clinical Use of Electronic Mail with Patients,* were published in 1998.[21] These guidelines were presented in a dual approach—as guidelines for effective communication with patients and risk management or medicolegal guidelines. The guidelines are summarized in Boxes 49-1 and 49-2.[22] Unfortunately, they do not satisfy many legal commentators, and several alternatives have been published as guidelines or decided in law review articles.[23]

Defining a turnaround time is essential for successful e-mail communication. The stated turnaround time must be conservative, however. If there is a chance that on busy days the recipient will check e-mail only once per day, the provider must not warrant that it will be checked more often than that. The AMIA guidelines envisioned a 2- to 3-day turnaround time for e-mail. Present practice indicates that e-mail has attained a next-day turnaround in most offices, and in many offices messages are processed on the day they are received. AMIA guidelines ask for provider assurances of privacy and security. There is a reasonable expectation of privacy when using e-mail, but the provider has no control over the security or the integrity of the e-mail communication and should make no assurances as to confidentiality or integrity or distinguish degrees of sensitivity of messages. The remainder of the communication guidelines is as valid today as in 1997.

Unfortunately the medicolegal guidelines have not fared as well in the ensuing years. Certainly informed consent and e-mail practice policies are as important today as when the guidelines were adopted, but the recommended content of those documents has changed with time. The essence of the informed consent agreement should be that the provider is making no assurances of e-mail confidentiality or security and that the patient desires that the communications of the types enumerated earlier be communicated by e-mail. Certainly the fact that the provider will make the e-mail transmission part of the record is still an essential part of the consent, but in these days of multiple providers and shifting personnel the hours of e-mail service are more important to detail than who will service the communication. Encryption

---

BOX 49-1. **SUMMARY OF COMMUNICATION GUIDELINES**

- Establish turnaround time for messages. Do not use e-mail for urgent matters.
- Inform patients about privacy issues. Patients should know:
  - Who besides addressee processes messages (1) during addressee's usual business hours and (2) during addressee's vacation or illness.
  - That message is to be included as part of the medical record.
- Establish types of transactions (e.g., prescription refill, appointment scheduling) and sensitivity of subject matter (e.g., human immunodeficiency virus infection, mental health) permitted over e-mail.
- Instruct patients to indicate category of transaction in subject line of message for filtering (i.e., "prescription," "appointment," "medical advice," "billing question").
- Request that patients include their name and patient identification number in the body of the message.
- Configure automatic reply to acknowledge receipt of messages.
- Print all messages, with replies and confirmation of receipt, and place in patient's paper chart.
- Send a new message to inform patient of completion of request.
- Request that patients use autoreply feature to acknowledge reading provider's message.
- Maintain a mailing list of patients, but do not send group mailings in which recipients' names are visible. Use blind carbon copy feature in software.
- Avoid anger, sarcasm, harsh criticism, and libelous references to third parties in messages.

BOX 49-2. **MEDICOLEGAL AND ADMINISTRATIVE GUIDELINES**

- Consider obtaining patient's informed consent for use of e-mail. Written forms should:
  - Itemize terms in communication guidelines.
  - Provide instructions for when and how to escalate to phone calls and office visits.
  - Describe security mechanisms in place.
  - Indemnify the health care institution for information loss caused by technical failures.
  - Waive encryption requirement if any at patient's insistence.
- Use password-protected screen savers for all desktop workstations in the office, hospital, and home.
- Never forward patient-identifiable information to a third party without the patient's express permission.
- Never use patient's e-mail address in a marketing scheme.
- Do not share professional e-mail accounts with family members.
- Use encryption for all messages when encryption technology becomes widely available, user-friendly, and practical.
- Do not use unencrypted wireless communications with patient-identifiable information.
- Double-check all "To": fields before sending messages.
- Backup mail onto long-term storage at least weekly. Define "long-term" as the term applicable to paper records.
- Commit policy decisions to writing and electronic form.

---

has not become user friendly enough to be used in current provider-patient communications, and in the typical provider-patient situation no encrypted messages are sent. Also, the security of internal networks should never be compromised by allowing patients' e-mail accounts to be placed on the internal network (a possibility suggested in the AMIA white paper).

Other risk management suggestions

No single set of guidelines incorporates all of the issues that must be contemplated in the development of a comprehensive set of risk management guidelines, and some include questionable advice. For example, Speilberg[24] suggests that e-mail from patients is so sensitive that it should not be included in the patient's regular medical record. This recommendation is hard to take seriously because the message has been transmitted over an acknowledged insecure network and the patient has consented to its inclusion in the medical record. An edited compendium of the current recommendations is presented next.

Informed consent. The informed consent should emphasize that the provider can make no guarantees of confidentiality because the transmission could be monitored in transit but that e-mail may be a convenience for the necessary type of communication. The patient also should be warned that even a deleted message may be available to anyone else using the same computer. The types of acceptable e-mail communications should be enumerated, and there should be a blanket prohibition of any other type of communication. Unless the provider specifically wants to receive emergency communications via e-mail, emergency communications should be specifically prohibited and the proper procedures for notifying the provider of emergencies given. The fact that all e-mail communications will become part of the medical record should be noted. The informed consent should include a specific request from the patient that the patient desires e-mail for the enumerated types of communications. The consent also should contain a signed acknowledgment of the accuracy of the patient's e-mail address. Some commentators suggest adding an agreement that e-mail communications will be made only from terminals within the state; this is an attempt to avoid the licensure issues of medical practice across state lines.*

Written e-mail policies and procedures. Detailed e-mail policies and procedures should be written and distributed to all staff members. Those portions of the policies and procedures applicable to patients should become part of the provider's new patient brochure or should be distributed to patients at the time they request e-mail communication. The patient's receipt of that brochure or written policy statement should be documented in the patient's medical record. Placing the patient policies on an easily accessed Internet site is an additional method of ensuring that the patient has realistic expectations of the e-mail service. The patient-related policies and procedures should include the following:

1. Realistic hours. Although e-mail may be sent on a 24-hour basis, in most cases it is processed during business hours. Therefore reasonable hours during which e-mail will be accessed for processing and a cut-off time after which no messages will be accepted for processing must be set for each business day.

2. Reasonable turnaround time. Although same-day turnaround is rapidly becoming the norm, a turnaround time that is routinely possible in the specific provider's practice must be designated. If a 1-, 2-, or 3-day turnaround is the best that the office can guarantee, the staff should not promise more.

3. Specific provider and patient identification. Set a specific signature character set or logo to be included in each message from the provider. Request that patients use a simple designation in addition to their names in each communication.

4. Specific "subject" line categories. Specific wording in the subject listing on patients' messages allows for easier triage and helps direct the message to the proper individual in the provider office. The same use on the provider's messages reinforces the categories. Simple categories, such as "prescription," "laboratory," "information," "appointment," or "billing," are recommended.

*In Northern practices with a number of "snowbirds," e-mail is considered an ideal way for patients spending the winter in the South to keep in touch with their regular providers, and these practices tend to accept or ignore the possible risk.

5. Clear notice that only consent e-mail is accepted. There should be a clear notice that e-mail will not be accepted from patients who have not signed an e-mail informed consent form. The provider's e-mail software can be programmed to accept messages from only the e-mail addresses acknowledged on the informed consent.

6. Replies requested. Request that patients acknowledge receipt of provider communications. (On most e-mail programs this can be done by a single keystroke or two, and a copy of the message received will be included with the acknowledgment.) This acknowledgment provides complete documentation of the request, the action on the request, and the patient's notification of the action.

Policies and procedures for staff should include the following:

1. Receipt of all incoming messages from patients should be acknowledged. This lets the patient know the inquiry is being processed, prevents needless follow-up calls, and instills confidence in the system.

2. All patients should be informed when their requests are completed.

3. All patient messages, the replies thereto, and patient acknowledgments should be printed and placed in the patient's paper medical record or should be transferred into the patient's electronic medical record.

4. All e-mail programs have the ability to maintain an e-mail address list and make mass e-mail messages. These lists are convenient; however, they are prone to two types of errors. First, unless the computer operator is vigilant, it is easy to click on the name above or below the intended addressee. Therefore the addresses on the message must be double-checked on every transmission. Second, sending a message to the entire address book without adequate precautions will reveal the names of every patient on the list to every other patient on the list. This problem can be solved by using the blind carbon copy (bcc) feature on the e-mail program (e.g., select "View" and then "bcc" on Microsoft Outlook). A message about an office closure could be sent to every patient on the provider's list by addressing the message to the provider, one of the provider's personnel, or the hospital and transferring the entire patient list to bcc. Each patient would get the message, but none would be aware of any name but that of the addressee.

5. Closely related to address book problems is the proximity of the "reply" button to the "reply to all" button on most e-mail programs. Therefore all personnel must be carefully coached to watch that messages are sent only to the patient sender.

6. Patient e-mail messages must be protected from other patients visiting the provider's office. If there are

computer terminals in patient areas, they must be equipped with passwords or smart card protection standby or screen savers.

7. The use of headers and footers, marking the message as a privileged and confidential communication intended only for the designated recipient, on all outgoing messages should be considered. However, such messages attract the attention of those attempting to intercept messages during transmittal. Certain types of transmissions attract hackers more than others, and marking a message "secret" or "confidential" can turn a boring health care provider message into something worth a hacker's time to retrieve.

8. Iron-clad forwarding criteria must be established. The patient's consent should be secured for all forwarding or for all forwarding except to other treating providers or third-party payers. Personnel should be informed of the hazards relating to electronic data transfer without the patient's permission unless it is in the context of treating or collecting for treatment.

9. The policy and procedures statement should spell out exactly who is responsible for handling each type of triage category messages and who is responsible for entering the messages, replies, and acknowledgments into the patient's medical record.

10. The triage system should be developed with the entire staff and should be kept within the bounds of the office e-mail system. A simple and effective system can be worked out using only the patient ID and the one-word subject line headings.

11. Each and every e-mail message may become a written record and will remain a retrievable electronic message for the foreseeable future. Those writing messages should be discrete and should not "SCREAM" (i.e., write all-capital messages). Anger, sarcasm, demeaning or defamatory language, "emoticons,"* and attempts at humor should be avoided.

12. Templates should be developed for frequently asked questions or for frequently sent messages.

13. Graphics should be confined to necessary diagrams and aids to instructions. Graphics require a tremendous amount of memory, and the patient's computer may not be able to handle elaborate illustrations.

14. Many e-mail programs handle attachments with difficulty. The staff should ensure that the patient and the patient's e-mail program can handle attachments before sending needed information via attachment.

15. If in doubt about sending a communication via e-mail, the staff member should not do it. The technology should be adopted for only those tasks that the physi-

cian is certain about. Additional tasks can be added as the staff become comfortable with the technology and as the legal issues surrounding the medical use of the technology become clarified.

16. Finally, every message and the address line must be read before the "send" button is hit.

ADMISSIBILITY IN COURT

In general, e-mail as a part of the medical record is treated no differently from any other part of the paper or electronic medical record. It is treated as part of the business record and admitted into evidence as such. However, e-mail communications not part of the medical record or accounting records[25] face a problem of authentication.[26] Although each e-mail message contains the header described earlier, it is evidently easy for those with expertise to create anonymous messages, without header information, or to forge false header information. The creators of the Internet made no provision for authentication of e-mail when the program began and have added none since. There is also the problem of messages coming from compromised accounts when a hacker has accessed the account name and password. Such cases have come to court[27] but have not resulted in authentication challenges. From the cases thus far, it would appear that the header information, despite its ease of forgery, will, barring evidence to the contrary, serve as authentication for e-mail's admission. Jablon[28] compares the use of the header for authentication to the court's use of an oriental "Chop" mark for authentication.[29]

CONCLUSION

E-mail is a valuable communication tool replete with security flaws. Its use is a fact of life. Its efficiency demands that the health care provider learn to deal with his or her resistance to change and adopt its use. It can increase bonding between provider and patient by providing a superior tool to carry out routine but essential communication tasks. The key to its successful use lies in the use of well-crafted informed consents and e-mail guidelines.

This chapter deals with communications between the provider and patients where the provider-patient relationship was previously established and after an informed consent had been signed by the patient. The inadvertent establishment of a provider-patient relationship and resultant or potential malpractice situations are not discussed.

---

*Emoticons are various character groups used by e-mail users to convey emotion (e.g., the happy face indicated as :)).

ENDNOTES

1. Pub. L. 99-508 codified in various sections 18 U.S.C.
2. *Id.* §101(c)(6).
3. *See,* Rafoth, *Development of a Discharge Lounge: the Use of E-Mail to Facilitate the Quality Improvement Process,* 12(4) Am. J. Medical Quality 194-195 (1997); *see also,* Acuff, *Lightweight, Mobile E-mail for Intra-Clinic Communication,* Proceedings of AMIA 729-733 (1997); Worth & Patrick, *Do Electronic Mail Discussion Lists Act as Virtual Colleagues?* Proceedings of AMIA 325-329 (1997); Bergus et al, *Use of*

an E-Mail Curbside Consultation Service by Family Physicians, 47(5) Journal of Family Practice 357 (1998).

4. Good, *An E-Mail Education,* 35(2) Trial 28 (1999).

5. Mold et al, *Patient-Physician E-Mail Communication,* 91(6) Journal of Oklahoma Medical Association 331-334 (1998).

6. Ellis et al, *Use of Electronic Mail for Postoperative Follow up After Ambulatory Surgery,* 11(2) Journal of Clinical Anesthesia 136-139 (1999).

7. *See* Eysenbach & Diepgen, *Responses to Unsolicited Patient E-Mail Requests for Medical Advice,* 280(15) J.A.M.A. 1333-1335 (1998).

8. Roemer, *Letter to editor,* 282(8) J.A.M.A. 729 (1999).

9. *Id.; see also* Sherman, *Patients and E-Mail,* 98(3) W.M.J. 66 (1999).

10. *Id.*

11. Sherman, *supra* note 9.

12. Henkel, *E-Mail, Snail Mail, Phone or Fax,* 32(6) FDA Consumer 7 (1998).

13. Heusner, *The E-Mail Connection,* 82 Minnesota Medicine 22 (1999).

14. Kane et al, *Guidelines for the Clinical Use of Electronic Mail With Patients,* 5(1) Journal of the Medical Informatics Association 104 (1998).

15. *Id.*

16. Nordhaus-Bike, *Patient Relations: Get Well E-Mail,* 1(1) Hospital Health Network 14 (1999).

17. *See* Kluchi et al, *Using a WWW-Based Mail User Agent for Secure Mail Service for Health Care Users,* 37(3) Methods of Information in Medicine 247 (1998).

18. *See* Loscalso & Simmons, 35(2) Trial 20 (1999); Brienza, 35(7) Trial 112 (1999).

19. Mandl et al, *Social Equity and Access to the World Wide Web and E-Mail: Implications for the Design and Implementation of Medical Applications,* Proceedings of AMIA Symposium, 215 (1998).

20. Brienza, *supra* note 18.

21. Kane & Sands, *Guidelines for the Clinical Use of Electronic Mail with Patients,* 5(1) Journal of the American Informatics Association 104 (1998).

22. *Id.* at 106.

23. *See supra* note 13; Jurevic, *When Technology and Health Care Collide: Issues with Electronic Medical Records and Electronic Mail,* 66 U.M.K.C. Law Review 809 (1998); *See also,* Bernstein, *Why and How to Use Technology,* 33(1) Trial 93 (1997); Speilberg, *Online Without a Net,* 25 American Journal of Law and Medicine 267 (1999).

24. Speilberg, *supra* note 23, at 275.

25. *See* Cavenaugh, *Fax and E-Mail Qualify as "Documentary Evidence" for Sec. 274,* 29(4) The Tax Advisor 210 (1998).

26. *See* Jablon, *"God Mail": Authentication and Admissibility of Electronic Mail in Federal Courts,* 34(4) American Criminal Law Review 1387 (1997).

27. *Id.* at 1390-1391.

28. *Id.*

29. *See Zenith Radio Corp. v. Matsushita Electric Industrial Co.,* 505 F.Supp. 1190 (1980).

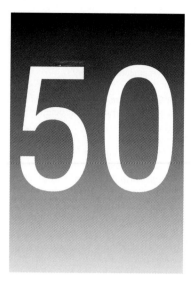

Human experimentation and research

CYRIL H. WECHT, M.D., J.D., F.C.L.M.

HISTORICAL BACKGROUND
BENEFIT VERSUS RISK RULE
CRIMINAL AND CIVIL LIABILITY
INNOVATIVE THERAPY
RADIATION EXPERIMENTS
QUESTIONABLE HUMAN RESEARCH AND EXPERIMENTATION PRACTICES
CONCLUSION

HISTORICAL BACKGROUND

Few subjects in the medicolegal field have raised as much widespread controversy since World War II as the question of human experimentation and clinical investigation. Exposés of activities by the Central Intelligence Agency (CIA), the Department of Defense, and other federal agencies involving the deaths of innocent victims, who were unknowing, involuntary guinea pigs, have raised many moral and ethical questions for the entire country. Ever since the Nuremberg trials after World War II, medical researchers and other professional scientific personnel involved in clinical investigation have been made aware of the medicolegal hazards and pitfalls of improper, illegal human experimentation. The Declaration of Helsinki and Codes and Guidelines adopted by the American Medical Association and other national professional organizations, as well as by the Department of Health and Human Services (DHHS), have emphasized the importance and necessity of having well-defined principles for all medical experimenters and researchers using human subjects in their studies.

The World Medical Association (WMA) addressed this controversial subject in 1949 at its meeting in London, at which time a rather strict International Code of Medical Ethics was adopted. It said in part: "Under no circumstances is a doctor permitted to do anything that would weaken the physical or mental resistance of a human being except from strictly therapeutic or prophylactic indications imposed in the interest of the patient." However, by 1954, the WMA had become uncomfortable with its commitment exclusively to the individual patient. That year, the organization adopted its "Principles for Those in Research and Experimentation," which, while warning that there must be "strict adherence to the general rules of respect of the individual," also explicitly recognized that experiments may be conducted on healthy subjects.

By 1964 the WMA had clearly abandoned the individual patient centered commitment of 1949 in a new set of recommendations, "because it is essential that the results of laboratory experiments be applied to human beings to further scientific knowledge and to help suffering humanity."

Today, not only the regulations of the WMA, but also those of the Nuremberg Code and the U.S. government justify a human experiment if the risks compare favorably with the foreseeable benefits to the subject or to others. Hence the Hippocratic tradition regarding human experimentation has been amended to include a concern for suffering humanity and, of course, for scientific progress.

Yet this same commitment to benefit society may also have opened the door for the type of experimentation that includes the injection of hepatitis virus into mentally retarded children, as occurred at Willowbrook State Hospital (see below). Thus a "Willowbrook" becomes possible once experimenters can convince themselves that the risks are outweighed by the possible benefits, including the potential benefits to people who were not included in the experiment.

Some scientific researchers have been irritated by the institution of codes and guidelines and continue to insist that they should be permitted to use their own best moral and ethical judgment as professional people. Although the majority of these persons would, of course, apply a high level of moral and ethical judgment, experience has demonstrated all too frequently that even highly experienced researchers can be carried away with a particular project and engage in activities that not only are in violation of the existing civil common law and criminal codes, but are in opposition to traditional medical morals and ethics. For all these reasons, it is essential that physicians and other scientists who directly or indirectly engage in any kind of experimentation or clinical investigation involving human beings be fully aware of all the legal ramifi-

cations and potential problems associated with this area of professional activity.

The late eminent Harvard Medical School anesthesiologist and medical ethicist, Dr. H. K. Beecher, claimed that human experimentation beyond the boundaries of medical ethics was being carried out to an alarming and dangerous degree by clinical investigators in the United States. He claimed that these investigators were more concerned with furthering the interests of science than with the good of the patient. He found 12 of 100 consecutively reported studies involving experimentation with human subjects, appearing in a highly respected medical journal in 1964, to be seemingly "unethical." Beecher concluded: "If only one fourth of them is truly unethical, this still indicates the existence of a serious situation." In the prestigious *New England Journal of Medicine,* he found 50 examples of unethical experimentation described or referred to in various articles.[1]

Government-sponsored experimentation

Medical experimentation on humans has a long history, but public concern over it is a comparatively recent development. One of the more spectacular recent examples of unethical human experimentation was partially revealed in June 1975 by the Commission on CIA Activities within the United States, the so-called Rockefeller Commission. In its chapter on domestic activities of the CIA's Directorate of Science and Technology, the Commission's report described some of the CIA projects involving drug experimentation on humans, noting that most of the records of such experiments had been destroyed. The report minimized the consequences of the experiments to the subjects involved, many of whom had not even been informed that they were subjects of an experiment. One of the CIA experiments was described more specifically, although still in casual, almost indifferent terms:

The Commission did learn, however, that on one occasion during the early phases of this program [in 1953], LSD was administered to an employee of the Department of the Army without his knowledge while he was attending a meeting with CIA personnel working on the drug project.

Before receiving the LSD, the subject had participated in discussions where the testing of such substances on unsuspecting subjects was agreed to in principle. However, this individual was not made aware that he had been given LSD until about 20 minutes after it had been administered. He developed serious side effects and was sent to New York with a CIA escort for psychiatric treatment. Several days later, he jumped from a tenth floor window of his room and died as a result.

The General Counsel ruled that the death resulted from circumstances arising out of an experiment undertaken in the course of his official duties for the U.S. Government, thus ensuring his survivors of receiving certain death benefits. The Director of Central Intelligence issued reprimands to two CIA employees responsible for the incident.[2]

As if to suggest that the experiment perhaps had nothing to do with the death, the report added a gratuitous footnote:

"There are indications in the few remaining Agency records that this individual may have had a history of emotional instability." The individual was not identified in the Commission's report.

The report went on to conclude that "it was clearly illegal to test potentially dangerous drugs on unsuspecting United States citizens," and recommended that "the CIA should not again engage in the testing of drugs on unsuspecting persons." Not a word about medical ethics, international codes, or anything else to indicate any genuine moral concern—not even a suggestion that the unknowing subjects of the experiments ought to be located and informed. This was how a prestigious governmental commission perceived its obligations and performed its duties.

Fortunately, the news media were not satisfied with this incomplete disclosure. The identity of the victim in the specific incident described by the Commission was soon determined to be Dr. Frank Olson, a civilian Army employee. His "history of emotional instability" consisted of visits to a New York psychiatrist, retained by the CIA, after he had been subjected to the CIA's drug experiment. When the detailed circumstances of the experiment and Dr. Olson's death became widely publicized, the President of the United States expressed public apologies to his widow and children. Ultimately, after a suit had been filed, the case was settled privately and quietly by a $2 million payment from the government.

Other examples of governmental drug experimentation on humans also came to public attention. One involved a 42-year-old hospital patient, Harold Blauer, who died in January 1953, approximately 2½ hours after receiving an injection of a mescaline derivative. (Mescaline is a hallucinogenic drug derived from a type of cactus plant and is similar to LSD in its effects on the mind.)

Blauer, along with an undetermined number of other patients, had been given injections of mescaline derivatives during the course of a 29-day project conducted by the New York State Psychiatric Institute under an Army contract. At no time was there knowledge on the part of any of the patients or their families as to the nature of the experiment, nor was any informed consent obtained.

Some comments by the acting Mental Hygiene Commissioner of New York State, Dr. Hugh F. Butts, after disclosure of the circumstances of Blauer's death, are especially relevant:

It was not uncommon practice at that time for medical and psychiatric researchers to use drug treatment without the detailed knowledge and special consent of patients. This was thought necessary to avoid false reactions. Such practices could not occur today because patients are protected by laws and regulations that have been specifically enacted to prevent such occurrences.[3]

After the public disclosures of the Olson and Blauer cases, the news media turned up numerous other instances of unethical experimentation with hallucinogenic drugs on unsuspecting human subjects involving several government agencies. At

least 7000 persons had been so treated by the U.S. Army alone. The Rockefeller Commission report had also alluded to experiments on "unsuspecting persons in normal social situations," on both the West and East Coasts during the 1950s and 1960s.[4]

Later, it was learned that the U.S. Atomic Energy Commission, predecessor to the Energy Research and Development Administration, sponsored and monitored various experiments from the 1940s through the 1960s on human subjects, including children, in which the subjects were exposed either to radiation or to the highly toxic metal plutonium. In the radiation tests, 79 inmates of the state penitentiary in Oregon, men and women, were exposed to doses of radiation to determine the effects on the reproductive organs. No follow-up studies had been performed in recent years, but as a result of the disclosure, prison officials agreed to conduct medical evaluations to detect adverse aftereffects.

In the plutonium exposure tests, 18 men, women, and children, all thought to be terminally ill, were injected with plutonium in amounts ranging from 2 to 145 times the maximum permissible dose under current standards. The subjects were not told what the substance was. The injections were performed between 1945 and 1947 at various hospitals in four different states. Astonishingly, although all the subjects were thought to be terminally ill at the time, three were still alive 40 years later.[5] Obviously, aside from the ethics of the experiment itself, such long survival of "terminally ill" patients raises serious questions about the ability of researchers to determine such conditions in their choice of subjects.

LSD

The Justice Department recently settled a lawsuit by nine Canadians who asserted that the CIA, unknowingly to them and their relatives, made them the subjects of mind-control experiments in the 1950s. The plaintiffs were patients of a psychiatrist who received money from the CIA to do research into drugs that could be used to control human behavior. According to government records, the nine plaintiffs were not told they were the subjects of experiments. They were subjected to heavy doses of the hallucinogen LSD, powerful electric shock treatment two or three times a day, and doses of barbiturates for prolonged periods of drug-induced sleep.

Documents that became public showed that the CIA had used private medical research foundations as a conduit for a 25-year, multimillion-dollar research program to learn how to control the human mind. Through a front organization called the *Society for the Investigation of Human Ecology,* the agency funneled tens of thousands of dollars to pay for an array of experiments that involved LSD, electroshock therapy, and a procedure known as *psychic driving,* in which patients listened to a recorded message repeatedly for up to 16 hours.

The Nuremberg Code

Of course, there is nothing new about medical experiments on humans. Galen founded the experimental science of med-

icine before 200 A.D., and there are references to medical experiments on human subjects in the oldest literature. Nonetheless, public awareness of ethical and legal problems posed by medical research involving human subjects did not coalesce until the post–World War II trials at Nuremberg, where more than 25 "dedicated and honored medical men" were accused of having committed war crimes of a medical nature against involuntary human subjects. According to Telford Taylor, chief prosecutor at the Nuremberg Military Tribunals, the defendants' "advances" in medicine were confined to the field of "thanatology," the science of death. Of the 25 defendants, only 7 were acquitted; 9 were sentenced to prison, and the remaining 9 were sentenced to death.

After it became known, through these trials, what the Nazis had done under the guise of medical and scientific research, there developed what has been referred to as the Nuremberg Code (see Appendix 50-1). The Nuremberg Code was the forerunner of the subsequent codes and guidelines that were adopted by different agencies and organizations in the ensuing decades. It addressed the question of what constitutes valid, legal, moral, and ethical experimentation. However, it did not explicitly deal with the subject of children. Probably nobody at that time thought it would be necessary. But it did deal with the subjects of consent, the voluntariness of consent, the right of a patient to withdraw if he or she wished, and the basic question of doing things in conformance with proper medical standards and safeguards. The Nuremberg Code prompted more interest and concern in these problems.

Declaration of Helsinki

In 1964, the World Medical Association promulgated a code that came to be known as the Declaration of Helsinki (Appendix 50-2). The Declaration of Helsinki was, in essence, adopted and given the imprimatur of the American Medical Association in November 1966. The AMA referred it to as *Ethical Guidelines for Clinical Investigation.* Earlier in 1966, the Public Health Service of the United States had issued some guidelines that were subsequently revised later in the year. Recently, the DHHS has also been attempting to draft some guidelines.

Children as subjects

Apart from international codes, there have also been a number of court decisions in this country bearing on the questions of ethical experimentation and informed consent, particularly in reference to children. Under existing case law, although it is often forgotten, a parent cannot say to a neighbor or friend or a research team of scientists: "Take one of my children and if you wish to do something that is not going to be beneficial or advantageous to him, go ahead and do it anyway because I, the parent, give you permission." A parent cannot legally do that. We are a nation governed by laws, and the law is clear in this regard. Neither parents, legal

guardians, administrators of homes and hospitals for retarded children, government officials, nor university research teams, individually or collectively, are empowered to ignore or circumvent a basic and important concept of Anglo-American law, namely, that you cannot commit an assault and battery on another human being.

In 1944 the U.S. Supreme Court, in *Prince v. Massachusetts,* stated: "Parents may be free to become martyrs themselves, but it does not follow they are free in identical circumstances to make martyrs of their children before they reach the age of full and legal discretion when they can make that choice for themselves."[6] *Prince v. Massachusetts* has never been overruled by a subsequent U.S. Supreme Court decision.

Some people refer to an earlier case in Mississippi, *Bonner v. Moran,*[7] in which a 15-year-old boy was apparently conned by an aunt into going to a hospital to give skin transplants for his cousin, the aunt's son, who had been burned. The boy did, but there was some question as to whether the mother of the donor really knew the facts of the treatment and the risks to her own son. She subsequently brought legal action against the hospital, but the court was far less than unequivocal in giving its opinion as to whether or not the mother could recover in damages. That case is sometimes quoted in defense of experimentation without consent, but the circumstances and facts were very peculiar and special for that case. There was good evidence to indicate that although the consent was not originally obtained from the mother, the procedure and risks were subsequently made known to her because the son went back repeatedly for more skin transplants and for treatment.

In any event, until such time as the Supreme Court definitively rules otherwise, or until the U.S. Congress enacts contrary legislation, the law prohibits experimentation on humans without informed consent. Furthermore, it is illegal to conduct experiments that are tantamount to assault and battery.

Rather than considering this subject as an academic or legalistic question, one should consider some specific examples. During and after World War II, physicians developed awareness that excessive oxygen could produce a condition known as retrolental fibroplasia (RLF) in children, which leads to blindness. In most instances, this condition was observed in premature infants who had been placed in an excessive quantity of oxygen. So it was decided to conduct an experiment, with no real informed consent from the parents and obviously not from the babies, in which one group of babies was placed in an excessive quantity of oxygen and another in an atmosphere with a much reduced amount of oxygen. Six of the babies became totally and permanently blind.[8]

Consider another experiment. Red blood cells are broken down in the liver of the human body. In some infants the liver fails to excrete bilirubin, the major degradation product in the breakdown of erythrocytes. Furthermore, in infants, unlike adults, bilirubin has the capacity to pass the blood-brain barrier and to precipitate in the brain a dangerous condition that can lead to permanent brain damage and, in some instances, death. Research had previously established that a chemical found in human breast milk seemed to alter, revise, or impede the biochemical processes within the liver by which bilirubin was normally excreted. The researchers wanted to see if that was also true in vivo. Therefore they prepared an experiment in which this chemical compound was given in significant dosages to babies. The experiment confirmed that there was a rather fast, quite substantial buildup of the bilirubin level in these children, with the possibility of subtle brain damage as a result. There was permanent brain damage in some of those children.[9]

In another situation, at Children's Hospital in Boston, there was great interest in the natural defense mechanisms of the human host in reaction to an organ transplant. Boston is a leader in the medical field, and Children's Hospital is one of its finest health care facilities. Yet here is what they did in designing and conducting an experiment. Without obtaining any kind of an informed consent (in most of the cases, it was questionable whether they even obtained a basic consent, that is, the traditional kind that sufficed before the concept of informed consent developed in the medical malpractice field in the early 1960s), they performed a thymectomy on babies and youngsters who were undergoing surgery for various cardiovascular problems. They took out the thymus gland, which is known to play a role in the body's immunological defense mechanisms. They then attached a piece of skin on these children from unrelated individuals to determine what the bodily reaction of the thymectomized child would be to the skin that had been placed on his or her body. This was very interesting and important research. But was there any possible danger to the thymectomized youngster? And did not the parents, at the very least, have the right to have an intelligent, informed discussion from the physicians about what the possibilities of subsequent damage might be?

At Willowbrook State Hospital, Staten Island, New York, some researchers wanted more information about hepatitis in an epidemiological environment. They reasoned that in such an institution, the patients might get hepatitis anyway at some time in the future. So they took retarded youngsters, with no informed consent and most probably without any kind of consent, and gave them orally a fecal extract containing hepatitis virus to see what the medical results would be. They also did a supplemental clinical investigation in which they directly injected hepatitis virus into still other retarded children.[10]

Here is yet another example. Linoleic acid is known to be an essential nutrient, the deprivation of which has been shown to produce serious problems in animals. The effects of its deficiency have also been noted clinically in children. Nevertheless, at the University of Texas at Galveston, from 1956 to 1962, 445 babies, without informed consent, were deprived of linoleic acid. Seven of those children are known to have died of conditions directly related to the deprivation of this essential nutrient. Many others became seriously ill

with a variety of dermatological conditions, pneumonia, and other problems.[11]

In Pennsylvania in 1973 there was an exposé of another deplorable situation at the Hamburg State Home and Hospital in Berks County. It was shown that retarded children, with no consent of any kind obtained from their parents, not even informed consent, were injected with a meningitis vaccine. The vaccine had not been approved by the FDA and was not on the clinical market, but it was given to these children nevertheless. Said the researchers at a later date, "We thought that the administrator of the hospital was the legal guardian for these children for all purposes, and he told us it was all right to go ahead and do it." After hearings before the Department of Health, Education, and Welfare and the Department of Justice in Harrisburg, the Commonwealth of Pennsylvania put an end to that experiment and to other similar experiments that had not received approval or that had not been reviewed by appropriate agencies and authorities.

Ethics and fetal research

For years, scientists who wanted to do research involving human embryos and fetuses have found themselves in a catch-22. They could do their work with impunity and receive federal funds for it, so long as an ethics advisory board approved their proposals. The catch is that the board does not exist, and has not existed for nearly a decade.

The research on fetuses has thrived, although it has remained in the ethical shadows. The testing of new methods for prenatal diagnosis or in vitro fertilization, among other things, has been financed with profits from infertility treatments and standard prenatal diagnosis. The research at issue involves either embryos, including those created by in vitro fertilization, or intact fetuses obtained from miscarriage or hysterotomy, an early form of cesarean birth.

The ethics board was originally created in 1974, partly in response to fetal research in the 1960s and 1970s, which took place without federal restrictions. Although many experiments were unremarkable, some were profoundly objectionable. In the early 1960s scientists at one university immersed 15 fetuses obtained from abortions in a salt solution to see whether they could absorb oxygen through the skin. One lived 22 hours. An experiment at another university examined the fetal brain's metabolism of glucose; the researchers used heads severed from live human fetuses.

At the same time, more researchers were working on in vitro fertilization, in which eggs removed from a woman's body are mixed with sperm and one or more resulting embryos are implanted in her uterus. To develop the method, research with human embryos was required. After the U.S. Supreme Court struck down most restrictions on abortion in 1973, Congress appointed a commission for the protection of human subjects and asked it to rule on fetal research.

The commission ruled that fetal research was permissible. But it also ruled that no one could subject a fetus to be aborted to any more risk than one that was to be carried to term. It was an extremely restrictive policy, the commission recognized, but there was an out: an advisory board would decide, on a case-by-case basis, when this "minimal risk standard" could be waived. However, the ethics board was dissolved before it had a chance to rule on any case, and the DHHS has declined to appoint a new one.

Adult experimentation

Of course, there have been similar problems in experiments with adults. Some of these have been widely publicized.

Between February 1945 and July 1956 at the Brooklyn Jewish Chronic Disease Hospital, injections of cancer cells were given to elderly hospital patients, with no actual or meaningful permission having been obtained from them or their families. Malignant tumor cells were injected directly into the veins of elderly people suffering from advanced parkinsonism, multiple sclerosis, and other kinds of severe neurological disorders. The principal researcher in that case was Dr. Chester M. Southam from Sloan-Kettering Institute, who subsequently had his license suspended temporarily by the state of New York. When asked why he had not injected himself in the experiments since he had said that it was quite safe, he replied: "Well, you know there is always a possibility of some harm and let's face it, there simply are not too many cancer researchers around."[12]

The infamous Tuskegee syphilis study, initiated and monitored by the U.S. Public Health Service, was not terminated until 1972. In Macon County, Alabama, some 400 black men with syphilis, of a total of 600 subjects in the study, were deliberately deprived of treatment from 1932 on, purportedly to study the effects of allowing the disease to take its natural course. At least 28 of these men, and possibly as many as 107, are known to have died as a result of the disease. It has been argued that in 1932, the cure for syphilis was ineffective and sometimes worse than the disease, but certainly this was not true in the 1950s, 1960s, and 1970s, during which time the "experiment was continued and regularly reported."

This incredible experiment was thoroughly evaluated and criticized extensively by a specially appointed committee. In the Final Report of the Tuskegee Syphilis Study Ad Hoc Advisory Panel, Department of Health, Education, and Welfare (Washington, D.C., 1973), one of the panelists, Jay Katz, M.D., stated:

In conclusion, I note sadly that the medical profession, through its national association, its many individual societies, and its journals, has on the whole not reacted to this (Tuskegee Syphilis) study except by ignoring it. One lengthy editorial appeared in the October 1972 issue of the Southern Medical Journal which exonerated the study and chastised the "irresponsible press" for bringing it to public attention. When will we take seriously our respon-

sibilities, particularly to the disadvantaged in our midst who so consistently throughout history have been the first to be selected for human research?[13]

In April 1997, President Clinton offered a formal apology to the families and the eight remaining survivors of the Tuskegee syphilis experiments, identifying the experiments as a "blight on the American record." In addition, the U.S. government has paid a total of $10 million in an effort to compensate the victims and family members for the incident.

Geriatric research

In Philadelphia in 1964 and 1965, 13 elderly nursing home patients died as a direct result of drug experiments conducted on behalf of one of the large pharmaceutical manufacturers. The experiment had two stages. One drug was used to induce nervous system disorders and then another was introduced to control them. Although the Food and Drug Administration (FDA) was aware of the experiment and prepared a report on it in 1967, the report was withheld for many years and not released until the Philadelphia Bulletin obtained it under the Freedom of Information Act.[14] There was much doubt as to whether informed consent had been obtained in this experiment.

Reporting on his observations from 50 field inspections by the FDA in 1972, Dr. Alan B. Listook, Medical Officer in the FDA's Bureau of New Drugs, stated the following:

We have seen consent forms of senile patients signed "X-(her mark)" and have found others executed posthumously. On one occasion, where the obtainment of consent was the major reason for the FDA to conduct an investigation, we visited the subjects of the study, and discussed their understanding of the document they signed. It turned out that the women were not fully aware that they were participating in an experiment of any kind. They were not aware that they had been given a medication which had not been proven to be safe and effective.[15]

More than 3 years later, exactly the same kind of problem was reported again in a study conducted at a "distinguished university hospital and research center," not otherwise identified.[16] According to this later study, of 51 pregnant women who had signed a consent form in an experiment on the effects of a new labor-inducing drug, 20 did not know they were the subjects of research, even after the drug had been administered, and did not learn of it until they were interviewed by the follow-up investigator. Most of the 51 women had not been aware that any hazards were involved and had been informed only that a "new" drug was being tested, and not that it was an experimental drug. Yet, their own private physicians referred many of these women to the hospital for study. Whether the private physicians were aware of the true nature of the experiment is not stated, but in any case, it is clear that having one's own physician is no safeguard in these matters.

The whole area of new drug investigations is a jungle from the standpoint of research ethics, quite apart from the specific question of informed consent. Again, a quote from the remarks of Dr. Listook is appropriate:

We have had examples of physicians submitting case reports recording the administration to subjects of much more new drug substance than was available to them. We have had police departments report the finding of case lots of investigational drugs by the roadside in trashcans.

On occasion we find records of months of treatment on an index card. We have looked at records of patients reported as having been treated for intractable angina and found no mention of heart disease, no electrocardiograms, and no noted treatment. We frequently find that laboratory results reported to the FDA cannot be substantiated by records in the physician's office or by contact with the clinical laboratory where the work was said to have been done.

In institutions such as mental hospitals or geriatric facilities, we often see therapy prescribed that makes a study impossible to interpret and thus invalid. Major tranquilizers are given during the study of psychoactive compounds; vasodilators are given during the study of drugs being evaluated for the same purpose. Investigational drugs are discontinued without the investigator's knowledge, and adverse reactions go unreported because of lack of communication or lack of awareness on the part of the ward staff.

I could quote horror stories about paroled inmates and discharged mental patients reported as being treated in situ for weeks after their release, of therapy duration and dosage and hospital clinical courses that did not approximate those reported. . . .

We have come across individuals who were able to care for patients in their offices while they were on extended European vacations. Others, while not quite so versatile, have been able to come up with large patient populations for the treatment of widely divergent types of disease. We have the internist who does a study on an antiobesity drug and a few months later is found to be using the same patients in the study of an antihypertensive agent. In our review of the case reports we find no hypertension reported in the first study.[17]

In view of such findings, it would seem that these researchers were not being meticulous about getting informed consent. Yet it is from this very area—the development of new drugs—that we most often hear the arguments being advanced that research must not be fettered and that those of us who insist on adhering to the law are obstructing scientific progress.

BENEFIT VERSUS RISK RULE

In situations in which there is no potential therapeutic benefit to the subjects, it is customary to distinguish four levels of human experimentation.[18]

1. Benefit is reasonably believed to exceed the risk to the patient, and the study involves a patient who consents to this low-risk diagnostic or therapeutic procedure by coming to the physician. The patient is given information and shows that it is understood. He or she is not a subject, but rather a patient, and the needs of the

patient come before any effort to gain knowledge. There is no legal problem in such a situation, except, of course, the one that physicians must contend with in all therapeutic situations, namely, obtaining an informed consent.

2. Benefit is reasonably considered to at least equal the risk, if not possibly exceed it. The patient is a volunteer. He or she may be a subject also, but if so, the relationship between the volunteer and the physician is made quite clear. At this level, we have a controlled experiment, but everyone knows what is happening, and there is definitely a strong possibility, in fact a probability, that the project may be of some therapeutic benefit to the patient.

3. The risk exceeds the benefit to the patient, but the risk is balanced by possible benefit to society. Here, the highest possible degree of informed consent is essential. Experiments in this field are still permissible, including those on children, provided the highest degree of informed consent is obtained from the patient or subject.

4. Risk exceeds benefit. The individual is either both the subject and the patient or purely just a subject. Consent from the individual either has not been obtained or has been obtained through deceit, the force of authority, or other improper means.

Usually, the last category is the issue. Because medical research trials commonly require that a convenient, stable subject population be monitored over weeks or months rather than days or hours, the medical scientist naturally turns to "captive" groups whose availability can be controlled. These groups include the following:

- Hospitalized or institutionalized patients
- Children
- Mentally abnormal persons
- Prisoners
- Persons under discipline (armed forces and police force)
- Laboratory assistants and medical students

In all these groups, factors are present that tend to make the individuals involved susceptible to pressures or influences that induce them to give their consent to experimentation. For example, prisoners hope for probation, soldiers for promotion, and students for higher grades. Use of such groups for medical experimentation is not invariably improper, but experiments conducted on such persons raise the question as to whether the consent obtained, if any, may have been the result of coercion or other influences that would place the project in Category 4.

In recent years, medical research in prisons has been prohibited in many states. The National Commission on Protection of Subjects has recently released its recommendations on allowable research on prison inmates. They are very stringent recommendations that would virtually eliminate such research from U.S. prisons.

This problem was particularly relevant in the case of children as experimental subjects. In the Hamburg State Home and Hospital case mentioned earlier, studies were initially undertaken without an informed consent. Indeed, there was no consent obtained at all. The physician in charge of the study "thought" that the administrator of the hospital was the legal guardian of these mentally retarded children!

Some time later, the physicians did send some kind of generalized consent form to the parents, and some of these were signed and returned. However, there is no question at all from a legal standpoint that this kind of consent is not a valid informed consent and would not hold up in the courts of Pennsylvania, even if the parents had been the subjects.

What if the pharmaceutical company involved with that meningitis vaccine believed it was essential to learn what the effects of that vaccine on children would be? Could that company, with its thousands of employees in this country and abroad, including all their research teams and top administrators, have gone to their employees and asked for volunteers?

Inasmuch as the meningitis vaccine that was being tested was of no direct therapeutic benefit to the children who were to receive it, even the parents within the pharmaceutical company could not have given a legal consent for their own children. Such experimentation would be considered assault and battery. And no one—even a parent—can give legal consent to have assault and battery committed on another human being.

Every one of these experiments on children involved subjects who did not have the necessary intellectual capacity to give a truly informed consent. They may have been legally adjudicated *non compos mentis,* or perhaps they merely had been socially and economically deprived to an extreme degree, but invariably they were incapable of giving an informed consent.

It is imperative that everyone in positions of authority within government, medical institutions, health care facilities, and custodial homes appreciate that no matter what the altruistic and projected humanitarian aspects of medical research may be, human beings cannot be subjected to medical experimentation without a proper informed consent having been obtained from them. In the case of minors (especially retarded children), elderly or senile persons who are suffering from serious diseases and do not have a full grasp of their mental faculties, or people who are imprisoned or otherwise subject to coercion, very serious moral and ethical principles must be carefully considered by the research team before undertaking any experiments that place the subjects at risk.

No legitimate reason or justification exists for further delay or governmental procrastination on this subject. There is absolutely no question from a legal standpoint that experiments of this nature are in violation of the law and are against basic concepts of medical morality and ethics. Physicians and scientists, as well as governmental officials in charge of hospitals, homes, and institutions of various kinds, should realize that the civil and criminal laws pertain to them, also.

CRIMINAL AND CIVIL LIABILITY

Although the *Hyman v. Brooklyn Jewish Chronic Disease Hosp.*[19] case makes mention of the "experimentation" question, it is of little value in ascertaining the legal guidelines for experimentation. The court confined itself to the narrow issue of whether a director of a membership corporation has a right to inspect the corporate records. In this case, the court held that possible corporate liability gives the director the right to inspection. As to the liability for the experimentation, the court ventures no unnecessary opinion. Assuming that experimentation is carried on under approved scientific techniques, it may be instructive to consider possible liabilities, viewing a researcher-subject relationship under criminal, tort, and contract law, recognizing that the categories are not always mutually exclusive.

Criminal liability, in the absence of statute, will attach when there is an intended harm constituting homicide or mayhem, or an unintended harm resulting from negligence by commission or omission of such character that it extends beyond ordinary negligence and is considered culpable negligence. If a volunteer dies during or as a result of "experimentation," the criminal liability, if any, would be for homicide—murder or manslaughter.

The Pennsylvania statute (typical of most states) defines the crime of murder as follows:

All murder which shall be perpetrated by means of poison, or by lying in wait, or any other kind of willful, deliberate and premeditated killing or which shall be committed in the perpetration of, or attempting to perpetrate any arson, rape, robbery, burglary, or kidnapping shall be murder in the first degree. All other kinds of murder shall be murder in the second degree. The jury before whom any person indicted for murder shall be tried, shall, if they find such person guilty thereof, ascertain in their verdict whether the person is guilty of murder of the first or second degree.

Murder is the unlawful killing of another with malice aforethought, express or implied.[20]

It is highly unlikely that a properly conceived and reliably approved research project undertaken by a competent specialist would qualify as an act of murder. If the research provides a strong possibility of death or severe injury, known in advance to the scientist in charge, malice may perhaps be implied. The statute provides a further definition: "Manslaughter, however, may be found without malice. Where the practice is such as to constitute a gross ignorance or culpable negligence or such a complete disregard of life or health, the courts have found voluntary or involuntary manslaughter."

Although no case involving experimentation that resulted in a conviction for voluntary or involuntary manslaughter can be found, it has been established that where such charges are brought, consent does not usually constitute a defense to criminal liability.

Professor Kidd of the University of California School of Law raises the question with specific reference to experimentation:

How far can one consent to serious injury to himself? The analogies are not close. Abortion, except for therapeutic reasons, is a crime, and the consent of the woman is no defense for the doctor. A person can not legally consent to his own death; it is murder by the person who kills him. . . . A person may not consent to serious injury amounting to a maim.[21]

In general, criminal negligence in a physician (experimenter) exists when the physician exhibits gross lack of competency, inattention, or wanton indifference to the patient's safety, either through gross ignorance or lack of skill. It is assumed that the same standards would be applicable to scientists engaging in human experiments: "In case of permanent injury or disease rather than death, the possible criminal charge would be mayhem. This crime at common law and by statute generally is also founded on malice and as such would be governed by the same considerations alluded to above."[22]

Basic to the law of torts, a second area of consideration as to the legal consequences of experimentation is the right of the individual to "freedom from bodily harm," so that any unauthorized invasion, or even threat, to the person constitutes grounds for liability. Consent is usually achieved through the use of a release, either written or oral, allowing the patient's person to be physically handled. In the normal physician-patient relationship, there usually is ample basis for finding informed agreement on the part of the patient for ordinary procedures by virtue of the recognized relationship between the parties. It is assumed that the physician is acting in good faith for the personal benefit of the patient who, by seeking professional assistance, may be assumed to consent to the treatment and diagnoses given. In an experimental situation, the inference of consent is not so easily drawn, and there seems to be more of a need for formal consent:

There is scant legal authority on this problem [but] . . . abundant expert testimony is usually available to show that subjecting a patient to experimentation without disclosure and consent is contrary to the customs of surgeons and thus negligent, even though there may be no technical slip in actual performance of the experiment.[23]

Specific to the problem of experimentation, tort liability may arise in cases of nontherapeutic, unnecessary, and legally questionable procedures involving criminal liability and public policy. For instance, in situations such as abortion and euthanasia, cases may be found in which, despite consent, the physician was held to tort liability. In none of these areas has there occurred experimentation by a scientist on humans for nontherapeutic reasons. In some states, a contract action is permitted on the theory breach of an implied agreement to treat with proper care and skill; the essence of the research contract lies in the complete understanding of the parties:

> The medical research procedure by definition and by nature is a deviation from normal practice, even though all the specific elements involved may be well established, simply because medical practice ordinarily does not encompass employment of human beings primarily for the advancement of knowledge. There is no implicit understanding that conventional methods will be used and that the patient will be released as soon as his condition warrants. Consequently, the researcher has a more specific responsibility for full disclosure of his purpose, method, and probable consequences. Achieving a meeting of the minds is a far more critical element in the research contract.[24]

Assuming there is a complete understanding, a research contract will probably provide a defense against liability in a reasonable execution of the contract obligation or performance of the experiment. However, such a contract is unlikely to serve as a complete bar to an allegation of negligence. The patient's own performance under the contract will not be the subject of a decree for specific performance by a court of equity as they are for "personal services."

In conclusion, it would seem that medical practice, generally conceived to be diagnosis, treatment, and care, is governed by state statute and supporting administrative licensing and regulatory bodies. Medical research experimentation on human subjects would appear to be outside the scope of these rules:

> Case law, insofar as it appears to recognize medically related activity, generally characterizes such research as experimentation and holds it to be outside legitimate medical practice. Reported cases have not yet considered modern controlled medical research as such, and have not yet established limits within which human research may be pursued. Cases which have involved conduct labeled experimentation have been decided basically on issues of disclosure or consent, negligence, lack of qualification, improper activity (quack procedures, medicines or devices) or unlicensed practice of medicine usually arising in cases of departure from accepted diagnosis, therapy or other practice.[25]

Despite the Nuremberg Code, the Declaration of Helsinki, the AMA Ethical Guidelines, and numerous other declarations of similar import, apparently many physicians, scientists, and governmental officials still think that because humane benefits may be derived from these experiments in later years, anything is justified today, particularly if the groups being used as guinea pigs consist of retarded children, senile persons, prisoners, or other unfortunate groups with various physical, psychological, or economic handicaps.

A special national commission has been proposed to review all the various facets of this sensitive, important, and complex matter. This group is to have a dual purpose: first, to establish basic principles and guidelines that would be uniformly applicable in all proposed projects involving human experimentation; and second, to consider, evaluate, and approve each new research proposal involving any kind of experimentation on humans. Legislation would have to be enacted to require that all such proposals be submitted and approved before being implemented. Membership in such a commission should necessarily be broad, extending beyond the medical and scientific professions, and all its decisions and records should be subject to public disclosure.

In 1982 the President's Commission for the Study of Ethical Problems in Medicine and Biomedical and Behavioral Research completed a 2-year examination of federal rules and procedures for conducting research with human subjects. The commission concluded that most government supervisory agencies have insufficient data on compliance, and a review of a few well-documented (and widely reported) cases of misconduct on the part of research scientists showed that government oversight can be improved. However, the public must keep a balanced perspective.

Because successful therapies for humans can be established only by tests on human subjects, medical progress depends on the participation of volunteers in research to test new therapies. The prerequisites for such experimentation include at least the following: a reasonable theoretical base for the belief that therapy may be useful; preliminary tests on nonhuman subjects; a careful weighing of the possible benefits and expected risks of the experimental therapy, as well as an assessment of the available standard therapies; and the genuine voluntary consent of the human subject.

The presidential commission's study demonstrates that federally funded institutions need well-defined procedures for responding to reports of misconduct, ranging from falsified data on patients/subjects' charts to conducting studies with drugs not cleared for tests on humans. Some procedures should protect from reprisal those who report their concern (the so-called whistle-blowers). Such procedures also should protect scientists accused of misconduct from publicity and loss of federal funds, at least until a preliminary finding is made that the accusations have some basis in fact. For the sake of all concerned, the institutional response should be prompt, thorough, and fair. The 23 governmental agencies and institutions involved in research on human subjects (e.g., the DHHS, the National Science Foundation) need clearly defined standards for investigations and sanctions.

INNOVATIVE THERAPY

To understand the concept of innovative therapy, it is useful to consider first the activities referred to as standard medical practice. The National Commission defined standard practice for the Protection of Human Subjects of Biomedical and Behavioral Research as "interventions that are designed solely to enhance the well-being of an individual patient or client and that have a reasonable expectation of success. The purpose of medical or behavioral practice is to provide diagnosis, preventive treatments, or therapy to particular individuals."[26]

The commission was established by Congress.[27] Its purpose was to conduct a comprehensive investigation and study to identify the basic ethical principles that should underlie the conduct of biomedical and behavioral research, evaluate existing guidelines for the protection of human subjects, and make appropriate recommendations to the Secretary of Health, Education, and Welfare concerning further steps, if any, to be taken.

The commission identified innovative therapies as a class of procedures that were "designed solely to enhance the well-being of an individual patient or client," but had not been tested sufficiently to meet the standard of having "a reasonable expectation of success." Innovative therapies have been defined as activities "ordinarily conducted . . . with either pure practice intent or with varying degrees of mixed research and practice intent that have been sufficiently tested to meet standards for acceptance or approval."

Dale H. Cowan[20] has stated that the difference between innovative and standard practices may be simply the difference between a beginning and an advanced level of the practice of medicine. However, as noted by R. J. Levine, in referring to the Belmont Report,[29] the attribute that defines innovative therapies is the "lack of suitable validation of [their] safety and efficacy," rather than their "novelty." A practice might not be validated because there is (1) a lack of sufficient testing to certify its safety and efficacy for an intended class of patients or (2) evidence that previously held assumptions about its safety and efficacy should be questioned.

In general, practices or therapies that are standard or accepted have risks and benefits that are known. Additionally, some basis exists for thinking that the benefits outweigh the risks. By contrast, the potential benefits and risks of innovative therapies are less well known and predictable. Consequently, their use exposes patients to a greater likelihood that the balance of benefits and risks may be unfavorable due either to the therapies being ineffective or entailing greater, possibly unknown, risks. Thus standard medical practice can be distinguished from innovative therapies on the basis of the extent of knowledge that exists regarding their likely risks and benefits.

The commission described experimentation or research as

an activity designed to test a hypothesis, permit conclusions to be drawn and thereby to develop or contribute to generalizable knowledge (expressed, for example, in theories, principles, and statements of relationships). Research is usually described in a formal protocol that sets forth an objective and a set of procedures designed to reach that objective.[30]

Levine defined research involving humans as

any manipulation, observation, or other study of a human being—or of anything related to that human being that might subsequently result in manipulation of that human being—done with the intent of developing new knowledge and which differs in any way from customary medical (or other professional) practice.[31]

The distinction between innovative therapy and experimentation can be drawn by focusing on the four levels of research listed previously. Like research, innovative therapy generally represents a departure from standard medical practice.

Federal regulations require that all research involving human subjects conducted by the DHHS, or funded in whole or in part by a grant, contract, cooperative agreement, or fellowship from DHHS, be reviewed by an institutional review board (IRB) established at each institution in which the research is to be conducted. The regulations define research as "a systematic investigation designed to develop or contribute to generalizable knowledge." The regulations further specify minimum requirements for the composition of IRBs and require that each institution engaged in research covered by the regulations must file a written assurance to the secretary of DHHS that "it will comply with the requirements set forth in [the] regulations."

To approve research by the regulations, IRBs must determine that a number of requirements are satisfied.

1. Risks to the subjects are minimized.
2. Risks to the subjects are reasonable in relation to anticipated benefits, if any, to subjects, and the importance of the knowledge that may reasonably be expected to result.
3. Selection of the subjects is equitable.
4. Informed consent will be sought from each prospective subject or the subject's legally authorized representative.
5. When appropriate, the research plan makes adequate provision for monitoring the data collected to ensure the safety of the subjects.

RADIATION EXPERIMENTS

In December 1993, the U.S. Department of Energy publicly disclosed that for the preceding 6 years it had ignored clear evidence of extensive illegal experiments conducted by distinguished medical scientists in the nation's nuclear weapons industry that took place over three decades after World War II, in which various groups of civilians were exposed to radiation in concentrations far above levels that are considered safe at this time. These experiments, conducted at government laboratories and prominent medical research institutions, involved injecting patients with dangerous radioactive substances, such as plutonium, or exposing them to powerful radiation beams. Allegedly, this work was undertaken to determine what the effect of radiation would be on soldiers and civilians if a global atomic war occurred. The experiments dealing with testing radiation on humans are listed in Table 50-1.

Other experiments of a similar nature took place at a state school in Fernald, Massachusetts, from 1946 to 1956, in which as many as 125 mentally retarded teenage boys were

TABLE 50-1. Radiation experiments on humans

Location(s)	Date	Those affected	Experiments
Vanderbilt University, Nashville	Late 1940s	About 800 pregnant women	Subjects were studied to determine the effect of radioactive iron on fetal development. A follow-up study of children born to the women found a higher-than-normal cancer rate.
Oak Ridge National Laboratory, Oak Ridge, Tennessee	Mid-1970s	Nearly 200 patients with leukemia and other cancers	Subjects were exposed to high levels of radiation. The experiments ended after a 1974 government to benefit the patients.
University of Rochester, Oak Ridge Laboratory, University of Chicago, and the University of California Hospital in San Francisco	1945-1947	18 people	Subjects were injected with high concentrations of plutonium, apparently without their informed consent. Many patients were chosen because medical specialists believed they suffered life-threatening illnesses.
Oregon State Prison	1963-1971	67 inmates	Prisoners' testicles were exposed to x-rays to help researchers understand the effects of radiation on production and function of sperm. The inmates signed consent statements indicating that they were aware of some of the risks, but the statements did not mention that radiation could cause cancer.
Washington State Prison	1963-1970	64 inmates	A similar study subjected prisoners to high levels of radiation. The purpose was to determine the minimum dose that would cause healthy men to become temporarily sterile.
Columbia University and Montefiore Hospital in the Bronx	Late 1950s	12 terminally ill cancer patients	Subjects were injected with concentrations of radioactive calcium and strontium-85, another radioactive substance, to measure the rate at which radioactive substances were absorbed into various human tissues.

From The Department of Energy, the Atomic Energy Commission, and Congress.

given radioactive iron and calcium in their breakfast cereal. Consent forms sent to the parents indicated that this study was intended to help researchers better understand human metabolism and nutritional needs. No mention was made that radioactive elements would be used.

Records from the Massachusetts Institute of Technology indicate that 23 pregnant women at the Boston Lying-In Hospital (now part of Brigham and Women's Hospital) were injected with radioactive iron in the early 1950s to allow researchers to study maternal-fetal circulation. In yet another experiment conducted around the same time at Massachusetts General Hospital, patients were given radioactive iodine to study thyroid function and body metabolism, even though the researchers acknowledged they did not know what the long-term effects would be.

Altogether, as of early 1994, U.S. government officials acknowledge that more than 30 experiments involving the use of radioactive materials or radiation, in which the subjects or their parents and guardians were not apprised of the true nature of the studies and therefore could not have given legally acceptable informed consent, took place during a three-decade period beginning in 1946. There may well have been more that are yet to be uncovered.

The government had previously resisted paying compensation to any of these individuals. However, from October 1991 to May 1993, the government spent $47.1 million to reimburse the legal expenses of the private corporations that operated its nuclear weapons plants. The present Energy Secretary, Hazel O'Leary, has proclaimed her definite intention to obtain compensation for all victims of these unethical experiments.

It is important to note that the General Accounting Office first disclosed some of these tests in 1986 in a report to Congress. However, when Representative Edward J. Markey of Massachusetts, chair of the congressional committee that reviewed this report, asked the government for more information and urged full disclosure of all such experiments, he was firmly and repeatedly rebuffed by both the Reagan and Bush administrations.

A senior official of the Atomic Energy Commission, in a 1950 memorandum to one of the prominent physician-scientists involved with some radiation experiments in the Boston area, observed that these medical experiments might have "a little of the Buchenwald touch." Thus it would appear that both the government officials and medical researchers who planned and conducted these radiation experiments were aware that these studies violated the 1947 Nuremberg Code, which was adopted after the Nazi war crimes trials and is regarded as the universal standard for experiments involving human beings.

Currently the U.S. government is aggressively pursuing settlement with the subjects of the Defense Department's radiation experiments in which the victims were unknowingly injected with uranium or plutonium. The federal government indicates that 16 of the 18 victims of the experiments have received a total of $6.5 million in compensation.

In addition, the Clinton administration seeks to expand the current 1990 Radiation Exposure Compensation Act to include the family members of 600 now deceased miners who worked in government-operated uranium mines. The proposed expansion resulted from a presidential advisory committee finding that the high level of exposure to radon experienced by the miners between 1947 and 1991 was due to the government's failure to adequately ventilate the mines.

QUESTIONABLE HUMAN RESEARCH AND EXPERIMENTATION PRACTICES

In addition to the large number of alleged illegal experiments involving radiation and radioactive compounds, several other highly controversial situations have been brought to light in the past few years involving research projects and experimentation, in which informed consent, official and academic guidelines, and other applicable legal and ethical considerations were ignored by the physicians, scientists, and officials in charge of those studies.

The Medical University of South Carolina was accused of testing pregnant women for illicit drug use without their consent and then transmitting that information to local law enforcement officials. This drug testing program was apparently adopted as a means of forcing drug-addicted women who were pregnant to stop using drugs by threatening them with jail if they refused to cooperate with the hospital's regimen of prenatal visits and also attend an established drug treatment program. Almost all the women in the program were African Americans, and several of them were actually arrested and prosecuted for illicit drug use as a result of the disclosure of this information by the university hospital to the police. Dr. Charles R. McCarthy, formerly chief of the Office of Protection of Research Risks at the National Institutes of Health, concluded that this project "fits the definition of an experiment." He indicated that federal rules regarding human experimentation require that subjects give informed consent before being made part of an experiment, and that the patient has the right to refuse to participate and still be given appropriate and necessary medical treatment.

The *Boston Globe* recently reported that the infamous Timothy Leary, the 1960s drug guru, gave inmates at the Concord State Prison in Massachusetts doses of psilocybin, a powerful hallucinogenic drug, without their knowledge or consent. This compound can produce hallucinations, perception distortion, and psychosis and is considered to be psy-

chologically addictive. These tests took place in the 1960s when Leary was a faculty member at Harvard University. He was eventually fired from his position at the prison by state officials, although not until these illegal tests had been under way for many years.

In late 1993 a rash of international articles reported that postmenopausal women were being impregnated with donated eggs fertilized with their husbands' sperm. In England, a 59-year-old woman gave birth to twins, and a 61-year-old Italian woman also gave birth after such a procedure. Numerous cases of a similar nature were also reported in France. Harvested eggs from aborted female fetuses were permitted to mature and then, via artificial insemination, were used to impregnate these elderly women. This experimental process, which had first been utilized in mice by Dr. Roger Gosden, a research scientist in Edinburgh, Scotland, has raised many ethical questions and has precipitated specific legislation in France and elsewhere that would ban the use of such a technique in postmenopausal women.

In the summer of 1993, two French physicians were charged with manslaughter in connection with the death of a child, who died after contracting Creutzfeldt-Jakob disease, a rare viral illness that attacks the brain after a long incubation period. Several other children were thought to have been afflicted also, but had not yet died. This disease, which is incurable and leads to rapid dementia and death, developed after the administration of pituitary gland extracts given to children who suffered from dwarfism. The pituitary glands had been acquired from 1983 to 1988 from corpses in Bulgaria and Hungary. Many of the deceased donors had been patients in psychiatric hospitals and infectious wards.

A current controversy with fascinating legal and ethical overtones is that of human cloning. Federally sponsored research dealing with in vitro fertilization (IVF) has been held in abeyance since 1980, but in 1993 the Clinton administration attempted to gain federal support for research on IVF and the resultant human embryos. The NIH Revitalization Act of 1993 nullified the requirement for ethics board scrutiny of IVF research proposals.

A scientific debate has yet to resolve the question of exactly what a clone is. Dr. Robert Stillman of George Washington University Medical Center reported his findings at a meeting in October 1993 of the American Fertilization Society. He claimed to have cloned human embryos, splitting single embryos into identical twins or triplets. Because human sperm can be frozen and used at a later date, it could be possible for parents to have a child, and years later use a cloned, frozen embryo to give birth to an identical twin, possibly as an organ donor for the older child. A technique has already been developed for making identical twins in animals (e.g., cattle) by dividing the embryo one or more times and letting the new clusters of cells develop into two genetically identical organisms.

In 1993 an internationally known medical researcher, Dr. Peter Wiernik, publicly admitted his role in having provided illegal injections of an experimental drug for 16 brain tumor patients in 1987, using them as human guinea pigs. Wiernik acknowledged a 5-year cover-up in an agreement worked out with federal prosecutors earlier in 1993, whereby he was demoted and reprimanded, but not subjected to criminal prosecution. The patients, all of whom were terminally ill and have since died, were told about the experimental nature of the drug, but were not informed that it lacked approval from the FDA. Wiernik had received FDA approval to use this drug, interleukin-2 (IL-2), in kidney cancer experiments. However, he gave leftover IL-2 to two neurosurgeons for treatment of patients with brain tumors. The FDA had never approved such treatments.

The FDA proposed a major change in the rules for reporting side effects from drug trials in 1993. This proposal came on the heels of publicly released information indicating that several people had died after having been given a new drug for hepatitis B in a series of experimental drug trials. A total of 5 of 15 patients who took the drug for 4 weeks or more died. It was determined in retrospect that five other patients in earlier experiments most probably died as a result of taking that same drug or its experimental predecessor. The drug involved was fialuridine; in the earlier experiments, it was a closely related drug, filacytosine. The scientists or the drug companies reported none of the deaths to the FDA, supposedly because the individuals conducting the experiments assumed that the drug had not caused the deaths.

In late 1993 articles appeared in newspapers throughout the world dealing with the use of cadavers in car crash tests at Heidelberg University in Germany. These experimental studies had been partly financed by the U.S. National Highway Traffic Safety Administration. Similar tests reportedly had been conducted at the University of Virginia and at the Medical College of Wisconsin, and also at Wayne State University in Detroit, the latter at the behest of the Centers for Disease Control and Prevention (CDC). Many questions were raised about whether an informed consent had been obtained by the legal next-of-kin before these corpses were used. The tests in Germany included the dead bodies of 200 adults and 8 children. German law permits the use of cadavers for research as long as the relatives' consent is obtained.

In 1976 John Moore, a 33-year-old man, was diagnosed with hairy-cell leukemia at the Medical Center of the University of California at Los Angeles (UCLA). His treating physician was Dr. David W. Golde, a hematologist and researcher at the UCLA Medical Center. A splenectomy was performed as part of the treatment. Golde recognized the commercial and scientific value of Moore's spleen and other bodily tissues and materials at the time he recommended the splenectomy. The spleen was taken to a hospital research unit to develop a cell line for commercial use. Golde and another researcher, Quan, then developed and patented a cell line

from Moore's cells that produced lymphokines, a genetic product of considerable commercial value. The two researchers, a pharmaceutical company, and UCLA entered into a contract with the Genetics Institute worth more than $330,000 for the products that would be developed from this patented cell line over a 3-year period.

After the splenectomy, Moore returned to the hospital on several occasions over 7 years at the request of Golde and had samples taken of his blood, skin, bone marrow aspirate, and sperm. These were done specifically for commercial and not therapeutic purposes. Moore was never informed at any time by Golde of these research activities, or of the commercial value of his cells. When Moore ultimately discovered that his cells had been used to develop this cell line, he sued the researchers, various companies, and UCLA. The trial court dismissed all the claims, but an intermediate appellate court reversed and held that Moore had stated a cause of action for conversion. On appeal, the California Supreme Court, two justices dissenting, reversed and held that Moore had no property interest in his cells and therefore no cause of action for conversion. However, the court unanimously held that Moore had set forth facts sufficient to state a cause of action for breach of fiduciary relationship and lack of informed consent against Golde for failing to disclose his research and commercial interest before the splenectomy and before the removal of Moore's other body tissues and blood in subsequent visits to UCLA. A petition for writ of certiorari to the U.S. Supreme Court was denied.

In 1994, after the publication of a series of articles on the plutonium injections, President Clinton appointed an advisory committee on human radiation experiments to investigate the matter and gave it access to thousands of secret documents. Jonathan D. Moreno, a biomedical ethicist at the University of Virginia, worked for the committee, and then went on to examine the broad history of experiments that the U.S. Government had secretly conducted on human subjects in the interest of national security from World War II through the Cold War.

During World War II, both military and civilian agencies sponsored numerous experiments with human subjects in connection with investigations of the new antibiotic penicillin, agents against malaria, and protections against poison gases. The subjects were conscientious objectors, prison inmates, hospital patients, students, and Army recruits. Most were volunteers who had been informed of the risks. But others participated without their consent, including tens of thousands of soldiers who were exposed to poison gases to test protective clothing and gas masks.

Despite the Nuremberg Code, the Atomic Energy Commission had no general policy governing experiments with human subjects. The Defense Department had a policy after 1953, at least for experiments in atomic, chemical, or biological warfare, but it was not widely disseminated.[32]

CONCLUSION

A discussion of the liability of a physician for experimental procedures including human research requires an initial examination of the two competing interests that must be balanced in any experimental situation. There is the obvious interest of the patient to be free from the abuses to which uncontrolled experimentation can lead—from the most grotesque examples of the atrocities of Nazi Germany to the violation of the rights of individuals to be free from becoming unwilling participants in any form of experimentation. The interest of the physician and the interest of society as a whole must be balanced against the interest of the individual. If physicians are limited strictly to previously established procedures, all innovation and progress in the field of medicine would cease. The courts have recognized both of these interests in attempting to deal with the problem of when the physician should bear the burden of the effects of experimental procedures.[33] They have laid down the principle that one who experiments with an innovative treatment is responsible for all the harm that follows. Later cases articulated the need for the advancement of medicine, and in these cases the court stated that it is a recognized fact that, if the general practice of medicine is to progress, a certain amount of experimentation must be carried on.

Complicating the problem of balancing these interests is the difficulty of defining experimentation.[34,35] Courts have confused judgmental decisions and experimentation. In the opinion of one court, a physician is presumed to have the knowledge and skill to use some innovation; yet courts have in the past mislabeled that area of permissible judgment as "experimentation." However, any time a physician's procedures do not follow accepted medical practice, he or she is moving in the direction of experimentation and the distinction between innovation and experimentation becomes blurred. On the other hand, the courts have determined that the mere fact of departure from the drug manufacturer's recommended dose does not make the departure an "experiment." A procedure does not rise to the level of an experiment if the physician has previously used the method successfully, the procedure has been described in the literature, and the choice has been reasonably and prudently calculated by the physician to accomplish the intended purpose. However, surely it is not enough that the intentions of the physician be reasonable to find that a previously unapproved procedure is not an experiment.

When drawing the line between experiment and judgment becomes difficult, the courts are likely to be influenced by the fact that no approved therapy is available. The physician then is faced with the choice of no treatment or innovation. And in examining the type of innovation chosen by the physician, the court will look at the rationale of the physician in making that choice and the extent to which that choice was a significant departure from previous standards of care.

Another factor that has been proposed as being important in deciding what is considered experimentation is the distinction between the curable and the terminally ill patient. It has been argued that the terminally ill patient with no hope of recovery from accepted medical procedures should be free to choose from any form of treatment and should not be restricted in his or her choice by laws that were designed to protect the patient from the risks of experimentation. A distinction between curable and terminally ill patients is not valid, however, when the protection of the rights of an individual from the use of experimental drugs is concerned. It has been held that a physician treating terminally ill patients with an unapproved drug may be subject to criminal penalties.[35] The U.S. Supreme Court has ruled that the Federal Food, Drug and Cosmetic Act, which restricts the use of experimental drugs, contains no exemptions for the terminally ill patient.[36]

Although a number of courts have recognized a legal right to recover for damages resulting from experimentation by the physician, no cases to date have actually turned on the issue of experimentation alone. The courts have seemed reluctant to base liability squarely on the issue of experimentation, perhaps because the issue of experimentation is composed of a number of elements. Instead, they have relied on a number of other legal theories for finding liability.

The first and most important is that of informed consent. One court has stated that without informed consent for an investigational procedure, a physician commits a battery.[37] Liability for experimental procedures has been predicated on the lack of informed consent of the patient in a number of cases.[38] In one case involving psychosurgery on a mental patient and a procedure that was totally novel and unrelated to any previously accepted procedure, lack of knowledge on the subject made a knowledgeable consent impossible.[39] However, most courts have accepted the idea that an informed consent is possible even when the knowledge surrounding the procedure is limited. Some believe absolute liability should be imposed on the physician for experimental procedures because they amount to abnormally dangerous activity under 402(a), Restatement (Second) of Torts. However, informed consent before the administration of an investigational drug amounts to voluntarily encountering a dangerous activity that bars recovery under 402(2).

If a physician adopts a method not recognized as sound by the medical community, the physician may be liable if it injures the patient in any way. Any variance from established standards can lead to liability. This "any variance" approach has been modified by most courts. It is generally recognized that where competent medical authorities are divided, a physician will not be held liable if he or she follows a form of treatment advocated by a considerable number in the profession. This represents the "respectable minority approach."[40]

It is important to consider whether the physician undertook a form of treatment that a reasonable and prudent member of the medical profession would undertake under the same or similar circumstances. This standard is an appropriate one, but in the area of experimentation there is a need for more specific guidelines to be articulated by the courts.[41] For example, the test might include factors such as (1) the qualifications of the physician in question to do the particular procedure involved, (2) the rationality of the procedure based on the extent of departure from accepted procedures and the indication of need for the procedure under the circumstances, and (3) the risk of the procedure versus the benefit to be derived from it.

A third legal theory used in experimentation cases is based on the patient's right of privacy. The right to control one's body is part of the right of privacy inherent in our Constitution. Experimentation has been considered a violation of this right.

The physician may be able to guard against liability for experimental procedures with a covenant not to sue. The patient agrees before treatment not to sue if injured as a result of the experimental treatment. When the procedure, although experimental, may have some value and represents a last chance for help, the physician may secure an agreement not to sue if the procedure is not helpful, provided the patient is fully advised.

In addition to the case law that has developed regarding experimentation, there is some federal and state statutory law in this area. Most important within the federal province is the Federal Food, Drug and Cosmetic Act and the regulations promulgated thereunder. These are designed to regulate the influx of new drugs in the market. Section 505(i) of the Act 42 exempts from premarketing approval drugs intended solely for investigational use if they satisfy certain criteria. Experimental drugs are available only to authorized investigators. At authorized institutions their use (as well as any experimental procedure) is subject to the IRB under the regulations of the DHHS. The board examines (1) the knowledge to be gained from the study, (2) prior experimental and clinical findings to determine the necessity and timeliness of using human subjects, (3) potential benefits to the subjects, (4) potential risks and procedures to minimize them, (5) confidentiality procedures, (6) the consent process, and (7) the proposed subject population.

The approval of a study does not mean that the investigator is then insulated from personal liability for harm suffered by the subjects in the study, but it substantially decreases the risk, especially with regard to liability based on failure to secure a subject's informed consent. These procedures are not universally mandated by law, but they apply when research is supported by DHHS funds or submitted to the FDA.

State statutes designed to protect subjects from the risks of experimentation tend to focus on specific matters rather than setting general guidelines for review of research.[43] These statutes regulate investigational drugs, fetal research, psychosurgery, confidentiality of information, and privacy. Only the state of New York statutorily requires institutional review committees for human research. Their function is basically the same as that of the IRB.[44] The state of Louisiana is the only state that defines the crime of human experimentation.[45] State statutes regulating human experimentation are a reasonable exercise of the state's police power.

ENDNOTES

1. H.K. Beecher, *Ethics and Clinical Research,* N. Engl. J. Med. 37ff (June 8, 1973). *See also* H.K. Beecher, *Experimentation in Man,* published as a report to the Council on Drugs of the American Medical Association, 169 J.A.M.A. 461-478 (1959) (republished by Charles C Thomas 1959).
2. Commission on CIA Activities within the United States, *Report to the President* (June 1975).
3. Associated Press dispatch, Washington, D.C. (Aug 13, 1975).
4. UPI dispatch, Salem, Oregon (Mar 4, 1976).
5. UPI dispatch, Washington, D.C. (Feb 22, 1976) (E. Delong).
6. *Prince v. Massachusetts,* 321 U.S. 158 at 170 (1944).
7. *Bonner v. Moran,* 126 F. 2d 121 (D.C. Cir. 1941).
8. Pappworth, *Human Guinea Pigs: Experimentation on Man* (1967).
9. The New Republic, Dec 3, 1966 at 10.
10. 288 N. Engl. J. Med., 755, 791, 1247 (1973).
11. Med. World News, 4 (April 13, 1973).
12. Med. World News, 6 (June 5, 1964); 151 Science 663 (1966).
13. Med. World News, 15 (Aug 18, 1972); Curran, *Legal Liability in Clinical Investigations,* 289 N. Engl. J. Med. 730 (1973).
14. The Philadelphia Bulletin 1 (Nov 16, 1975).
15. Hosp. Trib., 1 (May 14, 1973).
16. Barber, *The Ethics of Experimentation with Human Subjects,* 234 Sci. Am. 25 (Feb 1976).
17. Hosp. Trib., 1 (May 14, 1973).
18. *Human Experimentation,* Med. World News, 37ff (June 8, 1973).
19. *Hyman v. Jewish Chronic Disease Hosp.,* 206 N.E. 2d 3381 N.Y. (1965).
20. 18 Purdon's Statutes §2501 *et seq.;* 18 Pa. C.S.A. §2501 *et seq.*
21. Kidd, *The Problem of Experimentation on Human Beings: Limits of the Right of a Person to Consent to Experimentation on Himself,* 117 Science 211, 212 (1953).
22. *Id.*
23. *Id.*
24. *Id.*
25. *Id.*
26. The commission was established by Congress in Title II, Part A, §201(a) of the National Research Service Award Act of 1974, Pub. L. No. 93-348, 88 Stat. 142. The purpose of the commission was to conduct a comprehensive investigation and study to identify the basic ethical principles that should underlie the conduct of biomedical and behavioral research, evaluate existing guidelines for the protection of human subjects, and make appropriate recommendations to the Secretary of HEW concerning further steps, if any, to be taken. Id. at §202(a)(1)(A) (hereinafter referred to as *the commission*).
27. *Id.*
28. Dale H. Cowan, *Innovative Therapy versus Experimentation,* Tort and Insurance L.J. (Summer 1986).
29. National Commission, *The Belmont Report: Ethical Principles and Guidelines for the Protection of Human Subjects of Research,* DHEW Pub. No. (OS) 78-0012 (1978) (hereinafter referred to as the *Belmont Report*).
30. *Supra* note 26.
31. R.J. Levine, *The Boundaries between Biomedical or Behavioral Research and the Accepted and Routine Practice of Medicine, Belmont Report,* Appendix I, Paper No. 1, DHEW Pub. N. (OS) 78-0013 (1978).
32. J.D. Moreno, *Undue Risk: Secret State Experiments on Humans* (W.H. Freeman & Company 1999).
33. *Carpenter v. Blake,* 60 Barb. (N.Y.) 488, *rev'd on other grounds,* 50 N.Y. 696 (1872).
34. *Fortner v. Koch,* 272 Mich. 273, 261 N.W. 762 (1935).

35. *Brooks v. St. Johns Hickey Memorial Hosp.*, 269 Ind. 270, 380 N.E. 2d 72 (1978).
36. *People v. Privitera*, 23 Cal. 3d 697 (1979).
37. *U.S. v. Rutherford*, 582 F. 2d 1234, *cert. granted* 99 S.Ct. 1042, 439 U.S. 1127, *cert. denied* 99 S.Ct. 1045, 439 U.S. 1127, *revised*, 99 S.Ct. 2470, 442 U.S. 544, *on remand*, 611 F. 2d (1979).
38. *Gatson v. Hunter*, 121 Ariz. 33, 588 P. 2d 326 (1978).
39. *Ahern v. Veteran's Administration*, 537 F. 2d 1098 (1976).
40. *Kaimowitz v. Michigan Dept. of Mental Health* (Civil No. 73-19434-AW), Cir.Ct. Wayne Co., Mich. (1973).
41. *Colton v. New York Hosp.*, 414 N.Y.S. 2d 866 (1979).
42. *Fiorentino v. Wegner*, 272 N.Y.S. 2d 557 (1966).
43. Federal Food, Drug and Cosmetic Act, §501(i), 21 U.S.C. 335(i).
44. California Health and Safety Code §§24176-24179.5 and 26668.4.
45. New York Public Health Law 2440-2446 (Supp. 1976).
46. La. Stat. Ann. Title 14, 872 (1974).

GENERAL REFERENCES

A *Doctor's Drug Studies Turn into Fraud*, The New York Times, A1/Col 1 (May 17, 1999).

Rebecca Dresser, *Time for New Rules on Human Subjects Research?* Hastings Center Report, (Nov/Dec 1998).

Drug Trials Hide Conflicts for Doctors, The New York Times, A1/Col 1 (May 16, 1999).

Gregg Easterbrook, *Medical Evolution*, The New Republic 20-25 (March 1, 1999).

David M. Morens, *Should the Declaration of Helsinki Be Revised*, Letter to the Editor 341 N. Engl. J. Med. (1999).

Proposed Revisions to the Declaration of Helsinki: Will They Weaken the Ethical Principles Underlying Human Research? 341 N. Engl. Med. (1999).

Eileen Welsome, *Human Guinea Pigs*, The New York Times, Sunday Book Review, 28/Col 2 (Dec 12, 1999); provides a review of The Plutonium Files.

World Medical Association, *Declaration of Helsinki: Recommendations Guiding Physicians in Biomedical Research Involving Human Subjects*, 277 J.A.M.A. (1977).

APPENDIX 50 1   The Nuremberg Code

The Nuremberg Code provides as follows:

1. The voluntary consent of the human subject is absolutely essential. This means that the person involved should have legal capacity to give consent; should be so situated so as to exercise free power of choice, without the intervention of any element of force, fraud, deceit, duress, overreaching, or other ulterior form of constraint or coercion; and should have sufficient knowledge as to enable him to make an understanding and enlightened decision. This latter element requires that before the acceptance of an affirmative decision by the experimental subject, there should be made known to him the nature, duration, and purpose of the experiment; the method and means by which it is to be conducted; all inconveniences and hazards reasonably to be expected; and the effects upon his health or person which may possibly come from his participation in the experiment.

   The duty and responsibility for ascertaining the quality of the consent rest upon each individual who initiates, directs or engages in the experiment. It is a personal duty and responsibility which may not be delegated to another with impunity.

2. The experiment should be such as to yield fruitful results for the good of society, unprocurable by other methods or means of study, and not random and unnecessary in nature.

3. The experiment should be so designed and based on the results of animal experimentation and a knowledge of the natural history of the disease or other problem under study that the anticipated results will justify the performance of the experiment.

4. The experiment should be conducted as to avoid all unnecessary physical and mental suffering and injury.

5. No experiment should be conducted where there is a priori reason to believe that death or disabling injury will occur; except, perhaps, in those experiments where the experimental physicians also serve as subjects.

6. The degree of risk to be taken should never exceed that determined by the humanitarian importance of the problem to be solved by the experiment.

7. Proper preparation should be made and adequate facilities provided to protect the experimental subject against even remote possibilities of injury, disability or death.

8. The experiment should be conducted only by scientifically qualified persons. The highest degree of skill and care should be required through all stages of the experiment of those who conduct or engage in the experiment.

9. During the course of the experiment the human subject should be at liberty to bring the experiment to an end if he has reached the physical or mental state where continuation of the experiment seems to him to be impossible.

10. During the course of the experiment the scientist in charge must be prepared to terminate the experiment at any stage if he has probable cause to believe, in the exercise of good faith, superior skill and careful judgment required of him that a continuation of the experiment is likely to result in injury, disability, or death to the experimental subject.

From 1 and 2 *Trials of War Criminals before the Nuremberg Military Tribunals: The Medical Case* (U.S. Government Printing Office, Washington, D.C. 1948).

APPENDIX 50-2 The Declaration of Helsinki

The Declaration of Helsinki provides as follows:

It is the mission of the physician to safeguard the health of the people. His knowledge and conscience are dedicated to the fulfillment of his mission.

The Declaration of Geneva of The World Medical Association binds the physician with the words: "The health of my patient will be my first consideration" and the International Code of Medical Ethics, which declares that "Any act or advice which could weaken physical or mental resistance of a human being may be used only in his interest."

Because it is essential that the results of laboratory experiments be applied to human beings to further scientific knowledge and to help suffering humanity, The World Medical Association has prepared the following recommendations as a guide to each physician in clinical research. It must be stressed that the standards as drafted are only a guide to physicians all over the world. Physicians are not relieved from criminal, civil, and ethical responsibilities under the laws of their own countries.

In the files of clinical research a fundamental distinction must be recognized between clinical research in which the aim is essentially therapeutic for a patient, and the clinical research, the essential object of which is purely scientific and without therapeutic value to the person subjected to the research.

BASIC PRINCIPLES

1. Clinical research must conform to the moral and scientific principles that justify medical research and should be based on laboratory and animal experiments or other scientifically established facts.
2. Clinical research should be conducted only by scientifically qualified persons and under the supervision of a qualified medical person.
3. Clinical research cannot legitimately be carried out unless the importance of the objective is in proportion to the inherent risk to the subject.
4. Every clinical research project should be preceded by careful assessment of inherent risks in comparison to foreseeable benefits to the subject or to others.
5. Special caution should be exercised by the physician in performing clinical research in which the personality of the subject is liable to be altered by drugs or experimental procedure.

CLINICAL RESEARCH COMBINED WITH PROFESSIONAL CARE

1. In the treatment of the sick person, the physician must be free to use a new therapeutic measure, if in his or her judgment it offers hope of saving life, reestablishing health, or alleviating suffering.

   If at all possible, consistent with patient psychology, the physician should obtain the patient's freely given consent after the patient has been given a full explanation. In case of legal incapacity, counsel should also be procured from the legal guardian; in case of physical incapacity the permission of the legal guardian replaces that of the patient.
2. The physician can combine clinical research with professional care, the objective being the acquisition of new medical knowledge, only to the extent that clinical research is justified by its therapeutic value for the patient.

NONTHERAPEUTIC CLINICAL RESEARCH

1. In the purely scientific application of clinical research carried out on a human being, it is the duty of the physician to remain the protector of the life and health of that person on whom clinical research is being carried out.
2. The nature, the purpose, and the risk of clinical research must be explained to the subject by the physician.
3a. Clinical research on a human being cannot be undertaken without his free consent after he has been informed; if he is legally incompetent, the consent of the legal guardian should be procured.
3b. Consent should, as a rule, be obtained in writing. However, the responsibility for clinical research always remains with the research worker; it never falls on the subject even after consent is obtained.
4a. The investigator must respect the right of each individual to safeguard his personal integrity, especially if the subject is in a dependent relationship to the investigator.
4b. At any time during the course of clinical research the subject or his guardian should be free to withdraw permission for research to be continued. The investigator or the investigating team should discontinue the research if in his or their judgment, it may, if continued, be harmful to the individual.

From 67 Ann. Intern. Med. suppl. 7 at 74-75 (1967).

Glossary: selected health care and legal terminology

SAL FISCINA, M.D., J.D.
JANET B. SEIFERT, J.D.†

abandonment Termination of a physician-patient relationship by the physician without the patient's consent at a time when the patient requires medical attention, without making adequate arrangements for continued care.

abuse of process Use of legal mechanisms in a manner or for a purpose not supported by law. For example, pursuit of litigation based on little or no legal grounds, intended to harass and cause expense to the defendant. Damages may be recovered for expenses or loss incurred by a defendant as a result of abuse of process.

action Legal action, lawsuit.

affidavit Sworn statement for use in legal process.

affirmative defense An answer to a lawsuit that does not deny the alleged conduct or failure but asserts a legal basis to excuse or foreclose liability. Good Samaritan immunity or a statute of limitations defense are examples.

agent A person authorized by another, the principal, to act for or represent the principal. Agency relationships may include authority to exercise personal judgment.

allegation Asserted fact or circumstance that is expected to be proved by legal process.

allocated loss expense (ALE) See *expenses.*

amortized value See *investments.*

appeal A claim to a superior court of error in process or law by a lower court, asking the higher court to correct or reverse a judgment or decision. An appellate (appeals) court has the power to review decisions made in the trial court or a lower appellate court. An appellate court does not make a new determination of facts but examines the law and legal process as applied in the case.

battery Intentional and unauthorized physical contact with a person, without consent. For example, a surgical procedure performed without express or implied consent constitutes battery. Victims of medical battery may obtain compensation for the touching, even if no negligence occurred. A crime of battery may be defined differently.

bona fide Latin, meaning "good faith," that is, without deceit, fraud, simulation, or pretense.

borrowed servant Agent temporarily under the supervision, direction, and control of another. For example, an operating room nurse technically employed by a hospital may be borrowed by a surgeon in the operating room to perform certain tasks.

breach of contract Failure to perform a legal agreement. If a legally enforceable contract is established, performance of agreed promises may be compelled or adequate compensation for failure to perform may be required.

This glossary was taken in part from S. Fiscina & J.B. Seifert, *Legal Checkup for Medical Practice* (Mosby, St Louis 1997). Insurance and managed care terms contributed by James G. Zimmerly, M.D., J.D., M.P.H.
†Deceased.

burden of proof Responsibility of proving certain facts required to support a lawsuit. If the burden of proof is not met, the opposing side prevails on that point, even without a defense or response.

capitation Method of payment in which the provider receives a fixed prospective fee for each plan member serviced during a set period, regardless of the amount or type of services rendered to the member. Rates can be adjusted based on demographics or actuarial cost projections. It also refers to the per capita cost of providing a specific menu of health services to a defined population over a set period. Fee-for-service and prepaid medical groups usually receive in advance a negotiated monthly payment from the HMO, regardless of the amount of service rendered by the group.

captain of the ship doctrine A special agency relationship establishing liability for an employee's or agent's acts. This agency relationship imposes what is called *vicarious liability* on the one employing the agent. Initially used as an analogy in malpractice cases, it asserts that the surgeon in the operating room has total authority and full responsibility for the performance of the operating crew and the welfare of the patient. By this doctrine, the surgeon may be vicariously liable for the negligent act of any member of the surgical team. The doctrine is not accepted in every jurisdiction.

case law Legal principles applied to specific factual situations. Case law is drawn from judicial decisions in similar cases in a jurisdiction. Case law is used to make decisions that are based on precedent, the judicial principle that requires that similar cases be treated alike. Assembled case law principles are also called the *common law.*

case management (large case management) Planned approach to manage service or treatment to a member with a serious medical problem. Goal is to contain costs and promote more effective intervention to meet patient needs. Concurrent evaluation of the necessity, appropriateness, and efficiency of services and drugs provided to patients on a case-by-case basis, usually targeted at potentially high-cost cases.

cause Proximate cause. A reasonable connection between an act or failure alleged as negligence and an injury suffered by the plaintiff. In a suit for negligence, the issue of causation usually requires proof that the negligence of the defendant directly resulted in or was a substantial factor in the plaintiff's harm or injury.

cause of action Facts or circumstances that support a legal right to seek corrective action or compensation.

chargeback Payment by a pharmaceutical manufacturer to a wholesaler covering the difference between an institution's contract price for a drug and the wholesaler's book price.

civil action Legal proceeding by a party asking for correction or compensation, distinguished from a criminal action, which is brought by the state to punish offenses against public order.

civil liability Legal responsibility to compensate for losses or injuries caused by acts or failures to act. Compensation is awarded as monetary damages

paid by the defendant to the injured party. In contrast, criminal liability is the legal responsibility imposed by the state for violation of criminal laws. Consequences of criminal acts may include death, imprisonment, fines, and loss of property or privileges. Civil liability is limited to monetary damages; however, a single act may be both a criminal act and a civil wrong, also called a *tort*.

civil rights Enforceable rights of all citizens guaranteed by several amendments to the U.S. Constitution and laws passed recognizing specific liberties or privileges. Violation of another person's civil rights may result in criminal or civil penalties.

claim A demand to pay. A claim is a demand against a physician or hospital. It may or may not be insured under a policy, depending on the coverage afforded and the nature of the offense.

claims frequency The ratio of the number of claims reported in a period, such as a year, to the number of physicians insured—perhaps "per 100 physicians."

claims-made policy See *coverage.*

class Short for classification; a class is a subdivision of a "universe." To lump all insured persons into the same rate grouping would be to overcharge one subgroup (or class) and to undercharge another. In medical malpractice insurance, approximately 100 classes are based mostly on medical specialties. However, an insurer may have only seven rate groups, so each rate group contains several classes.

class action A legal action instituted by one or more persons on behalf of others in a similar situation. Class actions are used if many plaintiffs must prove the same allegations against the same defendant. An example would be litigation over responsibility for a plane crash with hundreds of victims.

clear and convincing evidence A level of persuasion required to support certain noncriminal legal actions. For example, involuntary civil commitment to mental treatment may require clear and convincing evidence of danger to self or others.

clinical indicator Measurable element in the process or outcome of care, the value of which suggests one or more dimensions of quality of care and is theoretically amenable to change by the provider.

closed panel Managed care plan that contracts with physicians on an exclusive basis to provide health services to members. Nonplan physicians are excluded from participation.

code Collection of laws in a jurisdiction or on a specific topic area arranged and indexed by subject, with revisions added to reflect the law currently in force. Each state's Code of Laws, the U.S. Code, and the Internal Revenue Code are examples.

coinsurance The percentage of a covered medical expense that a member must pay after any required deductible. The percentage of the cost of care paid by the patient as part of insurance coverage.

combined loss ratio The sum of (a) the ratio of losses and loss-adjustment expenses incurred to earning premiums and (b) the ratio of all other underwriting expenses incurred to written premiums.

common law See *case law.*

competitive medical plan (CMP) Health care organization that meets specific government criteria for Medicare risk contracting but that is not necessarily an HMO.

complaint Initial document filed by a plaintiff, also called a *pleading,* which begins a civil lawsuit. The complaint is intended to give the defendant notice of facts alleged in the cause of action on which the plaintiff bases a demand for corrective action or compensation.

confidential communication Medical information given to health care providers in the course of diagnosis and treatment of an illness or injury. Providers are entrusted with the duty to keep the information from disclosure to third parties, subject to existing requirements of statute and case law.

consent Agreement to accept the consequences of an action, such as to allow another person to do something or to take part in some activity. Express consent may be oral or written. Implied consent is agreement shown by signs or actions. An example of conduct showing that consent has been given for an injection or blood test is to roll up a sleeve and extend an arm for vein puncture. Taking part indicates consent to the risks of a game, such as hockey. Where no actual consent or refusal is possible (e.g., in the case of an unconscious person in an emergency situation), consent to others' actions to save life or limb is presumed. Consequences of actions taken without consent remain the burden of the individual acting without consent.

consortium Element of damages generally recoverable by one spouse for loss of company, services, and conjugal relations caused by the spouse's injury. Company, participation, counsel, and affection are consortium losses recoverable by other close family members in some jurisdictions.

consultation Request by an attending physician, generally to a specialist, for information, advice, diagnostic services, or therapy that is indicated or necessary for a patient's condition. A duty to consult may arise when diagnosis is uncertain, therapy is ineffective, or the patient requests a consultation. A consultation that is merely informative does not generally result in a relationship and duties between the consultant and the patient. Other consultations, which require that the consultant examine the patient or records or provide diagnostic or treatment services, may establish a duty to the patient separate from the consulting physician's. A referral is distinguished from a consultation because it involves transfer of responsibility for the care of the patient to the specialist. In many consultations the attending physician also retains some ongoing separate responsibility.

contention Earnest and vigorous assertion of legal significance and interpretation of facts or issues in a dispute.

continuous quality improvement (CAI) Method seeking to prevent problems from occurring, and if they do occur, to determine the underlying causes of the problem and then fix the process, not just the problem.

contract Agreement by two or more parties to exchange obligations. A contract depends on a similar mutual understanding of the terms of the contract and performance promised. A legally enforceable contract means that compensation for promises not kept can be compelled.

contributory negligence Affirmative defense in which a defendant contends that the plaintiff's negligence wholly or substantially caused the injury complained of by the defendant. The effect of plaintiff's negligence on liability or compensation varies among the states, depending on the timing and circumstances of the plaintiff's and the defendant's acts or failures to act.

copayments Predetermined amount of money a member pays for a specific service. A form of cost sharing in which the HMO member makes a nominal payment to the provider at the time of service, typically for office visits and prescription drugs.

cost-effectiveness analysis Method with underlying premises that, for any given level of resources available, the decision-maker wishes to maximize the aggregate health benefits conferred to the population of concern. Alternatively a given health benefit goal may be set, the objective being to minimize the cost of achieving it. The cost-effectiveness ratio is the ratio of costs to health benefits and is expressed, for example, as the cost per year per life saved or the cost per quality-adjusted year per life saved.

cost shifting Process by which insurers raise prices to some customers to cover discounts granted to other customers. Also, the process by which hospitals and other providers shift the costs of treating indigent patients to paying patients.

counterclaim Defendant's complaint against a plaintiff alleging obligation, failure, and damages for which compensation is demanded. For the counterclaim issues, the defendant is seen as having the burden of a plaintiff.

covenant Specific agreement or promise to act or refrain from acting in exchange for similar promises or payments. For example, a covenant not to sue one defendant may exchange relinquishment of that claim for a payment or a promise not to counterclaim. However, a specific covenant would not release all persons alleged to have a role in causing the injury and does not

accept the payment as full satisfaction for the injury. A covenant with one defendant therefore does not bar actions against others.

coverage The insurance afforded by the policy and the endorsements or riders attached to it.

I. Claims-made coverage—The claims-made policy covers only those claims that are reported during the term of the (annual) policy, regardless of when the incident occurred.

II. Occurrence coverage—This policy insures against all incidents that occurred during the term of the (annual) policy, no matter how many years later they are first reported.

criminal liability Responsibility imposed when a criminal statute, regulation, or ordinance is violated. Once criminal liability is established, consequences provided by criminal statute or sentencing codes are imposed. Criminal liability is the legal consequence imposed by the state for violation of criminal law—an offense against the public interest in safety and liberty—and is not directed toward compensating the losses of victims. Consequences of criminal acts may include death, imprisonment, fines, and loss of property or privileges.

damages Money receivable through judicial order by a person sustaining harm, impairment, or loss to person or property as the result of the intentional or negligent act of another. Damages may be compensatory, to reimburse a person for economic losses such as lost income and medical expenses. Other damages recoverable include noneconomic losses, such as pain and suffering or mental anguish, or hedonic damages awarded for the loss of life's enjoyment and aesthetic and other pleasures, such as music, athletics, sunsets, or children. Sometimes, token damages are awarded to demonstrate that a legally recognized error has been committed. So-called nominal damages can be awarded even if no actual economic or noneconomic losses are suffered. Punitive damages are those awarded to inflict economic punishment on defendants who have been found to act maliciously or in reckless disregard of others' rights.

decedent A person who has died and whose interests are involved in a legal proceeding.

deductible A set amount that beneficiaries must pay toward covered charges before insurance coverage can begin. Usually renewed annually.

defamation Intentional communication of false personal or business information that injures the reputation or prospects of another. Spoken defamation is slander; written defamation is libel. Truth is a defense to claims of defamation. Publication of true information may nevertheless violate duties of confidentiality or may be invasion of privacy.

deposition Part of pretrial process in which a sworn out-of-court statement is taken. In a deposition, a witness is asked questions and cross-examined. The statement may be admitted into evidence if it is impossible for a witness to attend in person. Deposition testimony also can be used to cross-question a witness at trial.

diagnosis-related group (DRG) Classification system that groups patients according to diagnosis, age, presence of comorbidity or complications, and other relevant data; used by Medicare and some private insurers to set reimbursement rates.

disclaimer Statement before or after disputed events that announces one party's stance and commitment regarding legal aspects of facts and circumstances in question. A disclaimer could be a statement that no warranties were intended or offered as part of contract terms or that risks of activities were not assumed by a party. Ordinarily a disclaimer of responsibility for future negligent conduct is not recognized by the law and would be ineffective as a defense.

discovery Pretrial activities in the litigation process to determine the essential questions and issues in dispute and what evidence each side will present at trial. Discovery is intended to narrow trial questions to the absolute minimum and to allow fair presentation of opposing evidence without surprise during trial. By discovery process, communications and disclosures also may facilitate out-of-court settlement.

drug utilization management Systemic effort to determine the most appropriate drug therapy, based on quality of care, outcomes, and cost.

drug utilization review Systemic review of frequency and usage of prescription drugs, typically on a per-member, per-month basis.

due care Level of reasonable and ordinary observation and awareness owed by one person to another in specific relationship or circumstances, such as a physician's duty of due care in attendance of patients. Due care anticipates and appropriately manages known, expected, or foreseeable events and complications of the patient's disease or treatment.

due process Level of fair method required by the U.S. Constitution in execution of governmental activities. Due process in legal proceedings must reflect both fair substance—the activity is appropriate and constitutional—and fair means—method of proceeding that provides parties involved the opportunity to present appropriate advocacy and evidence in any dispute or legal process.

earned premium See *premium*.

Employee Retirement Income Security Act of 1997 (ERISA) Comprehensive set of statutes, the provisions of which are found in federal labor codes and the Internal Revenue Code and govern nearly every aspect of operation of most employees' medical and pension plans. It was designed by Congress to supersede any and all state laws that relate to employee benefit plans.

EPO Exclusive provider organization.

evidence beyond reasonable doubt A level of persuasion required to support a judgment of criminal responsibility and consequent punishment.

exclusive provider organization (EPO) Organizational arrangements consisting of a group of providers who have a contract with an insurer, employer, third-party administrator, or other sponsoring group. It contracts with a payer to exclusively deliver plan benefits. The financial risk is borne largely by the payer and the plan members. There is more restrictive provider selection and credentialing process than with PPOs. Like PPOs, benefits are greater if plan providers are used. Unlike PPOs, the benefits are reduced dramatically or eliminated if plan providers are not used.

expenses

I. Loss expense
   A. Allocated loss expense (ALE)—That claim expense that can be allocated to a specific claim. This is almost 100% loss legal, that is, outside defense attorneys and expert witnesses.
   B. Unallocated loss expense (ULE)—The inside cost of running a claim department, including costs of employing supervisors and claim examiners, share of executive, heat, light, rent, and so forth.
II. Commissions—Percentage of premiums paid to brokers.
III. Taxes—The percent of written premium, paid to the state.
IV. Administration and overhead—Includes actuarial, legal, accounting, and investment service fees and so forth.

expenses incurred The expenses paid in a period, such as a year, plus the change in expense reserves. Equal to paid expenses less outstanding expense at the beginning of the period plus outstanding expenses at the end of the year.

experience A matching of premiums, losses, and expenses. May or may not include investment earnings, net profit, or both.

I. Calendar year experience—Combines the premiums earned in a year and the losses incurred in the year.
II. Accident year experience—Combines the losses that occurred in a year and the premiums earned on policies in effect during that year. Changes over time. See separate definitions of *premium* and *expenses incurred*.

experience rating A method of determining rates for health care benefits based on the group's past claims or health history.

expert witness Person invited to testify at a hearing or trial to bring special training, knowledge, skill, or experience to the proceeding where matters in legal dispute are beyond the average person's knowledge. Unlike a fact witness, who is compelled to testify because of involvement in the facts and circumstances of the dispute, an expert witness may be asked for an opinion about specific issues in the case. Fact witnesses testify about what was done,

written, or observed and what occurred. Experts educate the court about the scientific, medical, technical, or other specialized circumstances involved in the dispute. Experts are compensated for their time in court, usually at the rate of income they forego to give time to the court. Fact witnesses are not compensated.

federally qualified HMO An HMO that meets strict standards, including financial solvency and scope of coverage.

fee-for-service System of payment under which a fee is charged for each service provided on a retrospective basis. In contrast, most HMOs pay for services on a prospective, fixed-rate basis.

fiduciary A person in a position of confidence or trust who undertakes a solemn duty to act for the benefit of another who must trust the good intention and performance of the fiduciary. In a fiduciary relationship, virtually all the power reposes in the trusted fiduciary, and vulnerability lies with the beneficiary of the relationship. This disparity of knowledge and power imposes major duties on the fiduciary. Examples of fiduciary relationships are guardian and ward, parent and child, attorney and client, physician and patient, estate trustee and beneficiary, and other financial relationships. In contrast to the marketplace relationship, which may be largely "buyer beware," fiduciary relationships require that the fiduciary never act to the detriment of the trusting party, certainly not for personal gain or profit.

finder of fact In a trial, the jury, or in trials without juries, the judge. Conclusions of fact generally are not appealable. Appeals courts review findings of law, admissions of evidence, and application or interpretation of appropriate legal principles and laws.

formulary List of drugs for use by an HMO or hospital. An open formulary is a list of preferred drugs, but other drugs can be prescribed. A closed formulary requires permission for prescription of nonlisted drugs.

fraud Intentional misdirection, misinformation, or misrepresentation to another person that causes legal injury or loss to that person. Fraud is an intentional wrong, to be contrasted with negligent conduct causing loss. Examples of fraud in medical practice could be to mislead a patient about indicated procedures or therapies; to misstate diagnoses or treatment codes to falsely maximize reimbursement; or to conspire with patients to misstate injuries to obtain undeserved benefits.

free-standing plan Unbundled or separate health care benefits apart from the basic health care plan, usually dental or vision care. Employees are allowed to select or decline the separate benefit. This choice is often referred to as *cafeteria-type benefits.*

frequency See *claims frequency.*

gatekeeper The primary care physician must authorize all medical services, nonemergency hospitalizations, specialty referrals, and diagnostic workups. The insurer may not pay for services not approved by gatekeepers.

good faith Honest intent to avoid taking unconscionable advantage of another, even if technicalities of law might permit it.

Good Samaritan statute Law enacted by state legislatures to encourage physicians and others to stop and assist emergency victims. Good Samaritan laws grant immunity from liability for negligence to a person who responds and administers care to a person in an emergency situation. Statutes vary among the states regarding persons covered, the scene and type of emergency, and nature of conduct for which immunity is granted.

group-model HMO HMO staffing that occurs through contracting with multispecialty medical groups to provide services to plan members. Group is paid a set amount per patient to provide a specified scope of services and determines physician compensation. Physicians are not employees of the HMO but are considered a closed panel and are employed by the group practice. Practice may be in facilities owned by the group or HMO. Physicians generally are paid a fixed capitated amount for each individual enrolled in the HMO. Payments also may be based on costs rather than a set fee. Some groups may be allowed to provide service to patients outside the HMO. A closed panel HMO member may use only physician groups contracted with or employed by the HMO.

group practice without walls Network of physicians who have merged into one legal entity but continue to practice independently in their own office locations.

guardian Person appointed by a court to manage the affairs and to protect the interests of a person who is declared incompetent to manage personal affairs. Incompetence may be due to physical or mental status; guardians may be appointed to manage economic or personal matters, including medical treatment choices.

health maintenance organization (HMO) An organized system of care that provides health care services to a defined population for a fixed, prospective per-person fee. Members are not reimbursed for care not provided or authorized by the HMO. Organization that provides for a wide range of comprehensive health care services for a specified group of enrollees for a fixed, periodic prepayment.

health plan A plan, fund, or program "established or maintained" by an employer for the purpose of providing participants or their beneficiaries with medical, surgical, or hospital benefits in the event of sickness, accident, disability, death, or unemployment. An entity designed and marketed to furnish health-related services to entitled individuals for a premium. It must either furnish or arrange services or insurance coverage for enrollees.

health plan employer data and information set (HEDIS) A core set of performance measures developed by the National Committee for Quality Assurance. It provides a standardized format for reporting managed care entities' utilization review and quality assurance activities, including cost data. HEDIS enables plans and employers to more accurately evaluate and record the trends in health plan performance and use this information in a comparative manner. The performance measures cover the following areas: quality, access, patient satisfaction, membership, utilization, finance, and descriptive information on health plan management and activities.

holding A term for a specific conclusion made by a court in a case, which is used to support the court's final judgment in the case. A holding may be used to persuade later courts on the same point in similar cases.

IBNR Losses incurred but not reported. See *losses.*

immunity Protection given to certain individuals or entities that shields them from liability for certain acts. The individual or entity may be sued, but if immunity is established as an affirmative defense, no prosecution or trial of the dispute will be allowed. Examples of immunity include charitable or nonprofit hospitals granted charitable immunity, government agencies' complete or limited sovereign or governmental immunity, diplomatic immunity, immunity for reporting suspected child abuse, or immunity for peer review comment and activities.

in loco parentis Latin phrase for the status of one assigned by law to stand in the place of parents and exercise their legal rights, duties, and responsibilities toward a child.

incompetence Legal status of dependence on a natural or appointed guardian to make decisions and manage personal and business affairs. Incompetent persons cannot bind themselves by contract, cannot consent to or refuse medical treatment, and cannot be held to assume consequences of choices made. Parents are the natural guardians of children, who are legally incompetent until the age of majority or until emancipated. Legally recognized incompetent adults have appointed guardians. Medically, incompetence is the inability of a person to understand and manage personal affairs or to take responsibility for personal choices. Once this status or condition is legally recognized, a guardian is appointed to act in the person's place.

indemnity State of obligation to reimburse for losses. A person may indemnify another under the terms of an agreement that requires payment of specified losses under specified conditions. Insurance contracts are examples of indemnity agreements, as are hospital agreements to indemnify employed physicians in specific conditions of liability or defense.

indemnity benefit Insurance that pays the individual for medical services after the services are performed, usually on a fee-for-service basis.

independent contractor Person who agrees to perform tasks that are completed without direct supervision or control by the party employing the contractor. Ordinarily this arrangement and relationship shield the employer from liability for negligent acts of the independent contractor that occurred during the performance of the contracted work. Independent contractors are legally distinguished from employees, whose performance is supervised, directed, and controlled by the employer and for whose work the employer is vicariously responsible. Depending on the circumstances, a physician may be either an independent contractor or an employee in practice.

independent practice association (IPA) Organized system of care in which the HMO contracts with independent private practice physicians or an association of such physicians, who provide services to HMO members and other patients in their private offices. Physicians are paid on a negotiated per capita rate, flat retainer fee, or negotiated fee-for-service basis. Most specialty physicians are reimbursed on a discounted fee-for-service basis. When fee-for-service is used, frequently a portion of the payment is withheld as a method of risk sharing. Sometimes, primary care physicians are at financial risk for referral to speciality care and hospital admission.

informed consent A patient's agreement to permit diagnosis or treatment of an illness or injury based on the patient's knowledge of facts needed to choose whether or not to submit to the medical process considered. Informed consent is a patient's agreement to undergo a medical procedure after risks, benefits, alternatives, and consequences have been discussed and weighed.

injunction Court order commanding a person or entity to perform or to refrain from performing a certain act. Failure to obey an injunction may result in a citation of contempt of court and imprisonment until obedience is obtained. The person directed is said to be enjoined by such a court order.

Insurance services office (ISO) A large organization in New York City that gathers and processes the statistics of most insurance companies (not life) in the United States. ISO also publishes rate manuals for most lines of insurance (see line) in each of the states.

integrated delivery system (IDS) Combination of a full range of physician and other health services under one corporate entity.

interrogatories Part of pretrial discovery, interrogatories are formal written questions submitted to an opposing party to be answered before and in preparation for trial. These written answers are signed and affirmed as true by the party or witness in the suit.

invasion of privacy Violation of person's right to be free from unwarranted publicity and intrusions. The offense may be unauthorized dissemination of private information about the person or the publication of photographs or records without specific consent. Disclosure of a medical condition without legal justification or release could represent such a violation. Invasion of privacy is a tort, for which civil liability damages are awarded to compensate for mental suffering, humiliation, or other losses of the person whose privacy was violated.

investments
I. Interest—The interest received on bonds in the portfolio.
II. Maturity—Unlike stocks, bonds are debts that become due and payable at some time in the future, at which time they are said to *mature.*
III. Portfolio valuations
  A. Market value—The value at which a bond could be sold today. Fluctuates widely—inversely with general interest rates and directly with quality and other factors.
  B. Par value—The face amount (maturing amount) of each and all of the bonds.
  C. Price or purchase amount—The cost of the bonds; what was paid for them when they were purchased.
  D. Amortized value—A straight line indicating the trend from the date and amount of purchase to maturity at par. If a bond maturing in 10 years is bought at 90, its amortized value is 91 at the end of the first year, 92 at the end of the second year, and so on, regardless of the market values of the bonds at those times. Bonds of insurance companies are valued this way. If they were not, there would be many technical insolvencies when market values become abnormally depressed.
  IV. Realized capital gain (loss)—The difference between the purchase price of a bond and the amount for which it was sold. By selling the bond, or letting it mature at par, a gain or a loss is realized, which is measured in dollars.
  V. Unrealized capital gain (loss)—The difference between the purchase price of a bond and what it's worth now at market. The bond has not been sold or has not matured, so the gain or loss is unrealized.

joint and several liability Responsibility shared by a number of persons who are found to have contributed to a plaintiff's injury. Establishment of joint and several liability means that each or any one of those liable can be made to satisfy the whole loss to the plaintiff and must then sue the other liable parties for contribution to the payment.

joint venture Enterprise undertaking to carry out limited objectives, entered into by associates under circumstances in which all have an equal voice in directing the conduct of the enterprise. Each is the agent of the others; therefore the act of only one joint venturer is to be charged vicariously against the others. Some of the elements of joint enterprise are a contract, a common purpose, a community of interest, and an equal right to voice accompanied by an equal right to control.

judgment Official decision of a court about the respective rights and claims of the parties to an action or suit litigated and submitted for determination.

jurisdiction Geographic or subject matter limits to power and authority of courts and other government agencies and officers.

leading case Case decision in a specific jurisdiction dealing with specific facts and circumstances that have decided the same issues involved in a later case. A leading case is determinative of the same issues in subsequent cases unless distinctions from the leading case facts are established.

libel Written defamation by any type of communication or publication, including pictures.

line Line of insurance; a general kind of insurance, such as fire, auto, or workers' compensation. The Annual Statement blank provides for 29 lines of insurance and leaves a line blank for some specialty lines. It separates malpractice liability from other liability.

losses The most important statistic.
I. Losses paid—The losses paid on a body of policies. Calendar year losses paid (see *experience, I. Calendar year experience*) are the losses paid in a given period, for example, during 1999, on claims whenever occurred or reported but do not include loss adjustment expenses, which are separate. After a claim is paid, it is usually but not always closed. There are partial payments on claims that remain open. Indemnity payments are those made to claimants and do not include payments to defense attorneys (ALEs). Losses paid are indemnity payments only.
II. Losses outstanding—Losses that are unpaid and are represented by loss reserves.
  A. Case reserves—*Case* is a claims department term for "claim" or "file." Technically, a claim number accompanies a case. When a claim is reported and set up, it gets a claim number and a "case estimate"; that is, the claims department estimates the final liability of the claim, that amount goes into reserve, and liability is set up for its ultimate cost. The total of such estimates minus any amount paid thereon becomes the losses outstanding reserve for known cases.
  B. Losses incurred but not reported (IBNR)—Some claims are not reported promptly; others are reported late because the injury takes a long time to manifest. In any event, provision must be made for such claims, often reported 10 or more years after the event or injury. IBNR reserves, particularly for medical malpractice liability, are substantial and often exceed the reserves for known cases. They are calculated by the actuary and are based on past patterns of claims emergence, trended to the future.
  C. Loss adjustment expenses—See *expenses.*

III. Losses incurred—The sum of losses paid and losses outstanding, with reserves for both case estimates and losses IBNR. The estimated ultimate cost of a body of claims.

malice The performance of a wrongful act without excuse, with apparent intent to inflict an injury. Under some circumstances of conduct, the law will infer malicious intent from the evidence of the defendant's actions.

malicious prosecution Lawsuit or countersuit seeking damages that have been caused to a defendant by a civil suit filed by a plaintiff in bad faith and without probable cause. Ordinarily the countersuit may not be brought until the initial suit has been found meritless.

malpractice Professional misconduct or failure to properly discharge professional duties by failing to meet the standard of care required of a professional.

managed care Any system that integrates the financing and delivery of appropriate medical care by means of (1) contracts with selected physicians and hospitals that furnish a comprehensive set of health care services to enrolled members, usually for a predetermined monthly premium; (2) utilization and quality controls that contracting providers agree to accept; (3) financial incentives for patients to use providers and facilities associated with the plan; and (4) assumption of some financial risk by physicians. Delivery system approach that brings together different services and technologies simultaneously to affect price, volume, quality, and accountability with the goal of providing cost-effective health care. It is a process, not an end state, depending on the competitive environment and state and federal rules.

managed indemnity insurance Combines fee-for-service coverage with efforts to control hospital admissions, through preadmission certification, concurrent review, second surgical opinion, and mandatory outpatient surgery.

market value See *investments.*

material Influential and necessary. Material facts or issues concern the substance of the matter in dispute as distinguished from form.

maturity See *investments.*

medical foundation Entity that purchases the business and clinical assets of a physician group or services independent physicians, providing all the business and administrative support services needed to support the practice. In certain circumstances this arrangement may represent the prohibited corporate practice of medicine, although a special exemption may be available for medical foundations that accept payment for physician services.

medical risk contract Federal Medicare contract with HMOs or CMPs that pays a prospective monthly capitation payment for each Medicare member in the plan.

Medicare Select Federal program designed to introduce Medicare beneficiaries to managed care systems through prospective payment health insurance.

minor A person who has not yet reached the age determined by law for transactional capacity, that is, a legally incompetent person. Minors generally cannot be held responsible for their contracts or other civil actions; thus minors ordinarily cannot consent to their own medical treatment. An exception exists for emancipated minors, defined as persons substantially independent from their parents, supporting themselves, married, or otherwise on their own. A statute also may provide exceptions to legal incapacity to allow minors authority to consent to treatment for drug abuse, venereal disease, birth control, or pregnancy.

misrepresentation Words or conduct amounting to an assertion not in accordance with the existing facts or circumstances. A person who has reasonable grounds for believing that the representation is true makes an "innocent misrepresentation." A "negligent misrepresentation" is made when a person has no reasonable grounds for believing that the representation is true, even if the speaker believes it to be true. A "fraudulent misrepresentation" is made by a person who is aware of the falsity of the representation that causes the other party to enter an arrangement or an agreement or to rely to a detriment on the false representation.

motion Request to a judge for an order or a ruling.

multiple option plan Insurance plan offered by employers, with options, such as an HMO, a PPO, and indemnity coverage. Employees choose coverage annually during an open enrollment period.

multispecialty group practice Independent physicians group that is organized to contract with a managed care plan to provide medical services to enrollees. The physicians are employed by the group practice.

negligence Failure to exercise the degree of diligence and care that a reasonably prudent person would be expected to exercise under the same or similar circumstances. Failure that proximately causes an injury is recognized as a basis for compensation owed to the injured party.

network-model HMO (mixed model) Provider arrangement that contracts with a number of independent practice associations or group practices to provide physician services to HMO members. It can be either an open or closed panel. Physicians work out of their own offices and may see non-HMO patients. Multiple provider arrangement consisting of group, staff, or IPA structures in combination. Sometimes a network model will contract with a number of small primary physician groups and will reimburse them on a capitation basis. These groups are then responsible for providing compensation to member physicians. In other cases the network-model HMO may become more integrated by contracting with primary care groups, specialty care groups, and hospitals to reduce utilization risk to primary care physician groups by spreading the risk to other provider groups. May be either closed or open panels.

no-pay claims Claims closed without indemnity payment. Also known as *closed without payment* (CWOP). There may be some loss adjustment expense paid.

occurrence See *coverage.*

open-end HMO Organized hybrid entity that allows its members to use physicians outside the plan in exchange for additional personal financial liability. It is unique among HMOs in that it allows members to use providers outside the HMO network without referral by gatekeepers. Patients who do so are charged an additional copayment, deductible, or both.

open panel Managed care plan that contracts with private physicians to deliver care in their own offices to plan members. The physicians also may provide services to patients outside the plan.

opinion of the court An appellate court's outline of a case, which states the factual circumstances and the law applied to the case. The opinion also details the legal reasoning supporting the decision and any issues appealed as error. The court's opinion finally affirms, reverses, or remands (sends back for more action) the case appealed.

ordinance A rule established by the authority of the state. Generally this is an enactment by the legislative branch of a municipal corporation, such as a city council or equivalent body.

outcome management Method that seeks to control and improve the quality of care and quality of medical outcomes through a continuous process.

outcome measurement A tool, used to assess a health system's performance, that measures the outcome of a given intervention (e.g., death rates for a given procedure or days needed for recovery).

parens patriae Latin term describing the role of the state as the sovereign guardian of persons under the state's protection. It is the legal basis for the state's power to act to protect the health and welfare of persons who suffer from legal disabilities, such as minority or mental incapacity.

par value See *investments.*

party A legal person or entity. Party is a more general term than person and is useful because it can refer to organizations, groups, and legal persons, such as corporations and partnerships.

peer review Evaluation of the quality and effectiveness of a health care professional's services. Performed by physicians or other professionals who have training comparable to those being reviewed.

perjury Willful false testimony under oath and punishable as a crime.

physician hospital organization (PHO) Form of IPA group practice. PHO structures include medical service organization, group practice without walls, medical foundation, and integrated delivery system. Includes physicians outside the boundaries of a hospital's medical staff. Common IPA group practice arrangement in which hospitals and physicians organize for purposes of contracting with medical care organizations (MCOs). It is a legal entity formed and owned by one or more hospitals and physician groups to obtain payer contracts and to further mutual interests. The physicians maintain ownership of their practices while agreeing to accept managed care patients. It serves as a negotiating, contracting, and marketing unit. Typically provides for equal physician and hospital ownership and board representation. May contract with IPA-HMOs. Various PHO structures include management service organizations (MSOs), which are legal entities formed to provide administrative and practice management services to individual physicians or group practices, group practice without walls, medical foundations, and integrated delivery systems.

point of service (POS) plan Combination of HMO and PPO features in which a plan member can opt to use the defined managed care program or can go out-of-plan but pay the difference for nonplan benefits.

police power Authority granted to the state to restrain personal or property rights of persons within the state for the protection of public safety and health. Police power has limitations imposed by the U.S. Constitution and by state constitutions.

practice guidelines A specific, professionally agreed on recommendation for medical practice used within or among health care organizations in an attempt to standardize practice to achieve consistent quality outcomes. Practice guidelines may be instituted when triggered by specific clinical indicators.

practice standard Similar to a practice guideline, but it is stricter and requires specific actions to be taken.

preferred provider organization (PPO) Plan in which members receive a higher level of benefits at a lower cost when they choose physicians in the PPO network. Managed arrangements consist of a group of hospitals, physicians, and other providers who have contracts with an insurer, employer, third-party administrator, or other sponsoring group.

prepaid group practice Fixed, periodic payments made in advance by or on behalf of each plan member.

premium The money a policyholder pays for the policy.
  I. Written premiums—The sum total of all the premiums for all the policies written for a period (e.g., during 2000).
  II. Earned premium—That part of the premium for a policy that represents the expired part of the policy. If a policy has already run for 4 months, then one third of its premium is earned and belongs to the company and two thirds is unearned and refundable to the policyholder if he or she cancels. A proper matching of premiums, losses, and expenses to determine profit includes earned premiums, losses incurred, and expenses incurred.
  III. Unearned premium—Premium representing the unexpired part of a policy. Equals written premium minus earned premium. Can become a substantial item on the balance sheet of an insurance company and is carried as a liability because it is theoretically refundable.

preponderance of evidence A level of persuasion required to award judgment in civil actions for damages. For example, a plaintiff must produce a preponderance of evidence that a defendant failed a recognized duty and that proved losses were caused by the failure. Preponderance is a standard of better-than-equal evidence.

presumption An initial rational position of law, which can be challenged by evidence presented in legal proceedings. Examples are the presumption of innocence of the accused in a criminal trial, the presumption of legitimacy of children born in wedlock, or the presumption of competence in adult persons.

prima facie case Latin description for a complaint with supporting evidence that apparently supports all the necessary legal elements for a recognized cause of action. A prima facie case is sufficient to produce a verdict or judgment for the plaintiff until overcome by evidence in defense of the case.

primary care physician (PCP) Physician who delivers and manages health care; central to controlling costs and utilization.

privilege Exemption or immunity connected to a specific legal situation. For example, the physician-patient privilege is a rule of evidence by which communications made to a physician by a patient in the course of treatment may not be used as evidence in court. It is the patient's privilege to keep such information from disclosure; it is the physician's duty to resist attempts to compel disclosure. This privilege is conditional and usually subject to certain exceptions. The physician-patient privilege of confidentiality is recognized by statute in most states.

probable cause Evidence that would lead a reasonable person of ordinary intelligence to conclude that a cause of action is supportable in a civil lawsuit or that facts exist to prompt a search or an arrest in criminal matters.

probate court Court having jurisdiction over wills and supervision of decedents' estates. In some states, probate courts also have jurisdiction over minors, including the appointment of guardians.

realized capital gains See *investments*.

reasonable person Hypothetical person used as an objective test or standard against which a defendant's conduct in a negligence suit can be judged. The reasonable person is the figurative standard of care. For example, a standard of care in medical practice could be established by the answer to the question, "What would a reasonably knowledgeable and skilled physician be expected to have done under the circumstances described?"

referral care specialists (RCS) Physicians who provide specialty service on request from primary care physicians.

referral pool Capitation set aside for referrals or inpatient medical services. If utilization targets are met at the end of the year, PCPs may share what is left in the pool.

regulation A rule or order prescribed for the management of specific activities subject to government control. Regulations can be rules or orders issued by executive authority or by an administrative agency of government.

release An agreement to relinquish a right or claim against another person or persons, usually exchanged for a payment or a promise, called *consideration*. A signed release agreement indicates that a claimed injury has been compensated. A release is distinguished from a covenant not to sue by the element of satisfaction of the claim.

res ipsa loquitur Latin, meaning "the thing speaks for itself." It is a legal doctrine sometimes applied in a negligence action when the plaintiff has no direct evidence of negligence but the nature of the injury under the particular circumstances indicates to reasonable persons that such injuries do not occur in the absence of negligence. The doctrine is applicable to cases in which the defendant had exclusive control of what caused the harm to the plaintiff and the plaintiff could not have contributed to the injury. Use of the doctrine does not assure the plaintiff a judgment. After proof of the elements of res ipsa loquitur, the doctrine shifts to the defendant the burden to prove that conduct was reasonable and appropriate or that other mechanisms caused the plaintiff's injury.

rescind To nullify a contract by declaring the contract void. A rescinded contract is considered never to have existed. Rescission is distinguished from cancellation or termination, which release the parties to a contract from any additional or ongoing responsibilities, even if the contract terms are not fulfilled.

reserve A liability on the balance sheet for future payments (see *losses*.) There are reserves for unearned premiums, for losses and loss expenses unpaid, and for other expenses unpaid. The solvency of a company can be determined only after all reserves and other liabilities have been taken into account.

resource-based relative value scale (RBRVS) Method developed by the Health Care Financing Administration (HCFA) to redistribute physician payments to more adequately encourage the use of primary care physician services.

respondeat superior Latin, meaning "let the master answer." It is the legal doctrine that imposes vicarious liability on the employer for breaches of duties by employees. The duty is the employer's and is imposed if the employer engages others to perform tasks on the employer's behalf, which is work within the scope of employment. For example, a hospital is liable for the negligent acts of a nurse it employs if the acts occurred while the nurse was performing tasks within a nursing job description.

slander Spoken defamation about one person in the presence of another person that harms the slandered person's income, reputation, or character.

speciality HMOs Behavioral health, prescription drugs, and dental services, also known as *carve-outs or single-service entities.*

staff-model HMO Organized system of care in which physicians are salaried employees of the HMO and provide services only to HMO members. Providers are employees of the plan, not outside contractors, and service is provided in plan-owned and plan-operated offices. Tightest control over the practice pattern of physicians.

standard of care The measure of assessment applied to a defendant's conduct for liability determination, comparing what occurred with what an ordinary, reasonable, and prudent person would have done or not done.

stare decisis Latin, meaning "let the decision stand." This is the principle of case law that requires courts to apply the approach and rationale of previously decided cases to subsequent cases involving similar facts and legal questions. When a point of law has been settled by decision, it forms a precedent that is binding. Later decisions may distinguish their facts or circumstances to come to different results but otherwise must adhere to the rule of precedent. On rare occasion, precedent is rejected, and a new ruling case decision is adopted. Such a case is called a *landmark case.* Landmark case decisions have been made in civil rights, criminal law, abortion, and consumer law.

statute A written law enacted by the legislature to achieve a specified legislative objective. Statutes apply legislative prescriptions to some of the same factual situations dealt with by case law and administrative law. Generally, former case law governing the situation is no longer operative in situations in which a subsequent statute is applicable.

statute of limitations Laws that specify the permissible time interval between an occurrence giving rise to a civil cause of action and the filing of the lawsuit. Failure to file suit within the prescribed time is an affirmative defense. These time limits for filing suit vary among the states, even for similar legal actions. Most statutes of limitation have exceptions that stop the time from elapsing. Stopping the time is called *tolling the statute.* In malpractice actions the time allowed for bringing suit is stopped or does not begin to run until the party claiming injury first discovers or should reasonably have discovered the injury. Fraudulent concealment of an injury by the defendant tolls the statute. Prosecution of some crimes also is subject to a statute of limitations, which elapses while the perpetrator remains within the jurisdiction.

statutory accounting The system under which insurance companies must report to the state. Many businesses use generally accepted accounting principles (GAAP). Two major differences for joint underwriting associations (JUAs) are as follows: (1) under statutory accounting, the JUA may not "discount" its reserves to take into account the investment income they will earn before they are paid out, and (2) the JUA may not be given credit for its "equity" in the unearned premium reserve. This is the prepaid acquisition expense or commission paid to brokers. The unearned premium reserve, which is a liability, may not be reduced to reflect this prepaid expense.

stipulation Acknowledgment by a party of a specific fact or circumstance that will not be disputed in a case. One party may stipulate that a witness is qualified to testify or that a physician had been an employee of a facility at the time of disputed care. Stipulations save time and expense by removing certain issues from trial proceedings.

stop-loss arrangements Withheld arrangements to protect physicians from suffering severe financial loss if a few patients have catastrophic medical costs. Stop-loss is a type of insurance that provides protection from claims that are greater than a specific dollar amount per covered person. There are many different types of stop-loss arrangements, including:

I. Aggregate stop-loss insurance—Reimbursement for claims that exceed an aggregate limit within a specified time period. The limit is usually set at a percentage of expected claims and is expressed as a monthly amount multiplied by the number of insureds.

II. Specific stop-loss insurance—Protection against large individual claims by limiting the buyer's liability for any one insured person during a specified time. The specific stop-loss limit usually is expressed as a dollar amount.

strict liability Responsibility for harm caused by special activities or circumstances. This is liability without the need to prove a negligent act or failure. The proof of damages sustained by the plaintiff in connection with the situation and the involvement of the defendant support the finding of strict liability. Examples could be management by the defendant of inherently dangerous activities, placing a defective and dangerous product into commerce, or assembling hazardous substances or mechanisms.

subpoena A court order requiring a person to appear in court to give testimony or be punished for not appearing.

subpoena duces tecum Subpoena that requires a person to personally present to the court a specified document or property possessed or under the person's control.

tort Civil wrong in which a person has breached a legal duty with harm caused to another. To establish liability for a tort, an injured party must establish that a legal duty was owed to the plaintiff by the defendant, that the defendant breached that duty, and that the plaintiff suffered damage caused by the breach. Torts can be negligent or intentional.

unallocated loss expense (ULE) See *expenses.*

underwriting profit (loss) The amount left over after subtracting from earned premiums in a period the sum of losses and loss expenses incurred in the same period. Investment income is not taken into account; when it is, the result is called *operating profit* or *loss.*

unearned premiums See *premium.*

unrealized capital gains See *investments.*

vicarious liability Derivative responsibility for an agent's or employee's failures based on the defendant's employer-employee or principal-agent relationship. The responsibility is imposed because the ability to supervise, direct, and control employees to safeguard others lies with the employer.

waiver Intentional and voluntary agreement to forego a known claim or right. For example, a patient could waive the privilege of confidential communication, or a defendant could waive the right to challenge certain testimony. Sometimes a right may be unintentionally waived if it is not exercised in time. For example, the right to make or amend allegations and claims not disclosed in pretrial discovery and depositions may be considered waived by the court for failure to assert them in a timely manner.

wanton act Grossly negligent, malicious, or reckless conduct that implies a disregard for the consequences or for the rights or safety of others.

warranty Express or implied commitment or promise undertaken as part of a contract but aside from the central contract purpose. It is to be distinguished from a representation. A warranty is given contemporaneously with the contract agreement as part of the contract. A representation precedes and may be seen as an inducement to enter the contract. For example, a representation would be the disclosed indication for surgery; a warranty would be a promise of a specific result from the procedure.

wrap-around coverage HMO plan that, in some states, was prevented by state law from taking on financial risk for out-of-plan care and therefore joined with insurers to cover the out-of-plan portion of care. Such programs led to development of POS plans.

Case index

Subject index